Essentials of Nursing Informatics

Notice

Essentials of Nursing Informatics

FOURTH EDITION

Virginia K. Saba, EdD, RN, FAAN, FACMI

Distinguished Scholar, Adjunct
School of Nursing & Health Studies
Georgetown University
Washington, District of Columbia

Professor, Adjunct
Uniformed Services University
Bethesda, Maryland

Consultant, Informatics
Clinical Care Classification & Information Technology Systems
Arlington, Virginia

Kathleen A. McCormick, PhD, RN, FAAN, FACMI

Senior Scientist/Vice President
Science Applications International Corporation
Falls Church, Virginia

McGraw-Hill
Medical Publishing Division

New York • Chicago • San Francisco • Lisbon • London Madrid • Mexico City
Milan • New Delhi • San Juan • Seoul • Singapore • Sydney • Toronto

The *McGraw-Hill* Companies

Essentials of Nursing Informatics, Fourth Edition

This book was written by Kathleen McCormick in her private capacity. No official support or endorsement by Science Applications International Corporation (SAIC) is intended or should be inferred.

1 2 3 4 5 6 7 8 9 0   DOC/DOC   0 9 8 7 6 5

ISBN: 0-07-144197-2

This book was set in Vendome by International Typesetting and Composition, Inc.
The editors were Michael L. Brown and Karen Edmonson.
The production supervisor was Sherri Souffrance.
Project management was provided by International Typesetting and Composition, Inc.
The index was prepared by Susan G. Hunter.
RR Donnelley was the printer and binder.

Cataloging-in-Publication Data for this book is on file at the Library of Congress.

CONTENTS

CONTRIBUTORS

Patricia A. Abbott, PhD, RN, FAAN, FACMI
Assistant Professor and Codirector
PAHO/WHO Collaborating Center for Information and
    Knowledge Management
Johns Hopkins University School of Nursing
Baltimore, Maryland
> *Chapter 29: Data Mining and Knowledge Discovery*

Patricia E. Allen, EdD, RN
Associate Professor and Director
Center for Innovation in Nursing Education
Texas Tech Health Services Center School of Nursing
Lubbock, Texas
> *Chapter 33: Accessible, Effective Distance Education*
> *   Anytime, Anyplace*

Ida M. Androwich, PhD, RNC, FAAN
Professor and Director
Health Systems Management
Marcella Niehoff School of Nursing
Loyola University Chicago
Maywood, Illinois
> *Chapter 10: Incorporating Evidence: Use of Computer-based Clinical*
> *   Decision Support Systems for Health Professionals*

Myrna L. Armstrong, EdD, RN, FAAN
Professor
Texas Tech University Health Sciences Center School of Nursing
Texas Tech University-Highland Lakes
Marble Falls, Texas
> *Chapter 33: Accessible, Effective Distance Education*
> *   Anytime, Anyplace*

Jean M. Arnold, EdD, RN, BC
Self-Employed Nurse Educator
University of Phoenix-Tampa
Thomas Edison State College, Excelsior College
Bradenton, Florida
> *Chapter 33: Accessible, Effective Distance Education Anytime, Anyplace*

Dixie B. Baker, PhD, MS, BS
Vice President for Technology and Group Chief Technology Officer
Science Applications International Corporation
Redondo Beach, California
Chapter 15: Dependable Systems for Quality Care

Suzanne Bakken, RN, DNSc, FAAN, FACMI
The Alumni Professor of Nursing and Professor of
   Biomedical Informatics
Columbia University
New York, New York
Chapter 18: Advanced Terminology Systems

Amy J. Barton, PhD, RN
Associate Professor and Associate Dean for Clinical Affairs
University of Colorado at Denver and Health Sciences Center
Denver, Colorado
Chapter 34: Innovations in Telehealth

Asher E. Beckwitt, MA
Qualitative Analysis Research Consultant
Fenwick Library
Resource Collection Management Services
George Mason University
   Fairfax, Virginia
Chapter 35: Computer Use in Nursing Research

Carol J. Bickford, PhD, RN, BC
Senior Policy Fellow
American Nurses Association
Silver Spring, Maryland
Chapter 17: Theories, Models, and Frameworks

Molly Billingsley, EdD, MEd, MSN, RN,
Assistant Vice President
Operations Support
Georgetown University Hospital
Washington, District of Columbia
Chapter 20: Practice Applications

Patricia Flatley Brennan, PhD, RN, FAAN, FACMI
Moehlman Bascorn Professor
School of Nursing & College of Engineering
University of Wisconsin-Madison
Madison, Wisconsin
Chapter 31: Decision Support for Consumers

Robyn L. Carr, RGON
Director
Informatics Project Contracting and Associates
Waikato, New Zealand
Chapter 39: Pacific Rim

Barbara Carty, EdD, RN, FAAN
Coordinator
Graduate Nursing Informatics Program
New York University
New York, New York
Chapter 32: The Nursing Curriculum in the Information Age

Gail R. Casper, PhD, RN
Post-Doctoral Fellow
University of Wisconsin-Madison
Madison, Wisconsin
Chapter 31: Decision Support for Consumers

Marian L. Celli, MS, RN, BC, FHIMSS
Engagement Management
Cerner Corporation
Alexandria, Virginia
*Chapter 19: Implementing and Upgrading Clinical
    Information Systems*

Betty L. Chang, DNSc, RN, FNP-C, FAAN, FACMI
Professor Emerita
University of California
Los Angeles, California
Chapter 35: Computer Use in Nursing Research

Kathleen G. Charters, PhD, RN, CPHIMS
Assistant Professor
University of Maryland School of Nursing
Baltimore, Maryland
Chapter 9: PDA and Wireless Devices

Amy Coenen, PhD, RN, FAAN
Associate Professor
University of Wisconsin-Milwaukee
College of Nursing
Milwaukee, Wisconsin
Director of International Classification for Nursing Practice (ICNP)
International Council of Nurses
Geneva, Switzerland
Chapter 18: Advanced Terminology Systems

Hedy Cohen, MS, BSN, RN,
Vice President
Institute for Safe Medication Practices
Huntingdon Valley, Pennsylvania
Chapter 12: The Role of Technology in the Medication-Use Process

Ann M. Daddona, RN, BA
Clinical Systems Analyst
Siemens Health Care Solutions
Malvern, Pennsylvania
Chapter 21: Critical Care Applications

Mary Jo Deering, PhD
Director for Informatics Dissemination
National Cancer Institute Center for Bioinformatics
Rockville, Maryland
*Chapter 14: Electronic Health Record Systems: U.S. Federal
Initiatives and Public/Private Partnerships*

Connie White Delaney, PhD, RN, FAAN, FACMI
Dean and Professor
School of Nursing
University of Minnesota
Professor Emeritus
College of Nursing
The University of Iowa
Minneapolis, Minnesota
Chapter 16: Nursing Minimum Data Set Systems

Marina L. Douglas, MS, RN
Principal
Beacon Healthcare Consulting, Inc.
McLean, Virginia
*Chapter 19: Implementing and Upgrading Clinical
Information Systems*

Margareta Ehnfors, PhD, RN, DiplEdN, FACMI
Professor
Department of Caring Sciences
Orebro University
Orebro, Sweden
Chapter 38: Nursing Informatics in Europe

Anna Ehrenberg, PhD, RN
Assistant Professor, Post-Doctoral Fellow
Department of Health and Social Science
Dalarna University, Falun
Department of Caring Sciences
Orebro University
Orebro, Sweden
Chapter 38: Nursing Informatics in Europe

William Scott Erdley, DNS, RN
Clinical Assistant Professor
School of Nursing
State University of New York
Buffalo, New York
Chapter 2: Historical Perspectives of Nursing and the Computer

Ann Farrell, BSN, RN
Principal and Senior Consultant
Farrell Associates
San Francisco, California
Chapter 26: Vendor Applications

Veronica D. Feeg, PhD, RN, FAAN
Professor
George Mason University
Fairfax, Virginia
Chapter 35: Computer Use in Nursing Research

Linda F. Fischetti, MS, RN
Health Informatics Architect
Department of Veterans Affairs
Veterans Health Administration
Office of Information
Silver Spring, Maryland
*Chapter 14: Electronic Health Record Systems: U.S. Federal
Initiatives and Public/Private Partnerships*

Carole A. Gassert, PhD, RN, FACMI, FAAN
Associate Dean
Information and Technology
Director of Informatics
University of Utah College of Nursing
Salt Lake City, Utah
Chapter 11: Nursing Informatics and Healthcare Policy

Matthew C. Grissinger, RPh, FASCP
Medication Safety Analyst
Institute for Safe Medication Practices
Huntingdon Valley, Pennsylvania
Chapter 12: The Role of Technology in the Medication-Use Process

Thomasine D. Guberski, PhD, CRNP
Associate Professor
University of Maryland School of Nursing
Baltimore, Maryland
Chapter 9: PDA and Wireless Devices

David M. Haight, MSCS
Research Fellow
Health Systems Research Laboratory
Department of Industrial and Systems Engineering
University of Wisconsin-Madison
Madison, Wisconsin
Chapter 31: Decision Support for Consumers

Nora Hammell, MN, RN
Director
Nursing Policy
Canadian Nurses Association
Ottawa, Ontario, Canada
Chapter 37: Nursing Informatics in Canada

Kathryn J. Hannah, PhD, MScN, BScN, RN
President and CEO
HECS, Inc.
Professor, Adjunct
Department of Community Health Sciences
Faculty of Medicine
University of Calgary
Calgary, Alberta, Canada
Chapter 37: Nursing Informatics in Canada

Nicholas R. Hardiker, PhD, RN
Senior Research Fellow
Salford Health Informatics Research Environment
University of Salford
Salford, United Kingdom
Chapter 18: Advanced Terminology Systems

Michelle L. L. Honey, RGON, MPhil(Nursing), FCNA(NZ)
Senior Lecturer
School of Nursing
University of Auckland
Auckland, New Zealand
Chapter 39: Pacific Rim

Evelyn J. S. Hovenga, PhD, MHA, BAppSc, RN, FCHSE, FRCNA, FACHI, MACS
Professor
Health Informatics
Head School of Information Systems
Faculty of Informatics and Communication
Central Queensland University
Rockhampton, Queensland, Australia
Chapter 39: Pacific Rim

Kathleen M. Hunter, PhD, RN
President and CEO
K&D Hunter Associates, Inc.
Lithia, Florida
Chapter 17: Theories, Models, and Frameworks

Joyce Ernharth Johnson, RN, DNSc, FAAN
Senior Vice President
Operations and Chief Nursing Officer
Georgetown University Hospital
Washington, District of Columbia
Chapter 20: Practice Applications

Rosemary Kennedy, MBA, RN
Chief Nursing Informatics Officer
Siemens Medical Solutions
Malvern, Pennsylvania
Staff Nurse
Montgomery Hospital
Norristown, Pennsylvania
Chapter 21: Critical Care Applications

Margaret Ross Kraft, RN, PhD
Assistant Professor
Loyola University Chicago Niehoff School of Nursing
Reasearch Associate
Veterans Information Resource Center
Maywood, Illinois
*Chapter 10: Incorporating Evidence: Use of Computer-Based
Clinical Decision Support Systems for Health Professionals*

Mary Ann Lavin, ScD, RN, ANP, BC, FAAN
Associate Professor
Saint Louis University School of Nursing
Coordinator
Network for Language in Nursing Knowledge Systems (NLINKS)
St. Louis, Missouri
Chapter 24: Internet Tools for Advanced Nursing Practice

Sun-Mi Lee, PhD, MPH, RN, BC
The Catholic University of Korea College of Nursing
Seoul, Korea
Chapter 29: Data Mining and Knowledge Discovery

June R. Levy, MLS
Managing Director
CINAHL Information Systems
Glendale Adventist Medical Center
Glendale, California
Chapter 36: Computerized Information Resources

Heimar de Fatima Marin, PhD, MS, RN, FACMI
Professor in Nursing Informatics
Federal University of São Paulo
São Paulo, Brazil
Chapter 41: Nursing Informatics in South America

Kathleen A. McCormick, PhD, RN, FAAN, FACMI
Senior Scientist/Vice President
Science Applications International Corporation
Falls Church, Virginia
Chapter 1: Overview of Computers and Nursing
Chapter 28: Translation of Evidence into Nursing Practice: Evidence,
*   Clinical Practice Guidelines, and Automated Implementation Tools*
Chapter 42: Future Directions

Mary L. McHugh, PhD, RN, BC
Associate Professor
University of Colorado at Denver and Health Science Center
Denver, Colorado
Chapter 4: Computer Hardware
Chapter 5: Computer Software and Systems

Shirley M. Moore, RN, PhD, FAAN
Professor and Associate Dean for Research
Frances Payne Bolton School of Nursing
Case Western Reserve University
Cleveland, Ohio
Chapter 31: Decision Support for Consumers

Michael J. Morgan, PhD, NP
Deputy Health Officer
Wayne County Department of Public Health
Wayne, Michigan
Chapter 24: Internet Tools for Advanced Nursing Practice

Peter J. Murray, PhD, RN, MSc, CertEd, MBCS
Honorary Research Fellow in Health and Informatics
University College Winchester
Founding Fellow
Centre for Health Informatics Research and Development (CHIRAD)
Nocton, Lincoln, United Kingdom
Chapter 6: Open Source and Free Software

Lynn M. Nagle, PhD, MScN, BN,
Assistant Professor
University of Toronto
Senior Vice President
Technology & Knowledge Management
Mount Sinai Hospital
Toronto, Ontario, Canada
Chapter 37: Nursing Informatics in Canada

Ramona Nelson, PhD, RN, BC, FAAN
Professor
Slippery Rock University
Slippery Rock, Pennsylvania
Chapter 7: Data Processing

Susan K. Newbold, MS, RNBC, FAAN, FHIMSS
Doctoral Candidate
University of Maryland School of Nursing
CARING Founder and Board
Faculty, Excelsior College
Healthcare Informatics Consultant
Columbia, Maryland
Chapter 23: Ambulatory Care Systems

Marilyn M. Nielsen, MSN, RN
Implementation Consultant
McKesson Provider Technologies
Bloomington, Minnesota
Chapter 34: Innovations in Telehealth

Rolf Nikula, PhD, MI, RN, DiplNEd,
Research Fellow
Department of Caring Sciences
Orebro University
Orebro, Sweden
Chapter 38: Nursing Informatics in Europe

Alric M. O'Connor, RN
Principal
Open Source Medical Solutions
Silver Spring, Maryland
Chapter 6: Open Source and Free Software

Iris Ong, MA, BSN, RN
Clinical Analyst
Maimonides Medical Center
Brooklyn, New York
Chapter 32: The Nursing Curriculum in the Information Age

Hyeoun-Ae Park, PhD, RN
Professor
Seoul National University College of Nursing
Seoul, Korea
Chapter 40: Nursing Informatics in Asia

Donna Ambler Peters, PhD, RN, FAAN
Professor
St. Petersburg College of Nursing
Pinellas Park, Florida
Chapter 22: Community Health Applications

Sally J. Phillips, PhD, RN
Director
Bioterrorism Preparedness Research Program
Agency for Healthcare Research and Quality
Rockville, Maryland
Chapter 25: Informatics Solutions for Emergency Preparedness and Response

Diane S. Pravikoff, RN, PhD, FAAN
Director of Research and Professional Liaison
CINAHL Information Systems
Glendale, California
Chapter 36: Computerized Information Resources

Virginia K. Saba, EdD, RN, FAAN, FACMI
Distinguished Scholar, Adjunct
School of Nursing & Health Studies
Georgetown University
Washington, District of Columbia
Professor, Adjunct
Uniformed Services University
Bethesda, Maryland
Consultant, Informatics
Clinical Care Classification & Information Technology Systems
Arlington, Virginia
> *Chapter 1: Overview of Computers and Nursing*
> *Chapter 2: Historical Perspectives of Nursing and the Computer*
> *Chapter 22: Community Health Applications*
> *Appendix: Clinical Care Classification System Version 2.0*

Joyce Sensmeier, MS, RN, BC, CPHIMS, FHIMSS
Director of Informatics
Healthcare Information and Management Systems Society
Chicago, Illinois
> *Chapter 13: Healthcare Data Standards*

Sarah E. Sheehan, MLS
Education and Nursing Liaison Reference Librarian
George Mason University
Fairfax, Virginia
> *Chapter 35: Computer Use in Nursing Research*

Roy L. Simpson, RN, C, CMAC, FNAP, FAAN
Vanderbilt University and University of Kansas Medical Center
   Adjunct Faculty
Excelsior College, Trustee
Vice President
Nursing Informatics
Cerner Corporation
Kansas City, Missouri
> *Chapter 27: Administrative Applications of Information*
>   *Technology for Nursing Managers*

Diane J. Skiba, PhD, FAAN, FACMI
Professor and Option Coordinator
Health Care Informatics
University of Colorado at Denver and Health Sciences Center
Denver, Colorado
> *Chapter 34: Innovations in Telehealth*

Cynthia M. Struk, PhD, RN, PNP
Associate Vice President
Performance Improvement and Research
Visiting Nurse Health Care Partners of Ohio
Clinical Faculty
Case Western Reserve University Frances Payne Bolton
    School of Nursing
Cleveland, Ohio
> *Chapter 22: Community Health Applications*

Vida B. Svarcas, PhD, RN, BC
Director
Continuing Education Programs—Nursing and Health Professions
Cleveland State University
Division of Continuing Education
Adjunct Assistant Professor
School of Nursing
Cleveland, Ohio
> *Chapter 8: The Internet: A Nursing Resource*

Sheryl Lynn Taylor, BSN, RN
Product Director
Care Management Applications
QuadraMed
Reston, Virginia
> *Chapter 26: Vendor Applications*

Charlotte A. Weaver, PhD RN, MSPH
Adjunct Professor
School of Nursing
University of Kansas
Kansas City, Kansas
Chief Nurse Officer and Vice President of Patient Care Systems
Cerner Corporation
Kansas City, Missouri
> *Chapter 27: Administrative Applications of Information*
> *Technology for Nursing Managers*

Elizabeth Weiner, PhD, RN, BC, FAAN
Senior Associate Dean for Educational Informatics and
    Professor in Nursing and Biomedical Informatics
Vanderbilt University School of Nursing
Nashville, Tennessee
> *Chapter 25: Informatics Solutions for Emergency Preparedness*
> *and Response*

Lucy A. Westbrooke, RN, DipNg, GDipBus
IS Account Manager
Information Services
Auckland District Health Board
Epsom, Auckland, New Zealand
Chapter 39: Pacific Rim

Patricia B. Wise, RN, MA, MSN
Director of EHR Initiatives
Healthcare Information and Management Systems Society
Evans, Georgia
Chapter 3: Electronic Health Record from a Historical Perspective

Rita D. Zielstorff, MS, RN, FAAN, FACMI
Chief Nursing Officer and Director
Product Strategy and Management
Healthvision, Inc.
Waltham, Massachusetts
Chapter 30: Consumer and Patient Use of Computers for Health

PREFACE

In 2004, the United States entered into the decade of the electronic health record (EHR) as declared by the President of the United States and endorsed by the Secretary of Health and Human Services. This fourth edition includes many new authors and new concepts that are important in this new decade of the EHR. Forty-two chapters with several specialist authors have contributed to this fourth edition. Like the third edition, this book includes an international section that covers most continents and updates the state-of-the science in nursing informatics from around the world. This is a book for the new decade of the EHR. It includes chapters on EHR from the perspectives of the users, policy makers, vendors, and from a historical perspective describing the Davies Award winners from Health Information Management Systems Society (HIMSS). It also includes scenarios for the staff nurse and advanced users.

Updates on the history of nursing and the technologies impacting on the nursing profession are addressed. More focus on wireless devices and the Internet abound in this edition. In addition, updates on the traditional applications in practice, education, administration, and research are included. The experts of each chapter have updated their references and illustrations to meet current situations.

With a focus on information technology (IT) and standards by the Congress and the Secretary of Health and Human Services, chapters have been added that focus on these new initiatives. To keep the nursing profession in the forefront of these changes in healthcare IT and standards, more focus has been placed on the accomplishments of nursing informatics specialists in nursing standards, terminology, and reference terminologies at the national and international level. These IT and standards are emerging because of the needs to improve quality, insure safety, and measure outcomes and determine costs. With these new standards concerns for security of information have motivated the editors to include a new chapter on security. These new chapters have been added to educate nurses about these important forces of national concern.

Since September 11, 2001 nurses are working in new environments requiring information on preparedness, emergency response, and biodefense. A special chapter written by experts in public health, policy, and biodefense describes new resources for the nursing profession.

This book also includes more information for those nurses in primary care. As more nurses are prepared at the advanced practice level and are contributing toward the delivery of healthcare in rural and urban areas, more chapters have been added that focus on the resources needed by those nurses. A chapter on the web-based resources available includes valuable sites where nurses can turn to for aid in diagnosis, treatment, evidence, and prevention of common problems. Another chapter describes the new handheld devices that these primary care nurses find invaluable in working in today's new healthcare.

A challenge has been delivered to the country to prepare 6000 nurses in informatics for the next decade. This book is dedicated toward helping those nurses prepare for that new requirement.

Virginia K. Saba, EdD, RN, FAAN, FACMI

Kathleen A. McCormick, PhD, RN, FAAN, FACMI

ACKNOWLEDGMENTS

Authoring chapters for books is more demanding for our information technology authors who already have busy schedules. Because of the desire to teach what is known to others, our authors of this fourth edition have taken their precious time to prepare their chapters. Therefore, we thank them sincerely for sharing their knowledge and expertise.

We want to thank our publisher and editors Michael Brown and Karen Edmonson for their support and patience in the preparation of the book. Books do not become realities without the dedication of publishers and editors who promote the book within the publishing industry. Virginia and Kathleen thank you, Michael and Karen, for your perseverance.

We are driven to develop new editions to keep the nurses current and in the forefront at this critical time in the decade of the electronic health record mandated by the President of the United States and the Secretary of Health and Human Services. Our families have supported our efforts which often demanded time for the book rather than the family. Virginia's sister Bernice provided special nurturance and understanding of Virginia's commitment to compete the book. She also wants a special dedication to her nephew Michael Myers, deceased. Kathleen's sons have learned from the book experiences the value of being an author and Francis, Jr. is even focusing and dedicating his career to supporting authors. The book is also dedicated to Christopher who is learning the lessons of dedication and commitment to lifelong learning. Several authors have gone before us who gave us the courage to continue to add to the literature. A special dedication for my deceased surrogate mother and author Ellen Berman.

PART 1

Computers and Nursing

1

Overview of Computers and Nursing

Virginia K. Saba
Kathleen A. McCormick

OBJECTIVES

1. Introduce nursing informatics (NI) and clinical information systems (CIS).
2. Highlight new technologies and their applications in traditional and new environments of nursing.
3. Introduce the focus of each section and highlight new trends and content in this textbook.

KEY WORDS

nursing informatics
electronic health record
nursing standards
telehealth
biodefence systems

 ## Introduction

As we start the decade of the electronic health record (EHR) mandated by the president of the United States and the secretary of Health and Human Services (HHS), NI is moving to the forefront of the nursing profession and nursing information technology systems. Nurses are becoming computer literate and the nursing profession is implementing practice standards for its clinical care and data standards for its nursing information technology systems.

NI represents the transition of data and data information and knowledge into action. NI represents the practice, administration, community health, nursing education, and nursing research applications. It also addresses other new applications such as international aspects or peripheral to the field such as legal, consumer issues, or theoretical issues. This new edition also includes new content to demonstrate how IT supports nurses to improve quality, ensure safety, measure outcomes, and determine costs.

 ## Overview

There are 2.7 million nurses in the United States. They serve as the largest group of professionals that provide clinical care to patients and remain the consumer advocate. Recent survey data indicate that a growing number of nurses are qualified as information specialists. They may serve as administrators, researchers, educators, and community healthcare professionals, or work as computer information officers (CIOs), corporate executives in vendor companies, implementers of information technology, developers of systems, and consultants. This textbook brings to the nursing field and others interested in nursing, an overview of NI and nursing information technology systems that impact nursing and patient care. This textbook provides the updated, revised, and new chapters on the current issues and applications in the information technology field.

Nursing informatics is defined by the American Nurses Association (ANA, 2001) as:

> A specialty that integrates nursing science, computer science, and information science to manage and communicate data, information, and knowledge in nursing practice. Nursing Informatics facilitates the integration of data, information, and knowledge to support patients, nurses, and other providers in their decision-making in all roles and settings. This support is accomplished through the use of information structures, information processes, and information technology. (p. 46)

In the past 25 years, NI specialists emerged as a new specialty by the ANA. In 1981, there were approximately 15 nurses who identified this new specialty as their area of interest and expertise; in 1990 this number increased 500% to approximately 5,000 nurses; and by the year 2000 it increased approximately another 500%. However, by the year 2010, it is anticipated that the majority of nurses entering the profession will be computer literate. It is also anticipated that every healthcare setting—acute care hospital, academic school of nursing, large community health agency or healthcare setting where nurses function—will employ at least one NI specialist and will implement some type of a CIS.

A CIS is designed to support clinical nursing practice. It requires not only an understanding of professional nursing practice process but also technology that is the application for the science to function electronically.

CIS that adequately support nursing practice have not emerged over the past decades. Figure 1.1 provides an organizing framework and identifies some of the system components, influencing factors, and relationships that have not been fully considered in describing the complexity of nursing, a profession that relies so heavily on evidence, knowledge, and critical thinking. Consequently the requisite detailed analysis and design processes have never begun or have failed to generate the appropriate and diverse information system components

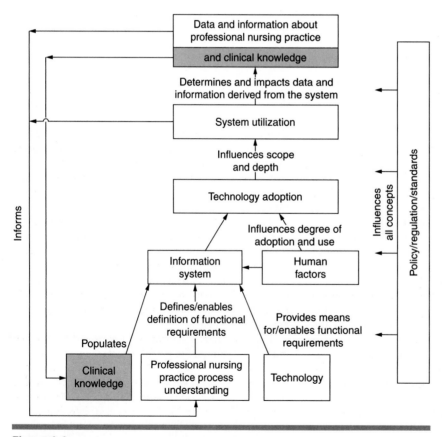

Figure 1.1
The organizing framework for clinical information systems: critical knowledge as the critical factor.
(Source: I.M. Adrowich, et al. (2003). *Clinical Information Systems: A Framework for Reaching the Vision.* Washington, DC: American Nurses Publishing.)

necessary for successful support for nurses and nursing practice (Androwich et al., 2003).

The increased interest in NI occurred because of the concerted efforts of several groups that promoted nursing as an integral part of the EHR systems being implemented in healthcare. The national and international professional nursing organizations began to endorse and approve data standards as separate or as an integral component of the EHR systems. Individual nurses began to demand CIS to document their care, regardless of where they worked and the vendors of the EHR systems began to include nursing care components in their systems.

Further, it was determined that the existing data standards and EHR systems primarily utilized medical, disease, and diagnostic assessment vocabularies and omitted the patient care aspects for an episode of illness. Thus, the users determined that nursing care data, CIS should be included as an integral component of their systems. Such a strategy has made the goal of nursing care an integral part of EHR systems.

A description of chapter sections follows.

 ## Section Overviews

Computers and Nursing

This book provides an updated historical overview of the events, activities, and initiatives related to NI. It also provides the names of key nurses and pioneers involved in these events. It includes national events and international events that have been critical to the field. The milestone table provides an excellent calendar for the NI field. This chapter includes an extensive list of references and a bibliography that highlight the field of NI.

New in this section is the chapter that documents the historical nature of the EHR from the Davies Award perspective. For the first time, the criteria for evaluating the technology and impact of notable EHRs in the country are documented. The issues and challenges remaining have been highlighted.

Two interrelated chapters address hardware and software. It is critical for a user to understand the concepts of hardware: "what is a computer" and/or a "computer system." Further, another chapter describes the concepts of software: "what makes the computer run" and/or a "computer system run." In each of the two chapters, historical landmarks and pioneers in their respective field of computer technology are described.

A new chapter is presented on open source. The basic concepts of open source are defined and a frame-work for understanding the uses and potential misuses of open source are described. Current open source technologies are presented and the authors have attempted to represent both European and American perspectives.

Updating the concept of data processing is a new focus on the structure of meta-analysis of data. The Internet chapter includes many new resources for nursing. The new chapter on personal digital assistant and wireless focuses on their characteristics and differentiates the different types available in the marketplace. Even though this is a changing and evolving technology, the author attempts to define a perspective of use for the nursing profession.

Also, new to this edition is an overview of the concept of decision support and examples of its use in healthcare. There are few examples of decision support in nursing and the author suggests the role of the nurses in informatics to further develop this area in the future.

Issues in Informatics

Healthcare policy has been rapidly evolving in the past 5 years and the author of that chapter has updated and described the changes in national health policy. From a public policy perspective, the author stresses the importance of complete and accurate data sets to monitoring patient status in shaping health. She stresses the need to continue to pursue the literacy of nurses in informatics. She describes some of the newest policy issues of the HHS trends.

The issues involved in patient safety are described by experts from the perspective of the role of technology in the medication use process. This new chapter contributes to the growing interest of the nursing profession in computerized patient order entry (CPOE) and bar coding. An important framework to understand the issues in medication delivery is presented by these experts in the field.

The new chapter on standards authored by a leader in the area updates the profession on the recommended standards from the National Center on Health and Vital Statistics (NCVHS) and the secretary of HHS. Because of the importance to the future of NI, the description of each of the standards has been thoroughly presented by the author.

The new chapter on national initiatives reiterates the importance of national policy and standards through the perception of two leaders in policy in the country. From their perspective in developing the national policies within the federal government, this chapter describes the current state of affairs and the future impacts of these new initiatives. More importantly, this chapter defines how these national policies, standards, and efforts are interrelated.

The new chapter on security is developed with a framework from a national leader in security who gives the U.S. healthcare system a report card on how it is doing with regards to security. This important new contribution provides a vision for future applications and sets a target to be attained by those working in NI.

The new chapter on minimum data set (MDS) provides an overview of the development and uses of the MDSs to be included in any EHR. It includes national and international uses and addresses the new initiatives such as the International Minimum Data Set project which is attempting to gain consensus around the world as to what the minimum nursing data elements should be.

Informatics Theory

The chapter on nursing informatics theory provides an update on theoretical overview of the new nursing specialty. This chapter also provides a brief description of all 13 terminologies for documenting nursing practice, recognized by the ANA.

The chapter on concept-oriented nursing terminologies provides an excellent update and overview of the reference terminology model approved by the International Standards Organization (ISO) as one of the first standards for a profession. This chapter also covers the different definitions, models, and core concepts of NI. In this chapter, the authors describe the key aspects of NI as it relates to the EHR.

The classic chapter on implementing and upgrading systems has been updated. Attention has included the concept of migrating legacy systems.

The new chapter on practice applications by practitioners in a busy and successful metropolitan hospital adds much new content to this chapter. They have maintained the historical points but expanded on the execution of nursing process into information systems, and integration of these principles with case management and decision supports. They have updated the literature for new concepts that are guiding the practice. These authors have given us their benefit/risk analysis of the future.

The chapter on critical care applications was revised and updated by new practitioners in the field. Many principles remain the same on how electronic monitoring systems function, but the content has been updated. They stress the need for integrated systems in the critical care environment and their connections to other areas

of the hospital or healthcare facility. The need for the EHR to follow the patients using the continuity of care format as the patient progresses and moves to medical surgical and ambulatory units is essential. The authors describe the newest electronic systems and how they function. Critical care systems are critical to the saving of lives and essential for all such units.

Community health includes an update and an overview of community health information systems including those required by the federal government. It provides a description of the Clinical Care Classification (CCC) system (previously known as the Home Health Care Classification [HHCC] system) classified by care components. It is used to document, code, and classify nursing and patient care for both the manual and EHR in community health and in all healthcare settings. The CCC Version 2.0 is presented in the Appendix of the book. The chapter also includes a description of a community health intensity rating scale (CHIRS), a tool designed to score intensity measures of community including school healthcare. It includes an overview of current community telehealth applications that are restructuring community health services.

Ambulatory care is covered in an updated chapter on the scope of ambulatory practice including the role of the nurse. The issues, financial benefits, administrative benefits, and regulatory and clinical benefits, are discussed. The role of the nurse using informatics concepts in ambulatory care discussed.

The new chapter on biodefense offers a fresh perspective on the role that nurses are taking in emergency preparedness and training. These leaders in systems to support biodefense and nursing training have defined issues and challenges for the next decade. There are many nurses in state, regional, and local governments who are immersed in the role of developing training and support in biodefense. This chapter is an important contribution in advancing the framework for needs in this field.

For many years, the book has not included a description of many vendor products in EHRs. The authors of this new chapter on vendor applications provide not only a theoretical framework for the integrated health record, but a perspective on nursing within the record. Through a survey of the major vendors, they provide insight into the offerings of the major vendors of EHRs.

Administrative Applications

The chapter on administrative applications reinforces the theoretical foundations of administrative applications in the past decade, but updates the chapter related to important workflow and challenges, chances and choices being made by nurse administrators. The authors have described how the shortage of nurses, the increasing demand for patient safety, and the need for visibility of nursing documentation is influencing the need for IT in managing and administrating today's healthcare environment.

Extensive literature updates have gone into reworking the chapter on evidence-based nursing and informatics. Experts working in the Agency for Health Care Research and Quality (AHRQ—formerly AHCPR) updated this chapter and included the process of gathering evidence-based information.

The chapter on data mining and knowledge discovery reiterates the theoretical concepts on data mining and knowledge discovery. A few examples of practice applications are given in this chapter. New references have been added to update the concepts.

Consumer Use of Informatics

This new chapter provides an overview on the innovative use of the Internet by consumers and patients. The communication between patients/consumers and healthcare providers is discussed as a mechanism for facilitating consumer satisfaction. Issues related to consumer use of the Internet are discussed.

An excellent theoretical framework and description of consumers making decisions has been updated. New references have been added to this chapter.

Educational Applications

The chapter on nursing curriculum in the information age provides an update on the educational applications including curriculum design. It provides an overview of technology applications in nursing education and how they are reshaping higher nursing education. The chapter describes the resources needed to move the nursing curriculum and nursing education into the information age. The author describes the strategies used to integrate information and computer technology into the nursing curriculum. She indicates that information technology in education will cut across departments and disciplines and will facilitate interactions and connectivity. Curriculum implications including faculty development, interactive learning, cognition, electronic communication, multimedia, and informatics are summarized and described as they relate to the NI curriculum.

The chapter on distance education expands the educational applications to learning at any time and in any place. The authors have been involved in distance education for several years and have first-hand knowledge of this innovative application. Programs of distance learning are flourishing especially Internet and Web courses. Since this field has changed so much, the authors provide perspectives on the past and the present uses and developments of this redesigned educational approach. They include an overview of the different strategies and support for the distance education learner and faculty including the electronic assistance required. Also, the legal, ethical, and copyright issues are addressed. The authors conclude with the need for further research on several critical issues.

The final educational chapter focuses on innovations in telehealth. The authors indicate that with the new advances in computing and communications technologies will impact on where we live, work, and interact with each other. They indicate that these technologies will affect not only the practice of healthcare, but also education and research. Their chapter describes in detail the new technological—telehealth—advances. They define "telehealth" and addresses data communication applications available for the user. They include all forms of electronic communication, electronic bulletin board, electronic networks, and video media. They describe the challenges and issues that need to be addressed in order to conduct successful telehealth educational programs.

Research Applications

The chapter on computer use in nursing research provides an update and a new approach to research applications. The authors focus on the differences between quantitative and qualitative research. They provide an overview of computer-based applications that facilitate and support the steps of the research process including data collection, data management and coding, data analysis, and results reporting. They compare and contrast selected computer software applications that are used including examples of specific applications that have been used in quantitative and qualitative research studies. They also discuss how the computer software can be used for the four major steps of the research process—data collection, data coding, data analysis, and dissemination of data results including meta-analysis. This research chapter widens the horizons of using technology for nursing research and for nurse researchers.

The second chapter in the research applications section focuses on computerized information resources. The two authors are officers of Cinahl Information Systems and are qualified to prepare this chapter on the online bibliographic retrieval systems and other literature and information resources used and needed by the nurses and other health professionals. They describe the content of a retrieval system as a database and identify the steps for choosing an appropriate database. They also highlight the steps in planning a search of the information using computer technology and boolean logic of the existing databases with nursing literature. They discuss the searching of the Internet for other nursing literature and information resources. They include the rationale for why all practicing nurses and professional nurses should identify the sources of information resources to stay professionally current.

International Perspectives

There is also much developing internationally in standards and EHRs. This section of the book allows the students and scholars of NI to gain an understanding of the leadership of nurses internationally in advancing the NI agenda. The Canadian Perspective defines how the MDS is advancing in Canada. The important advances in the Canadian Infohighway and the definitions of NI and educational goals are updated. The terminology challenges in Europe are updated and defined by new authors from the continent. They have updated descriptions of important projects that have obtained funding in Europe from the European Commission.

The chapter on Pan-Pacific represents Australia, New Zealand, and Hong Kong. The update of advances in standards, education, and organizations supporting NI are described. The information infrastructure that has developed to support healthcare and nursing has developed because of the government funding environment, the use of information systems for acuity and restoring, as well as workload. The role of nurses in standards development also allows the reader to appreciate the unique contributions the nursing profession is making in the Pacific Rim. They update the broader Asia innovations that are also taking place in Hong Kong.

A new chapter was added on the Asian perspective, focusing on current status of NI in South Korea, Japan, China, Taiwan, and Thailand. Each country provides an overview of its uses of informatics in clinical practice, education, and research including government initiatives and professional outreaches. Each country identifies

their historical milestones, changes, and trends that influence how their nurses embrace informatics such as government initiatives and international collaboration. Healthcare information and information technology have proceeded rapidly in these Asian countries.

The chapter on South America updates the development and the use of information systems in South America. They identify the use of information technology in practice. They also describe educational and distance learning initiatives in South America. They have begun impressive standard setting activities that are also described in this chapter. The authors have highlighted the *Nursing Informatics 2003 Symposium* held in Rio de Janeiro.

This new chapter on the future has been developed because there is so much new technology on the horizon resulting from developments in IT and the scientific revolution in basic biology. The emerging fields of genetics, genomics, and proteomics, and the changes in environmental factors are necessitating changes in looking at the future. Several of the futuristic predictions in the third edition are already realities, and others have not materialized. Advancing convergence of the Internet, telephony, and communication networks may allow visions of the future to be realized quicker in the next decade. Attention to a decade of the EHR, terminologies and standards will accelerate the use of IT in nursing providing nurses are involved in defining the vision, receive adequate funding, and demonstrate their impact on quality, outcomes, patient safety, and cost.

References

American Nurses Association Workgroup. (2001). *Scope and Standards of Nursing Informatics Practice.* Washington, DC: American Nurses Publishing.

Androwich, I.M., Bickford, C.J., Button, P.S., Hunter, K.M., Murphy, J., and Sensmeier, J. (2003). *Clinical Information Systems: A Framework for Reaching Vision.* Washington, DC: American Nurses Publishing.

McCormick, K.A., Sensemeier, J., Delaney, C., and Bickford, C. (2005). Introduction to informatics and nursing. In Joe Bronzino (Ed. in Chief), *Handbook of Biomedical Engineering* (3rd ed.). Boca Raton, FL: CRC Press.

2

Historical Perspectives of Nursing and the Computer

Virginia K. Saba
William Scott Erdley

OBJECTIVES

1. Highlight a brief historical perspective of nursing and computers.
2. List the major landmark events and milestones of nursing and computers.

KEY WORDS

computer literacy
computer systems
information systems
Internet
nursing informatics
data standards

The computer is the most powerful technological tool to transform the nursing profession prior to the new century. The computer has transformed the nursing paper-based records to computer-based records. Today and tomorrow, the computer and the Internet are essential for all settings where nurses function—hospitals, ambulatory care centers, health maintenance organizations, community health agencies, academic institutions, research centers, and schools of nursing.

"Computer" is an all encompassing term referring to information technology (IT), computer systems, and when they are used in nursing, refer to nursing information systems (NISs), nursing applications, and/or nursing informatics (NI). "NI" has emerged as a new term encompassing these technologies enabling nurses to manage health care and patient care more efficiently and effectively and, at the same time, make nurses more accountable.

Computers in nursing are used to manage information in patient care, monitor the quality of care, and evaluate the outcomes of care. Computers and networks are now used for communicating (sending/receiving) data and messages via the Internet, accessing resources, and interacting with patients on the World Wide Web (WWW). Nurses are increasingly involved with systems used for planning, budgeting, and policy-making for patient care services as well as enhancing nursing education and distance learning with new media modalities. Computers are also used to support nursing research, test new systems, design new knowledge databases, and advance the role of nursing in the health care industry.

Overview

This chapter is an update and a revised version of the chapter "Historical Perspectives of Nursing and the Computer" (Saba, 2001) published in the third edition, *Essentials of Computers for Nursing: Informatics for the New Millennium* (Saba and McCormick, 2001). Most of the previous details can be found in the third edition. However, this chapter provides a brief overview of the history of the computer since its introduction in the field of nursing based on six time periods leading to the present and highlighting several major nursing areas. It addresses the latest key issues related to data standards and significant landmark events. Also, this chapter presents a milestone table listing those events that influenced the introduction of computers into the nursing profession including the key "computer/informatics" nurse that directed the activity (Saba et al., 2000).

 ## Major Historical Perspectives of Nursing and Computers

Computer technology emerged in nursing in response to the changing and developing technologies in the health care industry and in nursing practice. It is analyzed according to (1) **six time periods**: prior to the 1960s, the 1960s, the 1970s, the 1980s, the 1990s and post-2000; (2) **four major nursing areas**: nursing practice, administration, education, and research; (3) **standards initiatives**: nursing practice, nursing data, and health care data standards; (4) **significant landmark events**; and (5) **major landmark milestone chart** listing those events that influenced the introduction of computers into the nursing profession including the key "computer/informatics" nurse that directed the activity.

Six Time Periods

Six historical perspectives of nursing and computers follow:

Prior to the 1960s   Starting in the 1950s, and as the computer industry grew, the use of computers in the health care industry also grew. During this time, there were only a few experts who formed a cadre of pioneers that attempted to adapt computers to health care and nursing. During this time the nursing profession was also undergoing major changes. The image of nursing was improving, nursing practices and services were expanding in scope and complexity, and the number of nurses was increasing. These events provided the impetus for the profession to embrace computers.

Computers were initially used in health care facilities for basic business office functions. These early computers used punch cards to store data and card readers to read computer programs, sort, and prepare data for processing. They were linked together and operated by paper tape and used teletypewriters to print their output. As computer technology advanced, the health care technologies improved.

1960s   During the 1960s the uses of computer technology in health care settings began to be questioned. Questions such as "Why computers?" and "What should be computerized?" were discussed. Nursing practice standards were reviewed, and nursing resources were analyzed. Studies were conducted to determine how computer technology could be utilized effectively in the health care industry and what areas of nursing should be automated. The nurses' station in the hospital was viewed as the hub of information exchange, the most appropriate center for the development of the computer applications.

During this period, computer technology advanced, while the number of health care facilities increased. The introduction of cathode ray tube (CRT) terminals, online data communication, and real-time processing added important dimensions to the computer systems, providing more accessible and "user-friendly" machines. Hospital information systems (HISs) were developed primarily to process financial transactions and serve as billing and accounting systems. However, a few HISs emerged that documented and processed a limited number of medical orders and nursing care activities. Vendors of computer systems were beginning to enter the health care field and market software applications for various hospital functions; however, because of technology limitations, lack of standardization, and diversity of paper-based patient care records, progress was slow.

1970s   In the 1970s, the inevitable continued integration of computers into nursing. Nurses began to recognize the value of the computer for their profession. During this decade, giant steps were taken in both dimensions: nursing and computer technology. Nurses recognized the computer's potential for improving the documentation of nursing practice, the quality of patient care, and the repetitive aspects of managing patient care. They assisted in the design and development of nursing applications for the HISs and other environments where nurses functioned. Interestingly, computer applications for the financial and management functions of patient care systems were perceived as cost-saving technologies. Further, several mainframe HISs were designed and developed, a few of which eventually became forerunners of a number of today's systems. Many of the early systems were funded by contracts or grants from federal agencies (National Center for Health Services Research, 1980).

During this period, several states and large community health agencies developed and/or contracted for their own computer-based management information systems (MISs). Generally, public health MISs provided statistical information required by local, state, and federal agencies for specific program funds, whereas home health agencies provided billing and other financial information required for reimbursement of patient services by Medicare, Medicaid, and other third-party payers.

1980s   During the 1980s, the field of informatics emerged in the health care industry and nursing. NI became an accepted specialty and many nursing experts entered the field. Technology challenged creative professionals and the use of computers in nursing became revolutionary. As computer systems were implemented, the needs of nursing took on a cause-and-effect modality; that is, as new computer technologies emerged and as computer architecture advanced, the need for nursing software evolved. It became apparent that the nursing profession needed not only to update its practice standards but also determine its data standards, vocabularies, and classification schemes that could be coded for the computer-based patient record systems (CPRSs).

During this period, many mainframe HISs emerged with nursing subsystems. These systems documented several aspects of the patient record; namely, order entry emulating the Kardex, results reporting, vital signs, and other systems that documented narrative nursing notes via word-processing packages. Discharge planning systems were developed and used as referrals to community health care facilities in the continuum of care.

In the 1980s, the microcomputer or personal computer (PC) emerged. This revolutionary technology made computers more accessible, affordable, and usable by nurses and other health care providers. PCs brought computing power to the workplace and, more importantly, to the point-of-care. PCs served not only as terminals linked to the mainframe computers but also as stand-alone systems (workstations). They were user-friendly and allowed nurses to create their own applications.

1990s   Beginning with the early 1990s, computer technology became an integral part of health care settings, nursing practice, and the nursing profession. The professional organizations identified initiatives that addressed IT and informatics. Policies and legislation were adopted promoting computer technology in health care including nursing.

The nursing profession became actively involved in promoting NI. In 1992, NI was approved by the American Nurses Association (ANA) as a new nursing specialty (McCormick et al., 1994). The demand for NI

expertise increased greatly in the workplace and other settings where nurses functioned, and the technology revolution continued to impact the profession.

The need for computer-based nursing practice standards, data standards, nursing minimum data sets, and national databases emerged concurrent with the need for a unified nursing language, including nomenclatures, vocabularies, taxonomies, and classification schemes. Nurse administrators demanded that the HISs include nursing care protocols and nurse educators continued to require use of innovative technologies for all levels and types of nursing and patient education. Also, nurse researchers required knowledge representation, decision support, and expert systems based on aggregated data.

The 1990s brought smaller and faster computers—laptops and notebooks—to the bedside and all of the point-of-care settings. Workstations and local area networks (LANs) were developed for hospital nursing units, wide area networks (WANs) were developed for linking care across health care facilities, and the Internet started to be used for linking across the different systems. The Internet made it possible for information and knowledge databases to be integrated into bedside systems.

In the 1990s, the Internet brought new cyberspace tools forming building blocks for increasingly sophisticated information technologies. By 1995, the Internet had moved into the mainstream social milieu with electronic mail (e-mail), file transfer protocol (FTP), Gopher, Telnet, and WWW protocols, which greatly enhanced its usability and user-friendliness (Saba, 1996; Sparks, 1996). The Internet began to be used for high performance computing and communication (HPCC) or the "information superhighway." Also, it facilitated data exchange between CPRSs across facilities and settings and over time. The "Web" became the means for communicating online services and resources to the nursing community. The Internet became an integral component of all IT systems, and the WWW used to browse the Internet and search worldwide resources (Nicoll, 1998; Saba, 1995b; Saba, 1996; Sparks, 1996).

Post-2000   The early years of the new millennium continued the torrid pace of hardware and software development and growth. This growth is reflected in healthcare and nursing, with developments such as wireless point-of-care, serious consideration for open source solutions, regional database projects, and increased IT solutions targeted at all healthcare environments. Further, clinical information systems became individualized in the electronic patient record (EPR) and patient specific systems considered for the lifelong longitudinal record or the electronic health record (EHR).

Information technologies continued to advance with mobile technology such as with wireless tablet computers, personal digital assistants (PDAs), and smart cellular telephones. The development and subsequent refinement of voice over Internet protocol (VoIP) promises to provide cheap voice communication for healthcare organizations. The prediction of smart cards were realized in Europe (Germany) where, a health "smart card" has been in existence since the early 1990s (Sembritzki, 2003).

The advancement of the Internet as well as the forces of labor shortage and cost containment continue to provide impetus for increased adoption and utilization of information technology in nursing and healthcare. The Internet has also provided a means for development of clinical applications. Critical care units are monitored remotely by health providers (eICU: *http://www.visicu. com/products/*, accessed April 22, 2004). Home health care has also increasingly partnered with information technology for the provision of patient care. Telenursing, a recognized specialty since the late 1990s, is increasing in popularity and providing patient care in an efficient and expeditious fashion.

Post-2000 also witnessed the continued impact of legislation on the U.S. healthcare industry. The Health Insurance Portability and Accountability Act of 1996 (HIPAA) was enacted to streamline health care transactions and reduce costs. Components of HIPAA specifically those portions related to the electronic collection and transmission now impact all federally required reimbursement data. Standardized transaction and code sets were selected to protect the security as well as ensure the privacy and confidentiality and were implemented in early 2004.

This legislation also recommended health care providers use a provider identification number (PIN) to maintain privacy and security of patient information (Appavu, 1999; Coate and McDonald, 2002). This new legislation has lead to several federal and private initiatives for health care technologies. The major ones include eHealth Initiative and Institute, Consolidated Health Information (CHI) initiative, the National Health Information Infrastructure (NHII) initiative, and several others continue to emerge. These organizations are all involved in promoting information technologies, standards, applications, systems, and laws that support effective health care and are described in other sections of this book.

Four Major Nursing Areas

This second section addresses the historical perspectives of nursing that shaped the need for computers, information technologies, and informatics. The focus is on these four major nursing areas: nursing practice, administration, education, and research. They are also described in the chapter "Historical Perspectives of Nursing and the Computer" (Saba, 2001) published in the third edition *Essentials of Computers for Nursing: Informatics for the New Millennium* (Saba and McCormick, 2001). However, this chapter highlights and updates new trends and issues that impact on "why computers."

Nursing Practice   Nursing practice has evolved and changed radically. It has become an integral part of the EHR. Computer systems with nursing and patient care data, nursing care plans are no longer separate subsystems of the computerized HISs, but rather integrated into one interdisciplinary patient health record in the EHR. The need for an interdisciplinary EHR resulted because of many initiatives proposed and promoted by the nursing profession as well as by other health care providers. They all require patient care data to track the care process. Further nursing practice data emerged with the introduction of several nursing terminologies that were recognized by the ANA as coded terminologies usable for the EHR. They are used to assess problems, document care, track the care process, and measure outcomes. Thus the electronic version of nursing practice—the computer—has revolutionized and transformed nursing practice.

Nursing Administration   Nursing administration in hospitals has also changed with the introduction of the computer that links nursing departments together. Most policy and procedure manuals are accessed and retrieved by computer. Further, workload measures, acuity systems, and other nursing department systems are online and integrated with the hospital or patient's EHR system or in separate nursing department systems. The Internet is being used by nurses to access digital libraries, online resources, and research protocols at the bedside.

Nursing Education   The computer has radically changed nursing education. Most universities and schools of nursing offer computer enhanced courses, online courses, and/or distance education. They are becoming universities without walls where students can attend a university anywhere in the world without being present. Campus-wide computer systems are available for students to communicate via e-mail, transfer data files, access the digital libraries, and retrieve online resources of millions of Internet WWW sites (Saba, 1996).

These new educational strategies require different methods of teaching. Today, most faculty members use the Internet to teach courses via the Web and communicate with their students via e-mail. They require new tools, techniques, and a full array of multimedia strategies to stimulate their students. The students on the other hand have to be more active and assume more responsibility for their education. Interactive teleconferencing courses also bring live classroom lectures via computer systems via digital telephone lines or satellite communication to remote sites. This "face-to-face" medium makes it possible for students to stay at home and work while attending classes in their own environments. Time, distance, and cost are no longer barriers to educational programs (Joos and Nelson, 1992; Saba, 2000).

Nursing Research   Nursing research provides the impetus to use the computer for analyzing nursing data. Software programs are available for processing both quantitative and qualitative research data. With the advancement of computer technology databases supporting nursing research emerged, principally for online searching and retrieving information from the electronic bibliographic literature systems or other databases that contain relevant health care content, such as drug data. These large databases are used for meta-analysis to develop evidenced-based practice guidelines (Saba et al., 1989). The Internet also provides online access to the millions of Web resources around the world which have increased the capabilities and expanded the field of nursing research.

Standards Initiatives

The third significant historical perspective concerns standards initiatives focusing on nursing practice standards, nursing data standards, and health care data standards as well as federal legislation that impact on the use of the computer into nursing. These standards have influenced the nursing profession and its need for computer systems, information technology, and terminologies to gain acceptance among the health care policy makers. The legislative acts during the early stages influenced significantly the use of the computer for collection of federally required data, reimbursement, measure quality, and evaluate outcomes. The historical details are also described in the chapter "Historical Perspectives of Nursing and the Computer" (Saba, 2001) published in the third edition *Essentials of Computers for Nursing: Informatics for the New Millennium* (Saba and McCormick, 2001). However, this section only highlights briefly the critical initiatives "to set the stage" for other sections in this edition.

Nursing Practice Standards   Nursing practice standards have been developed and recommended by the ANA, the official professional nursing organization. The ANA published The Standards of Clinical Nursing Practice (ANA, 1998) which focused not only on the organizing principles of clinical nursing practice but also the standards of professional performance. They recommended that the nursing process serve as the conceptual framework for the documentation of nursing practice.

Nursing practice standards have also been set by the Joint Commission on Accreditation of Hospital Organizations (JCAHO) which stressed the need for adequate records on patients in hospitals and practice standards for the documentation of care by nurses (Namdi and Hutelmyer, 1970). They also recommended acuity systems to determine resource use as well as required care plans for documenting nursing care (JCAHO, 1994). Further, they have included in their recent manual the required contents of an EHR, such as what data should be collected and how the data should be organized in the electronic database (Corum, 1993). These standards have evolved and continue to increase as the federal requirements evolve and/or are implemented.

Nursing Data Standards   Nursing data standards have emerged as a new requirement for the EHR. The original data elements and historical details are described in the third edition; however, for this fourth edition is it important to understand that currently there are 13 nursing terminologies that have been recognized by the ANA and which are described in other sections of this book. Several of these terminologies are in the public domain and usable by the general public such as the Critical Care Classification (CCC) system by Saba and colleagues (Saba, 1995a; 1997; 2002) (see detailed description in Chap. 21 and web site <*www. sabacare.com*>). There are other terminologies such as Nursing Information Classification (NIC) that requires a license fee to use. Each of the 13 terminologies was developed at different times, has different characteristics, and is used for documenting different aspects of nursing practice. Further, only one or two of these terminologies were developed and coded for computer processing, whereas the majority were designed for documenting nursing practice without any regard for computer processing which is why it has been so difficult to computerize them.

The ANA is responsible for the recognition of the terminologies and for determining if they have met the criteria to be included in the National Library of Medicine (NLM) Unified Medical Language Systems (UMLS) (Humphreys and Lindberg, 1992; Saba, 1998). Further, recently many of the nursing terminologies have also been integrated into SNOMED CT developed by SNOMED International (College of American Pathologists and American Veterinary Medical Association, 1998). Several aspects of SNOMED have recently been integrated into the UMLS. This new initiative has made it possible for many of the nursing terminologies in SNOMED CT and in the UMLS available to the public (Health Level Seven, 1999).

Heath Care Data Standards Organizations

It is critical to review the standards organizations that have emerged to either develop or recommend health care data standards that should be recommended to the federal government as required health care data standards. The major ones are listed below but also described elsewhere in this book.

The American National Standards Institute (ANSI) is a private nonprofit membership organization. It was instituted to coordinate and approve voluntary standards efforts in the United States. ANSI was combined with the Health Care Informatics Standards Board (HISB) to form ANSI-HISB to fulfill a request by the European standards coordinating organization (CEN TC/251) to represent the U.S. standards effort. Thus, the ANSI-HISB organization acts as one linking to the two major organizations in Europe, the European

Standardization Committee (CEN) and International Standards Organization (ISO).

American Society for Testing and Materials (ASTM): The ASTM E-31 Committee on Healthcare Informatics is an accredited committee that develops standards for health information and health information systems designed to assist vendors, users, and anyone interested in systematizing health information (Cendrowska et al., 1999; Hammond, 1994).

Health Level Seven (HL7) is an organization accredited by the ANSI, which was created to develop standards for the electronic interchange of clinical, financial, and administrative information among independent healthcare-oriented information systems. It grew out of efforts that involved multiple vendors to initiate open HISs (Agency for Health Care Policy and Research, 1999; Fitzmaurice, 1995; Hammond, 1994; Van Bemmel et al., 1997).

SNOMED International is another organization that serves as an umbrella of the structured nomenclatures, and its merger with the Read Codes from the National Health Service in the United Kingdom in 1999. Since the existing medical and disease condition nomenclatures are already indexed, the newly named SNOMED CT serves as the coding strategy and has become a national standard for the EHR aspects of which are integrated into the UMLS and available to the public.

The National Committee on Vital and Health Statistics (NCVHS) Workgroup on Computer-based Patient Records: This national workgroup was created to help the Department of Health and Human Services (DHHS) investigate and approve health care standards for the federal government to use to implement federal legislation (Chute et al., 1996). The Committee evaluated and recognized medical, nursing, and other health profession nomenclatures for the DHHS to the implement the HIPAA of 1996 (NCVHS, 1996). The NCVHS workgroup on CPRSs prepared a report for the DHHS recommending standards to implement the HIPAA legislation. They proposed standards for the electronic transmission of federally mandated reimbursement for Medicare and Medicaid patient services. They also recommended that the selected transaction and code sets primarily focus on privacy and security for the EHR. They have been involved in several other federal and national initiatives such as the Patient Medical Record Information (PMRI) which is the second phase of the HIPAA legislation.

Early Computer-Based Nursing Applications

Several computer-based nursing applications, developed before the mid-1970s as part of larger HISs, still exist. Each in its own way developed different nursing applications focused on documentation of nursing practice and management of patient care. These applications were designed for hospitals, ambulatory care settings, and community health agencies. Additionally, several significant nursing projects were conducted to improve nursing care documentation methodologies, which in turn could be computerized. These major nursing applications, which influenced the industry, were subsystems or components of early HISs focused on (a) early HISs, (b) early ambulatory care information systems, (c) early community health nursing information management systems, (d) early computer-focused nursing projects, and (e) early educational applications. They are described in detail in the chapter "Historical Perspectives of Nursing and the Computer" (Saba, 2001) published in the third edition *Essentials of Computers for Nursing: Informatics for the New Millennium* (Saba and McCormick, 2001).

Landmark Events in Nursing and Computers

Computers were introduced into the nursing profession over 35 years ago. Major milestones of nursing are interwoven with the advancement of computer and information technologies, the increased need for nursing data, development of nursing applications, and changes making the nursing profession an autonomous discipline. The major developments in the use of information technologies and nursing, and in the introduction of NI, were chronologically described by program effort, or by organizational initiative. The landmark events were described by the following categories: (a) early conferences, meetings, (b) early academic initiatives, (c) initial ANA initiatives, (d) initial National League for Nursing (NLN) initiatives, (e) early international initiatives, (f) initial educational resources, and (g) significant collaborative events.

The landmark events are also categorized and described in the chapter "Historical Perspectives of Nursing and the Computer" (Saba, 2001) published in the third edition *Essentials of Computers for Nursing:*

Informatics for the New Millennium (Saba and McCormick, 2001).

Major Landmark Milestones

In this edition, the major landmark milestones table has been outlined in Table 2.1. The milestone events are listed in chronological order including for the first time, the key NI pioneer or expert involved in the event. Many other events have occurred; however, this table represents the most complete history of the NI movement.

Summary

Computers, and subsequently information technology, emerged during the past five decades in the health care industry. Hospitals began to use computers as tools to update paper-based patient records. Computer systems in health care settings provided the information management capabilities needed to assess, document, process, and communicate patient care. As a result, the "man-machine" interaction of nursing and computers has become a new and lasting symbiotic relationship (Blum, 1990; Collen, 1994; Kemeny, 1972).

Computer applications in nursing and early computerized information systems that were described can be found in the chapter "Historical Perspectives of Nursing and the Computer" (Saba, 2001) published in the third edition *Essentials of Computers for Nursing: Informatics for the New Millennium* (Saba and McCormick, 2001). Many of these systems are considered to be forerunners of systems still used in hospitals, community health, and other health care settings. Also, several projects were described that influenced today's systems. Further, applications supporting nursing practice, administration, education, and research were highlighted.

The last section focused on landmark events in nursing and computers, including major milestones in national and international conferences, symposia, workshops, and organizational initiatives contributing to the computer literacy of nurses. The success of the conferences and the appearance of nursing articles, journals, books, and other literature on this topic demonstrated the intense interest nurses had in learning more about computers and information technologies. These advances confirmed the status of NI as a new specialty in nursing and provided impetus to transform nursing in the twenty-first century.

Table 2.1 Landmark Events in Computers and Nursing

Year	Title	Sponsor(s)	Coordinator/Chair NI Representative(s)	Site
1973	First Invitational Conference: Management Information Systems (MIS) for Public/Community Health Agencies	National League for Nursing (NLN) and Division of Nursing, Public Health Service (DN/PHS)	Goldie Levenson (NLN) Virginia Saba (DN/PHS)	Fairfax, VA
1974–1975	Five Workshops on MISs for Public/Community Health Agencies	NLN and DN/PHS	Goldie Levenson (NLN) Virginia Saba (DN/PHS)	Nationwide
1976	State-of-the-Art Conference in Management for Public/Community Health Agencies	NLN and DN/PHS	Goldie Levenson (NLN) Virginia Saba (DN/PHS)	Washington, DC
1977	First Research: State-of-the-Art Conference on Nursing Information Systems	University of Illinois College of Nursing	Harriet Werley Margaret Grier	Chicago, IL
1977	First undergraduate academic course: Computers and Nursing	The State University of New York at Buffalo	Judith Ronald	Buffalo, NY
1979	First Military Conference: Computers in Nursing	TRIMIS Army Nurse Consultant Team, Walter Reed Hospital	Dorothy Pocklington Linda Guttman	Washington, DC
1980	First Workshop: Computer Usage in Health Care	University of Akron School of Nursing, CE Dept.	Virginia Newbern (UA) Dorothy Pocklington (ARMY) Virginia Saba (DN/PHS)	Akron, OH
1980	First Computer book: Computers in Nursing	Nursing Resources	Rita Zielstorff, Editor	Boston, MA
1981	First Special Interest Group: Computers in Nursing (SIG-CIN)	SCAMC, Inc. Event	Virginia Saba, Chair	Washington, DC
1981	First National Conference: Computer Technology and Nursing	NIH Clinical Center, TRIMIS Army Nurse Consultant Team, and DN/PHS	Ruth Carlsen (NIH) Dorothy Pocklington (TRIMIS Army) Virginia Saba (DN/PHS)	Bethesda, MD
1981	First nursing sessions at Fifth Annual Symposium on Computer Applications in Medical Care (SCAMC)	SCAMC, Inc.	Virginia Saba Coralee Farlee	Washington, DC
1981	Early academic course: Computers in Nursing	Foundation for Advanced Education in Sciences (FAES) at NIH	Virginia Saba (DN/PHS) Kathleen McCormick (NIH)	Bethesda, MD

Year	Event	Organization	People	Location
1982	Study Group on Nursing Information Systems	University Hospitals of Cleveland, Case Western Reserve University and National Center for Health Services Research, PHS	Mary Kiley (UHC) Gerry Weston (NCHSR)	Cleveland, OH
1982	First Annual National Nursing Computer Technology Conference	Rutgers, State University of New Jersey, College of Nursing, CE Dept.	Gayle Pearson Jean Arnold	Newark, NJ
1982	First International Workshop: The Impact of Computers on Nursing	London Hospital, U.K. and IFIP-IMIA	Maureen Scholes Barry Barber	Church House Westminster, London and Harrogate, Yorkshire, England
1982	Second National Conference: Computer Technology and Nursing	NIH Clinical Center. TRIMIS Army Nurse Consultant Team, and DN/PHS	Ruth Carlson (NIH) Dorothy Pocklington (TRIMIS Army) Virginia Saba (DN/PHS)	Bethesda, MD
1982	First Newsletter: *Computers in Nursing*	School of Nursing, University of Texas at Austin	Gary Hales	Austin, TX
1982	First BU Workshop: Computers and Nursing	Boston University School of Nursing	Diane Skiba	Boston, MA
1982	PLATO IV—CAI Educational Network System	University of Illinois School of Nursing	Pat Tymchyshyn	Urbana-Champaign, IL
1983	First Nursing Papers at MED-INFO'83: Fourth World Congress on Medical Informatics	International Medical Informatics Association (IMIA)	Elly Pluyter-Wenting	Amsterdam, The Netherlands
1983	Third National Conference: Computer Technology and Nursing	NIH Clinical Center, TRIMIS Army Nurse Consultant Team, and DN/PHS	Carol Romano (NIH) Carolyn Tindal (TRIMIS Army) Virginia Saba (DN/PHS)	Bethesda, MD
1983	Second Annual Joint SCAMC Congress and IMIA Conference	SCAMC and IMIA	Nursing Papers	San Francisco, CA and Baltimore, MD
1983	New newsletter publisher: *Computers in Nursing*	J. Lippincott Corp.		Philadelphia, PA
1983	Early Workshop: Computers in Nursing	University of Texas at Austin	Sue Grobe, Chair	Austin, TX
1983	First Hospital Workshop: Computers in Nursing Practice	St. Agnes Hospital for HEC	Sue Newbold	Baltimore, MD
1983	First Nursing Model for Patient Care	TRIMIS Program Office	Karen Rieder Dena Nortan	Washington, DC

Table 2.1 Landmark Events in Computers and Nursing (*Continued*)

Year	Title	Sponsor(s)	Coordinator/Chair NI Representative(s)	Site
1983	IMIA initiated: Working Group 8 on Nursing Informatics	IMIA	Maureen Scholes, First Chair	Amsterdam, The Netherlands
1984	Fourth National Conference: Computer Technology and Nursing	NIH Clinical Center, TRIMIS Army Nurse Consultant Team, and DN/PHS	Carol Romano (NIH) Carolyn Tindal (Army) Virginia Saba (DN/PHS)	Bethesda, MD
1984	First Seminar on Microcomputers for Nurses	University of California at San Francisco, College of Nursing	William Holzemer	San Francisco, CA
1984	First nursing computer journal: *Computers in Nursing*	J. Lippincott Corp.	Gary Hales	Philadelphia, PA
1984	American Nursing Association (ANA) initiated: Council on Computer Applications in Nursing (CCAN)	ANA	Harriet Werley, Chair	Kansas City, MO
1984–1995	First *Directory of Educational Software for Nursing*	Christine Bolwell and National League for Nursing (NLN)	Christine Bolwell	New York, NY
1984	Second BU Workshop: Computers and Nursing	Boston University School of Nursing	Diane Skiba	Boston, MA
1985	NLN initiated National Forum on Computers in Health Care and Nursing	NLN	Sue Grobe, First Chair	New York, NY
1985	First Annual Seminar on Computers and Nursing Practice	NYU Medical Center	Patsy Marr	New York, NY
1985	First Invitational Conference: Nursing Minimum Data Set (NMDS) Conference	University of Illinois School of Nursing	Harriet Werley Norma Lang	Chicago, IL
1985	Early academic course: Essentials of Computers in Undergraduate /Graduate Programs	Georgetown University School of Nursing	Virginia Saba	Washington, DC
1985/1990	Early project: Continuing Nursing Education in Computer Technology	Southern Regional Education Board (SREB)	Eula Aiken	Atlanta, GA

Year	Event	Organization	People	Location
1985	Second International Symposium: Nursing Uses of Computers and Information Science—NI '85	IMIA/NI—Working Group 8	Kathryn J. Hannah, Evelyn J. Guillemin	Calgary, AB, Canada
1985	First Test Authorizing Program (TAP)	Addison-Wesley	William Holzemer	Menlo Park, CA
1986	Early Microcomputer Institute for Nurses	Georgetown University and University of Southwest Louisiana	Virginia Saba (GT), Dorothy Pocklington (USL), Diane Skiba (BU)	Washington, DC and Lafayette, LA
1986	Established first Nurse Educators's Newsletter: *Micro World*	Christine Bolwell and Stewart Publishing	Christine Bolwell	Alexandria, VA
1986	MEDINFO '86: Fifth World Congress on Medical Informatics	IMIA/SCAMC	Nursing Papers	Washington, DC
1987	International Working Group 8 Task Force on Education	IMIA/NI—Working Group 8 and Swedish Federation	Ulla Gerdin-Jelger, Kristina Janson, Hans Peterson	Stockholm, SW
1987	Initiated *Interactive Videodisc Software Programs*	American Journal of Nursing - Grants	Mary Ann Rizzolo	New York, NY
1987	Video disk for Health Conference: *Interactive Healthcare Conference*	Stewart Publishing	Scott Stewart	Alexandria, VA
1988	Recommendation no. 3: Support Automated Information Systems	Secretary's Commission on Nursing Shortage	Vivian DeBack	Washington, DC
1988	Priority Expert Panel E: Nursing Informatics Task Force	National Center for Nursing Research, PHS	Judy Ozbolt, Chair	Bethesda, MD
1988	Third International Symposium: Nursing Use of Computers and Information Science—NI'88	IMIA/NI—Working Group 8 and The Irish Nursing Board	Noel Daley, Maureen Scholes	Dublin, Ireland
1989	First Initiated Nurse Scholars Program	HBO and HealthQuest Corp.	Roy Simpson, Diane Skiba, Judith Ronald	Atlanta, GA
1989	MEDINFO '89: Sixth World Congress on Medical Informatics	IMIA	Nursing Papers	Singapore, Malaysia

Table 2.1 Landmark Events in Computers and Nursing (*Continued*)

Year	Title	Sponsor(s)	Coordinator/Chair NI Representative(s)	Site
1989	Invitational Conference: Nursing Information Systems	National Commission on Nursing Implementation Project (NCNIP), ANA, NLN, and NIS Industry	Vivian DeBack, Chair	Washington, DC
1989	ICN Resolution Initiated Project: International Classification of Nursing Practice (ICNP)	International Council of Nurses	Fadwa Affra (ICN)	Seoul, Korea
1990	Invitational Conference: State-of-the-Art of Information Systems	NCNIP	Vivian DeBack	Orlando, FL
1990	Formation of ANA Steering Committee on Databases to Support Nursing Practice	ANA	Norma Lang, Chair	Washington, DC
1990	First Annual European Summer Institute	International Nursing Informatics Experts	Jos Aarts	Amsterdam, The Netherlands
1990	Task Force on Nursing Information Systems	NCNIP, ANA, NLN, NIS Industry Task Force	Vivian DeBack	Project Hope, VA
1991	First Nursing Informatics Listserv	University of Massachusetts	Gordon Larrivee	Amherst, MA
1991	Formation of Combined Annual Special Nursing Informatics Working Group	AMIA / SCAMC Sponsors	Judy Ozbolt, First Chair	Washington, DC
1991	First WHO Workshop on Nursing Informatics	World Health Organization U.S. PHS	Marian Hirschfield (WHO) Carol Romano (PHS)	Washington, DC Baltimore, MD
1991	First Summer Institute in Nursing and Healthcare Informatics	University of Maryland School of Nursing (SON)	Carol Gassert Mary Etta Mills	
1991	First graduate program: Masters and Doctoral Specialty in Nursing Informatics	University of Maryland SON	Carole Gassert, Chair Barbara Heller, Dean	Baltimore, MD
1991	Fourth International Conference on Nursing Use of Computers and Information Science: Nursing Informatics—NI'91	IMIA/NI—Working Group 8	Evelyn S. Hovenga Joan Edgecumbe	Melbourne, Australia

Year	Event	Organization	Person	Location
1992	Second WHO Workshop on Nursing Management Information Systems	WHO	Marian Hirschfield (WHO) Carol Romano (PHS)	Geneva, Switzerland
1992	MEDINFO '92: Seventh World Congress on Medical Informatics	IMIA	Nursing Papers	Geneva, Switzerland
1992	ANA approved Nursing Informatics as a Nursing Specialty	ANA Database Steering Committee	Norma Lang, Chair	Washington, DC
1992	Virginia Henderson International Nursing Library (INL)	Sigma Theta Tau International Honor Society	Judith Graves	Indianapolis, IN
1992	ANA recognized four nursing vocabularies: HHCC, OMAHA, NANDA, NIC	ANA Database Steering Committee	Norma Lang, Chair	Washington, DC
1992	Read Clinical Thesaurus added nursing terms	Read Codes Clinical Terms Version 3	Ann Casey	London, U.K.
1992	Nursing Minimum Data Set Conference	Canadian Nurses Assoc.	Phyllis Giovanetti, Chair	Edmonton, AB, Canada
1993	Four ANA recognized nursing vocabularies integrated into UMLS	ANA Database Steering Committee and NLM	Norma Lang (ANA) Betsy Humphreys (NLM)	Washington, DC
1993	Virginia Henderson Electronic Library Online	Sigma Theta Tau International Honor Society	Carol Hudgings	Indianapolis, IN
1993	AJN Network Online via Internet	American Journal of Nursing Company	Mary Ann Rizzolo	New York, NY
1993	ANC postgraduate course: Computer Applications for Nursing	Army Nurse Corps	Army Nurse Corps	Washington, DC
1993	Formation of Nursing Informatics Fellowship Program	Partners Healthcare Systems	Rita Zielstorff, Chair	Boston, MA
1993	Alpha Working Paper of ICNP	International Council of Nurses	Fadwa Affara (ICN)	Geneva, Switzerland
1993	Denver Free-Net	University of Colorado Health Sciences Center	Diane Skiba	Denver, CO
1993	Priority Expert Panel E: Nursing Informatics Report: Nursing Informatics: Enhancing Patient Care	National Center for Nursing Research, NIH, PHS	Judy Ozbolt, Chair	Bethesda, MD

Table 2.1 Landmark Events in Computers and Nursing (*Continued*)

Year	Title	Sponsor(s)	Coordinator/Chair NI Representative(s)	Site
1994	ANA*NET online	ANA	Kathy Milholland	Washington, DC
1994	Nursing Educators' Workshops	Southern Council on Collegiate Regional Education and University of Maryland	Eula Aiken (SREB) Mary Etta Mills (UM)	Baltimore, MD, Atlanta, and Augusta, GA
1994	Next Generation Clinical Information Systems Conference	Tri-Council for Nursing and Kellogg Foundation	Sheila Ryan, Chair	Washington, DC
1994	Fifth International Conference on Nursing Use of Computers and Information Science: Nursing Informatics—NI'94	IMIA/NI—Working Group 8, ANA, and NLN Nursing Informatics Councils	Sue Grobe, Chair Virginia Saba, Vice-Chair	San Antonio, TX
1995	MEDINFO '95: Eighth World Congress on Medical Informatics	IMIA	Nursing Papers	Vancouver, BC, Canada
1995	First International NI TeleConference*	International NI experts: HIS, Australia; NI, New Zealand; NI, U.S.	Evelyn Hovenga, Australia Robyn Carr, New Zealand Sue Sparks, MD	Melbourne, Australia Auckland, New Zealand and Bethesda, MD
1995	First Combined NYU Programs on Nursing Informatics and Patient Care: A New Era	NYU Division of Nursing and NYU Medical Center	Barbara Carty (SON) Janet Kelly (MC)	New York, NY
1995	First Weekend Immersion in NI (WINI)	CARING	Susan Newbold Carol Bickfod Kathleen Smith	Warrenton, VA
1995	First CPRI Davies Recognition Award of Excellence Symposium	Computer-based Patient Record Institute	Intermountain Healthcare—Salt Lake City, UT Columbia Presbyterian MC—NYC Dept. of Veterans Affairs—Washington, DC	Los Angeles, CA
1995	CARING Web site	CARING	Susan Newbold	Baltimore, MD

Year	Event	Organization	People	Location
1996	ANA established: Nursing Information and Data Set Evaluation Center (NIDSEC)	ANA Database Steering Committee	Rita Zielstorff, Chair; Connie Delaney, Vice-Chair	Washington, DC
1996	Initiated: Nightingale Project—Health Telematics Education: Three workshops and two international conferences	University of Athens, Greece, and European Union	John Mantas, Chair (Athens Univ.); Arie Hasman, Co-Chair (The Netherlands)	Athens, Greece
1996	Initiated: TELENURSE Project	Danish Institute for Health and Nursing Research and European Union	Randi Mortensen; Gunnar Nielsen	Copenhagen, Denmark
1996	First Harriet Werley Award for Best Nursing Informatics Paper at AMIA	AMIA-NI Working Group	Rita Zielstorff	Washington, DC
1997	Invitational National Nursing Informatics Workgroup	National Advisory Council on Nurse Education and Practice and DN/PHS	Carol Gassert (DN/PHS)	Washington, DC
1997	ANA published: *NIDSEC Standards and Scoring Guidelines*	ANA Database Steering Committee	Rita Zielstorff, Chair; Connie Delaney, Vice-Chair	Washington, DC
1997	Sixth International Conference on Nursing Use of Computers and Information Science—NI'2000	IMIA/NI—SIG	Ulla Gerdin; Maryanne Tallberg	Stockholm, Sweden
1998	Initiated NursingCenter.com Web site	J. Lippincott Corp.	Maryanne Rizzolo	New York, NY
1998	MEDINFO '98: Ninth World Congress on Medical Informatics	IMIA	Nursing Papers	Seoul, South Korea
1999	Beta version of ICNP	International Council of Nurses	Fadwa Affara (ICN)	Geneva, Switzerland
1999	First Annual Nursing Vocabulary Summit	Vanderbilt University	Judy Ozbolt, Chair	Vanderbilt, TN
1999	Convergent Terminology Group for Nursing	SNOMED/RT International	Debra Konichek, Chair; Suzanne Bakken, Co-Chair	Northbrook, IL
1999	Inaugural Virtual Graduation: Postmasters: ANP Certificate Program	GSN, Uniformed Services University and VA TeleConference Network	Virginia Saba (USU); Faye Abdellah (USU Dean); Charlotte Beason (VA)	Bethesda, MD and eight Nationwide VA MCs
1999	First meeting: Nursing Data Standards Project for Central Organization (PAHO) Heimar Marin (Brazil) and South America	Pan American Health Organization (PAHO)	Roberto Rodriquez (PAHO); Heimar Marin (Brazil)	Washington, DC

Table 2.1 Landmark Events in Computers and Nursing (*Continued*)

Year	Title	Sponsor(s)	Coordinator/Chair NI Representative(s)	Site
2000	ICNP programme office established	International Council of Nurses	Amy Coenen (Univ. of WI at Mil) Dir.	Geneva, Switzerland
2000	Seventh International Conference on Nursing Use of Computers and Information Science—NI'2000	IMIA/NI-SIG	Robyh Carrr Paula Rocha	Auckland, New Zealand
2000	Eighteenth Annual International Nursing Computer and Technology Conference	Rutgers, State University of New Jersey, College of Nursing	Gayle Pearson	Arlington, VA
2000	Tenth Annual Summer Institute in Nursing Informatics	University of Maryland, School of Nursing	Pattie Abbott, Chair	Baltimore, MD
2000	AMIA 2000 Annual Symposium	AMIA	Nursing Papers	Los Angeles, CA
2000	Computer-Based Patient Record Institute (CPRI) 2000 Conference	CPRI	Nursing Papers	Los Angeles, CA
2001	AMIA 2001 Annual Symposium	AMIA	Pattie Brennan, President Susanne Bakken, Program Chair	Washington, DC
2002	ICNP Strategic Advisory Group established	ICN	Amy Coenen	Geneva, Switzerland
2002	Strategy Conference for Health IT and eHealth Vendors	Medical Records Institute (MRI)	Peter Waegemann	Palm Springs, CA
2002	AAN Conference: Using Innovative Technology	American Academy of Nursing	Margaret McClure Linda Bolton Nellie O'Gara	Washington, DC
2002	AAN Initiated: Expert Panel on Nursing Informatics	American Academy of Nursing	Virginia Saba, Chair Ida Androwich, Co-Chair	Naples, FL
2003	Eighth International Congress: Nursing Informatics – NI '2003	IMIA/NI-SIG	Heimar Marin Eduardo Marques	Rio de Janeiro, Brazil
2003	Finnish Nursing Informatics Symposium	Finnish Nurses Assoc (FNA), Siemens Medical Solutions	Kaija Sarento (FNA) Anneli Ensio (FNA) Rosemary Kennedy (Siemens)	
2003	First ISO Nursing Standard: Integrated Reference Terminology Model for Nursing	IMIA/NI-SIG and ICN	Virginia Saba (NI/SIG) Kathleen McCormick (NI/WG) Amy Coenen (ICN) Evelyn Hovenga (NI/SIG) Susanne Bakken (RT Chair)	Oslo, Norway

Year	Event	Organization	Person	Location
2004	Fourteenth Annual Summer Institute in Nursing Informatics	University of Maryland, School of Nursing	Mary Etta Mills, Chair Diane Covington, Co-Chairs	Baltimore, MD
2004	Twenty-second Annual International Nursing Computer and Technology Conference	The State University of New Jersey—Rutgers	Gayle Pearson	Arlington, VA
2004	MEDINFO 2004: Eleventh World Congress on Medical Informatics and AMIA Annual Symposium	IMIA/AMIA	Nursing Papers	San Francisco, CA
2004	First ICN Research and Development Centre	Deutschsprachige ICNP	Peter Koenig	Freiburg, Germany
2004	First Nursing Informatics Symposium at HIMSS	HIMSS	Joyce Seisemeier, Chair	Orlando, FL

AMIA/SCAMC conducts an annual symposium on computer applications in medical care in cooperation with numerous professional societies, governmental agencies, universities, and healthcare organizations including the ANA and NLN (1981 to present).

References

Agency for Health Care Policy and Research. (1999). *Current Activities of Selected Healthcare Informatics Standards Organizations: A Compilation.* Rockville, MD: AHCPR, U.S. DHHS.

American Nurses Association. (1998). *Standards for Clinical Nursing Practice.* Washington, DC. Appavu, S.I. (1999). Federal Administrative Simplification Law (PL 104-191/HIPAA) toward standardization of healthcare information. In *Proceedings of the 1999 Annual HISs Conference: Volume 3* (pp. 339–347). Chicago, IL: HISS Publications.

Blum, B.I. (1990). Medical informatics in the United States, 1950–1975. In B. Blum and K. Duncan (Eds.), *A History of Medical Informatics* (pp. xvii–xxx). Reading, MA: Addison-Wesley.

Cendrowska, T.J., Amatayakul, M., and Tessier, C. (1999). Standards in healthcare: Meeting industry's needs by using ASTM standards. In *Proceedings of the 1999 Annual HISS Conference: Volume 3* (pp. 433–442). Chicago, IL: HISS Publications.

Chute, C.G., Cohen, S.P., and Campbell, K.E. (1996). The content coverage of clinical classifications. *Journal of the American Medical Informatics Association* 3:224–233.

Clinical Information Technology Program Office, Coate, D., and McDonald, K. (2002). Projecting the budget impacts of HIPAA. *Healthcare Financial Administration* 56(2):42–28.

College of American Pathologists and American Veterinary Medical Association. (1998). *SNOMED International.* Northfield, IL: College of American Pathologtsts and American Veterinary Medical Association.

Collen, M.F. (1994). The origins of informatics. *Journal of the American Medical Informatics Association* 1(2):91–107.

Corum, W. (1993). JCAHO's new information management standards. *Healthcare Informatics* 10(8):20–21.

DeGoulet, P., Piemme, T.E., Reinhoff, O. (Eds.) (1992). In *MEDINFO 92: Proceedings of the Seventh World Congress of Medical Informatics* (pp. 1496–1500), Amsterdam, North-Holland.

Fitzmaurice, M.J. (1995). Computer-based patient records. In J. Bronzino (Ed.), *Biomedical Engineering Handbook* (pp. 2623–2634). Boca Raton, FL: CRC Press.

Hammond, W.E. (1994). The role of standards in creating a health information infrastructure. *International Journal of Bio-Medical Computing* 34:29–44.

Health Level Seven. (1999). *Catalog of HL7 Resources.* Ann Arbor, MI: Health Level.

Humphreys, B.L. and Lindberg, D.A.B. (1992). The unified medical language system project: A distributed experiment in improving access to biomedical information. In K.C. Lun, P. DeGoulet, T.E. Piemme, and O. Reinhoff (Eds.), *MEDINFO 92: Proceedings of the Seventh World Congress of Medical Informatics* (pp. 1496–1500), Amsterdam, North-Holland.

Joos, I. and Nelson, R. (1992). Strategies and resources for self-education in nursing informatics. In J. Arnold and G. Pearson (Eds.), *Computer Applications in Nursing Education and Practice.* New York: National League for Nursing Press.

Kemeny, J.G. (1972). *Man and the Computer.* New York: Charles Scribner.

McCormick, K.A., Lang, N., Zielstorff, R., et al. (1994). Toward standards classification schemes for nursing language: Recommendations of the American Nurses Association Database Steering Committee to Support Nursing Practice. *Journal of the American Medical Informatics Association* 1:422–427.

Namdi, M.F. and Hutelmyer, C.M. (1970). A study of the effectiveness of an assessment tool in the identification of nursing care problems. *Nursing Research* 19(4):354–358.

National Center for Health Services Research. (1980). *Computer Applications in Health Care*, Hyattsville, MD: (NCHSR Research Report Series, DHHS Pub. No. 80–3251).

National Committee on Vital and Health Statistics (NCVHS). (1996). *Report: Core Health Care Data Elements.* Washington, DC: GPO (Pub No. 1996-1722-677/82345).

Nicoll, L.H. (1998). *Nurses Guide to the Internet*, 2nd ed. New York: Lippincott.

Saba, V.K., Oatway, D.M., and Rieder, K.A. (1989). How to use nursing information sources. *Nursing Outlook* 37(4):189–195.

Saba, V.K. (1995a). Home Health Care Classifications (HHCCs): Nursing diagnoses and nursing interventions. In ANA Database Committee, *Nursing Data Systems: The Emerging Framework* (pp. 50–60). Washington, DC: ANA.

Saba, V.K. (1995b). A new nursing vision: The information highway. *Nursing Leadership Forum* 1(2):44–51.

Saba, V.K. (1996). Developing a home page for the World Wide Web. *American Journal of Infection Control* 24(6):468–470.

Saba, V.K. (1997). Why the home health care classification is a recognized nursing nomenclature. *Computers in Nursing* 15(2S):S69–S76.

Saba, V.K. (1998). Nursing information technology: Classifications and management. In J. Mantas (Ed.), *Advances in Health Education: A Nightingale Perspective.* Amsterdam: IOS Press.

Saba, V.K. (2000). *Distance Education Using Teleconferencing.* Bethesda, MD: Uniformed Services University of the Health Sciences.

Saba, V.K., Carr, R., Sermeus, W., and Rocha, P. (Eds.) (2000). *Nursing Informatics 2000: One Step Beyond:*

The Evolution of Technology and Nursing. Auckland, New Zealand: Adis.

Saba, V.K. (2001). Historical perspectives of nursing and the computer. In V.K. Saba and K.A. McCormick (Eds.), *Essentials of Computers for Nurses: Informatics for the new Millennium* (pp. 9–46). New York: McGraw-Hill.

Saba, V. (2002). Nursing classifications: Home Health Care Classification System (HHCC): An overview. *Online Journal of Issues in Nursing.* Available at *http://nursing world.org/ojin/tpc7/tpc7_7htm*

Saba, V.K. and McCormick, K.A. (2001). *Essentials of Computers for Nurses: Informatics for the new millennium.* New York: McGraw- Hill.

Sembritzki, J. (2003). Your medical history all on a smart card. *ISO Bulletin. http//www.iso.ch,* last accessed 07.05.04.

Sparks, S. (1996). Use of the Internet for infection control and epidemiology. *American Journal of Infection Control* 24(6):435–439.

Van Bemmel, J.H. and Musen, M.A. (Eds.) (1997). *Handbook of Medical Informatics.* The Netherlands: Springer-Verlag.

Electronic Health Record from a Historical Perspective

Patricia B. Wise

OBJECTIVES

1. Describe the Nicholas E. Davies Program.
2. Name the four key criteria sections of the Davies application.
3. Name and describe one feature of an electronic health record (EHR) implementation that has not changed over time.
4. Describe an external factor that has impacted EHR implementation.
5. Describe several of the commonalities found in all Davies winners.

KEY WORDS

Nicholas E. Davies Award of Excellence
electronic health record
CPR project evaluation criteria
Organizational Davies
Primary Care Davies
Public Health Davies

Introduction to Davies

The Computer-based Patient Record Institute (CPRI), a nonprofit membership organization founded in 1992, was a unique organization representing all stakeholders in healthcare, focusing on clinical applications of information technology. CPRI was among the first nationally based organizations to initiate and coordinate activities to facilitate and promote the routine use of computer-based patient records (CPRs) throughout healthcare.

A CPRI Workgroup on CPR Systems Evaluation developed the CPR project evaluation criteria in 1993. These criteria, drawn together with input from national experts and volunteer members, formed the basis of a self-assessment that could be used by organizations and outside reviewers to measure and evaluate the accomplishments of CPR projects. The four major areas of the initial criteria—management, functionality, technology, and impact—provided a framework through which to

view an implementation of computerized records. The criteria also provided the foundation for the Nicholas E. Davies Award of Excellence Program.

The Davies program, named for Dr. Nicholas E. Davies, an Atlanta-based physician, president-elect of the American College of Physicians, and a member of the Institute of Medicine (IOM) committee on improving the patient record, was killed in a plane crash just as the IOM report on CPRs was being released. Modeled after the Baldridge award, this national program is intended to award and bring to national attention excellence in the implementation of computerized medical records. The program is founded on the belief that healthcare organizations benefit when collective experiences and lessons learned are shared. During its 10-year existence, the Davies program has had four criteria revisions and seen its terminology updated from computerized patient record to electronic medical record (EMR) and today's EHR. CPRI merged with HOST in 2000, followed by a consolidation of CPRI-HOST with Healthcare

Table 3.1   Nicholas E. Davies Award Winners

ORGANIZATIONAL

1995
Intermountain Health Care, Salt Lake City, UT
Columbia Presbyterian Medical Center, New York, NY
Department of Veterans Affairs
1996
Brigham and Women's Hospital, Boston, MA
1997
Kaiser Permanente of Ohio, Cleveland, OH
North Mississippi Health Services, Inc, Tupelo, MS
Regenstrief Institute for Health Care, Indianapolis, IN
1998
Northwestern Memorial Hospital, Chicago, IL
Kaiser-Permanente Northwest, Portland, OR
1999
Kaiser-Permanente, CO
Queens Medical Center, Honolulu, HI
2000
Harvard Vanguard Medical Associates, Boston, MA
VA Puget Sound Health Care System, Washington, DC
St. Vincent's Hospital, Westchester County, NY and NY,
NY (commendation)
2001
University of Illinois at Chicago Medical Center, Chicago, IL
The Ohio State Medical Center, Columbus, OH
2002
Maimonides Medical Center, Brooklyn, NY
Queens Health Network, Queens, NY
2003
Cincinnati Children's Hospital Medical Center Cincinnati,
OH
2004
Evanston Northwestern Healthcare Evanston, IL

PRIMARY CARE

2003
Cooper Pediatric, Duluth, GA
Evans Medical Group, Evans, GA
Roswell Pediatrics, Alpharetta, GA
2004
North Fulton Family Medicine, Cumming, GA
Old Harding Pediatric Associates, Nashville, TN
Pediatrics @ the Basin, Pittsford, NY
Riverpoint Pediatrics, Chicago, IL

PUBLIC HEALTH

2004
Pennsylvania National Electronic Disease Reporting System
Harrisburg, PA
South Dakota Department of Health Electronic Vital
Records and Screening System
Pierre, SD
Utah Statewide Immunization Information System
Salt Lake City, UT

Information and Management Systems Society (HIMSS) in 2002. Throughout the multiple transitions the program has survived and flourished. Today, under HIMSS management, the Davies Award of Excellence is offered in three categories: Organizational or Acute Care first offered in 1995, Ambulatory since 2003, and Public Health, which was initiated in 2004. See Table 3.1 for the names of Davies award winners.

In its first 9 years of existence the Organizational Davies has awarded 19 organizations. Throughout the decade much has remained the same in organizations that have successfully implemented electronic records while at the same time differences have been noted. This chapter will look at the characteristics of winning organizations: the characteristics that have prevailed over time, while exploring the changing technologies and speed of implementation.

What's the Same?

How They Define the Effort

The 19 Organizational Davies winners located throughout the country started and completed their implementations at different times and in different departments of their facility, under different types of leadership. On the surface it would appear they have little in common. A closer look, however, reveals that these organizations have much in common. Prior to the onset of effort, the winning organizations have clearly made the EHR a key component of the strategic vision. Recognized organizations know and understand that healthcare is an information business. A first year winner, the Veteran's Health Administration (VHA), whose mission is to provide high-quality healthcare for America's veterans, made the development of an EHR a major long-term goal (Curtis, 1995). Brigham & Women's Hospital (BWH), a 1996 winner, decided in 1989 to redevelop their information systems, moving the computer from its role as a reporter of requested facts to an integral tool in the healthcare process. The BWH vision encompassed the establishment of a new technical platform that would serve as the base to provide the processing power and scalability envisioned for the future (Teich et al., 1996). More recently, Maimonides Medical Center located in Brooklyn, New York, turned to the EHR in response to managed competition. In 1996, in New York's deregulated reimbursement system, Maimonides goal to expand rapidly into an integrated delivery system placed the EHR at the core of its new business model. At the time this vision seemed remote since Maimonides was still dependent on the 1960s legacy keypunch-based mainframes (Beltran et al., 2002). Maimonides Chief Executive Officer (CEO) Stanley Brezenoff and Chief Operating Officer (COO) Pamela Brier backed their vision with commitment of one-third of the medical center's capital budget for 7 years to realize the goal (Beltran et al., 2002). As Harvard Vanguard was formed in 1997, the vision encompassed a multisite, multispecialty group practice whose EHRs linked to its practice management system (Crowell et al., 2000).

The EHR implementation in all winning organizations was a clear part of the strategic vision and defined by remarkably similar organizational goals and objectives. The Veterans Affairs (VA) Puget Sound Health Care System (VA Puget Sound), a 2000 Davies winner, delineated several key objectives: improving the accessibility and availability of clinical information, support of integrated care delivery across two different sites, and maximizing improvements in quality care through the use of order entry and order checks and reminders (Payne, Torell, and Hoey, 2000). Strikingly similar were the project objectives of Queens Health Network (QHN), Queens, New York, a 2002 winner, which were shared by all the medical staff and administration. Those included improved quality of patient care through timely access to patient information, improved documentation of clinical data throughout the continuum of care, and the integration of clinical information from a variety of legacy systems (Carr, 2002). The 2003 Davies winner, Cincinnati Children's Hospital Medical Center (CCHMC), made optimizing patient safety, followed by optimizing consistency in care as their top two strategic objectives, which took precedence in the planning, design, and implementation of the EHR at CCHMC (Jacobs et al., 2003).

How is the Effort Organized?

The implementation of an EHR is a daunting effort. A common element to all Davies winners is the shared belief that information management is a key tool to the clinical and business processes of the hospital. Without exception, one or more of the senior executives realizes the importance of the EHR initiative and champions the effort. The champion is absolutely necessary to ensure continued funding and appropriate resources needed for the project to realize success. The planning process requires the skills of financial and operational adminis-

trators as well as clinicians from all departments working closely with information technology professionals. Project leaders did not necessarily come from the Information Services Department. Success with implementation requires integrating the system with the business of care delivery. Owners of the business, the clinicians, must be directly involved and engaged throughout the planning and implementation cycles. Nurses need to participate in design review, serve as champions, and provide local resources to ensure the planned implementation will enhance their ability to care for the patient. Centralized planning is desired; however, Davies winners that have rolled out implementations across multiple sites have repeatedly advised that all implementation is local and local clinicians must be engaged in order to achieve success.

Many Davies applicants described similar evolutions in the governance of the EHR system implementation. Throughout each phase there was representation of key stakeholders. Nurses, physicians, and clinical support staff led the needs analysis effort to ensure clinical quality. Due to the technologies involved, the selection process or design phase required input from not only clinicians but also from information system specialists. The contract negotiation phase was guided by hospital administration and information systems personnel with close oversight of the financial, technical, and legal implications. The early portion of system implementation, usually consisting of hardware and software installs was led by personnel from information systems.

The VA Puget Sound formed a steering committee whose members included the chief of medicine, surgery, nursing, mental health, and ambulatory care. In turn, each department nominated members for two special groups of users, Clinical Users and Super Users. The Clinical Champions were approximately 20 physicians, nurses, and other allied health professionals who were advocates of the project and willing to lead discussions and provide presentations and education sessions for other members of their profession. Super Users were a larger group whose members received more training and worked closely with the developers in planning system changes and improvements. The Super Users additionally served as local resources for the colleagues, answering questions, and providing on the spot training (Payne, Torell, and Hoey, 2000). A consistent characteristic of winning organizations is the customer service and constant consideration of the impact of the system on the end user. Consider the needs not only of large clinical departments but also those of small niche services. Consider the impact to patient care not only during the busiest hours, but also during weekend and night-time hours. No EHR implementation can be successful without the buy-in from the clinicians throughout the facility, in all departments and on all shifts. Another characteristic of Davies winners has been the active pursuit of feedback from all users. Winning organizations have employed user-inclusive design for feedback or have developed "help" buttons that allow clinicians to instantly communicate frustrations or suggestions for design improvement.

Change Management

Many Davies winners stressed the importance of operational planning for the EHR implementation. To maximize success, it must be recognized that the forthcoming implementation will bring about a culture of change. The positive effect of this upcoming change must be echoed by medical, nursing, and administrative leadership. New systems necessitate new standard operating procedures. New policies and procedures must be considered, written, and tested before they "go live."

At CCHMC, several weeks of live implementation planning preceded the arrival of the EHR in any patient unit. Clinical advocates from the respective units performed usability tests. In the case of CCHMC, these tests revealed that the time it took to perform the frequent documentation of various clinical data such as vital signs was unacceptable. Consequently, CCHMC pursued a critical care documentation system that allowed for multiple close interval entries (Jacobs et al., 2003).

Strong end-user support for new systems was a key factor for success. Ohio State University Health System (OSUHS) treated this as an organizational effort and responsibility. All available personnel were required to support each phase. Roving support personnel termed "red coats" responded to user calls for help around the clock (Ahmed, Teater, and Bentley, 2001). Just-in-time training was done by specialty or department at Maimonides Medical Center. All system documentation was deployed prior to implementation including test plans, training manuals, user manual, system specifications, and physician pocket reference guides. Development of downtime procedures and user access policies were included in all the system training (Beltran et al., 2002).

Maimonides as well as other Davies winners learned early on that process redesign was required to achieve the desired efficiency and results. It was necessary to achieve agreement from physicians and nurses on standard orders, practice protocols, and decision support rules for measurable improvements in patient outcomes

(Beltran et al., 2002). Getting clinicians to use an EHR as part of their day-to-day work is one of the most significant hurdles that had to be overcome by successful Davies applicants. Maimonides, a 2002 winner, decided not to call their clinician classes "training." Instead, announcements featured an educational offering designed to show physicians and nurses how to navigate the Internet and the Maimonides Intranet. After completing this 2-hour introduction level class, caregivers eagerly signed up for the next level. Their self-perceived stigma of not knowing how to use a PC and perform simple navigation had been alleviated (Beltran et al., 2002). At the University of Illinois at Chicago Medical Center (UICMC) extensive efforts were made from the onset to establish that the EHR was "owned" by clinicians and not the Information Technology Department. The priorities for implementation became driven by what the clinicians believed would generate the most value, both for themselves and their patients (Keeler, 2001).

QHN noted in their application that resistance at all levels of the organization to the EHR was being confronted and transformed. At a steering committee meeting, one chief of service complained that the business of an academic medical center was to teach physicians to practice medicine, not to practice typing. This was challenged by a counterpart who asserted that the skills required of any twenty-first century healthcare personnel, including nurses and physicians must include mastery of the computer (Carr, 2002). Clinicians at all levels and from all departments must become partners in the technology process.

At some point in the planning for the EHR implementation all Davies winners came to the realization that the electronic media is intrinsically different from paper. Electronic media is interactive. The term "hard copy" illustrates the difference; paper is tangible and static, electronic information is fluid and reactive. Manual paper processes cannot simply be transferred to the electronic media. An institutional EHR implementation forces an examination of the underlying work processes. The EHR will act as a catalyst for the development of clinical practice standards across services and departments from one campus to another within the organization. Although the QHN delivers more babies than any other provider in Queens, clinical practices between providers and even from site to site differed despite adherence to nationally recognized practice standards. At Queens it took an extensive discussion among several clinicians to define the algorithm to electronically calculate estimated date of confinement, with each caregiver having a slightly different and preferred methodology backed by academic resources, to obtain this date (Carr, 2002).

Impact to Value

Documenting the impact of an EHR is very difficult at best and impossible for some organizations. The system impacts an organization in subtle ways, such as avoidance of a medication error, and directly through nonduplication of an ordered test. Throughout this past decade of Davies winners, the application process has included a documentation of impact and value to the implementing organization. Value has never been assumed and winning applicants justified their clinical systems. Winners highlighted their successes based on value to the care processes. From 1995 to 2001 applicants were asked to provide examples of impact derived for the organization from the EHR. As applications were evaluated, great emphasis was placed on the organization's ability to demonstrate positive impact. Davies applicants were encouraged to provide quantitative examples of benefits that had been obtained against costs that had been incurred to help guide and direct expectations in other settings. Organizations with longstanding EHR efforts were not exempt. Dr. Clem McDonald from Regenstrief described "the unremitting pressure to show value." (McDonald et al., 1997). Organizations with a research orientation such as Intermountain Health Care (IHC), Brigham, and Regenstrief demonstrated proof of value through research and publications. These early Davies winners have contributed significantly to the body of research on the power and importance of clinical decision support to improve the process of healthcare and patient safety (McDonald et al., 1997).

During the first years of the Davies program, all winning organizations cited improvement in care documentation. Quality of care enhancements through avoidance of medication error, increased appropriateness of care interventions, and compliance with managed care and disease management protocols were obtained by all organizations. Additional quality impact was noted in improved continuity of care as medical records and plans of care were available in detail for residents on call or weekend triage nurses.

Organizations applying for the Davies award in 2002 and beyond faced revised criteria in which the impact section had been changed to value. Healthcare facilities were expected to document the business case of the EHR. Maimonides faced an uphill battle as the organization moved toward an EHR. Before 1996,

technology investments at Maimonides had not provided measurable results. No return on investment (ROI) could be documented. The perception was that technology offered little or no value. Maimonides Medical Center (MMC) realized that traditional cost-benefit justifications did not fully measure the value of clinical applications. What dollar amount was equal to improved patient outcome and satisfaction, increased efficiencies in the delivery of care, and accurate immediate access to patient and care information? Since metrics are needed to measure success, an interdisciplinary team was created prior to each technology initiative to identify benchmarks and savings to be realized from the new initiative (Beltran et al., 2002).

Maimonides used Eclipsys' strategic investment model to measure the business value of its projects. This computer model aligns business goals with the appropriate technology solution. The model then provides balanced decision-making criteria including tangible and intangible benefits and risks. The resulting analysis provides net present value, internal rate of return, payback periods, and ROI for each system (Beltran et al., 2002). Using this model, Maimonides has since 1996, realized a 9.4% ROI, a 3.84 year payback, and positive net cash flow by year 4. Partially contributing to this ROI have also been capital reimbursements, grant awards, and partial revenue from the medical center's length of stay reduction. Additional ROI was achieved in the radiology department, where picture achieving communication system (PACS) and voice recognition have produced savings of over $10.5 million over 5 years from savings in film, film jackets, and transcription (Beltran et al., 2002).

The QHN and Medical Board were cognizant that the value of the EHR technology must be demonstrated. They determined that for their organization success, and indirectly the business case would be measured by the improvement of processes that impact patient care; improved access to patient information, complete legible clinical documentation, and timely and accurate patient data at point of service. Process improvements were measured by analyzing different tools, their actions, and effects on patient care. One example of this was the nutritional screening tools with decision support that were made available for nurses and other clinicians in ambulatory care (Carr, 2002).

Online documentation by physicians and nurse practitioners has clearly enhanced the value of the Queens EHR. Queens Hospital Center, a component of the QHN, reported a 50% decrease in the number of pharmacist interventions in medication orders in the ambulatory setting because of system alerts, and improved legibility and completeness of prescriptions. At Elmhurst Hospital, an acute care facility of QHN, the completion in the EHR of patient problem lists, orders/referral for mammography, Pap smears, and diabetic retinal examinations had reached 100% by 1999 (Carr, 2002). Three months prior and 6 months after EHR implementation, QHN measured compliance with Joint Commission of Healthcare Organization (JCAHO)-mandated summary list completion which included patient diagnoses, procedures, allergies and adverse drug reactions, and patient medications. All elements of the summary list were required to be complete in order for compliance to be achieved for any individual record. Implementation of the EHR led to noteworthy and sustainable improvements with a jump from 3.7 (3 months prior to EHR) to 100% (6 months after conversion from paper to electronic records) (Carr, 2002).

The 2003 Organizational Davies winner, CCHMC, also centered the business justification on process improvement as the driver for technological change. Immediately after successful EHR implementation, the institution began to see significant benefits in targeted processes(Jacobs et al., 2003). In recent years, CCHMC believed patient safety was a cornerstone of quality. Through institutional committees such as Medication Safety, Patient Safety, and Risk Management deficiencies in the area of patient safety had been noted. These deficiencies at times were related to inconsistency of care between providers. Though not unique to CCHMC, problems with poorly written illegible written orders were commonplace. The CCHMC formulary lists 3,770 medications. Of these 470 were designated "high alert" due to their narrow window for therapeutic use or widespread frequency. Prior to EHR implementation, age-adjusted dose range checking limits were established for all 470 of these high-alert medications to include minimum and maximum single dose, maximum total daily dose, minimum and maximum frequency. As a result of the EHR implementation, clinicians at CCHMC now generate complete, unambiguous, legible orders that include clinician contact name and pager number on all orders (Jacobs et al., 2003).

Still Expensive

A commonalty shared by all Davies Organizational winners is the cost of their EHR implementation: expensive. This trait continues even today. Over the years of the Davies program, organization after organization has set aside multiple millions from their capital budgets to finance the cost of the infrastructure, hardware, and software all needed for an EHR implementation. Difficult to calculate but consistently present are the employee hours lost from patient care for the planning process, design phase, testing, and educational needs all required to support a successful implementation.

Focus on Decision Support

The functionality of an EHR is the result of the data it captures and the assistance it provides to all members of the healthcare team. An integral component of the EMR is its ability to offer clinical support in the provider's decision-making process. Previously, computerized systems delivered results reporting and reviewing. The pioneering visionaries recognized the value of real-time alerting, reminding, and protocol support. Davies winners have consistently recognized that decision support takes two forms. The first can be seen in applications that are designed to facilitate best practices through evidence-based clinical practice guidelines, electronic order protocols, electronic order defaults, allowable order specific elements. The second type of decision support is found in alerts and reminders that warn clinicians about patient variables (Ahmed, Teater, and Bentley, 2001). A multidisciplinary team at OSUHS developed guidelines that were incorporated into order protocols that were incorporated into provider order entry (POE). In addition, more than 400 electronic order protocols that address safety, quality, standardization, and cost with embedded alerts and reminders are also available in POE (Ahmed, Teater, and Bentley, 2001). At Maimonides, the power of advanced knowledge-based prompting and decision support can be seen in the perinatal EMR which capitalized on bedside workstations to deliver real-time point of care decision support. Since 99% of perinatal data can be entered via structured database fields rather than using free text, the ability of the system to analyze and assess is greatly enhanced. The system continuously assesses recorded documentation and generates menus automatically tailored to the current clinical situation (Beltran et al., 2002).

■ What's Different?

Where Winners Obtained Systems

In the first years of the Davies, winning organizations had spent years in the development of their award winning systems. The three organizations honored in the first year of the program all developed their own systems. IHC in Utah was the practice site for a visionary group of clinicians and scientists. Around 1965 they began experimenting with the process of applying computer technology to the provision of care. From these early experiments came the creation of an integrated, rules-based patient centered information system entitled HELP (health evaluation through logical processing) (Grandia et al., 1995). Throughout the late 1970s and early 1980s the HELP system was expanded until 1985 when it became apparent that an enterprise-wide clinical information system (CIS) was needed. A 5-year budget of $50 million was set aside for the creation of this system which was based on a creation of an enterprise-wide data repository fed by IHC's clinical, financial, and managed care plan systems.

Columbia Presbyterian Medical Center received a first year award for their CIS which was built as a central hub that enabled clinical systems on disparate platforms to share patient data. The hub consisted of a series of concentric layers handling a variety of requests from the various client applications to either store or retrieve data (Johnson et al., 1995). Network integration was accomplished by establishing connectivity to the token ring or Ethernet (Johnson et al., 1995).

Also honored in the first year of the Davies program was the VHA for a CPR that was based on Decentralized Hospital Computer Program (DHCP), a comprehensive system covering medical management, fiscal and clinical functions (Curtis, 1995). The DHCP served as the fundamental information system for the VHA's medical care network supporting 171 medical centers, 450 outpatient clinics, and 131 nursing homes (Curtis, 1995). As part of their commitment to provide high-quality healthcare to the veterans of the United States, a major goal of this system was to share and exchange data, first throughout the VHA, then with other federally based healthcare facilities, and finally with private sector organizations (Curtis, 1995). Despite funding at $1.2 billion for a 12-year life cycle from 1983 to 1994, there was no major EMR acquisition in VHA. Due to the necessity of keeping all options open for future growth, the VHA considered it vital to maintain a high degree of both vendor and platform independence. Consequently, systems procurements for the DHCP were open acquisitions with requests for proposals (RFP) written in terms of generic performance requirements with the result that most major hardware vendors were represented in the various incremental procurements (Curtis, 1995).

Second year award winner BWH developed Brigham integrated computing system (BICS) with the help and participation of a large number of their clinicians. These clinicians spent a portion of their time on system development and the remainder on clinical practice (Teich et al., 1996). This project was an ambitious redevelopment of the hospital's information system that dated back to 1989. One of the project's goals was to change the computer's role in the healthcare process. Instead of assuming the traditional computer role of results reporting, the computer would become an active partner in promoting optimal quality of care, reducing adverse events, and reducing costs (Teich et al., 1996). For more than 20 years, Harvard Vanguard Medical Associates had utilized an automated medical record system (AMRS) which had become outdated. This Boston-based clinician led multispecialty group practice, a 6th-year Davies winner, tried self-development, and then codevelopment, before implementing their current system which was purchased from a vendor (Crowell et al., 2000).

All winners since 2000 have implemented commercially sold multicomponent systems procured from a variety of vendors with Maimonides choosing multiple vendors. This modified best-of-breed approach met physician and departmental needs while conforming to the medical center's interfacing, hardware, software, and operating standards.

The technology employed in the system affects the ability to meet user expectations, including a wide variety of functional and organizational needs, reliability, response time, and scalability. The Davies program has shown that there is no single best technology solution. Awardees have been successful using a wide range of approaches in implementing systems. Over the years these have included several cases of completely homegrown systems based on different technology platforms, a mainframe-based vendor solution, homegrown systems with commercially procured document imaging, homegrown results management integrated with a commercially purchased clinical system, and complete purchase from a vendor of an EMR (Metzger et al., 1999).

Time to Get There

As more healthcare organizations purchase commercially available EMRs the timeline from initial planning, through purchase, training, and successful implementation shortens. For early Davies winners like the VHA, Brigham & Women's, and Regenstrief Institute for Health Care (1997 Davies winner), the EMR was part of a strategic plan that took more than a decade to realize. The Regenstrief institute was founded in 1969 in Indianapolis, Indiana, on the belief that industrial engineering principles could be applied to healthcare. Under the leadership of Clement McDonald, the vision of a longitudinal, integrated, acute, and ambulatory care record that provided information for clinical decision support and other applications developed over three decades (McDonald et al., 1997). At North Mississippi Health Services (NMHS) development started in the late 1970s when the Information Services Department and a consultant interviewed users to determine needs and wants for the most far-reaching medical system available. By the end of 1997 the clinical information stored in their EMR was available at approximately 120 different locations within their healthcare delivery system (Bozeman et al., 1997).

Recent winners have shortened the timeline. The two winners of the 2001 Davies award, the UICMC and the Ohio OSUHS each spent 7 years in the planning and implementation of their commercially procured systems (Keeler et al., 2001). CCHMC placed the development of a robust information technology infrastructure in their 1995 organizational strategic plan. The following years saw a dramatic increase in the development of the Information Services Department and accompanying increase in network infrastructure to support the vigorous development and implementation of clinical systems (Jacobs et al., 2003). By March 2000, CCHMC had completed the implementation of an enterprise-wide PACS system, and by December 2002 the EMR was implemented on 13 inpatient care units (Jacobs et al., 2003).

External Agenda

Factors external to healthcare organizations helped to accelerate the timeline for adoption of EMRs. In 1993, the driving force for developing an advanced CIS at Queens's Medical Center in Honolulu, Hawaii, was the onset of healthcare reform and managed care. Survival of Queens necessitated a seamless integrated healthcare system. Clinical and administrative leaders of Queens convened a planning committee from which emerged the vision held by all physicians, nurses, and allied health professionals that a CPR was essential to improve care (Davis et al., 1999). The EMR at UICMC was initially developed to mitigate concerns that the organization's legacy patient care information system was not Y2K compliant (Keeler et al., 2001). For Heritage Behavioral Health Center of Decatur, Illinois, the impetus was felt in the mid-1990s when competition for service contracts increased. Heritage found itself poorly prepared with an outdated back office system. An agency-wide, point of service information system would give the organization a competitive edge in quality-based, effective clinical

services. The focal point of this information system was to be an EMR that supported the delivery of care (Wilkinson et al., 2001). The EMR at QHN in Queens, New York, was seen as key to the strategic position of Queens in the competitive healthcare marketplace of New York. The EMR was viewed as essential to the development of an effective infrastructure from which to support the reorganization of care, design of quality measures, streamlined reporting processes, and the cornerstone of evidence-based medicine to improve management of chronic disease (Carr, 2002).

Technology

The technology behind each EMR affects the ability to meet user demands for rapid response, system reliability, future growth, and customization. Throughout the decade of Davies, new technologies have emerged and are being incorporated into the systems being deployed today. The technology at any Davies winner is difficult to precisely replicate due to data capture. The unique interfaces, user agreements, cultural changes, workflow revisions and window and menu customizations tend to make each EMR unique.

Document imaging systems have been incorporated into many EMRs as a key component of a transition strategy as an organization moves from a paper-based to an electronic system. First seen in the earliest Davies winners as a means to organize paper components of the medical chart, these systems have emerged as a key technology to capture paper originating from outside the system and stray clinical documentation.

A PACS has been deployed with a great degree of user acceptance and satisfaction in the last several Davies winners. This technology makes diagnostic quality images available wherever high resolution monitors are found; in the emergency room, intensive care units (ICUs), and ambulatory surgeries.

At Queens in New York, users are issued an electronic key at training and must chose a password that is changed every 3 months. Both the physical device (key) and electronic password are required to sign onto the system every time. This process taking about 5 seconds, requires the use of the plastic key which contains encrypted user file and security access information (Carr, 2002).

Wireless technology had made a significant impact on 1999 winner, Queens of Hawaii. Mobile wireless workstations in the ICUs were key to improving team function. Wireless ICU workstations that could be wheeled about and used in the patient's rooms improved clinician efficiency and the quality of patient care (Davis, 1999).

Hardware for the EMR has seen significant change over the past decade. IHC, a first-year Davies winner, imitated their system on serial terminals that were migrated to Intel-286-based personal computers. Today, high-speed work stations with flat panel monitors help manage work flow and clinical communications in all recent Davies winners. Fiber-optic cables facilitate communications within and to remote locations of the organization.

Davies Pool of Applicants

In the early years of the Davies program, only a few healthcare organizations had successful EMR implementations of sufficient scope and implementation to apply for the award. Despite "raising the bar" through three criteria revisions since the debut of the award, applications have steadily increased as more organizations realize the value of the EMR. Review of current applications reveals that numerous organizations have begun implementation of their system and will be ready to apply for the award in the next few years. To date, the Davies has not yet been awarded to a community hospital. Though many are close, no community hospital has successfully and fully implemented POE.

The Davies award program has widened in the past 2 years to include primary care practices and public health agencies. The Davies Primary Care Award was initiated in 2003, followed by the Davies Award for Public Health in 2004. Three primary care practices were awarded in 2003, an additional four practices in 2004. Three public health agencies were recognized in the inaugural year. Their implementations are remarkably different though equally successful and speak with dedication to the principles outlined in the criteria for all Davies; management, technology, functionality, and value.

Summary

The Nicholas E. Davies Program, founded by CPRI in 1993 awards excellence in EHR implementation. Organized into three different categories, the award program has recognized 20 healthcare organizations, 7 primary care practices, and 3 public health initiatives. Applicants for the award answer questions outlined by the project evaluation criteria. These questions are focused on the four broad areas of management, functionality, technology, and value. A review of award receiving applications reveals that some characteristics of winning organizations remain unchanged over the past decade while other characteristics are remarkably different.

Reference

Ahmed, A., Teater, P., and Bentley, T. D. (2001). The design and implementation of a computerized patient record at the Ohio State University Health System—a success story. In *Proceedings of the Seventh Annual Nicholas E. Davies CPR Recognition Symposium.* Chicago, IL: HIMSS.

Beltran, J., Cassera, F., Daurio, N., et al. (2002). Maimonides Medical Center makes a quantum leap with advanced computerized patient record technology. In *Proceedings of the Eighth Annual Nicholas E. Davies EMR Symposium.* Chicago, IL: HIMSS.

Bozeman, T. E., Harvey, K., Jarrell, I., et al. (1997). The development and implementation of a computer-based patient record in a rural integrated health system. In *Proceedings of the Third Annual Nicholas E. Davies CPR Recognition Symposium.* Bethesda, MD: CPRI.

Carr, D. M. (2002). Queens Health Network Healthcare Information System: A model for electronic physician order entry. In *Proceedings of the Eighth Annual Nicholas E. Davies EMR Symposium.* Chicago, IL: HIMSS.

Crowell, M., Lopez, R., Cochran, D., et al. (2000). The journey to a CPR in a large multi-specialty group practice. In *Proceedings of the Sixth Annual Nicholas E. Davies CPR Recognition Symposium.* Bethesda, MD: CPRI-HOST.

Curtis, C. (1995). A computer-based patient record emerging from the public sector: The decentralized hospital computer program. In *Proceedings of the First Annual Nicholas E. Davies CPR Recognition Symposium.* Bethesda, MD: CPRI.

Davis, D. C., Moriyama, R., Tiwanak, G., et al. (1999). Clinical performance improvement with an advanced clinical information system at the Queen's Medical Center. In *Proceedings of the Fifth Annual Nicholas E. Davies CPR Recognition Symposium.* Bethesda, MD: CPRI.

Grandia, L. D., Pryor, T. A., Wilson, D. F., et al. (1995). Building a computer-based patient record system in evolving integrated health system. In *Proceedings of the First Annual Nicholas E. Davies CPR Recognition Symposium.* Bethesda, MD: CPRI.

Jacobs, B., Lykowski,G., Mahoney, D., et al. (2003). Improving the quality and safety of care through implementation of an integrating clinical informatics system. In *Proceedings of the Ninth Annual Nicholas E. Davies EMR Recognition Symposium.* Chicago, IL: HIMSS.

Johnson, S. B., Forman, B., Cimino, J. J., et al. (1995). A technological perspective on the computer-based patient record. In *Proceedings of the First Annual Nicholas E. Davies CPR Recognition Symposium.* Bethesda, MD: CPRI.

Keeler, J. (2001). The Gemini Project: University of Illinois at Chicago Medical Center. In *Proceedings of the Seventh Annual Nicholas E. Davies CPR Recognition Symposium.* Chicago, IL: HIMSS.

McDonald, C. J. ,Tierney, W. M., Overhage, J. M., et al. (1997). The three legged stool: Regenstrief Institute for Health Care. In *Proceedings of the Third Annual Nicholas E. Davies CPR Recognition Symposium.* Bethesda, MD: CPRI.

Metzger, J., Simpson, N., Underwood, C., et al. (1999). Lessons from the First Four Years. In *Proceedings of the Fifth Annual Nicholas E. Davies CPR Recognition Symposium.* Bethesda, MD: CPRI.

Payne, T. H., Torell, J., and Hoey, P. (2000). Implementation of the computerized patient record system and other clinical computing applications at the VA Puget Sound Health Care System. In *Proceedings of the Sixth Annual Nicholas E. Davies CPR Recognition Symposium.* Bethesda, MD: CPRI-HOST.

Teich, J. M., Glaser, J. P., Beckley, R. F., et al. (1996). Toward cost effective quality care: The Brigham integrated computing experience. In *Proceedings of the Second Annual Nicholas E. Davies CPR Recognition Symposium.* Bethesda, MD: CPRI.

Wilkinson, G. (2001). Award for behavioral health: Heritage Behavioral Health Center, Inc. In *Proceedings of the Seventh Annual Nicholas E. Davies CPR Recognition Symposium.* Chicago, IL: HIMSS.

PART **2**

Computer Systems

4

Computer Hardware

Mary L. McHugh

OBJECTIVES

1. List the key hardware components of a computer and the four basic operations of the central processing unit (CPU).
2. Describe how power is measured for computers.
3. Describe common computer input, output, and storage devices.
4. Discuss the history of computers.
5. Describe the three classes of computers and key functionality of each class.
6. Describe computer network/communications devices and functionality.

KEY WORDS

information systems
computer science
software
hardware

Hardware

Computer **hardware** is defined as all of the physical components of the machine itself. The basic hardware of a computer includes the electronic circuits, microchips, processors, and the motherboard itself inside the computer housing. In addition, hardware typically includes devices that are peripheral to the main computer box such as input and output devices including the keyboard, mouse, printer, fax, and storage components such as the hard drive, Universal Serial Bus (USB) drive, floppy drives, tape drives, and so on. Typically, computer systems are composed of many different component parts that enable the user to communicate with the computer, and with other computers to produce work. The group of required and optional hardware items that are linked together to make up a computer system is called its configuration. When computers are sold, many of the key components are placed inside a rigid plastic housing or case, which is called the **box**. What can typically be seen from the outside is the box (Fig. 4.1) containing the internal components, and the peripherals such as a keyboard, mouse, speakers, monitor, and printer.

A computer is a machine that uses electronic components and instructions to the components to perform calculations and repetitive and complex procedures, process text, and manipulate data and signals. Computer technology has evolved from huge electronic calculators developed with military funding during World War II to palm-sized information-processing machines available to virtually everybody. Today, computer processors are encountered in most areas of people's lives. From the grocery store to the movie theater; from infusion pumps to physiologic monitors; from the bedside alarm clock to the automobile accelerator, computer processors are employed so widely that the late twentieth century can accurately be described as the beginning of the information age.

Computer hardware advances during the late 1900s have made possible many changes to the health care industry. The first operations to be modified were special administrative functions such as finance, payroll, billing, and nurse staffing and scheduling support. Later, the computer allowed fantastic changes in the practice of radiology and imaging, allowing noninvasive visualization of the human body that heretofore could only be performed in surgery (Asirvatham, 2003; Beets-Tan and Beets, 2004). Computers are now pervasive throughout the health care industry. Their applications are expected to continue to expand and thereby improve the quality of health care while at the same

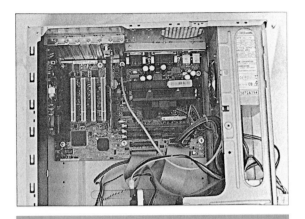

Figure 4.1
Computer box with components loaded.
(Reproduced, with permission, from Rosenthal M. (1999).
Build Your Own PC (p. 82). New York, NY: McGraw-Hill.)

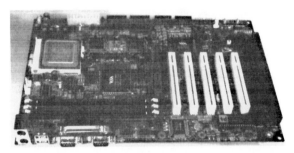

Figure 4.2
Motherboard with CPU, chips, and slots.
(Reproduced, with permission, from Pilgrim A. (2000). *Build
Your Own Pentium III PC* (p. 34). New York, NY: McGraw-Hill.)

time reducing some costs. Most important, the applications of computers to health care will greatly expand the diagnostic and therapeutic abilities of practitioners and broaden the options available to recipients of health care. Additionally, telemedicine is now being used to reduce the impact of distance and location on accessibility and availability of health care (Wang et al., 2004; Debnath, 2004; Marcin et al., 2004). None of these changes could have happened without tremendous advances in the machinery, the hardware, of computers.

This chapter covers various aspects of computer hardware: components and their functions, classes of computers, and their characteristics and types. It also highlights the functional components of the computer and describes the devices and media used to communicate, store, and process data. Major topics addressed include basic computer concepts and classes and types of computers, components, and computer communications. To understand how a computer processes data, it is necessary to examine the component parts and devices that comprise computer hardware.

Computer Hardware Fundamentals

The box of any computer contains a **motherboard** (Fig. 4.2). The motherboard is a thin, flat sheet made of a firm, nonconducting material on which the internal components—printed circuits, chips, slots, and so on—of the computer are mounted. The motherboard is made

of a **dielectric** or nonconducting plastic material, and the electric conductions are etched or soldered onto the bottom of the board. The motherboard has holes or perforations through which components can be affixed (Fig. 4.3). Typically, one side looks like a maze of soldered metal trails with sharp projections (which are the attachments of the chips and other components affixed to the motherboard). On one side can be seen the microchips, wiring, and slots for adding components. The specific design of the components—especially the CPU and other microprocessors—is called the computer's architecture.

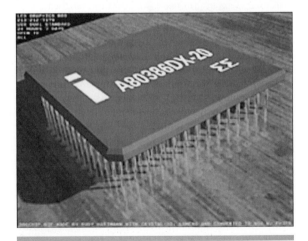

Figure 4.3
CPU chip attached to motherboard.
(Courtesy of James C. Miller.)

A computer has four basic components, although most have many more added-on components. At its most basic, a computer must consist of a CPU, input and output controllers, and storage media.

Central Processing Unit

The CPU is the "brains" of the computer. It consists of at least one arithmetic and logic unit, a control unit, and memory. The arithmetic and logic units control mathematical functions such as addition and subtraction and functions that test logic (boolean) conditions, such as, "Is this number being read equal to or greater than 4?" The control unit carries out the machine language functions called **fetch, execute, decode,** and **store.** For an extremely simplified example, when a command is given to add two numbers, the control unit "fetches" the instruction and numbers from their storage locations and decodes the instruction so that the proper operations can be performed. These are called the fetch and decode cycles. Then the control unit initiates the execute cycle, which sends the instruction to the arithmetic and logic unit. Finally, the control unit initiates the store cycle, which places the result of the instruction in a memory location. Memory includes the locations of the computer's internal or main working storage. Memory consists of registers (a small number of very high-speed memory locations), random access memory (RAM), which is the main storage area in which the computer places the programs and data it is working on, and cache (a small memory storage area holding recently accessed data).

Memory

There are two types of memory in the main memory of a computer. They are read only memory (ROM) and RAM.

Read Only Memory   ROM is a form of permanent storage. This means that data and programs in ROM can only be read by the computer, and cannot be erased or altered. ROM generally contains the programs, called firmware, used by the control unit of the CPU to oversee computer functions. In microcomputers, this may also include the software programs used to translate the computer's high-level programming languages into machine language (binary code). ROM storage is not erased when the computer is turned off.

Random Access Memory   RAM refers to working memory used for primary storage. It is volatile

(changeable) and used as temporary storage. RAM can be accessed, used, changed, and written on repeatedly. It contains data and instructions that are stored and processed by computer programs called applications programs. RAM is the work area available to the CPU for all processing applications. The computer programs, which are stored on diskettes, on the hard drive, or on CD-ROM (compact disk, read only memory), are not permanent parts of the computer itself. They are loaded when needed, and they can be altered. The contents of RAM are lost whenever the power to the computer is turned off.

Input and Output

To do work, the computer must have a way of receiving commands and data from the outside and a way of reporting out its work. The motherboard has slots and circuit boards that allow the CPU to communicate with the outside world. Input and output devices are wired to a **controller** that is plugged into the slots or circuit boards of the computer. Some devices can serve as both input and output devices. Such devices as the hard drive on which most of the programs people use as well as their personal data are stored, the disk drive and CD on which people store most of their personal data, and more recently, the USB disk serve to both receive and send information to the computer.

Input devices   These allow the computer to receive information from the outside world. The most common input devices are the keyboard and mouse. Others commonly seen on nursing workstations include the touch screen, light pen, voice, and scanner. A touch screen is actually both an input and output device combined. Electronics allow the computer to "sense" when a particular part of the screen is pressed or "touched." A light pen is a device attached to the computer that has special software that allows the computer to sense when the light pen is focused on a particular part of the screen. For both the touch screen and light pen, software interprets the meaning of that screen location to the program. Voice systems allow the nurse to speak into a microphone to record data. Many other input devices exist. Some devices are used for security and can detect users' fingerprints, retinal prints, voiceprints, or other personally unique physical characteristics that identify users who have clearance to use the system. In health care computing, some medical devices serve as input devices. For example, the electrodes placed on a patient's body provide input into the computerized physiologic monitors.

Output Devices   These allow the computer to report its results to the external world. Output can be in the form of text, data files, sound, graphics, or signals to other devices. The two most obvious output devices are the monitor (display screen) and printer.

Storage Media

Storage includes the main memory but also external devices on which programs and data are stored. The most common storage devices include the hard drive, diskettes, and CD-ROMs. The hard drive and diskettes are magnetic storage media. The CD-ROM is a form of optical storage. Optical media are read by a laser "eye" rather than a magnet (Columbia Encyclopedia, 2003).

Hard Drive   The hard drive is a peripheral that has very high speed and high density (Fig. 4.4). That is, it is a very fast means of storing and retrieving data as well as having a large storage capacity in comparison with the other types of storage.

Diskettes   The diskette drive allows input and output from a diskette, which is a round magnetic disk encased in a flexible or rigid case (Fig. 4.5). It allows the user to transport data and programs from one computer site to another.

CD-ROM   The CD-ROM is a rigid disk that holds a much higher density of information than a diskette and

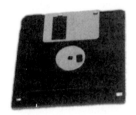
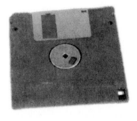

Figure 4.5
Diskette with write protect slot.
(Reproduced, with permission, from Pilgrim A. (2000). *Build Your Own Pentium III PC* (p. 165). New York, NY: McGraw-Hill.)

has a much higher speed (Fig. 4.6). Until the late 1990s, CD-ROMs were strictly input devices. However, new technology developed by Phillips Corporation permitted the development of a new type of CD that could be written on by the user. These are called CD-RWs.

USB Disk   As demands for higher and higher density transportable storage rise, the popularity of the USB disk has also risen. A USB disk is actually a form of a small, removable hard drive that is inserted into the USB port of the computer. There are many names for it including pen drive, thistle drive, pocket disks, and so forth.

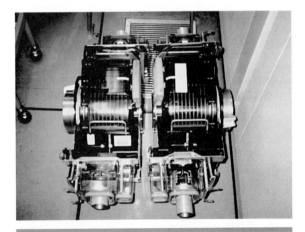

Figure 4.4
Hard disk platters from an IBM mainframe computer.
(Courtesy of Akos Varga.)

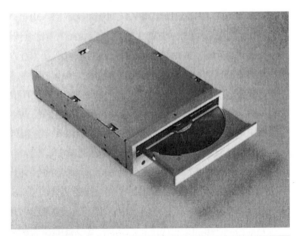

Figure 4.6
CD-ROM drive.
(Reproduced, with permission, from Mitsumi.)

This is a device that can store 64 megabytes (MB) for about $20 for the home user to over 4 gigabytes (GB) (for about $1,000). It is highly reliable unlike floppy diskettes, is a read-write device like floppies, and small enough to transport comfortably in a pants pocket. The device plugs into the back of a computer box's USB port (one needs to have a USB drive installed) and instead of saving to hard drive or CD-ROM or floppy, the user simply saves to the USB disk. Since the USB disk can store so much data in a package so much smaller than a CD-ROM, the convenience makes it worth the higher price to many users Of course, as the popularity increases, prices are dropping.

Other Output Devices As computers became more standard in offices during the 1990s, more and more corporate and individual information was stored solely on computers. Even when paper backup copies were kept, loss of information on the hard drive was usually inconvenient at the least and a disaster at worst. Diskettes could not store large amounts of data, so people began to search for economical and speedy ways to backup the information on their hard drive.

Other output devices developed to help with the backup problem included magnetic tape drives and Zip drives. Magnetic tape drives run magnetic tape which is similar to the tape in any music tape player. In the 1980s and early 1990s, magnetic tape drives were a popular way to back up hard drive data, but today are obsolete for home computer use.

Zip drives are more similar to ordinary floppy disks, but are of higher capacity. In 1996, Iomega Corporation won the *Byte* magazine's Readers' Hardware Choice Award for its development of a removable, 100-MB (100 million-byte) hard drive and disk product. This product, called a **Zip drive** greatly streamlined the backup process for personal computer (PC) users. Later, the company introduced its "Jaz" drive, which stores 1 GB (1 billion bytes) of information.

Zip and Jaz drives have been a popular way for diligent home users to back up data files during the mid to late 1990s. Unfortunately, these drives were not inexpensive, and many users did not have them. Then in the late 1990s, the price of home CD-ROMs that could be written on dropped dramatically. Writable CD-ROMs became generally available on home computers. Even people who were not diligent enough to purchase a Zip or Jaz drive could quickly back up their personal data files on the high density CD-ROMs, which were originally released only in the write-once form. However, a write-many version was available fairly soon for those

who wished, although these were more expensive than the write-once versions.

The write-many versions have the advantage of being rewritable whereas the cheaper CD-ROMs can only be written on once. However, the price of CD-ROMs has dropped so dramatically that even if rewritable CD-ROMs were not available, price would not be a barrier. Of course, rewritable CD-ROMs are now fairly inexpensive and so Zip and Jaz drives are no longer so important as backup devices as was the case in the 1990s.

Computer Power

The terms **bits** and **bytes** refer to how the machine stores information at the lowest, or "closest to machine registers and memory," level. Computers do not process information as words or numbers. They handle information in bytes. A byte is made up of 8 bits.

Bits and Bytes

A "bit" (**b**inary dig**it**) is a unit of data in the binary numbering system. Binary means two, so a bit can assume one of two positions. Effectively, a bit is an on/off switch—on equals the value of 1 and off equals 0. Bits are grouped into collections of eight, which then function as a unit. That unit describes a single character in the computer, such as the letter A or the number 3, and is called a "byte."

A byte looks something like this:

0	0	0	0	1	1	0	0

There are 255 different combinations of 0 and 1 in an 8-character (or 1-byte) unit. That forms the basic limit to the number of characters that can be directly expressed in the computer. Thus, the basic character set hardwired into most PCs contains 255 characters. In the early days of PCs, this was a problem because it severely limited the images that could be produced. However, with the advent of graphics cards and additional character sets and graphics that the new technology allowed, virtually any image can be produced on a computer screen or printed on a printer. Even without graphics cards, additional character sets can be created by means of programming techniques. The size of a variety of computer functions and components is measured by how many bytes they can handle or store at one time (Table 4.1).

Table 4.1   Meaning of Storage Size Terms

Number of Bytes	Term	Formula (≈ means approximately)	Approximate Size in Typed Pages or Other Comparison
1,024	1 kilobyte (K)	$2^{10} \approx 1,000$	One-third of a single-spaced typed page
1,048,576	1 megabyte (M or MB)	$2^{20} \approx 1,024^2$	600-page paperback book
1,073,741,824	1 gigabyte (G or GB)	$2^{30} \approx 1,024^3$	Approximately 1 billion bytes or an encyclopedia
1,099,511,627,776	1 terabyte (T or TB)	$2^{40} \approx 1,024^4$	Approximately 1 trillion bytes
1,125,899,906,842,624	1 petabyte (PB)	$2^{50} \approx 1,024^5$	None available
1,152,921,504,606,846,976	1 exabyte (EB)	$2^{60} \approx 1,024^6$	About 10 to the 18th power bytes
1,180,591,620,717,411,303,424	1 zettabyte (ZB)	$2^{70} \approx 1,024^7$	None available
1,208,925,819,614,629,174,706,176	1 yottabyte (YB)	$2^{80} \approx 1,024^8$	None available

Main memory, which includes the ROM on the motherboard in today's computers, is very large as compared to that of even 10 years ago. Since the size of memory is an important factor in the amount of work a computer can handle, large main memory is another key measure in the power of a computer. In the early 1970s, the PCs on the market were typically sold with a main memory of between 48 and 64 K . In the late 1990s, the size of main memory in computers sold to the public increased rapidly, and by the end of 1999, most computers were advertised with between 32 and 128 MB of main memory.

Another important selling point of a computer is the size of the hard drive that is installed in the box. The first drives sold for microcomputers in the 1970s were external devices that stored about 1,500 K. At that time, few home computers had internal hard drives. When the user turned on the computer, they had to be sure the operating system (see Chap. 5, "Software") diskette was in the disk drive, or the computer could not work. This architecture severely limited the size and functionality of programs. Therefore, consumer demand for hard drives was such that their size grew exponentially while at the same time cost of hard drive storage decreased exponentially. By late 1999, home computers typically sold had between 6 and 20 GB of space on the hard drive. Applications programs have

become so large that both the main memory and especially the hard drive storage space have had to increase exponentially. The typical hard drive sold with a microcomputer in 1990 was 80–100 MB while the hard drives advertised in 1999 typically ranged from 6 to 20 GB.

Computer Speed

Earlier in the discussion about the CPU, it was noted that the basic operations of the CPU are called cycles (fetch, decode, execute, and store cycles). It takes time for the computer to perform each of these functions. The CPU speed is measured in cycles per second which are called the **clock speed** of the computer. One million cycles per second is called one **megahertz** (MHz). CPU speeds are very fast, and today's computers perform many millions of cycles per second. For example, the original IBM PC introduced in 1981 had a clock speed of 4.77 MHz (4.77 million cycles per second). In the late 1990s, Intel Corporation introduced its Pentium III processor, which had clock speeds of 550 MHz. Today, PC speeds are timed in billions of cycles per seconds, or gigahertz (GHz).

In general the higher the clock speed possessed by the CPU, the faster and (in one dimension) the more powerful the computer. However, clock rate can be misleading, since different kinds of processors may perform a different amount of work in one cycle. For example, general purpose computers are known as complex instruction set computers (CISCs) and their processors are prepared to perform a large number of different instruction sets. Therefore, a cycle in a CISC computer may take longer than that for a specialized type of computer called a reduced instruction set computer (RISC). Nonetheless, clock speed is one important measure of the power of a computer.

Overview of Descriptive Terms Used in Computing

The computer is generally described in terms of several major characteristics that have been generally explained—automatic, electronic, and general purpose—as well as in terms of speed, reliability, and storage capacity. The computer is **automatic** because it is self-instructed; that is, it automatically processes data using computer programs called software. The computer is **electronic** because it uses microelectronic components etched on silicon chips for its circuitry. This means that its basic building blocks are microminiaturized. The computers discussed so far are **general purpose** machines, because the user can program them to process all types of problems and can solve any problem that can be broken down into a set of logical sequential instructions. Special purpose machines designed to do only a very few different types of tasks have also been developed. An example of a special use computer is the RISC computer described above. The computer is also characterized by its **speed** and split-second processing of large amounts of data, its **reliability** due to the silicon circuitry, and its ability to **store** large amounts of data that can be retrieved quickly.

The computer is also described by its **architecture,** which refers to the design of the individual hardware components and to the microprocessor used. A key characteristic of a computer is its hardware platform, or simply, its platform. The two main types of platform in the commercial PC market are the IBM and Apple Macintosh platform. The two are not compatible, and without a translator, one computer cannot read the other's diskettes.

History of Computers

The first true digital computer, called the Colossus Mark I, was built in 1943 with funding from the U.S. Military and used in airplane design and other complex engineering applications. At the same time, Bell Laboratories was working on development of a computer, as were two scientists at the University of Pennsylvania, J. Presper Eckert and John Mauchly, later founders of Eckert-Mauchly Corporation.

The prototype World War II military computers were very different from today's computers. First, they were big. A computer with much less power than an ordinary desktop computer of the 1990s took up an entire room. Second, there were relatively few operations they could perform as compared to today's computers. Essentially, they were giant and complex mathematical calculators. Third, they were difficult to program. In fact, they were programmed by the scientists getting to the back of the computer and changing the wires. This approach was slow, tedious, and impractical for a commercial machine.

After the war, Eckert and Mauchly produced the first vacuum tube computer, the electronic numerical integrator and computer, more commonly known as the ENIAC (Weik, 1961). In 1950, the Remington Rand Corporation bought Eckert and Mauchly's company (Unisys, date unknown) and 1 year later began to market the first large scale commercial computer system, called the UNIVAC-I (Anonymous, 2004). In 1955, the Sperry Corporation merged with Remington Rand, forming the giant Sperry Rand Corporation. That year, the very first commercial application was run when General Electric processed its payroll on a UNIVAC computer, and the age of business computing was born. The American business establishment recognized the value of this machine that could do thousands of repetitive, mathematical calculations. In response, companies such as Bell Labs, National Cash Register (NCR), Burroughs, and IBM began to develop their business computer products. Today, these early computers are called **first generation computers.**

The Univac and other first generation computers used vacuum tubes in their design. Those computers ran hot and thus required a great deal of cooling. Vacuum tubes got hot easily, and when they got hot, they failed regularly. Given that those computers used many vacuum tubes, and the high (and random) failure rate of vacuum tubes, the early computers were a real challenge to keep operational.

For the first generation of computers, the speed of the main processor was measured in access speeds (how fast the CPU could access commands entered through punched cards). Access speeds were measured in thousandths of a second (milliseconds). First generation computers were physically huge (one computer took up a large room), but their power was much less than that of the average desktop computer of the 1900s. Main memory was less than 10 K of storage.

Second generation computers were introduced in the late 1950s. They included the IBM 1401 and 1620. They used transistors instead of vacuum tubes. This meant less heat, improved reliability, and much greater speeds. Second generation CPU access speeds were measured in millionths rather than thousandths of a second (microseconds). They still were quite large, but transistors were smaller and more durable than vacuum tubes. They also allowed for the development of much more powerful computers.

Third generation computers were introduced in the mid-1960s. These used microminiature, solid state components. Third generation CPU access speeds were measured in billionths of a second (nanoseconds). The IBM 360 and 370 were the classic computers in this generation. They had about 110 K of main memory, and it was this generation in which hard disk drives were introduced. These hard disks were not encased in protective plastic cases, so they were very vulnerable to dust. Any magnetic media is vulnerable to dirt, even the diskettes used today. However, today the hard drives are much better protected against dust than was the case in the 1960s. That is why pictures of computer rooms taken during the third generation era often show people in surgical type garb. They were trying to keep the failure rate down by keeping the computer room as clean as possible.

The Rise of the Modern Personal Computer

In November 1972, Intel Corporation introduced the first commercial microprocessor, called the Intel 8008 (Maxfield and Brown, 1997). This invention made the PC, or microcomputer, possible. Shortly thereafter, two teenaged boys named Steve Jobs and Steve Wozniak who shared an intense interest in electronics bought a microprocessor for $25 and built a very simple computer they called the "Apple" (MIT, 1996). Like Henry Ford's dream of bringing automobiles to everyone, Jobs had a passionate dream of bringing computers to everybody. They failed to interest Wozniak's employer, Hewlett-Packard (HP) Corporation, in their idea to build a small computer that people could have and use in their homes (Mesa, 1997). At that time, according to legend, HP executives could not imagine why anyone would want such a machine in the home. They were focused on business computing, with its billing and payroll processing, and people's home finances simply did not require such power. Not to be refused, the two Steves decided to pursue their dream anyway. They began building the machines in Steve Jobs' garage, and in May of 1976, they introduced their first computer at a meeting of the Homebrew Computer Club, at which

Paul Terryl, president of the Byte Shop chain, ordered 50 computers (Mesa, 1997). At the time, Steve Jobs was 21 years old and Wozniak was 26. The Apple Computer Company and the first PC were born. In 1999, Steve Jobs was chairman and CEO of Pixar, the computer animation studio that won an Academy Award for its work on the motion picture, "Toy Story." The home page of Pixar may be found at *http://www.pixar.com* (Fig. 4.7).

At the same time that Jobs and Wozniak were working in the garage, IBM introduced the first fourth generation mainframe, the IBM 370 (Watson, 1999). This was the first mainframe family that had printed circuits. This computer was so fast that the old measurement of speed was deemed unsuitable. Since a CPU processes instructions (which the CPU fetches, decodes, executes, and stores), the new CPU's speed was measured by the speed with which it could process instructions, rather than accesses. Fourth generation computer CPU speeds were (and still are today) measured by instructions per second that they can process. The IBM 370's CPU speed was measured in millions of instructions per second (MIPS). Today's mainframes are measured in billions of instructions per second (BIPS) or giga-instructions per second (GIPS).

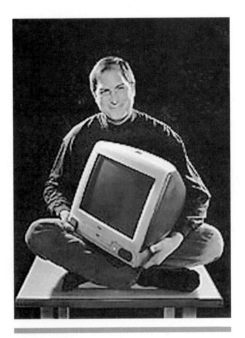

Figure 4.7
Stephen Jobs.
(Courtesy of Apple Computer, Inc.
Photographer: Moshe Brakha.)

Supercomputers

The first supercomputer was developed by a computer engineer named Seymour Cray (The Franklin Institute, 1999). Cray had been one of the architects of the UNIVAC (Bell, 1997). He left UNIVAC in 1957 to join in the development of a new company, Control Data Corporation (CDC), and continued his processor development work throughout the 1950s and 1960s. His work at CDC culminated in the production of the CDC 7600, a computer 10 times more powerful than the CDC 6600, often called the first supercomputer.

Shortly thereafter, Cray and CDC parted ways over the development of a whole new concept in computer architecture that Cray wished to pursue. Unwilling to invest in this new concept, CDC did not agree to work with Cray to produce it. Therefore, in 1972, Cray decided to go into business for himself so that his dream could be realized (Breckenridge, 1996). The new company, Cray Research, in Minnesota was the result of this split. Cray Research's first product was the Cray-I supercomputer. Most consider the Cray-I to be the first true supercomputer, since its architecture was innovative and its power was orders of magnitude greater than anything that came before it. In 1989, history repeated itself, and Cray left Cray Research to open a new company in Colorado Springs. That company went bankrupt, some say due to a combination of reduced need for supercomputing due to the end of the Cold War and Cray's unwillingness to compromise speed for compatibility with other computer technology. Sadly, Cray was involved in a terrible accident and died on October 5, 1996, at the age of 71 from severe head injuries. At the time of his death, Cray was a vital, energetic, and creative man who had just founded yet another new company dedicated to the advancement of computer power and speed (Bell, 1997). Cray was truly a genius. Certainly the Father of Supercomputing, in many ways Cray was instrumental in the development of the modern digital computer (Breckenridge, 1996; Bell, 1997) and it will never be known what further advances already in his mind were lost with him.

Classes of Computers

Three broad classes of computers exist: the analog computer, the digital computer, and the hybrid computer. Analog computers handle continuous input data, such as are found in the continuously changing electric patterns of the heartbeat. Digital computers handle input that comes in at discrete points in time, such as the workload measured at 10 o'clock in the morning. The hybrid computer—as suggested by its name—is a computer that is able to process both kinds of signals.

Analog Computer

The analog computer operates on continuous physical or electrical magnitudes, measuring ongoing continuous analog quantities such as voltage, current, temperature, and pressure. Selected physiologic monitoring equipment, which accepts continuous input/output signals, is in the analog class of computers. An example of these machines in the clinical setting include heart monitors and fetal monitors. An analog computer handles data in continuously variable quantities rather than breaking the data down into discrete digital representations.

Digital Computer

The digital computer, on the other hand, operates on discrete discontinuous numerical digits using the binary numbering system. It represents data using discrete values for all data. Its data are represented by numbers, letters, and symbols rather than by waveforms such as on a heart monitor. Most of the computers used in the health care industry for charting and decision support are digital computers.

Hybrid Computer

The hybrid computer, as its name implies, contains features of both the analog and the digital computer. It is used for specific applications, such as complex signal processing and other engineering-oriented applications. It is also found in some monitoring equipment that converts analog signals to digital ones for data processing. For example, physiologic monitors that are able to capture the heart waveform and also to measure the core body temperature at specific times of the shift are actually hybrid computers. Some physiologic research projects can make use of hybrid computers that have analog ability to capture waveforms of physiologic monitors (i.e., ECG, EEG, and so forth) and convert them into digital format suitable for analysis.

Types of Computers

Today, four basic types of computers are generally recognized. Each type of computer was developed as the computer industry evolved, and each was developed for a different purpose. The basic types of computers include the supercomputer, the mainframe, the microcomputer, and the handheld. They differ in size, composition, memory and storage capacity, processing time, and cost. They generally have had different applications and are found in many different locations in the health care industry.

Supercomputers

The largest type of computer is the supercomputer. A supercomputer is a computational-oriented computer specially designed for scientific applications requiring gigantic amounts of calculations. The supercomputer is truly a world class "number cruncher." The supercomputer is designed primarily for analysis of scientific and engineering problems and for tasks requiring millions or billions of computational operations and calculations. It is found primarily in areas such as defense and weaponry, weather forecasting, and scientific research. The supercomputer is also providing a new source of power for the high-performance computing and communication (HPCC) environment.

Mainframes

The mainframe computer is the fastest, largest, and most expensive type of computer used in corporate America for processing, storing, and retrieving data. It is a large multiuser central computer that meets the computing needs—especially the large amount of repetitive calculations of bills, payroll, and the like—of a large organization. A mainframe is capable of processing BIPS and accessing billions (GB) of characters of data (Figs. 4.8 and 4.9). Mainframes can serve a large number (hundreds) of users at the same time. In many settings, hundreds of terminals (input and output devices that may or may not have any processing power of their own) are wired directly onto the mainframe. Typically, there are also phone lines into the computer so that remote users can gain access to the mainframe. As compared with a desktop PC, a mainframe has an extremely large memory capacity and fast operating and processing time, and it can process a large number of functions (multiprocessing) at one time.

Microcomputers (Personal Computers or PCs)

While mainframe computers provide critical service to the health care industry, microcomputers are being used for an increasing number of independent applications as well as serving as a desktop link to the programs of the mainframe (Fig. 4.10). Hospital nursing departments are using PCs to process specific applications such as

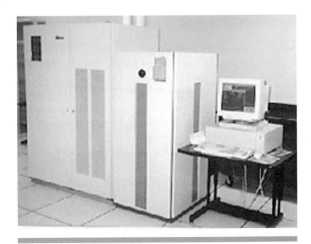

Figure 4.8
Hitachi 2 mainframe computer.
(Reproduced, with permission, from Wright State University, Dayton, OH.)

patient classification, nurse staffing and scheduling, and personnel management applications. Microcomputers are also found in educational and research settings, where they are used to conduct a multitude of special educational and scientific functions. Desktops are replacing

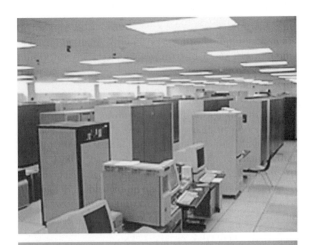

Figure 4.9
IBM mainframe computer room at Virginia Polytechnic and State University, circa 1996.
(Reproduced, with permission, from Virginia Polytechnic and State University, Blacksburg, VA. *http://black-ice.cc.vt.edu.* Photographer: Valdis Kletnieks.)

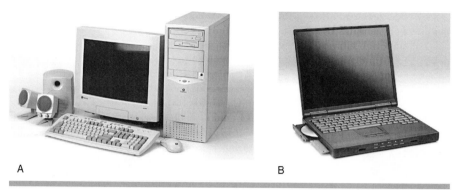

A   B

Figure 4.10
Gateway desktop (A) and notebook (B) computers.
(© 2000 Gateway, Inc. Photos courtesy of Gateway, Inc.)

many of the mainframe attributes. Desktops can serve as stand-alone workstations and can be linked to a network system to increase their capabilities. This is advantageous, since software multiuser licensing fees are usually less expensive per user than having each user purchase his or her own copy.

Microcomputers are also available as portable, laptop, notebook, and handheld computers. Handheld computers are now portable and laptop versions are smaller than the standard desktop microcomputer. The notebook microcomputer is generally 81/2 in. × 11 in. and weighs approximately 4 lb.

Handheld Computers

Handheld computers are small, special function computers, although a few "full function" handheld computers were introduced in the late 1990s. Even though of smaller size than the standard desktop microcomputer, some have claimed to have almost the same functionality and processing capabilities as the standard desktop microcomputer. However, they are limited in their expansion possibilities, their ability to serve as full participants in the office network, and the peripherals they can support. More popular are the palm-sized computers, including personal digital assistants (PDAs), which are the smallest of the handheld computers. The PDA is a very small special function handheld computer which provides calendar, contacts, and note-taking functions, and may provide word processing, spread sheet, and a variety of other functions (Hyperdictionary, 2004). They are invaluable to the busy professional who must travel and wishes to conduct some work at

home or on the road (Figs. 4.11, 4.12, and 4.13). They are particularly useful in that they can synchronize the user's office calendar with the calendar on the handheld computer when one or the other has had appointments added or changed. The current trend is that cell phones are adding functionalities and are combining the functions of cell phone and palm-sized computer in one convenient package.

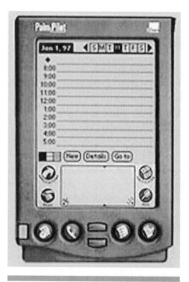

Figure 4.11
Palm Pilot.

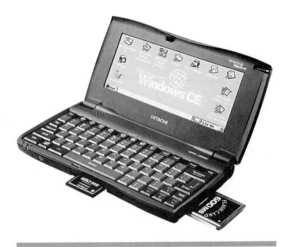

Figure 4.12
Hitachi handheld computer.
(Reproduced, with permission, from Hitachi America,
Ltd., *www.hitachi.com/*.)

 Common Hardware Peripherals

Keyboard

The keyboard is the most common input device. It is similar to the keyboard of a typewriter and is connected

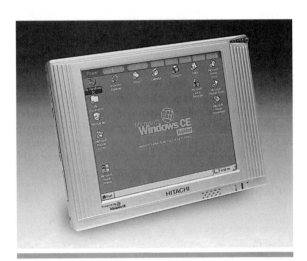

Figure 4.13
Hitachi handheld PC.
(Reproduced, with permission, from Hitachi America, Ltd.,
www.hitachi.com/.)

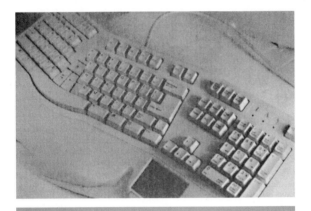

Figure 4.14
Ergonomic keyboard with touch pad.
(Reproduced, with permission, from Pilgrim A. (2000). *Build Your Own Pentium III* (p. 305). New York, NY: McGraw-Hill.)

to the box with a cord (Fig. 4.14). There are several different types of keyboards; however, regardless of type they all have similar sections of keys: (1) typewriter keys, (2) function keys, (3) numeric keypad, (4) cursor keys, (5) toggle keys, and (6) special operations keys. Carpal tunnel syndrome has been a severe problem for many people whose jobs require them to spend many hours a day typing on a keyboard. In response, several different styles designed to reduce the incidence of carpal tunnel have been introduced.

The **typewriter key** section is the largest and contains keys that follow the standard QWERTY arrangement of keys of a standard typewriter. (The term represents the first six letters in the first alphabetic row.) The **function keys** (F1–F12) are **software-specific**; that is, they are programmable, since their function is dependent on the software program being processed. For example, the function key F10 is used to retrieve a file in one word processing package and to save in another. Generally, a template is provided for the function keys that defines how the keys are used for the specific software package. Three other keys on the keyboard labeled **Shift, Ctrl,** and **Alt** expand the function keys by being used in combination with them to carry out other commands.

The **numeric keypad** is a second set of numeric keys that are placed differently on the keyboard than the alphabetic keys. The numeric keypad is a separate rectangle-shaped calculator-type section that enables the user to enter numeric data more efficiently. This section of keys can be converted to represent other keys, including moving the cursor in four directions, just by turning on the **Num Lock key**. The four **cursor keys** are used to direct the position of the pointer on the display monitor. They control the movement: **up** ($\uparrow$), **down** ($\downarrow$), **right** ($\rightarrow$), and **left** ($\leftarrow$) over the display screen. The **toggle keys** are those that have a dual purpose. When a toggle key is pressed once, the function is **on**, and when pressed a second time it is **off**. The major toggle keys include **Num Lock, Caps Lock, Scroll Lock,** and **Insert/Typeover.**

There are also **special operations keys** that are unique to the microcomputer and are used to make the keyboard easy to manipulate. The **Home** and **End** keys bring the cursor to the beginning or end of a line, **Print Screen** prints the screen display or saves it to the clipboard as a snapshot, **Esc** (escape) interrupts or cancels a function, a **Tab** key moves the cursor to predetermined set tabs, the **Del** key deletes text, and a **space bar** inserts blank spaces in a line. The **Enter** key performs a variety of functions depending on the context of the program. It sends information to the computer, such as during sign-on procedures, in word processing it creates a new paragraph, and it can be used to create a blank section in a document.

Monitor

The monitor is a display screen component of a terminal that allows the user to see images, programs, commands the user sends to the computer, and results of the computer's work (output). Similar to a television screen, the monitor can show colors, animation, text, and virtually anything that the computer can produce. Up to a point, larger screens are desirable on monitors, because people spend so much time looking at monitors that eye strain is common. Most PCs today come with monitors from 14 to 21 in., although larger screens are available. The resolution or clarity of the monitor screen is related to the number of dots, **pixels**, on the screen. Customers can order anything from a 14 in. viewing screen with $1{,}024 \times 768$ pixels to 21 in. screens with a resolution of $1{,}600 \times 1{,}280$ pixels. As pixel count rises, the sharpness and clarity of images and colors on the screen improve.

Mouse and Trackball

The mouse was introduced with the microcomputer as a new type of input device to replace moving the arrow keys on the keyboard. It is a hand-controlled mechanical device that electronically instructs the cursor to move across the video display screen. It resembles a bar

of soap with a tail. As the user slides the mouse across a desktop pad, a ball on the bottom of the mouse senses the motion and transmits it to the cursor (pointer) on the screen. The cursor moves in conjunction with the mouse. The mouse has at least two buttons and sometimes a roller at the top. The left button is used primarily to (1) select the icon, (2) activate a process, and (3) implement a function to be performed. The right button is a special function button, and its function is dependent on the program. A mouse requires a certain amount of space on a desk, and it is associated with carpal tunnel and wrist fatigue. Additionally, the mouse often "runs" off the pad and must be repositioned to work. The trackball was developed for people who prefer a stationary device. Similar to a mouse, the trackball has the ball on the top, and movement of the cursor is controlled by the fingers rolling the ball in place.

Floppy Disks/Diskettes and CD-ROMs

The floppy disk, commonly called a diskette, and the CD-ROM are another form of secondary storage or auxiliary memory. They serve as both input and output media. They are largely used by microcomputers. Data are read and written, using disk drives in the same manner as with magnetic tapes and magnetic disks or CD readers and burners. A floppy diskette turns a read/write head similar to a phonograph record to transfer electronic impulses between the diskette and memory. Each diskette has a disk window, which exposes the area on the magnetic surface where the data can be retrieved or stored. A write-protect slot is also cut near the top of the jacket. Covering the slot (or sliding the slot cover to the closed position) renders the diskette unavailable to the writing head. Thus, nothing can be erased or written onto the disk (see Fig. 4.7).

A floppy disk is a flexible mylar plastic oxide-coated disk thinly covered with magnetic spots. It is available in $3\frac{1}{2}$ and $5\frac{1}{4}$ in. sizes, though $5\frac{1}{4}$ in. floppy disks are rarely seen these days. The $3\frac{1}{2}$ in. diskette is encased in a hard plastic case that is sturdy and easier to store. The $5\frac{1}{4}$ in. diskette can hold 360 K to 1 MB of data, and the $3\frac{1}{2}$ in. diskette can hold 1.55 MB (double density) to 2.0 MB (high density). Each floppy disk is sectioned into concentric rings or tracks ranging from 9 to 15 and each track is divided into sectors ranging from 40 to 48 or 80 to 96. Sectors store the smallest unit of data. Tracks and sectors are used to provide the addresses of fields of data. The procedure to mark the tracks and sectors is called formatting. Formatting is done at the factory, but when a user wishes to completely erase a diskette, it is wise to reformat the disk to ensure that no sectors are lost to hidden files.

The CD-ROM can store around 640 MB of data (Foldoc, 2004), and is therefore a much more useful medium for the larger data, text, and graphics files that many users wish to store and move from computer to computer today. Multimedia applications tend to be large, so CD-ROMs are more convenient for storage of multimedia presentations than are diskettes.

Touch Pad and Mouse Button

The touch pad was developed by the makers of laptop computers for use in place of the mouse. A mouse is not practical for use in an airplane or other travel location. The touch pad is a flat, rectangular depression on the keyboard that senses pressure and movement of the user's finger. The user simply drags the finger around the touch-pad to move the cursor on the screen. A slight tap on the touch pad works as double-clicking the left mouse button or pressing the "Enter" key on the keyboard.

Light Pen/Touch Screen

A light pen is a photosensitive device that responds to light images when placed against a monitor screen. When the pen comes in contact with the display screen it highlights the item and sends data to the computer. Touch screens involve the use of a special filter on a monitor screen that allows the screen to "sense" the pressure of the user's finger on a particular position of the screen. That pressure can signal the computer to initiate an action (similar to a mouse click) or can function to let the user select a particular item on the screen, such as on a menu. Sensors on the screen pinpoint the X and Y axis location touched by a user.

Optical Character Recognition

Optical character recognition (OCR) is a specialized computer input medium that allows data to be read directly from a form or document. An electronic optical scanning device, a **wand reader**, or a bar code reader reads special marks, bar codes, numbers, letters, or characters. The scanner used in a grocery store uses a special type of OCR. Such a device converts the optical marks, characters, and bar codes into electrical signals that become computer input. OCR-readable codes include those outlined in areas on the answer sheet of the nursing state board examinations, which are filled in with pencil. The bar codes called universal product code symbols (zebra-striped bars) are another example. Ten bars, about 1 in. long, signify different numbers to code groceries or medical items. If read with a special scanning device, they become input into some hospital inventory systems, similar to the way product

codes read in the grocery check-out line become input into the store's inventory control system.

Magnetic-Ink Character Recognition

Magnetic-ink character recognition (MICR) is another medium for reading characters by computer. Here the characters are made of magnetized particles printed on paper. A MICR reader can examine the shape of the magnetic-ink characters and convert them into binary code for computer input. The most common example of a MICR is the magnetized characters imprinted on checks, which most banks use.

Voice Synthesizer

A voice synthesizer allows users to input data into the computer by speaking into a connected microphone. Also known as a speech synthesizer, it digitizes the sound for processing by the CPU. Although automatic recognition of the human voice is not yet perfected, voice input is used in situations requiring only a few spoken words, and it is becoming a common medium for all computer systems. The study of neural networks (many processors working in parallel in a single computer) offers one hope of improving the performance of voice recognition technology.

Imaging

The field of computer imaging exploded in the 1980s and 1990s with the enormous development of medical imaging. Many of the advanced imaging technologies, such as computerized axial tomography (CAT scans) and magnetic resonance imaging (MRI) are computer-enhanced imaging technologies. Several different types of image input devices are available that primarily transform images from various types of graphics into digital form, which the computer can accept, represent on the screen, and process. Many types of graphic images on paper such as x-rays can be scanned as computer input and/or digitized for computer use.

Digital Versatile Disk

While DVD began as digital video disk, it is now commonly and more correctly referred to as digital versatile disk to better reflect its capabilities of playing audio and multimedia as well as video. A DVD looks and feels like a CD-ROM but holds much more information and contains many more multimedia features. DVD technology is in the process of replacing most CD-ROM technology.

The technology was developed to support high resolution and dense applications such as placement of motion pictures on CDs.

Printers

The printer, the most important output device, converts information produced by the computer system into printed form, rendering data in the binary code into readable English. The major types of printed output include printed hard copy (paper), microfilm (microfiche), photographs, and graphic copy. The printer's output, known as **hard copy**, is output produced on paper. Most printers sold today are laser printers or jet printers—either inkjet or bubble-jet printers. Laser printers offer a substantial increase in output quality and speed over the jet printers. The laser printer's engine is composed of an integrated system of electronic and chemical parts that work together with optical processes to produce the printed image. The laser printers generally use fonts or typefaces as their printing elements, making documents look like they were typeset. They are also used for printing graphic images and illustrations. The inkjet and bubble-jet printers fire small bursts of ink on the paper. The principal difference between bubble-jet printers and other inkjet printers is that bubble-jet printers use special heating elements to prepare the ink, whereas inkjet printers use piezoelectric crystals to ionize the ink.

Modems

The modem is a communication device used to connect a terminal with a mainframe or another computer. A modem (**mo**dulating and **dem**odulating device) translates digital data into waves (analog) for transmission over the communication lines to the computer system and converts the waves back to their original digital form for input into the computer. Modems connect the user with a remote computer's CPU, enabling communication through telephone lines. By dialing the remote computer's modem, data can be both sent and received from outside sources. Modems, therefore, facilitate the function of both input and output devices and link remote computers to networks of computers. Modems are described by the rate of communication transmission or line transfer called the bits per second (bps) rate. 57 K is a common modem speed in late 1990s models. Most modems sold for PCs are actually **fax-modems**, which can send documents over the phone or network lines to be downloaded via fax machine at a distant site. The computer programs for fax-modem communication can save the fax as a data file for editing and storage.

They also can save the graphics/images using OCR technology and convert them into text files for storage.

Basics of Computer Network Hardware

A network is a set of cooperative interconnected computers for the purpose of information interchange. The networks of greatest interest include local area networks (LANs), wide area networks (WANs), and the Internet, which is a network of networks. A LAN usually supports the interconnected computer needs of a single company or agency. The computers are physically located close to each other, and generally, only members of the company or agency have legitimate access to the information on the network. WANs support geographically dispersed facilities, such as the individual grocery stores in a national chain. A subset of WANs include the metropolitan area networks (MANs) that support and connect the many buildings of local governmental agencies or university campuses.

The most important components of network hardware are the **adapter or interface card**, **cabling**, and **server**. The most important concepts in network hardware are **architecture** and **topology**. Note that much of the information in this section was generated with the assistance of on-line computer dictionaries and encyclopedias such as those offered by the following:

1. Infostreet.com, 18345 Ventura Blvd., Tarzana, CA 91356 and their "Information Please" on-line resource, which is located at *http://www.infoplease.com/*

2. The "What is" resource located at: *http://whatis.techtarget.com/*

3. The on-line dictionary, encyclopedia, and thesaurus information provided through the Dictionary.com Company located at *http://www.dictionary.com/*.

Network Hardware

The role of hardware in a network is to provide an interconnection between computers. For a computer to participate on a network, it must have at least two pieces of hardware:

1. *Network adapter or network interface card.* A network interface card (NIC) is a computer circuit board or card that is installed in a computer so that it can be connected to a network. PCs and workstations on LANs typically contain a NIC specifically designed for the LAN transmission technology, such as

Ethernet. NICs provide a dedicated, full-time connection to a network. Most home and portable computers connect to the Internet through modems on an as-needed dial-up connection. The modem provides the connection interface to the Internet service provider.

The oldest and still most commonly used "network interface" (or "adapter card") is an Ethernet card. But there exist other options such as arcnet, serial-port boards, and so on. Most of the time, the choice of NIC depends on the communication medium.

2. *Communication medium (cabling).*   The "communication medium" is the means by which actual transfer of data from one site to another takes place. Commonly used communication media include twisted pair cable, coaxial cable, fiber-optics, telephone lines, satellites, and compressed video. Most of the time, the choice of a communication medium is based on the following.

   (a) *Distance.*   Relatively short distances are required for compressed video and coaxial cables. For much longer distances, fiber-optics, telephone lines, and satellite transmission are used. For shorter distances where video is needed, coaxial cable and compressed video are used.

   (b) *Amount of data transfer.*   Large amounts of data (especially video) are best handled with coaxial cables and compressed video and through satellite communications (satellite and compressed video are very expensive). Smaller amounts of data or serial (nonvideo) streams are best handled through the other wire types, such as twisted pair copper wire and optical fiber, and are less expensive.

   (c) *How often the transfer is needed.*   Coaxial works best for locally wired networks that are used constantly by a very limited number of users. Telephone wires work well for the relatively high usage public networks (like the Internet) but are more likely to get overloaded when many users try to use the system at the same time. Consider, for example, the busy Internet or phone lines getting clogged up when a tornado or hurricane has struck a community.

   (d) *Availability.*   Availability depends on cost, transmission speed, number of users (who might clog up the system), weather conditions (satellites), and so on.

Telephone Line Communications

Specialized phone lines called integrated services digital network (ISDN) lines are used to carry communications across phone lines. ISDN is a set of communication standards for optical fibers that carry voice, digital, and video signals across phone lines. There are a variety of types of ISDN connections, each having a different bandwidth. The bandwidth controls how fast the signals can be transmitted across the phone lines. The first was DS0, which stands for "digital service—zeroth level," that transmitted at 64 kilobytes per second. Today, those have been replaced with **T-Lines**, which are used to handle the high-speed transmissions needed for network communications. The American Bell Telephone Company introduced the T-carrier system in the 1960s because increasing phone usage was overloading the DS lines. There are four bandwidths available for T-lines, ranging from the 1.54 megabytes per second (Mbps) speed and 24 channels of the T-1 line to the 274.1 Mbps speed and 4,032 channels of a T-4 line. Many Internet service providers still pass information through T-1 lines. However, with the increasing use of the Internet, more and more problems with slow transmission have created demand for even faster lines. The T-3 line has a transmission speed of 447.36 Mbps, and most large ISPs have had to move their customers to T-3 lines in order to provide adequate customer service. Some users, dissatisfied with the speed limitations of their own home phone line have purchased fractional T-1 line service. Fractional T-1 line service involves the rental of some portion of the 24 channels in a T-1 line.

Cable Modem

For many people, telephone modems have proven much too slow a medium for their Internet connection and many have moved to cable modem for their home Internet connectivity. Cable modem uses the same type of connection that cable TV uses. The interesting thing is that TV uses very little of the bandwidth of a cable connection, so the same cable that brings a user cable TV can be used to bring high-speed Internet service. A coaxial cable can carry hundreds of megahertz but the cable TV takes up only about 6 MHz. The Internet connection takes up only about 2 MHz upstream and about 5–6 downstream (Franklin, 2004). Thus, even with both TV and Internet connections, the household cable line is far from overloaded.

In general, the user will have to add an external cable modem box to the computer configuration. That cable box contains a tuner, a demodulator, a modulator, a MAC, a CPU, and network hardware. The tuner receives the signals and it then passes them to the demodulator. The demodulator takes radio and analog information and converts it to digital data, performs data correction functions, checks for problems in transmission, and finally, passes the signal onto the modulator. The modulator works with upstream traffic to convert the digital signals into radio frequency signals. The MAC, sitting between the upstream and downstream components, acts as an interface between the various parts of the network protocols.

A cable modem can serve up to 1,000 users at a time, although at that point performance may begin to degrade. Should that happen, all the cable network company need do is to simply add a new channel and half the number of users per channel (Franklin, 2004). A cable network can achieve speeds of up to 30–40 megabits per second, which is far faster than the maximum speed of a telephone modem connection.

Servers

The concept of a server is very important when networks are discussed today. For a network to exist, there must be a server. Most networks today use the client/server approach. In a pure client/server approach, one computer is the core or server computer that receives requests from the client (user) computer and fulfills those requests. For example, when the user requests a site on the Internet, the server receives the request, decodes it, and sends the link onto the correct Internet address.

1. In general, a server is a computer program that provides services to other computer programs in the same computer **or in other computers on a network**.

2. The computer that runs the server program is also frequently referred to as "the server" (although the server computer may contain a number of server and client programs).

3. In the client/server programming model, a server is a program that awaits and fulfills requests from client programs in the same or other computers. A given application in a computer may function as a client with requests for services from other programs and a server or requests from other programs.

Architecture

In informatics, architecture refers to overall physical structure, peripherals, interconnections within the computer, and its system software, especially the operating system. Computer architecture can be divided into five fundamental components: input/output, storage, communication, control, and processing. These are also called the computer's subsystems. When networks are discussed, architecture refers to how communication among the various computers in the network is accomplished. Broadly speaking, there are two types of network architectures.

1. **Broadcast.** Here the communication is done by transmitting the same information to all the computers in the network that are expected to respond to it. This is typically used in LANs.

2. **Point-to-point.** The computer for which information is intended is identified first, and the communication is only to that particular computer. This is typically used in "dial-up" networking, such as an individual who dials up the network through his or her internet service provider.

Topology

Topology defines how the network computers in a LAN are interconnected within a physical area and describes their physical interconnection. Several possible topologies are the following:

1. *Bus.*   A bus is a network topology or circuit arrangement in which all the node computers are directly attached to a line. Therefore, all communications travel through each of the node computers. Each computer has a unique identity and can recognize the transmissions sent to it. In this fashion all computers are connected in parallel to each other. The big advantage of this topology is that if one computer fails, other computers still can access the information. This structure is decentralized. (Note: The term "bus" is also used in computer hardware. In that context, it usually refers to an expansion slot on the motherboard of the computer.)

2. *Star.*   This is a centralized structure where all computers are connected through a central computer, called the server. If this central computer fails, information cannot be sent or received by any of the computers connected to this server.

3. *Ring.*   Originally, all LAN computers were connected in a ring fashion with wires or cables that directly connected all the computers together. If one computer failed, none of the computers could communicate and share the resources. That topology has been replaced by the **token ring** network protocol. Token rings work by having the server pass a marker, or "token," to the computer that is next in line to communicate. No computer can send or receive data unless it is the target of the token. In this way, collisions between two workstations that wish to transmit information at the same time are avoided. It should be noted that, generally, the token is passed so

rapidly that the LAN users may never know they had to wait. A token ring structure can support networks in which the computers are up to 124 miles apart.

(a) *Hub: A form of ring topology.* A hub consists of a "backbone," or main circuit, attached to a number of outgoing lines. Each of the outgoing lines can support a number of ports to which devices can be attached. Generally, hub LANs are used for a relatively small number of connected workstations. In the hub, all computers are connected to a central hub processor that contains the networking software and provides for communication among the various computers on the network. For a computer to talk to one or more of the other computers on the network, it must first go through the hub.

(b) *Arcnet.* Another type of ring technology used for LANs is arcnet. It uses what is called a "token-bus" system for managing line sharing among all the users on the network. It works well for LANs in which all the links are physically near each other (each cable can go only 2,000 feet, but the total span can be up to 20,000 feet). While not as powerful as some other topologies, it is by far the least expensive.

Summary

This chapter described computer hardware, including both internal and peripheral hardware. It explained the fundamental components of a computer and provided a simple overview of how computers function at the machine level. It offered a brief history of the development of computer hardware and of some of the people who played major roles in the computer industry. It also described computer classes, characteristics, and types. It outlined the four major functions of a computer: input, output, processing, and storage. The most common peripheral hardware was introduced and described. Finally, it presented basic concepts of computer networks and the hardware necessary to support networks.

References

Anonymous. (Downloaded, 2004). *The Univac.* The Computer Science Club: UC Davis. University of California at Davis: Computer Science Museum. *http://wwwcsif.cs.ucdavis.edu/~csclub/museum/items/univac.html*

Asirvatham, S., Bruce, C., and Friedman, P. (2003). Advances in imaging for cardiac electrophysiology. *Coronary Artery Disease* 14(1):3–13.

Beets-Tan, R. and Beets, G. (2004). Rectal cancer: Review with emphasis on MRI imaging. *Radiology* 232(2):335–346.

Bell, G. (1997). *The Seymour Cray Lecture Series.* University of Minnesota. *http://research.microsoft.com/_users/gbell/_craytalk/sld001.htm*

Breckenridge, C. (Downloaded, 2004). *A Tribute to Seymour Cray. Keynote Presentation at Supercomputing '96, November 19, 1996. http://www.cgl.ucsf.edu/home/tef/cray/tribute.html*

Columbia Encyclopedia. (2003). Optical disks. *The Columbia Encyclopedia* (6th ed.). New York: Columbia University Press.

Debnath, D. (2004). Activity analysis of telemedicine in the UK. *Postgraduate Medical Journal* 80(944):335–338.

Foldoc: Online Computer Dictionary. (2004). CD-ROM. *NightFlight.* Oakland, CA. *http://www.nightflight.com/foldoc-bin/foldoc.cgi?Compact+Disc+Read-Only+Memory*

Franklin, C. (Downloaded, 2004). How cable modems work. In *How Stuff Works.* HSW Media Networks. *http://www.howstuffworks.com/cable-modem.htm*

Hyperdictionary. (2004). *PDA.* Webnox Corporation. *http://www.hyperdictionary.com/dictionary/Personal+Digital+Assistant*

Marcin, J., Schepps, D., Page, K., Struve, S., Nagrampa, E., and Dimand, R. (2004). The use of telemedicine to provide pediatric critical care consultations to pediatric trauma patients admitted to a remote trauma intensive care unit: A preliminary report. *Pediatric Critical Care Medicine* 5(3):251–256.

Massachusetts Institute of Technology (MIT). (1996). *The Lemelson-MIT Awards: Invention Dimension. http://web.mit.edu/invent/www/inventorsI-Q/_apple.html*

Maxfield, C. and Brown, B. (1997). *Bebop Bytes Back.* Madison, AL: Doone Publications.

Mesa, A. (1997). *Apple History Timeline.* The Apple Museum. *http://www.applemuseum.seastar.net/*

The Franklin Institute. (1999). *Seymour Cray. http://sln.fi._edu/_tfi/exhibits/cray.html*

Unisys Corporation. A *Brief Historical Overview. http://www.unisys.se/presentation/nyckelh._htm*

Wang, S., Goss, H., Lee, S., Pardue, C., Waller, J., Nichols, F., Adams, R., and Hess, D. (2004). Remote evaluation of acute ischemic stroke in rural community hospitals in Georgia. *Stroke* 35(7):1763–1768.

Weik, M. (1961). *The ENIAC Story.* Washington, DC. (Reprinted from the January–February 1961 issue of O R D N A N C E. The *Journal of the American Ordnance Association.*) *http://_ftp.arl.mil/~mike/comphist/eniac-story.html*

Computer Software and Systems

Mary L. McHugh

OBJECTIVES

1. Define the difference between computer software and computer hardware.
2. Identify the two categories of software and discriminate between the two for purpose and functionality.
3. List the categories of programming languages and identify at least one example of each.
4. Identify key requirements for software designed to support nursing practice.
5. Define the term "system," and describe how the term applies to the field of computers.
6. Identify the five defining attributes of a system and define the meaning of each.
7. Discuss computer information systems (IS) and their subsets: management information systems (MIS) and hospital information systems (HIS).
8. List the most common administrative and clinical modules in an HIS.
9. Define the term "network," and describe the two essential components of network technology.

KEY WORDS

software
information systems
computer science
networks

 ## Computer Software

Software is the general term applied to the instructions that direct the computer's hardware to perform work. It is distinguished from hardware by its conceptual rather than physical nature. Hardware consists of physical components, whereas software consists of instructions communicated electronically to the hardware. Software is needed for two purposes. First, computers do not directly understand human language, and software is needed to translate instructions created in human language into machine language. At the machine level, computers can understand only binary numbers, not English or any other human language.

Second, packaged or stored software is needed to make the computer an economical work tool. Users could create their own software every time they needed to use the computer. However, writing software instructions (programming) is extremely difficult, time-consuming, and, for most people, tedious. It is much more practical and economical for one highly skilled person or programming team to develop programs that many other people can buy and use to do common tasks. Software is supplied as organized instruction sets called "programs," or more typically as a set of related programs called a "package."

For example, several prominent software companies sell their own version of a package of programs that are typically needed to support an office computer, including a word processor, a spread sheet, a graphics program, and sometimes a database manager. Programs translate operations the user needs into language and instructions that the computer can understand. By itself, computer hardware is merely a collection of printed circuits, plastic, metal, and wires. Without software, hardware is nonfunctional.

Brief History of Computer Programming and Software

The idea of having computer programs stored on a hard drive and brought into memory at the user's command has its roots in the 1800s, long before the first true computer was invented. Augusta Ada Byron, Countess of Lovelace (1816–1852), a mathematician and coresearcher with Charles Babbage (1791–1871), first described the concept of a stored computer program (Toole, 1992). Babbage was a late nineteenth century mathematician and inventor (Charles Babbage Institute, 2004). He "invented" (but never built) a device that he named the "analytical machine." Babbage's son finally built his machine in 1910 but was never able to make it work reliably (Fig. 5.1). However, the concept of a machine that could perform mathematical functions stimulated the thinking of other scientists and mathematicians about how to build such a machine and how instructions could be communicated to the machine. In her

writings about Babbage's concept of an analytical engine, Countess Lovelace theorized the use of automatic repetitious arithmetic steps that the analytical engine would follow to solve a problem, namely, the "loop concept" (Falbo, 2000). This concept gave her the title of the "first programmer" in computer history. However, it was Robert Von Newmann (1888–1976) who proposed that both data and instructions could be stored in the computer and that the instructions could be automatically carried out. The stored program concept was subsequently implemented as a major concept in the evolution of the computer.

Programs often require data as input. Today, people take for granted that computers will process huge amounts of data; however, it was not always feasible to handle large datasets. In the case of management of very large collections of data, necessity was truly the mother of invention. As part of the development of the new nation, America's founders decreed that a census of the population be taken every 10 years, the first of which commenced on August 2, 1790. The order was more difficult to carry out than anticipated. It took over 9 months to gather and process the 1790 census information, and there were only about 3.8 million people in the United States at the time. There were simply no machines to help with data collection or collation—they had not been invented yet! By the 1860 census, it was apparent that the manual methods of processing the census were inadequate. Unless the number of questions was severely limited, it would take more than 10 years to process the 10-year census data (Dunne, 2004). Some type of machine was needed if the constitutional requirement for a census was to be fulfilled successfully.

Ultimately, the development of data processing machines was taken from the field of textiles. Jacquard blouses, so popular in women's better clothing stores, were made possible by an invention of a weaver from France, Joseph Jacquard (Maxfield and Brown, 1998). Jacquard invented the Jacquard loom, a device that used blocks of wood with holes drilled in such a way that the threads to be woven into cloth could form a "program," or set of machine instructions, to the loom (Fig. 5.2). The instructions varied the way the cloth was worked by the loom so that a particular design (such as flowers or birds) would be produced in the fabric; that is, the weave produced images without changing the thread color or type.

In 1881, Herman Hollerith (1860–1929), a 19-year-old graduate of the Columbia School of Mines, was employed as a special agent by the U.S. Census Bureau (Austrian, 1982; Dunne, 1994). Recognizing the problem

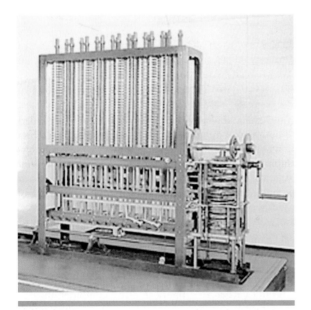

Figure 5.1
Babbage's analytic machine.

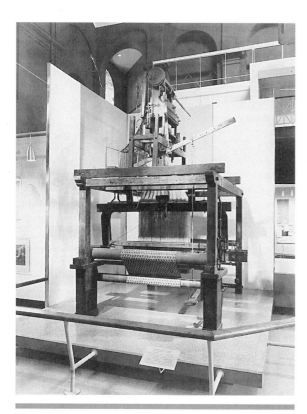

Figure 5.2
The Jacquard loom.
(Smithsonian Institution Photo No. 45599.)

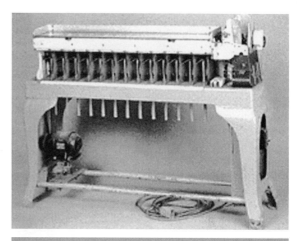

Figure 5.3
Hollerith's counting machine.

with trying to process such massive amounts of data, Hollerith used Jacquard's idea but developed a machine that could read punched cards and tabulate the results. In 1884, Hollerith patented his machine and punched card system (Austrian, 1982) (Fig. 5.3). Hollerith's ideas were so successful that he formed a company called Tabulating Machine. Eventually, after several changes of ownership and name changes, the company became International Business Machines, more popularly known as IBM. The punched card method of entering programs (software) and data into computers continued to exist until the late 1960s (Dunne, 1994). In many computing centers, some punched card use continued until around 1980. After that time, keypunch machines and punch card readers were withdrawn from computer centers.

In any history of computer programming, a remarkable woman known as "The Mother of Computing" should be acknowledged (Women's International Center, 2004). Rear Admiral Grace Murray Hopper was born in New York in 1906 (Lee, 1987). She obtained a degree in mathematics and physics, Phi Beta Kappa from Vassar in 1928, and her PhD in mathematics in 1934. In 1941, she offered her services to her country by enlisting in the U.S. Naval Reserve. On active duty throughout World War II, she was assigned to the Bureau of Ordinance Computation at Harvard University, where she worked with the first digital computer, the Mark I, and its successor, the Mark II. Dr. Hopper was perhaps the world's most expert programmer of early computers. During her long career, she greatly advanced the power of computers through her innovations in computer programming and program languages (Fig. 5.4). She is said to have written the third program ever on the Mark I, which was the first large-scale, digital computer in history. In 1946, the navy returned Hopper to inactive duty, but they recalled her to active duty in 1967 during the Vietnam War. Her brilliance with computers was considered irreplaceable by the military, and she continued to serve her country until she retired a second time in 1986 at the age of 79. Throughout her career, she developed many of the concepts and mathematical foundations of computer programming science.

A major activity in program testing is **debugging**, which means checking the program to ensure that it is free of error. This term was coined by Grace Hopper.

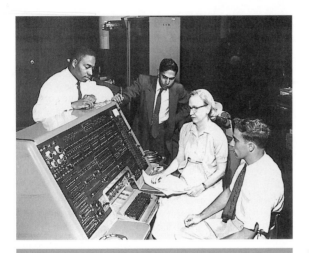

Figure 5.4
Rear Admiral Grace Hopper, PhD, and colleagues.
(Smithsonian Institution Photo No. 83.4878.)

In 1945, when working at Harvard on the Mark II computer, her program crashed. On examination of the computer, she discovered that a moth caught in the machine had caused the crash. To correct the problem and get the system working again, she "debugged" the computer. As a result, the term was used to refer to any correction of a computer programming error.

Admiral Hopper was widely known not only for her accomplishments in computer programming language development but also for her extraordinary vision and wit. She was the early force behind the idea that computer programming languages should become more English-like. She recognized that obscure assembly and machine-like programming languages limited access to the computer and therefore the utility of the machines. Her work on programming languages in the early 1950s formed the foundation for the first truly English-like language, the **Common Business-Oriented Language** (COBOL). COBOL was considered the first "universal" programming language and is still used in many older (legacy) business applications. In an age when the focus was on bigger rather than on more friendly computers, she quipped, "In pioneer days they used oxen for heavy pulling, and when one ox couldn't budge a log, they didn't try to grow a larger ox. We shouldn't be trying for bigger computers, but for more systems of computers." (Schieber, 1987). She recognized that a better approach would be to have many computers working independently

and together so that more work could be accomplished. Today, the Internet, the network of networks, might be viewed as the realization of Grace Hopper's early vision of computing. It is appropriate that this section be closed with another of her quotes: "Life was simple before World War II. After that, we had systems." (Schieber, 1987).

■ Types of Software

There are two basic types of software: system software and applications software. System software "boots up" (starts up and initializes) the computer system; controls input, output, and storage; and controls the operations of the application software. Applications software includes the various programs that users require to perform day-to-day tasks. They are the programs that support the actual work of the user. Some users claim a third type of software called utility programs. These are programs that are used to help maintain the system, clean up unwanted programs, protect the system against virus attacks, access the World Wide Web (WWW), and the like. Sometimes it can get confusing as to whether programs are utility programs or system software because system software packages today usually include a variety of utility programs with the basic system software packages.

System Software

System software consists of a variety of programs that control the individual computer and make the user's application programs work well with the hardware. System software consists of a variety of programs that initialize, or boot up the computer when it is first turned on and thereafter control all the functions of the computer hardware and applications software. System software helps speed up the computer's processing, expands the power of the computer by creating cache memory, reduces the amount of confusion when multiple programs are running together, "cleans up" the hard drive so that storage is managed efficiently, and performs other such system management tasks.

Basic Input Output System

The first level of system control is handled by the basic input output system (BIOS) stored on a read only memory (ROM) chip on the motherboard. The software on the BIOS chip is the first part of the computer to function when the system is turned on. It first searches for an operating system (OS) and loads it into the random access memory (RAM). Given that the BIOS consists of a set of instructions permanently burned onto a computer chip, it is truly a combination of hardware and software. Programs on chips are often called "firmware," because they straddle the line between hardware and software. For this reason, many computer engineers make a distinction between firmware and software. From that perspective, the OS is actually the first level of system software.

Operating Systems   OSs are actual software, loaded from the hard drive into RAM as soon as the computer is turned on. While the firmware cannot be upgraded without changing the hardware chip, the OS can be upgraded or entirely changed through software. The user simply deletes OS files from the hard drive and installs a new OS from a CD-ROM or floppy diskettes or perhaps downloads it from the Web or another site. Most users purchase a computer with the OS already installed on the hard drive. However, the OS can be purchased separately and installed by the user. OSs handle the connection between the central processing unit (CPU) and peripherals. (The connection between the CPU and a peripheral or a user is called an "interface.") The OS manages the interfaces to peripheral hardware, schedules tasks, allocates storage in memory and on disks, and provides an interface between the machine and the user.

One of the most critical tasks (from the user's perspective) performed by the OS involves the management of storage. In the early computers, there were no OSs. Every program had to explicitly tell the CPU exactly where in RAM to locate the lines of program code and data to be used during processing. That meant the user had to keep track of thousands of memory locations, and be sure to avoid writing one line of code over another active line of code. Also, the programmer had to be careful that output of one part of processing did not accidentally get written over output from another part of processing. As can be imagined, the need for management of storage consumed a great deal of time and programming code, and it produced many errors in programs. Since those errors had to be discovered and corrected before the program would run correctly, the lack of an OS made programming enormously time-consuming and tedious. In comparison, programming today—while still a difficult and time-consuming task— is much more efficient.

User Interfaces

Disk Operating System   The OS also provides a basic interface between the user and the hardware and software. There are two types of OS user interface: the interface provided by a disk operating system (DOS) and a graphical user interface (GUI) provided by OSs such as Microsoft Windows. Essentially, DOS OSs present a blank screen to the user, and the user submits typed commands.

DOS OSs were first designed for mainframe computers and replicated the procedures programmers used under manual OSs. They were an extension of the move away from dependency on human operators and tedious memory allocation programming requirements. When OSs were first developed for mainframes, they permitted tremendous advances in productivity in the computer department. However, just about everybody associated with the computer department at that time was a programmer. They all knew the syntax (wording and sequencing of commands). Thus, the need to type in long, non-English-like commands was not viewed as a great burden.

As computers became more popular and their applications became more useful to the general population, the need to learn DOS's obscure syntax became a real issue in office and home computing. Business people, office support personnel, and home users may have wanted to use computers for document preparation, financial management tasks, games, and other personal applications; however, they very much did not want to learn programming. Unfortunately, some programming skills had to be acquired to use the DOS interface effectively. During the late 1970s and early 1980s, a great proportion of the potential market for PCs was lost because of people's extreme resistance to using systems with such a poor user interface.

Graphical User Interface   In 1979, Steve Jobs of Apple Computers made a strategic decision to abandon the DOS interface and move to a GUI system for a new product to be called the Macintosh. The idea came as a result of his visit to the Xerox laboratory, where he saw the GUI that had been developed for a system that never really succeeded in the popular computer market. In 1984, the Macintosh with the first commercially available GUI was introduced. This was the "computer for everybody," and the PC market exploded. Although the GUI did not eliminate the need for users to spend time learning new programs, it did bring closer to reality the ideal that computers could become "self-teaching" devices. People could begin to use computers with minimal training, using built-in tutorials and online answers to common questions. Bill Gates, founder and CEO of the Microsoft Corporation, quickly recognized the need to provide a GUI product and immediately began development of Windows, the GUI for the IBM PC platform. The popularity of GUIs is a function of their use of pictures rather than typed narrative commands.

A GUI OS supports use of graphic images called "icons" to represent commands to the computer. Each icon image is designed to look like the physical representation of the operation the user wishes to employ. For example, a small image of a printer is used to symbolize the command to print a page or document. Rather than typing in commands such as "PRINT FILE," the user simply clicks the mouse button on the printer icon, and the print command is executed.

There are far too many commands needed for running most application programs for all commands to be represented by icons. Therefore, GUI OSs also support the operation of **menus**. Similar to menus in restaurants, the GUI menu provides a narrative list of common commands, or operations that the computer can execute. Rather than typing out a command, the user simply clicks the mouse button on the menu item desired, and the command represented by that menu word is executed. In complex programs that have hundreds or thousands of commands, the GUI supports **nested menus**.

Nested menus are submenus and sub-submenus; that is, the user clicks on a menu item, and instead of executing a command, the computer presents another menu of choices. (The submenu is fit, or nested, inside the main menu.) Clicking on a menu choice on a submenu might bring forth yet another menu. The process proceeds until the actual operation to be executed is listed. The nested menu format permits a virtually unlimited number of command options to be presented to the user, who never needs to remember the proper wording and order of a command in order to execute it.

Utility Programs   In addition to the operating system, there are a variety of other system programs available to the user. Some are called **utility** programs, and are designed to enhance the functions of the OS or perhaps to add facilities that the basic OS does not offer. These include programs that provide algorithms (formulas) for efficiently sorting a large set of numbers or character-based items, copying files or parts of files, security programs, and the like.

Language Translation Utilities   People and computers do not speak the same language. At the machine level, computers only understand binary. Human beings do not speak binary. Consequently, it is very difficult to write a program in the machine's language. Translation programs are needed to convert instructions written in

an English-like language into binary. These types of translation programs are called **assemblers, compilers,** or **interpreters.** Originally, they were all machine-dependent; that is, a compiler written for an IBM 360 mainframe computer could not work on a Hitachi mainframe computer. Even worse, a program written to work with one compiler could not work on a computer with a different compiler, even if the programming language was the same. With the advent of portable translators, that limitation has been at least partially overcome. Translation programs today are often 90% or more portable among different computer platforms. However, when buying a compiler, one still needs to purchase the version that has been customized to the user's computer platform.

The World Wide Web and Web Browsers   The WWW is a sort of network system utility program for the Internet. It provides a protocol for document transfer across the Internet. A Web browser is a utility program that allows the user to access the Web and the materials available through the Web. Prior to the advent of the WWW, commands to access and transfer documents throughout the Internet required users to know the command syntax of the Unix OS. While Unix is still the OS of the Internet, its command language is about as obscure to the average reader as machine language.

The Internet is a system of data and voice lines routed through dedicated servers to create a network of networks; that is, it consists of linkages that allow users from one computer network to access the documents and files available on another network. The trick in developing a network is figuring out how to make documents stored on one platform available to networks that use entirely different platforms. Early in the development of computer communications, utility programs called file transfer protocols (FTPs) were developed to allow files to be ported from one computer to another and from one network to another.

While the original Internet was an extremely useful system to programmers and scientists who could construct commands in the Unix syntax, it was time-consuming to use. In 1989, Tim Berners-Lee, a scientist at CERN, Switzerland's laboratory for particle physics, originated the idea of having a protocol that would be standard for all documents and sites on the Internet (Berners-Lee and Fischetti, 2000) (Fig. 5.5). In this way, use of the Internet would be greatly facilitated not only for programmers, but for just about everybody who might want to use it. In August of 1991, CERN released the first WWW software.

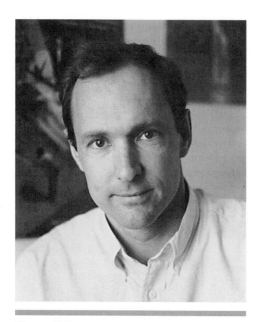

Figure 5.5
Tim Berners-Lee.
(Courtesy Donna Coveney/MIT.)

Berners-Lee conceived the WWW as a system utility program that requires all users to adhere to a standard set of text retrieval protocols (i.e., a standard command syntax for transfer of text from one computer to another). This set of protocols is called the **hypertext transfer protocol** (HTTP). "Hypertext" refers to the facility that permits a standard text-linking command to be incorporated into documents. Text linking occurs when content in one document refers to another document, and the user can click on the linking text and have the protocol automatically move the user from the first document to the linked document (Berners-Lee and Fischetti, 1999). The WWW also needed to have a standard addressing system, so that every document would have only one address. This addressing system is called the universal resource locator (URL). Finally, it needed a way to have documents formatted so that colors, fonts, spacing, tables, and images could be created and transmitted across the Internet. The language developed for the Internet is called HTML, which stands for Hypertext Markup Language. HTML allows document creators to format their text.

Although the WWW was an enormous advance, it still lacked one utility necessary to making the Web a household tool for everyone; it lacked a user-friendly GUI. This problem was addressed through the release of Mosaic, a GUI interface for the Web developed by the National Center for Supercomputing Applications (NCSA) at the University of Illinois, Champagne-Urbana campus. Mosaic was largely developed by Marc Anderson who later founded Netscape, one of the two most popular Web browsers.

Applications Software

Applications software includes the various programs people use to do work, process data, play games, communicate with others, or watch multimedia programs on a computer. Unlike system and utility programs, they are written by or for system users. When the user orders the OS to run an application program, the OS transfers the program from the hard drive, diskette, or CD-ROM into RAM and executes it.

Application programs are written in a particular programming language. Then the program is "compiled" (or translated) into machine language so the computer can understand the instructions and execute the program. Originally, programs were written for a specific computer and could only run on that machine. However, the science of programming languages and their translation eventually advanced to the point that programs today can generally be "ported" (or transferred) across many machines. This advance permitted programmers to develop programs that could be used on a class of machines, such as the IBM type or Macintosh (the two are still generally incompatible). This advance opened a whole new industry, since programs could be marketed as off-the-shelf software packages.

Programming Languages

A programming language is a means of communicating with the computer. Actually, of course, the only language a CPU can understand is binary or machine language. While it is certainly possible for programmers to learn to use binary—some highly sensitive defense applications are still written in machine language—the language is painfully tedious and inefficient of human resources, and its programs are virtually impossible to update and debug. Since the invention of computers, users have longed for a machine that could accept instructions in everyday human language. Although that goal largely escapes the industry, a variety of English-like languages have been developed.

Generations and Levels of Programming Languages

Programming languages are divided into five generations, or sometimes into three levels. The term "level" refers to how close the language is to the actual machine. The first level includes the first two generations of programming languages: machine language and assembly language. The second level includes the next two generations: high-level procedural and nonprocedural languages. The third level (and fifth generation) is natural language.

The low-level languages are machine-like. Machine language is, of course, binary. It consists of strings of zeros and ones and can be directly understood by the computer. However, it is difficult to use and to edit.

Machine Language   Machine language is the true language of the computer. Any program must be translated into machine language before the computer can execute it. The machine language consists only of the binary numbers 1 and 0, representing the **on** and **off** electrical impulses. All data—numbers, letters, and symbols—are represented by combinations of binary digits. For example, the number 3 is represented by eight binary numbers (00000011), and 6 is represented by 00000110. Traditionally, machine languages are machine-dependent, which means that each model of computer has its own unique machine language.

Assembler Language   Assembler language is far more English-like, but it is still very close to machine language. One command in machine language is a single instruction to the processor. Assembler language instructions have a one-to-one correspondence with a machine language instruction. Assembler language is still used a great deal by system programmers and whenever application programmers wish to manipulate functions at the machine level. As can be seen from Fig. 5.6, assembly language, while more English-like than machine language, is extremely obscure to the nonprogrammer.

Third Generation Languages   Third generation languages include the procedural languages and were the beginning of the second level in programming languages. Procedural languages require the programmer to specify both what the computer is to do and the procedure for how to do it. These languages are far more English-like than assembly and machine language. However, a great deal of study is required to learn to use these languages. The programmer must learn the words the language recognizes, and must use those words in a rigid style and sequence. A single comma or letter out of place will cause the program to fail, or "crash."

```
PRINT_ASCII PROC
        MOV DL, 00h
        DL MOV CX, 255
PRINT_LOOP:
        CALL WRITE_CHAR
        INC DL
        LOOP PRINT_LOOP
        MOV AH, 4Ch
        INT 21h ;21h
PRINT ASCII       ENDP
```

Figure 5.6
Assembler language lines of code.

The style and sequence of a language are called its "syntax." FORTRAN and COBOL are examples of early third generation languages.

A third generation language written specifically for use in health care settings was MUMPS (Massachusetts General Hospital Utility Multi-Programming System). MUMPS was originally developed to support medical records applications at Massachusetts General. MUMPS offers powerful tools to support database management systems; this is particularly useful in any setting in which many users have to access the same databases at the same time. Therefore, MUMPS is now found in many different industries such as banks, travel agencies, the stock exchange, and of course, other hospitals. Originally, MUMPS was both a language and a full OS; however, today most installations load MUMPS on top of their own computer's OS.

Today, the most popular computer language for writing new OSs and other system programs is called C. (It was named after an earlier prototype program called simply B.)

Two important late third generation languages are increasing in importance as the importance of the Internet grows (see Chap. 4, "Computer Hardware"). They include the visual programming languages and Java. Java was developed by Sun Microsystems to be a relatively simple language that would provide the portability across differing computer platforms and the security needed for use on a huge, public network like the Internet. The world community of software developers and Internet content providers has warmly received Java. Java programming skills are critical for any serious Web developer.

Visual Programming Languages As the popularity of GUI technology grew, several languages were developed to facilitate program development in graphics-based environments. Microsoft Corporation has marketed two very popular such programs: Visual BASIC (Beginners' All-purpose Symbolic Instruction Code) and Visual C11. These programs and their "cousins" marketed by other companies have been used for a variety of applications, especially those that allow users to interact with electronic companies through the Internet.

Fourth Generation Languages Fourth generation languages are specialized application programs that require more involvement of the user in directing the program to do the necessary work. Some people in the computer industry do not consider these to be programming languages. Procedural languages include programs such as spreadsheets, statistical analysis programs, and database query languages. The difference between these languages and the earlier generation languages is that the user specifies **what** the program is to do, but not **how** the program is to perform the task. The "how" is already programmed by the manufacturer of the "language" program. For example, to perform a chi-square calculation in FORTRAN, the user must specify each step involved in carrying out the formula for a chi-square and the data on which the operations are to be performed. In Statistical Package for Social Sciences (SPSS), a statistical analysis program, the user enters a command (from a menu of commands) that tells the computer to compute a chi-square statistic on a particular datasheet. The formula for chi-square is already part of the SPSS program; the user does not have to tell SPSS how to calculate the chi-square.

Fifth Generation Languages Fifth generation or third level languages are called natural language. In these types of programs, the user tells the machine what to do in the user's own natural language or through use of a set of very English-like commands. Ideally, voice recognition technology is integrated with the language so that voice commands are recognized and executed. True fifth generation languages are emerging. True natural language recognition, in which any user could give understandable commands to the computer in his or her own word style and accent is being performed at the beginning of the twenty-first century. However, natural language systems are clearly in the future of personal computing. The great difficulty is, of course, how to reliably translate natural, spoken human language into a language the computer can understand.

To prepare a translation program for a natural language requires several levels of analysis. First, the sentences need to be broken down to identify the subject's words and relate them to the underlying constituents of speech (i.e., parsed). The next level is called semantic analysis, whereby the grammar of each word in the sentence is analyzed. It attempts to recognize the action described and the object of the action. There are several computer programs that translate natural languages based on basic rules of English. They generally are specially written programs designed to interact with databases on a specific topic. By limiting the programs to querying the database, it is possible to process the natural language terms.

■ Common Software Packages for Microcomputers

The most common package sold with computers is a standard office package. The standard office package includes a word-processing program, a spreadsheet, a presentation graphics program, and some form of database management system. The two most commonly used programs are e-mail systems and word processor. In fact, some people purchase a computer with only an OS, word processor and an Internet browser and sign up for their e-mail account and use little else. Another very common product is a desktop publisher. Most of these common programs have to be written in two versions: one for the IBM PC platform and one for the Macintosh. Typically, software packages are sold on CD-ROM, although some are still available on floppy disks and many software companies are now marketing their products through the Internet and customers download the software directly through the Internet from the vendor's Internet site.

■ Software Package Ownership Rights

Protecting ownership rights in software has presented a challenge to the computer software industry. A program sold to one customer can be installed on a very large number of machines. This practice obviously seriously harms the profitability of software development. If programs were sold outright, users would have every right to distribute them as they wished; however, the industry could not survive in such market conditions. As a result, the software industry has followed an ownership model more similar to that of the book publishing industry than to the model used by vendors of most commercial products.

When a commercial product is sold, the buyer cannot use the product or resell it or loan it to a friend if so desired. The product sold is a physical product that can be used only by one customer at a time. Copying the product is not feasible. However, intellectual property is quite a different proposition; what is sold is the idea. The medium on which the idea is stored is not the product. However, when the PC industry was new, people buying software viewed their purchase as the physical diskette on which the intellectual property was stored. Software was expensive, but the diskettes were cheap. Therefore, groups of friends would often pool money to purchase one copy of the software and make copies for everyone in the group. This, of course, enraged the software vendors.

As a result, copyright laws were extended to software so that only the original purchaser was legally empowered to install the program on his or her computer. Any other installations were considered illegal copies, and such copies were called pirate copies. Purchasers of software do not buy full rights to the software. They purchase only a license to use the software. Individually purchased software is licensed to one and only one computer. An exception can be made if the individual has both a desktop and a laptop. Fair use allows the purchaser to install the software on all the machines he or she personally owns—so long as the computers are for that user's personal use only. Companies that have multiple computers that are used by many employees must purchase a separate copy for each machine, or in some cases they may purchase a "site license." A site license is a way of buying in bulk, so to speak. The company and software vendor agree on how many machines the software may be used on, and a special fee is paid for the number of copies to be used. Additional machines over the number agreed on require either an increase in the allowable sites—and payment of the higher site-license fee, or separate copies of the software may be purchased. What is not permitted, and is, in fact, a form of theft, is to install more copies of the software than were paid for.

Common Software Useful to Nurses

In most hospitals, software used by nurses includes admission, discharge, and transfer (ADT) systems that help with patient tracking, and medication administration record (MAR) software. Increasingly, hospitals have added charting software that computerizes at least some parts of the nursing record. In addition, quality and safety groups such as the Leapfrog group consider a computer physician order entry (CPOE) system to be so important that they list it as a separate item on their quality checklist. Additionally, nurses may have the support of computer based systems for laboratory and radiology orders and results reporting, a computerized patient acuity system used to help with nurse staff allocation, and perhaps there may be a hospital e-mail system used for at least some hospital communications. Increasingly, nurses are finding that they are able to build regional, national, and international networks with their nursing colleagues with the use of chat rooms, bulletin boards, and listservs on the Internet.

Chat Rooms

Chat rooms are like electronic conference calls. Multiple users can send and receive messages at the same time. Some chat rooms are private and require a password to enter. Others are open to the public. All members of the chat room can see all the messages posted, just as all people at a party can hear all the conversations near them. The strengths of chat room technology include the ability of many people to "meet" without having to leave their homes. Distance does not matter with a chat room. The person the user is "chatting" with can be at another computer in the same room, or halfway around the world. Chat room technology is real-time technology; that is, messages disappear once they scroll off the screen unless they are printed or otherwise explicitly saved. Chat rooms have their dangers. Users can remain anonymous, and anybody can participate in a public chat room. There have been cases where pedophiles have used chat rooms to become acquainted with children and to entice them into face-to-face meetings. The general rule in a public chat room is, "Let the buyer beware."

Electronic Bulletin Boards

An early form of computer conferencing involved electronic bulletin boards. Even today this form of communication is very popular. As with chat rooms, some are public and some private; however, most are private. They are called by different names, depending on the terminology used by the software creator. They may be called discussion boards, listservs, or electronic forums but they all work in similar ways. This technology creates space where users can post a message. In the better software, the messages can be posted according to user-defined or system administrator-defined categories. For example, there may be a discussion on CPU technology and problems, another discussion about peripherals, and so forth.

Electronic discussion boards or forums are an important technology in distance courses offered through the Internet. These programs are accessed entirely at the user's convenience. Most of these programs separate the discussion into discrete "topics" or "forums" so that the discussion board is more organized. They let the user define a new topic of discussion when appropriate, add a new item to an existing topic, or respond to an item placed by another user. The strengths of this technology are that the items are organized according to topic, and they remain available until the conference organizer explicitly removes them. Unlike chat rooms, users access the board at their own convenience and can take time to formulate a response.

Listservs

The least powerful version of an electronic bulletin board is a listserv. This program functions more like an electronic mailing list than a true discussion board. When a user posts a message to the board, it is merely e-mailed to all members of the conference. The software may or may not store all the messages in an accessible archive so users can review all the entries at one time. A user can respond to an item on the listserv by posting a new item. Some users find the listserv technology inconvenient because e-mailboxes can get filled up with messages the user does not need to view immediately. Limiting one's own access to the messages on a listserv to the times that are personally convenient is not possible. The messages arrive whenever other members send them.

Computer Programming

Computer programming refers to the process of writing a computer program, which is a series of instructions written in proper sequence to solve a specific problem. A program primarily encompasses the program instructions and is generally written by a computer programmer.

The five major steps in writing any computer program are as follows:

- Problem definition (functional specifications)
- Program design
- Writing the code and program documentation
- Alpha testing
- Beta testing and program documentation

Problem or Functions Specification

Defining the problem to be solved or the functions to be performed by the program is the most critical step in programming. It requires that the problem or task be very precisely defined and the procedures to be performed by the program be perfectly understood. In essence, the problem definition must analyze and outline in detail the scope of the problem and all the elements needed to solve it. For example, a very simple problem definition for the cost of a nursing visit might read as follows: "Calculate the cost of nursing visit 'C' by totaling cost of nurse 'A' and cost of supplies 'B.'"

Program Design Specifications

Once the problem/task is precisely specified, the process for solving the problem must be designed. There are generally two types of specifications involved in program creating. The first is the set of functional specifications that identifies all the functions the program is to perform. This should include a narrative description of the functions of the system and a graphical representation of the system's process flow. This is used to ensure that both the system designer and the people who have contracted for the designer's services share the same understanding of the planned system. The second set of specifications (called "specs") is the design specifications. The design specs are the instructions given to the programmer. Design specs may be highly technical and are not typically viewed by the customers. They are prepared by the system analyst after consultation with the customer about the functional specs. The system analyst, an expert in both analysis and design, is typically a person with expertise in programming. It is the analyst's job to ensure that the programmer's instructions not only fully meet the functional specs, but also help the programmer prepare a program that runs smoothly and consumes no more of the computer's processing power than necessary.

Program Preparation

Program preparation, the actual writing (or coding) of the program, entails translating the design specifications into the programming language to be used. The program instructions (algorithms) must be coded in detail and in logical sequence so that the program can process data correctly. The programming language selected must not only be appropriate for processing the problem but must be translated by the computer for which it is written. The language rules must be followed precisely, because a single coding error can stop the program from running or cause program malfunction. The process of error correction so that the program runs is called "debugging."

Documentation

Two types of documentation must be produced during programming. First, the program itself should be designed in a highly structured, top-down manner, and the lines of code should be liberally sprinkled with explanatory statements. These statements are not part of the program itself; however, they clearly identify what program modules or individual lines of code do in the program. Program documentation also includes a narrative manual of instructions to system administrators who will have to maintain the program after the initial programming is completed. A well-documented program is easier to edit, easier for other programmers to support, and easier to debug. The second type of documentation that must be produced is the user's manual. The user's manual provides clear directions and examples of how to make the program work as intended. It should also provide suggestions for how to proceed when users cannot get the program to function as they expect. The process of manual development proceeds throughout several stages of the programming process, including code preparation, program testing, and program implementation.

Program Testing

Alpha Testing   Program testing occurs during and after coding. Two types of testing are performed. First, the programming team and system analysts carefully desk check the program in a process called "alpha testing." This process is also called "desk checking." The purpose of alpha testing is to see if all the processes appear to be functioning as specified in the flow charts, functional specifications, and design specs.

Beta Testing   The second level of testing is called "beta testing." In beta testing, the program is installed in the actual user environment, and further programming of screen formats and other user interface functions is performed. Documentation adequacy is examined. Some users are trained to use the system. Users begin the final testing phase by entering real data and checking that the system products are accurate and complete. During initial beta testing, the system implementation process is

begun. Usually, only one unit or workstation is brought online and only for the purpose of system testing. During beta testing, users should actually perform both the old manual procedures and the new computer program. In that way, when the new program fails to perform exactly as required (and virtually all new programs need further debugging during beta testing), the work of the organization is not compromised.

Program Implementation

Program implementation is the final step in programming. In this phase, the program is implemented throughout the beta site. All the users are trained, and the full day-to-day data load is imposed on the system. At this point, there will still be bugs, but the problems should be relatively minor. However, sometimes when the large amount of data that the system must handle on a daily basis are entered, and the full range of program functions is called, new problems arise. Programmers must be readily available to solve these problems at any time of the day or night. This step is where user-related problems are most likely to be discovered. When users who are perhaps not favorable to making a system change—and are perhaps not naturally talented in the use of computers—begin to use the system on a daily basis, new problems will arise. When these problems are solved and the beta site is up and running smoothly, then—and only then—is the program ready to be sold in the consumer market.

A final caution for users of software packages. Users may design screens and report formats, but they must be aware that all copyrights remain with the software package creators. Any plans to distribute designed screens or report formats must first be cleared with the vendor of the program.

Computer Systems

Every functioning computer is a system; that is, it is a complex entity, consisting of an organized set of interconnected components or factors that function together as a unit to accomplish results that one part alone could not. At a minimum, a computer must have at least four components to function. These minimum components are a power source, a CPU, a peripheral to allow input, and a peripheral to permit output. Of course, computers typically have more than four components. "Computer system" may refer to a single machine (and its peripherals) that is unconnected to any other computer. However, most health professionals use computer systems consisting of multiple, interconnected computers that function to facilitate the work of groups of providers and their support people in a system called a **network**. The greatest range of functionality is realized when computers are connected to other computers in a network or, as with the Internet, a system of networks.

The use of systems in computer technology is based on system theory. System theory and its subset, network theory, provide the basis for understanding how the power of individual computers has been greatly enhanced through the process of linking multiple computers into a single system and multiple computer systems into networks.

System Theory

System theory provides the conceptual basis for understanding complex entities that consist of multiple interrelated parts working together to achieve a desired result. Such entities are called **systems**. A system, by its nature, is not random; it is orderly and predictable in its functioning. If a system begins to exhibit unpredictable behavior, one of two conditions pertain. Either the system is malfunctioning for some reason internal or external to the system itself, or the observer does not fully understand the system and thus a proper result is misinterpreted as incorrect (unpredicted). The key concepts of system theory are parts, interaction (among the parts), interdependency (among the parts), input, output, processing, feedback, and control. The primary propositions of the theory are the following:

1. A system takes in input on which to perform processes.

2. The processes performed by a system on input result in system output.

3. The processes in a system are subject to control forces.

4. Feedback is the key mechanism of control in a system.

5. A system's parts interact in such a way that the parts are interdependent with respect to the system's processes.

6. Impingement on one part in a system will produce effects on the system's processes and may produce distortions on other parts of the system. A corollary to this proposition is the following.

7. Distortion in one part of a system may be a symptom of a problem in another component. (This is called a secondary malfunction.)

8. Thus, correction of a malfunctioning part will correct the system functioning only if the malfunction was a primary malfunction and not a secondary malfunction.

9. Effects on the system's processing function will affect the system's output.

10. A system is more than the sum of its parts. Thus, while a system can be broken down into its component parts, if this is done, the system no longer exists. Corollaries to this proposition are the following:

    (a) The functioning of a system is different than the functioning of its separate parts.

    (b) The output of each separate part, even if combined, does not equal the output of the system.

    (c) When combined into a system, the component parts form an entirely new entity.

System Elements

A system consists of the following six elements: the system's set of interdependent parts, input to the system, system processes, output of the system, system control, and feedback.

Interdependent Parts

The most defining attribute of a system is that its parts interact to conduct some process. Without the interaction, the system process could not occur. Therefore, in the production of the system's process, the parts are interdependent. Each acting alone could not perform the system's process. In computer systems, the process involves mathematical, logical, or data transfer operations requiring interaction among the CPU, RAM, and ROM chips and the motherboard's power source.

Input

Input is any factor from the external environment that is taken into the system. Input in a computer system may serve to initiate system functioning, as when the machine is turned on and the OS is loaded into RAM. It may consist of data that the system is to process. In living systems, input may consist of energy from the sun, nourishment, or stimulation, or it might be information needed to survive, function, or enjoy life. However, by itself, input is just inert substance or data. The system must act on input if it is to get use from it.

Process

Process is the activity of the system. A system performs process on its inputs to produce outputs, or create some sort of result. (Survival is the result of the processes of a living system.) Process in a computer system can be seen in the example of a presentation graphics system. The hardware, software, and peripherals constitute the interdependent parts. The commands entered by the user, the numerical data for a graphic, and the alphanumeric characters used for title, labels, and notations on the graph constitute the input. The system sends the translated data and commands to the CPU, which performs the ordered operations (processes) on the input to create a graphic image (e.g., pie graph and bar graph). Then the graphic package further processes the instructions to produce whatever output is ordered by the user of the system.

Output

Output is any product or waste produced as a result of system process. Not all processes produce a visible, external product. (The result of life processes may be homeostasis, energy, movement, or feedback within the living system.) However, in many of the systems people work with—such as manufacturing systems—the purpose of the system is to produce output. For example, the output of the manufacturing process at Ford Motor Company is composed of automobiles, trucks, and specialty vehicles. For computer systems, output is the reason the system was created or purchased. Typical computer system output includes electronic data transmission from the main memory to a hard or floppy disk, paper reports, or data transmissions (such as information exchange through the Internet).

For example, many users today have word processors and presentation graphics program packages. The output from the presentation graphics system might be an electronic file stored on the hard drive or on a portable floppy disk. It might be an image printed in either black and white or color on a piece of paper or a transparency; or it might be that same image printed onto color 35-mm film for processing into a color slide. Output from a word processor is usually a professionally formatted and printed text document.

Control

"Control" refers to any component or activity that serves to prevent or correct problems or errors in the system's input, process, or output. A system must function within rules and procedures that keep it functioning smoothly. These rules and procedures constitute a system's **control** operations. Process means activity. Activity must have some beginning and end point, or else the system goes out of control. Cancers are an example of an out-of-control function in a person's body. Cells that need to regrow as part of healing from injury must stop growing once repair is accomplished. When cells continue to grow without control, the result is eventually fatal. Control is an essential function of any system.

In computer systems, a variety of control facilities exist within the OS. Most application programs also incorporate control functions to help the user avoid erroneous results. Control in computers functions by checking, validating, and verifying input and output data and by checking for and flagging certain conditions during processing. An example of a processing error is division by zero. Such an operation is impossible, and whenever such a problem is detected, processing is terminated and an appropriate error message is displayed on the screen or printout.

A good application program will have special programming that creates "error traps" to detect certain kinds of errors. For example, most word processor programs automatically detect words that are misspelled. In such a program, the concept, "misspelled" means that the word has no match in the word processor's dictionary and therefore is not recognized by the program. The user is notified that the system does not recognize the word (by a change in color of the word on the screen, by underlining, or in some other way). Data entry programs for some statistical analysis programs may detect impossible values. The way they do this is that during creation of the data entry screen, the developer identifies upper and lower numerical limits or acceptable/unacceptable characters for the type of data to be stored in that variable. Any value that does not fit the defined acceptable codes is considered an "out-of-range" value. Then any time a data entry person enters an out-of-range value, processing stops, and a warning message is issued.

Feedback

Feedback is output from one part of a system process that serves as input to another part of a system process. Feedback is a special case of control. Feedback within a system is typically used as part of a system's self-regulation function. For example, in human beings, body temperature is regulated by a feedback system. A falling core temperature stimulates temperature-sensitive neurons in the hypothalamus. In response, the hypothalamus (in conjunction with certain higher brain centers) activates a number of temperature response mechanisms, most obviously the shivering response. Shivering consists of rapid muscle movements—and muscle movement produces heat. The heat is disseminated and raises the body temperature; that, in turn, changes the sensations to the hypothalamus temperature-sensing neurons. (This is a much-simplified picture and only a small part of the temperature-regulatory feedback system in a human being.)

In a computer system, feedback components are important functions of the OS and utility programs. The user will experience the results of feedback if a "save" command orders the system to store a file on a diskette that is already full. The OS checks the diskette, and the discovery of a "full" condition initiates a subroutine (small program module used repeatedly). The subroutine stops the processing and issues a message to the user that the command has failed because the disk is full.

A clinical computing example of feedback is the ventilation rate in a mechanical ventilator set at "demand." The processor in the ventilator detects its own activity, and based on the timing of the last activity, it initiates or does not initiate another breath. That is, it has a timer that keeps track of the most recent breath taken by (or delivered to) a patient. The ventilator is set to deliver a breath if a certain amount of time has elapsed since the last breath. If the patient's breathing rate is such that each breath is taken prior to the "deadline," the system does not initiate forced inspiration. Otherwise, the machine initiates a breath. In this way, the ventilator controls the rate at which it delivers breaths to the patient—neither too fast nor too slow for optimal oxygenation.

 ## Classification of Systems

There are two types or classes of system, closed systems and open systems.

Closed Systems

A closed system is defined as a system with the following characteristics: differentiation, isolation, independence, and self-sufficiency (sometimes called self-containment or self-regulation). A closed system is clearly differentiated from all other systems and factors in its environment. Its boundaries are clearly defined and rigid. Therefore, it is easy to tell just where the system begins and ends and what is part of the system and what is not part of the system.

By definition, a closed system has sealed boundaries that separate it from the rest of the environment. Access to the system is highly restricted, because the only inputs acceptable to the system are inputs from another part of itself. System outputs are actually forms of internal communication; that is, the output of one part of the system serves as input to another part of the system in a feedback loop. In this sense, a closed system is self-contained.

A closed system has to be self-sufficient, because any input from the external environment is a threat to the integrity of a closed system. It must therefore be able to provide for all its energy and processing requirements without going outside its boundaries. Furthermore, it cannot need an external source to help rid it of its output or waste products. Due to the need for an energy source, it may be that no system is ever truly closed; however, some systems are sufficiently isolated that it makes conceptual sense to consider them closed. More typically, a closed system has a closed feedback loop as its major process. Outside energy is still required to power the system.

For example, animal habitats often function as closed systems. When the boundaries of the environment are breached, and animals from other systems intrude on the formerly closed system, animals originating in the closed system often cannot compete, and they become extinct. A closed system such as an animal habitat must isolate itself from, rather than accommodate to, outside influences.

A nursing example of a closed system could be an intravenous hypertension control system (Fig. 5.7). The components of the system include the patient's intravenous line and fluid with the antihypertensive medication, the electronic sphygmomanometer, the volumetric pump, and the programmed computer processor (the CPU) that controls the system. In such a system, the computer is programmed to initiate a blood pressure (BP) reading at determined time intervals. At the proper time, the CPU sends a command to the sphygmomanometer to take a reading through the arterial line. The value is returned to the CPU, where it is compared to a preset critical value. The processor determines whether or not the reading is above the critical value. If not, it does nothing until its clock indicates that it is time for another measurement. If the BP is above the critical value, it sends an instruction to the volumetric pump to deliver the correct dose of antihypertensive medication. In reality, a system such as described would

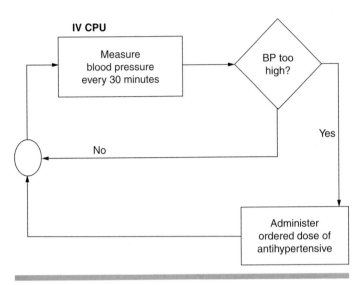

Figure 5.7
Closed system with feedback loop.

never be completely closed. There would always be an alarm system to warn the nurse if the medication was ineffective or if the BP fell too low or rose too high, or of other problems requiring system maintenance.

Open Systems

Open systems are systems that exhibit integration, fluid or fuzzy boundaries, and interaction with their environments (Markas, 2002). They need not be self-regulating, although they might exhibit that facility. They are fundamentally different from closed systems. An open system overlaps other systems and may be a subsystem within a larger system. Consequently, it is often difficult to determine whether a particular process belongs to a specific system or to a related system. In fact, it can be quite easy to iteratively redefine a system's borders whenever an interaction with another system occurs. The interaction is viewed as a new system function. Taken to extremes, the redefinition continues until the entire universe is included in the system.

For this reason, it is sometimes very difficult to identify the borders or boundaries of an open system. The boundaries are permeable to external influences rather than sealed against them. Open systems fundamentally require the energy of input from the external environment. All living creatures are examples of open systems.

They must acquire nourishment from their external environment or die. Unlike closed systems, open systems exhibit change with respect to both internal and external processes. Since they interact with their environment, open systems may not appear to have any clearly identifiable boundaries. However, it is important to define boundaries because any system is defined as much by its boundaries as it is by its processes (Fig. 5.8).

An open system may exhibit self-regulation. More commonly, however, an open system expands until it bumps up against another system's boundary, and the second system takes action to protect itself against the encroachment of the first system. Closed systems are often described as fixed or static. This description is fundamentally flawed, because closed systems do have processes. Therefore, they exhibit some degree of internal fluidity. The change must be with internal processing, however, not through interaction with the external world. From that perspective, to an outsider, the closed system appears to be static and unchanging.

Computer Systems

The term "computer system" is used to describe the set of peripherals, computer "box," and software that together perform computing functions for one or more users. The actual devices that comprise a computer

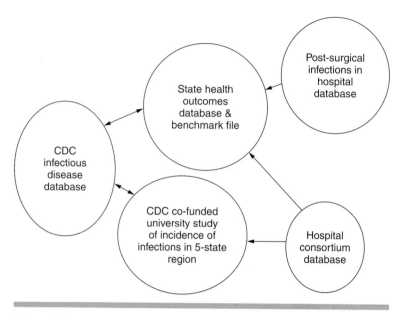

Figure 5.8
Open system interactions.

system depend on the needs of the user. Typically, most users need a keyboard and mouse or trackball for input. Many also use a joystick for games or drawing programs. Peripheral devices that have grown in popularity as use of the Internet has increased include a modem, scanner, microphone, and video camera. Application software usually includes an "office" package that includes word processor, spread sheet, presentation graphics and database programs, an Internet browser, and a Web authoring program such as Front Page or Lotus Notes.

The term "computer system" is vague and could refer to anything from a hand-held personal computer to an organization's entire network of computers. In most nursing settings, nurses work with what is known as an information system and, in hospitals, a HIS.

Information Systems

An information system is the collection and integration of various pieces of hardware and software and the human resources that meet the data collection, storage, processing, and report generation needs of an organization. For most large health care organizations, the software requirements are varied and complex. The hardware must always be purchased to fit the software

requirements. As a result, most large organizations must retain a sophisticated IS department to construct, maintain, and interface the various—and sometimes incompatible—hardware and software necessary to support the work of the organization. When an organization is so large and its computing requirements so diverse that the organization simply cannot obtain a single system to meet all its needs, the result is usually a hodge-podge of incompatible software and hardware platforms. The IS department must program and maintain the software interfaces that let the systems work together. The key pieces of an information system are the hardware, software, and the database or databases in which the organization's data are stored.

Information System Types

IS are found almost everywhere in health care, including hospitals, clinics, community health agencies, research facilities, and educational institutions. Their configuration, power, and functions vary widely depending on how they are used and the type of work performed in the organization. There is a wide range of IS in health care facilities that provide different functions. They have different titles/names, which overlap depending on the context in which they are used. The major ones to be described include MIS, bibliographic retrieval systems, stand-alone systems, transaction systems, physiologic monitoring systems, decision support systems, and expert systems.

Management Information Systems   An MIS provides managers information about their business operations. A MIS is defined as an organized system for managing the flow of information in an organization in a timely manner. Its primary use is assisting in the decision-making processes. The MIS in a health care facility may be integrated with a large, HIS, or it might be a stand-alone system. Most MIS systems have programs that support strategic planning, management control, and operations support.

"Strategic planning" refers to the policy decisions made by the top-level team of administrators. Strategic planning is the work that seeks to position the organization with respect to its customers and competitors. The management control function refers to the program and personnel decisions made by middle-level managers, supervisors, and head nurses. They need information to measure performance standards and to control, plan, and allocate resources. The operations control support functions provide data and information to the first line managers. For example, unit managers need information on the state of the unit budget, on occupancy and workload, and on overtime hours spent. They need information on incident reports, infection rates, and other clinical indicators of care quality. They need the type of information that helps them manage the unit in such a way that patient care is effectively and efficiently carried out.

A health care MIS typically provides information that can be used to generate the balance sheet and cash flow reports, help the finance department gather information for other financial reports, and track inpatient occupancy rates by unit or department, clinic visits, procedures, and so forth. It also usually has programs that will allow management to analyze trends in the data and project future business given current trends and other assumptions. However, most MIS databases supplement internal data with data from external, local, regional, and national databases. Many organizations join private organizations that share buying power and information useful to management.

Increasingly, health care organizations are joining each other into private consortia. The purpose is the collection of information from all members so that averages and ranges of performance data can be used for benchmarking purposes. The University Hospital Consortium in Oakbrook, Illinois, is one such organization (University Hospital Consortium, 2004). Hospital consortia provide their members with a variety of reports that supplement, and sometimes help managers interpret, their own internal organizational data.

Bibliographic Retrieval Systems   A bibliographic retrieval system is a retrieval system that generally refers to bibliographic data, document information, or literature. Such a system is primarily used to store and retrieve data and not to conduct any computations per se. The textual data are input and stored and are available for retrieval in a user-friendly format that is easy to read and understand. The system is designed to provide bibliographic data on journal articles, books, monographs, and textual reports. It generally contains the full citations, keywords, abstracts, and other pertinent facts on the documents in the database. An example of a bibliographic retrieval system is CINAHL MEDLINE, developed and published by the National Library of Medicine (NLM). In the late 1990s, NLM made MEDLINE, along with a friendly user interface, Grateful Med, available free online to anyone who wishes to use it. MEDLINE may be accessed at the NLM URL: *http://igm.nlm.nih.gov/*. The user simply clicks on the word MEDLINE, which is the first choice on the left-hand side of the screen in the "Select Database to Search" menu.

Stand-Alone, Dedicated, or Turnkey Systems   A stand-alone system is a special purpose system. It is developed for a single application or set of functions. A patient classification system is an example of a stand-alone system. Most stand-alone systems are described by their purpose, such as a pharmacy or laboratory system or an imaging system in the radiology department. Until recently, most turnkey systems ran on a microcomputer or PC. However, during the 1990s, most vendors of large HIS changed their design strategy. Formerly, most vendors deliberately designed their systems to be unique rather than easily integrated with other systems. Due to customer demand and the realization that a hospital's needs were simply too large for any one vendor to support completely, most HIS vendors made real efforts to make their products more "friendly" to other products. Advances in networking science have also changed the technology available for transporting information across different products and platforms. Eventually, most organizations should be able to freely move their data from one system to another electronically.

Transaction Systems   A transaction system is used to process predefined transactions and produce predefined reports. It is designed for repeated operations using a fixed list. From this list, displayed on a computer terminal, a user selects the names of transactions to be processed. A computer program is written so that it can be used repeatedly to process the same type of transactions and generate the same type of reports or products. The computer programs and the list of transactions are retained in storage and retrieved as needed.

An inventory system is an example of a transaction system. It is used to monitor the distribution of items as well as to update and reorder supplies. These kinds of operations are repetitious and always processed in the same manner. A standard list of items is initially developed. Inventory systems usually have information about vendors and prices, track inventory, and can generate automatic reorders when stock on hand drops below a certain level. Typically, inventory control systems produce a set of management reports that helps management keep track of which items are increasing in demand so they can take advantage of volume discounts. The transactions can also be summarized and reports developed to produce monthly bills, prepare order vouchers, and summarize the inventory status for any given time period. In this type of system, the computer program is specifically written to process the transactions (raw data). Grocery store scanners are linked to a transaction-based inventory control system.

Pharmacy, laboratory, and admission/discharge/ transfer systems are also forms of transaction systems. Transaction systems can also be designed to process routine medical or nursing orders and permit clinicians to update the orders in real time. This activity is done to ensure that the orders once entered are current in the system. The updating of medical and nursing orders can also be summarized for documenting care plans, change of shift reports, discharge summary, quality review, research studies, and so forth.

Physiologic Monitoring Systems   Physiologic monitoring systems are widely used in hospital patient care units, in surgery, and more and more commonly, in private homes. The heart monitor was one of the first physiologic monitors used by nurses. Primarily due to the heart monitor, survival rates for hospitalized myocardial infarction patients increased by about 30% in the early 1970s. In the labor and delivery unit, mothers'

uterine contractions and fetal heart rate are routinely monitored so that complications can be recognized and addressed without delay. Brain waves are monitored in seizure and sleep disorders units. Intraventricular pressure is monitored in neurologic intensive care units for patients at great risk of cerebral aneurysm rupture.

All of these devices are a form of an oscilloscope. An oscilloscope is an electronic device that senses electric impulses and converts them into waveforms on a monitor screen. On the screen, the impulses are represented by a light cursor (a point on the screen that is bright as compared with the darker background). The cursor moves from left to right across the screen at a timed rate (i.e., moves a defined number of centimeters across the screen per second). When the monitor is not connected, the cursor travels at the bottom edge of the usable screen in a straight line, and this line is called the **baseline**. The strength of the impulse deflects the cursor vertically. Thus, when a positive or negative impulse occurs in the human body being monitored, the cursor is deflected up or down from the baseline. As the impulse ebbs, the cursor returns to the baseline (Fig. 5.9).

Physiologic monitoring systems are being used more frequently to measure and monitor continuous automatic physiologic findings such as heart rate, BP, and other vital signs. Monitoring systems provide alarms to detect significant abnormal findings when personnel are needed to provide patient care and save lives.

Decision Support Systems   A decision support system is a computer system that supports some aspect of the human decision-making process. Decision support systems work with the user to support, but not replace, human judgment in a decision-making situation (Brennan and McHugh, 1988). Decision-making systems also exist, and these tend to be closed systems that function on internal feedback loops. Decision support systems may model the decision process. This type of system guides the user in a highly structured approach

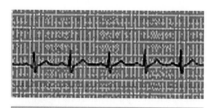

Figure 5.9
An ECG.

that helps identify the salient components of the problem (Brennan and McHugh, 1988).

Certain types of analytic modeling systems may also be considered as decision support systems. Business and engineering applications for decision support include linear programming, computer simulation modeling, trend analysis, and forecasting. Although some merely consider these tools to be analysis tools, others consider them to be decision support systems, since they are used to analyze the outcomes of a variety of possible decisions. Still another form of decision support system is an **optimization** program. Optimization programs take all the information about a problem situation and generate a variety of possible solutions. Then each solution is **implemented** (usually simulated in a computer), and the results of the implementation for each solution are compared. Then the optimization program selects the best solutions based on the outcomes. In an optimization problem, several variables exist such that as one improves, another deteriorates. The difficulty is in producing a solution that jointly maximizes the benefits while minimizing the negative consequences. Nurse staffing is a good example of an optimization problem. If high levels of nursing hours are provided, costs of idle time rise. As staffing levels are lowered, more and more patient care needs are neglected. Since both nurse supply and patient acuity vary, however, a perfect staffing level does not exist, so the real challenge is to determine the optimal staffing level for an organization (McHugh, 1997). Other decision support systems provide expert advice to the user.

Expert Systems   An expert system is a computer system containing the information and decision-making strategies of an expert to assist nonexperts in decision-making (Marakas, 2003). An expert system is designed for users to simulate the cause and effect reasoning that an expert would use if confronted with the same situation in a real live environment.

The heart of an expert system has two parts: (1) a knowledge base containing facts and data pertinent to the problem area and (2) an inference engine programmed to replicate the reasoning and decision-making strategies of expert clinicians. The format for decision-making allows the rule, "What if?—then..." rule of logic. This approach is used to draw inferences about the problem posed by the user so that a solution or possible solutions to the problem can be provided. The inference system is based on a method of reasoning that can be either inductive or deductive. Expert systems can be used for assisting practitioners to implement clinical practice guidelines.

Artificial Intelligence Systems   An artificial intelligence (AI) system is a system that attempts to model human reasoning processes. The field is concerned with symbolic inference and knowledge representation. Symbolic inference is concerned with deriving new knowledge from known facts and the use of logical inference rules. An example of an inference rule is "if A > B and B > C, then A must be greater than C." Knowledge representation is the field concerned with devising ways to represent and use abstract knowledge and then store those representations and use rules in a computer system. Once abstract phenomena can be represented, and the rules about how to combine facts about phenomena can be determined and programmed into the computer, then new facts can be added as they are discovered. Then the computer can replicate the human process of developing new knowledge by combining new facts with existing knowledge patterns to generate new facts and understandings.

A true AI system can also track the accuracy of its predictions and judgments and alter its own decision-making rules, based on new knowledge it generates for itself. This capacity replicates the human power to reason under conditions of uncertainty. AI is a subject that sheds light on the nature of thinking by simulating the process of reasoning. Programs have been devised to solve typical mental problems in an effort to demonstrate that the reasoning process follows a systematic series of rules.

Pattern recognition and problem solving are important aspects of AI. People have longed for computers that they could talk with rather than having to rely on slow and inconvenient methods of data entry such as typing. Unfortunately, understanding natural human language has proven to be a most difficult task, requiring a much higher degree of intelligence than simple serial processing.

Natural Language Systems   A natural language system is a system that can understand and process commands given in the user's own natural, spoken language. It does not require the user to learn a special vocabulary, syntax, and set of programming rules and instructions. Natural language requires the computer to understand a wide range of words, speech styles (accents), syntax, and sentence structures. Some computer programs are marketed to accept and process natural language input. They consist of relatively crude matching technique methods to process the input. The newer natural language systems are used to recognize and process human speech (voice) and/or handwriting.

Hospital Information Systems

An HIS, sometimes called a medical information system (MIS) or patient care system (PCS), provides support for a wide variety of both administrative and clinical functions. The purpose of an HIS is to manage information needed to facilitate daily hospital operations by all health care personnel. Administrators manage financial budgets and establish charges for services; physicians diagnose, treat, and evaluate patient conditions; nurses assess, plan, and provide patient care; other personnel provide ancillary services; and a variety of other personnel support the delivery of patient care services.

An HIS is usually a large package of programs, and it is often purchased from a single vendor. While the hospital may own programs that were not supplied by the HIS vendor, the difficulties of integrating programs from multiple vendors can greatly raise the cost of operating the HIS department. Therefore, most hospitals try to keep the number of different products to a minimum.

HIS Configurations

An HIS can use several different computer system configurations. The most common configuration uses a mainframe computer with hardwired terminals or workstations. Users are able to work directly with the mainframe through an interactive interface and real-time processing. Another, and increasingly popular, configuration employs a local area network (LAN). The HIS software is either on the mainframe or on a network server. Users access the HIS through their office PC and the network connections.

Many HIS configurations consist of multiple separate systems that are either linked through a network or, in some cases, may not be electronically linked at all. Many hospitals' configurations include dedicated IS for special purposes, such as nurse staffing, pharmacy, or laboratory systems (Collen, 1983; Shortliffe and Perreault, 1990; Wiederhold and Perreault, 1990).

Program Modules Available in an HIS

Programs typically offered in an HIS include a wide variety of administrative applications (modules) such as admission and discharge, patient tracking, finance, payroll, billing, budgeting support, inventory, and management reporting programs. Clinical support programs are increasingly being viewed as critically important modules in an HIS. As a result, vendors have increased the number and quality of the clinical support tools available in commercial HIS packages.

Administrative applications refer to the support of the administrative functions of patient care. They generally include budgeting and payroll, cost accounting, patient billing, inventory control, bed census, and medical records. These are the same systems that are available in almost any MIS. For nursing administration, a variety of administrative support systems are available commercially as part of an HIS, as partially integrated systems, or as completely stand-alone systems. Patient classification systems are one of the most popular modules for nursing administration. These systems support the process of assigning nursing staff to units and patients. They function by evaluating the acuity of patients in a particular unit and determining the number of nurses needed to care for that group of patients. Many of these modules can produce a variety of specialized operations reports. Other supports for upper and middle management include staff scheduling and budget support modules.

Semiclinical Modules

Two modules in a HIS support both administrative and clinical operations. These are the ADT and order entry systems. The ADT module monitors and sometimes controls the flow of patients in a hospital from admission to discharge. The ADT module may automatically prepare the midnight census and activity reports. Admissions and discharges constitute the hospital's patient census, which is a key factor in billing and future planning for how to best deploy hospital resources.

Another "semiclinical" module is the order-entry-results-reporting (OE) module. OE is almost always available in a HIS. Order entry means that staff can enter laboratory, pharmacy, and radiology orders online. Results reporting means that the lab, pharmacy, and radiology can enter the results into the computer system and have those results available to the nursing unit. Some are "paperless systems" in which all results are reported and posted to the chart electronically. Others may post the results online, but paper reports are still generated and manually posted to the patient chart.

Clinical Support Modules

Charting Systems   Support for nurse charting is highly variable. However, during the 1990s, most vendors greatly upgraded their clinical record products and most vendors now offer some form of online charting. Usually included are the medication administration reports, admission assessment, shift assessments, special assessments (e.g., neurologic assessments and labor records), at least some elements of the nursing care plan (such as nursing diagnosis and interventions), vital signs records, wound care, and hygienic care records. Some provision is usually made for online progress notes.

Unfortunately, there is still a major stumbling block to computerizing the record of nursing care. The lack of a universally implemented standard nursing language continues to impede both the development effort and the market success of the systems that are available. Worse, for the profession of nursing, it impedes efforts of nurses to document the outcomes—and therefore the value of nursing care. This problem is not a function of lack of nursing nomenclatures. The American Nurses Association has recognized such nomenclatures as the Home Health Care Classification (HHCC), the Nursing Intervention Classification/Nursing Outcomes Classification (NIC/NOC), North America Nursing Diagnosis Association (NANDA), the Omaha and Grobe systems (Carroll-Johnson and Paquette, 1994; McCloskey and Bulechek, 1996; Grobe, 1996; Martin, 1996; Saba, 1992; Keenan et al., 2003; Barton, et al., 2003).

Point-of-Service Systems　A point-of-service (POS) or point-of-care system is a special type of clinical system. A POS system uses a hand-held or bedside PC to ensure that data are entered at the point at which they are collected. In other types of clinical systems, the placement of workstations may create a problem for nurses. Typically, workstations have been located at the nurses' station, or in a separate physician's charting room; however, patient data are not collected at those locations. This situation forces the nurse to record information on a "scrap" sheet and later transcribe it to the computer record. This approach produces several suboptimal conditions. First, it is costly to record the same data twice. Second, there is a certain amount of error whenever data are transcribed from one place to another. Third, there is a greater potential that the scrap sheet and the data it contains could be lost or misplaced. Fourth, if the scrap sheet is lost, there is a potential for compromise of patient confidentiality. Fifth, there is always a delay between the time data are collected and the time those data show up on the chart. Finally, the remote workstation approach virtually guarantees idle nursing time because only one person can use the workstation at a time, and there is always competition for access to the workstations. POS systems eliminate all of these problems.

A POS system is designed to save time by recording critical clinical data such as patient assessment, drug administration, vital signs, and so forth, as they are administered by the provider of the service. It also provides immediate access to key patient information to all care providers involved with the patient. It can retrieve the patient's care plan, latest vital signs, or medication administered. A point-of-service system is generally installed in a direct patient care unit, such as the intensive or critical care units, but can be also found in patient care units in a facility where an HIS is installed (Massengill; 1993; Wiederhold and Perreault, 1990).

Laboratory, Pharmacy, and Radiology Modules

Laboratory, pharmacy, and radiology support programs are needed by all hospitals. A typical laboratory system, for example, includes a laboratory test request, generates the specimen labels, tracks the specimen through the various laboratory stages, generates the results, and communicates the findings to patient's medical record. Pharmacy systems track medication orders and changes in orders. They often have drug interaction warning programs, dosage calculators, and other supports for the pharmacy function. They generally include a computer-stored database of the Physician Drug Reference (PDR) Manual, which provides a knowledge base for the pharmacists. Radiology systems are usually separate products developed by companies that specialize in diagnostic computer imaging systems. Ideally, they can be linked with the HIS in such a way that the pictures (digitized versions of the radiographic studies) and radiologist report can be viewed at the bedside or unit workstation.

■ Network Systems

A network is a set of interconnected computers that, through hardware and software technology, work cooperatively for the purpose of information and application program interchange. This definition identifies two essential factors for any network: (1) **hardware** (see Chap.4), including a physical (electronic) connection (card in the computer) and a physical linkage that permits data and information to be transferred back and forth between the computers in the network (typically coaxial or twisted wire cables) and (2) network communication **software** that allows different computers to make sense of the electronic signals and data streams sent back and forth across the wires. The purpose of the hardware and software configuration is to facilitate the transmission of information across different types of computers and computer platforms throughout the system.

Network systems are key to the effective functioning of most hospital computer systems and of many home health, visiting nurse, and clinic computer systems. Increasingly, private and public networks are being used to support the operations of large corporations, educational institutions, governmental operations, and virtually all areas of the economy. Given their importance, it is important that students of informatics science gain an understanding of the fundamental concepts of network science.

The central concept of network science is **cooperation**. All computers in a network must function in an interdependent way. Merely connecting two computers with a wire does not produce a network. In fact, it might not produce any communication. Communication implies mutually understandable interactivity. Simply sending electronic signals from one computer to another does not necessarily mean that the receiving computer can make any sense of the signal. A network, therefore, must have software that can **interpret** the signals it receives. At a minimum, a network must have a set of communication rules. The rules are written into system software programs called **protocols** or networking software.

Networks offer enormous advantages to companies and to individual users. For companies, networking computers often saves money in storage, software purchase prices, reduction of costs attributable to errors in the data, and human time and efficiency.

Efficiencies Related to Storage and Data Integrity

In a HIS, many departments often must use the same data items. Storing the same information in multiple computers increases the cost of storage and may increase the organization's costs of maintaining accurate records. Consider a major hospital that has many inpatient departments and outpatient clinics. Every department in which care or services are provided needs a patient's identifying information. Storing that patient's identifying information in only one record that can be accessed by all the departments means that storage space is conserved. Even more important, patients may visit multiple departments and clinics over time. Since people's identifying information sometimes changes, the information should be changed *in every instance in which it has been stored*. This might include hospital admissions, pharmacy, laboratory, several clinics, the billing department, medical records, and so on. Patients may move from one residence to another. When information is stored in multiple computers, updates almost never reach all the various storage sites if multiple different systems store the information in multiple places rather than in a single master patient file. Thus, the integrity (accuracy and currency) of data in at least some of the departmental computers is compromised. In a network system in which data are stored in a central location and shared with remote workstations, the networks not only save storage space dollars, they can improve the accuracy of the data in the institution's database.

Software Savings

Many health care organizations have a LAN in which most of the workstations use "desktop office" software (e.g., Microsoft Office and Corel Office). If the organization had to individually purchase the "desktop office" software for each workstation, the purchase cost might be prohibitive. Even worse, each user might select a different brand, and workers might not share work efficiently. As a result, the major software vendors offer what is called a "site network license." When a site license is purchased, the cost per workstation is considerably less than the cost of purchasing the same number of software packages individually.

As an added advantage, the cost of maintaining the software is significantly reduced. This is because only one copy of the software is actually stored on the server. The network version of the software allows each user to access and use the same program. Then, if a problem arises, the HIS department can determine quickly if the problem is encountered everywhere in the network (a program problem) if only one user is experiencing problems (local problem). Problem diagnosis is facilitated. If a program bug is found and must be corrected, it is corrected in only one place.

Savings in Human Time and Efficiency

In many cases, multiple departments in an organization need the same information. When networks allow all of the departments to use the same information, only one has to collect and enter the data. Networks also facilitate the work of groups within an organization. One can initiate a document, and others can add to the document, edit it, and print it. Electronic mail (e-mail) on networks greatly reduces human dependence on real-time communication devices such as telephones.

With e-mail, the worker can stop to review messages at a convenient time rather than stopping work in progress to answer a phone. This also reduces stress and anxiety. Stress and anxiety do not constitute states of mind compatible with efficient performance.

Network Functions

Some of the functions performed by networks include (1) file transfer (from one computer to another), (2) information availability (e.g., data and text files can be simultaneously received by more than one recipient at the same time), (3) resource sharing (e.g., programs and data are available to all users simultaneously), (4) online transactions (e.g., grocery stores use computer networks for their charging and inventory control programs attached to the laser scanners at the checkout stand), (5) provision of a powerful communication medium among widely separated employees who may use different computer platforms, (6) interactive environment, (7) education and entertainment (sharing privately or publicly developed educational offerings, games, movies, recordings, and so forth.), and (8) e-mail.

Network Security

The data or information on a network is a valuable property to its owner. Loss or damage to health care data can be costly and can create serious legal liability for a facility that loses critical patient care data or other business data and communications. For example, if a baby is later diagnosed with brain damage, and the labor and delivery record is damaged or destroyed, how shall the facility defend itself against a malpractice suit?

Modern security practices weave layers of physical, administrative, electronic, and encrypted security around valuable data. In the early days of computing, data security was not a major concern; however, the physical safety of the computer itself was quite important. The vacuum tubes were vulnerable to heat and dirt. Therefore, mainframe computer systems required a closed, air-conditioned environment. They generally were not connected to the outside world, however. They certainly were not connected in any way to other computers, and computer expertise was extremely rare. To steal data from a mainframe computer, one would need physical access to the computer itself. One would also need an in-depth knowledge of machine language. Today, neither physical access nor obscure programming knowledge is necessary to break into another's computer.

Networks have simultaneously opened up enormous opportunities to share knowledge and to engage in a variety of malicious and sometimes criminal activities. Physical security remains an important factor, but electronic security is even more important. It is difficult to produce the requisite security with a group of networked personal computers and a large cohort of highly sophisticated computer users throughout the world.

During the 1980s, several trends combined to make data security a major concern. First, computers became the hub of most modern businesses. They became the storehouse for inventory payroll, employee information, design, and manufacturing documents. Due to the sensitivity and value of the information, computer installations have become very attractive targets for thieves, disgruntled employees, vandals, and industrial espionage agents. Second, the trend toward networking and open communications led computer makers to adopt common standards for data communication and storage. It became easy to view a file created on an IBM mainframe on a PC. Finally, most large computers became connected to some kind of networking system, either by LAN or modem. Sensitive corporate data came within the reach of anyone clever enough to get it.

In the 1990s, a new criminal, the hacker, emerged. Originally used to describe anyone who was a "clever programmer," the term is now almost exclusively applied to people who illegally break into computers belonging to someone else. Some hackers do it for profit or for hire as a form of corporate or international espionage. But many others break into computer systems purely for the challenge. Many older mainframe computers were designed with few security measures beyond password protection. In some cases, all computers with the same OS were shipped with the same maintenance password. If an administrator did not change the maintenance password, a savvy hacker had an unobstructed ride into the system. (This happened to the Mayo Clinic in the 1980s, because nobody bothered to change that system password. Unfortunately, the system password was widely published on hacker bulletin boards.)

Password protection can be enough security for most systems, provided that people give their passwords the proper handling and respect. In nursing, it is absolutely essential that all personnel know there is a policy of severe punishment for disclosing one's password to anyone else and that the policy is rigidly followed. Failure to enforce the rules in one case makes it legally difficult to enforce the rules when others break them. Lax security actually leads people to believe security violations are "naughty" or even acceptable rather than helping them understand that these may be criminal acts. The Health Insurance Portability and Accountability Act (HIPAA) of 1996 has made the security of private health records even more critically important and nurses and nursing administrators are expected to know their responsibilities under the law. The standards have been published and are readily available on the Internet through the Centers for Medicare and Medicaid Services (2002).

An administrative security program focuses on passwords, access rights, and personnel issues. System administrators have to work with managers to ensure that only people with a current need to access information are on authorization lists. The HIS department needs to be sure people know that writing their computer passwords down on a desk calendar or a note taped to their monitors is a serious security violation! The fact is that most intrusions into computer systems involve a compromised password. Passwords should be more than five characters long, random, frequently changed, and protected in order to provide effective security. The most sophisticated electronic security systems are useless without good administrative security practices. Unfortunately, few people can remember such passwords and must have a mnemonic password—which is more easily compromised. Physical security devices also exist, and they can be much more reliable than software methods. They include fingerprint and handprint readers, retinal scanners, and the like. They are the best security available but are very much more expensive and there are serious issues with interoperability (compatibility across the multiple systems in use in most hospitals) and reliability and so are hard to sell to cost-conscious managers (Vijayan, 2004). However, they may be much more useful in a clinical setting where many users must sign on to the same workstation and who do not have time for time-consuming password routines.

Electronic security techniques are designed to keep hackers away from important data. These techniques operate at different levels, but generally they recognize and accredit the source of the data. Starting with connections from outside the LAN, many modems can receive a call and, on command, dial back the caller at a prestored number to foil a would be intruder. Modems can also use incoming caller ID, an optional telephone company feature, to identify calls as coming from an authorized telephone number. Similarly, network OSs can recognize the embedded addresses of network adapters and associate certain maximum privileges with specific adapter.

In wide area networks (WANs), particularly those with Internet connections, specialized routers, called **firewalls**, carefully inspect each incoming packet of information, looking for authorized source addresses and rejecting any unknown addresses or even suspicious packets. A skillful and determined hacker can generate packets with some correct authorized source information, so sometimes illegal packets are only detected by their process and intent. There is quite a complete discussion of firewalls at the following URL: *http://www. interhack.net/pubs/fwfaq/* (Robertson, Curtin, and Ranum, 2004).

Encryption is another layer of protection. Encryption means that the data are converted into a cipher, or a code of some kind. Even if it is intercepted, the hacker probably cannot break the code and read the material. Sometimes data are compressed into smaller packets for more economical storage. Interestingly, compression techniques, often used during data transmission and file storage, act as a primitive form of encryption. It takes a lot more effort to hijack compressed data. Beyond compression, serious encryption systems obscure even the volume of information being transmitted and stored. Some OSs and electronic mail systems encrypt files during storage, and all commercial-quality network OSs offer encryption of passwords. Several companies offer encryption modules for routers so that all of the data passing between networked sites is, in practical terms, totally private.

The threat to data exists even in small companies. The larger the monetary stakes, the higher the threat. Good administrative security practices are a must for every organization. We can and should scale electronic protection schemes to match the value of the information and the threat—both to the information and to the organization if the information is compromised.

Types of Networks

Local Area Network   A LAN is a data network intended to serve a single building or a group of buildings in close proximity to each other. Due to the restricted physical area served by the LAN, the connections among the machines on the network are by means of physical wiring. That is, the communications do not have to go through telephone lines or satellite transmission technology. This direct wiring between the machines is called **hard wiring**, and machines on the network are said to be "hard wired" into the system. Due to hard wiring, very fast data transmission rates are made possible by LAN technology.

Wide Area Network A WAN is a system of connected computers spanning a large geographical area, often a continent or country. This network is usually constructed with serial lines, telephone lines, satellites, and FDDI (fiber-optic distributed data interface) cables for WANs. It can also be constructed by connecting LANs.

The Internet

The Internet is a network of networks. It might be visualized as widest of WANs. The Internet is a collection of thousands of networks linked by a common set of technical protocols that make it possible for users of any one of the networks to communicate with or use the services located on any of the other networks. These protocols are referred to as Transmission Control Protocol over Internet Protocol, or TCP/IP. The package of TCP/IP protocols is sometimes called the TCP/IP protocol suite. The Internet began in 1968 with the Advanced Research Projects Agency Network (ARPANET). ARPANET began as a network designed to link certain U.S. Defense Department computers with university computers on campuses performing defense-related research. Today, ARPANET has been subsumed by the National Science Foundation Network (NSFNET), which also includes such networks as the Australian Academic and Research Network (AARNet), the NASA Science Internet (NSI), the Swiss Academic and Research Network (SWITCH), and about 10,000 other large and small, commercial and research, networks. To be part of the Internet, a network must be based on the TCP/IP protocol.

There are other major WANs that are not based on the TCP/IP protocols and are thus often not considered part of the Internet; however, it is possible to communicate between them and the Internet via electronic mail because of mail gateways that act as "translators" between the different network protocols involved.

Navigating the Internet In order to enter the Internet, the user must have an Internet service provider (ISP) and a Web browser. Most large hospital, corporate, and university computer departments have their own Internet address (node), and serve as an ISP to their faculty and staff. Private home users typically purchase ISP services from public companies like America Online (AOL) or Sprint.. During the late 1990s, cable companies developed the technology to let users access the Internet directly from their cable provider. Increasingly, users are seeking services from a cable television provider both because cable modem transmissions are

often faster than transmissions through private telephone lines and because this produces one less bill to pay at the end of the month. Recently, telephone companies have begun to offer bundled services that include home telephone, cell phone, cable, and Internet access all for one monthly fee.

To search the Internet efficiently, a search engine is essential. Today, most of the popular search engines are supported not by user fees, but by advertising. Some popular search engines and their addresses are the following:

1. Altavista. Created by Digital Computer Corporation for scientific searches, this is a highly effective and efficient engine. URL: *http://altavista.com*

2. Yahoo! Originally developed by graduate students Jerry Yang and David Filo at Stanford University. Yahoo is now a privately owned and operated commercial company. URL: *http://www.yahoo.com/*

3. Google. One of the most popular and most highly advertised. URL: *http://www.google.com*

4. 37.com. This is a **metacrawler**. A metacrawler is a search engine that searches for the requested term or phrase on more than one other search engine. URL: *http://37.com*

5. Go2net is another Webcrawler. URL: *http://www.go2net.com/search.html*

Web Browsers A Web browser is a program that is used to visit Web pages. The two most well-known web browsers are Netscape Navigator (part of the Netscape Communicator package) and Microsoft Internet Explorer. Other browsers are available as well but are not as popular. A Web browser has features that allow the user to download and print documents on the Internet; to view the source document, which includes the program codes that format the document; to save images found on the Internet; and to perform a variety of other useful functions. It is the user's window into the Internet. Prior to the development of Web browsers, about the only people who could use the Internet were programmers and other sophisticated users. They had to understand DOS commands, because the user's interface with the Internet was not graphical.

How Does a Web Browser Work? A Web browser is a software program or set of programs that allows users of the Internet to communicate and send/receive files, sound, and graphics. It works by using a special protocol called HTTP. Documents on the Internet contain special instructions (written in HTML) that tell the browser how to display the document on the user's screen. The instructions may include references (hyperlinks) to other Web pages, text color and position, locations for various images contained in the document, and where to position them. Some Web pages may use layout instructions contained in separate documents called style sheets.

World Wide Web   The WWW is a hypertext-based, distributed information system created by a team of researchers led by Dr. Tim Berners-Lee at CERN in Switzerland. Users may create, edit, or browse hypertext documents. The clients and servers are freely available. This is a subset of the Internet that uses a combination of text, graphics, audio, and video (multimedia) to provide information on almost every subject imaginable.

Hypertext Markup Language   HTML is the language used to create hypertext documents. It is a subset of the Standardized General Markup Language (SGML) and includes mechanisms to establish hyperlinks in one

document that take the user to the address of other documents. With HTML you can build Web pages. It is basically a formatting language. Table 5.1 presents a sample of HTML codes designed to format text on a Web page.

Hypertext and Hyperlinks   Hypertext is a document, written in HTML, which contains automated links (hyperlinks) to other documents, which may or may not also be hypertext documents. Hypertext documents are usually retrieved using the WWW. A hyperlink pointer within a hypertext document points (links) to another document, which may or may not be a hypertext document. Hyperlinks are usually a bright blue color (although the person who designs the Web page may change the color). Hyperlinks are also often underlined as well, and often, when the reader places the cursor on the hyperlink, it changes color to be sure the user knows the text is a hyperlink. Hyperlinks are usually documents placed on other sites on the Internet. Clicking on these links activates the necessary protocols and pulls up the chosen site.

Table 5.1   HTML Formatting Codes Generated in Microsoft Front Page

```
<html>
<head>
<meta http-equiv="Content-Type" content="text/html; charset=iso-8859-1">
<title>Module 2</title>
<meta name="GENERATOR" content="Microsoft FrontPage 3.0">
<meta name="Microsoft Theme" content="none">
</head>
<body>
<h1 align="center"><font color="#FF0000">Module 2</font></h1>
<h1 align="center"><font color="#FF0000">Structured System Analysis</font></h1>
<p ALIGN="CENTER"> 
Structured System Analysis</p>
<p align="left">    Structured system analysis (SSA) incorporates
a set of strategies and techniques designed to improve the probability that the
final system designed or purchased actually meets the users, needs for system
support. The process is useful not only in the computer system design and
selection process. The philosophy that underlies SSA has proven so durable and
effective that many managers find that using it improves the success rate of
their decisions in a variety of managerial as well as computer system situations.
SSA is so important that failure to use an SSA model in computer system selection
virtually guarantees some degree of failure of the whole project.</p>
</font>
</body>
</html>
```

Glossary of Internet Terms

Address: The location of an Internet resource. The address identifies the type of agency. The most commonly encountered are nonprofit organizations (.org), companies (.com), governmental bodies (.gov), and educational institutions (.edu). An e-mail address may take the form of jones@someclinic.com. A Web address looks something like *http://www.charityhospital.org*.

Applet: An applet is a little application program that can be downloaded over a network and launched on the user's computer. Java applets can perform interactive animations, immediate calculations, or other simple tasks without having to send a user request back to the server. Applets make it possible for a Web page user to interact with the page.

Bandwidth: A measurement of the volume of information that can be transmitted over a network at a given time. Think of a network as a water pipe—the higher the bandwidth (the larger the diameter of the pipe), the more data (water) that can pass over the network (through the pipe).

Browser: A program run on a client computer for viewing WWW pages. Examples include Netscape, Microsoft's Internet Explorer, and Mosaic.

Cache: A region of memory where frequently accessed data can be stored for rapid access. A cache (pronounced "cash") is a place to store something more or less temporarily.

CGI: Common gateway interface—the specification for how an HTTP server should communicate with server gateway applications.

Chat: A system that allows for online real-time communication between Internet users. Since it is a real-time activity, chat discussions disappear as they scroll off your screen. Also, everybody has to be online at the same time.

Client: A program (like a Web browser) that connects to and requests information from a server.

Cookies: The collective name for files stored on your hard drive by your Web browser that hold information about your browsing habits, like what sites you have visited, which newsgroups you have read, and so forth. Many view cookies as an invasion of privacy.

Dial-up Connection: A connection to the Internet via phone and modem. Connection types include Point-to-Point Protocol (PPP) and Symmetric List Processsor (SLIP).

Direct Connection: A connection made directly to the Internet—much faster than a dial-up connection.

Discussion Group: A particular section within the USENET system typically, though not always, dedicated to a particular subject of interest. Also known as a newsgroup. A class discussion board is an example of a discussion group.

Domain: The Internet is divided into smaller sets known as domains, including .com (business), .gov (government), .edu (educational), and others. The WSU domain is an educational domain; thus the .edu at the end of all its server names.

Domain Name: A domain name is the Internet name or identifier of a company, university, or other entity on the Internet.

Download: The process of copying data file(s) from a remote computer to a local computer. The opposite action is upload, where a local file is copied to a server.

FTP: File transfer protocol—a set of rules for exchanging files between computers via the Internet.

Gateway: Computer hardware and software that allow users to connect from one network to another.

Home Page: The first or entry level page in an individual's or institution's Web site. Typically, the home page is the default page that is located at the user's URL address.

HTTP: Hypertext transfer protocol—a set of instructions for communication between a server and a WWW client.

ISDN Line: A category of leased telephone line service, allowing transfer rates of 128 kilobytes per second over the Internet. No longer too expensive for home users (around $50 per month plus 1 cent a minute), but still more commonly found in business environments. (See T1 line.)

IP Address: IP address—every computer on the Internet has a unique identifying number, like 191.1.24.2.

Link: Another name for a hyperlink.

Mirror Site: An Internet site set up as an alternate to a busy site; it contains copies of all the files stored at the primary location.

Mosaic: One of the first graphical WWW browsers, developed at NCSA.

Network: A system of connected computers exchanging information with each other. A LAN is a relatively small form of a network in comparison with the Internet, a worldwide network of computers.

Online: When you are on a computer, especially when connected to the Internet, you are online.

Online Service: Another name for an ISP. Companies such as AOL, CompuServe, Prodigy, and the Microsoft Network provide content to subscribers and usually connections to the Internet.

Page: An HTML document or Web site.

Point of Presence: In the Internet, the location of a device that serves as an access point or gateway into the Internet is called a point of presence, or POP. When users need to get a new e-mail address working, they have to identify their computer's POP server to the e-mail program so it knows where to send the mail. Every POP server has a unique Internet address.

Protocol: An agreed on set of rules by which computers exchange information.

Router: When two computers in different networks need to exchange information, they must be connected through a common computer. This is called a router. A router is a device (or it may be software installed in a server computer) that determines the next network point to which a packet should be forwarded toward its destination. The router is connected to at least two networks that need to exchange information (same protocol). It is the job of the router to determine which way to send each information packet. To accomplish its mission, a router must develop and maintain a table of available routes, cost, and distance. The router applies an algorithm to these data to determine the fastest and lowest-cost path for each information packet. A router must be located at any juncture of networks (gateway).

Server: One-half of the client-server protocol, it runs on a networked computer and responds to requests submitted by the client. Your WWW browser is a client of a WWW server.

Site: A single Web page or collection of related Web pages. A site has a URL.

SMTP: Simple Mail Transfer Protocol—a protocol dictating how e-mail messages are exchanged over the Internet.

Telnet: A protocol for logging onto remote computers from anywhere on the Internet.

Upload: To copy a file from a local computer connected to the Internet to a remote computer. Opposite is download.

URL: Uniform resource locator—the method by which Internet sites are addressed.

References

Austrian, G. (1982). *Herman Hollerith: Forgotten Giant of Information Processing*. New York: Columbia University Press.

Barton, A., Gilbert, L., Erickson, V., Baramee, J., Sowers, D., and Robertson, K. (2003). A guide to assist nurse practitioners with standardized nursing language. *CIN: Computers in Nursing* 21(3):128–133.

Berners-Lee, T. and Fischetti, M. (2000). *Weaving the Web: The Origin, Design and Ultimate Destiny of the World Wide Web by Its Inventor*. San Francisco, CA: Harper Books.

Brennan, P. and McHugh, M. (1988). Clinical decision-making and computer support. *Applied Nursing Research* 1(2):89–93.

Bulechek, G. and McCloskey, J. (1996). *Nursing Interventions Classification (NIC)* (2nd ed.). St. Louis, MO: Mosby.

Carroll-Johnson, R. and Paquette, M. (Eds.). (1994). Classification of Nursing Diagnoses: *Proceedings of the Tenth Conference*. Philadelphia, PA: Lippincott.

Centers for Medicare and Medicaid Services. (2002). *Health Insurance Portability and Accountability Act (HIPAA)—Administrative Simplification*. http://www.cms.hhs.gov/hipaa/hipaa2/default.asp

Charles Babbage Institute. (2004). *Who Was Charles Babbage?* Center for the History of Informational Technology. http://www.cbi.umn.edu/exhibits/cb.html

Collen, M. F. (1983). The function of a HIS: An overview. In O. Fokkens, et al. (Eds.), *MEDINFO 83 Seminars* (pp. 61–64). Amsterdam: North-Holland.

Dunne, P. E. (2004). *Mechanical Aids to Computation and the Development of Algorithms*. http://www.csc.liv.ac.uk/~ped/teachadmin/histsci/htmlform/lect1.html

Falbo, C. (2000). Augusta Ada Byron, Countess of Lovelace. *Math Odyssey 2000*. Champlain, IL: Stipe Publishing.

Grobe, S. (1996). The nursing intervention lexicon and taxonomy: Implications for representing nursing care data in automated patient records. *Holistic Nursing Practice* 11(1):48–63.

Keenan, G., Stocker, J., Barkauskas, V., Treder, M., and Heath, C. (2003). Toward collecting a standardized nursing data set across the continuum: Case of adult care nurse practitioner setting. *Outcomes Management* 7(3):113–120.

Lee, J. (1987). Grace Murray Hopper. *Annals of the History of Computing* 9(3):273.

Marakas, G. (2003). *Decision Support Systems in the 21st Century* (2nd ed.). Upper Saddle River, NJ: Prentice Hall.

Martin, K. (1996). The Omaha System: A model for describing practice. *Holistic Nursing Practice* 11(1):75–83.

Massengill, S. (1993). The four technologies of the electronic patient record. In *Conference Proceedings: Toward an Electronic Patient Record '93* (pp. 92–94). Newton, MA: Medical Record Institute.

Maxfield, C. and Brown, A. (1998). *Bebop Bytes Back*. Madison, AL: Maxfield & Montrose Interactive.

McHugh, M. (1997). Cost effectiveness of clustered versus unclustered unit transfers of nursing staff. *Nursing Economics* 15(6):294–300.

Robertson, P., Curtin, M., and Ranum, M. (2004). *Internet Firewalls: Frequently Asked Questions*. *http://www.interhack.net/pubs/fwfaq/*

Saba, V. (1992). The classification of home health care nursing diagnoses and interventions. *Caring* 11(3): 50–57.

Schieber, P. (Downloaded, July 15, 2004). The wit and wisdom of Grace Hopper. *OCLC Newsletter*, No. 167, March/April, 1987. *http://www.cs.yale.edu/~tap/Files/hopper-wit.html*

Shortliffe, E. H. and Perreault, L. E. (Eds.). (1990). *Medical informatics: Computer Applications in Health Care*. Reading, MA: Addison-Wesley.

Toole, B. A. (1992). *Ada: The Enchantress of Numbers*. Sausalito, CA: Strawberry Press.

University Hospital Consortium (UHC). (2004). *The University Hospital Consortium: An Overview*. *http://www.radsci.ucla.edu:8000/uhc/description.html*

Vijayan, J. (2004). Corporate America slow to adopt biometric technologies. *Computerworld* 38(32):1, 45.

Wiederhold, G. and Perreault, L. E. (1990). Hospital information systems. In E. H. Shortliffe and L. E. Perreault (Eds.), *Medical Informatics: Computer Applications in Health Care* (pp. 219–243). Reading, MA: Addison-Wesley.

Women's International Center. (Downloaded, July 1, 2004). Grace Hopper: Mother of the Computer. *WIC Biography Series*. *http://www.wic.org/bio/ghopper.htm*

6

Open Source and Free Software

Peter J. Murray

Alric M O'Connor

OBJECTIVES

1. Describe the basic concepts of open source software (OSS) and free software (FS).
2. Describe the differences between open source and free software, and proprietary software, particularly in respect of licensing.
3. Discuss why an understanding of differences is important in a healthcare context and where a migration from proprietary to open source and free software is being considered.
4. Describe some of the open source applications in current use, both healthcare-specific and for general office/productivity use.
5. Introduce some of the organizations and resources available to assist the nurse interested in exploring the potential of open source software.

KEY WORDS

open source software
free software Linux

 Introduction

Most nurses use OSS/FS (Table 6.1) on a daily basis, but without even realizing it.[1] Everybody who sends e-mail or uses the Web uses OSS/FS most of the time, as the majority of the hardware and software that allows the Internet to function (Web servers, file transmission protocol [FTP] servers, and mail systems) are OSS/FS. Many popular Web sites are hosted on Apache (OSS/FS) servers, for example, Amazon, Google, and Yahoo. While free software (as defined by the Free Software Foundation [FSF]; Table 6.2) has existed since the mid-1980s, the GNU is Not Unix Project (GNU)/Linux operating system (Table 6.1) has been developing since the early 1990s, and the open source initiative (OSI) (Table 6.2) definition of open source software has existed since the late 1990s; it is only more

recently that widespread interest has begun to develop in the possibilities of OSS/FS within health, healthcare and nursing, and in particular within nursing informatics (NI) and health informatics.

Today's nurses have an ever-increasing choice of possible software solutions to meet their computing and networking needs (Dravis, 2003), but many nurses have only a vague understanding of what OSS/FS are and their possible applications and relevance to nursing and NI. This chapter aims to provide a basic understanding of the issues, as it is only through being fully informed about the relative merits, and potential limitations, of the range of proprietary software and OSS/FS, that nurses can make informed choices, whether they are selecting software for their own personal needs or for a large healthcare organization. This chapter will provide an overview of the background to OSS/FS, explaining the differences and similarities between open source and free software and introducing some particular applications such as the GNU/Linux operating system. Licensing issues will be addressed in some depth as, at this point in time, they are exercising the minds of many, and issues such as the interface of OSS/FS and

---

[1]The abbreviation OSS/FS (open source software/free software) will be used in this chapter when the discussion refers to any component or mixture of open source and/or free software, including the GNU/Linux operating system, except where there needs to be a specific description or a distinction made between the variants.

Table 6.1 Some Common Acronyms and Terms

A number of acronyms are used to denote a combination of free software and open source software. OSS/FS is the term that is used for preference in this chapter; others include the following:

OSS—open source software

OSS/FS—open source software/free software

FOSS—free and open source software

FLOSS—free/libre/open source software

GNU—GNU is Not Unix Project (a recursive acronym)—a project started by Richard Stallman that has turned into the FSF to develop and promote alternatives to proprietary Unix implementations.

GNU/Linux or Linux—the complete operating system including the Linux kernel, the GNU components, and many other programs. GNU/Linux is the more accurate term because it makes a distinction between the kernel—Linux—and much of the software which was developed by the GNU Project in association with the FSF.

proprietary software, or use of OSS/FS components are not fully resolved. Some commonly available and health-care-specific applications will be introduced, with a few examples being discussed, and some of the organizations working to explore the use of OSS/FS within healthcare and nursing, and additional resources, will be introduced.

The chapter will conclude with a case study of what many consider the potential "mother of OSS/FS health-care applications," Veterans Health Information System and Technology Architecture (VistA) (Tiemann, 2004) (see footnote 1).

 ## OSS/FS—The Theory

Background

While we use the term "open source" (and the acronym OSS/FS) in this chapter, we do so loosely (and some would argue, incorrectly) to cover several concepts, including open source software, free software, and GNU/Linux. Each of these concepts and applications has their own definitions and attributes (Table 6.2). The two major philosophies in the OSS/FS world, i.e., the FSF philosophy and the open source initiative (OSI) philosophy, are today seen by many as separate movements with different views and goals, but often working together on specific practical projects (FSF, 2002a).

The key commonality between FSF and OSI is that the source code is made available to the users by the programmer. Where FSF and OSI differ is in the restrictions placed on redistributed source code. FSF is committed to no restrictions, so that if you modify and redistribute free software, as a part or as a whole of aggregated software, you are not allowed to place any restrictions on the openness of the resultant source code (Wong and Sayo, 2003). The basic differences between the two movements seem to be that the free software movement's fundamental issues are ethical and philosophical, while for the open source movement, the issue of "whether software should be open source is a practical question, not an ethical one . . . 'Open source is a development methodology; free software is a social movement.'" (FSF, 2002a)

OSS/FS is contrasted with proprietary or commercial software, again the two terms often being conflated but strictly needing separating. Proprietary software is that on which an individual or company holds the exclusive copyright, at the same time restricting other people's access to the software's source code and/or the right to copy, modify, and study the software. Commercial software is software developed by businesses or individuals with the aim of making money from its licensing and use. Most commercial software is proprietary, but there is commercial free software, and there is noncommercial non-free software.

OSS/FS should also not be confused with freeware or shareware. Freeware is software that is offered free of charge, but without the freedom to modify the source code and redistribute the changes, so it is not free software (as defined by the FSF). Shareware is another form of commercial software, which is offered on a "try before you buy" basis. If the customer continues to use the product after a short trial period, or wishes to use additional features, they are required to pay a specified, usually nominal, license fee.

Free Software Definition

Free software is defined by the FSF in terms of four freedoms for the software user, i.e., to have the freedom to use, study, redistribute, and improve the software in any way they wish. A program is only free software if users have all of these freedoms (Table 6.2).

Confusion around the use and meaning of the term "free software" arises from the multiple meanings of the word "free" in the English language. In other languages there is less of a problem, with different words being used for the "freedom" versus "no cost" meanings of "free"—most notably the French word "libre." The "free" of free

Table 6.2 Free Software and Open Source Definitions

Free Software

The term free software is defined by the FSF (*http://www.gnu.org/philosophy/free-sw.html*)

Free software is a matter of the users' freedom to run, copy, distribute, study, change, and improve the software. More precisely, it refers to four kinds of freedom for the users of the software:

- The freedom to run the program for any purpose (freedom 0)
- The freedom to study how the program works and adapt it to your needs (freedom 1). Access to the source code is a precondition for this
- The freedom to redistribute copies so you can help your neighbor (freedom 2)
- The freedom to improve the program and release your improvements to the public so that the whole community benefits (freedom 3). Access to the source code is a precondition for this

A program is free software if users have all of these freedoms

Open Source Software

The term open source is defined by the open source initiative (OSI)

(*http://www.opensource.org/docs/definition_plain.php*)

The Open Source Definition (OSD) Version 1.9

The following sections appear as annotations to the OSD and are not a part of the OSD

Introduction

Free Redistribution

The license shall not restrict any party from selling or giving away the software as a component of an aggregate software distribution containing programs from several different sources. The license shall not require a royalty or other fee for such sale.

Source Code

The program must include source code, and must allow distribution in source code as well as compiled form. Where some form of a product is not distributed with source code, there must be a well-publicized means of obtaining the source code for no more than a reasonable reproduction cost—preferably, downloading via the Internet without charge. The source code must be the preferred form in which a programmer would modify the program. Deliberately obfuscated source code is not allowed. Intermediate forms such as the output of a preprocessor or translator are not allowed.

Derived Works

The license must allow modifications and derived works, and must allow them to be distributed under the same terms as the license of the original software.

Integrity of the Author's Source Code

The license may restrict source code from being distributed in modified form only if the license allows the distribution of "patch files" with the source code for the purpose of modifying the program at build time. The license must explicitly permit distribution of software built from modified source code. The license may require derived works to carry a different name or version number from the original software.

Rationale: Encouraging lots of improvement is a good thing, but users have a right to know who is responsible for the software they are using. Authors and maintainers have reciprocal right to know what they are being asked to support and protect their reputations.

No Discrimination Against Persons or Groups

The license must not discriminate against any person or group of persons.

Rationale: In order to get the maximum benefit from the process, the maximum diversity of persons and groups should be equally eligible to contribute to open sources. Therefore we forbid any open source license from locking anybody out of the process.

No Discrimination Against Fields of Endeavor

The license must not restrict anyone from making use of the program in a specific field of endeavor. For example, it may not restrict the program from being used in a business, or from being used for genetic research.

(Continued)

Table 6.2 Free Software and Open Source Definitions (*Continued*)

Distribution of License

The rights attached to the program must apply to all to whom the program is redistributed without the need for execution of an additional license by those parties.

License Must Not Be Specific to a Product

The rights attached to the program must not depend on the program being part of a particular software distribution. If the program is extracted from that distribution and used or distributed within the terms of the program's license, all parties to whom the program is redistributed should have the same rights as those that are granted in conjunction with the original software distribution.

License Must Not Restrict Other Software

The license must not place restrictions on other software that is distributed along with the licensed software. For example, the license must not insist that all other programs distributed on the same medium must be open source software.

Rationale: Distributors of open source software have the right to make their own choices about their own software.

License Must Be Technology-Neutral

No provision of the license may be predicated on any individual technology or style of interface.

Rationale: This provision is specifically aimed at licenses which require an explicit gesture of assent in order to establish a contract between licensor and licensee. Provisions mandating so-called "click-wrap" may conflict with important methods of software distribution such as FTP download, CD-ROM anthologies, and Web mirroring; such provisions may also hinder code reuse. Conformant licenses must allow for the possibility that (a) redistribution of the software will take place over non-Web channels that do not support click-wrapping of the download and (b) the covered code (or reused portions of covered code) may run in a non-GUI environment that cannot support popup dialogues.

---

software is defined in terms of "liberty, not price," and to understand the concept, one needs to think of "free" as in "free speech," not as in "free beer" (FSF, 2002b). Acronyms such as FLOSS (free/libre/OSS—a combination of the above two terms emphasizing the "libre" meaning of the word free), or OSS/FS, are increasingly used, particularly in Europe, to overcome this issue (International Institute of Infonomics, 2002).

Open Source Software Definition

Open source software is any software that satisfies the open software initiative's definition (OSI, 2004; Tiemann, 2003). The open source concept is said to promote software reliability and quality by supporting independent peer review and rapid evolution of source code, as well as making the source code of software freely available. In addition to providing free access to the programmer's instructions to the computer in the programming language in which they were written, many versions of open source licenses allow anyone to modify and redistribute the software.

The open source initiative (OSI) has created a certification mark, "OSI certified." In order to be OSI certified, the software must be distributed under a license that guarantees the right to read, redistribute, modify, and use the software freely (OSI, 2004). Not only must the source code be accessible to all, but also the distribution terms must comply with 10 criteria defined by OSI (see Table 6.2 for full text and rationale).

OSS/FS Development Models/Systems

The development models of OSS/FS are said to contribute to its distinctions from proprietary software. Shaw et al. (2002) state that as OSS/FS has been "developed and disseminated in an open forum,' then it 'revolutionizes the way in which software has historically been developed and distributed." A similar description, in a United Kingdom government report, emphasizes the open publishing of source code and that development is often largely through voluntary efforts (Peeling and Satchell, 2001).

While OSS/FS is often described as being developed by voluntary efforts, this description may belie the professional skills and expertise of many of the developers. Many of those providing the volunteer efforts are highly skilled programmers who contribute time and efforts freely to the development of OSS/FS. In addition, many OSS/FS applications are coordinated through formal groups, for example, the Apache Foundation coordinates development of the Apache HTTP (hypertext transfer protocol) server.

OSS/FS draws much of its strength from the collaborative efforts of people who work to improve, modify, or customize programs, believing that they must give back to the OSS/FS community so others can benefit from their work. The OSS/FS development model is unique and is facilitated by the communication capabilities of the Internet that allow collaboration and rapid sharing of developments, such that new versions of software can sometimes be made available on a daily basis.

The most well-known description of the distinction between OSS/FS and proprietary models of software development lies in Eric Raymond's famous essay, "The cathedral and the bazaar" (Raymond, 2001). Cathedrals, Raymond says, were built by small groups of skilled workers and craftsmen to carefully worked out designs. The work was often done in isolation, and with everything built in a single effort with little subsequent modification. Much software has traditionally been built in a similar fashion, with groups of programmers working to strictly-controlled planning and management, until their work was completed and the program released to the world. In contrast, OSS/FS development is likened to a bazaar, growing organically from an initial small group of traders establishing their structures and beginning business. The bazaar grows in a seemingly chaotic fashion, from a minimally functional structure, with later additions or modifications as circumstances dictate. Likewise, most OSS/FS development starts off highly unstructured, with developers releasing early minimally functional code and then modifying their programs based on feedback. Other developers may then join, and modify or build on the existing code; over time, an entire operating system and suite of applications develops, evolves, and improves continuously.

The bazaar method of development is said to have been proven over time to have several advantages, including the following:

- Reduced duplication of efforts through being able to examine the work of others and through the potential for large numbers of contributors to use their skills. As Moody (2001) describes it, there is no need to reinvent the wheel every time, as there would be with commercial products whose code cannot be used in these ways

- Building on the work of others, often by the use of open standards or components from other applications

- Better quality control; with many developers working on a project, code errors (bugs) are uncovered quickly and may be fixed even more rapidly

- Reduction in maintenance costs; costs, as well as effort, can be shared among potentially thousands of developers (Wong and Sayo, 2003)

Choosing OSS/FS or Not

Proposed Benefits of OSS/FS

OSS/FS has been described as the electronic equivalent of generic drugs (Bruggink, 2003; Surnam and Diceman, 2004). In the same way as the formulas for generic drugs are made public, so OSS/FS source code is accessible to the user. Any person can see how the software works and can make changes to the functionality.

As OSS/FS can be obtained royalty free, it is less expensive to acquire than proprietary alternatives. This means OSS/FS can transform healthcare in developing countries just as the availability of generic drugs have.

This is one of several benefits that are proposed for OSS/FS and that form the basis of the aims and objectives of several of the groups currently working to promote OSS/FS within the health domain (see the groups' Web sites for further lists of proposed benefits). Other OSS/FS benefits include lack of proprietary lock-in, which can freeze out innovation, while OSS/FS projects tend to support open standards and provide a level playing field, expanding the market by giving software consumers greater choice (Dravis, 2003).

Besides the low cost of OSS/FS, there are many other reasons why public/private organizations are adopting OSS/FS, including security, reliability/stability, and developing local software capacity. Many of these proposed benefits have yet to be demonstrated or tested extensively, but there is growing evidence for many of them, and we will address some of them in the next section.

Issues in OSS/FS

There are many issues in the use of OSS/FS that we cannot address here in detail. Some are emerging issues that, as in any new field of endeavor, will not be resolved for a number of years, but some are issues that nurses exploring, using, or intending to use OSS/FS need to be aware of and to decide whether they apply to or need to influence the decisions that they make. These include, not necessarily in any order of importance:

- Licensing
- Copyright and intellectual property
- TCO
- Support and migration
- Business models
- Security and stability

Licensing and copyright will be addressed in the next section, but the other issues will be covered briefly here, before concluding the section with a consideration of a brief description of a strategy for choosing OSS/FS (or other software, as the issues are pertinent to any properly-considered purchase and implementation strategy).

Total Cost of Ownership (TCO)   TCO is the sum of all the expenses directly related to the ownership and use of a product over a given period of time. The popular myth surrounding OSS/FS is that it is always "free" as in "free of charge." This is true to an extent as most OSS/FS distributions (Red Hat, SuSE, Debian, and so on) can be obtained at no charge from the Internet; however, copies can also be sold.

No true OSS/FS application charges a licensing fee for usage, thus on a licensing cost basis OSS/FS applications are almost always cheaper than proprietary software. However, licensing costs are not the only costs of a software package or infrastructure. It is also necessary to consider personnel costs, hardware requirements, migration time, changes in staff efficiency, and training costs, among others. Without all of this information, it is impossible to really know which software solutions are going to be the most cost effective. There are still real costs with OSS/FS, specifically around configuration and support (examples are provided in Wheeler, 2003a; Wong and Sayo, 2003).

Wheeler (2003a) lists the main reasons why OSS/FS comes out cheaper, including

- OSS/FS costs less to initially acquire because there are no license fees

- Upgrade and maintenance costs are typically far less due to improved stability and security

- OSS/FS can often use older hardware more efficiently than proprietary systems, yielding smaller hardware costs and sometimes eliminating the need for new hardware

- Increasing numbers of case studies using OSS/FS show it to be especially cheaper in server environments

Support and Migration   Making an organization-wide change from proprietary software can be costly, and sometimes the costs will outweigh the benefits. Some OSS/FS packages do not have the same level of documentation, training, and support resources as their common proprietary equivalents, and may not fully interface with other proprietary software being used by other organizations with which an organization may work (e.g., patient data exchange between different healthcare provider systems).

Migrating from one platform to another should be handled using a careful and phased approach. The European Union (EU) has published a document entitled the "IDA Open Source Migration Guidelines" (European Communities, 2003b) that provides detailed suggestions on how to approach migration. These include the need for a clear understanding of the reasons to migrate, ensuring that there is active support for the change from information technology (IT) staff and users, building up expertise and relationships with the open source movement, starting with noncritical systems, and ensuring that each step in the migration is manageable.

Security and Stability   While there is no perfectly secure operating system or platform, factors such as development method, program architecture, and target market can greatly affect the security of a system and consequently make it easier or more difficult to breach. There are some indications that OSS/FS systems are superior to proprietary systems in this respect, and the security aspect has already encouraged many public organizations to switch or to consider switching to OSS/FS solutions. The French Customs and Indirect Taxation authority, for example, migrated to Red Hat Linux largely because of security concerns with proprietary software (International Institute of Infonomics, 2002).

Among reasons often cited for OSS/FS better security record is the availability of the source code (making it easier for vulnerabilities to be discovered and fixed). Many OSS/FS have a proactive security focus, so that before features are added, the security considerations are considered and a feature is added only if it is determined not to compromise system security. In addition, the strong security and permission structure inherent in OSS/FS applications that are based on the Unix model are designed to minimize the possibility of users being able to compromise systems (Wong and Sayo, 2003).

OSS/FS systems are well known for their stability and reliability, and many anecdotal stories exist of OSS/FS servers functioning for years without requiring maintenance. However, quantitative studies are more difficult to come by (Wong and Sayo, 2003).

Security of information is vitally important in the health domain, particularly in relation to access, storage and transmission of patient records.

The advocates of OSS/FS suggest that it can provide increased security over proprietary software, and a report to the U.K. government saw no security disadvantage in the use of OSS/FS products (Peeling and Satchell, 2001). Even the U.S. government's National Security Agency (NSA), according to the same report, supports a number of OSS/FS security-related projects. Stanco (2001) considers that the reason NSA thinks that free software can be more secure is that when anyone and everyone can inspect source code, hiding backdoors into the code can be very difficult.

In considering a migration to OSS/FS, whether it is for everyday office and productivity uses, or for health-specific applications, there are some commonly-encountered challenges that one may face. These challenges include the following:

- That there is a relative lack of mature OSS/FS desktop applications
- Many OSS/FS tools are not user-friendly and have a steep learning curve
- File sharing between OSS/FS and proprietary applications can be difficult.

As OSS/FS applications mature and the user community grows many of these challenges should be overcome.

Choosing the Right Software: The Three-Step Method for OSS/FS Decision-Making

Whether one is working with OSS/FS or commercial/proprietary tools, choosing the right software can be a difficult process, and a thorough review process is needed before making a choice. A simple three-step method for OSS/FS decision-making can guide organizations through the process and works well for all kinds of software, including server, desktop, and Web applications (see Surman and Diceman, 2004 for full detail).

Step 1   Defining the needs and constraints. Needs must be clearly defined, including those of the organization and of individual users. Other specific issues to consider include range of features, languages, budget (e.g., for training or integration with other systems), the implementation time frame, compatibility with existing systems, and the skills existing within the organization.

Step 2   Identifying the options. A short list of three to five software packages that are likely to meet the needs can be developed from comparing software packages against the needs and constraints listed in the previous phase. There are numerous sources of information on OSS/FS packages, including recommendations of existing users, reviews, and directories (e.g., OSDir.com and OpenSourceCMS.com.) and software package sites which contain promotional information, documentation, and often demonstration versions that will help with the review process.

Step 3   Undertaking a detailed review. Once the options have been identified, the final step is to review and choose a software package from the short list. The aim here is to assess which of the possible options will be best for the organization. This assessment can be done by rating each package against a list of criteria, including quality, ease of use, ease of migration, software stability, compatibility with other systems being used, flexibility and customizability, user response, organizational buy-in, evidence of widespread use of the software, and the existence of support mechanisms for the software's use. Hands-on testing is key and each piece of software should be installed and tested for quality, stability, and compatibility, including by a group of key users so as to assess factors such as ease of use, ease of migration, and user response.

Making a Decision

Once the review has been completed, if two packages are close in score, intuition about the "right" package is probably more important than the actual numbers in reaching a final decision.

Examples of Adoption or Policy Re: OSS/FS

OSS/FS has moved beyond the closed world of programmers and enthusiasts. Governments around the world have begun to take notice of OSS/FS and have launched initiatives to explore the proposed benefits. There is a significant trend toward incorporating OSS/FS into procurement and development policies, and increasing numbers of cases of OSS/FS recognition, explicit policy statements, or procurement decisions. There are over 70 existing or proposed laws mandating or encouraging OSS/FS around the world (Wong and Sayo, 2003).

A survey from The MITRE Corporation (2003) showed that the U.S. Department of Defense (DoD) used over 100 different OSS/FS applications. The main conclusion of their study (The MITRE Corporation, 2003) was that OSS/FS software was used in critical roles, including infrastructure support, software development, research, and that the degree of dependence on OSS/FS for security was unexpected.

In 2000, the (U.S.) President's Information Technology Advisory Committee (PITAC, 2000) recommended that the U.S. federal government should encourage OSS/FS use for software development for high-end computing. In 2002, the U.K. government published a policy (Cabinet Office, 2002), being updated in 2004, that it will "consider OSS solutions alongside proprietary ones in IT procurements," "only use products for interoperability that support open standards and specifications in all future IT developments" and "explore further the possibilities of using OSS as the default exploitation route" where research and development (R&D) software has been government funded. Similar policies have been developed in Denmark, Sweden, and The Netherlands (European Communities, 2003a; Wong and Sayo, 2003).

European policy encouraging the exploration and use of OSS/FS has been consequent on the European Commission's *eEurope2005—An Information Society for All* initiative (European Communities, 2004) and its predecessors, with their associated action plans. These have encouraged the European Commission and member states of the EU to "promote the use of open source software in the public sector and e-government best practice through exchange of experiences across the Union."

In addition, the EU has funded research and development on health-related OSS/FS applications as well as encouraging open standards and OSS/FS where appropriate in wider policy initiatives. In Germany, the Parliament now uses Linux servers and the city of Munich is migrating over 14,000 desktop machines to Linux, while police forces are also migrating to Linux, citing increased security considerations as well as reduced costs among the determining factors.

In other parts of world, Brazil and Peru are among countries whose governments are actively moving toward OSS/FS solutions, for a variety of reasons, including ensuring long-term access to data through the use of open standards (i.e., not being reliant on proprietary software that may not, in the future, be interoperable), and cost reduction. The South African government has a policy favoring OSS/FS, Japan is considering moving e-government projects to OSS/FS, and pro-OSS/FS initiatives are in operation or being seriously considered in Taiwan, Malaysia, South Korea, and other Asia Pacific countries.

Open Source Licensing

In this section, we can only briefly introduce some of the issues of software licensing as they apply to OSS/FS, and will include definitions of licensing, some of the types of license that exist, and how licenses are different from copyright. While we will cover some of the legal concepts, this section cannot take the place of proper legal counsel, which should be sought when reviewing the impact of licenses or contracts.

Licensing is defined, for example, by Merriam-Webster (2004) giving the user of something permission to use it; in the case here, the something is software. Most software comes with some type of licensing, commonly known as the End User Licensing Agreement (EULA). If you have installed software, you have probably seen one. The license may have specific restrictions related to the use, modification, or duplication of the software. The Microsoft EULA, for example, specifically prohibits any kind of disassembly, inspection, or reverse engineering of software (Zymaris, 2003). Most licenses also have statements that limit the liability of the software manufacturer toward the user in case of problems that may arise in the use of the software. Again, using Microsoft as an example (solely because most readers are likely to use or have used at least one Microsoft product), the EULA removes any recourse to claims for damages arising from use of the product (Zymaris, 2003).

From this working definition of licensing, and some examples of what can be found in a EULA, we can examine copyright. While licensing gives a person the right to use software, with restrictions in some cases, copyright is described as the exclusively-granted or owned legal right to publish, reproduce, and/or sell a work (Merriam-Webster, 2004). The distinctions between ownership of the original work and rights to use it are important, and there are differences in the way the two issues are approached for proprietary software and OSS/FS. For software the "work" means the source code, or the statements made in a programming language. In general, the person who creates a work owns the copyright to it and has the right to allow others to copy it or deny that right. In some cases the copyright is owned by a company with software developers working for that company usually having statements in their employment contracts that assign copyright of their works to the company. In the case of OSS/FS, contributors to a project will often assign copyright to the managers of the project.

Based on this brief introduction to copyright and licensing, we can now examine what open source licensing means and what impacts it may have on a user or a business. Most software manufacturing companies hold the copyright for software created by their employees. In financial terms, these works are considered intellectual property, meaning that they have some value. For large software companies, such as Oracle or Microsoft, intellectual property may be a large part of their capital assets. The open source community values software differently, and OSS/FS licenses are designed to facilitate the sharing of software and to prevent an individual or organization from controlling ownership of the software. The individuals who participate in OSS/FS projects generally do realize the monetary value of what they create; however, they feel it is more valuable if the community at large has open access to it and is able to contribute back to the project.

A common misconception is that if a piece of software, or any other product, is made freely available and open to inspection and modification, then the intellectual property rights (IPR) of the originators cannot be protected, and the material cannot be subject to copyright. The open source community, and in particular the FSF, have adopted a number of conventions, some built into the licenses, to protect the IPR of authors and developers. One form of copyright, termed "copyleft" to distinguish it from commercial copyright terms, works by stating that the software is copyrighted, and then adding distribution terms. These are a legal instrument giving everyone the rights to use, modify, and redistribute the program's code or any program derived from it but only if the distribution terms are unchanged. The code and the freedoms become legally inseparable, and strengthen the rights of the originators and contributors (FSF, 2001).

Types of OSS/FS License

There is a large and growing number of OSS/FS licenses that exist. Table 6.3 shows some of the more common ones, while fuller lists of various licenses and terms can be found in Wong and Sayo (2003) and on the FSF and OSI

Web sites. The two main licenses are the GNU General Public License (GPL) and the Berkeley system distribution (BSD)-style licenses. It is estimated that about 75% of OSS/FS products use the GNU GPL (Wheeler, 2003b), and this license is designed to ensure that user freedoms under the license are protected in perpetuity, with users being allowed to do almost anything they want to a GPL program. The conditions of the license primarily affect the user when it is distributed to another user (Wong and Sayo, 2003). BSD-style licenses are so named because they are identical in spirit to the original license issued by the University of California, Berkeley. These are among the most permissive licenses possible, and essentially permit users to do anything they wish with the software, providing the original licensor is acknowledged by including the original copyright notice in source code files and no attempt is made to sue or hold the original licensor liable for damages (Wong and Sayo, 2003).

Here is an example from the GNU GPL that talks about limitations:

In no event unless required by applicable law or agreed to in writing will any copyright holder, or any other party who may modify and/or redistribute the program as permitted above, be liable to you for damages, including any general, special, incidental, or consequential damages arising out of the use or inability to use the

Table 6.3   Some Common OSS/FS Licenses

GNU GPL: A free software license and a copyleft license. Recommended by FSF for most software packages. *www.gnu.org/licenses/gpl.html*

GNU Lesser General Public License (GNU LGPL): A free software license, but not a strong copyleft license, because it permits linking with non-free modules. *www.gnu.org/copyleft/lesser.html*

X11 license: A simple, permissive noncopyleft free software license, compatible with the GNU GPL. This license is sometimes called the "MIT" license, but that term is misleading, since MIT has used many licenses for software. *http://www.x.org/ Downloads_terms.html*

Modified BSD license: The original BSD license, modified by removal of the advertising clause. It is a simple, permissive noncopyleft free software license, compatible with the GNU GPL. *http://www.xfree86.org/3.3.6/COPYRIGHT2.html#5*

W3C Software Notice and License: A free software license and is GPL compatible. *www.w3.org/Consortium/Legal/2002/ copyright-software-20021231*

MySQL database license *www.mysql.com/products/licensing/faq.html*

Apache License, Version 1.0: A simple, permissive noncopyleft free software license but incompatible with the GNU GPL. *www.apache.org/LICENSE-1.0*

GNU Free Documentation License: A license intended for use on copylefted free documentation. It is also suitable for textbooks and dictionaries, and its applicability is not limited to textual works ("books"). *www.gnu.org/copyleft/fdl.html*

Public domain: Being in the public domain is not a license, but means the material is not copyrighted and no license is needed. Public domain status is compatible with the GNU GPL.

Further information on licenses is available at *www.gnu.org/philosophy/license-list.html* and *www.opensource.org/licenses*

program (including but not limited to loss of data or data being rendered inaccurate or losses sustained by you or third parties or a failure of the program to operate with any other programs), even if such holder or other party has been advised of the possibility of such damages. (FSF, 1999)

Like the Microsoft EULA, there are limitations relating to liability in the use of the software and damage that may be caused, but unlike the Microsoft EULA, the GPL makes it clear what you can do with the software. In general, you can copy and redistribute it, sell or modify it. The restriction is that you must comply with the parts of the license requiring the source code to be distributed as well. One of the primary motivations behind usage of the GPL in OSS/FS is to ensure that once a program is released as OSS/FS, it will remain so permanently. A commercial software company cannot legally take a GPL program, modify it, and then sell it under a different proprietary license (Wong and Sayo, 2003).

In relation to using OSS/FS within a healthcare environment, as with use of any software, legal counsel should be consulted to review any license agreement made; however, in general terms, when using OSS/FS there are no obligations that would not apply to using any copyrighted work. Someone cannot legally take a body of work, the source code, and claim it as their own. The licensing terms must be followed as with any other software.

Perhaps the most difficult issue comes when integrating OSS/FS components into a larger infrastructure, especially where it may have to interface with proprietary software. Much has been said about the "viral" nature of the open source license, which comes from the requirement of making source code available if the software is redistributed. Care must be taken that components utilized in creating proprietary software either utilize OSS/FS components in such a way as to facilitate distribution of the code or avoid their use. If the component cannot be made available without all of the source code being made available, then the developer has the choice of not using the component or making the entire application open source. Some projects have created separate licensing schemes to maintain the OSS/FS license and provide those vendors that wish to integrate components without making their product open source. MySQL, a popular open source database server offers such an option (Table 6.3).

Many OSS/FS licenses have yet to be tested in legal terms, and at the time of writing, there is a legal dispute over some of the code currently in the Linux operating system kernel. SCO Group LLC has claimed that IBM illegally put some of their Unix source code in the Linux kernel and that SCO own the copyright to that code, having purchased it from Novell. Most in the open source community feel that SCO has nothing to support their case and have made many requests for SCO to identify the offending code so it can be removed from the Linux kernel. SCO, so far has allowed only those willing to sign very restrictive nondisclosure agreements to view the offending code. This is likely to be a long legal battle, but it did originally have a chilling effect on businesses that were considering using OSS/FS, specifically Linux. Concerns have subsided somewhat since there is no clear proof that SCO can win the case and some companies, such as Red Hat, have offered some indemnification, in case SCO does win. The best resource for information regarding the SCO case can be found at GrokLaw.net.

Other than this particular case, the GPL has never been tried in court. There have been instances where an individual or organization has done something that appears to be a violation of the GPL, but generally pressure from the community has either lead to a clarification of the issue or correction of the problem. The FSF has provided a way for smaller projects to get legal support, and they ask that the developer assign copyright of the software to them so that they can enforce it.

Licensing is a complex issue; we have only touched on some of the points, but in conclusion, the best advice is always to read the license agreement and understand it. In the case of a business decision on software purchase or use, one should always consult legal counsel; however, one should remember that OSS/FS licenses are more about providing freedom than about restricting use.

OSS/FS Applications

Many OSS/FS alternatives exist to more commonly-known applications. Not all can be covered here, but if one thinks of the common applications that most nurses use on a daily basis, these are likely to be:

- Operating system
- Web browser
- e-mail client
- Word processing or integrated office suite
- Presentation tools

For each of these, OSS/FS applications exist. Using OSS/FS does not require an all or nothing approach (Dravis, 2003) and much OSS/FS can be mixed with proprietary software and a gradual migration to OSS/FS is an option for many organizations or individuals. However, when using a mixture of OSS/FS and proprietary or commercial software, incompatibilities can be uncovered and cause problems whose severity must be assessed. Many OSS/FS applications have versions that will run on non-OSS/FS operating systems, so that a change of operating system, for example, to one of the many distributions of Linux, is not necessarily needed. Most OSS/FS operating systems now have graphical interfaces that look very similar to Windows or Apple interfaces.

Operating Systems: GNU/Linux

A GNU/Linux distribution (named in recognition of the GNU Project's significant contribution, but often just called Linux) contains the Linux kernel at its heart and all the OSS/FS components required to produce full operating system functionality. GNU/Linux is a term that is increasingly used by many people to cover a distribution of operating systems and other associated software components. However, Linux was originally the name of the kernel created by Linus Torvalds, which has grown from a one-man operation to now having over 200 maintainers representing over 300 organizations (Tiemann, 2003).

A kernel is the critical center point of an operating system that controls central processing unit (CPU) usage, memory management, and hardware devices. It also mediates communication between the different programs running within the operating system. The kernel influences performance and the hardware platforms that the OSS/FS system can run on, and the Linux kernel has been ported to run on almost any computing architecture, including the Playstation 2, XboX, mainframes, cell phones, and personal digital assistants (PDAs). The Linux kernel is OSS/FS, licensed under the GNU GPL.

Over time, individuals and companies began distributing Linux with their own choice of OSS/FS packages bound around Linus' kernel; the concept of the "distribution" was born, which contains much more than the kernel (usually only about 0.25% in binary file size of the distribution). There is no single Linux distribution, and many commercial distributions and freely available variants exist, with numerous customized distributions that are targeted to the unique needs of different users (Table 6.4). While all distributions contain the Linux kernel, some contain only OSS/FS materials, while others additionally contain non-OSS/FS components, and the mix of OSS/FS and other applications included and the configurations supported vary. The Debian GNU/Linux distribution is one of the few distributions that is committed to including only OSS/FS components (as defined by the open source initiative) in its core distribution.

Web Browser and Server: Apache and Mozilla

While for most people their focus may be on their client end use of applications, many rely on other, server side

---

Table 6.4 Some Common Linux Distributions

Debian (*http://www.debian.org/*): Debian GNU/Linux is a free distribution of the Linux-based operating system. It includes a large selection of prepackaged application software, plus advanced package management tools to allow for easy installation and maintenance on individual systems and workstation clusters.

Mandrakelinux (*http://www.mandrakelinux.com/en/*): Available in multiple language versions (including English, Swedish, Spanish, Chinese, Japanese, French, German, Italian, and Russian). Mandrakelinux was first created in 1998 and is designed for ease of use on servers and on home/office systems. It comes with KDE, Gnome, Window Maker, Enlightenment, and other graphical interfaces. It provides ease of use for both home/office and servers.

Red Hat (Enterprise) (*http://www.redhat.com/*): Red Hat Enterprise Linux is a high-end Linux distribution geared toward businesses with mission-critical needs.

Red Hat (Community) (*http://fedora.redhat.com/*): Fedora Core is Red Hat plan to develop a complete, general purpose operating system exclusively from FS. The distribution was created to replace low-end, consumer versions of Red Hat Linux.

SuSE (*http://www.suse.com/*): SuSE, now a subsidiary of Novell, was fist developed in 1992. It is a popular mainstream Linux distribution.

Knoppix (*http://www.knopper.net/knop*): A full-featured Linux distribution, based on Debian, that boots from a CD includes the latest versions of KDE and OpenOffice. It can be used on PCs without actually installing it, so it is ideal for demonstrations of Linux.

applications, to function. Web browsing is a prime example where both server and client side applications are needed. Web servers, such as Apache, are responsible for receiving and fulfilling requests from Web browsers. An OSS/FS application, the Apache HTTP server, developed for Unix, Windows NT, and other platforms, is currently the top Web server with 70% of the market share (over twice of its next-ranked competitor), and has dominated the public Internet Web server market ever since Apache grew to become the #1 Web server in 1996 (Wheeler, 2003a,b; NetCraft Ltd., 2004). Apache was developed in early 1995 and is an example of an OSS/FS project that is maintained by a formal structure, the Apache Software Foundation.

Mozilla is an OSS/FS graphical Web browser, designed for standards compliance, and with a large number of browser features, including support for Hypertext Markup Language (HTML) 4.0, CSS 2, JavaScript, and Java. It aims to continue Netscape Communicator as an open project and is maintained by the Mozilla Foundation and employees of several other companies, as well as contributors from the community. Mozilla is released under the NPL/MPL (Netscape/Mozilla Public Licenses) which has similarities to the GNU GPL and BSD-style licenses.

E-mail: Sendmail (E-mail Server)

The Internet as we know would not exist without e-mail and OSS/FS has been among the primary drivers. An e-mail server's function is to deliver user e-mail to its destination, and Sendmail began development in 1982 at the University of California, Berkeley, as a project to enable e-mail routing between different servers (Dravis, 2003). Sendmail is now the market leader in Internet-based e-mail systems, at 42% of all e-mail servers.

Word Processing or Integrated Office Suite: Open Office (Office Productivity Suite)

While OSS/FS products have been strong on the server side, OSS/FS desktop applications are relatively new and few. Open Office (strictly OpenOffice.org), which is based on the source code of the formerly proprietary StarOffice, is an OSS/FS equivalent of Microsoft Office, with most of its features. It includes a full-featured word processor, spreadsheet, and presentation software. One of the advantages for considering a shift from a Windows desktop environment to Open Office is that it reads most Microsoft Office documents without problems and will save documents to many formats, including Microsoft Word (but not vice versa).

This makes the transition relatively painless and Open Office has been used in recent high profile switches from Windows to Linux. Open Office has versions that will run on Windows, Linux, and other operating systems. (Note that the text for this chapter was originally written using OpenOffice.org Writer, the word processing package within the OpenOffice.org suite.)

The word "PowerPoint' has become almost synonymous with software for making conference or other presentations—even as a teaching tool. The OpenOffice.org suite contains a presentation component, Impress, which produces presentations very similar to PowerPoint; they can be saved and run in OpenOffice format on Windows or Linux desktop environments, or exported as PowerPoint versions.

Some Other OSS/FS Applications

BIND (domain name system [DNS] server)—BIND or Berkeley Internet Name Domain, is an Internet naming system. Internet addresses, such as google.com or openoffice.org, would not function if not for DNS. These servers take these human-friendly names and convert them into the computer-friendly numeric Internet Protocol (IP) addresses and vice versa. Without these servers, users would have to memorize numbers such as 202.187.94.12 in order to use a Web site.

The BIND server is an OSS/FS program developed and distributed by the University of California at Berkeley. It is incensed under a BSD-style license by the Internet Software Consortium. It runs 95% of all DNS servers including most of the DNS root servers. These servers hold the master record of all domain names on the Internet.

Perl—Practical Extraction and Reporting Language (Perl) is a high-level programming language that is frequently used for creating CGI (common gateway interface) programs. Started in 1987, and now developed as an OSS/FS project, it was designed for processing text and derives from the C programming language and many other tools and languages. It was originally developed for Unix and is now available for many platforms. Perl modules and add-ons are available to do almost anything leading some to call it the "Swiss Army chainsaw" of programming languages (Raymond, 2003).

PHP—PHP stands for PHP Hypertext Preprocessor. The name is an example of a recursive acronym (the first word of the acronym is also the acronym), a common practice in the OSS/FS community for naming applications. PHP is a server-side, HTML-embedded scripting language used to quickly create dynamically-generated Web pages. In an HTML document, PHP script (similar syntax to that of Perl or C) is enclosed within special PHP tags. PHP can perform any task any CGI program can, but its strength lies in its compatibility with many types of relational databases. PHP runs on every major operating system, including Unix, Linux, Windows, and Mac OS X and can interact with all major Web servers.

LAMP—The Linux, Apache, MySQL, PHP (LAMP) architecture has become very popular in the industry as a way of cheaply deploying reliable, scalable, and secure Web applications (the "P" in LAMP can also stand for Perl or Python). MySQL is a multithreaded, multiuser, SQL (Structured Query Language) relational database server, using the GNU GPL. The PHP-MySQL combination is also a cross-platform, i.e., will run on Windows as well as Linux servers.

OSS/FS Healthcare Applications

It is suggested that in healthcare, as in many other areas, the development of OSS/FS could provide much-needed competition to the current relatively closed market of commercial, proprietary software (Smith, 2002), and so encourage innovation but at the same time promoting interoperability, due to OSS/FS conforming more to standards and the source code being open to inspection and adaptation. This, it is suggested, would lead to lower cost, higher quality systems that are more responsive to changing clinical needs.

OSS/FS could also solve many of the problems that health information systems currently face, including lack of interoperability and vendor lock-in, costs and difficulty of record and system maintenance given the rate of change and size of the information needs of the health domain, and lack of support for security, privacy, and consent. A number of OSS/FS projects exist that seek to develop systems that will address some or all of these issues. In the case study, we will look at one project, probably the largest and most sophisticated and furthest developed, i.e., VistA. Here we will briefly examine some of the other projects that currently exist, some of which have been in development for over 10 years. Many share commonalities in trying to develop components of electronic health records (EHR) and several (e.g., CARE2X, Trusted Open Source Records for Care and Health [TORCH]) have online demonstration versions that can be explored.

openEHR

http://www.openehr.org

The openEHR Foundation is an international, not-for-profit organization that is working toward the development of interoperable, lifelong EHRs. However, it is also looking to reconceptualize the problems of health records, not in narrow IT implementation terms, but through an understanding of the social, clinical, and technical challenges of electronic records for healthcare in the information society. The openEHR Foundation was created to enable the development of open specifications, software, and knowledge resources for health information systems, in particular EHR systems. It publishes all its specifications and builds reference implementations as OSS/FS. It also develops "archetypes' and a terminology for use with EHRs.

FreeMED

http://www.freemed.org

FreeMED is the flagship product of the FreeMED Software Foundation. It is the result of many years of work in developing an OSS/FS electronic medical record (EMR) and billing system, which focuses on the needs of physicians and healthcare providers. Commercial support for FreeMED is available through the Foundation's network of Value-Added Distributors (VADs).

OpenEMR

http://www.openemr.net

openEMR is a free, open source medical clinic practice management (PM) and EMR application. OpenEMR offers a range of functions, including Practice Management features for patient scheduling and patient demographics; online EMRs; prescription writing capability with ability to e-mail or print prescriptions; HL7 support to parse HL7 messages; and ability to generate Health Insurance Portability and Accountability Act of 1996 (HIPAA)-compliant files for electronic billing.

CARE2X

http://www.care2x.com

CARE2X is one of the few OSS/FS projects to have been originated by a nurse (Elpidio Latorilla, a surgery nurse). It aims to develop a practical, integrated healthcare information system (HIS), and is designed to integrate the different information systems existing in healthcare organizations into one single efficient system. It aims to overcome the interoperability problems of many existing, or legacy systems and claims to be able to integrate almost any type of services, systems, departments, clinic, processes, data, communication, and so on that exist in a hospital.

The CARE2X Integrated Healthcare Environment integrates data, functions, and workflows in a healthcare environment. It is currently composed of four major components, each of which can also function individually: HIS, hospital/healthservice information system; PM, practice (GP) management; CDS, central data server; and HXP, Health Xchange Protocol.

Among other projects:

- TORCH (*http://www.openparadigms.com*) is a Web-enabled EHR application that aims to be scalable up to multisite practices. It has been in development since 2002 and grew out of a PM system, FreePM which itself started in 1997;

- Open Infrastructure for Outcomes (OIO— *http://www.txoutcome.org/*) is a system to facilitate the creation of flexible and portable patient/research records. The OIO server is a Web-based data management system that manages users, patients, and information about patients, while the OIO library is a metadata repository that facilitates the sharing of metadata between users and between OIO servers. The OIO library also hosts a public/open content database of open source medical software projects and related documents.

- Open Source Cluster Application Resources (OSCAR—*http://oscar.sourceforge.net*) is a Web-based family practice system supporting the needs of care delivery, teaching, and research. OSCAR is based on more than 10 years of experience with the MUFFIN PM system. OSCAR includes evidence-based decision support tools for family practice.

EU-Funded Projects

The EU has, through its R&D framework programs, funded a number of OSS/FS projects, including the following:

- SPIRIT (*http://www.euspirit.org*): SPIRIT aims to provide a virtual community and meeting place,

and include resources and services for best practice open source news and software for healthcare. The intention is to accelerate the uptake of OSS/FS and facilitate OSS/FS-based regional healthcare solutions, so supporting the delivery of better citizen-centered care in Europe and around the world.

- SMARTIE (*http://www.smartie-ist.org*): The goal of SMARTIE is to offer a comprehensive collection or "suite" of selected medical software decision tools, ranging from clinical calculators (i.e., risk factor scoring) up to advanced medical decision support tools (i.e., acute abdominal pain diagnosis).

- openECG (*http://www.openecg.net*): openECG seeks to consolidate interoperability efforts in computerized electrocardiography at the European and international levels, encouraging the use of standards. The project aims to promote the consistent use of format and communications standards for computerized ECGs and to pave the way toward developing similar standards for stress ECG, Holter ECG, and real-time monitoring.

- Open Source Medical Image Analysis (OSMIA) (*http://www.tina-vision.net/projects/osmia.php*) is a project designed to provide an OSS/FS development environment for medical image analysis research in order to facilitate the free and open exchange of ideas and techniques.

- PICNIC (*http://picnic.euspirit.org*): PICNIC was designed to develop the next generation regional healthcare networks to support new ways of providing health and social care. The aim is to prepare regional healthcare providers to implement the next generation, secure, user-friendly, healthcare networks and to make the European market for telematics healthcare services less fragmented. The region's development of scenarios on new forms of patient-centered delivery of care is supported.

- A new project "FOSS: Policy Support" (FLOSSpols—*http://flossproject.org/flosspols*) was launched in March 2004, which aims to work on three specific tracks: government policy toward OSS/FS; gender issues in open source; and the efficiency of open source as a system for collaborative problem-solving; however, it should be noted that many of these are R&D projects only and not guaranteed to have any lasting effect or uptake beyond the life span of the project.

Organizations and Resources

A growing number of organizations exist to explore and, where appropriate, advocate the use of OSS/FS within health, healthcare, and nursing. We will briefly describe the major organizations that currently exist (see Table 6.5 for further detail).

Open Source Health Care Alliance (OSHCA) is probably the oldest of the organizations, having been formally established in Summer 2000 at a meeting in Rome, Italy, although informal meetings and electronic discussion on the need for such an organization had been ongoing for some time. It holds an annual conference, has an e-mail discussion list open to anyone interested in supporting the aims and work of the organization, and is currently upgrading its Web site.

National (in all countries) and international health informatics organizations seem to have awoken late to the need to consider the potential impact of OSS/FS. The International Medical Informatics Association (IMIA) established an Open Source Health Informatics Working Group at its General Assembly meeting in October 2002. It aims to work both within IMIA and through encouraging joint work with other OSS/FS organizations to explore issues around the use of OSS/FS within healthcare and health informatics. It organized the first of a series of think-tank meetings near Winchester, United Kingdom in February 2004 (Murray, 2004) and maintains mailing lists and a Web site.

To date, few nursing or NI organizations have sought to address the implications of OSS/FS from a specific nursing perspective. The first nursing or NI organization to establish a group dealing with OSS/FS issues was the Special Interest Group in Nursing Informatics of IMIA (IMIA-NI). Established in June 2003, the IMIA-NI Open Source Nursing Informatics (OSNI) Working Group has many aims congruent with those of the IMIA OSWG, but with a particular focus on addressing nursing-specific issues where they are identified and providing the nursing contribution within multiprofessional or multidisciplinary domains. The group will provide a forum for exploring the potential of OSS/FS within nursing and NI, and will share lessons, knowledge, insights, ad so on with the wider nursing and NI communities worldwide.

Among the aims of the IMIA-NI OSNI Working Group are the following:

- To play a leading role in informing the nursing profession around the world about the potential of, and developments within, OSS/FS. A large part of the role and activities of the group over the period 2003–2006 is centered on informing and consulting with the nursing profession. The group is also involved in international activities to identify priorities for the exploration of OSS/FS (Murray, 2004). Part of its activities will be to produce an "open source for dummies' primer aimed at nurses and other health professionals, and to facilitate this, has moved its Web site to run on an OSS/FS content management system (CMS), PostNuke.

- To critically examine some of the claims, and develop recommendations and creative solutions. The group will, in particular, seek to develop links between nurses in more developed countries and those in less developed countries to share information, ideas, and solutions, and to help in the development of NI worldwide.

Summary

This chapter has provided a necessarily brief introduction to OSS/FS. While we have tried to explain the underlying philosophies of the two major camps, only an in-depth reading of explanations emanating from each can help to clarify the issues.

Many of the issues we have addressed are in a state of flux, therefore we cannot give definitive answers or solutions to many of them, as debate and understanding will have moved on. As we have already indicated, detailed exploration of licensing issues is best addressed with the aid of legal counsel. Readers wishing to develop a further understanding of OSS/FS are recommended to read, in particular, the International Open Source Network's (IOSN) Free and Open Source Software (FOSS) Primer (Wong and Sayo, 2003). Additional resources are identified in Table 6.6.

Table 6.5 Some Healthcare-Specific OSS/FS Organizations

Web site: *www.amia.org/working/os/main.html*

Secretary/contact: Ignacio Valdes— ivaldes@hal-pc.org

Web site: *www.chirad.info/imiaoswg*

Chair/contact: Dr. Peter Murray—*peter@open-nurse.info*

Web site: *www.osni.info*

Chair/contact: Dr. Peter Murray—*peter@open-nurse.info*

Web site: *www.oshca.org*

Contact: Joseph Dal Molin—*dalmolin@e-cology.ca*

Table 6.6   Information and Resource Web Sites

Linux Medical News—*www.linuxmednews.com*

The leading news resource for health and medical applications of OSS/FS. The site provides information on events, conferences and activities, software development, and any other issues that contributors feel is relevant.

SourceForge—*sourceforge.net*

SourceForge is the largest repository and development site for open source software. Many healthcare applications and other OSS/FS applications use it as the official repository of their latest versions.

 Case Study/Scenario

VistA (Veterans Health Information System and Technology Architecture)

VistA itself is not strictly open source or free software, but is released in the public domain; however, it has been promoted by many OSS/FS organizations and individuals, and some suggest it is the "mother of all healthcare applications" (Tiemann, 2004).

VistA is widely believed to be the largest integrated HIS in the world. It was originally developed and maintained by the U.S. Department of Veterans Affairs (VA), for use in veterans' hospitals, so it is public domain. Its development was based on the systems software architecture and implementation methodology developed by the U.S. Public Health Service jointly with the National Bureau of Standards. It is designed to provide a high-quality medical care environment for the country's military veterans. VistA is in production today at hundreds of healthcare facilities across the country from small outpatient clinics to large medical centers. The software is currently used by the Indian Health Service and a number of other healthcare organizations around the world. It is currently used by over 10,000 users in hospitals and clinics worldwide, including 170 veteran hospitals.

The name "VistA" dates back to 1994, when the project that had previously been known as the Decentralized Hospital Computer Program (DHCP) was renamed.

VistA has a proven track record of supporting a large variety of clinical settings and medical delivery systems, within facilities ranging from small outpatient-oriented clinics to large medical centers with significant inpatient populations and their associated specialties, such as surgical care or dermatology. Hospitals and clinics in many countries depend on it to manage such things as patient records, prescriptions, laboratory results, and other medical information. It contains, among other components, integrated hospital management, patient records management, and medical imaging systems.

Versions of the VistA system are in active use in the U.S. Department of Defense Military Health System, the U.S. Department of Interior's Indian Health Service, and internationally, including, for example, the Berlin Heart Institute of Germany (Deutsches Herzzentrum Berlin, Deutschland), and National Cancer Institute of Cairo University in Egypt.

The use of VistA has been proven to improve patient treatment outcomes in many ways, including by reducing medical errors and by ensuring that clinicians can easily access all clinically relevant patient information.

The use of VistA helps demonstrate some of the proposed benefits of OSS/FS. The costs associated with the acquisition and support of an HIS can indirectly affect the quality of healthcare provided by limiting the availability of timely and accurate access to electronic patient records. One solution is to lower the cost of acquiring an HIS by using a software stack consisting of open source, free software (OSFS). Since VistA is in the public domain and available through the U.S. Freedom of Information Act (FOIA), software license fees are not an issue with regard to its deployment.

Two projects associated with and deriving from VistA are WorldVistA and OpenVistA. WorldVistA was formed as a U.S.-based nonprofit organization, committed to the continued development and deployment of VistA. It aims to develop and support the global VistA community, through helping to make healthcare IT more affordable and more widely available both within the United States and internationally. WorldVistA extends and improves VistA for use outside its original setting through such activities as developing packages for pediatrics, obstetrics, and other hospital services not used in veterans' hospitals. WorldVistA also helps those who choose to adopt VistA successfully master, install, and maintain the software.

Historically, running VistA has required adopters to pay licensing fees for the systems on which it runs: the programming environment (Massachusetts General Hospital Utility Multi-Programming System [MUMPS]) and the operating system underneath (such as Microsoft Windows or VMS [Virtual Memory System]). OpenVistA will help its adopters eliminate these fees by allowing VistA to run on the GT.M programming environment and the Linux operating system, both of which are open source and free. By reducing licensing costs, OpenVistA frees up money to be spent on medicine, medical professionals, and other resources more likely to directly improve patient care. Like all WorldVistA projects, the OpenVistA project not only provides adopters with the software itself but also transfers knowledge and expertise and builds long-term mutual support relationships between adopters and the rest of the worldwide VistA community.

The complete OpenVistA package comprises:

- GNU/Linux operating system GT.M, an implementation of the Standard M programming system (M = MUMPS)VistA

- EsiObjects, a standards-compliant, object-relational, database management, and interoperability system

- Information on VistA, OpenVistA, and WorldVistA, and software downloads are available at a number of Web sites, including the following:
  - *http://www.va.gov/vdl/*—VistA Documentation Library
  - *http://www1.va.gov/vista_monograph/*— VistA Monograph
  - *http://sourceforge.net/projects/worldvista/*— latest versions of OpenVistA software
  - A description of the historical development of VistA is available at *http://www.worldvista. org/vista/history/index.html*

References

Bruggink, M. (2003). *Open Source in Africa: Towards Informed Decision-Making*. The Hague, The Netherlands: International Institute for Communication and Development (IICD). *http://www.comminit. com/africa/ma2004/sld-1495.html*

Cabinet Office. (2002). *Open Source Software: Use Within UK Government, Version 1*. London: Cabinet office, e-Government Unit. *http://e-government.cabinetoffice. gov.uk/assetRoot/04/00/28/41/04002841.pdf*

Dravis, P. (2003). *Open Source Software: Perspectives for Development*. Washington, DC: Global Information and Communication Technologies Department, The World Bank. *http://www.infodev.org/symp2003/ publications/OpenSourceSoftware.pdf*

European Communities. (2003a). *Cases of FlOSS Recognition or Adoption in Government and Public Administrations*. Brussels: European Commission, Directorate-General Information Society. *http://europa. eu.int/information_society/activities/opensource/cases/ index_en.htm*

European Communities. (2003b). *The IDA Open Source Migration Guidelines*. Morden, Surrey: Netproject Ltd. and Interchange of data between Administrations, European Commission. *http://europa.eu.int/ ISPO/ida/export/files/en/1618.pdf*

European Communities. (2004). *e-Europe Action Plan 2005*. Brussels: European Commission, Directorate-General Information Society. *http://europa.eu. int/information_society/eeurope/2005/all_about/action_ plan/index_en.htm*

Free Software Foundation (FSF). (1999). *GNU General Public License*. *http://www.gnu.org/copyleft/gpl.html*

Free Software Foundation (FSF). (2001). *What is Copyleft?* *http://www.gnu.org/copyleft/copyleft.html*

Free Software Foundation (FSF). (2002a). *Why 'Free Software' is Better Than 'Open Source'*. Boston, MA: Free Software Foundation. *http://www.gnu.org/ philosophy/free-software-for-freedom.html*

Free Software Foundation (FSF). (2002b). *The Free Software Definition*. Boston, MA: Free Software Foundation. *http://www.gnu.org/philosophy/free-sw.html*

Goetz, T. (2003). Open source everywhere. *WIRED*, 11:11, November, 158–167, 208–211. *http://www.wired. com/ wired/archive/11.11/opensource.html*

International Institute of Infonomics. (2002). *Free/Libre and Open Source Software: Survey and Study: FLOSS Final Report*. University of Maastricht, The Netherlands: International Institute of Infonomics. *http://www.infonomics.nl/FLOSS/report/index.htm*

LeBlanc, D.-A., Hoag, M., and Blomquist, E. (2001). *Linux for Dummies*, 3rd ed. New York, NY: Hungry Minds.

Merriam-Webster. (2004). *Merriam-Webster OnLine*. *http://ww.webster.com*

Moody, G. (2001). *Rebel Code: Inside Linux and the Open Source Revolution*. Cambridge, MA: Perseus Publishing.

Murray, P. J. (2003). Open source and free software— what's in it for nurses? *ITIN* 15:1, 15–20. *http://www. bcsnsg.org.uk/itin15/Vol 15 issue 1 March 2003 research.pdf*

Murray, P. J. (2004). Open Steps, release 1.0. *Report of a Thinktank Meeting on Free/Libre/Open Source Software in the Health and Health Informatics Domains*, Marwell, February 2004. *http://www.peter-murray.net/chiradinfo/ marwell04/marwellreportv01.htm*

Murray, P., Shaw, N., and Wright, G. (2002). Open source and health informatics: Taking forward the discussions. *British Journal of Healthcare Computing and Information Management* 19(5):14.

Netcraft Ltd. (2004). *June 2004 Web Server Survey*. *http://news.netcraft.com/archives/web_server_survey.html*

Open Source Initiative (OSI). (2004). *The Open Source Definition, Version 1.9*. *http://www.opensource.org/ docs/definition.php*

Peeling, N. and Satchell, J. (2001). *Analysis of the Impact of Open Source Software*. Farnborough: QinetiQ Ltd. *http://www.govtalk.gov.uk/interoperability/egif_ document.asp?docnum=430*

President's Information Technology Advisory Panel (PITAC). (2000). *Developing Open Source Software to*

Advance High End Computing. Arlington, VA: National Coordination Office for Computing, Information, and Communications. *http://www.itrd.gov/pubs/pitac/pres-oss-11sep00.pdf*

Raymond, E. S. (2003). *The Jargon File, Version 4.4.7. http://www.catb.org/~esr/jargon/html/S/Swiss-Army-chainsaw.html*

Raymond, E. S. (2001). *The Cathedral and the Bazaar: Musings on Linux and Open Source By An Accidental Revolutionary* (Rev. ed.). Sebastopol, CA: O'Reilly and Associates.

Shaw, N. T., Pepper, D. R., Cook, T., Houwink, P., Jain, N., and Bainbridge, M. (2002). Open Source and International Health Informatics: Placebo or panacea? *Informatics in Primary Care* 10:1:39–44.

Smith, C. (2002). *Open Source Software and the NHS: A White Paper. http://www.nhsia.nhs.uk/text/pages/features/i_250202.asp*

Stanco, T. (2001). *World Bank: InfoDev Presentation. http://lwn.net/2002/0117/a/stanco-world-bank.php3*

Surman, M. and Diceman, J. (2004). *Choosing Open Source: A Guide for Civil Society Organizations.* Toronto, Canada: Commons Group. *http://commons.ca/articles/fulltext.shtml?x=335*

The MITRE Corporation. (2003). *Use of Free and Open-Source Software (FOSS) in the U.S. Department of Defense, Version 1.2.04. http://www.microcross.com/dodfoss.pdf*

Tiemann, M. (2003). *How Open Source Works. http://www.siia.net/software/webcasts/03-13-03/default.asp*

Tiemann, M. (2004). Open Source: The solution in many countries. *Presentation at HIMSS Annual Conference and Exhibition 2004*, Orlando, FL.

Wheeler, D. A. (2003a). *Why Open Source Software/Free Software (OSS/FS)? Look at the Numbers!. http://www.dwheeler.com/oss_fs_why.html*

Wheeler, D. A. (2003b). *Make Your Open Source Software GPL-Compatible. Or Else. http://www.dwheeler.com/essays/gpl-compatible.html*

Williams, S. (2002). *Free as in Freedom: Richard Stallman's Crusade for Free Software.* Sebastopol, CA: O'Reilly and Associates.

Wong, K. and Sayo, P. (2003). *Free/Open Source Software: A General Introduction.* Kuala Lumpur, Malaysia: International Open Source Network (IOSN). *http://www.iosn.net/downloads/foss_primer_current.pdf*

Zymaris, C. (2003). *A Comparison of the GPL and the Microsoft EULA. http://www.cyber.com.au/cyber/about/comparing_the_gpl_to_eula.pdf*

Recommended Readings and Webliography

Cox, A. (1999). *The Risks of Closed Source Computing. http://www.ibiblio.org/oswg/oswg-nightly/oswg/en_US.ISO_8859-1/articles/alan-cox/risks/risks-closed-source/index.html*

DiBona, C., Ockman, S., and Stone, M. (Eds.) (1999). *Open Sources: Voices From the Open Source Revolution.* Sebastopol, CA: O'Reilly & Associates.

Murray, P. J. and Wright, G. (2003a). Open source and its implications for nursing informatics. *Tutorial Presented at NI2003, 8th International Congress of Nursing Informatics*, Rio de Janeiro, Brazil.

Murray, P. J. and Wright, G. (2003b). Open source and free software: The potential for applying open source solutions to health informatics problems in education, research and practice. *Tutorial Presented at 2003 Fall Symposium of AMIA (American Medical Informatics Association)*, Washington, DC. *http://www.chirad.info/chiradat/amia2003/t27index.htm*

Pandaveine, Y. (2000). *Open Source Resources Webpage. http://homeusers.brutele.be/ypaindaveine/opensource/inventory.html*

SDNP (2001). *Open Source, Linux and Their Importance for Developing Countries: A Very Brief Introduction. http://www.sdnp.org.gy/whyopen.html*

Stallman, R. M. (2002). *Free Software Free Society: Selected Essays of Richard M. Stallman.* Boston, MA: GNU Press/Free Software Foundation.

Wright, G. and Murray, P. J. (2002). Open source: Global issues. *Presentation at MIST2002 (Medical Informatics Symposium in Taiwan 2002)*, Taipei, Taiwan. *http://www.chirad.info/chiradat/mist2002/mist2002index.htm*

CHAPTER 7

Data Processing

Ramona Nelson

OBJECTIVES

1. Describe the relationship between the data to wisdom continuum and database systems.
2. Explain file structures and database models.
3. Describe the purpose, structures, and functions of database management systems (DBMSs).
4. Outline the life cycle of a database system.
5. Explain concepts and issues related to data warehouses in healthcare.
6. Describe the knowledge discovery in databases process (KDD) including data mining.

KEY WORDS

database
data warehouse
knowledge discovery in databases (KDD)
data mining

Nurses are knowledge workers providing care to individuals, families, and communities in the data/information intensive environment of modern healthcare. They are continually collecting data about their clients and their clients' environment. The data are organized and processed, producing information about client needs and potential interventions. Using an extensive nursing knowledge database, the information is interpreted. Nurses then use their knowledge, judgment, and wisdom to develop a plan. The goal of this plan is to provide caring cost-effective quality care to individuals, families, groups, and communities.

In modern healthcare, the process of moving from data collection to implementing and evaluating an individualized plan of care is highly dependent on automated database systems. This chapter introduces the nurse to concepts, theories, models, and issues necessary to understand the effective use of automated database systems.

Defining Data, Databases, Information, and Information Systems

Data are raw uninterrupted facts that are without meaning. For example, a patient's weight is recorded as 140 lb, without additional information this fact or datum cannot be interpreted. The patient could be a young child who is overweight or an adult who is several pounds underweight. When data are interpreted, information is produced. While data are meaningless, information by definition is meaningful. For data to be interpreted and information produced, the data must be processed. This means that the data are organized so that patterns and relationships between the data can be identified. There are several approaches to organizing data.

Some common approaches include sorting, classifying, summarizing, and calculating. For example, students will often take all of their notes and handouts from their nursing classes and organize them into folders. The folders can be located on a personal computer, placed in a box, deposited in a file cabinet, or stored in some other media. Each folder is used for a different topic. The data in the folders can be organized by nursing problems, interventions, medical diseases, cell biology, or drugs, to name but a few classifications for the information. Sometimes it is difficult to decide which folder the notes should be stored in. Students may make a copy of the notes and store it in both folders or may put the notes in one folder and a cross-reference note in the other folder. In the process of organizing the data/information a database has been created.

Another common example of a database is a checkbook used to store everyday financial data. Each number by itself means nothing; however, if the owner of the checkbook is careful to capture each entry and correctly calculates as money moves in and out of the account, the final number will summarize the current status of the checking account. This information can be very meaningful to the owner of the checkbook. If these same data are captured in a money management software package, a number of reports can be generated from these dates.

A database is an organized collection of related data. Placing notes in folders and folders in file cabinets is one example of creating a database; however, a database can be organized and stored in many different formats. A common paper example is the phone book. A much more complex example can be a patient's medical record. Each of these databases can be used to store data and to search for information. The possibility of finding information in these databases depends on several factors. Four of the most important are the following:

1. How the data are named (indexed) and organized
2. The size and complexity of the database
3. The type of data within the database
4. The methodology or tools used to search the database

The systematic approach used to name, organize, and store data in a database has a major impact on how easy it is to find information in the database. The phone book is organized alphabetically by name. This makes it very easy to find a phone number if you know the person's name and very difficult to find a person's name if you start with the phone number. A large database can be more difficult to search than a small database. The size of a database is determined not only by the amount of data in the database, but also by the number and complexity of the relationships between the data. For example, the phone book may be for a large city and require two volumes, while the patient's chart may reflect an overnight observational visit at the hospital. While the phone book may be larger, there are a minimum number of relationships between the data. Data in the patient's chart can be organized in an infinite number of ways. A wide range of caregivers will see different relationships and reach different conclusions from reading the same chart.

Information systems are used to process data and produce information. The term "information system" is often used to refer to computer systems, but this is only one type of information system. There are manual information systems as well as human information systems. The most effective and complex information system is the human brain. People are constantly taking in data and processing that data to produce meaning.

At the beginning of this chapter, there was a reference to a patient weighing 140 lb. Most people when they read that sentence begin to fill in the "missing data" or start to list their additional questions. This piece of datum is being structured and organized to produce meaning. However, each person starts with a different conceptual framework. As a result, no two people will process data in exactly the same way. While computers offer more consistency, they cannot deal with the wide range of complex data that the human mind can interpret. In healthcare, you are working with a combination of manual, automated, and human information processing systems. This offers both the advantages and disadvantages of each of these systems as well as a multitude of interface problems.

Types of Data

When developing automated database systems, each data element is defined. As part of this process, the data are classified. There are two primary approaches to classifying data in a database system. First, they are classified in terms of how these data will be used by the user. This is sometimes referred to as the conceptual view of the data. For example, the data may be classified as financial data, patient data, or human resource data. The conceptual view of the data has a major impact on how the data are indexed. Second, data are classified by their computerized data type. For example, data can be numbers or letters or a combination of both. This classification is used to build the physical database within the computer system. It identifies the number of spaces needed to capture each data element and the specific functions that can be performed on these data.

Computer-Based Data Types   Alphanumeric data include letters and numbers in any combination; however, the numbers in an alphanumeric field cannot perform numeric function. For example, an address is alphanumeric data that may include both numbers and letters. A social security number is an example of alphanumeric data made up of numbers. It makes no logical sense to add or perform any other numerical functions on either addresses or social security numbers.

The number of spaces that can be used for an alphanumeric field must be identified for the computer system. Memo is a specific type of alphanumeric data with increased spaces and decreased indexing options.

Numeric data are used to perform numeric functions including adding, subtracting, multiplying, and dividing. There are several different formats as well as types of numeric data. The number of digits after the decimal or the presence of commas in a number are examples of format options. Numeric data can be long integer, currency, or scientific.

Date and time are special types of numeric data with which certain numeric functions are appropriate. For example, two dates could be subtracted to determine how many days, months, and/or years are between the two dates. However, it would not make sense to add together several different dates.

Logic data are data limited to two options. Some examples include YES or NO, TRUE or FALSE, 1 or 2, and ON or OFF.

Conceptual Data Types Conceptual data types reflect how users view the data. These can be based on the source of the data. For example, the lab produces lab data, and the x-ray department produces image data. Conceptual data can also be based on the event that the data are attempting to capture. Assessment data, intervention data, and outcome data are examples of data that reflect event capturing.

One of the major advantages of an automated information system is that each of these data elements can be captured once and used many times by different users for different purposes. For example, a patient with diabetes mellitus has an elevated blood sugar level. This datum may be used by the physician to adjust the patient's insulin dose and used by the nurse in a patient education program. These basic data elements can also be aggregated and summarized to produce new data and information that may be used by a different set of users. This is referred to as "data collected once, used many times." Figure 7.1 gives an excellent example of this concept.

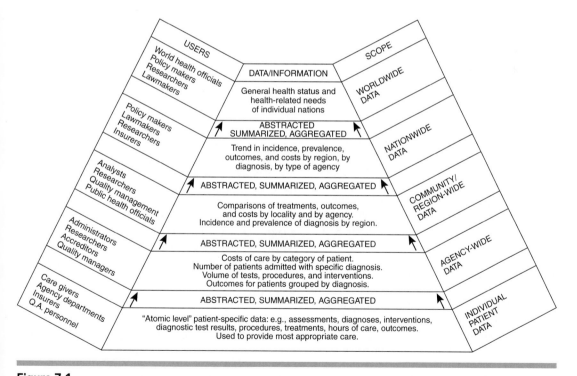

Figure 7.1

Examples of uses of atomic-level patient data collected once, used many times.

(Reprinted, with permission, from Rita D. Zielstorff, Carole I. Hudgings, Susan J. Grobe, and The National Commission on Nursing Implementation Project Task Force on Nursing Information Systems; Next-generation nursing information systems, 1993; American Nurses Publishing; American Nurses Foundation/American Nurses Association, Washington, DC).

Database Management Systems

DBMSs are computer programs used to input, store, modify, process, and access data in a database. Before a DBMS can be used, the DBM software must first be configured to manage the data specific to the project. This process of configuring the database software is called database system design. Once the software is configured for the project, the database software is used to enter the project data into the computer. A functioning DBMS consists of three interacting parts. These are the data, the DBMS configured software program, and the query language used to access the data. Some examples of DBMS in everyday life include computerized library systems, automated teller machines, and flight reservation systems. When these systems are being used, the data, the DBMS, and the query language interact together. As a result, it is easy to confuse one with the other.

Earlier in this chapter, a database was created for class notes. The notes and handouts are the data. The folders and file cabinet are the DBMS. The labels on the folders and the file cabinet are the database system design. It is possible to remove all the notes and to put new data that are unrelated to course work in the DBMS or to put the notes into a new set of folders and files. In either case, the folders and files would need to be relabeled.

The user knows how the data are organized and how to look for specific pieces of information. This makes it possible for the user to find information in the files. With a manual system, the index and query language are usually in the user's head; however, there are problems storing and finding data with a manual system. The user can forget how they classified and stored specific data. If there are two or more users the classification system becomes ever more inconsistent. Putting the data in sometimes requires duplicate copies. Once data have been stored, it is not unusual to forget where it is stored or to forget about the data completely. Automated DBMSs deal with many of these problems.

Advantages of Automated Database Management Systems   Automated DBMSs decrease data redundancy, increase data consistency, and improve access to all data. These advantages result from the fact that in a well-designed automated system all data exist in only one place. The datum is never repeated.

Data redundancy occurs when the same data are stored in the database more than once. Making a copy of class notes to store the same notes in two different folders is an example of data redundancy. In healthcare, there are many examples of data redundancy. Patients, as they are assessed by different healthcare providers, will complain that they have answered the same questions over and over. Often nurses will need to chart the same data on different forms in a patient's medical record. In a well-designed automated DBMS, the data are recorded once and accessed from this single location each time they are needed.

When the same data are stored in different manuals or automated databases, a second problem emerges. The data become inconsistent. As different users working with different databases update or change data, they do not always consistently record it in the same format. Once the data are inconsistent, it can be impossible to know the correct data. Two examples from education and healthcare may make this clearer. Many departments within a university maintain their own database with student information (i.e., address, phone number). Some of the databases are manual, and some are automated. When a student changes address, it is not unusual for that student to receive mail from the university at both the old and new address.

When a patient is admitted to a hospital, different caregivers will ask the patient to identify all medication he or she was taking at home. Sometimes the patient will list only prescription medications; other times the patient will include over-the-counter drugs taken on a routine basis. Sometimes the patient will forget to include a medication. As these different lists are recorded in different sections of the medical record, inconsistency occurs. In an automated DBMS, each caregiver is working with the same list each time the data are reviewed. With an automated DBMS, access to data becomes much easier. The database management software program uses a structured approach to organize and store data. The same software uses a query language, making it possible for the computer to do the work of searching for the data. This structured approach for storing data uses fields, records, and files.

Fields, Records, and Files

Figure 7.2 demonstrates the terms field, record, and file. Each of the blocks or cells in the table is a field. The top row lists the field names. The field name for the third column is L-name. Field names usually reflect the type of data that are stored in the related fields. For example, L-name refers to last name. In rows 2 through 5, each cell includes a field attribute. A field attribute is the specific datum for that field for that record. Each row

ID	F-NAME	L-NAME	ADDRESS-1	ADDRESS-2	CITY	ST
01	Betty	Smith	SRU, School of Nursing	20 North St	Pgh	PA
02	Leslie	Brown	DBMS Institute	408 Same St	NY	NY
03	Dori	Jones	Party Place	5093 Butler St	Any	VA
04	Glenn	Clark	Univ of Study	987 Carriage Rd		

Figure 7.2
Examples of files, records, and fields.

represents a record. For example, row 2 is the record for Betty Smith. Each row is assigned a primary identifier. A primary identifier is unique to that record. No other record in the database will have that identifier. In this table, the field name for the unique identifier is ID. The ID datum for each of these records is a unique number.

All the records in the table constitute a file. In a DBMS, there are several tables or files. A file is defined as a set of related records that have the same data fields. A database consists of several files. The DBMS can then search across the tables or files to find data related to any one entity in the database. The unique identifier is in each record in each file. It is the unique identifier that is used to tie the files together when searching across tables.

In summary, a database is made up of files, files are made up of records, records are made up of fields, and fields contain data. There are several different types of data, as discussed earlier that can be inserted in each field. The key datum used to tie the tables together and make it possible to search the total database is the unique identifier.

Types of Files

Within a DBMS, there are two basic types of files. These are the data files, as described in the previous section, and the processing files that direct the computer activities. On a personal computer, it is easy to see a list of the files that are stored on the computer. For example, on a computer using one of the Windows operating systems, click on My Computer. Then click on any of the disk drives. At this point, a list of files and folders will usually be displayed. If folders are displayed, simply open the folders by clicking on them. The name for each file will be displayed. Depending on the way the computer has been configured to display the files, there may also be additional information including the size, type, and date the file was created. Each of these files serves one of two basic purposes. There are files that direct the computer on how data are to be processed, and there are files that store data.

Processing Files

Executable files consist of a computer program or set of instructions that, when executed, causes the computer to open or start a specific computer program or function. These are the files that tell a computer what actions the computer should perform when running a program. For example, running a SET-UP.EXE file will tell the computer to begin installing the related computer program on the computer. On a personal computer, most executable files end with the extension EXE.

Command files are a set of instructions that perform a set of functions as opposed to running a whole program. For example, command files are used to boot or start the operating system when a computer is turned on. On a personal computer, some of the key command files include AUTOEXEC.BAT and CONFIG.SYS. The extension BAT indicates that the file is a specific type of command file called a batch file. A batch file contains a set of operating system commands. For example, a batch file may tell the computer to open or start a virus-checking program when the computer is booted.

Data Files

Data files contain data that have been captured and stored on a computer using a software program. Many times the extension for the file identifies the software program used to create the file. For example, a document created in Microsoft Word will have the extension DOC. Sometimes the extension indicates the format, especially if it is a standard format used across several computer programs. For example, a word processing document can be saved as "text only." This means that formatting specific to the software program is stripped off. In this case, the standard extension is TXT.

The master index file contains the unique identifier and related indexes for all entities in the database. An example is the identification file for all patient records in a healthcare system. In most cases, a master file will contain additional information that can be used to

ensure the identity of the entity. In a master index for
patient files, the additional information may include the
patient's birth date and social security number.

Database Models

A database system provides access to both the data in
the database and to the interrelationship within and
between the various data elements. Building a database
begins by identifying these data elements and the relationships that exist between the data elements. The
American National Standards Institute (ANSI)
Standards Planning and Requirements Committee
(SPARC) model has proven effective since the 1970s.
The ANSI/SPARC model identifies three views or models of the data elements and their relationships. These
three views are the users' view, the logical view, and the
physical view (Whitehorn, 2000). The first model and
the first step in building the database is to understand
the data and the data relationships from the users' perspective. This is referred to as the external or user
model. The users' view is the wish list of requirements
that the user will have for the database. It is the list of
functional specifications describing the queries, reports,
and procedures that can be produced by the database.
The user model is then used as a guide for structuring
the physical database within the computer. The common ground between the users' view and the physical
view is the conceptual model.

Conceptual Models

A conceptual model includes a diagram and narrative
description of the data elements, their attributes, and
the relationships between the data. It defines the structure

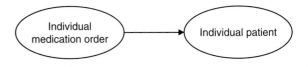

Figure 7.3
One-to-one relationship.

of the whole database in terms of the attributes of the
entities (data elements) relationships, constraints, and
operation. For example, there may be a database system
to manage patient medication orders. With each individual order, there will be several data elements. The
data elements include the specific medication, the dose,
the time and frequency of administration, the route of
administration, and any specific directions for administering the medication. Each medication order is an individual order written for one patient. This is referred to
as a one-to-one relationship. A one-to-one relationship
is diagrammed in Fig. 7.3.

While there is only one order, each order can result in
several administrations of the medication. For example,
an order for amoxicillin 500 mg q 8h × 10 days would
result in the medication being administered 30 times.
This is a one-to-many relationship. A one-to-many relationship is diagrammed in Fig. 7.4.

While Fig. 7.4 demonstrated a one-to-many relationship, a simpler form of this type of diagram is demonstrated in Fig. 7.5. Note that in Fig. 7.5 the first box,
Medication Order, includes the word "Frequency" while
the second box, Medication Administration, includes the
word "Time." It is the relationship between frequency
and time that creates the one-to-many relationship.

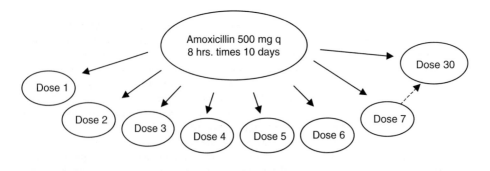

Figure 7.4
One-to-many relationship.

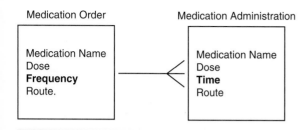

Figure 7.5
Simpler form diagramming the one-to-many relationship.

Data in a database may also have many-to-many relationships. For example, a patient may have several caregivers and each caregiver may have several patients or clients.

When completed, the conceptual data model will include a diagram of all data elements, the definition and attributes of each datum, and all relationships between data. The definitions and the description of each data attribute are used to create the data dictionary. For nursing, this has been a major challenge. Many of the data elements including nursing diagnosis, interventions, and outcomes have not been included in the data dictionaries of DBMSs used in healthcare. Nursing has had difficulty identifying and defining data elements in a format that can be used in an automated system.

In the last few years, there have been several major accomplishments in the development of nursing languages. It is now imperative that nursing leaders share these developments with database system developers in healthcare. One example of this sharing is the Nursing Information & Data Set Evaluation Center (NIDSEC) established by the American Nurses Association (ANA). NIDSEC was established to review, evaluate against defined criteria, and recognize information systems from developers and manufacturers that support documentation of nursing care within automated nursing information systems (NIS) or within computer-based patient record (CPR) systems (ANA: NIDSEC, 2004).

Conceptual data models for healthcare systems are usually very large and include several pages. Even when planning a small database for personal use developing the conceptual model is an important step. There are several questions that can be helpful in thinking through this process.

1. How will the database be used? What kind of information or output will be expected from the system? This includes both online queries and written reports.

2. What data elements need to be in the database to produce the desired output? What are the attributes of each data element? What type of data are the data elements, and how much space does each data element require? For example, a first name is an alphanumeric data type. The largest name in the database may require 25 character spaces.

3. What are easy to remember logical names for each of the data fields?

4. What approach will be used to create a unique identifier for each record in the database? Is each table designed so that there is a unique identifier for each record?

5. Is each of the tables designed so that there are no unnecessary overlapping data, and yet there are common data fields so that searches can include several tables?

Once developed, the conceptual data model provides the foundation for the physical data model.

Structural or Physical Data Models

The physical data model includes each of the data elements and the relationship between the data elements, as they will be physically stored on the computer. There are four primary approaches to the development of a physical data model. These are hierarchical, network, relational, and object-oriented. The initial database models were hierarchical and network. The relational and object-oriented are much more common today.

Hierarchical   Hierarchical databases have been compared to inverted trees. All access to data starts at the top of the hierarchy or at the root. The table at the root will have pointers called branches that will point to tables with data that relate hierarchically to the root. Each table is referred to as a node. For example, a master index might include pointers to each patient's record node. Each of the patient record nodes could include pointers to lab data, radiology data, and medication data for that patient. The patient record nodes are called parent nodes, while the lab, medication, and radiology nodes are called child nodes. In a hierarchical model, a parent node may have several children nodes, but each child node can only have one parent node.

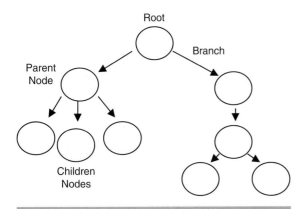

Figure 7.6
Hierarchical database model.

Figure 7.6 demonstrates a hierarchical model and the related terminology.

Hierarchical models are very effective at representing one-to-many relationships; however, they have some disadvantages. Many data relationships do not fit the one-to-many model. Remember the class notes that were put in two folders. In addition, if the data relationships change, this can require significant redesign of the database.

Network Model   Network models developed from hierarchical models. In a network model, the child node is not limited to one parent. This makes it possible for a network model to represent many-to-many relationships; however, the presence of multiple links between data does make it more difficult if data relationships change and redesign is needed.

Relational Database Models   Relational database models consist of a series of files set up as tables. Each column represents an attribute, and each row is a record. Another name for a row is "tuple." The intersection of the row and the column is a cell. The datum in the cell is the manifestation of the attribute for that record. Each cell may contain only one attribute. The datum must be atomic or broken down into its smallest format. For example, a blood pressure reading would be broken down into the systolic and the diastolic reading. Because of this limitation, the relationships represented are linear and only relate one data element to another.

A relational database joins any two or more files and generates a new file from the records that meet the matching search criteria. Figure 7.7 includes two related tables:

Table A

ID	L-NAME	F-NAME	SEX	B-DATE
12	Smith	Tom	M	01-23-73
14	Brown	Robert	M	02-01-77
13	Jones	Mary Lou	F	12-12-54
15	Yurick	Edward	M	04-04-38

Table B

ID	DX-1	DX-2	DX-3	DX-4
12	MI	CVA	GLACOMA	PVD
14	CVA	HEPATITIS C	COLITIS	UTI
13	DIABETES M	ANGINA	CVA	GOUT
15	CERF	AMENIA	GLACOMA	PEPTIC ULCER

Table C

ID	L-NAME	F-NAME	DX-1	DX-2	DX-3
12	Smith	Tom		CVA	
14	Brown	Robert	CVA		
13	Jones	Mary Lou			CVA

Figure 7.7
Relational database.

Table A and Table B. Both tables include the patient's ID number. This is the common field by which the tables can be joined. By joining these two tables, it is possible to create a new table that identifies all patients who have a diagnosis of **cerebral vascular accident** (CVA). For example, Table C is created by the DBMC in response to the query, "List all patients with a diagnosis of CVA."

While a relational database consists of multiple tables, it is possible to build a simple database with one table. This type of database is a flat file. An Excel spreadsheet is an example of a flat file. This approach is good if you have a relativity small amount of data and simple questions. For example, Excel can be used to calculate grades, convert the final number grades to letter grades, and then fill in a table with the number of A, B, C, D, and F's.

Object-Oriented Model   An object-oriented database was developed because the relational model has a limited ability to deal with binary large objects or BLOBs. BLOBs are complex data types such as images, sounds, spreadsheets, or text messages. They are large nonatomic data with parts and subparts that are not easily represented in a rational database. In object-oriented databases the entity as well as attributes of the entity are stored with the object. An object can store other objects as well. In the object-oriented model, the data definition includes both the object and its attributes. For example, amoxicillin is an antibiotic. All antibiotics have certain attributes or actions. Because amoxicillin is an antibiotic, it can be stored in the object antibiotic and inherit the attributes that are true of all antibiotics. The ability to handle nonatomic complex data and inheritance attributes are major advantages in healthcare computing.

Database Life Cycle

The development and use of a DBMS follow a systematic process called the life cycle of a database system. The number of steps used to describe this process can vary from one author to another. In this chapter, the life cycle process will be described in five steps. While the process of developing a DBMS moves forward through these steps, there is a recursive pattern to the development. Each step in the process provides the developer(s) with new insights. As these new insights occur, it is sometimes necessary to make modifications in previously completed steps of the process.

Initiation

Initiation occurs when a need or problem is identified and the development of a DBMS is seen as a potential

solution. This initial assessment looks at what is the need, what are the current approaches, and what are the potential options for dealing with the need. For example, the Staff Development Department in a home health agency may want to automate their staff education records. The current approach is to maintain an index card for each staff member. The index card lists all the programs attended by the individual staff member. When the card gets full, a second card is stapled to the first card. When the department needed to know how many total hours of staff development education had been provided monthly by each branch office for the last year, the department was required to pay staff several hours of overtime to review the cards and collect these data. The department had a computer with a DBMS software program; however, no one in the department knew how to use the program or structure the data for a database program. A decision was made to request assistance in designing a database from the Information Services Department. The nurse who organized most of the reports for the department attended in-service classes and worked with the database administrator from the Information Services Department. Now the Staff Development Department was ready to start planning for their automated DBMS.

Planning and Analysis

This step begins with an assessment of the users view and the development of the conceptual model. What are all the information needs of the department and how is the information used? This includes the internal and external uses of information. External needs for information come from outside the department. What are all the reports that the department produces? What are the requests for information that the department has been unable to fill? What information would the department like to report but has not reported because it is too difficult or time-consuming to collect the data? Internally what information does the department use in planning and/or developing educational programs? How does the department evaluate the quality of individual programs or its overall performance? How does the department evaluate the performance of individual faculty? By understanding the informational needs of the department, it is possible to identify data and the data relationships that will need to be captured in the DBMS. Diagrams and narrative reports will be used to describe the data elements, their attributes, and the overall ideal information flow in the conceptual model. A well developed conceptual model based on a careful assessment of the user's needs will be a major advantage for the database administrator. The conceptual model provides the framework for the physical model developed by the database administrator.

 Detailed Systems Design

The detailed systems design begins with the selection of the physical model: hierarchical, network, relational, or object-oriented. Using the physical model, each table and the relationships between the tables are developed. At this point, the data entry screens and the format for all output reports will be carefully designed. The users in the department must validate the data entry screens and output formats. It is often helpful to use prototypes and screen shoots to get user input during this stage. Revisions are to be expected.

Implementation

Implementation includes training the users, testing the system, developing a procedure manual for use of the system, piloting the DBMS, and finally "going live." The procedure manual outlines the "rules" for how the system is used in day-to-day operations. For example, what is the procedure for recording attendance at individual classes, and when is the attendance data to be provided to the data entry clerk? In going live with a database system, one of the difficult decisions is how much previous data must be loaded into the DBMS. The initial request that stimulated the development of the DBMS would have required at least 1 year of previous data to be loaded into the automated database system.

Evaluation and Maintenance

When a new database system has been installed, the developers and the users can be very anxious to immediately evaluate the system. Initial or early evaluations may have limited value. It will take a few weeks or even months for users to adjust their work routines to this new approach to information management. The first evaluations should be informal and focus more on troubleshooting specific problems. Once the system is up and running and users have adjusted to the new information processing procedure, they will have a whole new appreciation of the value of a DBMS. At this point, a number of requests for new options can be expected.

Common Database Operations

DBMSs vary from small programs running on a personal computer to massive programs that manage the data for large international enterprises. No matter what size or how a DBMS is used, there are common operations that are performed by all DBMSs. There are three basic types of data processing operations. These include data input, data processing, and data output. The relationship between these operations is demonstrated in Fig. 7.8.

Data Input Operations

Data input operations are used to enter new data, update data in the system, or change/modify data in the DBMS. Data are usually entered through a set of screens that have been designed for data entry. A well-designed

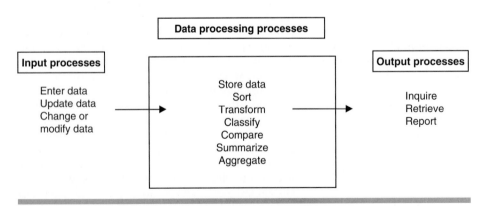

Figure 7.8
Common data processing operations.

screen will discourage data entry errors. In addition, the program can be designed to alert the user to potential errors or to prevent obvious data entry errors. It may not accept data that are out of range. For example, if someone tried to enter a blood pressure of 60/180, the system would issue an error message. The error message can be in the form of a sound or a text message on the screen. It is important that text messages are clear and help the user correct the error.

Sometimes data are entered that are unusual but could be correct. For example, a drug dose could be higher than normally recommended for that drug. In these cases, the system may be designed to offer an alert and request that the user reenter the data to confirm its accuracy. It is important to evaluate how the alert should function. For example, if this is a clerical office dealing with numerical data, there may be no problem with having the clerk reenter the data; however, if this is an intensive care unit, where drug doses are often higher than the recommended dose in textbooks, requiring busy caregivers to repeatedly reenter data may not be a good idea.

One of the most common errors involves inconsistent data entry formats. For example, one user may use all capitals when entering text data. Another user may use a combination of capitals and lowercase letters. If the DBMS is case-sensitive, this inconsistent data entry will have a major impact on query results. When data entry errors are of major importance, programs can be designed for double entry of all data. The first and second entries of the data are compared, and if there is a difference, the system issues an alert. With this approach, the user usually is required to reenter data. This type of an approach is more likely to be used with a research study as opposed to a clinical unit.

Database systems also let the user update, modify, or change data that has been previously entered into the system. Depending on the design of the DBMS, the original data may be overwritten and lost, or the original data may be saved in a separate file. With patient data, it is important to be able to track all data modifications. This should include who changed the data, what were the original data, and what modification was made to the data. It may also include why the data were changed.

Data Processing Processes

Data processing processes are DBMS-directed actions that the computer performs on the data once entered into the system. It is these processes that are used to convert raw data into meaningful information. These include common database functions discussed previously in this chapter. In large databases these are processes referred to as online transaction processing (OLTP). OLTP are defined as real-time processing of transactions to support the day-to-day operation of the institution.

Data Output Operations

This section includes online and written reports. The approach to designing these reports will have a major impact on what information the reader actually gains from the report. Reports that are clear and concise help the reader see the information in the data. On the other hand, poorly designed reports can mislead and confuse the reader.

The development of a database system within a department serves two important purposes. First, both the developers and the users create a new level of knowledge and skill. Second, as individual departments develop databases, institutional data are being created; however, if each department develops its individual database system, in isolation, islands of automation are then developed.

 ## The Development of Data Warehouses

Healthcare institutions have been automating their processes and developing databases since the mid-1960s. In most institutions, this process began in two areas, the financial department and in departmental systems. Some of the oldest and most developed departmental systems are in the labs, radiology, medical records, and cardiac departments. Initially, these systems developed as islands of automation that were focused on the operational needs of the individual department. The development of these systems and the interfaces between these systems were strongly influenced by the free-for-service approach to financing healthcare.

Room charges are a primary concern in a financial system for a hospital information system (HIS). For financial systems to function, they needed to track patients. When admission, discharge, and transfer (ADT) modules were added to the financial systems, this automated the process of room charges. However, in a hospital there are a number of other services that involve charges. Most of these services originate with a physician order. This stimulated the development of order entry systems. For most institutions, the financial system with charges and billing was closely tied to the ADT and order entry systems. In many cases, the same vendor offered these applications and interface problems were minimal. However, the order entry systems needed to interface with departmental systems.

One of the first approaches was to simply have the computer generate a printed copy of the order requisition in the department. This was then manually entered into the department system. Developing a computer interface with the department where the order entry system on the clinical units could "talk to" the department systems was a problem. Because the departmental systems had been developed independently, they used different naming and coding structures. The databases reflected different architectures. This was true for systems developed by the same vendors and was even more of a problem for systems that had been developed by different vendors.

Think back to the example of organizing class notes. What if several students agreed to share their class notes, but they maintained their notes in their own room and had their own filing system? Some of the students may have organized the content by courses, while others may have organized it by years, and still others set up their total filing systems by topic. Because the notes were stored in individual rooms, each student who wanted to use another student's notes would need to send a request to the other student(s).

Attempts to share data by building interfaces across automated systems in healthcare institutions shared many of the same problems as the student example. In healthcare institutions where interfaces needed to go from the order entry system to **all** departments, the problem was compounded. Of course, any change or update to any of the department computer programs required that changes be made to the interface. This could impact any of the other departmental systems.

While order entry systems automated the manual process for charging, which was a major advantage for the financial department, the results-reporting module of these systems proved to be very valuable to caregivers. The results-reporting module sent information back to the clinical units with the results of various tests and examinations. This was especially useful for lab results. Without automation, stat lab results had to be phoned back to the clinical units and manually dictated. Online lab results made it possible for nurses and doctors to make clinical decisions based on the latest information; however, each department system that could send results back to the clinical units functioned

independently. Users had to learn how to use each system, and there was no way that the results from different departments could be viewed in an integrated fashion. The departmental systems were used to meet the day-to-day operational needs of the institution. Data were not stored on a long-term basis. Due to systems' storage requirements, the data in the systems were usually purged within a set number of days after the patient left the hospital.

In the late 1980s and early 1990s, a number of changes stimulated the development of the data warehouse concept. Computer systems became much more powerful. Database theory and products were much more sophisticated. Users were becoming computer-literate and developing more requirements. A core of healthcare informatics leaders had developed. The Institute of Medicine issued its report on the CPR (Dick and Steen, 1991). The move away from fee-for-service to managed care created a new set of information needs. Systems no longer needed to track the charges for services but now needed to report the actual cost of providing health services. Historical data within the computer systems took on a new value. Analyzing historical data for the institution required that data from each of the systems be collected and stored in a common storage system called a data warehouse.

A data warehouse is defined as a large collection of data imported from several different systems within one database. The source of the data includes not only internal data from the institution but can also include data from external sources. For example, data related to standards of practice could be imported into a data warehouse and used to analyze how the institution achieved a variety of goals related to these standards. Smaller collections of data are referred to as data marts. A data mart might be developed with the historical data of a department or a small group of departments. A data mart can also be developed by exporting a subset of the data from the data warehouse.

Bill Immon, the father of the data warehouse concept, defined a data warehouse as a subject-oriented, integrated, time variant, nonvolatile collection of data used to support the management decision-making process (Lambert, 1999). In healthcare, management includes management of the client/patient as well as the healthcare institution. While operational databases use current data to support the day-to-day operation of the institution, a data warehouse uses historical data to discover new relationships within the data. These new relationships can support decision-making and strategic planning.

Purposes of a Data Warehouse

The development of a data warehouse requires a great deal of time, energy, and money. An organization's decision to develop a data warehouse is based on several goals and purposes. Because of its integrated nature a data warehouse spares users from the need to learn several different applications. For example, a warehouse no longer requires healthcare providers to access the lab reporting system to see lab work and use a different application with a different interface to view radiology results. When users are viewing several different applications there are several different "versions of the truth." These can result from looking at the database at different times as well as the use of different definitions. For example, the payroll database may show a different number of nurses on staff than the automated staffing system. That is because the payroll would include nurses in administrative positions; however, the staffing system may only include the nurses assigned to patient care.

These types of definitions are decided in building the warehouse and provide a more consistent approach to making decisions based on the data. A data warehouse makes it possible to separate the analytical and operational processing. With this separation the architectural design of the data warehouse is designed to support decisional information needs. The user can slice and dice the data from different angles and at different levels of detail (Humphries, Hawkins, and Dy, 1998).

Functions of a Data Warehouse

The management of a data warehouse requires three types of programs. First the data warehouse must be able to extract data from the various computer systems and import that data into the data warehouse. This is a key point for nursing. If nursing data are not in the various computer systems or do not exist in any standardized format, they cannot be extracted and imported into the data warehouse. Nursing data are not limited to the data that nurses generate but include all the data that nurses use for client care, administration, research, and education.

Furthermore, the data definitions that were established in the original computer systems must now be revised so that the data from the different systems can be integrated. For example, does the data definition for patient problem(s) include all problems identified by all professional caregivers, or is it limited to the medical diagnosis?

Second, the data warehouse must function as a database able to store and process all of the data in the database. This includes the ability to aggregate the data and process the aggregated data. For example, the operational database systems used to manage the institution on a day-to-day basis do not usually offer the opportunity to look at data over time, yet a data warehouse supports integration of data and the analysis of trends over time. The individual data elements that are imported into the warehouse are referred to as primary data. The aggregate data produced by the warehouse database system are referred to as secondary data or derived data.

Third, the data warehouse must be able to deliver the data in the warehouse back to the users in the form of information.

Information from a data warehouse is used for decision support systems and executive information systems. These systems show the "big picture" as well as trends over time. For example, the data in a data warehouse may demonstrate that patients with diabetes who attend a diabetic education class increase their number of clinic or office visits. The data may also demonstrate that these same patients show a decrease in their number of hospitalizations and an overall decrease in cost of care. In reviewing these data, the patient manager may need to "drill down" into the data. Does this summary apply to all patients, or are there select groups of patients who are gaining this benefit? It may be that adolescents do not demonstrate this benefit and that a different approach is needed for this group of patients.

Data from a data warehouse can be used to support a number of activities including (AHIMA, 1998):

1. Decision support for caregivers at the point of care
2. Outcome measurements and quality improvement
3. Clinical research and professional education
4. Reporting to external agencies, e.g., Joint Commission on Accreditation of Health Care Organizations
5. Market trend analysis and strategic planning
6. Health services management and process reengineering
7. Targeted outreach to patients, professionals, and other community groups

Quality of the Data

In a data warehouse, data are entered once but used by many users for a number of different purposes. As a result, the quality of the data takes on a whole new level of importance. In addition, the concept of data ownership changes. When dealing with a department information system, the department is usually seen as owning the data and being responsible for the quality of that data. For example, one might expect nurses to be responsible for the quality of data in a nursing information system.

However, when one is responsible for the data in a data warehouse, the concept of a data steward is more appropriate. A data steward does not own the data but ensures its quality. He or she is the "keeper of the data," not the "owner of the data." The data steward must work with the departments that generate the data to ensure the quality of the data coming into the warehouse. In addition, the data steward is responsible for working with caregivers and administrative personnel to develop naming standards, entity and attribute standards, rule specifications, data security specifications, and retention specifications (Imhoff, 1998).

Data to Knowledge (D2K)

Rapid advances in data capture and storage have resulted in huge increases in the amount of data that can be stored in a data warehouse. Traditional analyses of these data using human experts who manually analyze the data are no longer adequate (ALG, 2004a). The process of extracting information and knowledge from large-scale databases has been referred to as knowledge discovery and data mining (KDD) or D2K applications. AGL used this approach to coin the term Image to Knowledge (I2K) when referring to the mining of imaging data. While some authors use the term data mining and D2K interchangeably, others consider data mining one step in the D2K process. D2K uses powerful automated approaches for the extraction of hidden predictive information from large databases. These approaches make it possible to automate the prediction of trends and patterns as well as the discovery of previously unknown trends (Thearling, 2004).

D2K begins by carefully assessing the questions that users need answered. Without a clear objective data mining can produce an overload of data as opposed to information or knowledge. The second step is to prepare the data. The data must be selected, cleaned, and transformed into a consistent format. With clinical data this is a major process. For example, an MI or a myocardial infarction must be identified as the same event.

Once the data have been prepared, data mining processes can be applied to the data. There are a variety of data mining methods. These methods have been grouped into three types of data mining processes including data modeling, data discovery, and deviation detection. See Table 7.1 (ALG, 2004b). For example, if one was using data modeling to analyze medication errors the third step in the D2K process would be to

Table 7.1   Data Mining Processes

Approach	Description	Examples of Methods
Predicting	Discovering variables that predict or classify a future event	Decision tree Neural networks
Discovery	Discovering patterns, associations, or clusters within a large dataset	Apriori fractionalization
Deviation	Discover the norm via pattern recognition and then discover deviations from this norm	Scatterplots Parallel coordinates

build a model that would answer medication questions using known data. The model would include a number of variables that could influence the number and type of medication errors within an institution. Some variables include staffing ratios, number of medications to be given, presence of new or novice staff, and number of new medications. This information is used to build a model that predicts when medication errors can be expected to increase or decrease. The model is then applied to real data where the number and type of errors are known. Adjustments are made to the formulas and assumptions in the model until the model is able to predict the correct results.

The final step in the D2K process is to interpret, evaluate, and use the data mining results within the institution. In our example, once the model has been adjusted to predict correct results, it is then installed and issues an alert if a situation is developing where medication errors can be expected to increase.

The D2K process has been formalized in the cross industry standard process for data mining or the CRISP-DM model for data mining. While the CRISP-DM model is an international cross industry model it is now being applied to data mining within healthcare (Hogl et al., 2001). The CRISP-DM model describes the life cycle of a data mining project in six phases:

1. Understanding the business

2. Understanding the data

3. Data preparation

4. Modeling

5. Evaluation

6. Deployment

Key to this model is the idea that data mining requires individuals who are expert in data mining processes as well as individuals who are expert in understanding the business and data. For data mining to be successfully used in nursing, nurses who understand current issues in managing nursing data must be involved in the project. To date there have been few uses of data mining in nursing (Berger and Berger, 2004); however, Abbott's work with long-term care and Goodwin's research with preterm birth both demonstrate the potential of data mining for nursing (Abbott, 2000; Goodwin, 2001).

 The Nursing Context

This chapter began with a discussion of database concepts and ends with a discussion of how knowledge can be mined from huge data sets in a large data warehouse.

The basic concepts presented are not unique to nursing but as demonstrated by the Abbott and Goodwin research have a major impact on nursing. The context for understanding this impact can be seen in the data to wisdom continuum (Nelson, 2002) (Fig. 7.9).

The continuum begins with data, the raw facts. As the data are named, collected, and organized, it becomes information. By discovering the meaningful facts in the information and the relationships between the facts a knowledge base is built. By understanding the knowledge and the implications of that knowledge nurses are able to manage a wide range of human health problems. The appropriate and ethical use of knowledge to manage human problems is termed wisdom.

Databases and data mining makes possible to view, analyze, and understand new patterns and relationships. But understanding the implications of these patterns and relationships requires nursing wisdom. For example, the

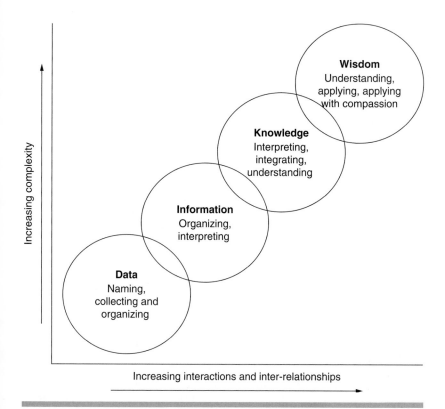

Figure 7.9
The Nelson data to wisdom continuum.
(Reprinted with permission from Englebardt, S. and Nelson, R. (2002). *Health Care Informatics: An Interdisciplinary Approach*. Figure 1-4, p. 13, Elsevier.)

CRISP-DM model of data mining requires experts who understood the business and the data. It is at the level of wisdom one becomes concerned with the ethical use of information and knowledge. Understanding the ethical implications of the new knowledge is termed infoethics (Layman, 2003).

Summary

This chapter describes data processing. The focus of the chapter is on understanding concepts and issues necessary to effectively use database systems in healthcare. The chapter began by discussing the difference between data and information. The process of using an information system to produce information from data was described. The chapter explained data structures and models. The purpose(s), structures, and functions of automated database systems are reviewed. The life cycle of an automated database system is outlined. Building on an understanding of databases the chapter explores concepts and issues related to data warehouses and knowledge discovery within large datasets. The chapter concludes by describing how an understanding of databases is key to understanding the data to wisdom continuum in nursing.

References

Abbott, P. (2000). The challenge of data mining in large nursing home data sets. *ITIN* 12:9–14.

AHIMA. (1998). Data resource administration: The road ahead. *Journal of AHIMA-Practice Briefs* 69–10. http://library.ahima.org/xpedio/groups/public/documents/ahima/pub_bok1_000057.html

Automated Learning Group (ALG). (2004a). *About ALG.* http://alg.ncsa.uiuc.edu/do/aboutAlg

Automated Learning Group. (2004b). *ALG D2K Toolkit Users Manual.* Located May 2004 at http://alg.ncsa.uiuc.edu/tools/docs/d2k/manual/index.html

ANA:NIDSEC. (2004). *Nursing Information Data Set Evaluation Center.* Located at http://nursingworld.org/nidsec/index.htm

Berger, A. and Berger, C. (2004). Data mining tools for research and knowledge development in nursing. *CIN* 22(3):123.

Dick, R.S. and Steen, E.B. (1991). *The Computer-Based Patient Record: An Essential Technology for Health Care.* Washington, DC: National Academy Press.

Goodwin, L., Iannacchione, M.A., Hammond, W.E., Crockett, P.W., Maher, S. and Schlitz, K.C. (2001). Data mining methods find demographic predictors of preterm birth. *Nursing Research* 50(6):340–345.

Hogl, O., Muller, M., Stoyan, H., and Stuhlinger, W. (2001). Using questions and interests to guide data

mining for medical quality management. *Topics in Health Information Management* 22(1):38.

Humphries, M., Hawkins, M., and Dy, M.C. (1998). *Data Warehousing: Architecture and Implementation.* Upper Saddle River, NJ: Prentice Hall.

Imhoff, C. (1998). Ensuring data quality through data stewardship. *DM Review.* http://www.dmreview.com/issues/1998/apr/apr98index.htm

Lambert, B. (1999). Data warehousing fundamentals: What you need to know to succeed. *DM Review.* http://www.datawarehouse.com/resources/articles/

Layman, E. (2003). Health informatics: Ethical issues. *Health Care Manager* 22(1):2–15.

Nelson, R. (2002). Major theories supporting health care informatics. In S. Englebardt and R. Nelson (Eds.), *Health Care Informatics: An Interdisciplinary Approach.* St. Louis, MO: Mosby.

Thearling, K. (2004). *An Introduction to Data Mining: Discovering the Hidden Value in Your Data Warehouse.* Accessed May 2004, from http://www3.shore.net/~kht/text/dmwhite/dmwhite.htm

Whitehorn, M. (2000). Models help database users and builders work together. *IT Week (UK)* V3(i38):36.

Zielstorff, R., Hudgings, C. Grobe, S., and NCNIP. (1993). *Next-Generation Nursing Information Systems: Essential Characteristics for Professional Practice.* Washington, DC: American Nursing Publishing.

Bibliography

Andersen, C.M. and Emery, L.J. (1998). Interdisciplinary team teaching of database management. *Occupational Therapy in Health Care* 11(2):45.

Arthur, P. (1997). Demonstrating value through information management: Database decision support for physical therapy practice. *Resource* 27(1):12.

Banerjee, K. (1998). Is data mining right for your library? *Computers in Libraries* 18(10):28–31.

Beck, C.T. (1996). The practical computer: Use of a meta-analytic database management system. *Nursing Research* 45(3):181.

Bedard, Y. and Henriques, W.D. (2002). Modern information technologies in environmental health surveillance: An overview and analysis. *Canadian Journal of Public Health. Revue Canadienne de Sante Publique* 93(Suppl. 1):S29–S33.

Brossette, S.E., Sprague, A.P., Hardin, J.M., Waites, K.B., Jones W.T., and Moser, S.A. (1998). Association rules and data mining in hospital infection control and public health surveillance. *Journal of the American Medical Informatics Association* 5(4):373–81.

Burch, J., Strater, F.R., and Grudnitski, G. (1983). *Information Systems: Theory and Practice* (3rd ed.). New York: Wiley.

Burnard, P. (1996). Using a database for managing interview data. *Professional Nurse* 11(9):578.

Button, P.S. (1997). Computers in practice: Challenges and uses-using standardized nursing nomenclature in an automated careplanning and documentation system. In M.J. Rantz, et al. (Eds.), *Classification of Nursing Diagnoses: Proceedings of the Twelfth Conference, North America Nursing Diagnosis Association* (p. 327). Glendale, CA: CINAHL Information Systems.

Callan, K. (2000). Preparing for a decision support system. *Topics in Health Information Management* 21(1):84–90,

Carpenter, I. (1997). Addressing the problems of care services for the elderly with a database of primary clinical data. *British Journal of Healthcare Computing & Information Management* 14(10):16.

Catrambone, C. (1995). Creating database links between nursing diagnoses and nursing activities. *Issues* 16(1):8.

Chang, B.L. (1993). CARIN system–database for Bayes' Theorem applications. . . computer-aided research in nursing. *Western Journal of Nursing Research* 15(5):644.

Cheek, J., Gillham, D., and Mills, P. (1998). Using clinical databases in tertiary nurse education: An innovative approach to computer technology. *Nurse Education Today* 18(2):153.

Cheung, R.B., Moody, L.E., and Cockram, C. (2002). Data mining strategies for shaping nursing and health policy agendas. *Policy, Politics, & Nursing Practice* 3(3):248–60.

Chu, S.C. and Thom, J.B. (1997). Database issues in object-oriented clinical information systems design. In U. Gerdin, et al. (Eds.), *Nursing Informatics: The Impact of Nursing Knowledge on Health Care Informatics. . .Proceedings of NI'97, Sixth Triennial International Congress of IMIA-NI, Nursing Informatics of International Medical Informatics Association* (p. 376). Amsterdam, The Netherlands: IOS Press.

Coenen, A. and Wake, M. (1996). Developing a database for an international classification for nursing practice. *International Nursing Review* 43(6):183.

Courtney, R. and Rice, C.A. (1995). Using an encounter form to develop a clinical database for documenting nurse practitioner primary care. *Journal of the American Academy of Nurse Practitioners* 7(11):537.

Crothers, D., Ramachandran, S., and Giles, P. (1997). Measuring clinical performance: Database effectiveness in a coronary heart disease prevention programme. *British Journal of Healthcare Computing & Information Management* 14(8):19.

Cullen, P.P. (2001). Feature selection methods for intelligent systems classifiers in healthcare. Chicago, IL: Loyola University of Chicago Ph.D. (p. 247)

del Hoyo-Barbolla, E. and Lees, D. (2002). The use of data warehouses in the healthcare sector. *Health Informatics Journal* 8(1):43–46.

Delaney, C. and Moorhead, S. (1995). The Nursing Minimum Data Set, standardized language, and health care quality. *Journal of Nursing Care Quality* 10(1):16.

Denwood, R. (1996). Data capture for quality management nursing opportunity. *Computers in Nursing* 14(1):39.

Dillon, W.P. and Arenson, R.L. (2002). Design and applications of a multimodality image data warehouse framework. *Journal of the American Medical Informatics Association* 9(3):239–254

Dobrzykowski, E.A. and Nance, T. (1997). The Focus On Therapeutic Outcomes (FOTO) Outpatient Orthopedic Rehabilitation Database: Results of 1994–1996. *Journal of Rehabilitation Outcomes Measurement* 1(1):56.

Elfrink, V. (2001). A look to the future: How emerging information technology will impact operations and practice. *Home Healthcare Nurse* 19(12):751–757, 785–786.

Enkin, M.W. (1995). Effective care in pregnancy and childbirth: The Cochrane Pregnancy and Childbirth Database. *Journal of Perinatal Education* 4(4):23.

Epstein, I. (2001). Using available clinical information in practice-based research: Mining for silver while dreaming of gold. *Social Work in Health Care* 33(3/4):15–32.

Fisk, J.M., Mutalik, P., Levin, F.W., Erdos, J., Taylor, C., and Nadkarni, P. (2003). Integrating query of relational and textual data in clinical databases: A case study. *Journal of the American Medical Informatics Association* 10(1):21–38.

Forgionne, G.A., Gangopadhyay, A., and Adya, M. (2000). Cancer surveillance using data warehousing, data mining, and decision support systems. *Topics in Health Information Management* 21(1):21–34.

Forgionne, G.A., Gangopadhyay, A., and Adya, M. (2000). Cancer surveillance using data warehousing, data mining, and decision support systems. *Topics in Health Information Management* 21(1):21–34.

Friedman, D.J., Anderka, M., Krieger, J.W., Land, G., and Solet, D. (2001). Accessing population health information through interactive systems: Lessons learned and future directions. *Public Health Reports* 116(2):132–141.

Gooch, P.M. (1996). Databases: Hom-Inform bibliographic database and information service for homoeopathic literature. *Complementary Therapies in Medicine* 4(1):63.

Goodwin, L.K. and Iannacchione, M.A. (2002). Data mining methods for improving birth outcomes prediction. *Outcomes Management* 6(2):80–85.

Goodwin, L. (1997). Data mining for improved patient care outcomes. *Tar Heel Nurse* 59(4):21.

Guyer, S. (2000). Clinical data repositories: An overview. *Nursing Case Management* 5(1):2–12.

Hoffman, P. (2001). Developing & using management reports under PPS. *Caring* 20(11):6–8.

Horton, B.J., Revak, G.R., and Jordan, L.M. (1994). The computer database for nurse anesthesia education programs. *AANA Journal* 62(3):234.

Hudson, R. and Bowen, C. (1997). Clinical audit database. *Health Visitor* 70(6):223.

Hutson, C. and Lichtiger, E. (2001). Mining clinical information in the utilization of social services: Practitioners inform themselves. *Social Work in Health Care* 33(3/4):153–161.

Jacobson, T. (1996). Standardized ET nursing database: Imagine the possibilities. *Journal of WOCN* 23(1):5.

Jacox, A. (1995). Practice and policy implications of clinical and administrative databases. In *An Emerging Framework: Data System Advances for Clinical Nursing Practice* (p. 161). Washington, DC: American Nurses Association Publications.

Johns, M. (2001). *Information Management for Health Professionals*. New York: Delmar Publishers.

Jones, J.K. (2001). The role of data mining technology in the identification of signals of possible adverse drug reactions: Value and limitations. *Current Therapeutic Research, Clinical & Experimental* 62(9):664–672.

Joos, I., Whitman, N.I., Smith, M.J., and Nelson, R. (2000). *Computers in Small Bytes*. New York: Jones and Bartlett.

Kuehn, A.F. (1998). Establishing an advanced practice nurse database: A four-phase comprehensive study. *Missouri Nurse* 67(3):12.

Lang, N.M., Hudgings, C., Jacox, A., et al. (1995). Toward a national database for nursing practice. In *An Emerging Framework: Data System Advances for Clinical Nursing Practice*. Washington, DC: American Nurses Association Publications.

Lange, L.L. and Jacox, A. (1993). Using large data bases in nursing and health policy research. *Journal of Professional Nursing* 9(4):204.

Lee, F.W. (1996). Technology–how to use entity-relationship diagrams in developing personal database systems. *Journal of American Health Information Management Association* 67(2):42.

Liao, S. and Lee, I. (2002). Appropriate medical data categorization for data mining classification techniques. *Medical Informatics & the Internet in Medicine* 27(1):59–67.

Loebl, D., Willems, B., and Nordin, M. (1995). Database analysis of injury patterns in an institution for developmental disabilities. *Journal of Occupational Rehabilitation* 5(3):169.

Marlett, J.D. and Cheung, T. (1997). Perspectives in practice. Database and quick methods of assessing typical dietary fiber intakes using data for 228 commonly consumed foods. *Journal of the American Dietetic Association* 97(10):1139.

McDaniel, A.M. (1997). Developing and testing a prototype patient care database. *Computers in Nursing* 15(3):129.

Melillo, K.D. and Futrell, M. (1995). A guide for assessing caregiver needs: Determining a health history database for family caregivers. *The Nurse Practitioner* 20(5):40.

Mirabito, D.M. (2001). Mining treatment termination data in an adolescent mental health service: A quantitative study. *Social Work in Health Care* 33(3/4):71–90.

Moseley, L.G. and Mead, D.M. (1993). Good relations: The use of a relational database for large-scale data analysis. *Journal of Advanced Nursing* 18(11):1795.

Myers, D.L., Burke, K.C., Burke, J.D., Jr., and Culp, K.S. (2000). An integrated data warehouse system: Development, implementation, and early outcomes. *Managed Care Interface* 13(3):68–72.

Mylod, D.E., and Kaldenberg, D.O. (2000). Data mining techniques for patient satisfaction data in home care settings. *Home Health Care Management & Practice* 12(6):18–29.

Neumann, L. (2003). Streamlining the supply chain. *Healthcare Financial Management* 57(7):56–62.

Ohrn, A. and Rowland, T. (2000). Rough sets: A knowledge discovery technique for multifactorial medical outcomes. *American Journal of Physical Medicine & Rehabilitation* 79(1):100–108.

Oliveira, J. (2001). The balanced scorecard: An integrative approach to performance evaluation. *Healthcare Financial Management* 55(5):42, 44–46.

Orton, J.A., Jacobson, J.T., and Haug, P.J. (2003). Automation of performance measures reporting. *Journal for Healthcare Quality* 25(5):21–27.

Oyri, K. (1997). Workload measurement in the ICU. In U. Gerdin, et al. (Eds.), *Nursing Informatics: The Impact of Nursing Knowledge on Health Care Informatics. . . Proceedings of NI' 97, Sixth Triennial International Congress of IMIA–NI, Nursing Informatics of International Medical Informatics Association* (p. 512). Amsterdam, The Netherlands: IOS Press.

Ozbolt, J.G. (1995). From minimum data to maximum impact: Using clinical data to strengthen patient care. *Advanced Practice Nursing Quarterly* 1(4):62.

Ozbolt, J.G., Fruchtnicht, J.N., and Hayden, J.R. (1994). Toward data standards for clinical nursing information. *Journal of the American Medical Informatics Association* 1(2):175.

Pheby, D.F.H. and Thorne, P. (1994). The Medical Data Index (MDI) dependency module: A shared database to assist discharge planning and audit. *Journal of Advanced Nursing* 20(2):361.

Picella, D.V. (1996). Use of relational database program for quantification of the CNS role. *Clinical Nurse Specialist* 10(6):301.

Pohlmann, B. (1995). The Department of Veterans Affairs experience: Development of a database for the patient problem list. In *An Emerging Framework: Data System Advances for Clinical Nursing Practice* (p. 185). Washington, DC: American Nurses Association Publications.

Reynolds, J.P. (1996). Are you ready to join an outcomes database? *PT–Magazine of Physical Therapy* 4(10): 36, 67.

Ribbons, R.M. and McKenna, L.G. (1997). Facilitating higher order thinking skills in nurse education: A prototype database for teaching wound assessment and management skills. In U. Gerdin, et al. (Eds.), *Nursing Informatics: The Impact of Nursing Knowledge on Health Care Informatics. . . Proceedings of NI'97, Sixth Triennial International Congress of IMIA–NI, Nursing Informatics of International Medical Informatics Association* (p. 389). Amsterdam, The Netherlands: IOS Press.

Roberts, D.J. (1995). Databases. AMED: A bibliographic database for complementary medicine and allied health. *Complementary Therapies in Medicine* 3(4):255.

Rock, B.D., Beckerman, A., Auerback, C., et al. (1995). Management of alternate level of care patients using a computerized database. *Health & Social Work* 20(2):133.

Rodrigues, R.J. (2000). Information systems: The key to evidence-based health practice. *Bulletin of the World Health Organization* 78(11):1344–1351.

Ross, B.A. (1994). Use of a database for managing qualitative research data. *Computers in Nursing* 12(3):154.

Rozic-Hristovski, A., Hristovski, D., and Todorovski, L. (2002). Users' information-seeking behavior on a medical library Website. *Journal of the Medical Library Association* 90(2):210–217.

Saar-Tschansky, M., Pliskin, N., Rabinowitz, G., Tschansky, M., and Porath, A. (2001). Monitoring quality of health care with relational patterns. *Topics in Health Information Management* 22(1):24–35.

Sainz, A. and Epstein, I. (2001). Creating experimental analogs with available clinical information: credible alternatives to "gold-standard" experiments? *Social Work in Health Care* 33(3/4):163–183.

Scally, J.T., McCullough, C.A., Brown, L.J., and Eppinger, R. (1999). Computers in clinical care. Development of the Crash Injury Research and Engineering Network. *International Journal of Trauma Nursing* 5(4):136–138.

Scheese, R. (1998). Data warehousing as a healthcare business solution. *Healthcare Financial Management* 52(2):56–59.

Schermer, J., Geisler, E., and Vang, P. (1995). Nursing Thesis Database Project: A cooperative venture for nursing faculty and computer science professionals. *Computers in Nursing* 13(2):50.

Schoech, D., Fitch, D., MacFadden, R., and Schkade, L.L. (2002). From data to intelligence: Introducing the intelligent organization. *Administration in Social Work* 26(1):1–21.

Shams, K. and Farishta, M. (2001). Data warehousing: Toward knowledge management. *Topics in Health Information Management* 21(3):24–32.

Shams, K. and Farishta, M. (2001). Data warehousing: Toward knowledge management. *Topics in Health Information Management* 21(3):24–32.

Sieler, P. and Adams, J. (1998). Using a database to integrate technology into the curriculum. *Nursing Standard*. http://www.nursing-standard.co.uk/

Simpson, R.L. (1998). Technology: Nursing the system. A NIDSEC primer: Part 2—setting the standards. . . *Nursing Informatics and Data Set Evaluation Center. Nursing Management* 29(2):26–27, 29.

Sokol, L., Garcia, B., Rodriguez, J., West, M., and Johnson, K. (2001). Using data mining to find fraud in HCFA health care claims. *Topics in Health Information Management* 22(1):1–13.

Stajano, F. (1998). *A General Introduction to Relational and Object Oriented Databases: (ORL technical report TR-98-2.)*. http://www.uk.research.att.com/~fms/

Stead, W.W., Miller, R.A., Musen, M.A., and Hersh, W.R. (2000). Integration and beyond: Linking information from disparate sources and into workflow. *Journal of the American Medical Informatics Association* 7(2):135–148.

Urden, L.D. (1996). Development of a nurse executive decision support database: A model for outcomes evaluation. *Journal of Nursing Administration* 26(10):15.

Warren, J.J. and Hoskins, L.M. (1995). NANDA's nursing diagnosis taxonomy: A nursing database. In *An Emerging Framework: Data System Advances for Clinical Nursing Practice* (p. 49). Washington, DC: American Nurses Association Publications.

Welton, J.M. (1997). Development of a computerized database for a nursing quality management team. In U. Gerdin, et al. (Eds.), *Nursing Informatics: The Impact of Nursing Knowledge on Health Care Informatics...Proceedings of NI'97, Sixth Triennial International Congress of IMIA–NI, Nursing Informatics of International Medical Informatics Association* (p. 82). Amsterdam, The Netherlands: IOS.

Wiggers, T.B. (1996). Educators' corner: Use of a computer database to facilitate management of hematology teaching slides. *Clinical Laboratory Science* 9(1):10.

Zisselman, M.H., Allen, D., Cutillo-Schmitter, T.C., et al. (1998). The minimum data set and psychotropic drug use in nursing home residents. *Annals of Long Term Care* 6(7):199.

The Internet: A Nursing Resource

Vida B. Svarcas

OBJECTIVES

1. Describe the way in which the Internet originated.
2. Identify protocols that make use of the Internet possible.
3. Name specific functions which the Internet supports.
4. Explore the customs used with Internet communication.
5. Outline the steps in evaluating information obtained on the Internet.
6. List the benefits and drawbacks to Internet use.
7. Discuss how consumer use of the Internet has changed healthcare delivery.
8. Identify how you can use the Internet both professionally and personally.

KEY WORDS

Internet
World Wide Web
electronic mail
search engines
Web resources

In the years since its inception, the Internet has had a tremendous impact on society, changing the way we communicate, conduct business, obtain information, and manage our lives. While Internet use is still concentrated in the more developed areas of the world, it has served to globalize our thinking. From the comfort of one's home or office, a person can quickly and easily access information from around the world. Often, the user is not even aware of the location of the information source. In a sense, the world has become smaller, as we communicate in real time with people on the other side of the globe.

The technology behind the Internet is at the same time logical and simple in theory and complex and constantly being updated in practice and application. As nurses, we need to understand the overall structure of the Internet, and then learn how to best use this tool for our work. We do not need to have a degree in mechanical engineering to drive a car; however, we do need to have a basic understanding of how it operates and know how to use the features important to us. When we drive a rental car or buy a new hybrid model, there is a period of learning and adjusting. The same is true with learning about and staying abreast of changes in computer technology.

The Internet can be simply described as a network of computer networks. It provides the ability for computers attached in some way to one of the wires or cables on the system to send and receive information from other computers on the network, regardless of their location or type. The openness and worldwide dimensions of the Internet have the power to democratize communication and level the playing field of access to information.

In practical reality, the Internet has only been used broadly for less than 20 years. When we consider the degree to which this technology has changed society in such a short time, we can begin to appreciate the importance of becoming more familiar with it and learning to use it to our best advantage.

These rapid changes in the exchange of information are readily apparent in the healthcare disciplines. Health has always been a key area of both interest and need for people, so it is not surprising that the Internet is filled with an ever-growing number of sources of healthcare information. Since the information is easily accessible, patients often come to healthcare professionals with a sizable amount of information about their conditions or concerns. How accurate and complete this information is becomes a matter that nurses and other healthcare professionals need to address. This has changed the way in which we interact with patients. Not only are we assessing health status and teaching, but we are correcting misinformation, reassuring patients who have misinterpreted what they have found, and answering questions about new trends and treatments that have suddenly found a new audience.

Nurses are also finding the Internet to be a constant source of up-to-date professional information. The Net provides access to information that previously was available only in large medical and nursing libraries. Nursing professionals eagerly embraced the opportunity to use the Internet to network with colleagues all over the world, sharing their knowledge and learning from each other, thus broadening the body of nursing knowledge. They are also searching the Internet for information about approaches to specific nursing situations. The sheer scope of the Internet and speed of the spread of information will cause nursing care standards to expand from community and regional to national and international.

These changes are creating new issues and challenges for nursing as well as providing many benefits. The goal of this chapter is to provide a basic understanding of the Internet and examine how we, as nurses, can use this tool to help us professionally and personally.

The History of the Internet

The Internet might never have come about, or at least would have been much longer in appearing, if in 1957 the Russians had not jolted the United States out of its complacency by launching Sputnik. The result was the creation of the Advanced Research Project Agency (ARPA) by President Eisenhower. Housed in the Pentagon with the Department of Defense (DoD), ARPA worked with the RAND Corporation's think tank to solve the problem of how U.S. authorities could communicate after a nuclear war (Gromov, 1998; Leiner et al., 1998). These individuals realized that no matter how thoroughly a conventional system such as the telephone network was protected, the switching and wiring would be vulnerable to attack.

The result was to devise a network that had no central authority and would be assumed at all times to be unreliable. To facilitate this, they devised a system known as "packet switching," which was invented by Paul Barran (Berners-Lee, n.d.). The packets would be the result of dividing messages into smaller pieces, each individually addressed. The route that each packet took to its destination would be dependent on the availability of routing at the nanosecond it was being transmitted. Thus, packets from the same message could be switched to different routes. When all of the packets arrived at their destination, the receiving computer would reassemble the packets, and do a little arithmetic to arrive at a checksum. This would be compared with the checksum originated by the sending computer. If they did not agree, a resend would be requested from the originating computer.

If part of the network were gone it would not make any difference; the packets would bounce from node to node until they found a route to their destination. It was not a very efficient delivery system, but one that was and still is rugged, a fact that was evident in the earthquake in Los Angles in 1994, when communication was quickly reestablished via the Internet.

Dr. J.C.R. Licklider was chosen in 1962 to lead the research to improve military use of computer technology. This visionary moved ARPA's work from the private sector to universities. His brainchild was first put into operation in the fall of 1969 and named ARPANET, after its DoD Pentagon sponsor the ARPA (Gromov, 1998). The first node was installed at the University of California, Los Angeles. Within a few months, other nodes were established at Stanford Research Institute, University of California, Santa Barbara, and the University of Utah. Not only did this system provide protection against an interruption in communication, but it provided a convenient service to scientists and researchers, allowing them to share what were then scarce computer resources.

Others also felt a need to share computer resources, resulting in the development of many additional networks. Each network, however, used a different method for sending and receiving transmissions with the result that it was impossible for the various networks to communicate with each other. To solve this problem, it was necessary to develop communication standards or protocols.

The first steps to this outcome were taken in 1973 by Vint Cerf and Bob Kahn, leading to the creation of the Transmission Control Protocol and the Internet Protocol (TCP/IP). Any computer or network that agreed to use these protocols could join ARPANET. The brand name of the computer, its content, and even its ownership were irrelevant. This decentralized structure together with standard communication methods made expansion easy. By the mid-1980s, many networks had adopted the standards, and a world Internet became a reality. However, it was not until the mid-1990s that the commercial networks such as CompuServe and Prodigy became a part of the Internet. Prior to this, users of these networks could only communicate with those using the same service.

As one would expect, there is much information available online about the history of the Internet. A very interesting site (*http://www.isoc.org/internet/history/ cerf.shtml*) to visit is "*A Brief History of the Internet and Related Networks*" since it is written by the individuals who were part of creating the Internet. Other excellent sites in addition to those cited in this section are indexed by the Internet Society (ISOC) (2002) at *http://www.isoc.org/internet/history/index.shtml*.

Who Controls the Internet?

Today, the connection of all major networks to the Internet represents the pinnacle of computer communication. The Internet itself has no owners, censors, bosses, board of directors, or stockholders. In principle, any computer or network that obeys the protocols, which are technical, not social or political, can be an equal player. It is an example of a true, modern, functional anarchy. It does, however, have voluntary groups that develop and coordinate standards, resources, and day-to-day issues of operation (MacPherson, 1997).

The overall organizing force is the **ISOC** (*www. isoc.org*), an international, nonprofit, professional membership organization with no governmental allegiances. It is comprised of over 150 organizations and 16,000 individual members that represent over 180 nations throughout the world. The society works to maintain standards, develop public policy, provide education, and increase membership. In recent years, there has been a push to promote standards, especially for the Web, which will enable users with special needs to make full use of the Internet. For many sources of information regarding special needs access, see *http://www.isoc.org/ isoc/access/*.

The Technology Behind the Internet

We have mentioned earlier that it was standardized communication protocols that enabled the Internet to function. A protocol, in plain English, is just an agreed on format for doing something. On the Internet, protocols determine how data will be transmitted between two devices, the type of error checking that will be performed, how data compression, if any, is accomplished, how the sending computer will signal that it has finished sending a message, and how the receiving computer will signal that it has received a message (Webopedia, n.d.).

As a user, your only concern should be that the software and hardware you are using supports the protocols of the computer or device with which you wish to have your computer communicate. To make it easy for all computer users to use the Internet, most computers sold already have software that supports these protocols installed.

The main protocols on which the functioning of the Internet is dependent are referred to as TCP and IP. Each of these protocols performs a different job. The TCP allows computers to connect to a network and exchange data. This protocol carries out the task of breaking messages into the small packets, which was described earlier. The IP is a lower level protocol, which is responsible for making decisions about these packets and routing them. TCP makes certain that the packets, also called datagrams, are all received and are in the correct order. When packets are lost or reordered, TCP will detect this and retransmit and/or reorder the packets as necessary. TCP presents an abstraction to user applications, which allows them to exchange streams of data without worrying about the lower level network issues, such as bit errors or packet loss (Kurose and Ross, 2001).

Other protocols used on the Internet include hypertext transmission protocol (HTTP), which supports the World Wide Web (WWW); file transmission protocol (FTP), which permits users to send all types of electronic files over the Internet; and Telnet, which allows users to access a distant computer as though they were sitting in front of it. For information about the many other protocols that exist, see *http://webopedia.internet. com/Internet_and_Online_Services/Internet/Internet_ Protocols*.

The Domain Name System (DNS)

In order for the computers on the Internet to perform the tasks required, they have to have a way of identifying each other. The Internet's DNS permits us to give globally unique "names" to networks and computers. There are several benefits to this system. First, a name is easier to remember than the long string of numbers that makes up an IP address, which is assigned to each computer on the network. Another benefit is that a name allows for a change of physical location that is transparent to the user. For instance, a computer could be moved from one city to another without changing names, and someone using the Internet would not notice the move.

The pioneer in the protocols that allow the DNS to work was Paul Mockapetris (Berners-Lee). A series of characters (usually letters) makes up each domain name. These strings, called "labels," are separated by dots. The right-most label in a domain name is referred to as its "top-level domain" (TLD).

Top-Level Domains (TLDs)

Each country, as of 2003, has a two-letter TLD. For example, Canada is .CA, Great Britain is .UK, Germany is .DE, and Switzerland is .CH. You can obtain all of the country codes at *http://www.iana.org/cctld/cctld-whois.htm*. In addition, there is a special TLD .ARPA where Internet infrastructure databases are located.

The other TLDs are shown in Table 8.1. The names in bold were the original seven TLDs in the 1980s. Four of these were restricted to certain purposes, while the others could be registered without restriction. Seven new TLDs were selected in November 2000, and introduced during the following 2 years. Four of these (.biz, .info, .name, and

.pro) are unrestricted, while three (.aero, .coop, and .museum) have specific purposes. For more information on the new TLDs see the InterNIC site (InterNIC FAQs on New Top-Level Domains, 2002) at *http://www.internic. net/faqs/new-tlds.html*. As the Internet expands, expect that more TLDs will be added (ICANN, 2003; Salamon, 2004). Currently .com is the largest domain accounting for about 33% of all hosts. The fastest growing appears to be .net, increasing at the rate of 45% annually (Center for Next Generation Internet, 2001).

Some computer names have more than one dot in them. This too is part of the DNS. Each of the top-level domains has delegated responsibility to groups within their domain who may have further delegated naming responsibility. The actual name of the computer, called the "fully qualified domain name," reads from left to right, beginning at the lowest level and ending in the TLD name. If you see a computer name of "peds.nursing.xyz.edu," you would know that the educational institution "xyz" named the computer for the nursing area "nursing," while the nursing group named the computer for the pediatric area, "peds." This is another example of the distributed responsibility characteristic of the Internet. Please note that if after the universal resource locator (URL) there is a forward slash (/) and more names, these refer to the path to the particular document and the name of the document.

Interestingly, and perhaps not surprising in our current culture, is the demand to obtain rights to a particular domain name. When for-profit thinking is applied to the workings of the Internet, as opposed to the original intent of sharing knowledge, the result is often conflict. There have been multiple lawsuits over rights to domain names (Gleick, 2004).

As mentioned earlier, no one owns the Internet. So how does this assigning of names take place? There have been several groups who have taken on this responsibility. Currently, this task is being done by the Internet Corporation for Assigned Names and Numbers (ICANN). ICANN was created in October of 1998 to be responsible for the technical coordination of the Internet. It is a nonprofit, private-sector corporation, which is a coalition of business, academic, technical, and user communities. ICANN has assumed the technical functions previously handled by other groups, including the Internet Assigned Number Authority (IANA). Basically ICANN coordinates assignment of identifiers that must be **globally unique** for the Internet to operate. These include domain names, IP addresses, and protocol parameter and port numbers. ICANN also oversees the root server system (ICANN, 2004).

Table 8.1   Current Top Level-Domain Names

.AERO	For the air transport industry
.BIZ	For businesses
.COM	Commercial/business organizations
.COOP	For cooperatives
.EDU	Restricted to 4-year degree granting institutions in North America
.GOV	Restricted to the U.S. federal government
.INFO	For all uses
.INT	Restricted to organizations that were established by international treaty
.MIL	Restricted to the U.S. Military
.MUSEUM	For museums
.NAME	For individuals
.NET	For network resources
.ORG	For nonprofit organizations*
.PRO	For professions

Note: The original TLD names are in bold.
*Originally intended as a miscellaneous category for organizations that were not educational institutions, commercial entities, governmental agencies, or network providers, the .org TLD has become open and unrestricted. Management of the .org domain was transferred to the Public Interest Registry (PIR) on January 1, 2003. The PIR was created by the ISOC.

The home page of ICANN (*http://www.icann.org/*) has a link to a special page with introductory information, an excellent glossary, and good background information if you are looking for more details about how Internet naming is handled.

 ## How Large is the Internet?

Results from the domain survey, which sought to discover every host on the Internet, were released by the Internet Software Consortium on March 15, 2001, from data collected during January of the same year. The survey indicated that at that time, the Internet had over 109 million hosts in 230 countries. It is not possible to compute the number of actual people using the Internet due to the unlimited number of network gateways and the fact that many computers are used by more than one individual. The growth rate of the Internet is estimated to be between 46 and 67% annually. If this rate of growth continues, it is projected that in mid-2005, the Internet would have over one billion hosts. The Internet Software Consortium estimates that the Net is growing worldwide at the amazing rate of 63 new hosts and 11 new domains per minute (Center for Next Generation Internet, 2001).

Use of the Internet—Then and Now

Even though the original purpose for creating networks was intended to be computer sharing, it did not take long for users to realize that they could also send messages to one another. Indeed, they became far more enthusiastic about this function than the original one. The first e-mail software appeared in 1972. Like today's e-mail software, it allowed users to list, selectively read, file, forward, and respond to messages. During the next decade, e-mail was the largest network application (Leiner et al., 2003).

The e-mail software was made freely available to anyone who wanted it, which was typical of the atmosphere of the Internet in its first two decades. The people involved developed applications that they freely shared with others. These applications could be software for any purpose, files of information, or pictures. To share these items, host computers became "anonymous FTP" sites. Anyone connected to the Internet could use the FTP protocols to connect to the host computer and download any of the available files. This involved learning some commands, which by itself was not difficult. Finding what one wanted, however, was.

Most information about available files was spread by word of mouth, particularly e-mail, although there was a file locator software called Archie that allowed searching of these sites. Several sites around the world served as Archie sites; they pooled the information from their searches and made it available to users at other sites. The Archie sites were extremely busy, which made it difficult to use them. Another difficulty with FTP was that users could only see the name of the file, which often was not indicative of the contents. It was also impossible to look at the file before downloading it. Still, many useful things were shared by FTP, and it kept the spirit of sharing on the Internet alive.

The next improvement in finding resources on the Internet was the Gopher system developed at the University of Minnesota. Like most networks, it was based on a client server model. Under this system, a client computer is one that has software that allows it to retrieve files from a distant computer, while a server is a computer that has software that allows it to respond to a client by sending a requested file (Thede, 1999a). A computer can be both a client and a server, although most computers have only client software.

The Gopher system provided users a menu of items available on Internet servers globally. Users entered the number of their selection, and the file contents were sent to the user's computer, where the user could then read the contents. It was possible to bookmark the file, a process in which one sets a pointer to that file so it can be easily accessed again, or download the file to one's own computer, where it could be accessed without using the Internet. Search programs called Veronica and Jughead allowed users to search the global indices for subjects of interest. Gopher, however, only supported text files. The ability to click on an item and retrieve information about that item as is now possible with the WWW has made Gophers fairly extinct. Many Gopher databases are now Web sites (Webopedia). Gopher pages can be accessed on the WWW and every now and then while using the Web one accesses a document that looks like a typewritten page and has no links, an indication that it is probably an old Gopher document.

File Transfer Protocol

The FTP was mentioned above as the method used by early Internauts (a moniker for users of the Internet) to upload files to and download files from distant computers. FTP used the Internet's TCP/IP protocols for the transfer of data. Uploading a file refers to the process of moving a file from the user's computer to another computer, while downloading is the transfer of a file from another computer to the user's computer, regardless of the physical distance between the two computers. This protocol is still in use today for exchange of data, but most use is transparent to the user. When you use the Web to download a file to your computer, the browser is giving commands to an FTP program behind the scenes. FTP is also used to upload or post files to a Web site. There are programs available that make this task easy, unlike in the early 1990s when individuals had to enter commands to accomplish these tasks.

Telnet

Telnet, mentioned earlier as one of the protocols used on the Internet, is a terminal emulation program that is part of the TCP/IP protocols. Telnet allows a connecting computer to behave like a terminal for a distant computer regardless of the type of computer that is either the target or originator of the Telnet session. A log in and a password are required to begin a Telnet session. Once connected, the user of the client computer is able to perform any functions as if entering the commands directly on the server, no matter how separated in distance the two computers may be. Although not as common as it used to be, some Internet service providers (ISPs) use Telnet behind the scenes to connect their subscribers to proprietary forums or the Internet. Telnet is also often used to control Web servers remotely (Webopedia).

Usenet News and Online Forums

There are several types of discussion groups on the Internet: newsgroups, online forums, and mailing lists. Newsgroups are a sort of worldwide bulletin board system that is accessed using software called a newsreader. Most WWW browsers contain a newsreader that tracks the messages that you have read and can be set up to allow you to easily access new messages. It also allows you to post a message to the group. There are newsgroups on almost every topic. They were originally organized hierarchically under seven main headings, but with the explosion of the Internet there are now more upper level headings.

Online forums are often set up by organizations to allow members, or anyone, depending on how the forum is organized, to share ideas. They often require that a user register and either create or be given a password, which is used to access the site. Forums were originally accessed by Telnet, but today they are usually accessed through a Web site.

Messages on both forums and newsgroups are organized by the subject entered by the poster. This same subject is also automatically assigned from the subject line when a reply to a subject is made. This type of organization is called threading, and it allows users to select the topics for which they will read messages and to read all of the messages on a given topic in the order they were received or from latest to earliest. Mailing lists are widely used and will be discussed further in this chapter.

E-mail

One of the most popular uses for the Internet remains the ability to send and receive electronic mail or e-mail. The number of e-mail users is growing rapidly. Many individuals have more than one e-mail address, using each for different purposes. You rarely see a business card without an e-mail address any more. Most colleges and universities provide an e-mail address for all students, faculty, and staff. Many employers provide e-mail addresses to their employees; however, employees should be aware of policies regarding the use of company e-mail for private purposes. If you obtain your Internet access through an ISP, you often can have many e-mail addresses for that account. Many companies are providing free e-mail address with a specified amount of space, charging a fee for larger amounts of storage. The most popular of these include Netscape, Yahoo, and Hotmail.

The Anatomy of an E-mail Address

Recall that the Internet works because all computers that are connected use the same protocol. Therefore, all e-mail addresses follow the same format. An e-mail address has two parts, separated by the "@" sign. The first part is what may be called the user name, user ID, or login name. Some organizations let users select their user name, while others assign them based on a system such as first initial and last name or first name dot (a period) last name. You may find such symbols as an underline (_), a hyphen (-), or even the percent sign (%) or pound sign (#) in the user name. What you will not find are spaces.

In the e-mail address in Fig. 8.1, the user name is "Clara.Barton." The characters after the user name are the name of the computer that assigned the user name. In Fig. 8.1, this name is "RedCross.org." Notice the last three letters of the computer name. They are assigned to the computer under the DNS previously discussed. The domain name of the computer in Fig. 8.1 is "org,"

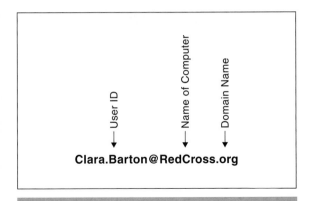

Figure 8.1
An E-mail Address.

indicating that this address is for a computer in a nonprofit organization. Currently, most e-mail addresses are not case-sensitive; that is, whether you use a capital letter or a lowercase letter will not affect the address. Omitting any characters, or typing just one incorrectly, however, will.

Using E-mail

To send and receive e-mail, besides having an account on the Internet that provides an e-mail address and having a computer, you need communication software. Computers purchased in the last few years have communication software included as part of the operating system. Additionally, most of the WWW browsers (software programs that allow you to use the WWW) have built-in e-mail programs. There are also other e-mail packages available; some are available free, and most can be downloaded from the Internet.

The functions that e-mail software provide vary with the package, but all permit a user to receive and read a message, send a reply, initiate a new message, forward a received message to someone else, and organize received messages in folders. The steps for accomplishing each task vary from program to program. There is a "help" option which provides online assistance and information about the specifics of e-mail software and is available for all of the major packages. As the use of the Web becomes more widespread, more and more e-mails are sent as Hypertext Markup Language (HTML) format. This results in larger file sizes. If your e-mail program only accepts text messages, you may not be able to read all or part of an HTML formatted message. Some distri-

bution sites give you the choice of format in which you would like messages sent. If your space availability is limited, you may want to stay with text format, but that prevents you from viewing the graphics and other special formatting allowed by HTML.

E-mail communication is different from either telephone or face-to-face communication. On the telephone, you can hear voice inflections, and in face-to-face communication, you can see and hear the other individual. E-mail is also different from a written letter in that it is often done "on the fly" and is usually posted immediately after finishing. For these reasons, some customs and e-mail common sense apply.

Many people have learned the hard way that e-mail is not considered private as is mail delivered by the post office. Nor is any e-mail sent from an account on a business or educational computer protected from oversight by an administrator. This may hold true even if the user has been told that his or her e-mail is private (Atkins, 1998; Zetter, 2004). Records of what you send can exist in many places besides your hard drive. Additionally, it is very easy for a recipient to forward a message you send to someone else either accidentally or on purpose. To avoid embarrassing moments, or worse, think carefully before you send any e-mail message. Never send something you would be ashamed of someone other than the intended recipient seeing. If something makes you angry, do not post an immediate reply. If you feel strongly about something, write a reply, save it, let time pass, and then edit it before sending it.

Use of Emoticons and Abbreviations

To make up for the inability of message recipients to accurately judge the mood of the sender, the practice of typing characters available on a standard keyboard to form a "picture" was begun. These small icons called emoticons or smileys are often used to denote a mood. They were originally intended to be viewed by tilting your head to the left. For example, saying something jokingly is often denoted with the icon :-). If you tilt your head you can see a sideways smiling face. The use of emoticons has become almost an art form; thousands have been suggested to be viewed both with your head tilted as well as in line with the text. Just do a search and you will be surprised at the volume. Emoticons originated when e-mail programs were only text based. Some newer programs allow you to type text, which is converted to a graphic emoticon. The most common emoticons can be seen in Table 8.2. While emoticons can help convey your message, overuse will only muddle it.

Table 8.2   Samples of Emoticons

Icon	Meaning
:-)	Smiling; joking, happy
;-)	Winking smiley
:-(	Sad
:-X	My lips are sealed
:-*	Sending a kiss
:-O	Surprised
:-D	Very happy; laughing
:-p	Tongue sticking out

Given that most electronic communication is done quickly at the keyboard, abbreviations are often used in e-mail and other messaging applications. Table 8.3 has some examples. Both emoticons and abbreviations should be used cautiously; if the recipient of the message does not understand the symbol or the abbreviation, communication is lost.

E-mail Etiquette

When sending e-mail, you should show the same consideration that you would show when writing to anyone. Given the nature of e-mail, there are a few additional things that should be considered. Using all

Table 8.3   Some Commonly Used Abbreviations

Acronym	Meaning
AFK	Away from keyboard
BTDT	Been there done that
BTW	By the way
CTS	Changing the subject
DQMOT	Do not quote me on this
FTF	Face to face
FWIW	For what its worth
HTH	Hope this helps
IMHO	In my humble opinion
LOL	Laughing out loud
OTOH	On the other hand
WYSIWYG	What you see is what you get

capital letters is considered "shouting"; additionally it is about 50% harder to read than the traditional upper and lowercase text. Get into the habit of always using a subject for your e-mail. This helps the recipient, who may have 50 or more messages to read, to decide if your message needs to be read right away or if it can wait until she or he has more time. Additionally, there are people who just delete any message that does not have a subject, especially in the last few years as e-mail is being used to spread viruses. If you are writing to someone who might not recognize your address, you should use a subject, which clearly indicates the reason for the e-mail. No longer can you just use "Hi," "Info," "As requested," or even "Important." Due to the previous common use of these subjects, e-mail which is infected with a virus often uses subject lines such as these.

Another custom is that all messages should be signed; assuming that the recipient will know who you are leads to problems. If you have received e-mail you may have noticed that some of the messages have rather lengthy signatures, perhaps a full identification of the sender, plus even an icon created on the keyboard or a saying. These are not typed in for every message or even pasted in. These users have learned how to use a signature file. A signature file contains the information that you want added automatically. Some e-mail programs will add it to every message that you send, others will give you a choice of when to use it. At a minimum, a signature file should include your name and e-mail address; at a maximum, it should not be longer than six lines. Some organizations also add some information about the company to all e-mail sent through the company's server. With the passage of the *Health Insurance Portability and Accountability Act of 1996 (HIPAA)*, many healthcare organizations are also including confidentiality statements at the end of each e-mail.

Many e-mail programs allow you to set an option that will automatically send a reply to each e-mail that is sent to you. This is usually used when you will not have access to a computer for a period of time. It lets people know that they are not being ignored and has become an accepted standard in many organizations. In many healthcare organizations, it also provides information about who to contact during your absence. This is a useful feature except when you are subscribed to one or more lists, where it can cause problems described later in this chapter. For more details about online etiquette, see the comprehensive list by Arleen Rinaldi (1998), "The Net: User Guidelines and Netiquette" at *http://www.fau.edu/netiquette/net/*.

Organizing Received Files

Once you start using e-mail, you will find that you want to keep some of the messages that you receive. E-mail packages provide a way to create folders and transfer a received message to them. This allows you to keep your "inbox" or mailbox area clear for messages that you still have to attend to and allows you to keep messages you may want in the future in an organized manner. Get into the habit of organizing your saved messages. As we try to use less paper, it becomes more important to be able to find a particular e-mail when you need it. Most packages will also allow you to sort mail by date, by size, and by sender. This is a very helpful feature when searching for a particular e-mail or when "cleaning out" your mailbox. Most programs also have a "search" function that will help locate a particular document. This comes in handy if you do not remember who sent you the e-mail or when.

File Attachments

All e-mails used to be plain text files. A plain text file, often referred to as an ASCII file, can be read by all e-mail software and all word processors. Text files, however, have no formatting; that is, text placement cannot be determined by the individual who created the file, nor can this individual add any attributes such as boldface or italics. For most e-mail communication, this is not a problem. Sometimes, however, you may wish to send someone a file that will preserve the formatting. Newer programs allow you to do this. However, it is often more convenient to send a file created by a word processor or other application program. These programs create what are called proprietary files, or a file format that can only be read by the program that created it. After you create such a file, you can send it to the recipient by attaching it to an e-mail. Your e-mail software "help" function will guide you to discover how your e-mail package fulfills this function. When you attach a file, the recipient must have the same software package to read the file that you used to create the file. If you send a Word Perfect file to a Word user, the Word user will not be able to read it. Before sending a file attachment, check to be sure your recipient will be able to read it.

As the practice of using attachments gains popularity, it brings with it many advantages as well as dangers. Almost any type of file can be sent as an attachment, the limits being those of the e-mail software. People these days send spreadsheets, pictures, files of scanned documents, and programs. If you are in a rush for something, this is really a benefit. However, many viruses are also sent as attachments. Be cautioned **never to** open an attachment, even if it is from someone that you know, unless you were expecting it or you have run a virus scan. Many individuals' computers have been crippled because they opened an attachment out of curiosity.

Cautions and Suggestions

As more and more people use e-mail and it becomes easier to send mail to multiple addresses with just a few keystrokes, individuals who do not always have the original goals of the Internet in mind find ways of using this tool for other than honorable reasons. The virus hidden in an attachment mentioned above is one example of this maliciousness. Less serious, but nonetheless irritating is something called "spam." This word describes unwanted e-mail, from an unknown source, often with the intent of selling something. Spam or junk e-mail, fills up your mailbox and takes time to delete. Even though people do not recognize the address from which spam originates, many are afraid to not open an e-mail on the chance that it contains something they really want to see.

One strategy suggested some years ago to eliminate junk e-mail (spam) was to charge a small fee for sending an e-mail. While originally dismissed as being contrary to the free spirit of the Internet, the idea resurfaced again in early 2004. The idea is obviously attractive to ISPs, as it would be a new source of revenue, but has a large opposition and could lead to legitimate e-mail not being delivered (Hansell, 2004).

If you are sending an e-mail message to more than one person, consider putting all the addresses on the blind copy line, especially if the people do not know each other. There is much useful information sent via e-mail and since it is so simple to just forward a message to a friend, many people enjoy forwarding received messages to large numbers of people. As this practice continues, the list of recipients remains in the e-mail. Not only does it make is harder for a later recipient to scroll down to the meat of the message, this practice also makes all those e-mail addresses available to anyone who has received the message. Since we know e-mail is not private, there are some who look to collect e-mail addresses for spam or similar reasons. Do go ahead and forward e-mail, but spend the few seconds it takes to block and delete unneeded parts before pressing "send."

Finally, be aware that some companies sell e-mail addresses. If you like a lot of mail, this is not a problem, but if your mail space or time is limited, you may want to be careful about whom you give your e-mail address to. Most reputable Web sites will tell you that they do not share addresses and will even give you the choice of opting out of getting other promotional messages from them. Some people set up a secondary e-mail address with a nickname and give that out. This way they know that the mail they really want will come to their primary address and they can check the secondary address less frequently and be less hesitant of deleting messages without opening them.

Lawrence Lessing, a law professor at Stanford, warns us that the Internet is having an impact on the concept of privacy. Once something is recorded on the Web, on any document, list, or in a blog, it becomes permanent record (Hockman, 2004).

Mailing List

E-mail communication between individuals led to a desire to be able to send one message to many people to enable group discussions. To enable this, mailing list software was developed in the early 1980s. It was Eric Thomas, however, in 1986, who created the first software that automated many of the functions necessary to maintain a list (Webopedia). Reflecting the ambiance of the Internet at the time, the software was free to anyone who wanted to use it. It was called Listserv after the earlier manual product, a name that is often used to denote any mailing list, even though today there are several other software products that manage mailing lists.

Mailing lists are set up to provide an arena for discussion on a specific topic (Bowers, 1997). They are "owned" by an individual who manages the day-to-day affairs of the list. Although the term "owner" is used, the owner pays no money to manage the list and in most cases receives no remuneration for this chore. The owner is responsible for taking care of error messages or messages that cannot be delivered, handling requests from members who have not learned how to use the automated functions of the list or who for other reasons are unable to carry them out, and for handling any disputes that degenerate into "flame wars." A flame war is a series of flames, or ill-considered, knee-jerk expressions of anger that are insulting.

When one subscribes to a list, one receives all messages that other members send to the list. A reply to a list message is automatically sent to the list, not to the individual who sent the message. Subscriptions are free, but thoughtful list members assume responsibilities that make the life of the owner easier.

Mailing lists have found many uses. They enable nurses from the entire world to communicate. On lists, students as well as graduate nurses can and do get into discussions with faculty, deans, and other nursing leaders. Ideas are explored, and individuals find solutions to situations and new ideas for approaching a situation. Many teachers open a mailing list for their class to enable students to ask and answer questions of the teacher and their classmates. They are also being used as support groups for people with chronic illnesses, such as asthma or cancer. Some organizations now use them to keep their members informed.

List Fundamentals

Mailing lists have two addresses. One is the address of the software that manages the list. This address is used to subscribe to the list, unsubscribe, or use some of the functions that the software makes available. The functions that are available vary with the software that manages the list, but typically include such things as accessing the archives of the list, getting a list of other subscribers, receiving all list messages in one "digest" version each day, and temporarily stopping the list e-mail if you are going to be away for an extended time. Once you are subscribed to a list, you will receive a message automatically sent by the software that contains information about the functions that are available and how to use them. It is important to save this welcome message so that it can be referred to when needed. It will be important when you would like to use any of the available functions or want to unsubscribe from the list. The simplest way is to file such messages in a folder specifically created for that purpose, so that you can find them easily when you need the information. One folder named "List Info" or "Subscriptions" will serve this function for all such reference messages you receive.

The second address for a mailing list is the one that subscribers use to post a message to the mailing list. That is the only purpose that this address has, although it is the address that subscribers use most frequently. Sending a message to be posted on the list is done the same way as sending a message to an individual. Most users "lurk," or just read list messages for a few days or weeks, to gain a feel for the list, before posting a message. If you want to respond to a message on the list, you can do so using the "reply" function. Again, check with the instructions you receive when you join. People still make mistakes, and some lists have changed the way they operate to compensate for this. For example, because so many people were hitting "reply," which sent the response to everyone subscribed to the list, when they only intended to reply to the author of the message, some lists are now requiring the use of the "reply to all" function when one desires to post a message to the entire list.

Finding a List

There were some individuals who tried to maintain Web sites with lists of mailing lists. The job was daunting since the number of mailing lists increases so rapidly. The software that is used to operate the majority of lists, most often referred to as Listservs, is from L-Soft International, Inc. This company has an automatically generated searchable database of Listserv lists that can be accessed at *http://www.lsoft.com/catalist.html.* It contains information about almost 70,000 public lists on the Internet, and allows you to search by several variables, such as country, area of interest, or size of list. Just by searching for the key word "nursing" on one occasion, there were 89 returns—that is Listservs that had a match to that word. Some lists have only a handful of members, while others number in the thousands. Some general interest lists have hundreds of thousands of subscribers. Obviously, the more specialized the topic, the smaller the numbers. Since this database is automatically generated, it is always up to date. In checking the site, it was amazing to see that in a span of 2 weeks, the number of lists indexed increased by 600 (June 2–16, 2004). Another resource for finding a forum for discussion on nursing issues can be accessed at *http://nursing.buffalo.edu/mccartny/nursing_discussion_ forums.html.*

This site will make you aware of various nursing discussion groups and mailing lists.

List Etiquette

List etiquette follows that for e-mail, with some added features that reflect the nature of lists. Remember that any message that you post to a list will be sent to **all** members of the list. Thus, you do not want to use the reply functions to send a personal message to a message received via the list. Instead, initiate a new message using the private e-mail address of the poster, which is found on the "From line." Also, do not add unnecessary traffic to the list with replies that do not really contribute to the discussion. A message of "me too" or "I agree" by itself serves no purpose; remember how many peoples' time you are affecting by sending a reply.

When you do reply to a posting, make sure you either use the "reply with history" function or clearly indicate the topic or question you are reacting to. Since there are often many topics of conversation going on simultaneously, and people around the world read e-mails at different times, help the list members' understanding of your response by putting it in context.

When sending a message, use descriptive subjects; not all list members are interested in everything on the list, and on a busy list members often choose what to read based on the subject. If you are initiating a new subject, do not use the reply function, because it will pick up the original subject and be misinterpreted; instead use a new message. Another important reason for using a descriptive subject is that this field is used to organize the list archives.

Avoid sending file attachments—not everyone can read them and they can also be a source of viruses. For these reasons many people discard them. Because members subscribe using a great variety of computers, messages should only be sent in text format. If the default in your e-mail program is to send Hypertext messages, turn this off in the mail section of preferences.

If you will be unable to read your e-mail messages for a while, either unsubscribe from a list or, if the mailing list software permits, use the "nomail" function. If your e-mail software supports the ability to generate an automatic reply stating when you will be gone and when you will return, do not use it when you have a subscription to a list. The message that it generates will create a loop in which messages bounce back and forth, creating hundreds of messages that fill subscribers' mailboxes and causing problems for other subscribers as well as the list owner.

These items are common sense when one considers how mailing lists and e-mail work. The most important item is a "Do." Do share your information and knowledge, and do ask questions. A good list has member participation. A mailing list is one venue where you can speak out and everyone will listen. Lists are helping nurses share information and learn from each other more quickly and easily.

■ The World Wide Web

There is much to affirm that the WWW is not just some passing trend, but an integral part of the world today. Among them are honors for the inventor of the WWW, Tim Berners-Lee. He was named as one of the top 20 thinkers of the twentieth century" by Time magazine, and was given the *Knight Commander of the Order of the British Empire* honor. On the occasion of his knighthood, Sir Tim told the BBC that "the original idea of the Web was that it should be a collaborative space where you can communicate through sharing information." (BBC News, 2003).

To many the WWW has come to symbolize the Internet, despite the fact that it is only one part of the Net. However, except for e-mail, today most people interact on the Internet using a WWW browser. A browser is a client program that translates files to the image you see on the screen. Just as with IPs, in order for the Web to work, all users must use standard protocols. For the WWW, these standards include HTTP. Before the browser interprets it, a WWW file is text that contains what are called tags that tell the browser how to display the file. Figure 8.2 shows the text that a browser receives and Fig. 8.3 shows how the browser uses the tags to display the information. In Fig. 8.2, the tags are what is enclosed between the less than signs (<) and greater than signs (>). These tags and many others comprise HTML, which is used to format documents for the Web. The term "Hypertext" refers to the ability to link information in a document to another. Therefore, a single source can provide the user an interface to many other sources of information. There are many choices in browsers, all of which can navigate the Web. The most common proprietary browsers today are Netscape and Explorer. Others are designed by programmers who participate in the open source community. These include Mozilla and Opera.

Origin of the World Wide Web

To many it may seem as if the WWW suddenly appeared in the last half of the 1990s. Like most things on the Internet, its history is very short. It was first proposed in 1989 by Tim Berners-Lee while working at CERN, the European Particle Physics Laboratory in Geneva, Switzerland, with Robert Cailliau. The first prototype appeared in 1990 with a subsequent release in 1991. It was, however, 1992 before the first browser was released to the public as freeware and that year there were 50 Web servers (Gromov, 1998). By the end of 1995, there had been improvements in browsers, and there were 73,500 Web servers all over the world. Today, Web servers number in the millions. The speed with which the WWW has gone from a proposal to full acceptance is indicative of the speed of change that the Internet is creating in society.

How the World Wide Web Functions

Like Gopher, the Web is built on the client/server model common to most networks. A software program called a browser allows any computer to be a Web client. A computer that functions as a server has special software that allows it to receive, interpret, and send to the client

```
<HTML>
<HEAD>
<TITLE>Mailing Lists</TITLE>
</HEAD>
<BODY TEXT="#000000" BGCOLOR="#FFFFC0" LINK="#0000FF" VLINK="#800080"
ALINK="#FF00FF">
<P>After confirming your subscription you will receive information about the list. KEEP
THIS INFORMATION. It gives useful items such as the address to use to post to the list,
how to unsubscribe from the list and other functions that the software provides such as setting
your mail to nomail when you will temporarily be unable to read your mail, and where the
archives for the list are located.</P>
<CENTER><A  HREF="INFO.htm">Return to the main INFO page</A></CENTER>
</BODY>
</HTML>
```

Figure 8.2
A WWW file before interpretation.

After confirming your subscription you will receive information about the list. KEEP THIS INFORMATION. It gives useful items such as the address to use to post to the list, how to unsubscribe from the list and other functions that the software provides such as setting your mail to nomail when you will temporarily be unable to read your mail, and where the archives for the list are located.

Return to the main INFO page

Figure 8.3
The WWW file from Figure 8.2 as interpreted by a browser.

computer the requested file. The Web's use of HTTP enables the transmitting and interpretation of all types of files, not just text.

The use of Hypertext is obviously central to the Web's functioning. Invented by Ted Nelson in the 1960s, Hypertext is a type of system, which permits objects to be linked to one another. An object can be almost anything—text, a picture, or a program. On your screen, a link is somehow differentiated by its appearance. For example, a link which is text is often underlined and blue. When you move your cursor over a link, the cursor's appearance changes to a hand. Clicking on a link will take you to whatever document the link is pointing to. It can be another Web page, a text document, a sound file, a video clip, or a graphic image (Webopedia).

In order for a browser to display a link, it first needs to contact the server named in the link, in other words, the place where the item sought resides. This process is possible because all computers, and therefore servers on the Internet have a specific IP address. This address for a Web site is called an URL. An URL contains the name of the computer where the document you are seeking is located along with other specifics to locate it. Web URLs start with "http." This indicates the transmission protocol being used. The standard server side port number for http is port 80. When establishing the TCP connection to the server, the client computer knows to contact the server via port 80. Following that, you will see a colon (:) and two forward slashes (//). Sometimes the next entry is "www," and sometimes the name of the computer follows. Figure 8.4 shows an imaginary URL with the parts labeled. As with the Internet, standards are essential to functioning of the Web.

Tim Berners-Lee currently heads up the WWW Consortium (W3C), which he founded in 1994. The main purpose of this international group is to promote open standards for the WWW and to work toward universal access (Hall, n.d.).

What Makes the World Wide Web Valuable?

One of the reasons that the Web has been so enthusiastically embraced by people is due to the fact that it functions similarly to the way people think. Humans do not think in a linear mode. Rather they make associations—linkages. This was clearly explained by Dr. Vannevar Bush in a seminal article he published in the July 1945 issue of *The Atlantic Monthly* (Bush, 1945). The article

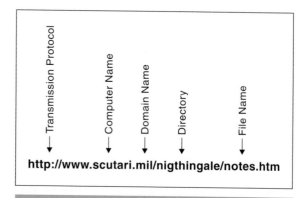

Figure 8.4
Anatomy of a URL.

was titled "As We May Think" and describes his vision of a program which could imitate the human linking of ideas. He called this program "memex." Dr. Bush was Director of the U.S. Office of Scientific Research and Development. The entire article, which is fascinating reading, can be accessed from *The Atlantic Monthly* Web site (*http://www.theatlantic.com/unbound/flashbks/computer/bushf.htm*).

Having access to the WWW opens the world to you. You can use libraries throughout the world, regardless of their hours of operation. It is just as easy to access information on a computer in Hong Kong as it is on one across the street. One can search library catalogs, databases, indexes of journals and dissertations, and use a search engine to find other resources available on the Net. Additionally, many print journals have an online presence that varies from just the table of contents, to abstracts, to the full text of some articles. More and more completely online journals are being established, including several for nursing, most of which are free. Most major newspapers also have Web sites that permit you to read recent articles, see today's front page, and search for topics of interest. Some even offer the option of being notified by e-mail when news about a particular subject is released. You can check your hometown paper when away or see how a particular newspaper handles a current event. A wonderful portal to a great deal of information is the Internet Public Library (2004), whose URL is *http://www.ipl.org*. This site, which is a public service of the University of Michigan School of Information, contains links to magazines and newspapers throughout the world, links to sites on a wide breadth of topics, and several search options.

For nurses, the Web makes professional information easily accessible. For example, while the practice of nursing and the issuance of licenses are controlled by individual state boards of nursing, they work together via the National Council of State Boards of Nursing (NCSBN) for many purposes, including development of the NCLEX examinations. Find your state board's Web address at *http://www.ncsbn.org/regulation/boardsofnursing_boards_of_nursing_board.asp*. From each state board's Web site you can access your state's Nurse Practice Act, rules governing nursing practice, continuing education (CE) requirements, and usually the various forms you might need to change your name, address, or obtain a duplicate license. If you are planning to move to another state, you can find the information you need to obtain a license from that state board's site ahead of time so you do not have to interrupt your practice.

Many nursing organizations provide information to their members via the Internet. The American Nurses Association (ANA), Sigma Theta Tau International (STTI), the National League for Nursing (NLN), and many specialty organizations have extensive Web sites that are visited not only by members, but by other health professionals, the media, and the public.

Nurses can obtain CE from organizations that post courses on the Web. Online CE offers many benefits including no travel, lodging, or meal costs as well as the ability to complete the offering on your own timetable (Plank, 1998). Many CE sites provide the ability to print the course certificate as soon as you successfully complete the course and pay the fee. As technology improves, these CE programs are moving from just reading text and answering questions to including audio and video clips and interaction with others taking the same course. Universities are also using the Internet to provide credit courses. This began initially as a way to bring higher education to those living far from a university, but is now becoming almost expected in some areas.

There are excellent tutorials available online, not only for using the various features of the Internet, but also for nursing. Easy access is also provided to information about National Institute of Health (NIH) grants. The NIH has a large Web presence as do other federal agencies. The U.S. Food and Drug Administration (FDA) has a large searchable site, *www.fda.gov*, which provides up-to-date information not only about prescription medications, but also foodborne illness, dietary supplements, medical devices, vaccines, cosmetics, and other products with health implications. One can find information about specific hospitals, products that one wishes to buy, the weather for any place in the world, and generally any topic that one wishes to know more about.

The amount of information being placed on the Internet is also growing. There are various groups who see the value in putting historical documents on the Web to make them more accessible to students, researchers, and the general public. More and more of these are being created each day (BBC News, 2004).

Project Gutenberg (Project Gutenberg, 2004) has, through the use of volunteers, made over 10,000 books available via the Internet. Begun in 1971, the goal of the project is to make electronic books easily and freely accessible. *Notes on Nursing: What It Is, and What It Is Not* by Florence Nightingale was released electronically in May of 2004. You can download the entire book from *http://www.gutenberg.org/etext/12439*.

The Internet as an Information Source

The Internet has changed the way we seek information and the quality of that information. For example, say you wanted to know how many people were living on our planet. Without the Internet, you could go to a library, locate a reference book, and hopefully locate a recent estimate in a short amount of time. If you had access to an encyclopedia, you could shorten your search time, but the information would not be as current. The Internet has eliminated the need for that effort. While online, you are able to do a search and find the answer to that question in just a minute or two, and the answer is specific and up to date. "According to the International Programs Center, U.S. Census Bureau (2004), the total population of the world, projected to 6/17/04 at 3:52:10 GMT (6/16/04 at 11:52:10 p.m. EDT) is 6,374,900,469."

In the example above, you could also have called a reference librarian on the phone and asked for the information. Increasingly, libraries are providing reference services not only by phone, but also via e-mail and 24-hour Internet chat services. However, not all questions can be answered that easily.

People tend to trust what is written, and librarians, among others, are concerned that consumers are not able to judge the accuracy of information they find, especially when it comes to seeking information about health issues. The head of the general reference area at the Cleveland Public Library is worried that people will not realize that the Web has no filter for the information that it makes available (Selingo, 2004).

The Chairman of the Internet Archive, Brewster Kahle, makes this sad comment, "The terrifying and wonderful observation about Google is that people these days are using it as an information resource of first resort. Unfortunately, many of them also believe if something's not on Google, it doesn't exist" (Hockman, 2004).

Searching the Web

While the Web provides access to an ever increasing body of information, this is not always a benefit. The Web is still vastly unorganized. Given the wide breadth of types of available information, this is not surprising. Having access to a tremendous amount of information on the Web creates some difficulties, especially if one is not able to search and sort quickly and systematically. As the number of Web sites increase, the potential number of sources to search also increase.

In 1994, one of the first Web search engines, the World Wide Web Worm (WWWW), was able to search 110,000 sources. Claims from top search engines 3 years later indicated that they were able to index nearly 100 million Web documents (Brin and Page, n.d.). That remarkable growth rate has continued, as has the number of queries handled daily by the various search engines available. What does this mean to the user?

There are many different programs that will search the Web to help you find information. They do not all search the same way. Some programs will only search within a Web site or organization. Others only search "approved" sources. How various search engines operate varies from engine to engine. Some look at titles and the first few lines of text, while others look at metastatements. A metastatement is text inserted into the source document by the author that is not placed on the screen by the browser and contains some key words about the document.

Deciding which type of search service to use should depend on the topic. There are two excellent sources that can help you select an appropriate search engine. One is a site maintained by Debbie and Damon Abilock (2004) located at *http://www.noodletools.com/*. The other is an article in PC *Magazine* by Sean Carroll (Carroll, 2004) available at *http://www.pcmag.com/ print_ article/0,1761,a=41018,00.asp*.

When searching for information, the completeness of a search does not necessarily bring about the desired results. For example, a search for the word "cancer" using several of the top search engines yielded the following results, in a mere fraction of a second no less:

Google	33,800,000
Alta Vista	9,058,171
Yahoo	32,800,000
MSN	6,874,950

Interestingly, the top results for each of these searches were different. It is clear that none of us has the time to read, much less look, at that many sites. It is a commonly accepted fact that the majority of search engine users never get past the first few pages of results (Selingo, 2004).

In addition to the growing amount of information available for searching, one of the reasons for the high number of results is that some commercial sites include certain words on their sites to increase the likelihood of being included in search results. Therefore, it is clear to see that the quantity of results is not as important as the relevance and placement of results.

Early search engines used the presence of key words to return results. With the proliferation of commercial sites coupled with the savvy of advertisers, this system is not as helpful as it had been. According to Nielsen//NetRatings. the top search engine currently is Google, followed by Yahoo, and MSN (MSNBC News, 2004). Google, a relative newcomer, was designed by two Stanford doctoral students, who had as their goal improving the quality and scale of Web search engines. They chose the name Google because it was a common spelling of googol, which is 10^{100}. Their new way of approaching the task yielded a search engine that returned much more precise results. Two main features used by Google are link structure and anchor text. Simply put, Google analyzes the hypertext links and their proximity to rank each Web page. It also looks at not only text, but the pages a link points to. Finally, it gives a higher weight to words which are more prominent, such as larger font, bold, or highlighted (Brin and Page, n.d.). For a more detailed and technical explanation of how this and other search engines work, as well as suggestions for more efficient use, see the links to supplemental documents found on the Google, Inc. homepage at *www.google.com*.

There are also specialized search services that will assist you in locating such things as e-mail addresses, regular and Web addresses for businesses, and even a map and driving directions from one location to another. The search engines also differ in how they request input to narrow or expand searches. For the best results, tailor your search request using the help that each search service provides. Some heavy Web users do not keep paper phone books, dictionaries, and other reference sources anymore, relying on the WWW for all their information. This might help keep a desk cleaner, but can be a real problem when there is a power outage.

When you come across a site that you find helpful, you may want to bookmark it so you can easily return to it. Browsers have a feature that allows you to not only save URLs in bookmark files, but also organize your bookmarks into folders. This makes it easier to find a site when you need it. You can even put the URLs to sites you visit very frequently in the browser's toolbar. Another helpful feature built into most browsers is called history. This keeps in memory the URLs you entered recently. You can see them by clicking on the arrow next to the current address on your browser. The settings function allows you to determine how long you would like the software to keep the history.

Cookies

A cookie is a piece of text information, which is placed on a client's browser by a Web site visited. The cookie is opaque, that is not understandable to the user. Cookies are used in software applications for many different reasons, which will not be discussed here. However, a brief mention of cookies is warranted as you will encounter them while browsing Web sites.

After a cookie is left by a Web site, the client's browser will put it on the hard drive when the computer is turned off so that it is available in the future. Depending on the setting, cookies can be set or retrieved at will. Because cookies contain real information, setting and retrieving cookies can pose a privacy issue. Browsers give you the option of being notified each time a cookie is set, refusing or accepting cookies, and clearing all stored cookies. Some sites will not let you proceed unless you have cookies enabled. For more details about cookies see *http://www.webopedia.com/DidYouKnow/Internet/2002/Cookies.asp*.

Evaluating Information from the Web

The fact that it is simple for anyone to publish on the Web, and that many search engines are not discriminatory in selecting from their databases, makes it important to all users on the Net to carefully evaluate information found.

A national telephone survey done by the Kaiser Family Foundation (KFF) and the Agency for Health Care Research and Quality (AHRQ) in early fall of 2000 revealed that while more Americans are using the Internet to obtain information, few trust the Net to provide accurate information. Just over a quarter (28%) of people surveyed said they would seek such information in the future. The full survey results are available at *http://www.ahrq.gov/qual/kffhigh00.htm*.

While strides have been made to rate Web sites, users are wise to be cautious and not automatically trust every source. Nurses should be aware of the importance of evaluating healthcare information for their own use as well as for helping patients interpret what they find.

Efforts have been expended by a number of organizations to assess the quality of health information on the WWW. Among them are Mitretek Systems and the Health Information Technology Institute (HITI), both nonprofit organizations, and the AHRQ, which is part of the U.S. Department of Health and Human Services.

Mitreteck's white paper (Ambre et al., 1997) put forth seven areas which should be considered when evaluating health information obtained on the Web. These were later revised and released in 1998 as a policy entitled *"Criteria for Assessing the Quality of Health Information on the Internet"* (Health Summit Working

Group, 1998). The criteria they identify include the following:

1. **Credibility**—What is the source of the information; how current is it; is it useful and relevant; what was the process for editorial review?

2. **Content**—To help judge accuracy, examine the hierarchy of evidence, presence of original sources. Are disclaimers provided?

3. **Disclosure**—What is the purpose of the site; who is sponsoring it, and what will the site owners will do with any information that they collect?

4. **Links**—What is the quality of the links provided?

5. **Design**—Is the site accessible, easy to navigate, and searchable?

6. **Interactivity**—Does the site allow for feedback and an exchange of information?

7. **Caveats**—Does the site clearly state its function? Is its purpose primarily information or it is trying to see products and/or services?

A 1995 conference in Switzerland of medical professionals from around the world who were concerned with the quality of information available on the Internet led to the development of the Health on the Net (HON) Foundation. The HON's Web site, *www.hon.ch*, was operational in March of 1996, and in 2002 HON was granted consultative status to the Economic and Social Council of the United Nations. The HON Code of Conduct for medical and health Web sites is located at *http://www.hon.ch/HONcode/Conduct.html*. The HON Foundation reviews Web sites for the adherence to these standards. HON also conducts worldwide surveys of Internet use related to health (Health on the Net Foundation, 2004).

Another organization that has published standards for heath Web sites is URAC. The acronym, which is used to identify the independent, nonprofit organization is taken from the original name of the organization, "Utilization Review Accreditation Commission." However, since 1996 as URAC expanded its work, just the acronym is used. URAC also does business as the "American Accreditation HealthCare Commission, Inc." Among its many different accreditation programs is one for Web site accreditation, which uses over 50 quality standards by which to evaluate sites. For more details on the standards and processes used, see *http://webapps.urac.org/websiteaccreditation/portal/consumer/Standards.asp*.

Health Internet Ethics, known as Hi-Ethics.Inc., is an organization concerned with the privacy, security, credibility, and reliability of health information available on the Internet. In May of 2000, Hi-Ethics released its 14 principles, which have been incorporated into URAC Web site accreditation. It is currently working on the second version of these principles and invites interested parties to participate. For more information see their home page at *www.hiethics.org*.

The National Quality Measures Clearinghouse (NQMC) is sponsored by AHRQ. Their Web site (*http://www.qualitytools.ahrq.gov/*) provides access to a large number of evidence-based quality measures and measure sets as well as recommendations for sites with quality information for healthcare professionals, providers, policy makers, and consumers.

Getting on the Information Superhighway

To access the Net, a computer must be able to connect to one of the networks that is part of the Internet. Originally this required either a modem, which made the connection via a telephone line, or a solid connection via an Ethernet or T1 line. New technology now makes it possible to be online while sitting in a park, restaurant, or airport. Most educational institutions, hospitals, and business provide a connection to the Internet. Most connect to the Internet with high speed lines such as ISDN (integrated services digital network) that can transmit knowledge at speeds from 64 to 128 kilobytes per second (Kbps) or T1 lines, which are capable of simultaneously carrying 24 channels of information at 64 Kbps (Thede, 1999b).

Another way to connect to the Internet is via digital subscriber lines (DSL). There are several different levels of DSLs rated by speed. These lines use sophisticated technology to pack data onto copper wire. DSL lines have speeds up to 32 megabytes per second (Mbps) (Webopedia). The ultimate connection is fiber-optic cable, which today transmits information at about 2 gigabytes per second (Gbps), although technically it is capable of speeds up to 250 Gbps per second.

ISPs are companies that provide access to the Internet for a monthly fee. They provide users with a software package, a user name, password, and access phone number. Many also make available one or more megabytes of space on their server for users to post Web pages. ISPs can also be called Internet access providers (IAPs).

There are many proprietary ISPs which individuals can choose from. The simplest use modem access. A modem is a device that translates computer output, which is digital, to an output that can be transmitted using the telephone line's analog signal and then converted back to a digital signal for the receiving computer. The price varies with the speed at which the modem can translate data, usually beginning at a rate of 28.8 Kbps. Some people now use cable modems, which use the television cable into a house. These modems transmit information that is downloaded very rapidly, but they upload information at the same speed as regular modems.

As people move larger amounts of information around the Net, they desire a connection which allows for faster transfer. Therefore, some ISPs are now making broadband available to individuals. These are wires which carry several channels of data at the same time, thereby increasing speed. The newest method of connecting to the Internet is called wireless fidelity or Wi-Fi, which uses radio waves (Webopedia). In many universities and hospitals, Wi-Fi technology allows access to the Internet without any "wire" connection. Radio waves travel through walls and floors; as long as you are within the range of the base station, you can be connected. In larger cities, there are specific areas that allow anyone with the proper equipment to access the Internet wirelessly. A nonprofit organization, the Wi-Fi Alliance (*http://www.wi-fi.org*), was established in 1999 to help assure reliable and compatible wireless services. While the setup of wireless hardware is being simplified, a recent article warned that users must be especially savvy to security issues when using Wi-Fi. Unless the data being sent via the radio waves in encrypted, you do not know who might be privy to that information (Associated Press, 2004). Some of the newer cell phones and personal digital assistants (PDAs) can now also connect to the Internet.

One very basic caution must be stressed. No matter what method you use to connect to the Internet, make sure that if you are entering any personal data, especially things such as credit card numbers when making purchase, that you do so only on a site you trust and that you have a **secure connection**. When using a browser, you will often see a graphic of a "lock" that is either open or closed at the bottom right or left hand corner of the screen. If the lock is open, your connection is not secure. Check the information provided by your software for details about this important security feature.

Finding and Evaluating an ISP

Most people today are aware of the large ISPs such as America Online and Microsoft Network, but there are many others. These large ISPs provide Internet access and many proprietary features such as chat rooms and games. Some, however, will not give direct access to a site in a URL without first connecting you to their version of the type of feature that URL represents. Also, they have many subscribers, and many find it difficult to get online in the evenings and weekends. They do, however, provide access from many areas of the world and may be the ISP of choice for those who access the Web from multiple points. To help find ISPs in your area see *http://www.thelist.com/*.

There are also many lesser known ISPs that often provide more flexibility in use as well as protection from "spam," or unsolicited e-mail that is sent from a phony address. Additionally, technical help is usually easily available via phone. Smaller ISPs often do not present the access problems that one can run into with the more well-known ISPs.

Depending on your location you may not have a choice of ISPs. If you do, there are several questions that you should ask of a potential ISP. Find out how many subscribers they have per modem; the more in excess of 20 the more busy signals you will get. Also ask what type of connection they have to the Internet. These can vary from a simple 56 Kbps to fiber-optic cable, all of which will affect the speed at which you can use the Internet. Getting a recommendation from someone who has used an ISP for over 6 months and is very satisfied is probably the best way to determine if the ISP is good.

Creating a Web Page

If you would like to do more than surf the Net, you can create a basic Web page without too much difficulty. All of the major office suites (Corel, Microsoft, and Lotus) provide the ability to publish documents and graphics to the Web, although the result is generally not polished. They do, however, make the information readable on the Web. Most of these products even provide the ability to insert links in the document. More advanced programs are now available as are classes in Web design. Some people joke that all you need to do is ask a 12-year old, but it take a little more effort than that.

Although using a word processor may be a good way to start a page, most people will want to modify the resulting HTML tags a little to get a desired effect. There are many online resources for learning HTML. An excellent place to begin is the site by Liam Quinn (1998) at *http://www.htmlhelp.com/reference/html40/olist.html*.

When one first looks at a document with the HTML tags such as the one in Fig. 8.2, it appears very difficult, but in truth it is not. Basic HTML can be learned in about

3 hours. There are also excellent HTML editors available, some of which are WYSIWIG (what you see is what you get); that is, you make your changes on the actual page just as you would to a word processing document, and the program automatically creates the code. These programs often provide some site management tools also. Examples are Adobe's Page Mill, Macromedia's Dreamweaver, and Microsoft's Front Page. Several of these allow a free 15–30-day trial period.

Home Page Design   A home page is the main page of a Web site. Generally, it serves as an index or table of contents to either other documents at that site or other sites. Some individuals have home pages for biographical information, or they may provide a list of links for a topic about which they are very interested. Whenever you see a URL with a tilde (~) in it, you are usually looking at the URL for an individual's home page.

Like all computer projects, the amount of time that one spends in planning a home page and any connected documents greatly reduces the amount of time that the construction takes. Saba (1996) mentions seven things that should be considered when building a home page: purpose, scope, structure, enhancements, links, forms, and maintenance.

Purpose and Scope   A Web site needs to have a focus. Decide on your purpose for creating the site is. If it is personal, is it to provide information about yourself, or about your interests? If for an organization, is the purpose to provide information for the group members or to showcase the organization? These decisions will determine what is on your page and how you organize it. One of the most difficult things about designing a Web page, especially if it is a site for a group, can be obtaining the necessary information. Some printed material that organizations want posted are copyrighted; be sure to clear up any copyright issues before posting information on a page.

Structure and Enhancements   How you place items on a page and the types of enhancements you use determine the usability of your page. Planning for the structure should start with your audience. Organize information in a logical way for them, not you. Look at other home pages and analyze how the ones that you find easiest to use are set up. Talk with some members of your potential audience to get their opinions. Be consistent in design throughout the entire site. If you place a link to return to the home page at the bottom of one

linked document, be sure that this placement is followed for all of the pages (Saba, 1996). Using paper to sketch the pages first will make this phase easier.

Be consistent in how you use color and fonts. The objective is to give the user a feel for the page so that she or he can pay attention to the content, not try to determine how to proceed. Remember that using too many colors or fonts can be distracting. Use colors for the text that contrast with the background color. If you use "wallpaper," or a design for the background, be sure that it does not detract from the readability of the information.

Many sites choose to use graphics or images, to enhance the site. Although they can add immeasurably to the looks of a site, they also increase download time. If the majority of your audience will be accessing your site from a home computer, give careful consideration to the size of the graphics; a long download time will decrease use. Also include alternative text for a graphic picture. This permits those who are accessing the site with a text browser or who have turned off their graphics display to decrease download time to know what the graphic is that they are not seeing. Copyright is also a consideration when using graphics. Before you use art on a site, be sure you know the copyright status. This holds true whether the clip art is from a software package or from the Web.

Links, Forms, and Maintenance   Links either within a site or to other sites are a hallmark of the Web. If you link to outside sites, they should relate to the purpose of the site. Providing a brief description of what a user can expect to find at a site prevents unpleasant surprises. Whether the links are internal or external they should be checked before posting and periodically after posting. Most of the HTML editors provide a way to check the links.

If the site is for an organization, you may wish to include a form to request more information, which users can download and mail, fax, or e-mail to the organization (Saba, 1996). It is also possible to design a form that users can use to enter information online, but this will require additional programming and the appropriate programs on the server. The use of the "mailto:" tag, which turns into a preaddressed e-mail message when the user clicks it, is another way to request information.

Many sites are started with a great deal of excitement and then left to fend for themselves, a result readily apparent to users. When planning a site, be sure to determine who will be responsible for updating the site and when. If provisions are made for a user to request information, it is imperative that requests are answered promptly.

Patient/Consumer Use of the Internet

Research conducted by NUA in January 2003 indicates that 46% of seniors in the U.S. have been Internet users for more than 5 years, while an additional 41% have been using the Internet for less than 5 years. That is a total of 87% on seniors online. Of these 70% use the Internet to search for health information (Jupitermedia Corporation, 2003). A similar survey reported by the BBC, found that 83% of seniors in the United Kingdom regularly use the Internet (BBC News, 2002).

As nurses we know that the number of possible health problems increases as individuals age. However, the rate at which seniors have embraced the Internet is still amazing, given that it did not exist for the greater part of their lives.

Many hospitals and insurance agencies, including the Federal government have Web sites set up for patients. Hospitals provide information about their hours and services, the ability to find a map or obtain directions, locate physicians and see their credentials, and learn about educational programs designed for the community. Organizations allow for the submission of information on online forms, the checking of healthcare benefits, and even encourage patients to order prescription medications online. These pharmacy sites include access to explanations about the uses of medications and provide for a way to obtain information and answers to questions from a pharmacist.

The Internet does provide a great deal of health information, and its usage is growing. However, the actual effect it is having on healthcare is still undetermined (Baker et al., 2003). On the other hand, the Web has been enthusiastically used for support and communication among people with various chronic diseases as well as mood disorders (Fogel, 2002; Lamberg, 2003; Mendelson, 2003).

Looking to the Future

As the Internet continues to become integrated into the lives of more and more people, government, corporations, and educators are working together to design the future. The Next Generation Internet (NGI) is a term used to describe this endeavor. The vision of those involved in this project is to make the Internet so reliable and transparent, that it is ingrained into life. They believe that the NGI will soon join services like basic plumbing and electricity as things we take for granted (IBM, n.d.). The U.S. government reported that the NGI

program had been completed and had met all of its goals except for the one related to speed of networking (1 terabyte per second [Tbps]). However, attainment of that goal is expected in the near future (Next Generation Internet Initiative, n.d.).

Another project currently under way to improve the Internet is called Internet2. This project has been undertaken by the University Corporation for Advanced Internet Development (UCAID), which is a nonprofit consortium led by universities. The aim of Internet2 is to develop advanced Internet technologies in research and education to support higher education. Over 120 universities in the U.S. are participating with partners in industry and government. There is a great deal of cooperation between the NGI and Internet2 groups (Next Generation Internet Initiative, n.d.a).

In March of 2004, the Nielsen//NetRatings reported that three quarters of all Americans have Internet access from their homes. This equates to over 204 million people and is an increase from a two-thirds penetration 1 year earlier (Silicon Valley Business, Inc., 2004).

Real-Time Communication

As technology increases the speed of transmission on the Internet, we are seeking other applications. These include the ability to send both audio and video data between two or more sites in what appears to be real time. This type of technology is being used for virtual meetings and has been enthusiastically accepted by educational institutions for distance learning. As the technical glitches are resolved, expect to see more use of these technologies.

Faster Speeds

Given the rate at which the Internet is growing and the technology supporting it is developing, the future is not that far off. For example, in March of 2004, researchers from North Carolina State University reported development of a new data transfer protocol. The Binary Increase Congestion TCP (BIC-TCP) has been tested and found to be able to transmit data at speeds that are 6,000 times faster than DSL and 150,000 times faster than modems (Science Blog, 2004).

Summary

The Internet has changed the way we communicate, gather information, and do business. It has changed the speed at which many tasks are accomplished. It has made our world feel smaller and minimized the differences of background, culture, and social class. There is no doubt that the Internet in an influential force on our society. Its amazing rate of growth—in the number of users, networks connected, and amount of information accessible, is evidence of it potential to further effect the way we live, work, and make decisions. No longer can any professional ignore the need to be familiar with at least the basic use of this technology.

The fact that the Internet and especially the WWW has made information available so quickly to anyone who seeks it, also adds additional responsibilities to our role as nurses. More and more consumers are turning to the Internet for information about their health. Although there is a great deal of excellent information available, consumers still need healthcare professionals to help them interpret and evaluate what they have read, and assist them in understanding how it relates to their health. We no doubt will find additional uses for the Internet in sharing information with our clients and each other.

As our world shifts to a knowledge economy, the ability to find and interpret information will be increasingly valued. It is no longer possible to grasp all of the knowledge that exists on any topic, as it increases so rapidly. The Internet provides us with an efficient way to search for and locate information we need when we need it. It is a wonderful information delivery tool. However, it is just that—a tool. Our ability to think, to ask the right questions, to interpret, integrate, and synthesize what we find is what leads to value and makes all the difference.

References

A Brief History of the Internet and Related Networks. (2001). Retrieved January 11, 2004, from *http://www.isoc.org/internet/history/cerf.shtml*

Abilock, D. and Abilock, D. (2004). *Information Literacy: Search Strategies*. Retrieved on March 28, 2004, from *http://www.noodletools.com/debbie/literacies/information/5locate/adviceengine.html*

Ambre, J., Guard, R., Perveiler, F. M., Renner, J., and Rippen, R. (1997). *White Paper: Criteria for Assessing the Quality of Health Information on the Internet*. Retrieved on April 1, 2004, from *http://hitiweb.mitretek.org/docs/criteria.html*

Americans as Health Care Consumers: Update on the Role of Quality Information. Highlights of a National Survey. (2000). Rockville, MD: Kaiser Family Foundation, and the Agency for Healthcare Research and Quality. Retrieved *http://www.ahrq.gov/qual/kffhigh00.htm*

Associated Press. (2004). *Wi-Fi Popularity Opens Security Holes*. Retrieved on June 1, 2004, from *http://www.cnn.com/2004/TECH/05/31/wi.fisecurity.ap/index.html*

Atkins, L. (1998). *Big Brother is Watching—and Reading Your Email. Cleveland Plain Dealer*, January 21,11B.

Baker, L., Wagner, T. H., Singer, S., and Bundorf, M. K. (2003). Use of the Internet and E-mail for health care information: Results from a national survey. *The Journal of the American Medical Association* 289(18):2400–2406.

BBC News. (2002). *Elderly Take Up Net Surfing*. Retrieved on May 16, 2004, from *http://news.bbc.co.uk/1/hi/sci/tech/1977823.stm*

BBC News. (2003). *Web's Inventor Gets a Knighthood*. Retrieved January 6, 2004, from *http://news.bbc.co.uk/1/hi/technology/3357073.stm*

BBC News. (2004). *19th Century News Going Online*. Retrieved on June 12, 2004, from *http://news.bbc.co.uk/go/pr/fr/-/2/hi/technology/3795631.stm*

Berners-Lee, T. (n.d.). *Frequently Asked Questions*. Retrieved on January 25, 2004, from *http://www.w3.org/People/Berners-Lee/FAQ.html*

Bowers, L. (1997). Constructing international professional identity: What psychiatric nurses talk about on the Internet. *International Journal of Nursing Studies* 34(3):208–212.

Brin, S. and Page, L. (n.d.). *The Anatomy of a Large-Scale Hypertextual Web Search Engine*. Computer Science Department, Stanford University. Retrieved March 26, 2004, from *http://www7.scu.edu.au/programme/fullpapers/1921/com1921.htm*

Bush, V. (July, 1945). *As We May Think. The Atlantic Monthly*. Retrieved on March 27, 2004, from *http://www.theatlantic.com/unbound/flashbks/computer/bushf.htm*

Bush, V. (July, 1945). *The Atlantic Monthly. As We May Think*, Vol. 176, No. 1;101–108.

Carroll, S. (2004). *How to Find Anything Online*. Retrieved June 14, 2004, from *http://www.pcmag.com/print_article/0,1761,a=41018,00.asp*

Center for Next Generation Internet. (2001). *Biannual Strategic Note: Internet Survey Reaches 109 Million Internet Host Level*. Retrieved March 21, 2004, from *http://www.ngi.org/trends/TrendsPR0102.txt*

Fogel, J. (2002). Internet use and advanced practice oncology nursing. *Topics in Advanced Practice Nursing eJournal*. Retrieved February 6, 2004, from *http://medscape.com/viewarticle/442738*

Gleick, J. (2004). *"Get Out of My Namespace."* New York Times. Accessed March 21, 2004, from *http://www.nytimes.com/2004/03/21/magazine/21NAMES.html*

Gromov, G. R. (1998). *History of Internet and WWW: The Roads and Crossroads of Internet History*. Retrieved January 22, 2004, from *http://www.netvalley.com/intvalold.html*

Hall, R. (n.d.). *History of the World Wide Web According to R. Hall.* Retrieved March 28, 2004, from *http://www.webdesignstuff.org/society/lecture_04_01_20/index.php*

Hansell, S. (2004). *Gates Backs E-mail Stamp in War on Spam.* New York Times Accessed on Feb. 2, 2004, from *http://www.nytimes.com/2004/02/02/technology/02spam.html*

Health on the Net Foundation. (2004). Retrieved on March 28, 2004, from *http://www.hon.ch*

Health Summit Working Group. (1998). *Criteria for Assessing the Quality of Health Information on the Internet.* Mitretek. Retrieved March 28, 2004, from *http://hitiweb.mitretek.org/docs/policy.pdf*

Hockman, D. (2004). In searching We trust. New York Times. *Retrieved March 15, 2004, from http://www.nytimes.com/2004/03/14/fashion/14GOOG.html*

IBM. (n.d.). *Next Generation Internet.* Retrieved May 31, 2004, from *http://www.ngi.ibm.com/ index.html*

ICANN. (2003). *Top Level Domains.* Retrieved March 21, 2004, from *http://www.icann.org/tlds/*

ICANN. (2004). *Welcome to ICANN.* Retrieved March 21, 2004, from *http://www.icann.org/new.html*

Internet Public Library. (2004). University of Michigan School of Information. Retrieved Jun 16, 2004, from *http://www.ipc.org*

Internet Society. (2002a). *All about the Internet: Internet Histories.* Retrieved on January 11, 2004, from *http://www.isoc.org/internet/history/index.shtml*

Internet Society. (2002b). *Internet Connectivity Access.* Retrieved on March 21, 2004, from *http://www.isoc.org/isoc/access/*

InterNIC FAQs on New Top-Level Domains. (2002). Retrieved on March 21, 2004, from *http://www.internic.net/faqs/new-tlds.html*

Jupitemedia Corporation. (2003). *eMarketer: Most US Seniors are Veteran Net Users. Retrieved March 30, 2004, from http://www.nua.ie/surveys/index.cgi?f=VS&art_id=905358703&rel=true*

Kurose, J. F. and Ross, K. W. (2001). *Computer Networking: A Top-Down Approach Featuring the Internet.* Boston: Addison Wesley Longman.

Lamberg, L. (2003). Online empathy for mood disorders: Patients turn to the Internet support groups. *Journal of the American Medical Association* 289(23):3073–3074.

Leiner, B. V., Cerf, V. G., Clark, D. D., et al. (2003). *A Brief History of the Internet.* Retrieved January 11, 2004, from *http://www.isoc.org/internet/history/brief.shtml*

MacPherson, K. I. (1997). Menopause on the Internet: Building knowledge and community on-line. *Advances in Nursing Science* 20(1):66–78.

Mendelson, C. (2003). Gentle hugs: Internet listservs as sources of support for women with lupus. *Advances in Nursing Science* 26(4):299–306.

MSNBC News. (2004). *Google Founders Sittin on $3 Billion Stakes.* From the Associated Press, posted May 21, 2004. Retrieved June 1, 2004, from *http://www.msnbc.msn.com/id/5033780/*

Next Generation Internet Initiative. (n.d.a). *Related Activity and Agency Servers.* Retrieved May 31, 2004 from, *http://www.ngi.gov/related/*

Next Generation Internet Initiative. (n.d.). *About the NGI.* Retrieved May 31, 2004, from *http://www.ngi.gov/*

Nursing Discussion Forums. (n.d.). Retrieved June 22, 2004, from *http://nursing.buffalo.edu/mccartny/nursing_discussion_forums.html*

Plank, R. K. (1998). Nursing on-line for continuing education credit. *The Journal of Continuing Education in Nursing* 29(4):165–172.

Project Gutenberg (2004). Retrieved June 1, 2004, from *www.gutenberg.org.*

Rinaldi, A. (1998). *The Net: User Guidelines and Netiquette.* Retrieved March 23, 2004, from *http://www.fau.edu/netiquette/net/*

Saba, V. (1996). Developing a home page for the World Wide Web. *American Journal of Infection Control* 24(6):468–470.

Salamon, A. (2004). *Top-Level Domains.* Retrieved March 21, 2004, from *http://www.dns.net/dnsrd/tld.html*

Science Blog. (2004). *New Protocol Could Speed Internet Significantly.* Retrieved on March 19, 2004, from *http://www.scienceblog.com/community/article2473.html*

Selingo, J. (2004). *When a Search Engine Isn't Enough, Call a Librarian.* New York Times. February 5, 2004. Retrieved February 6, 2004, at *http://www.nytimes.com/2004/02/05/technology/circuits/05libr.html?ex=1077097712&ei=1&en=b7f1de99614bb939*

Silicon Valley Business, Inc. (2004). *Three Out of Four American Have Access to the Internet, According to Nielsen//NetRatings.* Retrieved on March 18. 2004, from *http://www.prnewswire.com/cgi-bin/stories.pl?ACCT=SVBIZINK3.story&STORY=/www/story/03-18-2004/0002130511*

Thede, L. Q. (1999a). *Computers in Nursing: Bridges to the Future.* Philadelphia, PA: Lippincott Williams & Wilkins.

Thede, L. Q. (1999b). The Internet unraveled. *Orthopaedic Nursing* 18(2):32–42.

U.S. Census Bureau. (2004). *World POPClock Projection.* Retrieved June 15, 2004, from *http://www.census.gov/cgi-bin/ipc/popclockw*

Webopedia (n.d.). *The Only Online Dictionary and Search Engine You Need for Computer and Internet Technology Definitions.* Retrieved March 21, 2004, from *http://www.webopedia.com/*

Zetter, K. (2004). *E-mail Snooping Ruled Permissible.* Wired News 08:40 AM Jun. 30, 2004 PT. Retrieved July 1, 2003, from *http://www.wired.com/news/privacy/0,1848,64043,00.html*

Recommended Readings and Webliography

Adler, C. L. and Zarchin, Y. R. (2002). The "virtual focus group": Using the Internet to reach pregnant women on home bed rest. *Journal of Obstetric, Gynecologic, and Neonatal Nursing* 31(4):418–427.

Anthony, D. (1996). *Health on the Internet*. Cambridge, MA: Blackwell Science.

Anthony, D. (1998). Web worries . . . a major concern is over security and provision of relevant high quality information. *Nursing Standard* 12(43):28.

Bachman, J. A., and Panzarine, S. (1998). Enabling student nurses to use the information superhighway. *Journal of Nursing Education* 37(4):155–161.

Bagshaw, B. A. and Neill, K. M. (2000). Nurse practitioners on the Internet. *Clinical excellence for Nurse Practitioners* 4(4):245–249.

Bergren, M. D. (1999). Information technology. Create a virtual community: Start an Internet discussion list. *Journal of School Nursing* 15(5):24–28.

Brown, L. P., Bair, A. H., Meier, P. P., et al. (1998). Connecting points. Accessing on-line information at the National Institutes of Health: Highlights and practical tips. *Computers in Nursing* 16(4):198–201.

Buckman, J. (n.d.). *A History of Listservs*. Retrieved March 21, 2004, from *http://www.lyris.com/about/whitepapers/listserver_history.html*

Clark, D. J. (1998). Course redesign: Incorporating an Internet web site into an existing nursing class. *Computers in Nursing* 16(4):219–222.

Cobb, S. C. (2003). Comparison of oncology nurse and physician use of the Internet for continuing education. *Journal of Continuing Education in Nursing* 34(4):184–188.

Cragg, C. E., Edwards, N., Zhai, Y., Xin, S. L., Hui, D. (2003). Integrating web-based technology into distance education for nurses in China: Computer and Internet Access and Attitudes. *CIN* 21(5):265–274. Retrieved February 6, 2004, from *http://www.medscape.com/viewarticle/464290*

Davis, J. (Ed.), et al. (1998). *Health & Medicine on the Internet* (Professional ed.). New York: Chapman & Hall.

Denny, J. T., Ginsberg, S., Papp, D., Browne, G., Morgan, S., Kushiins, L., and Solina, A. (2002). Hospital initiatives in promoting smoking cessation: A survey of Internet and hospital-based programs targeted at consumers. *Chest* 122(2):692–698.

Estabrooks, C. A. (2003). The Internet and access to evidence: How are nurses positioned? *Journal of Advanced Nursing* 42(1):73–81.

Fawcett, J. and Buhle, E. L., Jr. (1995). Using the Internet for data collection. An innovative electronic strategy. *Computers in Nursing* 13(6):273–279.

Fleitas, J. (1998). Computer monitor. Spinning tales from the World Wide Web: Qualitative research in an electronic environment. *Qualitative Health Research* 8(2):283–292.

Frandsen, J. L. (1997). The use of computers in cancer pain management. *Seminars in Oncology Nursing* 13(1):49–56.

Gee, P. M. (1997). The Internet—a home care nursing clinical resource: Part 1. *Home Healthcare Nurse* 15(2):115–121.

Gibbs, M. A. (Ed.) (1997). *Mosby's Medical Surfari: A Guide to Exploring the Internet and Discovering Top Health Care Resources*. St. Louis, MO: Mosby.

Guard, J. R., Morris, T. A., Schick, L., et al. (1997). A community approach to serving health information needs: NetWellness. *Health Care on the Internet* 1(1):73–82.

Hamff, C. L. and Glaser, J. P. (1997). Internet policy and procedures for health care organizations: The approach of Partners Healthcare System, Inc. *Topics in Health Information Management* 17(4):40–61.

Henry, N. I. (1997). Getting acquainted with support and self-help groups on the Internet. *Health Care on the Internet* 1(2):27–32.

Hornstra, D. (2000). *Consumer Use of Websites. Presented at the Society for Healthcare Consumer Advocacy, September 2000*. Retrieved on February 28, 2004, from *http://hornstra.net/deb/SHCASanAntonioSeptember2000handout.pdf*

Jenkins, J. and Erdman, K. (1998). Web-based documentation systems. *Home Health Care Management & Practice* 10(2):52–61.

Kalsman, M. W. and Acosta, D. A. (2000). Use of the Internet as a medical resource by rural physicians. *Journal of the American Board of Family Practice* 13(5):349–352.

Kirkpatrick, M. K., Brown, S., and Atkins, T. (1998). Electronic education. Using the Internet to integrate cultural diversity and global awareness. *Nurse Educator* 23(2):15–17.

Klemm, P. and Nolan, M. T. (1998). Internet cancer support groups: Legal and ethical issues for nurse researchers. *Oncology Nursing Forum* 25(4):673–676.

Klemm, P., Reppert, K., and Visich, L. (1998). A nontraditional cancer support group: The Internet. *Computers in Nursing* 16(1):31–36.

Kolesar, M. S. (1997). Realizing the competitive advantage of the Internet. *Caring* 16(12):56, 58, 60.

Lakeman, R. (1997). Using the Internet for data collection in nursing research. Presented as a paper at a qualitative research conference for health researchers held at the Eastern Institute of Technology, Taradale, New Zealand, January 1997. *Computers in Nursing* 15(5):269–275.

Laws, J. (1998). Computer applications: Safety & health on the Internet. *Occupational Health & Safety* 67(4):25.

Lewis, A. (1998). Information technology in the next millennium: Five trends reshape home care's future. *Remington Report* 6(2):4–6.

Lybecker, C. J. (1998). Professionally speaking. Surfing the Net. *American Journal of Maternal Child Nursing* 23(1):17–21.

Mangan, P. (1998). Site perfect. *Nursing Standard* 12(39):22–25.

McKenzie, B. C. (1997). *Medicine and the Internet: Introducing Online Resources and Terminology*. New York: Oxford University Press.

Morris, D. A., Guard, J. R., Marine, S. A., et al. (1997). Approaching equity in consumer health information delivery: NetWellness. *Journal of the American Medical Informatics Association* 4(1):6–13.

Murray, P. J. (1996). Nurses' computer-mediated communications on NURSENET: A case study. *Computers in Nursing* 14(4):227–234.

Neray, P. (1997). End paper. Security on the Internet: Is your system vulnerable? *Nursing Management* 28(7):64.

Nicoll, L. H. (1994). An introduction to the Internet: History, structure, and access. Part 2. *Journal of Nursing Administration* 24(5):11–13.

Nicoll, L. H. (1998). *Computers in Nursing's Nurses Guide to the Internet*. Philadelphia, PA: Lippincott Williams & Wilkins.

Nicoll, L. H. (2000). Quick and effective website evaluation. *CIN* 3(3):8–9. Retrieved on May 23, from *http://www.mainedesk.com/website%20eval1.pdf*

O'Carroll, D. and McMahon, A. S. (1998). Research & development co-ordinating centre. *Nursing Standard* 12(38):32–33.

Oppenheimer, T. (2003). *The Flickering Mind*. New York: Random House.

Peterson, M. W. (2003). Patient use of the Internet for information in a lung cancer clinic. *Chest* 123(2):452–457.

Pomeroy, B. (Ed.) (1997). *A Beginner's Guide to the Internet and the World Wide Web*. San Diego, CA: Harcourt Brace Professional Publishing.

Puetz, B. E. (1997). Resume writing in a wired age. *RN* 60(2):28–31.

Ryan, J. M. and Southern, J. (1998). Soapbox. A&E nursing and the Internet. *Accident & Emergency Nursing* 6(2):106–109.

Schell, C. L. and Rathe, R. (1996). Geri Ann: Designing educational programs for the Internet. *Gerontology & Geriatrics Education* 16(4):15–25.

Scollin, P. (2001). A study of factors related to the use of online resources by nurse educators. *Computers in Nursing* 19(6):2449–2256.

Simpson, R. L. (1996). Technology: Nursing the system. Will the Internet supplant community health networks? *Nursing Management* 27(2):20;23.

Simpson, R. L. (1997). Technology: Nursing the system. Internet security concerns. *Nursing Management* 28(12):24–25, 27.

Sinclair, M. (1997). Education: Midwives, midwifery and the Internet. *Modern Midwife* 7(9):11–14.

Skiba, D. J. (1997). Intellectual property issues in the digital health care world. *Nursing Administration Quarterly* 21(3):11–20.

Sparks, S. (1996). Use of the Internet for infection control and epidemiology. *American Journal of Infection Control* 24(6):435–439.

Sparks, S. M. (1996). Using the Internet for urology nursing. *Urologic Nursing* 16(4):131–134.

Sparks, S. M. (1997). Using the Internet for nursing administration. *Journal of Nursing Administration* 27(3):15–20.

Swiatek-Kelley, J. (2000). Teaching cancer survivors hos to search the Internet. *Health Care on the Internet* 4(4):59–67.

Thede, L. Q. (2003). *Informatics and Nursing: Opportunities and Challenges* (2nd ed.). Philadelphia, PA: Lippincott Williams & Wilkins.

Thompson, T. and Penprase, B. (2004). RehabNurse-L: An analysis of the rehabilitation nurse LISTSERV experience. *Rehabilitation Nursing* 29(2):56–61.

Thorwaldson, J. (1997). "PAN Islands" experiment may be an answer to problem of Internet-access "have-nots." *Health Care on the Internet* 1(1):35–41.

Walker, G. D. and Burnham, L. D. (1997). Putting the Web to work. *Caring* 16(12):52–54.

Ward, R. (1997). Network. Implications of computer networking and the Internet for nurse education. *Nurse Education Today* 17(3):178–183.

Ward, R. and Haines, M. (1998). Don't get left behind—get on-line. *Practice Nurse* 16(3):164–166.

Wink, D. M. (1995). Electronic education. An introduction to nursing on the Internet. Part one. *Nurse Educator* 20(6):9–13.

Wink, D. M. (1996). Electronic education. An introduction to nursing on the Internet: Part two. *Nurse Educator* 21(1):8–12.

Wootton, J. C. (1997). The quality of information on women's health on the Internet. *Journal of Women's Health* 6(5):575–581.

WWWtools for Education. (n.d.). *Latest Articles*. Retrieved on March 28, 2004, from *http://magazines.fasfind.com/wwwtools/*

Xu, L., Khaled, H., and Rhee, I. (2004). *Binary Increase Congestion Control for Fast, Long-Distance Networks*. Presented at Infocom 2004. Retrieved on March 19, 2004 at *http://www.scienceblog.com/community/article2473.html*

Selected Consumer Websites

Black Women's Health Imperative,
http://www.BlackWomensHealth.org, Formerly the National Black Women's Health Project. Winner of several awards.

cancerfacts.com, *http://www.cancerfacts.com/* An award winning commercial site aimed at those whose lives are affected by cancer. Provides news, access to support groups, and links to other sites. Cookies must be enabled.

drkoop.com, *http://drkoop.com* A site for consumers with features on various health issues and an extensive search function. If you read the fine print at the bottom you will see that it is not associated with the former surgeon general.

HIV Stops With Me, *http://hivstopswithme.org* Information and support for individuals on HIV/AIDS.

KidsHealth, *http://kidshealth.org* Sponsored by the Nemours Foundation, this education site has sections designed for parents, kids, and teens. Choice of English or Spanish.

Lab Tests Online, *http://www.labtestsonline.net/* Searchable by tests, conditions and diseases, and screening for a broad range of lab tests. No values are provided, but explanations are given in easy to understand language. Site is easy to navigate.

Lung Cancer Online, *http://www.lungcanceronline.org/* Patient information and funding for research are the goals of this site of the Lung Cancer Online Foundation.

MayoClinic.com, *http://www.mayoclinic.com/* Search functions on many health topics, news articles, tools, and links for consumers sponsored by the Mayo Foundation for Medical Education and Research.

NetWellness, *http://netwellness.org* Health information for consumers is available on this site, which is cosponsored by the University of Cincinnati, The Ohio State University, and Case Western reserve University. There is an "Ask the Expert" section where individual can pose questions as well as search for and read the answers to previously posted questions. Included are many links, access to a health encyclopedia, and current news.

SeniorNet, *http://www.seniornet.org/php/* Designed for retirees, this site provides seniors the ability to chat on various topics of interest in addition to health-related issues. Online tutorials are available as is information about ways to adapt technology for those with motor or visual limitations.

teenwire, *http://teenwire.com* A site sponsored by Planned Parenthood Federation of America to provide sexual health information to teens. There is a section for parents and educators.

WebMD, *http://webmd.com* A commercial site with various sections for different audiences, including physicians, providers, and consumers.

9

PDA and Wireless Devices

Kathleen G. Charters
Thomasine D. Guberski

OBJECTIVES

1. Describe utilization of a personal digital assistant (PDA) in clinical care.
2. Apply principles of Health Insurance Portability and Accountability Act of 1996 (HIPAA) to the utilization of a PDA in clinical practice.
3. Analyze the usefulness of specific clinical applications for the PDA using a structured critique format.
4. Describe the key characteristics of a wireless device.
5. Apply the principles of HIPAA to the utilization of a wireless device in clinical practice.
6. List three advantages and three disadvantages of utilizing a wireless device in clinical practice.

KEY WORDS

personal digital assistant
PDA
wireless device
HIPAA
battery life
portability
clinical applications
case study

 ## PDA and Wireless Devices

As information technology evolves, the trend is to provide greater functionality using smaller computers. Individual use of information technology depends on a continuum along several dimensions: the desired physical size and characteristics of the hardware, the length of time a mobile device (computer that does not have to be plugged into an electrical outlet in order to use it) runs before requiring recharging, whether the computer functions as stand-alone or as part of a network, the availability of applications to support an individual's work, and the appropriate level of security. When evaluating information technology usefulness for an individual, all these factors are measured against the individual's workflow to determine what combination best supports their work. The question, "What works best for a nurse?" has no one right or wrong answer;

however, it is possible to come up with a best fit to meet a given nurse's needs.

 ## Continuum of Information Technology for Personal Computing

Desktop Computer versus Smartphone Physical Characteristics

The distinctions between different forms of computers are relative according to characteristics such as weight, display size, processing power, memory, storage capacity, and battery life. In general, a desktop computer is too heavy to hand carry, has a larger display, processing power measured in gigahertz (GHz), memory capacity up to gigabytes (GB), storage capacity up to GB, and is not designed to run on internal battery power (see Table 9.1). In contrast, a smartphone (a hybrid device combining

Table 9.1   Continuum of Physical Characteristics

Typical Dimension	Desktop	Notebook/Laptop	Tablet	PDA	Smartphone
Weight	25–50 lb	5–7 lb	3–4 lb	4–8 oz	4–7 oz
Screen size	15–20 in.	12–17 in.	10–14 in.	2–4 in.	2–5 in.
Processing power	2.4–3.2 GHz	800 MHz to 2.0 GHz	800 MHz to 1.3 GHz	126–400 MHz	130–400 MHz
Memory	128 MB to 2 GB	128 MB to 1 GB	128 MB to 1 GB	2–64 MB	8–64 MB
Battery life	None	1.5–3 hours	3–9 hours	6 hours to weeks	3–12 hours talk 240 hours standby

wireless telephone, e-mail, Internet access, and PDA organizer functions) is at the opposite end of the continuum. A smartphone represents a convergence between computing and communication. A smartphone fits in a shirt pocket, weighs ounces, has a 2 in. or slightly larger display, has processing power measured in megahertz (MHz), limited memory measured in megabytes (MB), limited storage capacity measured in MB, and can run on battery power in talk mode for 3 or more hours or on standby for up to 10 days before requiring recharging (see Table 9.1). Between the desktop computer and the smartphone are three stepping-stones.

Notebook/Laptop versus Tablet versus PDA Physical Characteristics

A notebook/laptop computer is light enough to hand carry, has a slightly smaller display, and slightly less processing power and storage capacity than a desktop computer (see Table 9.1); however, like a desktop, it is possible to add external devices to a notebook/laptop to enhance any shortcoming. The trade-off is that adding external devices increases the weight of the system. The most important difference between a desktop and a notebook/laptop is that a notebook/laptop is designed to run on battery power so that in addition to being portable, it can run without requiring access to an electrical outlet. This greatly enhances the ability of the user to have a computer available when traveling.

The next step in the progression to mobile computing is the tablet computer, a small light notebook computer with the ability to provide input using a stylus. The tablet is lighter, has a slightly smaller display, and slightly less processing power and storage capacity than a laptop (see Table 9.1). The most important difference between a notebook/laptop and a tablet is that the display allows use of a stylus for input on a tablet. Keyboard

and mouse input is possible but not necessary when using a tablet since the user may employ a stylus for writing or drawing (digital ink).

An even more mobile form of computer is the handheld. An example of a handheld computer is a PDA. Weighing in at 8 oz or less, it is small enough to fit in a shirt pocket (see Table 9.1). Features differentiating a tablet from a PDA include the size of the keyboard and lack of a mouse (Roseberry, n.d.). A PDA comes with a miniature keyboard and a stylus for data entry. It is possible to add an external portable keyboard for a PDA. The PDA has many characteristics in common with the smartphone (a hybrid of PDA and telephone), but tends to have a longer battery life since it need not support voice communication.

Battery Life

Mobile devices depend on batteries. The length of time a battery supports use of the device and the length of time it takes for the battery to recharge determine the usefulness of the device. Users are frustrated by limited battery life that does not support their workflow. There are different types of batteries, and depending on the individual battery characteristics (see Table 9.2), there are different strategies for extending battery life (see Table 9.3). Therefore, it is critically important to understand what type of battery is being used in order to get the best possible performance (Buchmann, 2001). Battery life has both hardware and software components, e.g., screen illumination algorithms for when to dim the screen to conserve the battery. Adding peripheral devices (e.g., external keyboards or memory cards) increases the workload of the battery. Strategies to achieve longer times between battery recharging include dynamic power-consumption-management procedures, power-aware applications for adaptive power management,

Table 9.2   Rechargeable Battery Characteristics

Characteristic	Lithium Ion (Li-Ion)	Lithium Ion Polymer (Li-Polymer)	Nickel Cadmium (NiCd)	Nickel Metal Hydride (NiMH)	Reusable Alkaline
Cost	High	Medium high	Medium low	Medium	Low[*]
Energy density	High	Medium high	Low	Medium low	Medium
Environmental considerations	Avoid venting with flame	Performs well in high ambient temperature[†]	Toxic metals	Friendly	Friendly
Overcharge tolerance	Very low	Low	Moderate	Low	Moderate
Recharge time	3 hours	3–5 hours	1-hour fast charge	2–4 hours quick charge	2–3 hours
Self-discharge rate	Medium low	Medium low	Medium high	High	Low
Storage	Store in charger[‡] or on a shelf at moderate temperature for up to 20 days		Store on a shelf; apply a topping-charge before use. Recharge after 30–60 days	Store on a shelf; apply a topping-charge before use. Recharge after 60–90 days	Store on a shelf for up to 10 years

[*]Cost per cycle is high compared to the other batteries listed.
[†]No danger of flammability.
[‡]No trickle charge, but may implement a topping charge periodically.

Table 9.3   Battery Life Strategies

Strategy	Lithium Ion (Li-Ion)	Lithium Ion Polymer (Li-Polymer)	Nickel Cadmium (NiCd)	Nickel Metal Hydride (NiMH)	Reusable Alkaline
To hasten death	Store for more than 6 months at full charge at elevated temperature	Store for more than 6 months at full charge	Leave in charger for days at elevated temperature and use occasionally for brief periods	Leave in charger for days at elevated temperature	Allow to discharge fully before recharging. Store at elevated temperature
To prolong life	Recharge after partial discharge	Recharge after partial discharge	Initial slow full charge followed by periodic full discharge (cycling) Avoid memory phenomenon (crystalline formations)	Initial rapid full charge followed by periodic full discharge (cycling). Avoid memory phenomenon (crystalline formations)	Recharge after partial discharge to 50% of original state

and energy-aware interfaces for reducing display demands on the battery (Bloom et al., 2004).

For mobile technology, the most common types are either some form of a lithium battery or some form of a nickel battery. Lithium batteries do not tolerate being stored for long periods at full charge. They perform best when recharged after a partial discharge. Nickel batteries do not tolerate being left for long periods on a trickle charge. They perform best when periodically fully discharged and then fully recharged (cycling). When nickel batteries are not properly handled, they develop a memory phenomenon where there is crystalline formation that interferes with the ability of the battery to fully recharge. Some mobile devices use alkaline rechargeable batteries, which perform best when allowed to discharge to half of their original charge, and then are recharged.

There are also different battery charger types (e.g., slow, quick, and fast) and a mismatch between battery type and charger will damage the battery and may create unsafe conditions (Buchmann, 2001). Rechargeable batteries may be used under a reasonably wide temperature range; however, recharging batteries should only be done at room temperature. Moderate temperatures produce better results and a safer environment.

PDA Operating Systems

The type of operating system determines in part the strategies for conserving energy in order to prolong battery life. The operating system for a computer determines many of the characteristics of the computer because the operating system controls how the hardware and the software work together. The two most commonly used operating systems for PDAs are Palm OS or Windows Mobile. Other less frequently used operating systems include Blackberry, Hiptop, Linux, and Symbian. The type of operating system must be compatible with the software the user adds to the computer or the software will not run properly.

Mobile Devices

Size and weight determine to what extent a computer is considered portable (see Table 9.4). Any computer system that can be hand carried or rolled around is a portable device. A desktop computer mounted on a wheeled cart or stand and plugged into a battery so it can be rolled from room to room is considered portable. Computers that are small and light weight enough to be hand carried are mobile devices. A laptop is considered mobile. The key to a mobile device is the nonbulky display. A computer that can be held in the palm of one hand and used with the other hand is a handheld device. A PDA is considered a handheld. The key to a handheld device is the miniature keyboard.

Note the trade-off in functions. A desktop computer has the least limitations in what it can do because it has the greatest capacity. A desktop computer has the largest display, most memory, greatest storage capacity, and a variety of ways to enter data (e.g., full keyboard, mouse, microphone, and touch-screen). As size gets smaller, there are corresponding limitations on what a computer can do. The most mobile devices are also the most limited in screen size, memory, storage space, and ways to enter data (i.e., primarily by stylus, with miniature keyboard access).

Desktop, notebook/laptop, tablet, and PDA computers may be used as a stand-alone device or as part of a network. (Smartphones, by definition, must be part of a cellular network.) The Institute of Electrical and Electronics Engineers (IEEE) establishes the rules that govern how networks work. A desktop computer typically is connected to the world through a metal wire cable (e.g., copper wire Ethernet following the IEEE 802.3 standard). An alternative way of connecting is through glass or plastic fiber-optic cable, which is more expensive and fragile than metal wire cable but has the advantage of greater bandwidth, which means a higher rate of data transmission (see Table 9.5).

Table 9.4   Continuum of Portability

Portability	Desktop	Notebook/Laptop	Tablet	PDA	Smartphone
Portable	No	Yes	Yes	Yes	Yes
Mobile	No	No	Yes	Yes	Yes
Handheld	No	No	No	Yes	Yes

Table 9.5   Continuum of Communication by Type of Connection to a Network

	Desktop	Notebook/ Laptop	Tablet	PDA	Smartphone
Hardwire connection					
Metal wire cable	Primary	Common	Common	Primary for synchronization	Possible
Fiber-optic cable	Rare	Rare	No	No	No
Wireless connection					
IrDA	No	No	Common	Primary	Possible
Bluetooth	Can add	Can add	Possible	Common	Common
Wi-Fi	Can add	Common	Common	Common	Possible
WiMAX	New technology— how it will be used remains to be seen				
Cellular	No	No	No	No	Primary

A PDA is designed to work both as a stand-alone computer and as a device that communicates with other computers. The most common way for a PDA to communicate with a computer is through a cable. The PDA may be placed in a synchronization cradle that both recharges the PDA battery and has a button that initiates a "hot synch" between the PDA and the computer. The person doing the synchronization has control over what is shared and in what direction (i.e., which device has precedence over the other). There are also cables that connect a PDA directly to a computer using the Universal Serial Bus (USB) port and no cradle is necessary. The synchronization process is initiated through software.

 Wireless Devices

For a computer to connect wirelessly there must be a physical component added to the device to enable wireless communication. Depending on what standard that device follows, there is also a requirement for a wireless access point to the network. It is possible to set up a desktop computer to connect wirelessly to a network, but that involves special hardware meeting specific standards for wireless communication (see the IEEE 802.11 series). With the right card added to the computer and a wireless local area network (WLAN), it is possible for a wirelessly enabled desktop computer to connect through an over-the-air interface to a network. The most common standard used for this is IEEE 802.11 that governs

how local area networks (LANs) connect wirelessly using wireless fidelity (Wi-Fi). Specific airwave GHz bands have specific communication standards (IEEE 802.11a, 802.11b, 802.11g, and 802.11i).

Notebook/laptop computers may come equipped to do both hardwired and wireless connections. A notebook/laptop computer may be plugged into a docking station that is hardwired (connected by a physical cable, the same as used for desktop computers) to the LAN. Growing numbers of notebook/laptop computers are also wireless enabled, most commonly using Wi-Fi following IEEE 802.11 standards to connect to a WLAN. Tablet computers typically are designed for both hardwire and two types of wireless connectivity. They often have an Ethernet port for metal cable connection to the LAN as well as both infrared (Infrared Data Association [IrDA], a standard for transmitting data using infrared light waves, requires a direct line of sight and devices must be within a few feet of each other) and Wi-Fi (following IEEE 802.11 standards).

A PDA typically communicates with the world through being plugged into a desktop computer by way of a cradle or a cable and synchronized, or through IrDA wireless connections. PDAs providing e-mail and Internet access typically do so using Wi-Fi (following the 802.11 standards) to connect to a WLAN. Bluetooth is an alternative standard, best used for connecting PDAs and cellular telephones for short intervals. Smartphones use cellular telephone technology for voice communication and may use any of the PDA communication protocols as well.

Why Use a PDA?

In the clinical practice setting, time is a precious commodity. Practices that allow a nurse to manage and organize time effectively and efficiently are valuable. One strategy for better use of time is to organize data and information so that it is readily available when needed. Most nurses would like to eliminate post-it notes and other small paper reminders and the multiple small reference books that fill (and fall out of) lab coat pockets. Nurses in the acute care setting would like to document data as they collect it, instead of writing data down one place and transcribing it into the health record at a later point in time. Nurses with the Visiting Nurses' Association gather information at the time of the visit and need to turn that information into an electronic version to support documentation requirements for billing and reimbursement. In primary care, nurses complain about the lack of time to accurately bill for office visits and procedures. Other clinic nurses would like a method to track patients. Lack of time to look up pertinent clinical information is a complaint often voiced by nurses in clinical practices.

One potential solution to manage and organize time is a paper-based daily planner. That helps solve some time management issues, but a paper-based daily planner does not address several other issues, especially availability of clinical information at the point of care. What if one small device that fits easily into the palm of a hand, or more importantly, in a lab coat pocket, could help nurses improve patient care by bringing information to the nurse at the point of care at the moment that information is most needed? That device is the PDA. Although PDAs share basic functions such as an address book, calculator, date book, memo pad, to do list, and security, the attractiveness of PDAs for nurses and other healthcare providers lies in the ability to customize the PDA's usefulness by applications specifically developed to assist healthcare providers in the clinical setting. The usefulness of the standard PDA applications in clinical practice as well as categories of specific clinical application software categories follow.

PDA Generic Functions and Their Application to Clinical Practice

The PDA evolved as an information technology to support personal information management. A PDA is a handheld computer that allows the user to organize and manage personal information. A PDA provides an address book, a calculator, date book, memo pad (for typed input), notepad (for hand-written input), to do lists, and a way to synchronize part or all of this information with another computer, to help the user organize their time and tasks (Carlson, 2000; Johnson and Broida, 2003; McPherson, 2002). The focus of generic PDA applications is to allow individuals to organize and manage their information, including their time, data, and money. Some PDAs can even provide voice recognition, take photos, and play music.

The *address book* is an always-alphabetical list that has fields for name, address, phone number, organization, e-mail, and other data. The entries can be categorized, however, as the nurse likes. This allows multiple categories such as attending physicians, nursing units, clinics, and staff members to be created.

The *calculator* is a basic function calculator, capable of basic mathematical operations. Calculators for specific medical calculations are available (see *Add-on Software*).

The *date book* allows the nurse to keep track of his or her schedule, from a daily, weekly, or monthly perspective. Reminder alarms can be set to alert the nurse to an upcoming event. Reoccurring events can be entered once and repeated multiple times. Some systems will allow providers to download their patient schedule.

The *memo pad* provides a place to compose memos, which can be synchronized with another computer. One use is to produce and edit project outlines. Many people use this function to download their written personalized "peripheral brains."

The *notepad* (the only function that responds to handwriting) is useful in jotting quick notes. Unlike other functions, the notepad allows the nurse to write directly on the screen in digital ink. It is useful for noting changes in patient conditions, changes in orders that occur on rounds, and taking notes at Continuing Education offerings.

The *to do list* allows the nurse to create multiple lists and keep track of tasks to be done daily, weekly, or monthly. Components of the lists can be prioritized by level of importance and/or due date. Unfortunately, only one list at as time can be viewed, so an overall view of multiple to do lists is not possible.

The infrared sharing of information (*beaming*) enables transmission of information or files from a PDA to another device without the use of cables. One way to use the beaming port is to beam information directly from the PDA to an IrDA-enabled printer. Another common use of beaming is to exchange electronic business cards.

Standard PDA functions supporting personal information management can readily be adapted to assist in professional activities management. The advantages for healthcare providers using the standard PDA functions include saving time through improved access to and management of information. Common examples include saving time and improving information management. Nurses save time looking up contact information when information for frequently contacted individuals is in one place, eliminating searching for beeper numbers and phone numbers in several sources. The ability to download a patient schedule into the date book saves time by enabling the provider to review test results prior to the patient encounter. The notepad feature is useful in keeping track of changes in patient orders during rounds.

 ## Add-on Software

Stand-alone and Synchronized

Several very useful applications that facilitate professional time management are available for the PDA. These applications may work as stand-alone programs with no need to connect to anything once they are loaded onto the PDA, e.g., a viewer for reading an e-book. Some applications require periodic asynchronous updating, e.g., a subscription with quarterly updates. Other applications are designed to connect to a WLAN each time they are launched, e.g., a wireless e-mail application. Typically, an application is downloaded to a computer and then during synchronization the application is put on the PDA. If the application requires periodic updating, it will prompt the user when it is time to load the update. If the application depends on connecting with a WLAN, it will seek out a WLAN when it is launched.

For example, an application loaded onto the PDA offers e-mail management capability. E-mail may be downloaded during synchronization and read at leisure. Responses may be composed on the PDA and when the device is synchronized, the responses will be sent. When the PDA has wireless capability and access to a WLAN, e-mail can be accessed by, and responses sent directly from the device in real time.

General Freeware, Shareware, and Commercial Applications

A PDA may be used for viewing information, or to perform office automation tasks (e.g., to create, view, and edit documents, spreadsheets, and databases), or to browse the Internet. There are three types of general applications: document and image viewers, office automation applications, and Web browsers.

Document viewers allow the user to download and read text files. Many publishers use special formats for their publications that require document viewers. Document viewers allow formatting, indexing of content, and special characters to be preserved when documents are downloaded. Some programs allow the viewer to bookmark sections of the document for quick reference. Most do not permit editing of a commercially purchased publication. Several document readers are available and many publishers specify which document reader must be used for their publication.

There is a PDA version of Adobe Reader for Palm OS or Acrobat Reader for Windows Mobile or Symbian operating systems available for free download (Adobe, 2004). The PDA version allows .pdf extension documents to be downloaded and read on a PDA. Although documents not specially formatted for the PDA can be opened using this application, formatting may not be preserved, making the document difficult to read. Other popular document readers, which are commercially available, include TealDoc (TealPoint Software, 2004) and Franklin Reader (Franklin, 2004). Palm OS also includes a document reader, eBook, that is used to read electronic versions of popular literature. One Hypertext Markup Language (HTML) document reader is iSilo (iSilo, 2004).

A *graphics viewer* for image viewing may be useful for individuals practicing in specialties where images are a basic requirement. Firepad Picture Viewer is a commercial application that may be downloaded and is useful for creating, viewing, and sharing images, videos, and multimedia presentations as well as acquiring free Internet images (Firepad, 2004). For PDAs without a camera function, Firepad Picture Viewer can also be used to download digital photos from the computer.

Office utilities allow the user to download, view, revise and upload documents to a computer. Documents To Go, shareware that is compatible with the Microsoft Office Suite, allows the user to view and revise on PDA Word documents, Excel spreadsheets, and PowerPoint presentations (DataViz, 2004; palmOne, 2004). Lotus Notes may be synchronized with supported PDAs (IBM, 2004). The Presenter To Go program allows the user to show a PowerPoint presentation directly from a PDA using a projector (Margi Systems, 2004). Printing programs, such as PalmPrint (Stevens Creek Software, 2004) are also available.

PDA database programs are available to read data files and can be used to create databases. Two common applications are HanDbase (DDH Software, 2004) and Jfile (Land-J Technologies, 2004). Filemaker Mobile 7 (Filemaker, 2004) allows multiple PDAs to synchronize with one central database, which is especially useful for remote data capture of research data that is aggregated in one central database.

Web browsers are another popular application for PDAs. These applications may also function as off-line HTML document readers. Content is provided, often free of charge to the subscriber, through a wide variety of channels (specially formatted Web sites). The content is updated regularly and provides news about a particular area or topic selected by the user. AvantGo (iAnywhere Solutions, Inc., 2004) allows the user to do an update as part of the synchronization process or using a wireless or Wi-Fi hot spot connection.

With these additional applications, a travel charger for the PDA, a backup memory card, and a portable keyboard, the PDA may function as a mobile office. A user so equipped may leave the laptop/notebook computer behind for short business trips. All the information and equipment needed to do a presentation can be available in a handheld.

Clinical Applications by Functional Categories

Once users discovered the effectiveness of a handheld device for managing personal information, they envisioned the usefulness of a PDA in supporting their workflow. Numerous applications that support healthcare professionals in their delivery of care are now available (e.g., Kiel and Goldblum, 2001). There are applications that support clinical care (e.g., medications, treatments, documentation, clinical decision-making), administrative functions (e.g., reporting), research (e.g., data collection), and education (e.g., presentations) (Health Sciences & Human Services Library, 2004). Available healthcare applications range from simple reference material (e.g., electronic books and journal articles), to interactive tracking databases (e.g., coding care delivery services for billing purposes), to highly sophisticated decision support systems (e.g., interactive clinical consultation applications).

Clinicians utilize their PDAs to support their workflow by having ready access to relevant information at the point of care. Clinical applications are the reason information is readily available. Because of its mobility, a PDA provides information and decision support at the point of care. PDA value to the clinician increases with wireless connectivity to clinical information sources at the point of care. The ability to quickly check on signs and symptoms that could indicate a medical emergency, review appropriate drug doses for a less familiar drug, check for drug interactions, review the latest evidence-based management guidelines for a particular problem, and utilize applications for differential diagnoses and clinical decision-making including management, all contribute to improving patient care. Available applications generally fall into one of three categories: clinical references, patient tracking, and billing and coding.

Clinical Applications by Category

Categories of *clinical references* include journals, general and specialty references, pharmacologic references, medical calculators, and clinical decision support tools for treatment and/or clinical consultation. PDA clinical references include applications that scan journals for specified topics, general and specialty practice electronic resources, pharmacology databases, medical calculators, and clinical decision-making applications. Clinical references account for most of the freeware and shareware healthcare applications for PDAs.

The amount of new patient care information available in journals can be overwhelming and often providers do not have the luxury of setting aside time each day for reading. The ability to access the Internet to find comprehensive clinically relevant information related to patient care is extremely valuable. Examples of PDA accessible information sources include POEMS (infoPOEM, Inc., 2004) and Clinical Evidence (BMJ Publishing Group, 2004). Journal Web sites can be used to access abstracts as well as full journal articles. Some Web sites such as JournalsToGo (Publicis eHealth Solutions, 2004), MDC Mobile (Mosby, 2004), and MD Consult/Pocket Consult (Elsevier, Inc., 2004) provide a journal scan service for PDAs. There is the ability to customize the selection of journals by area of interest. With some Web browsing services, MEDLINE searches are possible. Other Web sites such as Ovid (Ovid Technologies, 2004) allow the user to order searches on a particular topic and then deliver appropriate journal abstracts and articles to the PDA.

Most well-known healthcare references are commercially available in PDA format. Due to PDA memory limitations, some publishers condense reference texts while others remove pictures. In some texts, tables and figures are reduced in number. In others, content has been made more concise. When reducing the size of a reference, care is taken to include essential information. To address some limitations of the PDA, publishers are making their publications available on an expansion card. This makes more memory available for applications.

Specialty information is available in the form of standard text references such as the Nurses Manual of Laboratory and Diagnostic Tests (Skyscape, n.d.). Lippincott Williams & Wilkins (2004), Barnes and Noble (2004), and Skyscape (n.d.) provide examples of Web sites that have extensive listings of PDA healthcare titles. In addition to publishers, specialty organization and the federal government provide PDA resources and applications relevant for specialty practice. For example, the National Institutes of Health Web site, through the National Heart, Lung, and Blood Institute (NHLBI), provides electronic guidelines and PDA applications for the diagnosis and management of asthma, cholesterol, hypertension, and obesity (NHLBI, n.d.). The Centers for Disease Control and Prevention (CDC, n.d.) provides screen reader device text-only versions of documents such as the Childhood Immunization Schedule, STD Treatment Guidelines, and Guidelines for Management of Community Acquired Pneumonia. Evidence-based clinical practice guidelines, which support provider decisions about appropriate healthcare, provide the recommended course of action in specific situations. Guidelines are available from government agencies and professional organizations. The National Guideline Clearing House has links to multiple practice guideline sites (see Agency for Healthcare Research and Quality, 2004).

Other Web sites are sources of clinical practice information and are subscription based. PEPID (2004) has customized PDA programs available through subscription. The Clinical Awareness System (InfoPOEM, Inc., 2004) provides subscribers with a variety of evidence-based information tools, including the Cochrane Systematic Review abstracts. Merck Medicus (2004) provides subscribers with access to Mobile MerckMedicus and MEDLINE searches.

Pharmacology databases are probably the most frequently used PDA application. Many applications are available, including both freeware and subscription applications. All applications contain drug information for prescription drugs and some are bundled with additional applications that support clinical decision-making. Perhaps the most frequently used comprehensive pharmacology database is Epocrates Rx (Epocrates, Inc., 2004), which is available as both a free application and as a commercial expanded product. Epocrates Rx freeware includes adult and pediatric indications dosing, contraindications, adverse reactions, mechanism of action, and a program that allows the user to check for

drug interactions using a list of up to 30 drugs. Updated daily, the information is current. A more extensive version available by subscription is Epocrates RxPro, which includes the pharmacology database, alternative medicine information integrated into the pharmacology database, an infectious disease database updated quarterly, differential diagnosis applications, summary tables such as the Glasgow scale, and a medical calculator.

MobileMicromedex (Micromedex, n.d.) is available by subscription and many health sciences libraries hold a subscription so their authorized library users may access this application for free. MobileMicromedex contains both a pharmacology database, and in separate applications, toxicology information, alternative medicines and acute care information, and a decision support tool. Since each application can be downloaded separately, MobileMicromedex can be selectively used by each individual.

Lexi-Complete (Lexi-Comp, 2004) is a subscription that offers access to 15 databases related to drugs and clinical consultation. There is a separate Pediatric Lexi-Drugs application that is more extensive than any of the other pharmacology databases for pediatric patients. Lexi-Drugs, along with other drug references can be linked seamlessly to other applications such as Griffith's 5-Minute Clinical Consult (Lexi-Comp).

Although all drug reference programs list drug interactions, only Epocrates, Inc. (2004) applications allow the user to easily check for multiple drug-drug interactions. In a recent study, Barrons (2004) evaluated nine software applications for sensitivity, specificity, positive predictive value, and negative predictive value for clinically important drug interactions. The results indicate that iFacts (Skyscape, n.d.) and Lexi-interact (Lexi-Comp, 2004), two programs developed exclusively for the assessment of drug interactions, provided the best assessment of drug interactions. The highest scoring general drug information resource was MobileMicromedex (Micromedex, n.d.).

Medical calculator applications are available to assist providers who use standard formulas for calculation of body mass index (BMI), creatinine clearance, and so forth. Many are available as free downloads and may be included as a module in other applications. MedCalc (Medical Interactive Applications, n.d.) and MedMath (Cheng, 2004) are among the most popular for general use. In addition, special clinical applications calculators are widely available. Two examples are PregCalc (Medical Toolbox Software, 2001) and Stat Cholesterol (StatCoder.com, 2004).

Several drug database programs to aid in the selection of antibiotics are available and function as *clinical decision support* tools. The most frequently cited are ePocrates ID (infectious disease application) (Epocrates, Inc., 2004), the Johns Hopkins Antibiotic Guide (The Johns Hopkins University, 2004), the Sanford Guide to Antimicrobial Therapy (Antimicrobial Therapy, Inc., 2004), and Infectious Diseases Notes (PDA Medical Solutions, 2003). The earlier discussion of Epocrates RxPro covered Epocrates ID.

The Johns Hopkins Antibiotic Guide (The Johns Hopkins University, 2004) is marketed as a decision support tool, designed to bring clinicians information about the diagnosis and treatment of infectious diseases at the point of care. The application is free. Information in the application can be accessed by diagnosis, pathogen, or antibiotic. Once the search is initiated, categories of relevant information can be accessed. One drawback is that there is no hyperlink between the treatments suggested and detailed information about the specific antibiotic. Information about drug interactions, renal dosing, and other data are only available in the antibiotic section.

The Sanford Guide to Antimicrobial Therapy (Antimicrobial Therapy, Inc., 2004) is issued yearly and there is a PDA version of the book. Much of the information is presented in tabular form and the user can hyperlink between tables. Comprehensive drug information is not readily available. The PDA version is formatted for optimum display on the PDA screen. Several commonly used tables do not transfer well to the PDA and this could limit usefulness of the application.

Infectious Diseases Notes (PDA Medical Solutions, 2003) is also a combination drug database and clinical decision support tool. This application includes information on normal body flora and extensive information on microbiology and epidemiology as compared to the other applications.

Miller, Beattie, and Butt (2003) reviewed the above four infectious disease applications for completeness and accuracy. Miller et al. conclude that the applications reviewed contain the information that providers need at the point of care. They recommended the Johns Hopkins Antibiotic Guide because of the automatic updating of content, the rigorous review process, and the amount of detail on treatment and diagnosis.

Another decision support tool, TheraDoc Antibiotic Assistant (TheraDoc, Inc., 2004), is available for download from MerckMedicus (2004). Although the application is free, site registration is required. The user chooses a commonly found infection and then enters

data about the particular patient. The antibiotic of choice and the dose is generated for that particular case.

MDConsult through its mobile program offers FIRST Consult (Elsevier, n.d.), a clinical decision support tool. The application is designed to assist providers in the area of differential diagnosis by chief complaint. Once the problem has been translated into a medical condition, the provider can seamlessly navigate to tests. Information available includes the advantages and disadvantages of the test, normal and abnormal results, and their cause and factors affecting the test. When the drugs and other therapies section is accessed, detailed information about the drug is available without having to access another application.

In summary, PDAs can be optimized for clinical practice through the utilization of applications designed to support healthcare providers by providing ready access to journals and electronic resources, pharmacology databases, medical calculators, and clinical decision support tools. Bringing this information to the point of care should improve patient outcomes.

Patient tracking software is a handheld patient management tool that allows the provider to track a variety of patient information. Fields often included in the application include demographic information, physical examination findings, laboratory and other test results, clinical progress, and assessment notes. Entering data on each patient, especially in a busy office practice, can be time consuming if done on the PDA. This is often a reason cited not to use patient tracking software. Some time can be saved with the use of pull-down menus available on several programs for demographic information, names of common laboratory and other tests, and physical examination findings. An alternative to entering all data on the PDA is to enter data on the desktop and synchronize with the PDA. Many programs can be integrated with a desktop computer system. The ability to share patient information is most helpful for on-call coverage.

Several patient tracking programs are available as freeware or commercial products. PatientKeeper (PatientKeeper, n.d.) can be used exclusively on the PDA and is used to track basic patient information. Some customization by each user is possible. Another program is Patient Tracker, which is a combination desktop and PDA program. Information can be entered on either the PDA or the desktop, and synchronized (Handheldmed, Inc., 2004). A more limited application is the freeware Palm Patient (FreewarePalm, 2001). This application does not provide for beaming, printing, or billing.

One limiting factor with PDA patient tracking software occurs when there is a lack of communication with other hospital information systems such as the laboratory or x-ray department. Another limiting factor is when the clinical information system does not support PDA data sharing, so information cannot be downloaded to the PDA from other departments and the information must be entered by hand. Lapinsky et al. (2001) found that PDA users did not consider patient tracking valuable unless it was integrated with the hospital computer system.

Billing and coding applications are designed to document charges for patient visits, procedures, and medical diagnoses. The utilization of these applications may increase charges for practices. The applications allow coding of evaluation and management (E&M) charges, International Classification of Diseases (ICD) codes, and Current Procedural Terminology (CPT) codes. For example, PocketBilling (PocketMed, 2004) allows the user to customize the content. It uses a menu-driven format. Another application is STAT E&M coder in which the user is led through algorithms to determine the correct E&M billing (StatCoder.com, 2004). Billing and coding programs for patients seen in specialty practices are also available.

 ## HIPAA Implications

The HIPAA administrative simplification provisions include electronic transactions and code sets, security, unique identifiers, and privacy. If a computer has individually identifiable health information or protected health information stored on it, the person who maintains or transmits that information is responsible for reasonable and appropriate safeguards.

Asynchronous Communication and a PDA

A reasonable level of security for a PDA with individually identifiable health information is to have the device protected by having to enter an ID and password in order to use it. In case the PDA is lost or stolen, there should be an application that will wipe any information on the PDA in the event the user incorrectly enters an ID and password a set number of times. If the hardwire synchronization is between a protected PDA and a desktop computer that is secure (located in a locked room, protected by an ID and password to log on) that point-to-point transmission is secure. Users should be trained

by the organization in their responsibility for maintaining privacy and security of the data.

Synchronous Communication and Wireless Devices

All the considerations for asynchronous communication remain, but in addition, when a device is wireless enabled, the individually identifiable health information that is transmitted must be protected during the process of transmission as well as when it resides on a PDA or the receiving machine. This is typically done through encryption. The data exchanged is encrypted when it leaves and is decrypted when it arrives at its destination. Encryption and decryption take time, so system performance will be slower than if the data were not encrypted.

Evaluation of Clinical Applications

There are hundreds of applications available to support healthcare providers. Some problems exist. The quality of all applications is not equal. Not all applications are peer reviewed. Information may not be updated quickly, e.g., the standard for updating drug information may be a minimum of quarterly, but the vendor only provides annual updates. This is a serious deviation from the standard of practice. Some freeware applications collect information about users and make the information available commercially. Not all applications can be run from a memory card, limiting the amount of main memory available for other functions. When selecting applications, individuals need to consider how they choose to expend PDA memory and financial resources. Applications can be expensive. Individuals should consider purchasing a PDA version of the print reference they use most often. Most sites will allow the nurse to preview software prior to purchase. Some sites will allow the nurse to download a preview application or the entire application to use for a short time in order to evaluate usefulness before making a purchase. Some programs are available on CD-ROM as well as through a download. If the nurse should have a problem with the download or running the application, sites often provide technical support to assist in problem resolution.

A systematic approach to evaluating clinical applications starts with an understanding of the goal of the nurse selecting and using that software. The software selected must be compatible with the operating system of the PDA. Factors to consider include the amount of time and level of effort required to install and successfully run the application. There should be a way to install and back up the application. The human-computer interface should allow the user to comfortably view the information (it may be necessary to change the font size or color scheme to enhance the contrast). The user should be able to comfortably enter information (e.g., use a stylus and the keyboard for input). If the PDA "hangs" the user should be able to do a soft reset and not loose data. The user should have control over the synchronization process. The battery life should accommodate the user's workflow. The user should be able to get the information desired out of the application in the format desired. The benefit derived from using the application should offset the cost of the application.

Case Study: Integration of Information Technology into Clinical Practice

You have downloaded your clinic schedule for today onto your PDA. All the patients are familiar to you except for one who is new. Ms. AC arrives for her appointment. You open your PatientKeeper application and enter the following information during the visit. AC is a 35-year-old African American woman with a history of asthma for the past year, referred for care. She has few episodes of asthma but when she has difficulty breathing, she goes to the emergency room for care if it gets "real bad." She uses an albuterol inhaler and is now using it every 2 hours. She takes vitamin C 1 g and Ortho-Tri-Cyclen. For the past week she has had trouble sleeping at night because of the wheezing. She had a cough, producing yellow sputum, a frontal headache, and her chest hurts when she coughs. She has no drug allergies. On physical examination, she has a temperature of 100°F oral, a pulse of 92, and respirations of 22 minute, slightly labored. She has mild frontal sinus tenderness and a small amount of yellow nasal discharge. Her respiratory expansion is decreased. Lungs are resonant to percussion with inspiratory and expiratory wheezes throughout. There are diffuse rhonchi in the left lower lobe that did not completely clear with cough. The rest of the physical examination is unremarkable.

The question is: What are the current treatment options for this patient? You access the NHLBI asthma treatment guidelines on your PDA. You open the treatment of exacerbation section to evaluate the severity of her exacerbation and to review treatment recommendations. You decide to administer an albuterol treatment in the office and use your Epocrates Rx application to assess for drug interactions between her current medications and aerosolized albuterol. None were found. You

decide, based on the asthma treatment guidelines, she should receive a course of oral steroids for a week and will need to begin using a long-acting inhaler. You choose Singulair and, using Epocrates Rx, run a drug interaction check. There is an interaction that can result in hypokalemia. You order a potassium level. Your second diagnosis is sinusitis. You consider Amoxicillin and access the Johns Hopkins Antibiotic Guide to review the evidence-based practice guideline information. The preferred antibiotic, recommended by the Cochran Library, the CDC, and the Infectious Disease Society of America, is Amoxicillin. You run one more drug check and discover that Amoxicillin could decrease the effectiveness of the oral contraceptives. Based on the severity of her sinusitis symptoms, you decide to treat Ms. AC symptomatically with saline nasal irrigations, humidity, and a nasal decongestant. You schedule her to return in a few days. At the end of the day, you synchronize your PDA with your desktop, updating the databases.

References

Adobe. (2004). *Acrobat family home*. Retrieved October 18, 2004, from *http://www.adobe.com/products/acrobat/main.html*

Agency for Healthcare Research and Quality. (2004). *NGC–National Guideline Clearinghouse welcome*. Retrieved October 18, 2004, from *http://www.guideline.gov/*

Antimicrobial Therapy, Inc. (2004). *Sanford Guide*. Retrieved October 18, 2004, from *http://www.sanfordguide.com/*

Barnes & Noble. (2004). *Barnes & Noble.com*. Retrieved October 18, 2004, from *http://www.barnesandnoble.com/*

Barrons, R. (2004, February 15). Evaluation of personal digital assistant software for drug interactions. *American Journal of Health-Systems Pharmacists* 61(4):380–385.

Bloom, L., Eardley, R., Geelhoed, E., Manahan, M., and Ranganathan, P. (2004). Investigating the relationship between battery life and user acceptance of dynamic, energy-aware interfaces on handhelds. In S. Brewster and M. Dunlop (Eds.), *Mobile Human-Computer Interaction——Mobile HCI 2004*. Lecture Notes in Computer Science, 3160, 13–24.

BMJ Publishing Group. (2004). *Clinical Evidence*. Retrieved October 18, 2004, from *http://www.clinicalevidence.com/ceweb/conditions/index.jsp*

Buchmann, I. (2001). *Batteries in a Portable World: A Handbook on Rechargeable Batteries for Non-Engineers*. Retrieved October 15, 2004, from *http://www.buchmann.ca/*

Carlson, J. (2000). *Palm Organizers Visual Quickstart Guide*. Berkeley, CA: Peachpit Press.

Centers for Disease Control and Prevention. (n.d.) Retrieved October 18, 2004, from *http://www.cdc.gov/*

Cheng, P. (2004). *MedMath 2.01: A Medical Calculator for the PalmOS Platform*. Retrieved October 18, 2004, from *http://smi-web.stanford.edu/people/pcheng/medmath/*

DataViz, Inc. (2004). PDA *software, Palm software, Pocket PC Software Developed by Dataviz*. Retrieved October 18, 2004, from *http://www.dataviz.com/*

DDH Software, Inc. (2004). *DDH Software: HanDBase*. Retrieved October 18, 2004, from *http://www.ddhsoftware.com/*

Elsevier, Inc. (n.d.) *First Consult*. Retrieved October 18, 2004, from *http://www.mdconsult.com/firstconsult/evite.html*

Elsevier, Inc. (2004). *MD Consult: Clinical Information for Physicians*. Retrieved October 18, 2004, from *http://www.mdconsult.com/*

Epocrates, Inc. (2004). Epocrates: *The Leading Provider of Handheld and Web Based Clinical Reference Tools*. Retrieved October 18, 2004, from *http://www2.epocrates.com/index.html*

Filemaker. (2004). *Filemaker: Products: FileMaker Mobile 7*. Retrieved October 18, 2004, from *http://www.filemaker.com/products/mbl_home.html*

Firepad. (2004). *Firepad Palm Picture Viewer with Streaming Video and Multimedia Support: Mobile Media Software*. Retrieved October 18, 2004, from *http://www.firepad.com/*

Franklin. (2004). *Franklin Electronic Publishers: Dictionaries, Translators, Bibles*. Retrieved October 18, 2004, from *http://www.franklin.com/*

FreewarePalm. (2001). *PalmPatient*. Retrieved October 18, 2004, from *http://www.freewarepalm.com/medical/palmpatient.shtml*

Handheldmed, Inc. (2004). *Connect With the Future of Medicine Today*. Retrieved October 18, 2004, from *http://www.handheldmed.com/*

Health Insurance Portability and Accountability Act of 1996, Pub. L. No. 104-191. Retrieved October 18, 2004, from *http://aspe.hhs.gov/admnsimp/pl104191.htm*

Health Sciences & Human Services Library. (2004). *PDA Resources*. Retrieved October 18, from *http://www.hshsl.umaryland.edu/resources/pdainfo/res.html*

iAnywhere Solutions, Inc. (2004). *AvantGo*. Retrieved October 18, 2004, from *http://www.avantgo.com/*

IBM. (2004). *EasySync Pro*. Retrieved October 18, 2004, from *http://www.ibm.com/us/*

InfoPOEM, Inc. (2004). *InfoPOEMs: The Clinical Awareness System*. Retrieved October 18, 2004, from *http://www.infopoems.com/*

iSilo. (2004). *Welcome to the iSilo Website*. Retrieved October 18, 2004, from *http://www.isilo.com/*

The Johns Hopkins University. (2004). *Johns Hopkins Division of Infectious Diseases Antibiotic Guide*. Retrieved October 18, 2004, from *http://hopkins-abxguide.org/*

Johnson, D. and Broida, R. (2003). *How to Do Everything With Your Palm Handheld* (4th ed.). Emeryville, CA: McGraw-Hill/Osborne.

Kiel, J. M. and Goldblum, O. M. (2001). Using personal digital assistants to enhance outcomes. *Journal of Healthcare Information Management* 15(3):237–250.

Land-J Technologies. (2004). *Land-J Products Page: PalmOS Apps*. Retrieved October 18, 2004, from *http://www.land-j.com/palmapps.html*

Lapinsky S. E., Weshler J., Mehta S., Varkul M., Hallett, D. and Stewart, T. E. (2001). Handheld computers in critical care. *Critical Care* 5(4):227–231.

Lexi-Comp, Inc. (2004). *Providing Point of Care Knowledge for Today's Healthcare Professional*. Retrieved October 18, 2004, from *http://www.lexi.com/web/index.jsp*

Lippincott, Williams & Wilkins. (2004). *Welcome to LWW's PDA Products Store*. Retrieved October 18, 2004, from *http://www.lww.com/pda/*

Margi Systems. (2004). *Margi: Delivering Powerful Handheld Solutions*. Retrieved October 18, 2004, from *http://www.margi.com/*

McPherson, F. (2002). *How to Do Everything With Your Pocket PC* (2nd ed.). Berkeley, CA: McGraw-Hill/Osborne.

Medical Interactive Applications. (n.d.) *MedCalc: The Most Complete Free Medical Calculator*. Retrieved October 18, 2004, from *http://www.med-ia.ch/medcalc/*

Medical Toolbox Software. (2001). *Handheld Solutions for the Medical Workplace*. Retrieved October 18, 2004, from *http://www.medicaltoolbox.com/products/PregCalcPro/*

Merck Medicus. (2004). *MerckMedicus: Your Key to the Medical Internet*. Retrieved October 18, 2004, from *http://www.merckmedicus.com/pp/us/hcp/hcp_home.jsp*

Micromedex. (n.d.). *MobileMICROMEDEX*. Retrieved October 18, 2004, from *http://www.micromedex.com/products/mobilemicromedex/*

Miller, S. M., Beattie, M. M., and Butt, A. A. (2003, April 15). Personal digital assistant infectious diseases applications for health care professionals. *Clinical Infectious Diseases* 36(8):1018–1029.

Mosby. (2004). *Mosby's Drug Consult*. Retrieved October 18, 2004, from *http://www.mosbysdrugconsult.com/*

National Heart, Lung & Blood Institute. (n.d.). *Clinical Practice Guidelines*. Retrieved October 18, 2004, from *http://www.nhlbi.nih.gov/guidelines/*

Ovid Technologies. (2004). *Ovid*. Retrieved October 18, 2004, from *http://www.ovid.com/site/index.jsp*

palmOne. (2004). *PalmOne Formerly Palm, Inc.* Retrieved October 18, 2004, from *http://www.palmone.com/us/*

PatientKeeper. (n.d.) *Welcome to PatientKeeper*. Retrieved October 18, 2004, from *http://www.patientkeeper.com/*

PDA Medical Solutions. (2003). *Infectious Diseases Notes*. Retrieved October 18, 2004, from *http://www.pdamedsolutions.com/products/idn.htm*

PEPID. (2004). *Portable Healthcare Expertise*. Retrieved October 18, 2004, from *http://www.pepid.com/*

PocketMed. (2004). *Improving Patient Care Through Handheld Programming*. Retrieved October 18, 2004, from *http://www.pocketmed.org/*

Publicis eHealth Solutions. (2004). *JournalToGo.com: Delivers Medical Literature and News to Your Handheld Free of Charge*. Retrieved October 18, 2004, from *http://www.journaltogo.com/*

Roseberry, C. (n.d.) *Tablet PC or PDA: Comparison of Mobile Gadgets*. Retrieved October 18, 2004, from *http://mobileoffice.about.com/cs/mobilegear/a/pocketpcvspda.htm*

Skyscape. (n.d.) *Skyscape: Your Mobile Medical Library*. Retrieved October 18, 2004, from *http://www.skyscape.com/index/home.aspx*

StatCoder.com. (2004). *E&M, ICD-9, CPT Handheld Coding Tools: Free Clinical Software*. Retrieved October 18, 2004, from *http://www.statcoder.com/*

Stevens Creek Software. (2004). *A Leading Provider of Software Solutions for the Palm Computing Platform*. Retrieved October 18, 2004, from *http://www.stevenscreek.com/*

TealPoint Software. (2004). *Programs for PalmPilots*. Retrieved October 18, 2004, from *http://www.tealpoint.com/*

TheraDoc, Inc. (2004). *Antibiotic Assistant: Stand-Alone Model*. Retrieved October 18, 2004, from *http://www.theradoc.com/products/products_autonomic.html*

10

Incorporating Evidence: Use of Computer-Based Clinical Decision Support Systems for Health Professionals

Ida Androwich
Margaret Kraft

OBJECTIVES

1. Define computerized clinical decision support systems (CDSS).
2. Identify types of CDSS, their characteristics, and the levels of responsibility implicit in the use of each type.
3. Describe effects of CDSS on clinician performance and patient outcomes in healthcare.
4. Understand the features, benefits, and limits of CDSS.
5. Develop a future vision for CDSS within nursing.

KEY WORDS

clinical decision support
decision support systems
information systems
knowledge and cognition

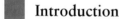

Introduction

Decision support systems (DSS) are automated tools designed to support decision-making activities and improve the decision-making process and decision outcomes. Such systems are intended to use the enormous amounts of data that exist in information systems to facilitate decision processes. A CDSS is designed to support healthcare providers in making decisions about the delivery and management of patient care. A CDSS program's goals may include patient safety and improved outcomes for specific patient populations as well as compliance with clinical guidelines, standards of practice, and regulatory requirements. Within the complexity of today's healthcare environment there is an increasing need for accessible information that supports and improves the effectiveness of decision-making and promotes clinical accountability and the use of best practices. Clinical tasks to which CDSS

may be applied include alerts and reminders, diagnostic assistance, therapy critiques and plans, medication orders, image recognition and interpretation, and information retrieval. The primary goal of CDSS is the optimization of both the efficiency and effectiveness with which clinical decisions are made and care is delivered (Tan and Sheps, 1998). The development of CDSS requires a huge financial and intellectual investment but also represents the potential to reduce care costs through improvement of the decision process at the point of care and to reduce the possibility of costly errors.

Clinicians depend on timely, reliable, and accurate information to make clinical decisions. Availability of such information depends on how data are collected, stored, retrieved, and transformed into meaningful information. Nursing decision support systems (NDSS) are tools that help nurses improve their effectiveness, identify appropriate interventions, determine areas in need of policy or protocol development, and support patient safety initiatives and quality improvement activities. Improving the efficiency and effectiveness of nursing practice supports the demand for more and more professional accountability for practice. Accuracy, timeliness, availability, format, and reliability of information are just as important to nursing as they are to other healthcare providers. Nurses as knowledge workers need access to current knowledge at the point-of-care delivery where it is useful: in clinics, at the bedside, in homes, offices, and in research that makes contributions to evidence-based nursing practice. Practicing nurses depend on clinical experience, evidence from research, available information resources, and patient preferences to make evidence-based decisions about care.

A CDSS includes a set of knowledge-based tools that can be fully integrated with the clinical data embedded in the computerized patient record (electronic health record) to assist providers by presenting information relevant to the healthcare problem(s) being faced. Ideally, the CDSS is available at the point of care with quick (real time) responses, requires minimal training, is easily integrated into the workflow of practice, and is user friendly. It should have a powerful search function that can access useful and reliable information from knowledge sources that may include electronic libraries, medical dictionaries, drug formularies, expert opinion, and patient database access. A CDSS is only as effective as its underlying knowledge base. Knowledge sources can provide simple facts, relationships, evidence-based best practices, and the latest in clinical research. CDSS may focus on treatment, diagnosis, or specific patient information. Systems may be passive, requiring the clinician to access the advice, or with a higher level of information processing, systems may be active, giving unsolicited advice.

The availability of reliable clinical information and the propagation and management of clinical knowledge within CDSS has the potential to transform healthcare delivery but it is important to remember that the clinical user's experience, understanding of context and knowledge base are not replaced but rather, supported in the decision-making process. Implementation of CDSS requires the development of a strategy built on an understanding of available CDSS tools, clinician readiness to adopt and use CDSS, and areas within the organization that carry significant risk to patient safety or of poor outcomes. Attention is paid to delivery of the right information at the right time and place to enable decision-making. CDSS is a "tool" system, not a "rule" system. In no way does a CDSS usurp the clinician's

decision-making role. Final decisions are always made by the clinicians who can accept or reject the CDSS information within the context of the healthcare situation.

■ Definition

A CDSS may be defined as any computer program that helps health professionals make clinical decisions. CDSS software has a knowledge base designed for the clinician involved in patient care to aid in clinical decision-making. Johnston et al. (1994) defined CDSS as "computer software employing a knowledge base designed for use by a clinician involved in patient care, as a direct aid to clinical decision-making." Sims et al. (2001) broadened the definition to "CDSS are software designed to be a direct aid to clinical decision-making, in which the characteristics of an individual patient are matched to a computerized clinical knowledge base and patient-specific assessments or recommendations are then presented to the clinician or the patient for a decision." Coiera (1994) discussed the role of CDSS as augmenting human performance and providing assistance for healthcare providers especially for tasks subject to human error. Whatever definition chosen, it seems clear that healthcare is being transformed through information and knowledge management and technology is being used to "tame data and transform information" (Berner, 1999). It is impossible for the unaided human mind to stay current when medical knowledge has exploded, the number of drugs has increased 500% in the last 10 years, and approximately 20,000 new articles appear in biomedical literature annually. The application of CDSS helps clinicians access and use what science has learned (*www. healthcommons.org/clinical.html*).

Expanded Use of CDSS

The rapid, exponential increase in the use of the Internet and the ability to store electronic data has proved to be a boon to the development of DSS (Negroponte, 1996). Randall Tobias, the former VP of ATT, is credited with saying that if the advances in power, storage capability, and cost of computers today were compared with the mainframes of the 60s and 70s, it would be like getting a Lexus for $2.00 that went 600 mph and used a thimble of gas. This means that the computer has virtually unlimited capacity for processing and storage of data. The human, on the other hand, has limited storage (memory) and processing power, but does have judgment, experience, and intuition. DSS integrate and capitalize on the strengths of both. Thus, three main purposes of a DSS are to

1. Assist in problem solving with semistructured problems

2. Support, not replace, the judgment of a manager or clinician

3. Improve the effectiveness of the decision-making process

Highly structured or deterministic problems, which can be solved with existing facts, and completely unstructured problems, which are highly dependent on values and beliefs, are generally not well suited for decision support.

 ## History of CDSS

Early Systems

Focus on Diagnosis One of the earliest known CDSS designed to support diagnosis of acute abdominal pain was developed by de Dombal in 1972 at Leeds University. This system used Bayesian theory to predict the probability that a given patient, based on symptoms, had one of seven possible conditions. The system was correct in its diagnosis in 91% of the cases compared to the physicians whose accuracy ranged from 65 to 80% depending on their experience in practice (Musen, Shahar, and Shortliffe 2001). By 1974, INTERNIST I was developed at the University of Pittsburgh to support the diagnostic process in general internal medicine by linking diseases with symptoms. Its medical knowledge base later became the basis of successor systems including quick medical reference (QMR). MYCIN, a rule-based expert system to diagnose and recommend treatment for certain blood infections was functional in 1976.

Many early expert systems were developed primarily for diagnosis of medical conditions and tended to use the "Greek Oracle" approach, where the DSS provided a solution from "on high," and the clinician entered information and passively awaited the solution. Miller and Masarie (1990) called instead for a "catalyst" approach whereby the DSS serves as a vehicle to provide guidance, but the user remains in control. In nursing, two early and well known systems, COMMES (Creighton online multiple modular expert system) (Evans, 1990) and computer-aided nursing diagnosis and intervention (CANDI) (Chang, 1988) were developed to assist nurses with care planning and nursing diagnosis.

Other CDSS Uses A series of systems addressing specific clinical issues were developed next. These included ONCOCIN developed for oncology protocol management at Stanford; CASNET developed at Rutgers University for diagnosis and treatment of glaucoma; and ABEL, an expert system developed at MIT that used causal reasoning to manage acid-base and electrolyte imbalance (*www.openclinical.org/dss.html on 3/22/2004*). Several websites addressing CDSS in routine clinical use with entries ranging from simple expert or knowledge-based systems to advanced systems capable of complex inferences are available. These sites contain links to specific CDSS (refer to Table 10.1 for an annotated listing of sample CDSSs).

Types and Characteristics of DSS

Types of DSS

Administrative and Organizational Systems Included in the field of healthcare decision support are systems that support organizational, executive/managerial, financial, and clinical decisions. Administrative systems, including those designed for finance or quality monitoring, generally support the business decision-making process. These systems encompass decision processes other than direct patient care delivery, and even if clinical in nature, such as quality improvement systems, are mainly used for strategic planning, budgeting, financial analysis, quality management, continuous process improvement, and clinical benchmarking. In these systems, decisions occur at the strategic, tactical, population or aggregate and operational levels, not at the individual level.

These systems tend to be batch-oriented in nature, i.e., not real time, mostly concerned with aggregations of many data elements largely for purposes of intelligence gathering. These systems tend to be unstructured, goal seeking/searching, and long range in nature. In contrast, CDSSs discussed in this chapter tend to be focused on real-time decision support, goal orientation, and intelligence gathering, and are designed to be used at the point of care by clinicians.

Integrated Systems More recently, healthcare agencies have begun to understand that combination systems offer optimal value to the organization. Such systems are able to support outcomes performance management by integrating operational data (the business side)—budgeting, executive decision-making, financial analysis, quality management, and strategic planning data—with clinical data (the clinical side)—clinical event tracking,

Table 10.1   A Sample List of Clinical Decision Support Systems

CDSS Sources	Descriptions
Clin-eguide	A point-of-care CDSS designed for integration with electronic health records that makes recommendations on diagnosis, management, and treatment of specific diseases
Clinical Pathway Constructor	Zynx Health's Web-based tool with a compendium of evidence-based guidelines. Available by subscription
CURE (Carotid U.S. Report Enhancement, Washington University, St. Louis)	Augments carotid ultrasound reports with treatment-specific prognostic information
DiagnosisPro	Contains a database of 9,000 diseases and drug terms and 16,000 symptoms, signs, lab, and x-ray findings linked with 120,000 relationships to suggest diagnoses and treatment
DXplain (Harvard/MIT/Mass General)	A system using a set of clinical findings including signs, symptoms, and lab data to produce a ranked list of diagnoses that might explain the clinical signs and symptoms
Healthaction (Health Development Agency [HAD])	A Web site that is a knowledge management service for primary care; shares approaches to reduce health inequalities and facilitated interactive learning exchange
HDP—The Heart Disease Program (MIT)	A system to assist in the diagnosis of cardiovascular disease
Iliad	A system that provides expert diagnostic consultation with more than 900 diseases and 1,500 symptoms; includes ICD-9 codes for each diagnosis
IMKI—Institute for Medical Knowledge Implementation	Has developed and maintains a library of medical knowledge applications and is developing a process for development, evaluation, and dissemination of CDSS rules
InfoRetriever (InfoPOEMS)	Contains seven evidence databases, clinical decision rules, practice guidelines, risk calculators, and basic information on drugs; can be loaded on a PDA
ISABEL	A diagnostic reminder system from the United Kingdom that covers the spectrum of pediatric medicine and is designed to integrate with electronic medical record (EMR) systems
LISA	A DSS for treatment of childhood acute lymphoblastic leukemia
Logiciana	MedicaLogic's electronic record system that checks medications and formulary compliance and includes clinical reminders and patient education material
MICROMEDEX	A system designed to provide clinicians with alerts, recommendations, and evidence-based references
Misys Insight	A open CDSS designed to work with a broad spectrum of clinical information systems
ORAD (oral radiographic differential diagnosis)	A system designed to evaluate radiographic and clinical features of patients with intrabony dental problems
Oxford Clinical Mentor (Oxford)	A U.K. electronic medical knowledge support system with details on more than 2,000 diseases cross-referenced with 26,000 commonly used terms and synonyms
PIER—physicians' information and education resource	American College of Physicians-American Society of Internal Medicine web-based DSS tool which combs medical literature and provides bullet lists under six different topics. Available to members only
PKC—Problem Knowledge Couplers (Weed, 1991)	A system of data capture and clinical guidance that provides decision and management support to clinicians

Table 10.1   A Sample List of Clinical Decision Support Systems (*Continued*)

CDSS Sources	Descriptions
PRODIGY—Prescribing rationally with decision support in genera-practice study	A U.K. initiative for evaluation of a prescribing practices in general practice
QMR—quick medical reference (University of Pittsburgh/first databank)	A system with a knowledge base of close to 700 diseases, signs, symptoms, and lab information to suggest relevant diagnosis
TheraSim CS-HIV (International Society of Infectious Diseases)	A system of clinical simulation, DES, and medical education technology for the management of HIV
TraumAID	A system of decision support for emergency center management of multiple trauma that produces diagnostic and therapeutic plans for patient management
VisualDx	An image-based system that serves as a reference to support diagnosis and treatment

Note: An excellent Web source for DSS information exists at *www.openclinical.org/dss.*

results reporting, pharmaceutical ordering and dispensing, differential diagnoses, real-time clinical pathways, literature research, and clinical alerts. The intent, the content, and the methods may differ but these two approaches to DSS (business and clinical) have common elements and the integration of the two can increase effective decisions (Perreault, 1999).

Characteristics of DSS

Just as there are many types of DSS, there are also a number of ways to examine the characteristics of a given DSS. These systems can be studied based on their structure, their organization, their content, or their purpose. Shortliffe (1990) uses function, mode of advice, consultation style, underlying decision-science methodology, and user-computer interactions to categorize systems. Teich and Wrinn (2000) examine DSS from the aspects of *functional and logical* classes and *structural elements*. They include in the *functional* class, feedback provided to the clinician, the organization of the data, the extent of proactive information provided, the intelligent actions of the system, and the communication method; the *logical* class includes substitute therapy alerts, drug family checking, structured entry, consequent actions, parameter checking, redundant utilization checking, relevant information display, time-based checks, templates and order sets, and profile display and analysis, rule-based event detection, and aggregate data trending. CDSS *structural elements* according to Teich and Wrinn include triggering, dispatching, rule logic,

process control, notification/acknowledgement, action choices, action execution, and rule editor.

Key CDSS Functions   Perreault (1999) organized key CDSS functions as:

> *Administrative*—support for clinical coding and documentation
>
> *Management of clinical complexity and details*— keeping patients on research and chemotherapy protocols, tracking orders, referrals, follow-up, and preventive care
>
> *Cost control*—monitoring medication orders and avoiding duplicate or unnecessary tests
>
> *Decision support*—supporting clinical diagnostic and treatment plan processes promotion of best practices, use of condition-specific guidelines, and population-based management.

If one were to classify CDSSs from an ontologic perspective (Tan and Sheps, 1998), DSSs could be divided into data-based (population-based), model-based (case-based), knowledge-based (rule-based), and graphics-based systems.

Data–based systems capitalize on the fundamental input into any intelligent system, data. They provide decision support with a population perspective and use routinely collected longitudinal, cohort, and cross-sectional databases. Population-based information is used to enhance clinical decision-making, "funnel" patients to medical care, and enhance medical practice. The development of technologies and techniques for OLAP (on line analytic processing) and for building and using data warehouses combined with the increased ability to store and process vast amounts of data effectively are allowing users to access data for decision support "at the speed of thought" (Dhar and Stein, 1997).

Model-based DSSs are driven by access to and manipulation of a statistical, financial, optimization, and/or simulation model. The data in this instance are compared to various decision-making and analytic models. A model is a generalization that can be used to describe the relationships among a number of observations to represent a perception of how things fit together. The models may be pathophysiologic, statistical, or analytic. Some model-based examples are linear programming, such as scheduling nurses or physicians or resource allocation, simulation, such as emergency department or operating room scheduling or provider profiling.

Rarely are new problems solved from scratch (Dhar and Stein, 1997). New information is compared to previously learned information and adjustments are made for the differences as a new solution is crafted. Genetic algorithms (GAs) and neural networks (NNs) are newer computation techniques that are evolving as problem solving solutions. GAs optimize solutions by using principles from Darwin's survival of the fittest evolutionary theory and attempting to "breed" better and better solutions. NNs build models by repeatedly sifting the data, searching for relationships, learning from mistakes, and constructing newer more accurate models (Dhar and Stein, 1997).

Knowledge-based systems rely on expert knowledge that is either embedded in the system or accessible from another source and uses some type of knowledge acquisition process to understand and capture the cognitive processes of healthcare providers. Much of what we consider evidence-based practice (EBP) refers to knowledge-based decision support. Yet there are many issues with maintaining current evidence in DSS. Sim et al. (2001) identify the policy and research challenges in developing and maintaining practice evidence in machine-readable repositories. They have coined a term, "evidence-adaptable CDSSs," to describe a new type of CDSS that has a knowledge base that is constantly updated with the most current evidence available and is viewed as both a goal and necessity.

Graphics-based systems take advantage of the user interface to support decisions by providing decision "cues" to the user in the form of color, graphical representation options, and data visualization.

Examples of CDSS Applications

Some examples of CDSS applications include the following:

1. Reminders and alerts which are computer tools for focusing attention such as "flags" for abnormal values

2. Therapy critiquing and planning as well as care maps, guidelines, protocols, and so on

3. Diagnostic assistance providing patient-specific consultations using diagnostic or management tools, such as Problem Knowledge Couplers (PKC) (Weed, 1991)

4. Lab systems with interpretation of measured values and automated preparation of reports as well as physician guidance as to which tests to order

5. Prescribing decision support such as drug advisory systems used for advising on drug-drug interactions, side effects, selecting most cost-effective drug

6. Clinical workstations with online literature, e-tools for calculation, patient guidelines

7. Image recognition and interpretation with capabilities of mass screening—e.g., mammography, assistance with expensive and complex investigations—e.g., MRI

8. Signal interpretation such as interpretive alarms for real-time clinical signals in intensive care unit (ICU), automated electrocardiogram (ECG) interpretation, retinal scans, and voice recognition

9. Natural language/speech recognition which offers interpretation of freely entered clinical notes and archiving to make electronically accessible in the future

10. Evidence-based quality improvement using up-to-date and consistent tools

11. Multitask tools for assessment, diagnosis, and management

CDSS have the ability to respond to recorded decisions that alter care (critiques of orders) and requests from decision makers (suggestion systems) by providing assistance in tasks subject to human error and tools to augment human performance.

Demand management centers (telephone call centers) often use decision tree logic (DTL) or rule-based logic (RBL) for patient management. DTL is useful for specific straightforward tasks. User training in the system is typically easily accomplished, but because DTL is often based on probabilities, the correct interpretation of the probabilities can be challenging for both developer and user. When cases are more complex with more variables to consider, DTL requires a tremendous amount of programming and often has limited data specificity and rigidness in solution options which may limit the value of the system. A simple example of DTL is if A, then B, if not A then C. In reality, knowing and interpreting Bayesian probabilities is not as straightforward. For example, we may know the probability of an MI in an overweight, highly stressed, 50-year-old man who smokes and is having chest pain, but we may not know the impact of a history of diabetes on his additional chances of having an MI.

RBL allows for complex decision capacities, is somewhat more flexible with answers, provides consistent outcomes, and is adaptable to change; however, it also tends to have rigid solutions and allows little or no clinician autonomy. A typical RBL statement would be if 1, 4, and 7 apply, then do A; if 2, 5, and 8 apply, then do B. Both DTL and RBL are forms of electronic algorithms using step-by-step problem solving and the evidence from which decisions are made comes from best practice guidelines. In a well-designed system, the clinician has an opportunity to override a solution with an explanation or justification.

The above CDSS distinctions are somewhat artificial and are increasingly blurring. A very simplistic, broad view of DSS is a "push-pull" distinction. In a "pull" system, the provider needs to take some action independent of the usual workflow in order to initiate a request for support from the system or to query the system for additional information; whereas, in a "push" system, the system automatically generates the alert in response to a clinician action such as a medication order for which the patient has reported an allergy.

Another useful framework for organizing thinking about clinical decision support system features has been proposed by Sim and Berlin (2003) (see Table 10.2). Their taxonomy for CDSS uses the following categories or axes:

1. Context
2. Knowledge and data sources
3. Workflow
4. Decision support
5. Information delivery

CDSS Impact on Clinicians and Clinical Decisions

Need for Evidence-Based Practice

There is growing pressure for clinicians including nurses to use knowledge at the point of care that is based on researched evidence. This became especially true after the Institute of Medicine (IOM) Report (2000) identified human error as a major source of patient care morbidity and mortality.

Studies have been designed to determine whether access to information in a variety of forms would impact patient care. One early study showed that MEDLINE access did have a significant effect on physician resolution of diagnostic and treatment problems (Lindberg et al., 1993). Gorman, Ash, and Wykoff (1994) found that availability of information at the time of a patient visit would definitely impact care. The use of CDSS to find and prevent errors related to gaps between optimal and actual practice can result in improved quality of care (Bates et al., 2001). Applications of CDSS suggest the ability to lessen the incidence of adverse drug events, nosocomial infections, and the inappropriate use of antibiotics. Prevention of prescription errors is seen as one of the most valuable and widely used functions of CDSS (Lippman, 2000). Bates et al. (2003) have determined that effective clinical decision support depends on CDSS speed, anticipation of information needs, real-time delivery, usability, simplicity, and the maintenance of the knowledge-based system. They also identified that successful use of a CDSS requires integration of the system with the user's normal workflow. CDSS must be designed to support clinician requirements rather than dictate clinician workflow practices and CDSS should actually help improve workflow.

Barriers to the Use of CDSS Systems

According to Sims et al. (2001), only about half of the treatments used for patient care in internal and family medicine are supported with evidence of efficacy. Bates et al. (2003) suggest that practice lags behind knowledge by several years. This lag could be shortened if not eliminated by the availability of current knowledge to support the decision-making process. A systematic review of CDSS studies (Hunt et al., 1998) showed that in 43 of 65 investigated studies some benefit was found in either the process of care or in patient outcomes. In instances where CDSS implementation has not been successful, barriers identified included lack of noticeable benefits, insufficient cost benefits, inadequate staff

Table 10.2   Sample Items from Sim and Belin CDSS Taxonomy (2003)

Category/Axis	Examples of Characteristics
Context: clinical setting	Outpatient
	Inpatient
Context: clinical task	Prevention/screening
	Diagnosis
	Treatment
	Drug dosing/prescribing
	Test ordering
Knowledge and data source: clinical knowledge source	National or professional society guidelines, well accepted standard, or adaptation of published RCTs or analytic reviews
	Clinician-developer
	System users involved in building knowledge base
Workflow: data input intermediary	Patient passive intermediary
	Physician active intermediary
	Non-physician clinician passive intermediary
Workflow: system user	Patient computer system user
	Physician computer system user
	Non-physician clinician computer system user
	Non-clinician staff computer user
	No direct system user or operator
Workflow: degree of workflow integration	Moderately to well integrated
	Allows for workflow flexibility
Decision support: recommendation explicitness	Explicit recommendation
	Implicit recommendation
Decision support: clinical urgency	Clinically urgent
	Clinically nonurgent
Decision support: response requirement	No response required
	Non-committal acknowledgment required
	Target decision maker required to indicate whether his/her decision is to comply with recommended action
	Target decision maker required to indicate whether his/her decision is to comply with recommended action, and if decision is not to comply, justification for not complying also required
Decision support: degree of customization	Generic
	Targeted
Information delivery: delivery format	Printed with chart
	Online computer-based record user session
Information delivery: delivery mode	Push
	Pull
Information delivery: interactive delivery/explanation availability	Interactive
	Noninteractive
	Explanation available
	Explanation not available

training, and lack of system support. Additional barriers to CDSSs include system costs and a lack of exposure to technology. Coiera (2003) cites a lack of congruence with work flow and the additional effort required by the user to fit the system into the usual care process as a barrier to use of CDSSs. Although it once may have been a factor in user reluctance to use automated decision support, it is no longer accurate to assume that poor utilization and lack of enthusiasm for systems by clinicians is due to discomfort with technology. Systems deemed by clinicians as beneficial will be used. The involvement of healthcare professionals in CDSS selection is essential to system acceptance. It is also important to consider how a CDSS will affect organizational culture, practice, and personnel attitudes.

The construction and upkeep of clinical protocols or guidelines is not easy or cheap. Often there are multiple authors, protocol selection (from a number of options) is not always straightforward, multiple protocols may be available, or there is a situation that demands a departure from protocol assumptions.

A significant, if not the most significant, requirement in CDSSs is precise vocabulary. It is unacceptable to have "fuzzy" vocabulary when implementing computerized guidelines, protocols, or algorithms (McCormick, 1998). Henry, in a classic article on DSS (1995), identified essential elements needed for an informatics infrastructure: (1) Standardized vocabularies to describe patient diagnoses, interventions, and outcomes; (2) computer-based methods to examine linkages among patient problems and characteristics, healthcare interventions, patient outcomes, and the intensity of care/resources and to examine practice variations; and (3) an integrated clinical information system where data required for quality improvement are both collected and returned to the provider during routine processes of patient care.

Evaluation of CDSS

Consequently, there is a need to evaluate CDSS with sound studies. The effect of CDSS on clinical outcomes currently remains uncertain without valid and generalizable findings. Sim et al. (2001) have identified as essential "ongoing iterative reevaluations and redesigns of CDSS to identify and amplify system benefits while identifying and mitigating unanticipated system errors/dangers." Basic questions to be answered include Does the design make sense? Will the system be accepted and successfully used in the setting? Does the system positively impact patient safety, efficiency, and effectiveness of care?

Increasing pressure to deliver quality care at the lowest possible cost has led to the implementation of CDSS to drive appropriate process improvement activities needed to achieve successful care outcomes (Healthcare Financial Management). Three key areas to assess in CDSS development are cost management, quality management, and information management. According to Coiera (2003) over 55 studies have been conducted to evaluate CDSSs. The studies examined process variables such as provider confidence in decision, patterns of care, adherence to protocol, efficiency/cost, and adverse effects. Overall in most studies where the variable was measured, improvement was demonstrated. Of the eight times that morbidity and mortality were studied, in only one case was an improvement detected.

One consideration in the evaluation of a system is the assessment of how a system handles continuous variables, like age. What if the literature (knowledge base) states that the patient must be 12 years of age to receive a given medication, and the patient is 1 day from being 12? One week? One month? Does the patient's weight make a difference? Needed is a series of probabilities outlining the risks at a variety of decision points.

Sittig (1999) cites the following five elements as necessary, but not sufficient for a real-time clinical decision support system.

1. *Integrated real-time patient database* which combines patient data from multiple sources, lab, radiology, pharmacy, admissions, nursing notes, and so on. This is needed to provide context for results interpretation.

2. *Data-drive mechanism* that allows event triggers to go into effect and activate alerts and reminders automatically.

3. *Knowledge engineer* who can translate the knowledge representation scheme used in the system so that the clinical knowledge in the system can be extracted and translated into machine executable logic.

4. *Time-driven mechanism* to permit automatic execution of programs at a specific time (e.g., at 3 p.m. or 4 hours after surgery) to alert provider to carry out a specific action or insure that the action had been completed.

5. *Long-term clinical data repository*—data collected over time from a variety of sources allowing a longitudinal patient record.

Knowledge and Cognitive Processes

Knowledge engineering is the field concerned with knowledge acquisition (extracting or eliciting knowledge from experts) and the organization and structure of that knowledge within a computer system. Building a knowledge-based or expert system requires an understanding of the cognitive processes of healthcare providers and how they deal with complexity. Most DSS take advantage of the research on human reasoning and decision-making.

How do nurses solve problems? Or even determine that there is a problem? What information seeking behaviors do nurses use? Is "intuition" really a case of statistical pattern recognition? When an expert nurse claims that the patient "just doesn't look right," is it intuition or do years of nursing experience place that patient three standard deviations from the mean of all the patients cared for? Answering these questions requires an understanding of the decision-making process, human diagnostic reasoning, and critical thinking. Nurses recognize various types of knowledge such as declarative knowledge and procedural knowledge. Declarative knowledge can be considered the "know what" or descriptive knowledge, procedural knowledge is the "know how" and the processes of reasoning and inference produce the "know why." Kassirer (1989) describes a number of methods of reasoning: rule-based, Bayesian, causal, probabilistic, decision-theoretic, possibilistic, commonsense, and case-based.

There are a number of cognitive limitations in the human reasoning process. These include belief systems that restrict information seeking, limited ability to retain and process information, a variety of risk aversion behaviors, a range of diverse intelligence, levels of motivation, and judgment and decision-making abilities. There are also perception blocks that detract from decision-making and information seeking such as delimiting the problem space, stereotyping, and having difficulty in isolating a given problem. The way a problem is formulated by the clinician has an impact on the solution that is selected.

In addition, a variety of methods have been used to elicit knowledge from expert clinicians. Some knowledge elicitation techniques require clinicians to "think aloud." Some use observations of clinician behavior in practice settings. Interviews with experts have been the most commonly used method of eliciting knowledge (Tan and Sheps, 1998). The expert clinician is directly asked in a structured interview to describe a typical case and how aspects of the case influence care decisions.

The advantages of this method are ease of use and the ability to draw out important information; however, a potential problem may be that the experts tend to say what they think they do, but may be unaware of what they actually do, or may be unable to break down their thought processes into steps. It is so natural for the expert to see the "big picture" that it is extremely difficult for them to be consciously aware of the discrete elements that comprise that picture. Benner (1984) described these phenomena in *Novice to Expert*.

Cognitive task analysis (CTA) refers to a set of methods that attempt to capture the skills, knowledge, and processing ability of experts in dealing with complex tasks. The goal of CTA is to tap into these "higher order" cognitive functions. This technique is often beneficial in comparing an "expert performance" with the performance of "less than experts" (Tan and Sheps, 1998). CTA attempts to identify pitfalls or trouble spots in the reasoning process of the beginner or intermediate level practitioner while comparing the reasoning process with that of the expert. In a study by Kushniruk et al. (1995) using nonexperts and experts, the nonexperts used more interventions such as ordering additional tests and tended to rely more on the test results. The experts, on the other hand, used increased assessment and were more apt to consider the context when determining a course of action.

Tan and Sheps (1998) describe a six-step approach to CTA as follows:

1. Identification of the problem to target in the analysis, e.g., pulmonary embolus (PE) with symptoms of shortness of breath, chest pain, and hemoptysis.

2. Generation of cases (decision tasks) that vary on key factors.

3. Observation of a record of an expert problem solving for the case using think aloud.

4. Observation of the novice and the intermediate problem solving.

5. Analyses of expert versus less than expert problem solving.

6. Recommendation of systems needs, design specs, and knowledge base components.

Computer-based techniques that use interactive tools are also used to assess decision-making. These tools have the advantage of not needing to interact directly with the clinician but often tend to be overly simplistic for complex decision analysis. Rating and sorting methods, borrowed from the social sciences and protocol analysis are other methods used. Each has advantages and disadvantages.

Miller and Gardner (1997) recommended adoption of a 0-3 risk-based review system for software where a 0 indicated systems providing factual content, and a 3 was a high risk, patient-specific system that was difficult to override by the clinician.

Responsibility of User: Ethical and Legal Issues

CDSS are considered similar to medical devices but the legal responsibility for treatment and advice given to a patient rests with the clinician regardless of whether a CDSS is used (Hunt et al., 1998). Still unknown are the legal ramifications of not following CDSS advice. Courts seem to believe that cost should have no role in clinical decision-making. Attempts to save money by reducing treatment below an undisputed standard of care are not acceptable. If a treatment plan is based on anything besides "sound medical consideration" it would most certainly be considered malpractice. Legal reasoning is more compatible with the old clinical decision paradigms based on anecdote, custom, and algorithms than with new statistical models (Poplin, 1999).

There seems to be no major adverse effect from the use of a CDSS; however, such systems must be developed with high standards of quality. The provision of erroneous information and/or incorrect guidance does have the potential for harmful impact. There must be some way to provide a high degree of assurance that a CDSS has been developed according to quality and safety standards. CDSS will be expected to comply with a "duty of care" if it is to become safely integrated into routine patient care. The knowledge base of healthcare changes frequently and often past practices are proven ineffective and perhaps even hazardous. Healthcare knowledge may also be based on professional judgment without objective scientific evidence. Therefore, the knowledge base of a CDSS must be as reflective as possible of the current state of professional and scientific opinion and evidence and must draw on traditional knowledge sources such as journals and texts to maintain currency.

Safe use of CDSS may include such techniques as limiting access, developing audit trails, monitoring use, and clinical hazard alerts. It is possible that a CDSS may be considered a specialized piece of clinical equipment requiring certification for use. Rector (2002) suggests that the risk of system harm should be weighted against the risks associated without the system.

CDSS documentation should address the purpose of the system, the population for which the application is intended along with inclusion/exclusion criteria, the context for use, the expected user skill level, evidence source(s), and review and update methods. Keeping a CDSS current requires a commitment of technical, professional, and organizational dimensions. A CDSS will be only as effective as the strength and accuracy of underlying evidence base. Requirements for CDSS to be methodologically rigorous include the availability of computer understandable clinical research databases, electronic medical records (EMR) with a standardized clinical vocabulary to ensure accurate communication, standardized interfaces, and use of newer technologies including wireless and speech recognition.

Implications for Future Uses of CDSS in Nursing

Increasing Inclusion of Patients   As hospital information systems began to develop patient portals that allow patients or their designated representatives access to their own medical records, CDSS systems of the future may also allow patient access to the knowledge base of the system. The computer can become a patient health medium with reference databases, library access for healthcare information, drug and disease management information, self-help programs, and advice about prevention available. Nursing needs to better understand the relationship between patient autonomy and well-being. Nurses advocate for increased patient control over decisions yet needs more evidence to support the association of this with positive health benefits.

CDSS applications can be developed for a spectrum of clinical users including nurses. No specific CDSS for nursing currently exists but the potential for future nursing applications is vast if certain basic issues are resolved. This includes definition of the nursing knowledge base and how nursing knowledge can be represented and how structure can be added to nursing knowledge. What clinical/nursing tasks are worth automating? The problem domain must be understood prior to CDS system design. Consideration should be given to support common clinical problems that comprise the greatest amount of clinical duties rather than the rare but more complex problems that may intuitively appeal to researchers and academics.

Dual Purpose of Documentation   Finally, we must balance the use of poorly designed or inadequately tested systems with individual clinicians being forced to make patient care decision-making without existing evidence at the point of care. We also need to find the balance between an individual and a population perspective. Every nurse must understand the dual purpose of documenting and capturing information in an automated manner, first that of improving care for the individual patient and second that of improving care for future populations of patients via aggregated information used for clinical decision-making.

Current evidence indicates that CDSS can improve patient care quality, reduce medication errors, minimize variances in care, improve guideline compliance, and promote cost savings. Wider adoption of such tools will support clinical care decisions through the provision of additional and current information at the time and place of care delivery while final decision authority will remain with the clinician. Although no one single CDSS is in widespread use, such systems whether simple or complex are becoming ubiquitous and research on their use is growing.

References

Bates, D., Cohen, M., Leape, L., Overhage, J., Shabot, M., and Sheridan, T. (2001). Reducing the frequency of errors in medicine using information technology. *Journal of the American Medical Informatics Association* 8(4):299–308.

Bates, D., Kuperman, G., Wang, S., Gandhi, T., Kittler, A., and Volk, L. (2003). Ten commandments for effective clinical decision support. *Journal of the American Medical Informatics Association* 10(6):523–530.

Benner, P. (1984). *From Novice to Expert: Excellence and Power in Clinical Nursing Practice*. Menlo Park, CA: Addison-Wesley.

Berner, E. (Ed.). (1999). *Clinical Decision Support Systems: Theory and Practice*. New York: Springer.

Chang, B. L., et al. (1988). CANDI: A knowledge based system for nursing diagnosis. *Computers in Nursing* 6(1):14–21.

Coiera, E. (1994). Designing for decision support in a clinical monitoring environment. In *Proceedings of the International Conference on Medical Physics and Biomedical Engineering—MPBE '94* (pp. 130–142).

Coiera, E. (2003). *Guide to Health Informatics* (2nd ed.). Oxford: Oxford University Press.

de Dombal, F. T., Leaper, D. J., Staniland, J. R., McCann, A. P., and Horrocks, J. D. (1972). Computer-aided diagnosis of acute abdominal pain. *British Medical Journal* 2(5804):9–13.

Dhar, V. and Stein, R. (1997). *Intelligent Decision Support Methods: The Science of Knowledge Work*. Upper Saddle River, NJ: Prentice Hall.

Evans, S. (1990). The COMMES nursing consultant system: A practical tool for patient care. In J. Ozbolt, et al. (Eds.), *Decision Support Systems in Nursing* (pp. 97–120). St. Louis, MO: C.V. Mosby.

Gorman, P., Ash, J., and Wykoff, L. (1994). Can primary care physicians' questions be answered using the medical journal literature? *Bulletin of the Medical Library Association* 82:140–146.

Henry, S. (1995). Informatics: essential infrastructure for quality assessment and improvement in nursing. *Journal of the American Medical Informatics Association* 2(3):169–182.

Hunt, D., Haynes, R., Hanna S., and Smith, K. (1998). Effects of computer-based clinical decision support systems on physician performance and patient outcomes: A systematic review. *Journal of the American Medical Association* 280:1339–1346.

Institute of Medicine: Committee on Quality of Health Care in America. (2000). In L. Kohn, J. Corrigan, M. Donaldson (Eds.), *To Err is Human*. Washington, DC: National Academy Press.

Johnston, M., Langton, K., Haynes, R., and Mathieu, A. (1994). The effects of computer-based clinical decision support systems on clinician performance and patient outcome: A critical appraisal of research. *Annals of Internal Medicine* 120:135–142.

Kassirer, J. P. (1989). Diagnostic reasoning. *Annals of Internal Medicine* 110:893–900.

Kushniruk, A. W., et al. (1995). An analysis of medical decision-making: A cognitive perspective on medical informatics. In R. Gardner (Ed.), *Proceedings of the Nineteenth Annual Symposium on Computer Applications in Medical Care*. (pp. 193–197).

Lindberg, D., Sioegel, E., Rapp, B., Wallingford, K., and Wilson, S. (1993). Use of MEDLINE by physicians for clinical problem solving. *Journal of American Medical Association* 269:3124–3129.

Lippman, H. (2000). Clinical decision support. *Hippocrates* 14(3). Available at http://www.hippocrates.com/archive/March2000/03 features/03cds.html.

McCormick, K. (1998). *Keynote Presentation at NANDA, NIC, NOC Conference*. St. Charles, IL.

Miller, R. and Gardner, R. (1997). Recommendations for responsible monitoring and regulation of clinical software systems. *Journal of the American Medical Informatics Association* 4(6):458–464.

Miller, R., and Masarie, F. (1990). The demise of the Greek oracle model for medical diagnosis systems. *Methods of Information in Medicine* 29:1–2.

Musen, M., Shahar, Y., and Shortliffe, E. (2001). Clinical decision support systems. In E. Shortliffe, L. Perrault (Eds.), G. Wiederhold, and L. Fagan (Assoc. Eds.), *Computer Applications in Healthcare and Biomedicine* (2nd ed.). New York: Springer-Verlag.

Negroponte, N. (1996). *Being Digital*. New York: Random House.

Perreault, L. and Metzger, J. (1999). A pragmatic framework for understanding clinical decision support. *Journal of Healthcare Information Management* 13(2).

Poplin, C. (1999). JNRM Clinical decision making, legal liability, and managed care. Downloaded on 3/22/2004, from *www.afip.org/Departments/legalmed/jnrm1999/managed.htm*

Rector, A. (2002). *Response to Quality and Safety of Clinical Decision Support Systems*. Draft V0.12 *openclinical.org* downloaded on 3/22/2004.

Shortliffe, E. H. (1990). *Medical informatics: Computer Applications in Health Care*. Reading, MA: Addison Wesley.

Sims, I., Gorman, P., Greenes, R., Haynes, B., Kaplan, B., Lehmann, H., and Tang, P. (2001). Clinical decision support systems for the practice of evidence-based medicine. *Journal of the American Medical Informatics Association* 8:527–534.

Tan, J. K. and Sheps, S. (1998). *Health Decision Support Systems*. Gaithersburg, MD: Aspen Publishers.

Teich, J. and Wrinn, M. (2000). Clinical decision support systems come of age. *MD Computing* Jan/Feb:43–46.

Toronto, A. F., Veasley L. G., Stephenson R. A mathematical approach to medical diagnosis:. Application to congenital heart disease, JAMA 177:177–83, July 22.

Weed, L. (1991). *Knowledge Coupling*. New York: Springer-Verlag.

www.healthcommons.org/clinical.html

Suggested Readings

Barnett, G. O., Cimino, J. J., Hupp, J. A., and Hoffer, E. P. (1897). DXplain: An evolving diagnostic decision-support system. *Journal of the American Medical Association* 258(1):67–74.

Bleich, H. L. (1969). Computer evaluation of acid-base disorders. *Journal of Clinical Investigation* 48(9): 1689–1696.

Collen, M. F., Rubin, L., Neyman, J., et al. (1964). Automated multiphasic screening and diagnosis. *American Journal of Public Health* 54:741–750.

de Dombal, F. T., Horrocks, J. D. Staniland, J. R., Guillou, P. J. (1971). Construction and uses of a "data-base" of clinical information concerning 600 patients with acute abdominal pain. *Proceedings of the Royal Society of Medicine* 64(9):978.

Gorry, G. A. and Barnett, G. (1968). Experience with a model of sequential diagnosis. *Computers and Biomedical Research, An International Journal* 1(5):490–507.

Gorry, G. and Barnett, G. (1968). Sequential diagnosis by computer. *Journal of the American Medical Association* 205(12):849–854.

Kingsland, L. C., Lindberg, D. A., and Sharp, G. C. (1983). AI/RHEUM: A consultant system for rheumatology. *Journal of Medical Systems* 7(3):221–227.

Larrabee, J. H. (1996). An emerging model of quality. *Image—The Journal of Nursing Scholarship* 8:353–358.

Ledley, R. S. and Lusted, L. B. (1959). Reasoning foundations of medical diagnosis. *Science* 130:9–21. (Reprinted in September, 1991, *MD Computing* 8(5):300–315.)

McDonald, C. J. (1976). Protocol-based computer reminders, the quality of care and the non-perfectibility of man. *New England Journal of Medicine* 295(24):1351–1355.

Miller, P. L. (1983a). Critiquing anesthetic management: The "ATTENDING" computer system. *Anesthesiology* 58:362–369.

Miller, P. L. (1983b). ATTENDING: Critiquing a physician's management plan. *IEEE Transactions on Pattern Analysis and Machine Intelligence (PAMI)* 5:449–461.

Miller, R. A., Pople, H. E., Jr., and Myers, J. D. (1982). Internist 1: An experimental computer-based diagnostic consultant for general internal medicine. *New England Journal of Medicine* 307(8):468–476.

Nelson, S. J., Blois, M. S., Tuttle, M. S., Erlbaum, M., Harrison, P., Kim, H., Winkelmann, B., and Yamashita, D. (1985). Evaluating RECONSIDER: A computer program for diagnostic prompting. *Journal of Medical Systems* 9(5–6):379–388.

Rothenberg, J. (1995). Ensuring the longevity of digital documents. *Scientific American* (Jan):42–47.

Shortliffe, E. H., Davis, R., Axline, S. G., Buchanan, B. G., Green, C. C., and Cohen, S. N. (1975). Computer-based consultations in clinical therapeutics: Explanation and rule acquisition capabilities of the MYCIN system. *Computers and Biomedical Research* 8(4):303–320.

Turban, E., Aronson, J., and Liang, T. (2005). *Decision Support Systems and Intelligent Systems* (7th ed.). Upper Saddle River, NJ: Prentice Hall.

Warner, H. R. (1961). Cardiology and Bayes? *Journal of the American Medical Association* 177.

Weiss, S., Kulikowski, C. A., and Safir, A. (1978). Glaucoma consultation by computer. *Computers in Biology and Medicine* 8(1):25–40.

PART 3

Issues in Informatics

11 Nursing Informatics and Healthcare Policy

Carole A. Gassert

OBJECTIVES

1. Consider the implications of policy on nursing informatics (NI) as a specialty.
2. Identify the impact of national trends and events that focus on information and information technologies on NI practice.
3. Discuss telehealth and NI.

KEY WORDS

informatics
information systems
public policy
health policy

To practice effectively in today's continually changing healthcare environment, informatics professionals need to be aware of existing and proposed healthcare policy. Policy is defined as a course of action that guides present and future decisions. That action is based on given conditions and selected from among identified alternatives. Healthcare policy is established on local, state, and national levels to guide the implementation of solutions for the population's health needs. Both existing conditions and emerging trends in the healthcare industry influence policy decisions. Policy decisions often establish the direction for future trends that impact informatics. NI professionals, therefore, need to become more cognizant of events and the healthcare policies that will affect their practice.

What a great time for NI professionals! The number of informatics programs for nurses has significantly increased, preparing more informatics nurse specialists to practice in the field and a number of trends and events have placed information technology (IT), information systems (IS), and informatics at the center of attention in healthcare. NI and trends and events influencing informatics will be discussed in this chapter. The events to be included are the nursing shortage, a concern for patient safety, national informatics initiatives, and delivery of services through telehealth. Each of these has significant impact on NI practice.

Healthcare Policy and Nursing Informatics as a Specialty

Nurses have contributed to the purchase, design, and implementation of IS since the 1970s. In 1992, the American Nurses Association (ANA) recognized NI as a specialty. Attempts in 1989 to be recognized as a specialty failed, but political forces within ANA supported the request when it was repeated in 1992. To be acknowledged as a specialty within nursing, informatics had to demonstrate a differentiated practice base, identify the existence of educational programs in the field, show support from nationally recognized organizations, and develop a research agenda (Panniers and Gassert, 1995).

The term NI first appeared in the literature in the 1980s (Ball and Hannah, 1984; Hannah, 1985; Grobe, 1988). The definition of NI has constantly evolved since that time, molded by the maturation of the field and influenced by health policy. In a classic article that described its domain, NI was defined as the combination of nursing, information, and computer sciences to manage and process nursing data into information and knowledge for use in nursing practice (Graves and Corcoran, 1989). Most recently, NI is described more broadly as " . . . a specialty that integrates nursing science, computer science, and information science to manage and communicate data, information, and knowledge in nursing practice. NI facilitates the integration of data, information, and knowledge to support patients, nurses, and other providers in their decision-making in all roles and settings. This support is accomplished through the use of information structures, information processes, and IT" (ANA, 2001, p. 17). Given the strong emphasis on evidence-based practice, integrated systems, and patient safety, future definitions may include some of this terminology.

The domain of NI is focused on data and its structures, information management, and the technology, including databases, needed to manage information effectively. Yet it also includes significant use of theory from linguistics, human-machine interface, decision science, cognitive science, communication, engineering, library science, and organizational dynamics. Because the knowledge base is so extensive, informatics nurses tend to develop expertise in one aspect of the domain. For example, informatics nurses working in acute care settings might focus on system selection and implementation, while informatics nurses employed in the research arm of vendor corporations develop expertise in data structures and databases. What is common among informatics nurses is that they have had strong clinical backgrounds but cease to deliver care directly to patients. They refocus their careers on the informatics domain of interest to provide indirect healthcare services.

Differentiated and Interdisciplinary Practice

A description of NI as a differentiated practice is given in the scope of practice and standards document (ANA, 2001). As the document emphasizes, NI brings an added dimension to nursing practice that focuses on knowledge and skill in information and information management techniques. Although all nurses must process information, informatics nurses demonstrate specialized knowledge of information and technology. This knowledge exceeds the ability to use technology that is expected of all nurses. Informatics nurses should assist with the development and implementation of technology tools for clinical practice, evaluation of the effectiveness of technological tools on nurses' work, and help prepare nurses to use information technologies.

NI practice differentiates itself from other areas of nursing practice but emphasizes its interaction with informatics disciplines such as mathematics, statistics, linguistics, engineering, computer science, and health informatics. In fact, NI has been described as one example of a specific domain of informatics that falls under a broader umbrella of health informatics (National Advisory Council on Nurse Education and Practice, 1997). Other examples of domain-specific informatics practices are medical informatics, dental informatics, and consumer informatics.

The NI community believes it is essential to practice within an interdisciplinary team. An example of interdisciplinary work is the Vocabulary Summit held annually at Vanderbilt University since 1999. Spearheaded by Judy Ozbolt, the summit brings together nursing and medical informatics vocabulary experts to explore how further language development in nursing can facilitate the integration of computerized languages among healthcare disciplines. Outcomes of these meetings have resulted in vocabulary standards work with the International Standards Organization (Ozbolt, 2000, 2001, 2003a,b).

NI supports national efforts, such as those outlined by the Pew Health Professions and Institute of Medicine (IOM) to increase interdisciplinary education (Pew Health Professions Commission, 1998; Greiner and Knebel, 2003). An interdisciplinary health professions education summit hosted by the IOM in 2002 produced a vision that "All health professionals should be educated to deliver patient-centered care as members of an interdisciplinary team, emphasizing evidence-based practice, quality improvement approaches, and informatics" (Greiner and Knebel, 2003, p. 45). An example of interdisciplinary education is the collaborative effort between the medical informatics (MI) and NI programs at the University of Utah. MI and NI faculty share teaching responsibilities in courses, serve jointly on student committees, work together on projects and share administrative decisions through an executive committee (Gassert and Gardner, personal communication, 2004). Because of these collaborative efforts administrators have assigned medical and NI to share space in a state-of-the-art interdisciplinary health sciences education building set to open on campus in fall 2005 (Peay, personal communication, January 7, 2004).

Preparation for Specialty Practice

To become a specialty, it was necessary for NI to show that educational programs are available to prepare nurses to practice in the field. Between 1988 and 1992, the Division of Nursing (DN), Health and Human Services Administration (HRSA), funded two Master's NI programs, University of Maryland (Heller et al., 1989) and University of Utah (Graves et al., 1995) and one doctoral program in NI at the University of Maryland (Gassert et al., 1992). Authorizing legislation passed in 1992 prevented the DN from funding other programs in NI, halting the implementation of additional NI specialty programs for several years. Finally, in 1997 an NI specialty program opened at New York University, and in 1998 a specialty program was implemented at Duquesne University in Pittsburgh. New Title VIII authorizing legislation was passed in 1998 and the DN was once again able to fund the start-up of NI programs. There is interest in opening additional informatics programs, but a scarcity of informatics faculty has limited the proliferation of NI programs. American Medical Informatics Association's (AMIA) president, Charles Safran, testified to the House Ways and Means Committee on June 17, 2004 that a new generation of physicians, nurses, and health professionals need to be prepared to lead the development, selection, and implementation of patient-centered health IS. Safran recommended that these professionals be prepared at the university level in applied clinical informatics (Safran, 2004). Hopefully his testimony will lead to increased opportunities to fund new informatics programs for nurses.

As the number of graduate NI programs increases, there will be a larger cadre of informatics nurses eligible for certification. The certification examination currently available through the American Nurses Credentialing Center is for a generalist in NI. From November 1995 through December 2003, 551 nurses have been certified as generalists in NI (ANCC, 2003). Some practicing informatics nurses have indicated that they will wait for the advanced level certification examination before they become certified. Perhaps it is time for the profession to develop a specialist level of certification for NI.

In her discussion of specialization, Styles included the need for identifying a research focus as one of the criteria for a specialty (Styles, 1989). NI researchers described seven areas needing scientific study in 1993 (National Center for Nursing Research, 1993). Even though the report was issued a decade ago, many of the same research needs still exist.

A final requirement for a specialty is representation by at least one organization. NI has the support of both nursing and multidisciplinary organizations. Within nursing, there is organizational support in the American Organization of Nurse Executives. Informatics councils previously existed within the ANA and the National League for Nursing, but these structures have become victims of budget cuts, certainly these cuts are examples of how policy impacts NI. Increasingly, multidisciplinary organizations encourage informatics nurses to become actively involved in their organizations to help solve informatics practice issues. Two examples are AMIA and the Health Information Management Systems Society; informatics nurses have served as president of both of these organizations. The field of NI has slowly expanded since 1992. It will be interesting to see how the current national focus on IT impacts the growth of NI as a specialty.

 ## Healthcare Policy Impact on Nursing Informatics Practice

Nursing Shortage and Nursing Informatics

Nursing has experienced a number of shortages in recent history. An older nursing workforce, a higher ratio of older associate degree graduates rather than their younger baccalaureate counterparts, the availability of more attractive career opportunities for women, decreased interest in nursing as a career, and difficult work environments make this shortage different from those previously experienced (Buerhaus et al., 2000; Auerbach et al., 2000; Staiger et al., 2000; HRSA, 2001; Berliner and Ginzberg, 2002). It is predicted that the shortage will result in a large deficit of nurses. In 2002 HRSA's National Center for Health Workforce Analysis found that a shortage projected for 2007 had already occurred by 2000. Unless something is done the shortage will rise from 6% in 2000 to 29% in 2020, or more than 800,000 nurses short of the number needed (HRSA, 2002). The Bureau of Labor Statistics (BLS) is predicting registered nurse positions will increase more than 600,000 between 2002 and 2012. To cover these new positions and replace retiring nurses 1.1 million more nurses are needed by 2012 (BLS, 2004).

Although these numbers differ it is clear that without intervention the healthcare industry is headed for a major crisis in the nursing workforce. At the same time the aging of the baby boomers will cause increased demand for hospital services (Berliner and Ginzberg, 2002; O'Neil, 2003). It is obvious this shortage will negatively impact the outcomes of patient care. Since a higher proportion and number of hours of care by registered nurses are related to better outcomes, the shortage of registered nurses is particularly worrisome (AACN, 2004; Kennedy, 2003; Needleman et al., 2002; Steinbrook, 2002; Stanton, 2004). Sensmeier and colleagues remind us that the intensity of the current shortage has caused it to be a public policy issue (Sensmeier, 2003).

Schools and colleges of nursing have shortened program lengths and instituted accelerated programs for those who already hold a baccalaureate degree in an attempt to increase nursing workforce numbers. The American Association of Colleges of Nursing (AACN) reports that in 2003 nearly 16,000 qualified applicants were turned away from entry-level baccalaureate programs primarily due to lack of faculty to supervise students (AACN, 2004). Nursing organizations have been actively advocating for increased federal funding to expand programs and increase loans, scholarships, and incentives to attract more young people into nursing. Other organizations, such as the American Academy of Nursing (AAN), have focused efforts on decreasing the demand side of nursing practice (McClure and Bolton, 2003). The academy believes that more efficient systems, including IT systems, must be created that will support care and lighten the workload load of nurses.

In 2002 the AAN Commission on Workforce launched a multiphase project to develop IT that will help support nurses in their day-to-day work, thereby reducing the demands of their jobs. In Phase I, interdisciplinary, creative thinkers were assembled to determine how technology could be used to facilitate nurses' work. Kennedy (2003) stated that healthcare and nursing would benefit from decision support technology, streamlined and integrated documentation support, measurement capability built into systems for determining intensity of care and outcomes, and workflow management tools. Bradley (2003) indicated that technology solutions should improve existing care processes and outcomes, increase access through the use of portable and handheld devices, incorporate Internet capability to overcome distance barriers of care and improve access to knowledge acquisition. Bradley also suggested that technological devices should be developed that would "optimize the working life span" of those individuals currently in nursing.

Given the average age of nurses is 45.2 (Spratley et al., 2000), technology devices would enable some nurses to stay in their careers longer. Sensmeier and colleagues (2003) added that wireless technology and personal digital assistants could support nurses' workflow by providing information at the point of care. These authors also advocate for using bar-coding of medications, use of speech recognition, and fine-tuning the user interface of systems to support nurses. Shabot (2003) feels that IS should support nurses by relieving them of all data gathering except for bedside assessments and notes.

As Phase II of the AAN technology project began, staff nurses from three hospitals in Virginia and California were asked to identify and/or verify the most difficult aspects of their practice and how technology would improve those tasks. As the project continues, systems will be designed, implemented, and tested to determine their effect on nurses' work.

Additional literature supports the integration of clinical information system capabilities to support nursing (Ball et al., 2003). These authors suggest that rules checking and "push" technology with clinical decision support systems would benefit all clinicians, including nurses. The additional integration of clinical data repositories, multidiscipline documentation, and point of care devices would help nurses access and share information in their work environments and finally nurses are migrating to organizations that have installed cutting-edge technology, making IS a marketing tool for attracting nurses (Priselac, 2003). The long list of recommendations for IT solutions designed to help nurses perform their work demonstrates how the public policy issue of the nursing shortage impacts NI. It is up to NI specialists to help design and implement IT systems that will finally assist nurses in their practice and to validate the results through research.

Patient Safety and Nursing Informatics

The IOM report issued in 1999, *To Err is Human: Building a Safer Health System* (Corrigan et al., 1999), has had a chilling and lasting effect on healthcare. Using data from two studies with large numbers of hospital admissions as a basis of analysis, the IOM determined that adverse events (injuries caused by medical management) occurred in 2.9 and 3.7% of admissions. When these percents were applied to the number of U.S. hospital admissions it was estimated that between 44,000 and 98,000 patients die each year from medical errors. Among other strategies the report recommended the implementation of computerized physician order entry (CPOE) systems requiring the prescriber to enter data directly into computer systems to reduce medication errors. This began a continuing discussion of IT and patient safety within healthcare.

A follow-up report, *Crossing the Quality Chasm: A New Health System for the 21st Century* (Institute of Medicine, 2001), strengthens the argument for using technology to improve patient safety. Although informatics professionals have talked for years about the advantages of using IT, these two reports elevated the discussion to the main stream of healthcare and the public in general. It is hard to pick up a healthcare article or report today that does not advocate the use of technology to improve patient care and safety.

Surveys confirm that concern for patient safety is the biggest factor driving IT (Anderson, 2004). Over 600 participants in *Health Data Management's* annual CIO survey from February 2004, list prevention of errors as the main reason for increasing IT budgets. Likewise, 47% of chief information officers who participated in the HIMSS' leadership survey in February 2004 specified that increasing patient safety would be their main focus in upcoming years (Goedert, 2004a).

Proposals to increase patient safety with IT have been made by a variety of groups. As an NI professional it is refreshing to see public-private efforts to move the implementation of IT forward but hopefully these organizations will communicate and share the results of their work. California law 1875, passed in 2003, applies pressure to hospitals to install IT to help healthcare professionals reduce errors. The Leapfrog Group, comprised of Fortune 500 companies and other large healthcare purchasers, lists CPOE as a strategy for improved patient safety (Chaiken and Holmquest, 2003).

The National Alliance for Health Information Technology (NAHIT) is a partnership of diverse healthcare leaders who are working to influence the use of technology to improve patient safety, quality, and efficiency (NAHIT, 2004). Members, assessed a substantial fee, are from provider-based organizations, technology companies, payers, the supply chain, and aligned stakeholders such as standards groups and government. During the next few years, this group plans to focus on the following: consensus-based standards, multiorganizational collaboration, an informed government, and best-practices knowledge for system implementation. Since the American Organization of Nurse Executives is a member of NAHIT, nursing will have input into group activities.

Connecting for Health (CFH), another public-private collaborative, was established by the Markle Foundation with additional support from the Robert Wood Johnson Foundation (CFH, 2004). The Markle Foundation is a private philanthropy that works to enable technology to improve people's lives. This group addresses barriers to developing an interconnected health information infrastructure and is concerned with reducing medical errors, improving the quality of care, lowering costs, and empowering patients. The steering group member list is an impressive gathering of IT business, government, and industry experts. To date CFH has obtained consensus on an initial set of data standards, developed case studies on security, and defined the electronic personal health record. Strategies to achieve their goal include policy development, research, supporting solutions, and

involving the public. NI specialists should follow the activities of public-private groups, such as NAHIT and CFH, and become involved in proposing technology solutions for improving patient safety.

National Informatics Initiatives and Nursing Informatics

Executive Order for National Interoperable Information System

Clinical information systems (CIS) were introduced in some form during the 1970s and informatics professionals have discussed the need for system improvement, integration, and wider dissemination since that time. Things have slowly progressed, but over the past 2–3 years CIS implementation has proliferated (Briggs, 2004). As indicated earlier, patient safety is one of the driving forces in increased clinical automation. Escalating healthcare costs and the availability of improved and cheaper CIS are additional driving forces.

National events have placed IS at the forefront of health policy. The impact of the first two IOM reports on patient safety has been discussed. An additional IOM report *Patient Safety: Achieving a New Standard for Care* (Aspden et al., 2003) states even more emphatically that electronic medical records, using standard data elements, are a critical tool to improve patient safety.

A 2001 report from the President's Information Technology Advisory Committee (PITAC) highlighted key issues in IT (PITAC, 2001). PITAC indicated that the United States lacks a broadly disseminated and accepted national vision for IT in healthcare and recommended the appointment of a senior IT person to provide strategic leadership. It was recommended this individual be assigned to the Department of Health and Human Services (DHHS, 2003).

On April 27, 2004, President George W. Bush issued an executive order "Incentives for the Use of Health Information Technology and Establishing the Position of the National Health Information Technology Coordinator" that has the potential to impact every healthcare entity, provider, and NI professional in the United States (Executive Order, 2004). Components of the order are (1) establish a national health information technology coordinator position; (2) work to develop a nationwide interoperable health IT infrastructure; and (3) develop, maintain, and direct implementation of a strategic plan to guide implementation of interoperable health IT in both public and private sectors. The inter-operable health IT should reduce medical errors, improve quality, and produce greater value for health-care expenditures. Guidelines for the infrastructure are (1) appropriate information is available at the time and place needed for medical decisions, (2) health quality is improved and evidence-based medical care is delivered, (3) healthcare costs are reduced, (4) more information is available to promote greater competition, (5) health information is exchanged, and (6) identifiable health information is secure and protected. The order makes it clear that adoption of the infrastructure initiative should not rely on federal resources or spending.

The executive order helped to thrust IT into the spotlight as an important political issue (Egan, 2004). The slow, quiet, and innovative changes in IT have given way to a flurry of activity as lawmakers influence policy about the use of IT. In June 2004, bipartisan House members formed a congressional caucus to influence issues surrounding IT. The caucus is expected to support policies such as financial incentives to increase the acceptance of IT by healthcare providers (House Caucus, 2004).

Various Washington leaders have proposed bills to support the purchase and implementation of IS. These modest bills will not be effective overall in supporting the purchase of IS but should raise questions about how much money is needed to accomplish the mandate. Unlike past years, the President's budget does include money for nationally integrated IS but informatics professionals, including nurses, recognize the amount would only fund a few demonstration projects. Secretary of Health and Human Services has proposed that half of the $1.2 billion annual fraud and abuse fines that are collected be used to help providers automate their practices and agencies implement IS. If this were to happen it would still take more than a decade to fund the building of an interoperable national health IS (Goedert, 2004b). Some experts believe that even if funding is not available, having IT proposed as a national solution to safety and biodefense will push IT forward in healthcare. Appointment of the first national health IT coordinator should have a significant impact on the health IT industry because there will be a single focal point for all federal efforts in health IT.

Incentives for provider acceptance will also be needed to move this initiative forward. According to regulations, physicians have been prevented from accepting IT from hospitals they are affiliated with but not working for, slowing their adoption of IT. The

Center for Medicare and Medicaid Services (CMS) has issued a final rule on physician self-referrals that creates exceptions for technology items or services furnished to physicians to enable their participation in a community-wide health IS (CMS, 2004a). Hopefully this exception will promote adoption of IT. Some suggest that such incentives are needed to assist physicians in caring for all of their patients, not just Medicare and Medicaid patients (Goedert, 2004b).

Secretary of Health and Human Services has stated that the federal government will not consider mandating that providers implement technology needed to create the national health infrastructure (Thompson, 2004). Even though Secretary Thompson has said mandates will not be used, the National Coordinator for Health IT, Dr. David Brailer, has warned that government would not wait long for the private sector to create a technology infrastructure in healthcare (Ihealthbeat, 2004a). He continually reminds audiences that everyday the infrastructure does not exist, 5–10 people die because needed information is not available or is unreadable.

Special interest groups may pressure the government to mandate use of computerized systems. The American Association of Retired Persons (AARP), 35 million members strong, supports mandatory electronic prescribing rules and federal efforts to increase adoption of CPOE (Novelli, 2004). Interestingly, "CPOE" increasingly stands for computerized practitioner order entry, language used by AARP. Such changes in language indicate the practice of nurse clinicians with prescribing authority needs to be accommodated by CPOE. Informatics nurses are well situated to describe nurse practitioner practice and design order entry systems for all practitioners.

All informatics professionals will need to help healthcare workers accept IT and push for implementation of CPOE. Informatics nurses have worked for years on implementation teams and are well positioned to continue to help get the national infrastructure in place. It will definitely take a collection of strategies, financial incentives, improved IT, and collaboration between public and private healthcare entities to accomplish the President's order.

National Health Information Infrastructure

Another national initiative that will impact NI is the National Health Information Infrastructure (NHII). This voluntary initiative, involving a three-stage process over 10 years, is intended to improve the effectiveness, efficiency, and overall quality of health and healthcare in the United States. The vision and process for building the NHII is outlined in a report "Information for Health: A Strategy for Building the National Health Information Infrastructure" released in November 2001 (National Committee on Vital Health Statistics, 2001). NHII calls for comprehensive knowledge-based networks that integrate clinical, public health, and personal health information to improve decision-making by having information available to providers. A national consensus conference was held in July 2003 to define the action steps needed to achieve an NHII (Yasnoff et al., 2004). A follow-up meeting in July 2004 wastitled "Cornerstones for Electronic Healthcare." Secretary Thompson announced that the first part of a national health IT plan would be delivered at the conference by the National Coordinator for Health IT. The report would launch the 2004 NHII conference. Conference tracks included personal health, governance, incentives, standards and architecture, confidentiality, ethics, privacy and access, measuring progress, population health, and clinical research (DHHS, 2004). Informatics nurses were invited to attend and offer input into the NHII plan. As representatives of the largest healthcare provider group, nurses who were experts in informatics needed to be among the stakeholders included in further delineation of the NHII.

Health Insurance Portability and Accountability Act (HIPAA)

HIPAA was passed in 1996 and is intended to improve public and private health programs by establishing standards to facilitate the efficient transmission of electronic health information (Public Law, 104-191, 1996). HIPAA preempts state law and payer-specific variations of data standards; and mandates input from private, standard-setting organizations. The law also designates financial penalties for noncompliance with standards related to specific transactions. To avoid further duplication of effort, the law requires the DHHS to adopt standards from those already approved by private standards-setting organizations.

HIPAA has significant impact on informatics; IT must be designed to comply with Title II of the act. Also known as administrative simplification, HIPAA requires the DHHS to establish national standards for electronic healthcare transactions; for national identifiers for providers, health plans, and employers; and for the

security and privacy of health data (DHHS, 2003). All of the requirements of HIPAA are expected to be in place by May 23, 2008 (CMS, 2004b). The timetable is as follows:

October 16, 2002—Electronic Healthcare Transactions and Code Sets—all covered entities (except small health plans)

April 14, 2003—Privacy—(except small health plans)

October 16, 2003—Electronic Healthcare Transactions—small health plans

April 14, 2004—Privacy—small health plans

July 30, 2004—Employer Identifier Standard— (except small health plans)

April 21, 2005—Security Standard—(except small health plans)

August 1, 2005—Employer Identifier Standard— small health plans

April 21, 2006—Security Standards—small health plans

May 23, 2007—National Provider Identifier— except small health plans

May 23, 2008—National Provider Identifier—small health plans

As rules are finalized they are put into effect. The final rule adopting the HIPAA standard unique health identifier was published by CMS in the *Federal Register* on January 23, 2004. Providers can begin applying for a national provider identifier on May 23, 2005 (CMS, 2003). In November 2004, under HIPAA administrative simplification, CMS expects to publish the proposed rules for a national health payer identifier and a format for standardized claims attachments. CMS also expects to release a final action rule for electronic submission of most Medicare claims in September 2006. This would replace the interim rule now in effect. In November 2006 home health agencies will be required to electronically report certain data. CMS has been pushing clients to submit electronic claims that comply with HIPAA. If claims are not HIPAA compliant, payment will be delayed for 13 days (Ihealthbeat, 2004b; Health Data Management, 2004).

The privacy rule of HIPAA was published in December 2000 and became effective in April 14, 2001 with a compliance date of April 14, 2003. In essence the regulation requires health plans, healthcare clearinghouses, and healthcare providers to protect and guard against the misuse of identifiable health information. In response to public comment, modifications were made to the rule. The privacy rule and other HIPAA regulations are having a tremendous impact on health informatics, including NI. For example, under HIPAA patients must be permitted to review and amend their medical records. Healthcare providers have expressed concern that accessing their records could cause patients increased anxiety. Ross and Lin (2003) have determined that there are benefits, such as enhanced doctor-patient communication, and only minimal risks in increasing access of patients to their records (Ross and Lin, 2003).

Implementation of the privacy standards has caused much confusion in healthcare. According to reports misunderstanding of HIPAA can prevent the sharing of needed information by healthcare providers. Informatics nurses are responsible for understanding and helping to implement the HIPAA regulations. They can help to explain the HIPAA regulations or point individuals to needed information resources. Informatics nurses are also in a position to research potential impact of regulations on patients and can impact regulations by offering comments during the public comment period after the rules are published.

National Agenda for Nursing Informatics

The DN, HRSA, is responsible for setting national policy to guide the preparation of the nursing workforce, including preparation in the area of NI. The DN recognized the importance of information management and technology long before the title NI was used to describe the field of practice and has funded projects focused in this area since 1972. During the 1970s, funding efforts focused on increasing awareness of the need for IS that could be used to support nursing practice and developing a nursing language that could be applied to public health settings. Funding during the 1980s and early 1990s enabled four different educational models to be developed for NI; two models focused on specialty practice in NI, and two models incorporated NI skills into administration and community health programs, respectively. In 1987 and since 1994, the DN has funded projects that either focus on distance learning methodologies or use them to deliver advanced nursing education. Faculty development in NI was the focus of funding for three regional compacts in 1996.

Although the DN has supported NI projects, the nursing workforce has continued to be deficient in informatics skills. As a result, in 1997 the DN convened the National Nursing Informatics Work Group (NNIWG) to make recommendations to the National Advisory Council for Nurse Education and Practice (NACNEP) for setting the nation's nursing informatics agenda (NIA) for nursing education and practice. There were 19 experts on NNIWG who identified NI needs from the perspectives of patient care settings, commercial business, government service, and nursing education. NNIWG members were experts in decision support, distance education, informatics education, IS, language and taxonomies, and telecommunications.

A nominal group technique was used to help NNIWG members identify NI needs and initiatives. Using a weighting scheme, NNIWG members prioritized items. The experts were then asked to suggest initiatives that would offer solutions for the identified informatics needs. Five initiatives were forwarded to NACNEP for consideration as a NIA.

NACNEP reviewed the recommended initiatives at their Spring 1997 meeting and approved them with minor changes. The advisory council's recommendations were sent to the secretary of DHHS as a National NIA. The council's report is titled *A National Informatics Agenda for Nursing Education and Practice, December 1997* and can be obtained from the DN (NACNEP, 1997). Even though NACNEP submitted their agenda to the secretary in 1997, the initiatives were reviewed in 2002 and still considered to be pertinent.

There are five assumptions considered by NACNEP to be a basis for all further discussion of NI initiatives:

Learners are students, faculty, and clinicians.

NI must be considered within an interdisciplinary context of partnerships and collaboration.

Efforts should target disadvantaged and underserved populations.

Initiatives should be responsive to other government funding priorities.

Collaboration among federal agencies and between federal and private entities is necessary.

Five key directions for informatics in nursing education and practice were recommended to the Secretary, DHHS in the NACNEP report. The recommendations are as follows:

Educate nursing students and practicing nurses in core informatics content.

Prepare nurses with specialized skills in informatics.

Enhance nursing practice and education through informatics projects.

Prepare nursing faculty in informatics.

Increase collaborative efforts in NI.

The existence of a national strategic direction for NI and the DN 1998 Title VIII authorizing legislation have enhanced the field of NI and the roles of informatics nurses. The 1998 legislation specifically named informatics as one of the seven priority areas for strengthening capacity and is consistent with the NIA's first strategic direction to include core informatics knowledge and skill in all undergraduate, graduate, and continuing education programs. Recognizing the need to identify core informatics skills and knowledge to be included in all educational programs. Staggers, Gassert, and Curran developed a research-based master list of NI competencies (Staggers et al., 2001; Staggers et al., 2002). If core content is included in educational programs, the nursing workforce increasingly will be prepared to use information technologies that have been or are being installed in healthcare delivery environments. This will decrease the length of time informatics nurses need to teach new graduates about IS in their work environments or eliminate the need for training altogether. Of concern, however, is how to improve core informatics skills and knowledge of practicing nurses who graduated several years ago. Innovative projects are needed to help this large population of nurses gain more competence in informatics.

The second strategic direction for NI is to increase the number of nurses with specialized skills in informatics. As stated before, amendments to the Public Health Service Act in 1992 prohibited the DN from funding more than the two initial graduate programs in NI. The 1998 legislation allowed the DN to fund additional NI graduate programs (Public Law 150-392, 1998). Having more opportunity to complete advanced informatics preparation has increased the number of NI specialists in practice, but more are needed (Safran, 2004). Having a larger cadre of NI specialists should increase nursing involvement in IS and IT design, purchase, and implementation. Because of their advocacy roles for patients, nurses should be able to address the information needs of patients and impact patient safety. Given the interdisciplinary nature and technological focus of informatics practice, it would be interesting to see unique models of NI programs emerge. One interesting model would be to develop collaborative educational programs that cut across traditional disciplinary lines. Schools of medicine, nursing, dentistry, and IS management could be full partners in these programs, collaborating to share financial burdens, decision-making, curriculum planning, teaching, and evaluation.

Collaborative programs could provide core informatics content to students from multiple disciplines and then allow students to apply knowledge within their individual professional domains. To make certain graduates have the necessary credentials to advance within their licensed professions, degrees should be awarded so that students retain their professional identify.

A third strategic direction for NI is to enhance nursing practice and education through informatics projects. There is a need to improve the informatics skills of the nursing workforce, particularly with nurses who have been out of school for a few years. Telehealth projects could be used to address this workforce issue. Informatics nurses need to work with academic and healthcare delivery entities to develop programs that use telehealth technologies to improve nursing workforce skills.

The fourth strategic direction for NI is to improve faculty skills in NI so that they in turn can promote the development of informatics competency in students. Unless faculty members have adequate computer knowledge and skills they are unlikely to require students to use IT as part of their assignments. Faculties are under tremendous pressures to deal with issues brought about by a rapidly changing healthcare environment. They are older, have larger classes, are required to bring in money to supplement their salaries, and are constantly asked to increase their scope of practice. To add the need to develop informatics skills might be overwhelming to some faculty members. Existing technology could facilitate innovative ways to meet the informatics needs of both faculty and students. Faculty could learn more advanced informatics skills through collaborative arrangements between schools of nursing or between a school of nursing and a department of IS management. Teleconferencing could be used for faculty to "attend" informatics courses offered on other campuses to improve their skills. Collaborative arrangements might also allow informatics nurse experts on one campus to educate students on another campus, thereby decreasing the unmet demand for faculty prepared to teach NI. This model would also decrease the stress placed on faculty members to increase their skills in so many important areas of healthcare all at once. Collaborative models need exploration to identify the best practices for faculty preparation in NI.

The fifth and final strategic direction is to increase collaborative efforts in NI. What is obvious in higher education is that the limited resources available will need to be used efficiently and economically. Many healthcare policy makers advocate that collaborative efforts are key to using resources wisely. Competitive educational models may need to be replaced by collaborative models, particularly in informatics.

The NIA also advocates collaborative efforts between federal agencies and among public and private organizations to identify and fund needed informatics research and projects. In 1998, the National Library of Medicine, National Heart, Lung, and Blood Institute, and the health informatics community collaborated to identify ways that information technologies could be used to accomplish the goals of the National Heart Attack Alert Program. Informatics nurses served on the planning committee for a 2-day conference that successfully identified projects for funding. A second example of collaboration between private and public organizations to advance NI is the Vocabulary Summit hosted by Vanderbilt University since 1999. Both the DN and AMIA's Nursing Informatics Working Group were among the initial financial supporters of this important meeting designed to advance work being done on nursing data structures. These are but two of the collaborative efforts that have occurred in NI.

Telehealth and Nursing Informatics

Telehealth services have been provided for about 50 years but telehealth remains an underutilized tool for nursing and NI. Telehealth is the use of electronic information and telecommunications technologies to support long-distance clinical healthcare, patient and professional health-related education, public health, and health administration. With the introduction of telehealth services tens of thousands of patients are accessing healthcare remotely from Arctic villages, Native American reservations, rural communities, prisons (Brantley et al., 2004) and in urban areas that are medically underserved in the United States. Many telehealth projects are supported by the government or universities. During 2003 and the first part of 2004, the federal government has spent about $88 million on telehealth projects (Telemedicine and Telehealth Grant, 2004).

Telehealth technologies are entering their third generation of evolution but the market for telehealth services remains relatively small. Factors advancing telehealth technology innovation are decreasing costs of telecommunication technologies, decreasing costs of telehealth devices and applications, resolution of interoperability issues, and convergence of telehealth and telecommunications technologies, IT, and the Internet. In spite of the advances in telehealth technologies, disjointed development, research, demand, and investment have produced the small telehealth market. The market that has been developed in telehealth has been independent of a national strategy or effort. Unfortunately telehealth provides such specialized tools it falls outside of the influence of groups like the American Medical Association and the Advanced Medical Technology Association (Brantley et al., 2004). Concerted effort must therefore be made to align telehealth with the mainstream of healthcare.

In addition there has been a significant disconnection between telehealth and informatics. Telehealth organizations such as the American Telemedicine Association are largely separate from informatics organizations, such as AMIA; the two entities need to become better aligned to promote development of integrated IS that seamlessly document telehealth events. This is especially true in view of the fact that both telehealth and information technologies face barriers of acceptance, reimbursement, and licensure. Efforts are being made to close the gap but until recently, documentation of telehealth events has frequently been independent of or isolated from IS. Since continued innovation in telehealth could significantly improve provider productivity and the quality of life for patients, informatics nurses need to become involved in both telehealth and informatics organizations to try to influence alliance building between the organizations.

In a 1997 report to Congress, the three major issues of reimbursement, licensure, and security were implicated in preventing widespread adoption and use of telehealth (Department of Commerce, 1997). In 2004 the Department of Commerce stated that not much has changed since the earlier report. HIPAA regulations have addressed issues of privacy of patient information and security standards will be effective from April 2005 but reimbursement and licensure issues still exist.

Although policy makers have suggested that state licensure regulations should not become barriers for practicing telehealth, delivering telehealth services across state lines remains an issue. The model suggested by the Federation of State Medical Boards to allow limited practice across state lines has been largely ignored. Nineteen states have passed laws requiring physicians to obtain full and unrestricted licenses to deliver interstate telehealth services, seven states issue special purpose licenses for telehealth practice. Three states license physicians for telehealth practice by rule making and 21 states do not specifically address licensure for telehealth practice (Center for Telehealth Law, 2002). In December 2003, the Center for Telemedicine Law and the Office for the Advancement of Telehealth (OAT) in HRSA assembled telehealth experts and state licensing board members to discuss options for eliminating interstate licensure barriers that impact telehealth practice. OAT also has a contract with the Federation of State Medical Boards for two regional pilot projects to test interstate licensure models, hopefully some that were proposed at the December workshop (Brantley et al., 2004).

On the other hand the National Council of State Boards of Nursing (NCSBN) has implemented a model of mutual recognition in which nurses obtain a state-based license that is nationally recognized and locally enforced (NCSBN, 2004). A nurse obtains one license in the state of residence and can practice in other states that agree to participate in the compact, a legal document that regulates business between two or more states, without obtaining additional licenses. Nurses remain accountable for their practice in states in which they are delivering services. States agree to recognize the nursing licenses of other states through the compact. Each compact state appoints a nurse licensure compact administrator to facilitate the exchange of information between the states relating to compact nurse licensure and regulation.

As of July 2004, 17 states have passed and implemented the Nursing Compact (Arizona, Arkansas, Delaware, Idaho, Iowa, Maine, Maryland, Mississippi, Nebraska, New Mexico, North Carolina, North Dakota, South Dakota, Tennessee, Texas, Utah, and Wisconsin). Three additional states have passed the compact, Virginia will implement it on January 1, 2005, but Indiana and New Jersey have not announced implementation dates. Over time more states are expected to pass the multistate compact. The Health Care Safety Net Amendments of 2002 provide incentive grants to state professional licensing boards to implement state policies to reduce barriers to telehealth. This should help states relook at licensure policies. Changes in interstate licensure are expected to support biodefense projects, but they will also help telehealth practice.

Lack of reimbursement has been identified as the key barrier to expanding telehealth practice. Brantley et al. (2004) indicate the sustainability of telehealth programs is dependent on third party reimbursement. Third party payers account for over 88% of all telehealth reimbursements. The telehealth community has generally believed that third party payers were very restrictive. Surveys by CTL and AMD Telemedicine, however, found that reimbursement issues are not as widespread as they were once thought to be. Seventy-two telehealth programs surveyed had billable services, more than half of these programs are receiving reimbursement from private payers. Payers are reimbursing in at least 25 states (AMD Telemedicine, 2003). Interestingly, Louisiana, California, Oklahoma, Texas, and Kentucky have passed legislation that mandates private payer reimbursement for telehealth services.

The Balanced Budget Act passed in 1997 mandated the first national reimbursement policy of telehealth services for Medicare recipients. Since January 1, 1999, physician and non-physician providers, including nurse practitioners, nurse midwives, and clinical nurse specialists, have been reimbursed for Medicare teleconsultation in rural health professional shortage areas. According to the 1997 act, the consultation had to be interactive, and an eligible provider had to present the patient to an eligible consulting provider. Store and forward technologies could not be reimbursed.

Telehealth providers felt the regulations as implemented were not inclusive enough to meet health needs in rural areas and voiced their concerns to CMS (formerly the Health Care Finance Administration) and Congress and asked for changes in the reimbursement policies. The Medicare, Medicaid, and SCHIP Benefits Improvement and Protection Act of 2000 (BIPA) changed some of the reimbursement policies. For example, an eligible provider no longer has to present the patient in the originating site. This ruling facilitates the increased use of telehealth in areas where specialists are not located. BIPA also expanded who could receive telehealth services and what services would be covered; clarified home care coverage; changed the payment methods, eliminating the fee-splitting and providing an origination fee; and allowed store and forward coverage in Alaska and Hawaii demonstration projects (CTL, 2001). Because CMS has proposed to establish a process for adding to or deleting from the list of telehealth services (Brantley, 2004), additional changes in telehealth reimbursement can be expected.

Informatics nurses must keep up to date on both licensure and reimbursement issues in telehealth. They will need to implement health policy as it is made and be certain that their systems comply with any regulations that pertain to interstate use of information technologies. Informatics nurses, while largely focused on IS, generally have failed to recognize the need to integrate telehealth technologies with existing IS. Telehealth and informatics professional groups have developed in isolation from each other. Informatics nurses need to help to integrate telehealth technologies and IS so that patient encounters became part of the computerized patient record and informatics issues such as standards and language are systematically addressed. Since telehealth technologies have such a tremendous potential to increase underserved populations' access to healthcare, it would be fantastic to see more nurse practitioners deliver their services using telehealth. Informatics nurses need to become more involved in telehealth and inform other nurses about uses of telehealth technologies.

Summary

In summary, NI is well established as a specialty within nursing. Current and proposed healthcare policy will impact NI in several ways. Given the emphasis on interdisciplinary practice, NI needs to broaden its educational and practice perspectives to include a more interdisciplinary focus. More graduate programs in NI have been established, but more are needed to prepare both practitioners and faculty in NI. Certification as a generalist in NI is currently available, but a specialist level of certification is needed to acknowledge more advanced informatics skills. Even though opportunities for specialty preparation in informatics are increasing, there is a tremendous need to improve the general informatics skills of nursing faculty, students, and clinicians. Collaborative efforts are needed to link schools so that informatics resources can be shared.

Informatics nurses need to embrace telehealth as part of informatics practice and work to reduce barriers imposed by licensure and reimbursement issues. NI can advocate for the use of telehealth technologies to increase the delivery of healthcare to underserved populations and finally, the NI community needs to become more aware of health policies that have been established or are under consideration to determine their effect on informatics practice. Issues need to be addressed through position papers, proposed regulations need to be reviewed and comments submitted if necessary, and funding agencies need to be encouraged to expand opportunities for informatics initiatives that include nursing.

References

American Association of Colleges of Nursing. (2004). *Strategies to Reverse the New Nursing Shortage.* Retrieved June 29, 2004, from *http://www.aacn.nche. edu/publications/positions/trishortage.htm*

American Nurses Association. (2001). *Scope and Standards of Nursing Informatics Practice.* Washington, DC: American Nurses Publishing.

American Nurses Credentialing Center. (2003). *ANCC Certificate Exam Results.* Retrieved July 7, 2004, from *http://www.ana.org/ancc/certification/cert/exams/ results/others.html*

AMD Telemedicine. (2003). *Private Payer Reimbursement Information Directory Survey.* Retrieved July 13, 2004, from *http://www.amdtelemedicine.com/private_payer/ about_survey.cfm*

Anderson, H. (2004). *Patient Safety Still Driving I.T. Demand. Health Data Management.* Retrieved June 29, 2004, from *http://www.healthdatamanagement. com/html/current/PastIssueStory.cfm?PostID=17317& PastMonth=April&PastYear=2004*

Aspden, P., Corrigan, J. M., Wolcott, J., and Erickson, S. M. (Eds.). (2003). Institute of Medicine, Committee on Data Standards for Patient Safety. *Patient Safety: Achieving a New Standard for Care.* Washington DC: The National Academies Press.

Auerbach, D. I., Buerhaus, P. I., and Staiger, D. O. (2000). Associate degree graduates and the rapidly aging RN workforce. *Nursing Economics* 18(4):178–184.

Ball, M. J. and Hannah, K. J. (1984). *Using Computers in Nursing.* Reston, VA: Reston Publishers.

Ball, M. J., Weaver, C., and Abbott, P. A. (2003). Enabling technologies promise to revitalize the role of nursing in an era of patient safety. *International Journal of Medical Informatics* 69:29–38.

Berliner, H. S. and Ginzbers, E. (2002). Why this hospital nursing shortage is different. *JAMA* 288(21): 2742–2744.

Bureau of Labor Statistics. (2002). Reprinted from the *Occupational Outlook Handbook (2004–05). Tomorrow's Jobs.* Retrieved June 30, 2004, from *http://stats.bls.gov/oco/pdf/oco2003.pdf*

Bradley, C. (2003). Technology as a catalyst to transforming nursing care. *Nursing Outlook* 51(3):S14–S15.

Brantley, D., Laney-Cummings, K., and Spivack, R. (2004). *Innovation, Demand and Investment in Telehealth.* U.S. Department of Commerce, Office of Technology Policy.

Briggs, B. (2004). Clinical Systems Move to the Head of the I. T. *Class,* Clinical information systems are the New I. T. darlings as provider organizations embrace the latest technology tools. *Health Data Management.* Retrieved June 29, 2004, from *http://www. healthdatamanagement.com/html/current/ PastIssueStory. cfm?PostID=17678&PastMonth=January&PastYear= 2004*

Buerhaus, P. I., Staiger, D. O., and Auerbach, D. I. (2000). Why are shortages of hospital RNs concentrated in specialty care units? *Nursing Economics* 18(3): 111–116.

Centers for Medicare & Medicaid Services. (2003). *HIPAA Administrative Simplification News.* Retrieved July 7, 2004, from *http://www.cms.hhs.gov/hipaa/ hipaa2/news/NewsReleaseFull.asp*

Centers for Medicare & Medicaid Services. (2004a). *CMS Issues Interim Final Rule Addressing Physician Self-Referrals.* Retrieved June 30, 2004, from *http:// www. cms.hhs.gov/media/press/release.asp? counter=985*

Centers for Medicare & Medicaid Services (2004b). *HIPAA Administrative Simplification Compliance Deadlines.* Retrieved July 11, 2004, from *http://www.cms.hhs.gov/hipaa/hipaa2/general/deadlines.asp*

Center for Telemedicine Law. (July 2002). *Medical Licensure Law Affecting Telehealth.* Retrieved July 7, 2004, from *http://www.ctl.org/assets/medLicensure.pdf*

Chaiken, B. and Holmquest, D. (2003). Patient safety: Modifying processes to eliminate medical errors. *Nursing Outlook* 51:S21–S24.

Connecting for Health, Markle Foundation. (2004). *Improving Health in the Information Age.* Retrieved July 7, 2004, from *http://www.connectingforhealth.org*

Corrigan, J. M., Kohn, L. T. and Donaldson, M. S. (Eds.). (1999). Institute of Medicine. *To Err is Human: Building a Safer Health System.* Washington, DC: National Academy Press.

Department of Commerce, National Telecommunications and Information Administration in Consultation with U.S. Department of Health and Human Services. (1997). *Telemedicine Report to the Congress.* Washington, DC.

Department of Health and Human Services. (2003). *General Overview of Standards for Privacy of Individually Identifiable Health Information.* Retrieved, June 30, 2004, from *http://www.hhs.gov/ocr/hipaa/guidelines/overview.rtf*

Department of Health & Human Services, Health Resources and Services Administration. (2004). *News Release, HHS to Present Plan on Transforming Health Care Through Information Technology at National Conference July 21.* Retrieved June 30, 2004, from *http://www.dhhs.gov/news/press/2004pres/20040625c.html*

Egan, C. (2004). Industry: Federal attention to health IT should spur progress. *IHealthBeat.* Retrieved July 7, 2004, from *http://ihealthbeat.org/index.cfm?action=dspItem&itemid=10397*

Executive Order. (2004). Retrieved from *http://whitehouse.gov/news/releases/2004/04/print/20040427-4.html*

Gassert, C. A., Mills, M. E., and Heller, B. R. (1992). Doctoral specialization in nursing informatics. In P. D. Clayton (Ed.), *Proceedings of the Fifteenth Annual Symposium on Computer Applications in Medical Care* (pp. 263–267). New York: McGraw-Hill.

Goedert, J. (2004a). *HIMSS Survey: Security, Safety Top Concerns. Health Data Management.* Retrieved June 29, 2004, from *http://www.healthdatamanagement.com/html/current/PastIssueStory.cfm?PostID=17313&PastMonth=April&PastYear=2004*

Goedert, J. (2004b). *Electronic Records: Will Washington Pay? Health Data Management.* Retrieve June 29, 2004, from *http://www.healthdatamanagement.com/html/current/PastIssueStory.cfm?PostID=17314&PastMonth=April&PastYear=2004*

Graves, J. R., Amos, L. K., Heuther, S., Lange, L. L., and Thompson, C. B. (1995). Description of a graduate program in clinical nursing informatics. *Computers in Nursing* 13(2):60–70.

Graves, J. R. and Corcoran, S. (1989). The study of nursing informatics. *Image: Journal of Nursing Scholarship* 21(4):227–231.

Greiner, A. C. and Knebel, E. (Eds.). (2003). Health professions education: The core competencies needed for health care professionals. In *A Bridge to Quality* (pp. 45–74). Washington, DC: The National Academies Press.

Grobe, S. J. (1988). Nursing informatics competencies for nurse educators and researchers. In H. E. Peterson and U. Gerdin Jelger (Eds.), *Preparing Nurses for Using Information Systems: Recommended Informatics Competencies* (pp. 25–33). New York: National League for Nursing.

Hannah, K. J. (1985). Current trends in nursing informatics: Implications for curriculum planning. In K. J. Hannah, E. J. Guillemin, and D. N. Conklin (Eds.), *Nursing Uses of Computers and Information Science* (pp. 181–187). Amsterdam, The Netherlands: Elsevier.

Health Data Management. (2004a). *Feds Plan New HIPAA Rules for Fall.* Retrieved July 7, 2004, from *http://www.healthdatamanagement.com/html/PortalStory.cfm?type=gov&DID=11694*

Health Data Management. (2004b). *Thompson: No Mandates for I.T. (2004).* Retrieved July 7, 2004, from *http://www.healthdatamanagement.com/html/PortalStory.cfm?type=gov&DID=11726*

Health Resources and Services Administration. (2001). HRSA National Survey Cites Slowdown in Number of Registered Nurses Entering Profession. *HRSA News* (Press Release). Retrieved February 15, 2001, from *http://newsroom.hrsa.gov/releases/2001%20Releases/nursesurvey.htm*

Health Resources and Services Administration. (2002). *Projected Supply, Demand, and Shortages of Registered Nurses: 2000–2020.* Retrieved June 30, 2004, from *ftp://ftp.hrsa.gov/bhpr/nationalcenter/rnproject.pdf*

Heller, B. R., Romano, C. A., Moray, L. R, and Gassert, C. A. (1989). Special follow-up report: The implementation of the first graduate program in nursing informatics. *Computers in Nursing* 7(5): 209–213.

House Caucus Focuses on Health I. T. (2004). Retrieved July 7, 2004, from *http://healthdatamanagement.com/html/portalstory.cfm?type=gov&DID=1171*

IHEALTHBEAT. (2004a). *Policy, IT Chief, Experts Outline Vision for Health IT.* Retrieved June 29, 2004, from *http://www.ihealthbeat.org/index.cfm?action=dspitem&itemID=103681*

IHEALTHBEAT. (2004b). *Medicare Delays Payment for Non-HIPAA Compliant Claims.* Retrieved July 7, 2004, from *http://www.ihealthbeat.org/ index.cfm?action=itemprint&itemID=104095*

Institute of Medicine, Committee on Quality of Health Care in America. (2001). *Crossing the Quality Chasm: A New Health System for the 21st Century.* Washington, DC: National Academy Press.

Kennedy, R. (2003). The nursing shortage and the role of technology. *Nursing Outlook* 51(3):S33–S34.

McClure, M. L. and Burnes Bolton, L. (2003). Using innovative technology to decrease the nursing demand and enhance patient care delivery. *Nursing Outlook* 51(3):S1.

National Advisory Council on Nurse Education and Practice. (1997). *A National Informatics Agenda for Nursing Education and Practice: A Report to the Secretary of the Department of Health and Human Services.* Rockville, MD: Department of Health and Human Services, Health Resources and Services Administration, Bureau of Health Professions, Division of Nursing.

National Alliance for Health Information Technology. (2004). *About Us.* Retrieved June 29, 2004, from *http://www.hospitalconnect.com/nahit/ about.html*

National Center for Nursing Research. (1993). Nursing *Informatics: Enhancing Patient Care.* Bethesda, MD: Department of Health and Human Services, National Institutes of Health, National Center for Nursing Research.

National Council of State Boards of Nursing. (2004). *Nurse Licensure Compact.* Retrieved June 30, 2004, from *http://ncsbn.org/nlc.index.asp*

Needleman, J., Buerhaus, P., Mattke, S., Stewart, M. and Zelevinsky, K. (2002). Nurse-staffing levels and the quality of care in hospitals. *New England Journal of Medicine* 346(22):1715–1720.

Novelli, W. D. (2004). AARP to press for healthcare IT initiatives. *Healthcare IT News.* Retrieved July 13, 2004, from *http://www.healthcareitnews. com/ newsarticleview.aspx?contentID=1123*

O'Neil, E. (2003). A strategic workforce framework for considering the use of technology to address the current and future shortage of nurses. *Nursing Outlook* 51(3):S2–S4.

Ozbolt, J. (2000). Terminology standards for nursing: Collaboration at the summit. *Journal of American Medical Informatics Association* 7(6):517–522.

Ozbolt, J. (2003a). Reference terminology for therapeutic goals: A new approach. In *Proceedings of the American Medical Informatics Annual Symposium*, pp. 504–508.

Ozbolt, J. (2003b). The Nursing Terminology Summit Conferences: A case study of successful collaboration for change. *Journal of Biomedical Informatics* 36(4–5):362–374.

Ozbolt, J., Adrowich, I., Bakken, S., Button, P. Hardiker, N., Mead, C., Warren, J., and Zingo, C. (2001). The Nursing Terminology Summit: Collaboration for progress. *Medinfo* 10:236–240.

Panniers, T. L. and Gassert, C. A. (1995). Standards of practice and preparation for certification. In B. R. Heller, M. E. Mills, and C. A. Romano (Eds.), *Information Management in Nursing and Health Care.* Springhouse, PA: Springhouse Corporation.

Pew Health Professions Commission. (1998). Executive summary. In *Recreating Health Professional Practice for a New Century.* San Francisco, CA: University of California, San Francisco.

President's Information Technology Advisory Committee, Panel on Transforming Health Care. (2001, February). *Transforming Health Care Through Information Technology.* Arlington, VA: Author.

Priselac, T. (2003). Information technology's role in improving practice environments and patient safety. *Nursing Outlook* 51(3):S11–13.

Public Law 104-191. (1996). *Health Insurance Portability and Accountability Act of 1996.*

Public Law 150-392. (1998). *Health Professions Education Partnership Act of 1998, Title VIII, Subtitle B, The Nursing Education and Practice Improvement Act of 1998.*

Ross, S. E. and Lin, C. T. (2003). The effects of promoting patient access to medical records: A review. *Journal of the American medical Informatics Association* 10(2):129–138.

Safran, C. (2004). Statement of Charles Safran, M. D., President, American Medical Informatics Association, Bethesda, MD. *Testimony Before the Subcommittee on Health of the House Committee on Ways and Means, June 17, 2004.* Retrieved on June 29, 2004, from *http://waysandmeans.house.gov/hearings.asp? formmode=view&id=1653*

Sensmeier, J., Raiford, R., Taylor, S., and Weaver, C. (2003). Improved operational efficiency through elimination of waste and redundancy. *Nursing Outlook* 51(3):S30–S32.

Shabot, M. (2003). Closing address: Breaking free of the past: Innovation and technology in patient care. *Nursing Outlook* 51(3):S37–S38.

Spratley, E., Johnson, A., Sochalski, J., Fritz, M., and Spencer, W. (2000). *The Registered Nurse Population. Findings from the National Sample Survey of Registered Nurses.* Washington, DC: Department of Health and Human Services.

Staggers, N., Gassert, C. A., and Curran, C. (2002). A Delphi study to determine informatics competencies for nurses at four levels of practice. *Nursing Research* 51(6):383–390.

Staggers, N., Gassert, C. A., and Curran, C. (2001). Informatics competencies for nurses at four levels of practice. *Journal of Nursing Education* 4(7): 303–313.

Staiger, D. O., Auerbach, D. I., and Buerhaus, P. I. (2000). Expanding career opportunities for women and the declining interest in nursing as a career. *Nursing Economics* 18(5):230–236.

Stanton, M. W. and Rutherford, M. K. (2004). *Hospital Nurse Staffing and Quality of Care*. Rockville, MD: Agency for Healthcare Research and quality. *Research in Action* 14:1–11.

Steinbrook, R. (2002). Nursing in the crossfire. *New England Journal of Medicine* 346(22):1757–1766.

Styles, M. M. (1989). *On Specialization in Nursing: Toward a New Empowerment*. Kansas City, MO: American Nurses Foundation.

Telemedicine and Telehealth Grant and Contract Awards for FY 2003/2004. (2004). Retrieved July 12, 2004, from *http://www.atmeda.org/news/newres.htm*

The White House Office of the Press Secretary. (1996). *Background on Clinton-Gore Administration's Next-Generation Internet Initiative*. Retrieved 2000, from *http://www.npr.gov/library/news/101096-2.html*

Yasnoff, W. A., Humphreys, B. L., Overhage, J. M., Detmer, D. E., Brennan, P. F., Morris, R. W., Middleton, B., Bates, D. W., and Fanning, J. P. (2004). A Consensus action agenda for achieving the national health information infrastructure. *Journal of the American Medical Informatics Association* 11(4):332–338.

12

The Role of Technology in the Medication-Use Process

Matthew Grissinger
Hedy Cohen

OBJECTIVES

1. Define the benefits and limitations of automated dispensing cabinets in healthcare and its application to the medication process.

2. Describe factors that will influence on the adoption of technology in healthcare.

3. Recognize the benefits and limitations of bar code-enabled point-of-care (BPOC) technology as it relates to overall efforts to reduce medication errors including errors using these systems.

4. Describe the challenges and rewards related to implementing a computerized prescriber order entry (CPOE) system.

5. Recognize the value of and a methodology for assessing an organization's readiness for implementing technology.

KEY WORDS

medication error
computer prescriber order entry (CPOE)
automated dispensing cabinet (ADC)
smart infusion pump delivery systems
bar code-enabled point-of-care technology (BPOC)
failure mode and effects analysis (FMEA)
high-alert medications

Introduction

Due to the numerous steps required in the care of patients, the healthcare industry is an inherently error-prone process that is fraught with opportunities for mistakes to occur. This concept was confirmed in the oft-quoted 1999 Institute of Medicine (IOM) report, *To Err is Human: Building a Safer Health System*, where the authors extrapolated that between 44,000 and 98,000 patients die each year in the United States from preventable medical error. These deaths were the results of practitioner interactions with "bad systems" (Kahn et al., 1999). The authors emphatically state that the healthcare industry must place safety as the number one national priority and work diligently toward this goal. One explicit recommendation emanating from the first of a series of IOM reports on healthcare is to improve the safety design of systems as is presently being employed in other high error-prone industries such as the aerospace and nuclear industry. These industries not only acknowledge and accept the notion that individuals will make errors from normal mental slips and lapses in memory, but recognize that enhancing safety system design through the use of technology is an invaluable tool in the prevention of potentially life-threatening mistakes.

Technology and Healthcare

Until recently, the majority of technology acquisitions have consisted of basic stand-alone computer systems, which were primarily used for data input to increase each department's efficiency with financial accountability measures. These computers were generally installed in the pharmacy, radiology, and laboratory departments, and could also be found in the administration and business offices. Each department was allowed to evaluate and purchase their own unique computer system preventing any integration of data or dissemination of critical patient information, which is indispensable in providing safe care (Leape, 1995). But even as improving technologies have emerged allowing for seamless integration of information to occur, most organizations have shown little interest or incentive to incur the huge costs associated with replacing their present nonintegrated computer systems. In fact, less then 10% of healthcare organizations have yet to incorporate any type of medication safety technology indicating that they have allocated their limited financial and human resources in other directions. However, if patient safety is to be acknowledged as a national priority as is recommend by the IOM panel, healthcare organizations will need to reevaluate the "cost" of this decision.

Influences on the Adoption of Technology

Consumers have become increasingly concerned that hospitals are less than safe following the numerous mass media reporting of medical mistakes, which have resulted in patient harm and deaths. In 1995, there were television and newspaper accounts that reported the tragic death of a patient from a preventable adverse drug event (ADE) due to an inadvertent administration of a massive overdose of a chemotherapy agent over 4 days. This particular error became a watershed event for patients, practitioners, and healthcare organizations alike, not only because it occurred at the world renowned Dana Farber Cancer Institute, but also because it happened to the prestigious Boston Globe healthcare reporter Betsy Lehman. How could a mistake of this proportion occur in a leading healthcare facility where each practitioner is specifically educated in the care and treatment of cancer patients? A root cause analysis of the error revealed that there was no malpractice or egregious behavior, but that excellent, conscientious, and caring pharmacists and nurses simply interpreted an ambiguous handwritten chemotherapy order incorrectly. In retrospect, had technology been available,

the physician would have entered the medication order into a CPOE system and this heartbreaking error would not have happened.

Unfortunately, this example is by far not an isolated case. According to a 1994 American Medical Association report, medication errors related to the misinterpretation of physicians' prescriptions were the second most prevalent and expensive claim listed on malpractice cases filed over a 7-year period on 90,000 malpractice claims between 1985 and 1992 (Cabral JDT, 1997). Also, it has been estimated in the outpatient setting that indecipherable or unclear orders resulted in more than 150 million telephone calls from pharmacists and nurses to prescribers requiring clarification, which not only is time-consuming for practitioners, but estimated to cost healthcare systems billions of dollars each year. Thus, the availability of critical clinical information needed at the point-of-care (during prescribing, dispensing, and administering) can not only improve time management and contribute to cost savings through improved utilization of medications, staff, and patient satisfaction, but most importantly reduce the incidence of error.

The first organized attempt to move acute-care organizations toward improving patient safety through technology began from an initiative by The Leapfrog Group. Composed of more than 150 private and public organizations providing healthcare benefits, this group felt that they had a significant financial investment in preventing errors for their employees, thus increasing productivity by contracting only with those hospitals that had hospital wide adoption of CPOE technology. Yet, a survey by The Leapfrog Group completed in 2003 showed that not only did this financial incentive result in no increase from the 2002 survey in the number of hospitals that had implemented CPOE, but there was also a drop of 17% in hospitals now fully committed to CPOE implementation before 2005 (Stefanacci, 2004). Another report from The Leapfrog Group, based on site visits to 12 nationally representative communities, showed that only 6.7% of hospitals in the 12 sites reported full CPOE implementation (iHealth, 2004). Since there is still a dearth of research on the effectiveness of CPOE on medication error prevention, other organizations such as the Joint Commission on Accreditation of Healthcare Organizations (JCAHO) and the National Quality Forum (NQF) are presently refraining from uniformly requiring its adoption.

While CPOE technology purchases seemed to have plateaued, interest in bar coding technology has dramatically increased due to the Federal Drug Agency's (FDA) February 25, 2004 ruling, which requires medications to have machine-readable bar coding. In an optimally acute-care bar coded environment, a nurse would scan his or her bar code identification badge at the beginning of each medication administration time, the patient's bar code identification band, and the intended drug's bar coded label with a bar code scanner. A mismatch between the patient, the drug packaging applied during manufacturing or repackaging, an incorrect time, dose, route, and the patient's medication record would trigger a warning, prompting the nurse to investigate the discrepancy before administering the medication. One of the first healthcare facilities to adopt bar code technology was the inspiration of a nurse at the Department of Veterans Affairs (VA) in Topeka, Kansas. Her insight resulted in a 74% improvement in errors caused by the wrong medications being administered, a 57% improvement in errors caused by incorrect doses being administered, a 91% improvement in wrong patient errors, and almost a 92% improvement in wrong time errors between 1993 and 1999. Presently, the VA is the only healthcare system that has fully adopted bar coding technology. Additional examples of evolving technology used to prevent medication errors include ADCs and smart infusion pumps. As more technology systems are introduced into healthcare, it is important that nurses understand their benefits and problems, and how technology will affect their practice. Also, it is important for nurses to understand that technology is a "tool" to assist them, not replace cognitive thought processes or basic nursing principles.

Computerized Prescriber Order Entry (CPOE)

Healthcare practitioners still communicate information in the "old fashioned way." It has been estimated that handwritten prescriptions are used 99% of the time to communicate orders. There are many factors that demonstrate the need for a shift from a traditional paper-based system that relies on the unaided mind to automated order entry, record keeping, and clinical care. These factors include accessing patient information spread across multiple organizations that may be unavailable, especially in large organizations and, therefore, medical care would be provided without pertinent patient information. The structure of the patient's record often makes it difficult to locate valuable information, illegible handwritten entries by healthcare practitioners, and for those patients with chronic or complex conditions, the records can increase to multiple volumes over many years. These problems result in a variety of communication breakdowns when providing healthcare to patients from the duplication of services, delays in treatment, increased

length of stay, and increased risk of medical errors. Additionally, human memory-based medicine can be inaccurate or not recalled.

Currently, practitioners rely heavily on the unaided mind, which has been proven to be unreliable, to recall a great amount of detailed information. Actually, only a portion of medical knowledge is ever loaded into the prescribers' minds and not all of this knowledge is retained. Also, much of the retained learned knowledge in healthcare quickly becomes obsolete with no assurance that they will acquire any new knowledge. Even if new knowledge is learned and retained, it is impossible for practitioners to integrate all knowledge with an infinite amount of patient data in a short period of time. Faced with knowledge overload, prescribers and other practitioners tend to fall back on clinical judgment rather than organized knowledge.

There are also many barriers that lead to ineffective communication of medication orders that include issues with illegible handwriting, use of dangerous abbreviations and dose designations, and verbal and faxed orders. Studies have shown that as a result of poor handwriting, 50% of all written physician orders require extra time to interpret. Sixteen percent of physicians have illegible handwriting (Cohen, 1999). Illegible handwriting on medication orders has been shown to be a common cause of prescribing errors and patient injury and death have actually resulted from such errors (Brodell, 1997; Cabral, 1997; ASHP, 1993). Illegible orders may also lead to delays in the administration of medications. In order to clarify these illegible orders, the healthcare practitioner's workflow is typically interrupted (Cohen, 1999).

The use of a CPOE system has the potential to alleviate many of these problems. CPOE can be defined as a system used for direct entry of one or more types of medical orders by a prescriber into a system that transmits those orders electronically to the appropriate department (AHA, 2000). But there are many other potential enhancements that even a basic CPOE system could offer to further enhance safe medication ordering practices including features unique to the acute-care setting, ambulatory care setting or both; allow for prescribers to access records and enter orders from their office or home; prescriber selectable standardized single orders or order sets; implementation of organization-specific standing orders based on specific situations such as before or after procedures; menu-driven organization-specific lists of medications on formulary and; passive feedback systems that present patient-specific data in an organized fashion such as test results, charges, reference materials and progress notes, or active feedback systems to provide clinical decision-making tools by providing specific assessments or recommendations through alerts and reminders or even therapeutic suggestions at the time the order is written.

CPOE systems offer many other advantages over the traditional paper-based system. They can improve quality, patient outcomes, and safety by a variety of factors such as increasing preventive health guideline compliance by exposing prescribers to reminder messages to provide preventive care by encouraging compliance with recommended guidelines, identifying patients needing updated immunizations or vaccinations, and suggesting cancer screening and diagnosis reminders and prompts. Other advantages include reductions in the variation in care to improve disease management by improving follow-up of newly diagnosed conditions, reminder systems to improve patient management, automating evidence-based protocols, adhering to clinical guidelines, or providing screening instruments to help diagnosis disorders. Order entry systems can improve drug prescribing and administration by improving antibiotic usage, suggesting whether certain antibiotics or their dosages are appropriate for use. Medication refill compliance can be increased using reminder systems to increase adherence to therapies. Drug dosing could be improved, especially for those medications whose dosing is based on laboratory results, such as heparin or warfarin, to maintain adequate anticoagulation control.

Many studies have demonstrated a reduction in ADEs. For example, one study by Bates et al. showed that serious medication errors were reduced by 55% and preventable ADEs were reduced by 17% (Bates et al., 1998). Another study has shown that non-missed-dose medication errors fell from 142/1,000 patient days to 26.6/1,000 patient days (Bates et al., 1999). The same study showed a reduction of nonintercepted serious medication errors from 7.6/1,000 patient days to 1.1/1,000 patient days. Errors of omissions would be reduced, such as failure to act on results or carry out indicated tests. Handwriting and interpretation issues would be eliminated. There would be fewer handoffs if the CPOE system was linked to information systems in ancillary departments which would eliminate the need for staff members to manually transport orders to the pharmacy, radiology department, and labs, resulting in fewer lost or misplaced orders and faster delivery time. The system has also eliminated the need for staff members in those departments to manually enter the orders into their information systems, reducing the potential for transcription errors (HIMSS, 2002). Medical data

capture and display would be improved, enabling a more comprehensive and accurate documentation by prescribers and nurses. Access to pertinent literature and clinical information to knowledge bases and literature sources would enable ready access to updated drug information. These obvious improvements to patient care would not only improve patient safety but also increase efficiency, productivity, and cost effectiveness. Currently, the cost of providing healthcare is rising while reimbursement for services is declining. It has been estimated that 14% of America's gross national product is spent on healthcare in the United States (Regnier, 2004). CPOE systems offer a variety of solutions to help reduce the cost in providing healthcare and making more appropriate utilization of services. Reductions in hospitalizations and decreased lengths of stay can be obtained from automated scheduling of follow-up appointments to reducing unnecessary diagnostic tests. Better use of formulary and generic drugs by providing feedback of prescribing charges and patterns to encourage prescribers to substitute generics medications for more expensive branded medications. Properly designed systems can show an improvement in workflow and time-saving measures for prescribers, if the program makes sense to the prescriber and follows a rational process while performing order entry, by improving the availability and responses to information regarding diagnosis and treatment. Savings related to the storage of paper medical records could be substantial, compared to the cost of storing computerized backup storage devices. Entering medication and diagnostic orders into a computer system would allow for instantaneous capturing of charges and therefore enhancing revenue. Costs associated with the use of transcription notes would be eliminated as well by using an electronic patient record system. Lastly, there is patient and user satisfaction. For example, the admission process for patients from the outpatient setting into an acute-care organization can be a cumbersome and time-consuming process. Electronic systems would improve communication, if connected to an outpatient clinical referral system, by decreasing the amount of time needed to complete the referral process in addition to providing important patient information such as patient allergies and diagnosis. The time spent searching for or organizing paper-based information would be substantially reduced, thus improving prescriber and nurse satisfaction as well. Despite the numerous advantages in obtaining and employing a CPOE system, healthcare organizations have still been reluctant to implement this form of technology.

In spite of the many documented benefits of using a computerized system, many roadblocks and safety issues exist. One primary area of concern revolves around the costs of implementation. Investing in a CPOE system is not analogous to purchasing software off the store shelf and it involves far more resources than spending money on a software package. Hospitals need a minimum infrastructure to support its use such as a fiber-optic backbone network; time, space, and manpower to provide adequate staff education and development; and workstations and high-speed Internet access. The process of selecting the vendor is a costly and difficult process, especially if a vendor cannot address the organization's specific needs. In addition, there may be additional staff needed to develop and program any organization-specific rules, guidelines, or protocols and to implement the system, plus providing ongoing support for any needed enhancements or changes to the system. It is also difficult to prove or demonstrate any quantifiable benefits or returns on investment because it is hard to accurately measure the actual costs of using paper-based records. Benefits such as provider convenience, patient satisfaction, and service efficiency are not easily captured on the bottom line in terms of increase in revenue, decrease in expense, or avoidance of expense. Add on top of this the competing priorities including other forms of automation to enhance medication safety such as ADCs or point-of-care bar coding systems that are currently on the market. Another challenge involves the integration of "legacy" systems, those that have been in institutions for many years, which already exist in healthcare organizations. There are many organizations that are risk averse, waiting to let others be the clinical pioneers before they invest in these systems. Finally, despite the prospects of enhanced workflow and reduction in medication errors, there are real and potential problems with even the best CPOE systems.

As previously mentioned, CPOE systems have demonstrated a reduction in ADEs. Unfortunately, unsafe prescribing practices and medication errors are still possible with these systems. For example, errors may occur due to the lack of integration between a CPOE system and the organization's pharmacy system. Instead of medication orders electronically transferred to the pharmacy, orders would be printed on paper, which would then require order entry by another individual. Medication administration records (MARs) derived from one system, which does not correlate with the other, lead to discrepancies in medication profiles as well as possible loss of double checks between drug distribution and administration if the electronic MARs come from CPOE and not from the pharmacy order entry system.

Some organizations, in fear of alienating prescribers, have an active CPOE system but the clinical order screening capability of warnings and alerts have been turned off. The capability to build rule-based safety enhancements are often available in the software but the actual rules such as prompts for prescribers to order potassium replacement for patients with lab results reporting below normal potassium levels, are not provided by the vendor nor are they programmed for use by organizations. Studies have shown those prescribers, using only the basic CPOE system alone, order appropriate medication doses for patients 54% of the time. By comparison, prescribers using the CPOE system with decision support tools prescribed appropriate doses 67% of the time. The addition of the decision support tools also increased the percentage of prescriptions considered ordered at appropriate intervals to 59%, from 35% with the basic CPOE system (Kaushal et al., 2001).

Errors in monitoring patient's response to therapy can occur if the laboratory system is not interfaced with medication order entry system. Complex and time-consuming order entry processes can often lead to practitioner frustration, possible increase in verbal orders, and another error-prone process in communicating medication orders. Computer issues such as error messages, frozen screens, slow access to information, and other issues lead to problems of accessing critical patient or drug information as well as adding to prescriber frustration. It is important to have the ability to access past patient histories, particularly previous ADEs and comorbid conditions, yet some systems are unable to access prior patient care encounters. Problems may arise if drug information updates are not performed on a timely basis or if this information is difficult to access. One key error reduction strategy is the ability to install user-defined warnings (e.g., "look-alike/sound-alike" drug name alert), yet some systems do not allow for this type of customization.

Medication errors such as wrong patient errors, when the wrong patient is selected from a menu list of similar patient names; wrong drug errors, when the wrong medication is selected from a list due to look-alike similarity in either the brand or generic name or orders intended for laboratory levels that are filled as medications can occur.

Even though a CPOE system is intended for use by prescribers, their presence in organizations will affect nursing and other personnel as well. CPOE systems will affect or even change the work of nurses in many ways, both negative and positive (AHA, 2000). First, like prescribers, these systems will require nurses to possess basic computer skills. Depending on the design of the system, nurses may find it difficult to know when new orders have been entered into the system, a special concern with respect to "STAT" or new orders. Nurses sometimes see off-site entry of orders by prescribers as detrimental because it reduces the opportunity to communicate information or ask questions face-to-face with prescribers with regards to the care of patients. In some situations, prescribers are reluctant to enter orders and use verbal orders as a way of "getting around" entering orders into the CPOE system and, in fact, nurses may end up entering verbal orders from prescribers.

But there are many beneficial aspects of these systems for nurses. Nurses may have more time with patients due to enhanced productivity due to a reduced frequency in contacting prescribers to clarify orders. Additionally, there would be reductions in time wasted in transcribing duplicate orders for the same medication or test; greater standardization of orders, lessening the need to understand and adhere to diverse regimens and schedules; improved efficiency when ordering tests or procedures, thus reducing time devoted to carrying out redundant orders; and less need to enter voice orders into the system as prescribers gain access to the system from other units and remote locations. Finally, orders would be usually executed faster, medications would be available more quickly and patients receive prompter care. It is important for healthcare administration and nurses to understand that for a CPOE system to work as intended, it must be used by prescribers.

Bar Code-Enabled Point-of-Care Technology

Nurses play a vital role in the medication-use process, ranging from their involvement in the communication of medication orders to the administration of medications. As nurses know well, the administration of medications can be a labor-intensive and error-prone process. One study showed that 38% of medication errors occur during the drug administration process (Leape et al., 1995). While about half of the ordering, transcribing, and dispensing errors were intercepted by the nurse before the medication error reached the patient, almost none of the errors at the medication administration stage were caught. In another study of medication administration errors in 36 healthcare facilities, Barker et al. found that some type of medication administration error occurred in almost 20% of doses of medications administered (Barker et al., 2002). In addition, nurses are burdened with larger patient loads and are caring for patients with higher degrees of acuity then ever before. To make matters worse, the number of medications that have reached the market has grown 500% over the last 10 years to

more than 17,000 trademarked and generic drugs in North America (ISMP, 2000). Rapid advances in technology have helped to make this process more efficient and safe. One form of technology that will have a great impact on medication safety during the administration process BPOC technology.

For more than 20 years bar code technology has clearly demonstrated its power to greatly improve productivity and accuracy in the identification of products in a variety of business settings, such as supermarkets and department stores. Proven to be an effective technology, it quickly spread to virtually all other industries. Yet, few organizations in the healthcare industry have embraced this valuable technology as a method to enhance patient safety. In fact, the results of the 2000 *ISMP Medication Safety Self-Assessment*, completed by 1,435 hospitals showed that only:

- 43% of hospitals had even *discussed* the possibility of bar code drug administration
- 2.5% used this technology in *some* areas of the hospital
- less than 1% had *fully implemented* it throughout the organization (Cohen and Smetzer, 2001)

In another study, the American Society of Health-System Pharmacists (ASHP) National Survey reported that approximately 2% of hospitals (excluding federal facilities) stated using bar-code technology (Pedersen et al., 2003). The reasons for these few numbers are varied and include the cost of implementation, inadequate systems, and lack of the number of medications that are packaged with bar codes.

For the healthcare industry, the potential affect of implementing bar-code technology to improve the safe administration of medications is enormous. As previously stated, the VA Healthcare System, a pioneer in the use of bar code technology, looked at their medication error rate based on the number of incident reports related to medication errors before and after implementations of the BPOC system. The study showed that following the introduction of the BPOC, reported medication error rates declined from 0.02% per dose administered to 0.0025%. This is almost a 10-fold reduction in errors over 8 years (Johnson et al., 2002).

BPOC can improve medication safety through several levels of functionality. At the most basic level, the system helps to verify that the right drug is being administered to the right patient at the right dose by the right route and at the right time. On admission, patients are issued an individualized bar code wristband that uniquely identifies their identity. When a patient is to receive a medication, nurses scans their bar coded employee identifier and the patient's bar code wristband to confirm their identity. The JCAHO, a nonprofit organization that is the nation's leading standards-setting and accrediting body in healthcare, has stated that a bar code with two unique, patient-specific identifiers will provide healthcare organizations a system that complies with the 2004 National Patient Safety Goal requirement of obtaining two or more patient identifiers before medication administration (JCAHO, 2004). Prior to medication administration, each bar coded package of medication to be administered at the bedside is scanned. The system can then verify the dispensing authority of the nurse, confirm the patient's identity, match the drug identity with their medication profile in the pharmacy information system, and electronically record the administration of the medication in an online MAR.

The use of an online MAR is likely to be more accurate than traditional handwritten MARs. Furthermore, the bar code scanner can enable nurses to have greater accuracy in recording the timing of medication administration, as the computer generates an actual "real-time" log of medication administration. Additional levels of functionality can include some of the following features:

- Increased accountability and capture of charges for items such as unit-stock medications.

- Up-to-date drug reference information from online medication reference libraries. This could include pictures of tablets or capsules, usual dosages, contraindications, adverse reactions and other safety warnings, pregnancy risk factors, and administration details.

- Customizable comments or alerts (e.g., look-alike/sound-alike drug names) and reminders of important clinical actions that need to be taken when administering certain medications (e.g., respiratory intubation is required for neuromuscular agents).

- Monitoring the pharmacy and the nurse's response to predetermined rules or standards in the rules engine such as alerts or reminders for the pharmacist or nurse. This includes allergies, duplicate dosing, over/under dosing, checking for cumulative dosing for medications with established maximum doses such as colchicines.

- Reconciliation for pending or STAT orders (i.e., a prescriber order not yet verified by a pharmacist). The ability of the nurse to enter a STAT

order into the system on administration that is linked directly to the pharmacy profile and prevents the duplicate administration of the same medication.

- Capturing data for the purpose of retrospective analysis of aggregate data to monitor trends (e.g., percent of doses administered late and errors of omission). However, this analysis should *not* be used to assess employee performance, especially if it could lead to punitive action.

- Verifying blood transfusion and laboratory specimen collection identification.

It is vitally important to its success that affected staff members, and specifically front-line nurses, are involved in all the decisions related to the purchase, education, and implementation of bar code technology. Before embarking on a BPOC implementation, it is critical to anticipate potential failures and develop contingency plans for unexpected results. Of course, a stringent testing phase should also be built into the system rollout phase using a technique such as FMEA to proactively address potential sources of breakdowns, workarounds, or new sources of medication errors.

One study noted five significant negative effects that occurred during the implementation of a BPOC system at VA hospitals that might create new paths to ADEs (Patterson et al., 2002). Negative effects include the following:

- Nurses were sometimes caught "off guard" by the programmed automated actions taken by the BPOC software. For example, the BPOC would remove medications from a patient's drug profile list 4 hours after the scheduled administration time, even if the medication were never administered. Therefore, if the patient returned from a procedure more than 4 hours after a scheduled medication administration time, the nurse would have no way of viewing if the ordered medication had or had not been administered.

- The BPOC seemed to inhibit the coordination of patient information between prescribers and nurses when compared to a traditional paper-based system. Before the BPOC was implemented, the prescriber could quickly review the handwritten MAR at the patient's bedside or in the unit's medication room.

- Nurses found it more difficult to deviate from the routine medication administration sequence with the BPOC system. For example, if a patient refused a medication, the nurses had to manually document the change in a time-consuming process since the medication had already been documented as given when it was originally scanned. Based on the organization's recommendation, the software was revised so that the nurse could easily document changes in BPOC by selecting the medication and choosing a drop-down menu option.

- Nurses felt that their main priority was the timeliness of medication administration because BPOC required nurses to type in an explanation when medications were given even a few minutes late. Particularly in long-term care settings, some nurses were observed to scan and prepour medications for unavailable patients so that they would appear "on time" in the computer record, thereby relying on memory to administer the medications in an unlabeled cup with opened, unlabeled medications when the patient returned to the unit.

- Nurses used strategies to increase efficiency that circumvented the intended use of BPOC. For example, some nurses routinely input a patient's social security number by typing the numbers rather than scanning the patient's bar code wristband, because typing seemed to be quicker. This is especially true if the nurse experiences difficulty in scanning the patient's bar code arm band (i.e., curvature of bar code on patient's wrist band on patients with small wrists, or damaged bar codes) (Patterson et al., 2002).

The interaction between nurses and technology at the bedside is important and must be continually evaluated for safety. As previously mentioned, nurses tend to develop "workarounds" for ineffective or inefficiently designed systems. One example includes nurses circumventing the normal procedures by removing or duplicating patient's bar code wristbands and scanning all of the patient's bar code wristbands and then scanning the corresponding medications for each patient while in the medication room prior to or after medication administration. Another workaround method includes the scanning of a surrogate bar code by having a sheet of paper with multiple bar codes of commonly used medications rather than the one unique medication package for each patient.

One medication error report caused by a workaround involved a mix-up with an order for digoxin elixir (used for congestive heart failure), which was a stocked on the unit as a 0.05 mg/mL, 60 mL multidose bottle (usual dose is 0.125–0.25 mg [2.5–5 mL]). The nurse not only misinterpreted the dose of digoxin elixir as 60 mL, but accidentally retrieved a bottle of *doxepin* (used for depression), which is available as 10 mg/mL (usual dose is 75–150 mg per day [7.5–15 mL]) from unit stock and attempted to administer what she thought was digoxin elixir. This error occurred because she scanned the bar code on the bottle, which generated an error window on the laptop computer screen stating "drug not on profile" and did not investigate the error. The system allowed the nurse to manually enter the wrong medication's national drug code (NDC) number (a medical code set that identifies prescription drugs and some over-the-counter products), ignoring the correct drug NDC number that had been entered by the pharmacy which appeared on the laptop screen and administered 60 mL of *doxepin* elixir. This allowed the nurse a method to bypass the check system and simply type in numbers and administer a drug, whether was the right or wrong ordered medication.

It is important to understand that the successful implementation of an effective BPOC system "forces" nurses to accept and change some of their long-held practices when administering medications to achieve a higher level of medication safety. When BPOC technology is used correctly, it forces nurses to always be compliant with the proper identification of patients, it documents real-time administration, acts as a double check, and the system does not allow the nurse to prepare medications for multiple patients at one time or prepour medications prior to the appropriate administration time.

One major issue initially hindering the widespread implementation of BPOC systems lies largely with the pharmaceutical industry's apparent unwillingness to adopt a universal bar code standard and apply a bar code consistently to the container of all medications, including unit-dose packages. But in February 2004, the FDA established a new rule that requires a bar code on most products in a linear format that meets the Uniform Code Council (UCC) or Health Industry Business Communications Council (HIBCC) standards. This bar code must not only contain the product's NDC number, but the expiration date and lot number are optional. The rule allows for a few exceptions, among them oral contraceptive dial packs, low-density polyethylene (LDPE) containers, radiopharmaceuticals, drug sample packages, and medical gasses (Cohen et al., 2004).

Further complicating the issue is the extended lag time between the launch of new medications and their availability (if ever) in unit-dose packaging. Additionally, unit-dose packaging for some established products have been discontinued. At this point, hospital pharmacies that employ bar code technology must repackage many medications and relabel each with a bar code. This can only be done at considerable cost in manpower and/or automated repackaging equipment. In addition, the chance of a medication error occurring is increased because doses must be taken from their original container and then repackaged or relabeled and there could be an error in the application of the correct bar code label or in choosing the wrong medication. One medication error report includes a scenario where a facility that utilized a bar code medication administration system for their inpatients where not all injectables used at the organization had manufacturer's bar codes on the vials or ampuls, pharmacy technicians had to generate computer printed bar codes for those products. Prior to the intubation of a patient, a vial of succinylcholine chloride with an incorrect dose label was discovered. The printed label read 20 mg/10 mL, whereas, the manufacturer's label read 20 mg/mL. Had the patient received the incorrect dose, it would have been 10 times the dose needed.

The use of BPOC systems can possibly introduce new types of medication errors. Although, due to the low incidence of organizations using BPOC and few medication errors reported, it can be hypothesized that some of the following types of errors could occur, especially if the system includes only the most basic of functionality:

- Omissions: After the patient's bar code armband and medication have been scanned, the dose is inadvertently dropped onto the floor. This results in a time lapse between the documentation that the medication was supposedly administered and the actual administration after obtaining of a new dose.

- Extra dose: An extra dose may be given when there are orders for the same drug to be administered by a different route. For example, if one nurse gives an oral dose and is called away and the covering nurse administers the dose intravenous (IV). The problem arises when there is no alert between profiled routes of administration indicating that the medication was previously administered by one route that is different than the second route.

- Wrong drug: In situations when the nurse administers a medication, which has not been labeled with a bar code.

- Wrong dose: In situations when the nurse has difficulty in scanning medication and proceeds to scan the medication twice. This results in a "double" dose when only one tablet is to be administered.

- Unauthorized drug: An order to hold a medication unless a lab value is at a certain level such as an aminoglycoside (i.e., elevated gentamicin drug level).

- Charting errors: Distinguish the indication for the administration of the medication (Tylenol 650 mg every 4 hours as needed for pain or fever).

- Wrong dosage form: Certain drug shortages may force a pharmacy to dispense a different strength or concentration (mg/mL) other than what is entered in the BPOC software.

Automated Dispensing Cabinets

Traditionally, hospital pharmacies provided medications for patients by filling patient-specific bins of unit-dose medications, which were then delivered to the nursing unit and stored in medication carts. The ADC is a computerized point-of-use medication-management system that is designed to replace or support the traditional unit-dose drug delivery system. The devices require staff to enter a unique logon and password to access the system using a touch screen monitor or by using finger print identification. Various levels of system level access can be assigned to staff members, depending on their role in the medication-use process. Once logged into the system, the nurse can obtain patient-specific medications from drawers or bins that open after a drug is chosen from a pick list (Table 12.1).

Many healthcare facilities have replaced medication carts or open unit-stock systems with ADCs. The results of an ASHP survey of 1,101 pharmacy directors showed that 58% of hospitals employed technology that totally redesigned the medication-management system from the traditional unit-dose dispensing system to a decentralized system utilizing ADC on patient care units. The rationales behind the wide acceptance of this technology are the following:

- *Improving pharmacy productivity*: The streamlining of the dispensing process due to the reduced number of steps from filling each patient's individual medications bins to filling a centralized station. It also has the potential to reduce time needed to obtain missing medications.

- *Improving nursing productivity*: The time spent gathering or obtaining missing medications can be reduced. Also, the turnaround time in obtaining newly ordered medications is decreased.

Table 12.1 Examples of High-Alert Medications Stored in Automated Dispensing Cabinets

Class/category of medications

- Adrenergic agonists, IV (e.g., epinephrine)
- Adrenergic antagonists, IV (e.g., propranolol)
- Anesthetic agents, general, inhaled, and IV (e.g., propofol)
- Chemotherapeutic agents, parenteral and oral
- Dextrose, hypertonic, 20% or greater
- Epidural or intrathecal medications
- Glycoprotein IIb/IIIa inhibitors (e.g., eptifibatide)
- Hypoglycemics, oral
- Inotropic medications, IV (e.g., digoxin, milrinone)
- Liposomal forms of drugs (e.g., liposomal amphotericin B)
- Moderate sedation agents, IV (e.g., midazolam)
- Moderate sedation agents, oral, for children (e.g., chloral hydrate)
- Narcotics/opiates, IV and oral (including liquid concentrates, immediate- and sustained-release)
- Neuromuscular blocking agents (e.g., succinylcholine)
- Radiocontrast agents, IV
- Thrombolytics/fibrinolytics, IV (e.g., tenecteplase)

Specific medications

- IV amiodarone
- Colchicine injection
- Heparin, low molecular weight, injection
- Heparin, unfractionated, IV
- Insulin, subcutaneous, and IV
- IV lidocaine
- Magnesium sulfate injection
- Methotrexate, oral, nononcologic use
- Nesiritide
- Nitroprusside, sodium, for injection
- Potassium chloride for injection concentrate
- Potassium phosphates injection
- Sodium chloride injection, hypertonic, more than 0.9% concentration
- Warfarin

Reducing costs: Increased pharmacist and nursing productivity, which frees them from time-consuming processes and allowing more time for patient and clinical interactions. There also is a reduction in inventory and containment costs associated with expired medications.

Improving charge capture: ADCs that are interfaced with the accounting department allow for the capture of all patient charges associated with administered medications.

Enhancing patient quality and safety: ADCs that have built-in decision support systems that warn users on drug-drug interactions, drug-allergy interactions, drug-lab interactions (requires a laboratory interface), drug-drug duplications, and so forth (CardinalHealth, 2003).

In addition, some systems allow for organization-specific, user-generated warnings to prevent medication errors such as warnings of potential errors from look-alike/sound-alike medication names. ADCs can also be used to comply with regulatory requirements by tracking the storage, dispensing, and use of controlled substances.

However, such systems cannot improve patient safety unless cabinet *design* and *use* are carefully planned and implemented to eliminate opportunities for wrong drug selection and dosing errors. More than 126 medication error reports involving the use of ADCs have been submitted to the U.S. Pharmacopeia/Institute for Safe Medication Practices (USP/ISMP) Medication Error Reporting Program (MERP). Some documented unsafe practices with the use of these devices include **the lack of pharmacy screening of medication order prior to administration,** which negates an independent double check of the original order. At a minimum, medication orders are screened by the pharmacy for the appropriateness of the drug, dose, frequency, and route of administration, therapeutic duplication, real or potential allergies or sensitivities, real or potential interactions between the prescription and other medications, food, and laboratory values, and other contraindications.

This is particularly problematic when medications, which are considered "high-alert" medications are stored in these devices.[1] For example, one medication error

---

[1]High-alert medications can be defined as medications that, when involved in medication errors, have a high risk of injury or death. There is no documentation that the occurrence of medication errors is more common with high-alert medications than with the use of other drugs but the consequence of the error may be far more devastating (Cohen, 2002). Examples of high-alert medications stored in ADCs can be found in Table 12.1 (ISMP will provide list as a side table).

occurred in a small hospital after the pharmacy was closed. An order was written for "calcium gluconate 1 g IV," but the nurse misread the label and believed that *each 10 mL* vial contained only 98 mg. Thus, she thought she needed 10 vials when actually each mL actually contained 98 mg, or 1 g/10 mL vial. A 10-fold overdose was avoided because the drug cabinet contained only six vials of calcium gluconate. Fortunately, this error was detected when the nurse contacted a pharmacist at home to obtain additional vials.

Choosing of the wrong medication from an alphabetic pick list is a common contributing factor in medication errors arising from medication names that look alike. For example, one organization reported three errors regarding mix-ups between diazepam and diltiazem removals from their ADC in their intensive care units. In one case, diazepam was given at the ordered diltiazem dose and in another case, a physician noted the amber color of the diazepam vial as the nurse was drawing up the dose (meaning to obtain diltiazem). The organization concluded that once the wrong drug was chosen, the cabinet seemed to "confirm" that the correct drug was chosen since the nurse assumed the correct drug was chosen from the menu and thought the correct drug was in the drawer that opened. The nurse "relied" on her ability to choose the right drug from the pick list and, in these cases, no physical check of the product was made or reading of the label was done.

High-alert medications placed, stored, and returned to ADCs are problematic. The process of placing and restocking medications into an ADC is primarily a pharmacy function. Unfortunately, studies have indicated that an independent double check (one individual supplies the cabinet with the medication and a second independent individual checks that the correct medication was placed into the correct location) does not occur. In one study only 56% of respondents reported that a pharmacist always checked the medications to be used to restock a cabinet before placement, 15% reported that this check process never takes place and over half the respondents (54%) never verify correct drug placement in cabinets after restocking. In addition, this survey reported that medications could be stocked or returned to stock by nursing accidentally into the wrong bins. Additionally, 96% of respondents reported that bar code technology is not used when stocking cabinet (Cohen et al., 1999a) to verify that the correct medication is placed into the correct bin in the ADC. Even when the bar code on a drug container is matched with the proper location of an ADC, loading the equipment is a manual operation. In one case, a patient had orders for both MS Contin (morphine sulfate *controlled* release) 15 mg tablets

and for morphine sulfate *immediate* release 15 mg tablets. A pharmacy technician loaded both medications in the ADC in the patient care unit. The person loading the medications inadvertently loaded the MS Contin in the pocket for the morphine sulfate immediate release and the morphine sulfate immediate release in the pocket for the MS Contin. Some doses of each medication were actually administered to a patient. Fortunately, the patient suffered no apparent adverse effects from this incident. A second nurse discovered the error when removing the medication for the next dose.

Another report involved the need to refill unit stock in an ADC with furosemide 40 mg/4 mL. A pharmacy technician pulled what was thought to be vials of furosemide 40 mg/4 mL from the stock in a satellite pharmacy and then, without a pharmacist double check, left the pharmacy and filled the ADC. A nurse on the unit went to the cabinet to fill an order for furosemide 240 mg. She obtained six vials out of the ADC and drew them into a syringe. After drawing up the sixth vial, the nurse noticed a precipitation. At that point, the nurse checked the vials to find that she had five vials of furosemide 40 mg/4 mL and one vial of phenylephrine 1% 5 mL. Both these medications are available in the same size amber vials with very little color or marking differentiation.

Storage of medications with look-alike names and/or packaging next to each other in the same drawer or bin is one of the root causes of more than half the errors reported through the MERP (Cohen et al., 1999b). A common cause of these mix-ups is what human factors experts call "confirmation bias," where a practitioner reads a drug name on an order or package and is most likely to see that which is most familiar to him, overlooking any disconfirming evidence. Also, when confirmation bias occurs, it is unlikely that the practitioner would question what is being read. This can occur both in the restocking process of the ADC and in the removal of medications. One example includes a situation where a physician asked for ephedrine, but a hurried nurse picked epinephrine from the ADC, drew up the medication into a syringe and handed it to the primary nurse who administered the epinephrine. The patient suffered a period of hypertension and chest pain but eventually recovered. In another example, a prescriber wrote an order for morphine via a patient-controlled analgesia (PCA) pump. Since the organization used a system allowing for "overrides" (the manual action taken to counteract or bypass the normal operation) of certain medications, the nurse removed a PCA syringe containing meperidine from the ADC. When pharmacy reviewed the override medication removals report the next morning, the error was discovered. The PCA pump still had the meperidine cartridge in place, but the pump settings were for morphine, resulting in an inappropriate dose.

The development of "workarounds" for ineffective or inefficient systems can be devastating to patient safety. The interaction between a nurse and technology is very important and often is not considered when various forms of automation, including ADCs, are purchased, installed, and employed on the nursing unit. When the device does not respond as expected, nurses will find various ways of working around the system to obtain medications. In the error previously mentioned, overrides were established by the organization that allowed nursing to obtain medications without the approval or review by a pharmacist. Overrides usually are needed with medications used in emergency situations. Unfortunately, ADCs that allow overrides also serve as an "extended" pharmacy in order to obtain and administer medications prior to delivery by the pharmacy. Additional error reports involving workarounds include the removal of medications using the inventory function (used to determine the number of doses on hand of a particular medication) to obtain medications for patients without pharmacy screening, removal of a larger quantity of medications than ordered for one patient, and removal of medications for multiple patients while the cabinet is open.

Regardless of an organization's steps to purchase or implement ADCs, the following issues should be considered to ensure safe medication practices:

- Consider purchasing a system that allow for patient profiling so pharmacists can enter and screen drug orders prior to their removal and administered. Also, consider purchasing a system that utilizes bar-code technology during the stocking, retrieval, and drug administration processes.

- Carefully select the drugs that will be stocked in the cabinets. Consider the needs of each patient care unit as well as the age and diagnoses of patients being treated on the units. If possible, minimize the variety of drug concentrations avoiding bulk supplies, and stock drugs in ready-to-use unit doses.

- Place drugs that cannot be accessed without pharmacy order entry and screening in individual matrix bins. Store all drugs that do not require pharmacy screening together so that access to these medications does not also allow access to other drugs, which do require pharmacy screening.

- Use individual cabinets to separate pediatric and adult medications.

- Periodically reassess the drugs stocked in each unit-based cabinet. As appropriate, remove low-usage medications and those with multiple concentrations.

- Remove only a single dose of the medication ordered. If not administered, return the dose to the pharmacy or ADC return bin and allow pharmacy to replace it in the cabinet.

- Develop a check system to assure accurate stocking of the cabinets. Another staff member from pharmacy or nurse on the unit can verify accurate stocking by having pharmacy provide a daily list of items added to the cabinet.

- Place allergy reminders for specific drugs, such as antibiotics, opiates, and nonsteroidal anti-inflammatory drugs (NSAIDs) on the cabinets (some systems allow staff to build alerts that appear on the screen when attempting to access the drug).

- Routinely run and analyze override reports to help track and identify problems.

"Smart" Infusion Pump Delivery Systems

Infusion pumps are primarily used to deliver parenteral medications through IV or epidural lines and can be found in a variety of clinical settings ranging from acute-care and long-term care facilities, patient's homes, and physician's offices. According to ECRI, a nonprofit organization that evaluates medical device safety, incidents involving infusion pumps typically result from the unintentional free flow of solution (when the solution flows freely under the force of gravity, without being controlled by the infusion pump). The delivery of an incorrect dose of a medication or incorrect rate of infusion of an IV solution can cause an error when programming the infusion pump (ECRI, 2002). Medication errors with infusion pumps can also occur due to incorrect, inappropriate, or miscalculation of an order for the medication. In addition, studies have shown that medications intended for IV or epidural use are involved in many serious mishaps. In a study of pediatric inpatients, IV medications were associated with 54% of potential ADEs and 60% of serious and life-threatening errors were associated with IV therapy (Kaushal et al., 2001). Infusion pumps with dose calculation software, sometimes referred to as "smart pumps," could reduce medication errors, improve workflow, and provide a new source of data for continuous quality improvement (CQI) by identifying and correcting pump-programming errors.

The administration of parenteral medications has traditionally been based on a calculation of a volume to be infused per hour of delivery. Infusion pumps are capable of delivering a wide range of delivery rates, ranging from 0.01 mL/h to as much as 1 L/h, which could result in the device being programmed all too easily in error to deliver a 10- or 100-fold overdose. Because of this wide range of settings, there are many possibilities for errors resulting from infusion-device programming. A medication may be inadvertently programmed to be administered as micrograms per kilogram per minute (mcg/kg/min) instead of micrograms per minute (mcg/min), a 24-hour dose may be delivered over 1 hour, or a missing decimal point or an additional zero may result in a 10-fold overdose. Infusion pumps are specifically designed to have maximum flexibility, so they can be used in multiple areas of the facility. Consequently, a pump used today for a 200-kg patient in the adult ICU may also be used on a 600-g premature infant. Errors of 10, 100, or even 1,000 times the intended dose can easily be programmed, since there are no limits in devices. Basically, the safe use of infusion pumps requires perfect performance by the practitioner programming the pump.

There are numerous published reports of fatal errors involving infusion pumps such as when a nurse attempted to program an infusion pump for a baby receiving total parenteral nutrition (TPN) by inputting 13.0 mL/h. The decimal point key on the pump was somewhat worn and difficult to engage. Without realizing it, the nurse programmed a rate of 130 mL/hr. Fortunately, the error was discovered within 1 hour. The baby's glucose rose to 363, so the rate of infusion for the TPN was decreased for a while and the baby was fine.

In other cases, morphine was entered as 90 mg/hr instead of 9.0 mg/hr, causing delivery of 10 times the intended dose. Nitroglycerin ordered to be administered in mcg/min was inadvertently programmed as mcg/kg/min, resulting in administration of 60 times the intended dose, and in a neonatal ICU, an infusion rate was reprogrammed from 3.2 to 304 mL/hr, when the intention was 3.4 mL/hr.

In addition, many of the tragic errors occurring with PCA pumps have resulted from incorrect programming of the drug concentration, leading to a factor of 10 overdoses. In terms of rate, any IV solution ordered for administration over a 24-hour period can be easily programmed incorrectly to infuse in 1 hour (Reves, 2004).

The common denominator in many of these and other cases was a single wrong entry or button pressed. The use of a "smart" infusion pump, programmed with patient and drug parameters, would have been able to recognize the error before the infusion even began since a practitioner would no longer have to rely on memory to determine correct dosing, or on keystroke accuracy to ensure correct programming. Instead, a practitioner could rely on the technology of the smart pump, which is programmed according to institution-established best practices.

The introduction of smart infusion technology has changed the paradigm of infusion therapy by removing the reliance on memory and human input of calculated values to a software-enabled filter to prevent keystroke errors in programming infusion devices for delivery of parenteral medications. Smart pumps can include comprehensive libraries of drugs, usual concentrations, dosing units (e.g., mcg/kg/min, units/h) and dose limits as well as software that incorporate institution-established dosage limits, warnings to the practitioner when dosage limits are exceeded and configurable settings by patient type or location in the organization (i.e., ICU, pediatric intensive care unit [PICU]). Such systems make it possible to provide an additional verification at the point-of-care to help prevent parenteral medication errors. Smart infusion systems can also integrate bar code technology to provide additional checks and balances in the drug administration process. This would ensure that the correct medication intended for parenteral administration is reaching the correct patient at the right dose, prior to the initiation of the infusion.

The software also enables the infusion system to provide an additional verification of the programming of medication delivery. The nurse receives an alert when the dose is below or above the organization's preestablished limits. Depending on the drug, these alerts can be warnings that must be confirmed or stops that require the nurse to reprogram the pump for a different infusion rate. The limits can be set as either "soft" (can be overridden) or "hard" (one that will not let the nurse go any further with either documenting the reason why the limit is overridden or a total reprogramming of the pump). The drug library in the system requires the practitioner to confirm the patient care area, drug name, drug amount, diluent volume, patient weight, dose, and rate of infusion. The system can allow organizations to configure unit-specific profiles, which include customized sets of operating variables, programming options, and drug libraries.

Access to transaction data from the infusion device is obtained by direct cable downloads to a desktop computer for quality-improvement efforts. CQI logs in the software record the near misses (programming errors) averted by the new system. Practitioners can use this tool to assess current practices and identify ways of improving safe use of medications. This provides data on transactions at the bedside that are not currently available with traditional infusion devices. For each safety alert, a record is generated of the time, date, drug, concentration, programmed rate, volume infused, and limit exceeded, as well as the clinician's response to the warning (i.e., continue at the current settings or change the programming). Similar data for infusions delivered with traditional settings for rate and volume are captured, along with other transactional data generated as a result of pump use (e.g., alarms, air in line). Thus, the system can be used to show whether potential infusion errors were detected and to assess current practice to determine if improvements can be made to optimize care and reduce costs.

Documented examples of errors prevented using "smart pump" technology have been published. For example, a physician in the emergency department wrote an order for Integrilin (eptifibatide) but inadvertently prescribed a dose appropriate for ReoPro (abciximab). The Integrilin infusion was initiated and continued for approximately 36 hours after the patient was transferred to a medical/surgical unit. During this time, the patient's mental status was deteriorating. At this point, the hospital was switching a "smart pump" infusion system, which performed a "test of reasonableness" before allowing the infusion to begin. As the nurse was transferring the infusion parameters from the old infusion system to this new system, safety software incorporated in the device alerted the nurse that there was a "dose out of range." The pump would not allow the nurse to continue until a pharmacist was called and the mistake was corrected.

In another case, a hospital's heparin protocol called for a loading dose of 4,000 units followed by a constant infusion of 900 units/hr. The loading dose was administered correctly, but the nurse inadvertently programmed the continuous dose as 4,000 units/hr. Since the pump limit for heparin as a continuous infusion was set at 2,000 units/hr, the infusion device would not start until the dose was corrected. In both of the cases these mistakes may have gone undetected without preprogrammed limits and patient harm might have resulted (Cohen et al., 2002).

To implement the "smart" pump infusion technology, use a proactive technique (FMEA) to assess for the risk of error to determine issues with IV drug administration. Establish a multidisciplinary team to determine best practices. This team should institute changes in policies and procedures that reflect the smart infusion technology is installed. Asking a nurse to choose from among many concentrations, dosing units, or remembering several possible drug names will increase the risk of error.

Therefore, standardization of IV-related policies and procedures, standardization of concentrations, dosing units (for example, mcg/min vs. mcg/kg/min) and drug nomenclature is essential. These items should be consistent with that used on the MAR, the pharmacy computer system, and the electronic medical record, if applicable.

Many drug references provide information on the maximum dose over a 24-hour period but do not provide the minimum and maximum doses that can be administered over 1 hour so the team should determine dosage limits for infusions and boluses based on current policy and practice, the literature, and common references used in pharmacy practice. In addition, there needs to be a determination of which dose limits require a "soft" or a "hard" stop. Existing best practices and policies and unit-based dosage limits should then be used to developed data sets based on patient care areas, for example, adult ICU, adult general care, PICU, pediatric general care, labor and delivery, and anesthesia. Different configurations were available for each area. Lastly, a procedure for the nursing staff to follow in the event a drug must be given which is not in the library or if a nonstandardized concentration has to be used (IHI, 2004).

The effective implementation of smart technology thus changes the role of the nurse from that of a looking for or memorizing data and rules to that of a clinical decision maker.

Implementation of Technology

Implementing any form of technology into a healthcare organization can be an imposing task. Many organizations have purchased various forms of automation, with little or inadequate planning and/or preparation, which can lead to errors as well as the development of serious problems. Therefore, it is vitally important to thoroughly plan for this process and to remember your goal is to improve clinical processes, which can be facilitated by technology. Foremost, the process will require total commitment from the organization's executive and medical leadership as well as all staff members who will be affected by the implementation. It is of utmost importance that the leadership sends a clear message that this is important to patient safety and that they provide their unwavering support and financial backing as the project evolves. Lacking this level of commitment will greatly increase the chance of failure.

Identifying physician champions at a very high level in the organization is crucial and involving them in the decision-making and planning process will help to persuade practitioners to "buy into" technology. In addition, identify an interdisciplinary team of key individuals who can collaborate on an effective and realistic plan for implementation, including front-line clinical staff. Do not forget to include important key players such as the chief information officer (CIO), information technology (IT), risk managers, medical staff, front-line practitioners, and other support staff who may interact directly with the technology (ASHP, 2001). The multidisciplinary implementation team will need to address the following issues:

■ Outlining goals for the type of automation to be implemented (e.g., to improve safety, decrease costs, eliminate handwritten orders). You may also outline primary and secondary goals. Knowing and prioritizing your goals and their relative importance will be very valuable during implementation of the system.

■ Developing a wish list of desired features and determining which one, given budgetary constraints, are practical. Find out about successes and failures by talking with or visiting individuals from other organizations who have implemented similar systems.

■ Investigating systems that are presently available. Determine whether the new system will interface with your current information systems and to what extent will customization be required.

■ Analyzing the current workflow and determining what changes are needed. This may include any changes that will occur in the current processes as well as the culture. A lack of fit with clinical process and practice can be a downfall because healthcare practitioners tend to resist process changes that produce inefficiencies, complicate their work, or do not provide clear benefits. Policies and procedures for both the implementation and ongoing use must be defined prior to rollout. There will be numerous workflow changes that must be carefully planned to address the multiple operational transitions during the rollout such as when each care area transitions from a paper-based system to an automated system, when patients are transferred from the automated units to areas with no automation, healthcare providers going from areas with automation to areas without automation, and as the implementation process grows from one area of the organization to other areas (CHCF, 2000).

■ Identify the required capabilities and configuration of the new system. If the system allows for the development of rules, protocols, guidelines, or drug dictionaries, individuals that will be affected by these changes need to develop these items before the system is implemented.

■ "Sell" the benefits and objectives of automation to staff. Do not try to justify the new system by promising that it will allow the institution to decrease the number of staff members, because it most likely will not. A good system, though, should enhance safety and improve efficiency by decreasing the number of repetitive and mundane tasks. You may see the number of steps in the medication-use process decrease, but the remaining steps will require highly educated, competent personnel who understand and can deal with the complexity and importance of those steps.

■ Development of an implementation plan. Set realistic timeframe expectations. Extensively test the system for accuracy and safety before implementation. Focus on efficiency and safety. Healthcare practitioners will not use a system, which is perceived as less efficient than the existing system.

Once the system has been implemented into the organization, there are still many issues that need to be considered. Plan on many years of system development and enhancement after the product is initially piloted. As soon as the system is installed, it is important to commit in a meaningful way to its continual monitoring and improvement. The healthcare environment is a dynamic one in which opportunities for new (and some old, but as yet unidentified) errors will likely arise. Identify key measures that will help you determine whether your systems are really improving safety and quality and reducing costs. Beware of cumbersome features that may provoke users to override features or develop workarounds with the system. Finally, do not be discouraged by initial dissatisfaction among staff members, and do not interpret initial negative reactions as failures.

Conclusion

Newt Gingrich, past U.S. Speaker of the House of Representatives remarks, "The fact is paper records kill. And the tragic thing is the deaths are avoidable" (Modern Healthcare, June 2004). As patient advocates, nurses have a responsibility to discuss their patient safety concern and speak up about the dangers associated with the current paper-based medication-use process.

Nurses also have the responsibility to become familiar with the availability of "safety" technology, the advantages and disadvantages, and to work in collaboration with other healthcare stakeholders in the search for new and innovative technologic solutions to improve patient safety.

References

AHA. (2000). *AHA Guide to Computerized Physician Order-Entry Systems*. http://www.hospitalconnect.com/aha/key_issues/medication_safety/contents/CompEntryA1109.doc

American Society of Health-System Pharmacists. (1993). ASHP guidelines on preventing medication errors in hospitals. *American Journal Hospital Pharmacists* 50:305–314.

Anonymous. (1979). A study of physicians' handwriting as a time waster. *Journal of American Medical Association* 242:2429–2430.

ASHP. (2001). *Computerized Prescriber Order Entry Systems*. http://www.ashp.org/patientsafety/genprinciples.cfm?cfid=11647716&CFToken=88898100

Barker, K. N., Flynn, E. A., Pepper, G. A., et al. (2002). Medication errors observed in 36 healthcare facilities. *Archives of Internal Medicine* 162(16):1897–1903.

Bates, D. W., et al. (1998). Effect of computerized physician order entry and a team intervention on prevention of serious medication errors. *Journal of American Medical Association* 280:1311–1316.

Bates, D. W., et al. (1999). The impact of computerized physician order entry on medication error prevention. *Journal of the American Medical Informatics Association* 6(4):313–321.

Brodell, R. T. (1997). Prescription errors. Legibility and drug name confusion. *Archives of Family Medicine* 6:296–298.

Cabral, J. D. T. (1997). Poor physician penmanship. *Journal of American Medical Association* 278:1116–1117.

CardinalHealth. (2003). *Health Care Technology: Innovating Clinical Care Through Technology*. http://www.pyxis.com/products/Automation_Pharmacies.pdf

CHCF. (2000). *A Primer On Physician Order Entry*. http://www.chcf.org/documents/hospitals/CPOEreport.pdf

Chertow, G. M., Lee, L., et al. (2001). Guided medication dosing for inpatients with renal insufficiency. *Journal of American Medical Association* 286:2839–2844.

Cohen, M. R. (1999). Preventing medication errors related to prescribing. *Medication Errors* 8.2.

Cohen, H. and Mandrack, M. M. (2002). Application of the 80-20 rule in safeguarding the use of high alert medications. *Critical Care Nursing Clinics of North America* 14:369–374.

Cohen, M. C. and Smetzer, J. L. (1999a). Survey of automated dispensing shows need for practice improvements and safer system design. *ISMP Medication Safety Alert!* 7(12).

Cohen, M. C. and Smetzer, J. L. (1999b). "Prescription mapping" can improve efficiency while minimizing errors with look-alike products. *ISMP Medication Safety Alert!* 4(20).

Cohen, M. C. and Smetzer, J. L. (2001). The supermarkets do it—so why can't we raise the "bar" in health care? *ISMP Medication Safety Alert!* 6(15).1.

Cohen, M. C. and Smetzer, J. L. (2002). "Smart" infusion pumps join CPOE and bar coding as important ways to prevent medication errors. *ISMP Medication Safety Alert!* 7(3).

Cohen, M. C. and Smetzer, J. L. (2004). *ISMP Medication Safety Alert!* 9(4):1.

ECRI. (2002). General-purpose infusion pumps. *Health Devices* 31(10):352–384. Plymouth Meeting, PA.

HIMSS. (2002). Gaining MD buy-in: Physician order entry. *Journal of Healthcare Information Management* 16(2):67.

iHealth. (2004). *Physician Problems, Lack of Incentives Hinder Standards Adoption*. http://www.ihealthbeat.org/index.cfm?Action=dspItem&itemID=100646

IHI. (2004). *Reduce Adverse Drug Events (ADEs) Involving Intravenous Medications: Implement Smart Infusion Pumps*. http://www.qualityhealthcare.org/IHI/Topics/PatientSafety/MedicationSystems/Changes/IndividualChanges/ImplementSmartInfusionPumps.htm

ISMP (2000). *A Call to Action: Eliminate Handwritten Prescriptions Within 3 Years*. http://www.ismp.org/MSAarticles/Whitepaper.html

Kohn, L., Corrigan, J., and Donaldson, M. (Eds.). (1999). *To Err is Human: Building a Safer Health System*. Washington, DC: National Academy Press.

Johnson, C. L., Carlson, R. A., Tucker, C. L., and Willette, C. (2002). Using BCMA software to improve patient safety in Veterans Administration Medical Centers. *Journal of Healthcare Information Management* 16(1):46–51.

Joint Commission on Accreditation of Healthcare Organizations. (2004). *2004 National Patient Safety Goals - FAQs* http://www.jcaho.org/accredited+organizations/patient+safety/04+npsg/04_faqs.htm

Kaushal, R., Bates, D. W., Landrigan, C., et al. (2001). Medication errors and adverse drug events in pediatric inpatients. *Journal of American Medical Association* 285:2114–2120.

Leape, L. L., Bates, D. W., Cullen, D. J., et al. (1995). Systems analysis of adverse drug events. *Journal of the American Medical Association* 274:35–43.

Modern Healthcare. (2004). 'Wired' Group Effort (Vol. no. 34, No. 26, p. 54). Chicago, IL: Crain Communications.

Patterson, E. S., Cook, R. I., and Render, M. L. (2002). Improving patient safety by identifying side effects from introducing bar coding in medication administration. *Journal of the American Medical Informatics Association* 9(5)540–553.

Pedersen, C. A., Schneider, P. J., and Scheckelhoff, D. J. (2003). ASHP national survey of hospital pharmacy practice in hospital settings: Dispensing and administration-2002. *American Journal of Health-System Pharmacy* 60:52–68.

Regnier, P. (2004). *Healthcare myth: We spend too much. http://money.cnn.com/2003/10/08/pf/health_myths_1/*

Reves, J. G. (2004). *"Smart Pump" Technology Reduces Errors. http://www.apsf.org/newsletter/2003/spring/smartpump.htm*

Stefanacci, R. (2004). Public reporting of hospital quality measures. *Health Policy Newsletter* 17(1):4.

13 Healthcare Data Standards

Joyce Sensmeier

OBJECTIVES

1. Discuss the need for data standards in healthcare.
2. Describe the standards development process.
3. Identify standards development organizations (SDOs).
4. Describe healthcare data standards initiatives.
5. Explore the business value of data standards.

KEY WORDS

standards
health data interchange
terminology
knowledge representation

Standards are critical components in the development and implementation of an electronic health record (EHR). The effectiveness of healthcare delivery is dependent on the ability of clinicians to access critical health information when and where it is needed. The ability to exchange health information across organizational and system boundaries, whether between multiple departments within a single institution or among a varied cast of providers, payers, regulators, and others is essential. A common set of rules and definitions, both at the level of data meaning as well as at the technical level of data exchange is needed to make this possible. In addition, there must be a sociopolitical structure in place that recognizes the benefits of shared information and supports the adoption and implementation of such standards.

This chapter examines healthcare data standards in terms of the following:

Need for healthcare data standards

Healthcare data interchange standards

Healthcare terminologies

Knowledge representation

Healthcare data standards development

Healthcare data SDOs

Healthcare data standards initiatives

Business value of data standards

Need for Healthcare Data Standards

Data standards as applied to healthcare include the "methods, protocols, terminologies, and specifications for the collection, exchange, storage, and retrieval of information associated with healthcare applications, including medical records, medications, radiological images, payment and reimbursement, medical devices and monitoring systems, and administrative processes" (Washington Publishing Company, 1998). In the domain of information management, standards can be further categorized as those that support the generic infrastructure and are not domain-specific, those that support the exchange of information and are domain-specific, and those that support activities and practices within a specific domain. Examples of the first type of standard would include equipment specifications such as processor type or network transmission protocols such as Ethernet or token ring. The second type of standard typically involves the specification of data structures and content and would include such standards as message formats and core data sets. The third type of

217

standard addresses the interpretation of that data as information, including how it should be acted on within a particular context. An example of this type of standard would be professional practice guidelines. It is the second class of standards, commonly described as data standards, that will be the focus of the following discussion as applied to healthcare.

Healthcare is fundamentally a process of communication. For much of history, verbal communication between a patient and a healthcare provider characterized this process. The temporal and physical proximity of the communicators provided ample opportunity to clarify any ambiguity regarding the intended meaning of what was being communicated.

Today, healthcare delivery is far more complex, and a single episode may frequently take place across multiple settings and involve numerous parties including patients and their social support system, providers working directly and indirectly with patients, administrators, and payers. In addition, the information about patients and their care is used not only for the direct care process but also for many other purposes including reimbursement, research, public health, education, policy development, and litigation.

It is this tremendous increase in the need for health information exchange that has driven the push for use of electronic information and management systems in the healthcare domain. However, while current information technology is able to move and manipulate large amounts of data, it is not as proficient in dealing with ambiguity in the structure and semantic content of that data. Data standards are an attempt to reduce the level of ambiguity in the communication of data so that actions taken based on the data are consistent with the actual meaning of the data.

While the term "data standards" is generally used to describe those standards having to do with the structure and content of health information, it may be useful to differentiate data, information, and knowledge. Data are the fundamental building blocks on which healthcare decisions are based. Data are collections of unstructured, discrete entities (facts) that exist outside of any particular context. When data are interpreted within a given context and given meaningful structure within that context, they become information. When information from various contexts is aggregated following a defined set of rules, it becomes knowledge and provides the basis for informed action (Saba and McCormick, 2000). Data standards represent both data and their transformation into information. Analysis generates knowledge, which is the foundation of professional practice standards.

Healthcare Data Interchange Standards

Data interchange standards address, primarily, the format of messages that are exchanged between computer systems, document architecture, clinical templates, user interface, and patient data linkage (Committee on Data Standards for Patient Safety, 2004). To achieve data compatibility between systems, it is necessary to have prior agreement on the syntax of the messages to be exchanged. The receiving system must be able to parse the incoming message into discrete data elements that reflect what the sending system wishes to communicate. In addition to a common message format, it is also necessary that the individual data elements be structured in a common way as well. Although there is a great deal of interest in the development of natural language processing capabilities, most health data exchange still involves coded, or structured, information. The following section describes some of the major organizations involved in the development of data interchange standards.

Message Format Standards

Four broad classes of message format standards have emerged in the healthcare sector: medical device communications, digital imaging communications, administrative data exchange, and clinical data exchange (Saba and McCormick, 2000). It should be noted that there is considerable overlap among standards development activities, and there may be more than one standard available for each of these classes.

The National Committee on Vital and Health Statistics (NCVHS) is the advisory committee established to make recommendations on health information policy to the Department of Health and Human Services (HHS) and Congress. As part of its responsibilities under the Health Insurance Portability and Accountability Act of 1996 (HIPAA), NCVHS was called on to "study the issues related to the adoption of uniform data standards for patient medical record information (PMRI) and the electronic exchange of such information." This public-private partnership has recommended that several message format standards be adopted for federal healthcare services programs including Health Level Seven (HL7) (v2.2 and later), Digital Imaging Communication in Medicine Standards Committee (DICOM), National Council for Prescription Drug Programs (NCPDP) SCRIPT and Institute of Electrical and Electronic Engineers (IEEE) 1073. The organizations that have developed these standards are profiled below.

Institute of Electrical and Electronic Engineers

The IEEE has developed a series of standards known collectively as P1073 Medical Information Bus (MIB), which support real-time, continuous, and comprehensive capture and communication of data from bedside medical devices such as those found in intensive care units, operating rooms, and emergency departments. These data include physiologic parameter measurements and device settings. These standards are used internationally. Current activities include efforts to develop standards that support wireless technology. The IEEE 802.xx suite of wireless networking standards, 802.11, 802.15, and 802.16, has stirred up developments in an otherwise sluggish communications market. The most widely known standard, 802.11, commonly referred to as Wi-Fi, allows anyone with a computer and either a plug-in card or built-in circuitry to connect to the Internet wirelessly through a myriad access points installed in offices, hotels, airports, coffeehouses, convention centers, and even parks, among other locations. Many healthcare organizations are currently evaluating and implementing wireless solutions that support point-of-care technology.

National Electrical Manufacturers Association

The National Electrical Manufacturers Association (NEMA), in collaboration with the American College of Radiologists (ACR) and others, formed the DICOM to develop a generic digital format and a transfer protocol for biomedical images and image-related information. The specification is usable on any type of computer system and supports transfer over the Internet. The DICOM standard is the dominant international data interchange message format in biomedical imaging. The Joint NEMA/The European Coordination Committee of the Radiological and Electromedical Industry/Japan Industries Association of Radiological Systems (COCIR/JIRA) Security and Privacy Committee (SPC) has recently issued a white paper which provides a guide for vendors and users on how to protect medical information systems against viruses, Trojan horses, denial of service attacks, Internet worms, and related forms of so-called "malicious software."

Accredited Standards Committee X12N/Insurance

Accredited Standards Committee (ASC) X12N has developed a broad range of electronic data interchange (EDI) standards to facilitate electronic business transactions. In the healthcare arena, X12N standards have been adopted as national standards for such administrative transactions as claims, enrollment, and eligibility in health plans, and first report of injury under the requirements of the HIPAA. Due to the uniqueness of health insurance and the policies for protection of personal health information from country to country, these standards are primarily used in the United States. HIPAA directed the secretary of the Department of HHS to adopt standards for transactions to enable health information to be exchanged electronically, and the Administrative Simplification Act (ASA), one of the HIPAA provisions, requires standard formats to be used for electronically submitted healthcare transactions. The American National Standards Institute (ANSI) developed these, and the ANSI X12N 837 Implementation Guide has been established as the standard of compliance for claim transactions.

National Council for Prescription Drug Programs

The NCPDP develops standards for information processing for the pharmacy services sector of the healthcare industry. This has been a very successful example of how standards can enable significant improvements in service delivery. Since the introduction of this standard in 1992, the retail pharmacy industry has moved to almost 100% electronic claims processing in real time. NCPDP's Telecommunication Standard Version 5.1 was named the official standard for pharmacy claims within HIPAA. NCPCP standards are forming the basis for electronic prescription transactions. Electronic prescription transactions are defined as EDI messages flowing between healthcare providers (i.e., pharmacy software systems and prescriber software systems) that are concerned with prescription orders. As with the X12N standards, the NCPDP standards are primarily used in the United States.

HL7 standards focus on facilitating the interchange of data to support clinical practice both within and across institutions. The major areas covered by the standard include medical orders; clinical observations; test results; admission, transfer, and discharge; document architecture, clinical templates, user interface, EHR, and charge and billing information. Since 1997, HL7 and ASC X12N have been collaborating on the development of a joint standard for claims attachments, with X12N supplying the transmission envelope and HL7 the internal message structure. The HL7 Board of Directors recently approved the electronic health record system (EHR-S) functional model to move forward as a draft standard for trial use. This draft standard consists of four distinct sections including an EHR-S functional overview, direct care, supportive, and information infrastructure. HL7 is widely supported by health information systems vendors worldwide and there are over a dozen foreign affiliates, which have adapted the basic standards for use in their particular settings.

Terminologies

A fundamental requirement for effective communication is the ability to represent concepts in an unambiguous fashion between both the sender and receiver of the message. Natural human languages are incredibly rich in their ability to communicate subtle differences in the semantic content, or meaning, of messages. While there have been great advances in the ability of computers to process natural language, most communication between health information systems relies on the use of structured vocabularies, code sets, and classification systems to represent healthcare concepts. Standardized terminologies enable data collection at the point of care, and retrieval of data, information, and knowledge in support of clinical practice. The following examples describe several of the major systems.

International Statistical Classification of Diseases and Related Health Problems: Ninth Revision and Clinical Modifications

The International Statistical Classification of Diseases and Related Health Problems: Ninth Revision and Clinical Modifications (ICD-9-CM) (World Health Organization, 1980) is the latest version of a mortality and morbidity classification that originated in 1893. The ICD-9-CM has been the sole classification used for morbidity reporting in the United States since 1979. It is widely accepted and used in the healthcare industry and has been adopted for a number of purposes including data collection, quality-of-care analysis, resource utilization, and statistical reporting. It is the basis for the diagnostic related groups (DRGs), which are used extensively for hospital reimbursement. ICD-9-CM is used primarily in the United States. Effective October 1, 2004 Medicare will no longer accept outpatient claims (including direct data entry [DDE]) with ICD-9 procedure codes. While ICD-9 procedure codes are the acceptable HIPAA code set for inpatient claims, Healthcare Common Procedure Coding System/Current Procedural Terminology (HCPCS/CPT) codes are the valid set for outpatient claims. Internationally, ICD-9 is used for death tabulation.

International Statistical Classification of Diseases and Related Health Problems: Tenth Revision

The International Statistical Classification of Diseases and Related Health Problems: Tenth Revision (ICD-10) (World Health Organization, 1992) is the most recent revision of the ICD classification system for mortality and morbidity, which is used worldwide. In addition to diagnostic labels, the ICD-10 also encompasses nomenclature structures. The U.S. version, ICD-10-CM, has yet to be broadly implemented in part due to its complexity; however, recent studies show migration to ICD-10-CM is supported by 83.6% of the health information management professional respondents who were the survey participants (AHIMA, 2003). A study of the costs and benefits of moving to the ICD-10 code sets determined that switching to both ICD-10-CM and IDC-10-PCS has the potential to generate more benefits than costs (Brahmakulam and Libicki, 2003).

Current Procedural Terminology, Fourth Revision

The Current Procedural Terminology, Fourth Revision (CPT-4) (American Medical Association, 1992) is a listing of descriptive terms and codes for reporting medical services and procedures. In addition to descriptive terms and codes, it contains modifiers, notes, and guidelines to facilitate correct usage. While primarily used in the United States for reimbursement purposes, it has, like ICD-9-CM, been adopted for other data purposes. Its use internationally has slowly increased.

Systemized Nomenclature of Human and Veterinary Medicine International, Clinical Terms

The Systemized Nomenclature of Human and Veterinary Medicine International, Clinical Terms (SNOMED) (College of American Pathologists, 1993) is a comprehensive, multiaxial nomenclature and classification system created for indexing human and veterinary medical vocabulary, including signs and symptoms, diagnoses, and procedures. It has gained increasing international acceptance as a standard for recording medical record information since its introduction in 1993. It is being used by a number of health professional specialty groups, and a subset of SNOMED is used in the DICOM imaging standard. SNOMED-CT is an inventory of medical and nursing terms and concepts for human and veterinary medicine arranged in a multihierarchical structure with multiple levels of granularity and relationships between concepts. NCVHS has recommended SNOMED-CT as one of several core terminologies to be adopted for federal healthcare service programs. The National Library of Medicine (NLM) and SNOMED have reached an agreement to use government funds to promote a common terminology in healthcare. Under the agreement the government will pay license fees for users of the terminology, thus removing some of the financial roadblocks to adoption of the SNOMED-CT-controlled clinical language in the U.S. HHS, the Department of Defense, and the Veterans Health Administration are also a part of the agreement.

LOINC Logical observation identifiers names and codes (LOINC) (Regenstrief Institute, 1994) provides a set of universal names and numeric identifier codes for laboratory and clinical observations and measurements in a database structure. The laboratory subset of LOINC was recommended for adoption by NCVHS. LOINC represents laboratory data in terms of names for tests and clinical observations. It is clear that such consistency in terminology is important for patient safety. Secretary Thompson recently announced additional standards for the electronic exchange of clinical health information to be adopted across the federal government as part of the Federal eGOV Health Information Exchange standards. These new standards include the use of LOINC to standardize the electronic exchange of laboratory test orders and drug label section headers.

RxNorm RxNorm is a clinical drug nomenclature produced by NLM, in consultation with the Food and Drug Administration (FDA), the Department of Veterans Affairs (VA), and HL7 SDO. RxNorm provides standard names for clinical drugs (active ingredient + strength + dose form) and for dose forms as administered. It provides links from clinical drugs to their active ingredients, drug components (active ingredient + strength), and some related brand names. To the extent available from the FDA, Nods (National Drug Codes) for specific drug products that deliver the clinical drug are stored as attributes of the clinical drug in RxNorm.

There are many more vocabularies, code sets, and classification systems in addition to those described above. The American Nurses Association has recognized the following nursing languages: Omaha System, Home Health Care Classification, Patient Care Data Set, Perioperative Nursing Data Elements, SNOMED-CT, International Classification for Nursing Practice, ABC Codes, LOINC, North American Nursing Diagnosis Association, Nursing Interventions Classification (NIC), Nursing Outcome Classification (NOC), nursing management minimum data set, and the nursing minimum data set (ANA, 2003).

Other domain-specific terminologies include Current Dental Terminology (CDT), International Medical Terminology (IMT), and Diagnostic and Statistical Manual of Mental Disorders (DSM-III-R) to name just a few. There have been a number of efforts to develop mapping and linkages among various code sets, classification systems, and vocabularies. One of the most successful is the Unified Medical Language System (UMLS) project undertaken by the U.S. NLM.

Unified Medical Language System There are specialized vocabularies, code sets, and classification systems for almost every practice domain in healthcare. Most of these are not compatible with one another, and much work needs to be done to achieve usable mapping and linkages between them. In 1986, the U.S. NLM began an ambitious long-term project to map and link a large number of vocabularies from a number of knowledge sources to allow retrieval and integration of relevant machine-readable information. Currently, the UMLS consists of a metathesaurus of terms and concepts from dozens of vocabularies; a semantic network of relationships among the concepts recognized in the metathesaurus; and an information sources map of the various biomedical databases referenced.

Data Content Standards

In addition to standardizing the format of health data messages and the lexicons and value domains used in those messages, there has been a great deal of interest in defining common sets of data for specific message types. The concept of a minimum data set is that of "a minimum set of items with uniform definitions and categories concerning a specific aspect or dimension of the healthcare system which meets the essential needs of multiple users" (Health Information Policy Council, 1983). A related concept is that of a core data element. It has been defined as "a standard data element with a uniform definition and coding convention to collect data on persons and on events or encounters" (National Committee on Vital and Health Statistics, 1996). Core data elements are seen as serving as the building blocks for well-formed minimum data sets and may appear in several minimum data sets.

As with vocabularies and code sets, there are many minimum data sets in place or under development. A recent survey of public and private sector efforts in the development of minimum data sets and core data elements reported on 17 such sets in use nationally (McCormick et al., 1997). The following are some brief examples of minimum, or core, data sets currently in use. As with code sets, professional specialty groups are the best source for current information on minimum data set development efforts. A number of SDOs, which develop messaging format standards such as HL7 and ASC X12N, have been increasingly interested in incorporating domain-specific data sets into their message standards.

National Uniform Claim Committee Recommended Data Set for a Noninstitutional Claim   The National Uniform Claim Committee (NUCC) was organized in 1995 to develop, promote, and maintain a standard data set for use in noninstitutional claims and encounter information. The committee is chaired by the American Medical Association, and its member organizations represent a number of the major public and private sector payers. The current NUCC data set forms the basis for the proposed noninstitutional claim and encounter standard proposed for national adoption under HIPAA (American Medical Association, 1997).

Standard Guide for Content and Structure of the Computer-Based Patient Record (ASTM E1384-96)   The American Society for Testing and Materials (ASTM) is one of the largest SDOs in the world and publishes over 9,000 standards covering all sectors in the economy. Committee E31 on Healthcare Informatics has developed a wide range of standards supporting the electronic management of health information. E1384-96 (American Society for Testing and Materials, 1996) provides a framework vocabulary for the computer-based patient record (CPR) content. It proposes a minimum essential content drawn from a developing annex of dictionary elements. It is used in conjunction with ASTM E1633-95, standard specification for coded values for the CPR (American Society for Testing and Materials, 1995). A new work item being proposed by the E31 subcommittee is the continuity of care record (CCR). The CCR is a core data set of the most relevant and timely facts about a patient's healthcare. It is to be prepared by a practitioner at the conclusion of a healthcare encounter in order to enable the next practitioner to readily access such information. It includes a summary of the patient's health status (e.g., problems, medications, allergies) and basic information about insurance, advance directives, care documentation, and care plan recommendations.

The Standards Development Process

The development and adoption of data standards is not only a technical process; it takes place within a sociopolitical context. Initially, there must be recognition that potential ambiguity exists at a level that would significantly impair communication and that this impairment is unacceptable within the social context. In healthcare, there is an increasing recognition that there exist significant opportunities to improve the quality of care provided and the outcomes associated with that care. It has also been recognized that any potential improvement in quality of care depends greatly on the ability to communicate healthcare information consistently, efficiently, and effectively. In its final report, the President's Information Technology Advisory Committee (2004) offered 12 specific recommendations for federal research and actions to enable development of twenty-first century electronic medical records systems.

At the core of such systems is the concept of a secure, patient-centered EHR that (1) safeguards personal privacy, (2) uses standardized medical terminology that can be correctly read by any care provider and incorporated into computerized tools to support clinical decision making, (3) eliminates the danger of illegible handwriting and missing patient information, and (4) can be transferred as a patient's care requires over a secure communications infrastructure for electronic information exchange (President's Information Technology Advisory Committee, 2004, p.1). Specific emphasis was placed on the need for developing a single set of data standards for the most common forms of clinical information.

Identification of a need for standardization, while necessary for development and implementation of standards, is not, in itself, sufficient. As with all things in life, there is never only one way to accomplish consistent communication of health information. Standards are resource-intensive to develop and to implement, particularly if an organization is already using a different way to do things. For this reason, widespread adoption of particular standards always involves "winners and losers" and so it becomes a political process.

While standards, when adopted, drive a consensus approach to data and information exchange and management, it does not follow that the development and adoption processes themselves are the result of a consensus-based methodology. There are primarily three ways in which standards are commonly developed and adopted: proprietary standards developed by vendors who hold a dominant position in the market, legislated standards developed by government organizations, and consensus-based standards developed by SDOs and adopted by virtue of their utility. An example of the first is CPT-4, developed by the American Medical Association and used for reimbursement of medical services and procedures. There are numerous examples of government-developed and government-mandated standards, such as the long-term care minimum data set required by the U.S. Centers for Medicare and Medicaid Services (CMS) to be reported for all long-term care residents in Medicare-certified long-term care facilities. An example of the third group is the messaging standards developed by the HL7 SDO and supported by a majority of health information systems vendors. Each of these approaches has its advantages and disadvantages.

Proprietary standards can often be developed quickly and are supported by available implementations and tools. If the developer can maintain a dominant market position, the standards can gain widespread acceptance quickly. Although proprietary standards can respond quickly to technologic changes, they can, paradoxically, also result in a delay in the adoption of new technologies as the creator of the standard wishes to gain a maximum return on the investment required to develop the standard in its current form. It may also not be responsive to changes in the environment, since it will reflect primarily the view of the creating organization and its market interests. Finally, in a sector as fragmented as healthcare, it is difficult for any organization to gain and retain the requisite dominant market position.

Legislated, government-developed standards are able to gain widespread acceptance by virtue of their being required by either regulation or in order to participate in large, government-funded programs, such as Medicare. Because government-developed standards are in the public domain, they are available at little or no cost and can be incorporated into any information system; however, they are often developed to support particular government initiatives and not be as suitable for general, private sector use. Also, given the amount of bureaucratic overhead attached to the legislative and regulatory process, it is likely that they will lag behind changes in technology and the general business environment.

Standards developed by SDOs are consensus-based and reflect the perspectives of a wide variety of interested stakeholders. They are generally not tied to specific systems. For this reason, they tend to be robust and adaptable across a range of implementations; however, most SDOs are voluntary organizations that rely on the commitment of dedicated individuals and organizations to develop and maintain standards. This often limits the amount of work that can be undertaken. In addition, the consensus process can be time consuming and result in a slow development process, which does not always keep pace with technologic change. Perhaps the most problematic aspect of consensus-based standards is that there is no mechanism to ensure that they are adopted by the industry, since there is usually little infrastructure

in place to actively and aggressively market them. This has resulted in the development of many technically competent standards that are never implemented.

Integrating the Healthcare Enterprise

Standards, while a necessary part of the solution, are not sufficient alone to fulfill the needs for interoperability. Integrating the healthcare enterprise (IHE) is an initiative that provides a detailed framework for implementing standards, filling the gap between standards, and their implementation (Wirsz, 2001). While IHE is not a standards body and does not create standards, it offers a common framework, available in the public domain, to understand and address critical integration needs. Vendors publish IHE integration statements to document the integration profiles supported by their products. Users can reference the appropriate integration profiles in requests for proposals, thus simplifying the systems acquisition process.

It is increasingly recognized that combining the strength of these initiatives and their approaches tends to minimize their weaknesses and can lead to significant gains for the healthcare sector as a whole. This melding of approaches is being achieved both at the organizational level by the development of coordinating bodies and consortia, and through the development of several national, government-directed initiatives.

Standards Coordination Efforts

It has become clear to both public and private sector standards development efforts that no one entity has the resources to create an exhaustive set of health data standards that will meet all needs. In addition to the various SDOs described above, the following organizations have been developed at the international, regional, and national levels to try and create a synergistic relationship between their member organizations. These larger organizations are involved in standards development across all sectors of the economy. Since many of the data standards issues in healthcare, such as security, are not unique to the healthcare sector, this breadth of scope offers the potential for technology transfer across sectors. The following is a brief description of some of the major international, regional, and national organizations involved in broad-based standards development and coordination.

International Organization of Standardization

The International Organization of Standardization (ISO) is an organization that develops and publishes standards internationally. ISO standards are developed, in large part, from standards brought forth by member countries, and through liaison activities with other SDOs. Often, these standards are further broadened to reflect the greater diversity of the international community. In 1998, ISO Technical Committee (TC) 215 on Health Informatics was formed to coordinate the development of international healthcare information standards, including data standards. Consensus on these standards will influence health informatics standards adopted in the United States and the interoperability of national and international health information exchange. This committee has recently published the first international standard for nursing titled *Integration of a Reference Terminology Model for Nursing*. This standard includes the development of reference terminology models for nursing diagnoses and nursing actions and relevant terminology and definitions for its implementation. The Healthcare Information and Management Systems Society (HIMSS) is the secretariat for ISO TC 215, as delegated by the ANSI. The United States Technical Advisory Group (TAG) determines the national position on standards being developed by this committee.

European Technical Committee for Standardization

In 1990, TC 251 on medical informatics was established by the European Committee for Standardization (CEN). CEN TC 251 works to develop a wide variety of standards in the area of healthcare data management and interchange. CEN standards are adopted by its member countries in Europe and are also submitted for development into ISO standards.

American National Standards Institute

The ANSI serves as the coordinator for voluntary standards activity in the United States. Standards are submitted to ANSI by member SDOs and are approved as American National Standards through a consensus methodology developed by ANSI. ANSI is also the U.S. representative to ISO and is responsible for bringing forward U.S. standards to that organization. In 1991, the ANSI Healthcare Informatics Standards Planning Panel was convened to act as a coordinating forum for both SDOs and other stakeholders in the area of health information standards. Rechartered as the ANSI Healthcare Informatics Standards Board (HISB) in 1996, ANSI HISB does not write standards but serves as a forum to identify needs and coordinate activities

related to healthcare information standardization. All of the major healthcare SDOs are HISB members, as well as a number of government agencies involved in health data standards, several major vendors of health information systems, and professional societies with an interest in healthcare information systems.

Object Management Group

While the organizations described so far are made up of voluntary SDOs, the Object Management Group (OMG) is representative of a different approach to standards development. OMG is an international consortium of over 800 organizations, primarily for-profit vendors of information systems technology, who are interested in the development of standards based on object-oriented technologies. While its standards are developed by private organizations, it has developed a process to lessen the potential problems noted above with proprietary standards. Standards developed in OMG are required to be implemented in a commercially available product by their developers within 1 year of the standard being accepted; however, the specifications for the standard are made publicly available. The OMG CORBAMed working group is responsible for development of object-based standards in the health information arena.

Health Insurance Portability and Accountability Act

Perhaps the single most important advance in the adoption of national health data standards was the passage in 1996 of HIPAA. It has been estimated that, on average, 26 cents of every dollar intended for healthcare is spent on administrative overhead. Administrative overhead includes such tasks as enrolling an individual in a health plan, paying health insurance premiums, checking insurance eligibility, getting authorization to refer a patient to a specialist, filing a claim for insurance reimbursement for delivered healthcare, requesting additional information to support a claim, coordinating the processing of a claim across different insurance companies, and notifying the provider about the payment of a claim. These processes involve numerous paper forms and telephone calls and many delays in communicating information between different locations, creating problems and costs for healthcare providers, plans, and insurers alike.

To address these problems, the healthcare industry has been attempting to develop standards to allow these transactions to be accomplished electronically, but it has been very difficult to get voluntary agreement from all of the competing parties involved to adopt a uniform set of such standards. Consequently, at the request of the industry, and with bipartisan support, Congress included the administrative simplification provisions (Title II, Subtitle F) in the HIPAA (Public Law 104-191, 1996), which was signed into law August 21, 1996. The industry estimates that full implementation of these provisions could save up to $9 billion per year from administrative overhead without reducing the amount or quality of healthcare services (Workgroup for Electronic Data Interchange [WEDI], 1993).

To make these savings in cost and administrative efficiency a reality, the law charges the U.S. secretary of HHS with establishing standards for a broad range of health information, including health insurance claims and encounters; health claims attachments; health insurance enrollment and eligibility; health identifiers for providers, health plans, employers, and individuals; code sets; and classification systems. To address concerns about the potential for abuse of electronic access to this type of information, the law also requires standards for the security and confidentiality of health information that might be associated with an individual. Civil and criminal penalties are prescribed for failure to use standards or for wrongful disclosure of confidential information.

The administrative simplification subtitle of the HIPAA represents the first time that the federal government has mandated health data standards on a national level. As can be seen from this very brief overview, this standards activity is likely to have a major impact on the development of electronic healthcare records beyond the administrative and financial realms. In today's world of quality-focused healthcare delivery, the line between administrative and clinical data is very blurred indeed. Although the transaction sets specified in this legislation are, perhaps, narrowly focused, the same cannot be said of the wide variety of supporting standards that must be adopted. Standards for such things as patient identifier, vocabularies, and electronic signatures have impact directly on anyone designing or implementing an electronic clinical system. In addition, the privacy and security legislation covers health information in the broad sense and will apply to any system handling personally identifiable information. Another important aspect of this legislation is that it preempts state law in most cases, thus establishing a consistent legal framework for electronic exchange of certain healthcare data.

As we continue to move toward compliance with all aspects of the HIPAA regulations, it is clear that the road has been rocky and full of both expected and unpredicted challenges. Clearly, the industry has made great progress over the past several years in its goal to achieve compliance and operationalize the HIPAA requirements, but recent survey results indicate that there is still much work to be done (Healthcare Information and Management Systems Society & Phoenix Health Systems, 2004).

National Committee on Vital and Health Statistics Subcommittee on Standards and Security

In addition to its focus on administrative and financial transactions, the administrative simplification provisions also begin the process of addressing the broader standards issues of electronic healthcare records in general. The subject of these recommendations and legislative proposals are set forth in Section 263 of the administrative simplification provisions of HIPAA. These provisions state that NCVHS

> (B) shall study the issues related to the adoption of uniform data standards for patient medical record information and the electronic exchange of such information;
>
> (C) shall report to the Secretary not later than 4 years after the date of the enactment of the Health Insurance Portability and Accountability Act of 1996 [August 2000] recommendations and legislative proposals for such standards and electronic exchange. (Public Law 104-191, 1996)

In order to meet this charge, the NCVHS formed the CPR Workgroup. This workgroup develops recommendations based on public hearings and input from informed stakeholders and domain experts. The workgroup has identified six major areas of interest (NCVHS, 1996):

1. Message format standards that contain PMRI. This area of focus includes message format syntaxes, document format standards, the role of information models to enable the development of message format standards, and the need to coordinate standards.

2. Medical terminology related to PMRI including data element definitions, data models, and code sets. This area of focus includes issues related to convergent medical terminologies, coordination and maintenance of vocabularies, coordination of drug knowledge bases, and other issues related to medical terminologies.

3. Business case issues related to the development and implementation of uniform data standards for

PMRI. This area of focus includes return-on-investment issues and the cost burden of vendors, SDOs, code set developers, and users to participate in the standards development processes.

4. National Healthcare Information Infrastructure (NHII). The vision of NHII and identification of issues related to it are being defined within the NHII workgroup of the NCVHS. The CPR Workgroup will identify the standards issues necessary to support this vision.

5. Data quality, accountability, and integrity related to PMRI. This area of focus includes data quality issues beginning with the initial capture or recording of data, the communication of data, the translation and encoding of data, and the decoding or presentation of data. It also includes the guidelines or standards for accountability and data integrity (e.g., accuracy, consistency, continuity, completeness, context, and comparability).

6. Inconsistencies and contradictions among state laws that discourage or prevent the creation, storage, or communication of PMRI in a consistent manner nationwide. Inconsistencies include laws for record retention, document authentication, access to records, and so forth.

In a report to the secretary of the U.S. Department of HHS, the CPR Workgroup stated that the lack of complete and comprehensive PMRI standards is a major constraint on the ability of our healthcare delivery system to enhance quality, improve productivity, manage costs, and safeguard data (NCVHS, 2000). In its recommendations the workgroup called on the government to take a leadership role in addressing these issues by accelerating the development, adoption, and coordination of PMRI standards. The committee has subsequently recommended two sets of PMRI standards including message formats and terminologies.

Consolidated Health Informatics

Another federal project that has great potential for furthering health data standards is the consolidated health informatics (CHI) initiative coordinated by the U.S. Department of Defense, the U.S. Department of VA, and the U.S. Department of HHS, Indian Health Service. The goal of this ambitious project is to develop and implement a standard means of exchanging and managing health information across federal health providers. It is not an attempt to develop a single federal EHR, but

rather, it is focusing on creating interoperability between health information systems in terms of how data are defined, structured, and exchanged. The Departments of HHS, Defense, and VA announced uniform standards for the electronic exchange of clinical health information to be adopted by the federal government. In the first phase, the agencies adopted a total of 20 standards including HL7 (multiple standards), NCPDP, IEEE 1073, DICOM, LOINC, SNOMED-CT, HIPAA, RxNorm, Human Gene Nomenclature (HUGN), and the Environmental Protection Agency's Substance Registry System.

Although this project is focused solely on federal healthcare providers, three factors increase its general interest and impact. First is the size of the population these organizations serve. Combined, these three organizations are the largest providers of healthcare in the United States by a considerable margin, both in terms of persons served and organizationally in terms of number of facilities and hospital beds. They are also geographically distributed throughout the United States and, in the case of the Department of Defense, in many parts of the world. This size makes them the largest purchaser of health information system technology in the United States, and any specifications developed for the CHI project will have a significant impact in the vendor community.

A second characteristic of the project extends this potential influence further. It was decided from the outset that the project would rely on standards-based solutions and that where standards did not exist, an effort would be made to foster their development through recognized SDOs. In addition, any technologies developed for this project are to be held in the public domain and will be available freely for use by other healthcare organizations, both public and private sector.

Finally, an explicit effort is being made to coordinate the CHI activities with those of the NCVHS CPR Workgroup. Key individuals participate in both initiatives, and it is hoped that the CHI experience can provide "real world" testing of some of the potential recommendations that the NCVHS will be making to the secretary and Congress.

Framework for Strategic Action

On April 27, 2004, President Bush called for widespread adoption of interoperable EHRs within 10 years and established the position of National Coordinator for Health Information Technology. Secretary Tommy Thompson appointed David Brailer, MD, PhD to serve in this new position. In fulfilling the requirements of the executive order, Dr. Brailer has submitted a report that outlines a framework for a strategic plan that will help the nation to realize a new vision for healthcare made possible through the use of information technology (Thompson and Brailer, 2004). These goals convey the vision for consumer-centric and information-rich healthcare.

Goal 1: Inform clinical practice
- Incentivize EHR adoption
- Reduce risk of EHR investment
- Promote EHR diffusion in rural and under-served areas

Goal 2: Interconnect clinicians
- Foster regional collaborations
- Develop a national health information network
- Coordinate federal health information systems

Goal 3: Personalize care
- Encourage use of PHRs
- Enhance informed consumer choice
- Promote use of telehealth systems

Goal 4: Improve population health
- Unify public health surveillance architectures
- Streamline quality and health status monitoring
- Accelerate research and dissemination of evidence

The Business Value of Data Standards

Clearly the importance of data standards to enhancing the quality and efficiency of healthcare delivery is being recognized by our national leadership. Reviewing the business value of defining and using data standards is critical for driving the implementation of these standards into applications and systems. Having data standards for data interchange and information modeling will provide a mechanism against which deployed systems can be validated (Loshin, 2004). Reducing manual intervention will increase worker productivity and streamline operations. Defining information exchange requirements will enhance the ability to automate interaction with external partners which in turn will decrease costs. Considering the value proposition for incorporating data standards into products, applications, and systems should be a part of every organization's information technology strategy.

Summary

This chapter discussed health data standards, organizations that develop them, the process by which they are developed, and examples of current standards initiatives. Data standards that deal with data communications include those describing common message formats and those that specify standardized code sets, classification systems, and vocabularies. Data standards that focus on the content of messages specify minimum data sets for specific purposes and commonly defined core data elements. A number of SDOs involved in the development of these types of standards were profiled.

A discussion of the standards development process highlighted the sociopolitical context in which standards are developed and the potential impact it has on the availability and currency of standards. The increasingly significant role of the federal government in influencing the development and adoption of health data standards is discussed. Several key initiatives, including HIPAA, CHI, and the framework for strategic action were described, and their potential impact was highlighted.

References

American Health Information Management Association. (2003). *ICD-10-CM Field Testing Project*. Chicago, IL.

American Medical Association. (1992). *Current Procedural Terminology* (fourth revision). Chicago, IL: AMA.

American Medical Association. (1997). *The National Uniform Claim Committee Data Set*. Chicago, IL: AMA.

American Society for Testing and Materials. (1995). *Standard Specification for Coded Values for the Computer-Based Patient Record E1633-95*. West Conshohocken, PA: ASTM

American Society for Testing and Materials. (1996). *Standard Guide for Content and Structure of the Computer-Based Patient Record E1384-96*. West Conshohocken, PA: ASTM.

Brahmakulam, I. and Libicki, M. (2003). *The Costs and Benefits of Moving to the ICD-10 Code Sets*. Arlington, VA: RAND Science and Technology.

College of American Pathologists. (1993). *SNOMED International: The Systemized Nomenclature of Human and Veterinary Medicine*. Northfield, IL: CAP.

Committee on Data Standards for Patient Safety. (2004). *Patient Safety: Achieving a New Standard for Care*. Washington, DC: Institute of Medicine.

Health Information Policy Council. (1983). *Background Paper: Uniform Minimum Health Data Sets*. Washington, DC: U.S. Department of Health and Human Services.

Healthcare Information and Management Systems Society & Phoenix Health Systems. (2004). U.S. Healthcare Industry HIPAA Survey Results: Summer 2004. Chicago, IL: HIMSS.

Loshin, D. (2004). The business value of data standards. *DM Review* 14(6):20.

McCormick, K.A., Renner, A.L., Mayes, R.W., et al. (1997). The Federal and private sector roles in the development of minimum data sets and core health data elements. *Computers in Nursing* 15 (2, Suppl.):S23–S32.

National Committee on Vital and Health Statistics. (1996). *Report of the National Committee on Vital and Health Statistics: Core Health Data Elements*. Washington, DC: Government Printing Office.

National Committee on Vital and Health Statistics. (2000). *Report to the Secretary of the U.S. Department of Health and Human Services on Uniform Data Standards for Patient Medical Record Information*. Washington, DC: Government Printing Office.

President's Information Technology Advisory Committee. (2004). *Revolutionizing Health Care Through Information Technology* Washington, DC: Government Printing Office.

Public Law 104–191. (1996). *Health Insurance Portability and Accountability Act of 1996*. Washington, DC: Government Printing Office.

Saba, V.K. and McCormick, K.A. (2000). *Essentials of Computers for Nurses: Informatics for the New Millennium* (3rd ed.). New York: McGraw-Hill.

Thompson, T.G. and Brailer, D.J. (2004). *The Decade of Health Information Technology: Delivering Consumer-centric and Information-rich Health Care. Framework for Strategic Action*. Washington, DC: Government Printing Office.

Washington Publishing Company. (1998). *Overview of Healthcare EDI Transactions: A Business Primer*. Frederick, MD.

Wirsz, N. (2001). IHE: Future directions. In P. Vegoda (Ed.), *Integrating the Healthcare Enterprise*. Chicago, IL: Healthcare Information and Management Systems Society.

Workgroup for Electronic Data Interchange. (1993). *WEDI Report*. Washington, DC.:WEDI.

World Health Organization. (1980). *International Classification of Diseases: 9th Revision: Clinical Modifications (ICD-9-CM)*. Geneva, Switzerland:WHO.

World Health Organization. (1992). *International Statistical Classification of Diseases and Related Health Problems (ICD-10)*. Geneva, Switzerland:WHO.

Web Sites

The field of data standards is a very dynamic one with existing standards undergoing revision and new standards being developed. The best way to learn about specific standards activities is to get involved in the process. All of the organizations discussed in this chapter provide opportunities to be involved with activities that support standards development and implementation. Listed below are the World Wide Web addresses for each organization. Most sites describe current activities and publications available and many have links to other related sites.

Accredited Standards Committee (ASC) X12. *http://www.disa.org* or *http://www.wpc.edi.com*

American National Standards Institute (ANSI). *http://www.ansi.org*

American Society for Testing and Materials (ASTM). *http://www.astm.org*

Consolidated Health Informatics (CHI). *http://www.whitehouse.gov/omb/gtob/health_informatics.htm*

Digital Imaging Communication in Medicine Standards Committee (DICOM). *http://www.nema.org*

European Technical Committee for Standardization Technical Committee 251 on Medical Informatics (CEN TC251). *http://www.centc251.org*

Health Insurance Portability and Accountability Act (HIPAA). *http://aspe.os.dhhs.gov/admnsimp*

Health Level Seven (HL7). *http://www.hl7.org*

Institute of Electrical and Electronic Engineers (IEEE). *http://www.ieee.org*

Integrating the Healthcare Enterprise (IHE). *http://www.himss.org/ihe*

International Standards Organization (ISO). *http://www.iso.org*

International Statistical Classification of Diseases and Related Health Problems (ICD-9, ICD-9CM, ICD-10). *http://www.cdc.gov/nchswww/*

National Committee on Vital and Health Statistics (NCVHS). *http://aspe.os.dhhs.gov/ncvhs*

National Council for Prescription Drug Programs (NCPDP). *http://www.ncpdp.org*

Object Management Group (OMG). *http://www.omg.org*

Office of the National Coordinator for Health Information Technology (ONCHIT). *http://www.hhs.gov/onchit/index.html*

Systemized Nomenclature of Human and Veterinary Medicine (SNOMED®) International. *http://www.snomed.org*

Unified Medical Language System (UMLS). *http://www.nlm.nih.gov/research/umls/*

14

Electronic Health Record Systems: U.S. Federal Initiatives and Public/Private Partnerships

Linda Fischetti
Mary Jo Deering

OBJECTIVES

1. Define the terms electronic health record (EHR), distinguishing it from the electronic health record system (EHR-S).
2. Summarize the history of use of health information technology (HIT) by federal health provider communities.
3. Discuss how federal agencies that do not provide direct patient care play a leadership role in healthcare.
4. Describe the creation of the office of the National Coordinator for Health Information Technology (ONCHIT).
5. Identify key public/private partnerships and the focus of their efforts.

KEY WORDS

electronic health record
electronic health record system
federal agencies
federal healthcare providers
public/private partnerships

In April 2004, the president of the United States issued an executive order that called for action to put EHRs in place for most Americans in 10 years. (White House, 2004) This order gave new momentum to efforts across the healthcare community to use HIT to improve healthcare. For over a decade, the Institute of Medicine (IOM) has been calling for the use of information technology (IT) to improve the efficiency, safety, and quality of the healthcare Americans receive in a series of groundbreaking reports (Dick, Steen, and Detmer, 1991, 1997; Kohn, Corrigan, and Donaldson, 2000; Corrigan, Donaldson, and Kohn, 2001; Corrigan, Eden, and Smith, 2003; Aspden et al., 2004).

Today, there is growing consensus that EHR-Ss, can meet clinical and business needs in healthcare by capturing, storing, and displaying clinical information when and where it is needed to improve treatment and to provide aggregated cross-patient data analysis. These systems can manage healthcare data and information in a way that is patient-centered and information-rich. Improved information access and availability can enable both the provider and the patient to better manage the patient's health by using capabilities provided by enhanced clinical decision support and customized education materials.

The involvement of nurses is critical to such efforts. Responsible for care coordination and promotion of wellness, nurses are often the patient's primary contact—and the final point in healthcare delivery where medical errors and other unintended actions can be caught and corrected. As the largest human resource in healthcare, nurses are drivers in organizational planning and process reengineering to improve the healthcare delivery system. Increasingly, nurses and nurse managers are turning to nurse informaticists for leadership as their profession works to bring IT applications into the healthcare environment.

After a brief overview and discussion of the definition of EHR-Ss, this chapter covers two main areas: federal initiatives and public-private partnerships. The description of federal initiatives focuses on agencies that provide direct care and those which use a variety of mechanisms to provide leadership toward an interoperable IT-enabled healthcare environment. The discussion of public-private partnerships includes groups newly formed to address issues of electronic connectivity, professional association that have done so as part of their attempts to serve their membership, and long established standards development organizations. The chapter concludes by highlighting progress to date and challenges nurse informaticists to take a more active role in future activities.

Overview

An early adopter of EHR-S, the U.S. government is currently advancing initiatives to accelerate the use of HIT in both the public and private sectors. Private groups have been instrumental in promoting awareness of the benefits of EHR-S across their memberships, including standards organizations that have developed standards for EHR-S architecture, messaging, and functions.

Both sectors have done considerable EHR-S innovation and some notable benchmark implementation over the past decade. This pioneering work has validated the IOM recommendations that HIT can provide proven, quantifiable improvements in safety, quality, and efficiency. Even with this success, however, there continues to be a sharp dichotomy within the healthcare community between early adopters who quickly grow to depend on the added knowledge and availability of information an EHR-S provides and those who have not embraced EHR-S implementation. For the latter group, potential barriers to adopting technology range from locating the initial capital investment or the systems that provide needed functions, to factors such as resistance to change and the time needed to transform organizational processes.

Federal initiatives continue to actively identify and target solutions that lessen the barriers and accelerate use of EHR-S. Development and implementation in conformance with existing and future standards activities are crucial to achieving interoperable systems.

 ## Defining Electronic Health Record Systems

The term EHR-S is often used interchangeably with computerized patient record, clinical information system, electronic medical record, and many others. Yet the choice of the words in the term EHR-S reflects the broader focus on the health of the consumer or patient and indicates that the EHR-S may be used by all participants in the process of achieving health, including all disciplines of clinicians, family caregivers, and the patient. As a term, EHR-S is recognized internationally.

By including the word system, the term forces a distinction between an EHR, which is a physical or logical (virtual) repository of data, and an EHR-S, which can be made up of one or more applications. The latter, the EHR-S, provides the components that support clinical and healthcare functions including business rules, procedures, and so forth by accessing the EHR to write and/or read patient data (ISO/TS 18308, 2004). At the time of this writing, the International Organization for Standardization (ISO) had drafted its standard for EHR definition, scope, and context, ISO 20514; the final version was expected in 2005 or 2006.

The IOM's 1991 definition of computer-based patient record system is currently the basis for domestic and international definitions of an EHR-S:

> The set of components that form the mechanism by which patient records are created, used, stored, and retrieved. A patient record system is usually located within a healthcare provider setting. It includes people, data, rules and procedures, processing and storage devices (e.g., paper and pen, hardware and software), and communication and support facilities. (Dick, Steen, and Detmer, 1991)

In its use of the word system, the IOM drew a visionary distinction between a dynamic system and a static record. This distinction continues in international definitions today and will likely become more useful in the United States as the domestic knowledge of EHRs and EHR-Ss grows.

Recently, the IOM modified this definition in its report, Key Capabilities of an Electronic Health Record System (2003), reiterating the new definition in a report on patient safety (Aspden et al., 2004). An EHR-S includes the following:

1. longitudinal collection of electronic health information for and about persons, where health information is defined as information pertaining to the health

of an individual or healthcare provided to an individual;

2. immediate electronic access to person- and population-level information by authorized, and only authorized, users;

3. provision of knowledge and decision support that enhances the quality, safety, and efficiency of patient care; and

4. support of efficient processes for healthcare delivery.

Federal Initiatives

Within the federal government, different departments exert different influences toward the common goal of an EHR for most Americans. Agencies providing direct healthcare offer evidence that the use of EHR-Ss across a multifacility enterprise is a realistic goal with measurable, repeatable positive outcomes. Other agencies provide leadership by offering monetary incentives; funding research, development, and demonstration projects; and shaping regulations and policy.

Government as Provider and Early Adopter

Federal agencies that provide direct care have been early adopters of EHR-S. The Veterans Health Administration in the Department of Veterans Affairs (VA) and the National Institutes of Health (NIH) in the Department of Health and Human Services (HHS) are two examples of the initiation of systems in the 1970s that were actively used by clinicians (Kolodner, 1997; *http://www.cc.nih.gov/dcri/index.html*). The Department of Defense (DoD) and the Indian Health Service (IHS) in the Department of HHS both acquired the VA's original clinical information system years ago, customizing it to meet their clinical and business needs (Kolodner, 1997).

Department of Veterans Affairs   The Veterans Health Information Systems and Technology Architecture (VistA) supports day-to-day clinical and administrative operations at local VA healthcare facilities. (VA 2004) Long a leader, VA dates its computerization efforts back to the early 1980s. In the 1990s, a graphic user interface was added to bundle all existing functions from VistA and present them in an interface that was easier for the clinical user. This new interface named the computerized patient record system (CPRS) provided a single place for healthcare providers to review and update a patient's health record and order medications, special procedures, x-rays, nursing orders, diets, and laboratory tests. Once

in a graphic environment, users quickly requested new functionality capitalizing on visual displays such as images and graphs. Currently CPRS supports 158 hospitals and 854 clinics in processing 865,000 orders, over a half a million progress notes (with discharge summaries), and 585,000 medications administered via VA's Bar Code Medication Administration per day (Perlin, 2004).

All aspects of a patient's record are integrated, including active problems, allergies, current medications, laboratory results, vital signs, hospitalizations, and outpatient clinic history. All electronic records are password protected to guarantee patient privacy. Other features include the following:

- A checking system that alerts clinicians if an order they are entering could cause a problem

- A notification system that immediately alerts clinicians to clinically significant events

- A visual posting system that alerts healthcare providers to issues specifically related to the patient on the opening of the patient's electronic chart, including crisis notes, adverse reactions, and advance directives

- A template system that allows the healthcare provider to automatically create reports

- A clinical reminder system that electronically alerts clinicians when certain actions, such as examinations, immunizations, patient education, and laboratory tests, need to be performed

- Remote data viewing to allow clinicians to see the patient's medical history at all the VA facilities where the patient was seen.

In 2004, VA began implementing MyHealtheVet as an Internet tool for personal health management. It permits veterans to voluntarily interact with subsets of their VistA health record and, ultimately, manage their own personal health record (PHR) (*www.myhealth.va.gov*).

Department of Defense   Within DoD, providers have had a computerized physician order entry capability that enables them to order lab tests and radiology examinations and issue prescriptions electronically for over 10 years. In January 2004, DoD began a worldwide rollout of the next generation system, the composite health care system II (CHCS II), a secure, scalable, patient-centric EHR-S. As of May 2004, CHCS II had more than 1.3 million patient encounters recorded in and available from its database (*www.dod.gov/releases/2004/nr20040511-1222.html*).

In addition, DoD's Pharmacy Data Transaction Service links military treatment facilities, mail order, and network pharmacies. This service enables providers at all military and civilian pharmacies to track nearly 400,000 daily medication transactions and to check for drug allergies and drug interactions. Because beneficiaries have come to rely more and more on the Internet for information and services, the department has developed Tricare Online, a secure Web portal through which its 8.9 million beneficiaries and physicians can access 18 million pages of verified health information and schedule appointments (*www.tricareonline.com*).

Indian Health Service   The IHS has long been a pioneer in using computer technology to capture clinical and public health data. Its Resource and Patient Management System (RPMS) was developed in the 1970s, and many facilities have access to decades of personal health information and epidemiologic data on local populations. Its primary clinical component, the patient care component (PCC), has been in place since the early 1980s. The next phase of clinical software development for IHS is IHS-EHR (*www.ihs.gov/CIO/EHR*). Many of its components are imported from the VA's CPRS and adapted to fit the business needs of the IHS clinical environments of care.

Government as Leader

Federal agencies that do not provide direct care are taking multiple approaches to promote use of EHR-S. These include decreasing the cost and risk of acquisition and providing incentives for their use. Other activities target the sharing of electronic data across and among systems to provide a patient-centric view of data across organizational boundaries and to make information available in a de-identified (all personal identifying data removed), aggregate form for population analysis and disease surveillance.

Federal activities are focused on the development and adoption of terminologies and standards, grants for community demonstrations of data exchange, and other pilot projects. The government is also pursuing the development of a public-private national health information network to facilitate EHR-S deployment.

Office of the National Coordinator for Health Information Technology

The executive order of April 2004, mentioned earlier in the chapter, created the ONCHIT to coordinate HIT efforts in the federal sector and to collaborate with the private sector in driving HIT adoption across the healthcare system. David Brailer, MD, PhD, was named to fill the subcabinet-level post. Steps outlined for coordinating public and private sector efforts included the completion and adoption of standards that allow medical information to be stored and shared electronically while assuring privacy and security, increased funding for demonstration projects on HIT to $100 million in FY 2005 (subsequently reduced by Congress), and the identification of opportunities where government supports, provides, or pays for healthcare to create incentives and opportunities for healthcare providers to use electronic records.

In July 2004, HHS Secretary Tommy Thompson and Dr. Brailer released a framework for strategic action. Intended to guide collaborative efforts to promote progress toward a consumer-centric and information-rich healthcare industry, the framework identified four goals to achieve the vision of using IT to improve healthcare delivery, as shown in Table 14.1.

The office of the national coordinator is positioned to bring together public and private entities for accelerating solutions to known problems. To assist in this collaborative effort, the strategic framework envisions a health information technology leadership panel, a private interoperability consortium for the development of a national health information network, private certification of HIT products, and demonstrations for community health information exchange. The national health information network is the technical infrastructure enabling national interoperability. Regional health information organizations are now being proposed at the community, regional, or state level, as mentioned in the discussion of the Agency for Healthcare Research and Quality (AHRQ).

The National Committee on Vital and Health Statistics

In 2000 and 2001, the National Committee on Vital and Health Statistics (NCVHS), which advises the secretary of HHS on health information policy, held a series of national hearings to develop a consensus vision of the National Health Information Infrastructure (NHII). In the resulting report, Information for Health, NCVHS (2002) presented the concept of an infrastructure that emphasizes health-oriented interactions and information-sharing among individuals and institutions, rather than simply the physical, technical, and data systems that make those interactions possible. It further defined the NHII as including the values, practices, relationships, laws, standards, systems, applications, and technologies that support all facets of individual health, healthcare, and population health. The NHII also encompasses tools such as clinical practice guidelines, educational resources for the public and professionals, geographic information systems permitting regional

Table 14.1   Goals of the Strategic Framework

Goal 1

Inform Clinical Practice: Informing clinical practice is fundamental to improving care and making healthcare delivery more efficient. This goal centers largely around efforts to bring EHRs directly into clinical practice. This will reduce medical errors and duplicative work, and enable clinicians to focus their efforts more directly on improved patient care. Three strategies for realizing this goal are:

Strategy 1: Incentivize EHR adoption
Strategy 2: Reduce risk of EHR investment
Strategy 3: Promote EHR diffusion in rural and under-
        sergved areas

Goal 2

Interconnect Clinicians: Interconnecting clinicians will allow information to be portable and to move with consumers from one point of care to another. This will require an interoperable infrastructure to help clinicians get access to critical healthcare information when their clinical and/or treatment decisions are being made. The three strategies for realizing this goal are:

Strategy 1: Foster regional collaboration
Strategy 2: Develop a national health information network
Strategy 3: Coordinate federal health information systems

Goal 3

Personalize Care: Consumer-centric information helps individuals manage their own wellness and assists with their personal healthcare decisions. The ability to personalize care is a critical component of using healthcare information in a meaningful manner. The three strategies for realizing this goal are:

Strategy 1: Encourage use of personal health records
Strategy 2: Enhance informed consumer choice
Strategy 3: Promote use of telehealth systems

Goal 4

Improve Population Health: Population health improvement requires the collection of timely, accurate, and detailed clinical information to allow for the evaluation of healthcare delivery and the reporting of critical findings to public health officials, clinical trials and other research, and feedback to clinicians. Three strategies for realizing this goal are:

Strategy 1: Unify public health surveillance architectures
Strategy 2: Streamline quality and health status monitoring
Strategy 3: Accelerate research and dissemination of evidence

Source: Thompson, T. and Brailer, D. (2004). *The Decade of Health Information Technology, Delivering Consumer-centric and Information-rich Health Care: Framework for Action.* Washington, DC: U.S. Department of Health and Human Services. Available at *http://www.os.dhhs.gov/healthit/documents/hitframework.pdf*

analysis and comparisons, health statistics at all levels of government, and many forms of communication among users. It is neither a system of systems, nor a centralized government database for storing personal health information. Health data and health information reside in myriad locations, connected within the framework of a secure network (NCVHS, 2002).

As envisioned by NCHVS, PHRs are a core component of the NHII, enhancing the ability of each individual to control his or her health data and the access by healthcare providers to those data. EHRs, including PHRs, are both *enabled by* the NHII, in the sense that their optimal use and effectiveness requires the comprehensive infrastructure, and *enablers of* the NHII, because of their capacity to store, organize, display, and exchange crucial health information. Thus, the NCHVS vision of the NHII has become accepted as the comprehensive concept of information linkages across all aspects of health and healthcare. Figure 14.1 presents a conceptual overview of the NHII, now moved organizationally to the ONCHIT.

Agency for Healthcare Research and Quality   In 2003–2004, AHRQ unveiled a major HIT portfolio, with grants, contracts, and other activities to demonstrate the role of HIT in improving patient safety and the quality of care. About $24 million funded new implementation grants for healthcare organizations; of this amount, $14 million was targeted for small and rural hospitals and communities. An additional $7 million supported new planning grants to provide communities and organizations with the resources to develop their HIT infrastructure; about $5 million of this amount was for rural and small communities. Grants to demonstrate the value—or return on investment (ROI)—derived from the adoption, diffusion, and use of HIT totalled approximately $10 million. The objective of these projects was to provide healthcare facilities and providers with the information they need to make informed clinical and purchasing decisions about using HIT. AHRQ also awarded the IHS $2 million in fiscal year 2004 toward the enhancement of the IHS EHR. Individual facilities were given flexibility in how they configured their EHR-Ss.

In addition, AHRQ funded demonstration grants to establish and implement interoperable health information systems and data sharing to improve the quality, safety, efficiency, and effectiveness of healthcare for patients and populations on a specific state or regional level.

In support of these grantees, AHRQ contracted over $18 million for a health information technology resource center to provide technical assistance, serve as a repository for best practices, and disseminate tools to help providers

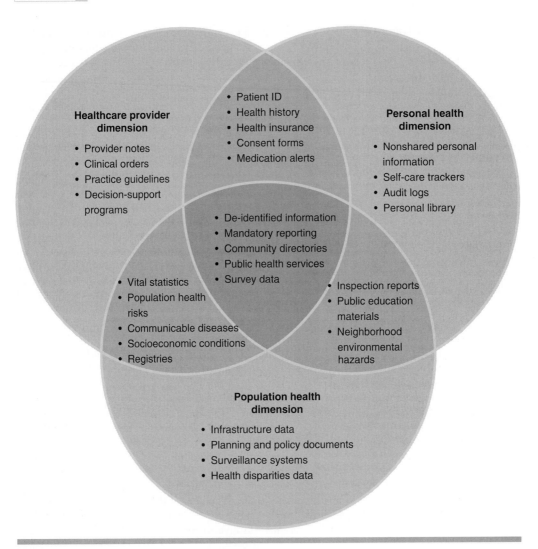

Figure 14.1
The three dimensions of the National Health Information Infrastructure and examples of their content.
(Source: National Committee on Vital and Health Statistics (2004). *Information for health: A strategy for building the National Health Information Infrastructure, report and recommendations.* Washington, DC: U.S. Department of Health and Human Services.)

explore the adoption and use of HIT to improve patient safety and quality of care. The center also supports EHRs collaboration among IHS sites and federally supported health centers, such as the Health Resources and Services Administration and the Centers for Medicare and Medicaid Services (CMS).

In 2004, AHRQ also funded five contracts of about $1 million per year for 5 years each for state and regional demonstrations of health IT. The five entities (Colorado, Indiana, Rhode Island, Tennessee, and Utah) must implement statewide data sharing and interoperability activities to improve the quality, safety, efficiency, and effectiveness of healthcare for patients and populations at discrete state or regional levels.

The state and regional grantees must involve wide variety of healthcare settings, including major purchasers of healthcare; significant payers, both public and private; and providers, including hospitals, ambulatory care facilities, home healthcare, and long-term care providers. They are also required to determine core clinical data elements for data exchange, using standards adopted by the Federal Consolidated Health Informatics (CHI) initiative where possible. The entities must determine core healthcare entities for data exchange and exchange 25% of this core care data in the first year, 50% in the second, and 100% in the third. By the end of the contracts, they must also report on financial, technical, organizational, personnel, cultural, and procedural lessons learned.

Centers for Medicare and Medicaid Services

Within HHS, the CMS has initiated several pilot projects to promote health IT. In May 2004, CMS awarded a $100,000 grant to the American Academy of Family Physicians (AAFP) for a pilot project to provide comprehensive, standardized EHR software to small- and medium-sized ambulatory care practices. By assessing the transition to EHRs in these practices, AAFP intends to learn more about what factors facilitate or hinder smooth adoption of the technology.

Several large pilot programs were authorized in the 2003 Medicare Modernization Act (MMA). The 3-year Care Management Performance Demonstration Program is intended to promote continuity of care, help stabilize medical conditions, prevent or minimize acute exacerbations of chronic conditions, and reduce adverse health outcomes, such as adverse drug interactions. Under this pay-for-performance program, physicians are using IT (such as e-mail and clinical alerts and reminders) and evidence-based medicine to meet the needs of beneficiaries. In another program, MMA called for the NCHVS to develop a national standard for electronic prescriptions, so that providers can share information on what medications a patient is taking and to be alerted for possible adverse drug interactions. Under MMA, the federal government is authorized to give grants to doctors to help them buy computers, software, and training to get ready for electronic prescribing.

At the end of 2004, CMS launched the Chronic Care Improvement Program (CCIP), with CCIP pilots that offer self-care guidance and support to chronically ill beneficiaries. The aim is to help beneficiaries manage their health, adhere to the plans of care given by their physicians, and assure that they seek or obtain medical care that they need to reduce their health risks. Although the use of health IT is not mandatory, CMS views CCIP as a significant opportunity to demonstrate innovative, integrative information infrastructures and communication technologies.

Public-Private Partnerships

A number of collaborative efforts are focused on the use of EHR-Ss and HIT to improve care. Among these private sector organizations are those formed specifically to address issues of connectivity, HIT, and standards development. Others are established standards development organizations; some are based in professional association, where they arose in efforts to serve their memberships.

The collaborations covered below represent only a portion of those underway. Given the current level of activity in this arena, the listing provided here will quickly become out of date.

Connecting for Health

A large private collaborative with federal participants supported by the Markle and the Robert Wood Johnson Foundations, Connecting for Health is addressing the barriers to development of an interconnected health information infrastructure. It brings together several dozen of the leading healthcare provider and payer organizations, HIT vendors, and representatives of federal and state agencies. The first phase of its work drove consensus on the adoption of an initial set of data standards, developed case studies on privacy and security, and helped define the electronic PHR (Markle, 2004).

More recently, in July 2004, Connecting for Health released an incremental "roadmap" that laid out near-term actions necessary to achieving electronic connectivity. To carry out its work, Connecting for Health organized several working groups focusing on understanding the business and organizational issues of community-based information exchange, the issues relevant to sharing electronic information with patients, and several aspects of technical interoperability. The initiative has identified key issues and opportunities for PHR development as well.

eHealth Initiative

The eHealth Initiative (*www.ehealthinitiative.org*) is an independent, nonprofit affiliated organization established to foster improvement in the quality, safety, and efficiency of healthcare through information and IT. Its membership brings together hospitals and other providers, practicing clinicians, community organizations, payers, employers, community-based organizations, HIT suppliers, manufacturers, and academic organizations. It is affiliated with the Foundation for eHealth Initiative, which shares its mission and provides funding for its initiatives.

The major program of the foundation for eHealth Initiative is *Connecting Communities for Better Health,* a nearly $4 million program that provides seed funding and technical support to multistakeholder collaboratives within communities (both geographic and nongeographic) that are using electronic health information exchange and other HIT tools to drive improvements in healthcare quality, safety, and efficiency. Funded under a cooperative agreement with the HHS Health Resources and Services Administration office for the advancement of telehealth, *Connecting Communities for Better Health* is implementing activities on a national, regional, and local basis that will lay the foundation for an interconnected, electronic, standards-based health information infrastructure to support patients, clinicians, and those responsible for population health (*http://ccbh.ehealthinitiative.org/communities/funded.mspx*).

Institute of Medicine

As an independent advisor to the nation with the goal of improving health, the IOM has championed the advantages of use of IT to improve healthcare since its 1991 foundational work, The computer-based patient record, which was revised and republished in 1997 (Dick, Steen, and Detmer, 1991, 1997). The IOM continues to illuminate the importance for the use of IT in healthcare. In the 2002 report, Leadership by Example: Coordinating Government Roles in Improving Health Care Quality, the IOM showcased federal programs and encouraged the development of an information infrastructure for the comparison of data to evaluate performance (Corrigan, Eden, and Smith, 2002). In summer 2003, at the request of HHS, the IOM issued a report, Key Capabilities of an Electronic Health Record System, Letter Report, which identified key functions of EHRs in four settings: hospitals, ambulatory care, nursing homes, and care in the community (PHRs). The report created a framework for identifying core functions of an EHR-S, along with the primary and secondary uses of these systems (Committee on Data Standards for Patient Safety, 2003).

Certification Commission for Health Information Technology

The Health Information and Management Systems (HIMSS, *www.himss.org*), American Health Information Management Association (AHIMA, *www.ahima.org*), and National Alliance for Health Information Technology (NAHIT, *www.nahit.org*) have joined together to establish the Certification Commission for Health Information

Technology (CCHIT) (HIMSS, 2004). The goal of this group is to support Goal 1, Strategy 2, "Reduce risk of EHR investment" of the strategic framework shown in Table 14.1. Twelve commissioners serve on the certification group, with two ex-officio (nonvoting members) representing the federal government.

Health Level Seven

An international, not-for-profit, volunteer standards organization, Health Level Seven (HL7, 2004) is known for its large body of work in the production of technical specifications for the transfer of healthcare data. This transport mechanism, known as messaging, is widely used domestically and internationally. As an organization, HL7 continues to have technical specifications for messages as the primary body of its work product but is changing to address additional technical solutions for the transport of healthcare data.

Supported by public and private groups, the HL7's EHR Technical Committee developed a draft standard for trial use, known as a DSTU, for EHR-Ss and made it available for public comment prior to being reballoted as a standard. Consistent with HL7 practice, if the trial period did not result in subsequent ballots, the draft status would expire at the end of a 2-year period of 2004–2006.

The draft received unprecedented preballot validation from over 1,000 individuals. The majority of the preballot outreach to industry was done with the EHR Collaborative (*www.ehrcollaborative.org*) to engage the clinical segment of healthcare. Participation by the clinical community resulted in significant improvements to the draft, producing a more useful ballot and moving the work much closer to its original goal of being a communication tool between clinical and technical segments of industry.

The HL7 EHR-S functional model contains a list of functions in three categories: direct care, supportive, and information infrastructure. The direct care functions are familiar to clinicians; contained in the user interface, these functions are needed to support direct care delivery. The supportive functions involve secondary use of the data captured via the direct care functions; these functions support enhanced functions for direct care and advanced information handling needs for the organization. The information infrastructure section is the "backend" of the system; unfamiliar to many clinicians, this is considered essential by informaticists and technical staff.

The act of customizing the HL7 EHR-S functional model is the creation of a profile. The types of profiles that can be created are defined by the user. As profile developed by clinicians to provide care to their patient population is called a use profile; a list of functions customized to describe a vendor product is called a product profile. As the scenario in Table 14.2 illustrates, this tool may be useful to nurse informaticists. The users of this tool are encouraged to provide feedback and participate in the continued maturation of this product (*www.hl7.org*).

Table 14.2 Developing a Use Profile with the Draft Standard for Trial Use: A Scenario

Step 1

With the help of a nurse informaticist, a small group of clinical subject matter experts generates a definition of the environment in which the EHR-S is to be used. The definition identifies existing legislative or organizational definitions of the environment (e.g., more than *x* number of clinicians) and states what is in and out of scope for that environment (e.g., long-term acute care vs. long-term subacute care).

Step 2

The clinical experts review the list of functions and prioritize each function as Essential Now, Essential Future, Optional, or Nonapplicable to each function. This produces a customized list of functions the clinical experts believe they need now or in the future.

Step 3

Using the list, the nurse informaticist prepares a "story board" that shows the work flow and clinical functions to be performed within that work flow and marks the clinical functions with the function identifier from the EHR-S DSTU.

Step 4

The nurse informaticist presents the story board to a larger group of clinicians who validate that it is comprehensive and accurately portrays the activities of the clinical environment.

Step 5

The final validated story board is used as a tool to communicate the clinical work flow integrated with the EHR-S functions needed to support the clinical environment or compare to a product profile for the selection of a product that is able to support the clinical environment.

 ## Looking to the Future

The year 2004 was a year of amazing growth, in federal initiatives and in public-private partnerships.

Federal agencies that had been early adopters of EHR-Ss continued to launch new programs and new capabilities; others offered new incentives to the healthcare community to embrace EHRs and the creation of the ONCHIT provided new leadership at a time public-private partnerships for common solutions were already increasing across federal and community environments.

Over the next 10 years, as the nation moves toward the goal of EHRs for most Americans, nurse informaticists will have increased opportunities to participate in the activities of these formative groups, using the growing body of tools available to them. This time of great change brings grand opportunities for nursing informaticists and the entire nursing profession.

 ## References

Aspden, P., Corrigan, J. M., Wolcott, J., and Erison, S. (Eds.). (2004). *Patient safety: Achieving a new standard for care* (pp. 3–17). Report of the committee on data standards for patient safety. Washington, DC: National Academy Press.

Committee on Data Standards for Patient Safety. (2003). *Key Capabilities of an Electronic Health Record System: Letter Report*. Washington, DC: National Academies Press.

Committee on Quality of Health Care in America. (2001). Using information technology. In J. M. Corrigan, M. S. Donaldson, and L. T. Kohn (Eds.), *Crossing the Quality Chasm: A New Health System for the 21st century* (pp. 175–192). Washington, DC: National Academy Press.

Corrigan, J., Eden, J., and Smith, B. (Eds.). (2002). *Leadership by Example: Coordinating Government Roles in Improving Health Care Quality*. Washington, DC: National Academy Press.

Dick, R., Steen, E., and Detmer, D. (Eds.). (1991). *The Computer-Based Patient Record: An Essential Technology for Health Care*. Washington, DC: National Academy Press.

Dick, R., Steen, E., and Detmer, D. (Eds.). (Rev. ed., 1997). *The Computer-Based Patient Record: An Essential Technology for Health Care*. Washington, DC: National Academy Press.

Health Information and Management Systems Society (HIMSS). (2004, September 1). *Certification Commission for Healthcare Information Technology Names Inaugural Slate of Commissioners*. Retrieved October 8, 2004, from *http://himss.org/asp/Content Redirector.asp?Contentid=547=97*.

Health Information and Management Systems Society (HIMSS). (2003). *Position Statement: National Health Information Infrastructure.* Retrieved June 21, 2004, from *www.himss.org/content/files/NHII_Fact_Sheet.pdf*

Health Level 7. (2004). *HL7 EHR System Functional Model and Standard: Draft Standard for Trial Use.* Release 1.0, July 2004. *www.hl7.org/ehr*

International Standard Organization, Technical Standard (ISO/TS) 18308. (2004). *Requirements for an Electronic Health Record Reference Architecture.* Retrieved October 7, 2004, from *www.iso.org/iso/en/CatalogueDetailPage*

Kolodner, R. M. (1997). Creating a robust multi-facility healthcare information system. In R. M. Kolodner (Ed.), *Computerizing Large Integrated Health Networks: The VA Success* (pp. 39–56). New York: Springer-Verlag.

Markle Foundation. *Connecting for Health Initiative.* Retrieved January 10, 2004, from *http://connectingforhealth.org/*

National Committee on Vital and Health Statistics (NCVHS). (2002). *Information for Health: A Strategy for Building the National Health Information Infrastructure. Report and Recommendations.* Washington, DC: U.S. Department of Health and Human Services. *www.ncvhs.hhs.gov/nhiilayo.pdf*

Perlin, J. (2004). *National Health Information Infrastructure: Cornerstones of Electronic Healthcare.* Reactor Panel—Federal Departments & Agency Heads.

Thompson, T. and Brailer, D. (2004). *The Decade of Health Information Technology, Delivering Consumer-centric and Information-rich Health Care: Framework for Action.* Washington, DC: U.S. Department of Health and Human Services. Available at *http://www.os.dhhs.gov/healthit/documents/hitframework.pdf*

U.S. Department of Defense. (DoD). (2004). *DOD Meets, Exceeds White House e-Health IT Standards.* News release No. 444-04, May 11. Retrieved from *www.dod.mil/releases/2004/nr20040511-1222.html*

U.S. Department of Health and Human Services, Centers for Medicare and Medicaid Services. *Chronic Care Improvement Program.* Retrieved June 21, 2004, from *www.cms.hhs.gov/medicarereform/ccip/*

U.S. Department of Health and Human Services, Indian Health Services. *Indian Health Service Electronic Health Record.* Retrieved from *http://www.ihs.gov/CIO/EHR/index.asp*

U.S. Department of Veterans Affairs. (2004). *VistA Monograph 2005–2006.* Retrieved March 25, 2005 *http://www1.va.gov/vista_monograph/docs/vista_monograph2005_06.pdf*

U.S. Department of Veterans Affairs. *My HealtheVet.* Retrieved October 7, 2004, from *http://www.myhealth.va.gov*

White House. (2004). *Incentives for the Use of Health Information Technology and Establishing the Position of the National Health Information Technology Coordinator.* Executive order dated April 27, 2004. Retrieved June 21, 2004, from *http://www.whitehouse.gov/news/releases/2004/04/20040427-4.html*

15

Dependable Systems for Quality Care

Dixie B. Baker

OBJECTIVES

1. To explain the relationship between dependability and health care quality and safety.
2. To identify and explain five guidelines for building dependable systems.
3. To present an informal assessment of the healthcare industry with respect to these guidelines.

KEY WORDS

dependable systems
dependability
security
patient safety
trustworthy systems

Introduction

The healthcare industry is undergoing a dramatic transformation from today's inefficient, costly, manually intensive, crisis-driven model of care delivery to a more efficient, consumer-centric, science-based model that proactively focuses on health management. This transformation is driven by several factors, most prominently the skyrocketing cost of healthcare delivery, the exposure of patient-safety problems, and an aging "baby boom" population that recognizes the potential for information technology (IT) to dramatically reduce the cost and improve the quality of care. Some of the key technologies that will enable this transformation to occur are identified in Table 15.1.

The electronic health record (EHR) will form the foundation for pervasive, personalized, and science-based care. Other key applications are clinical information systems (CIS) with integrated, outcomes-based decision support, clinical knowledge bases, computerized physician order entry (CPOE), electronic prescribing, consumer knowledge bases and decision support, and supply chain automation. The technologies that enable the transformation are largely state of the art and include enterprise application integration (EAI);

wireless communications; handheld and tablet computers; continuous speech recognition; new models for knowledge representation, integration, and interpretation; electronic sensor technology; radio frequency identification (RFID) tagging; and robotics. The functional capabilities these applications and technologies can provide are indeed impressive and can vastly improve the quality of healthcare delivery.

The International Council of Nurses (ICN) Code of Ethics for Nurses affirms that the nurse "holds in confidence personal information" and "ensures that use of technology...[is] compatible with the safety, dignity, and rights of people" (ICN, 2000). Fulfilling these ethical obligations is the individual responsibility of the nurse, who presumably has the ability and authority to ensure that personal information is protected and that technology is safe. As IT assumes a greater role in healthcare decision-making and in the provision of care, the nurse increasingly must rely on IT to help protect the patient's personal information and safety. Thus, ethical obligations drive requirements for system reliability, availability, confidentiality, data integrity, responsiveness, and safety attributes collectively referred to as dependability. Dependability is a measure of the extent to which a system can justifiably be relied on to deliver the services

Table 15.1   A Number of Technologies are Important in Transforming Care Delivery

Attributes of Transformed Healthcare	Technology Enablers
Medical decisions are based on the current state of medical knowledge interpreted within the context of the patient's complete health profile	Electronic health record (EHR)
	Electronic, outcomes-based clinical decision support
	Wireless communications
	Tablet personal computers (PCs), personal data assistants
	Continuous speech recognition
Current, synthesized clinical knowledge is available at the point of care	Clinical knowledge bases
	New models for knowledge representation, integration, and interpretation
Errors are detected before information is acted on. Orders and prescriptions are clear and unambiguous	Ambulatory and in-patient computerized physician order entry (CPOE)
	Electronic prescribing
Consumers are partners in their own care. Patients with chronic diseases and conditions are monitored continuously	Consumer knowledge bases
	Electronic sensors
	Wireless communications
	Radio frequency identification (RFID) tagging
	Decision support
	Home health systems
Equipment, supplies, patients, and delivery staff are accurately tracked and efficiently managed	RFID tagging
	Wireless communications
	Supply chain automation
Authorization, adjudication, inquiry, billing, and payment are handled electronically in real time	Standardized electronic transactions
	Rules-based decision support
	Enterprise application integration (EAI)
High-quality care is delivered to rural areas	High-quality communication services
	Robotics
	Telemedicine applications
Drugs are dispensed efficiently and safely	Robotics
	RFID tagging

expected from it. Dependability comprises the following six attributes:

1. **System reliability:** The system consistently behaves in the same way.

2. **Service availability:** Required services are present and usable when they are needed.

3. **Confidentiality:** Sensitive information is disclosed only to those authorized to see it.

4. **Data integrity:** Data are not corrupted or destroyed.

5. **Responsiveness:** The system responds to user input within an expected and acceptable time period.

6. **Safety:** The system does not cause harm.

Because dependability tends to be a property of the system as a whole, it cannot be retrofitted, but must be designed and built into the system from the outset and conscientiously preserved as the system evolves. Discovering dependability problems in an operational system often indicates that extensive—and expensive—changes to the system are needed.

When Things Go Wrong

Although we would like to be able to assume that computers, networks, and software are as dependable as our toasters and telephones, unfortunately that is not the case, and stories that have appeared in trade journals have documented this fact. One of the more dramatic examples is the cover story for the February 2003 issue of *CIO*, which relates in detail the occurrence and recovery from "one of the worst healthcare IT crises in history"—a catastrophic failure in the network infrastructure that supported CareGroup, one of the most prestigious healthcare organizations in the United States. The source of the problem ultimately was traced to network switches that directed network traffic over a highly overburdened and fragile network that was further taxed when a researcher uploaded a multigigabyte file into the picture archiving and communication system (PACS). The failure resulted in a 4-hour closure of the emergency room, a complete shutdown of the network, and 2 days of paper-based clinical operations—a true "retro" experience for many of the physicians who had never practiced without computers. Network services were not fully recovered until 6 days after the onset of the disaster (Berinato, 2003a).

CIO's report of CareGroup's experience was followed by additional reports of similar experiences. Covenant Health, based in Knoxville, TN, reported that the SQL Slammer worm attack invaded its six-hospital network through a single port connection with one of its trusted technology partners. Recovering from the attack took Covenant 12 hours, during which the hospitals resorted to manual operations. In March 2003, Kaiser Permanente learned how the lack of dependability can affect its business, when a power outage caused a prescription system to misprint labels on prescribed medications. To assure that the correct medications were delivered to patients, Kaiser was forced to contact 4,700 people to verify their orders. One month after the Kaiser incident, a new laboratory computer system at the Los Angeles County Medical Center overloaded, forcing the emergency room to turn away ambulances when they appeared at the door (Berinato, 2003b).

In August 2003, the Blaster and SoBig worm attacks invaded hospitals around the world. In Glasgow, Scotland, 10,000 computers used by city hospitals and emergency services were infected, and systems at one hospital were down for 15 hours. Nearly one-third of the computers at Baylor College of Medicine (about 2,100 machines) were infected by the Blaster and SoBig worm attacks. The cost to recover from the attacks exceeded $100 K and 2.5 days

of productivity were lost campus-wide due to system outages (Ausman, 2004).

The bottom line is that systems, networks, and software applications are highly complex, and the only safe assumption is that failures will occur. Thus, dependability is an essential factor in system planning and operations.

Guidelines for Dependable Systems

All computer systems are vulnerable to both human-created threats, such as malicious code attacks and software bugs, and natural threats, such as hardware aging and earthquakes. In the gray area between these lie system incompatibilities, such as the incompatibility between Intel's Centrino mobile chip set and virtual private networking client software, which caused notebook and laptop personal computers (PCs) to experience "blue-screen" system crashes (System crashes, 2003).

Removing all system vulnerabilities is not practical—particularly given complex, heterogeneous environments where software and hardware changes are a part of routine operations. A more practical approach to attaining dependability is to build *tolerant* systems—systems that anticipate problems; that detect faults, software glitches, and intrusions; and that take action so that services can continue and data are protected from corruption, destruction, and unauthorized disclosure. In this section we discuss five fundamental guidelines that can help increase the dependability of healthcare systems.

Guideline 1: Architect for Dependability

A fundamental principle of system architecture is that an enterprise system architecture should be developed from the bottom up so that no critical component is dependent on a component less trustworthy than itself. Figure 15.1 illustrates this dependency relationship. At the bottom of the architecture are the physical and logical networks that support the enterprise and provide the "pipes" that carry data from system to system. One or more computers are connected to this network, and the software foundation of each computer is an operating system that is responsible for managing all of the resources in the computer system. Running on top of the operating system are a number of software applications. In this figure, we show applications that perform functions that support security and patient safety. At the top is the user interface—the screen the user sees as she or he runs the applications (Fig. 15.1).

We chose to illustrate security and safety applications to make an important point: while these applications provide

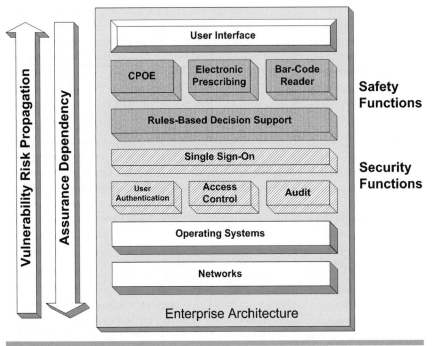

Figure 15.1

System architecture must be viewed in terms of the dependencies critical to system dependability.

services that are critical to assuring patients' privacy and safety, these services are only as dependable as the operating systems, networks, and other system services on which they depend. A corollary is that any vulnerabilities that exist in the networks, operating system, and other services that support the applications will propagate up to the applications, creating vulnerabilities for them as well. In particular, operating systems and networks provide system-level security functions that are critical to assuring that individuals, systems, and applications can access only those resources for which they are authorized, and that they can perform only those actions they are authorized to perform. These security functions play a huge role in achieving dependability.

Single-point dependencies should be avoided or eliminated. That is, no single component should be capable of bringing the system down should that component fail. Distributed architectures can tolerate failures more easily than large, centralized systems. Redundancy and failover should be incorporated for all critical components. Finally, complexity should be minimized throughout the

architecture. The simplest design and integration strategy will be the easiest to understand, to maintain, and to recover in the case of a failure or disaster.

Guideline 2: Anticipate Failures

Unfortunately, minimizing complexity is more easily said than done. Consistent with Moore's law (Moore, 1965), the speed of processors is doubling every 18 months, while the cost for that computing power is halving within the same time period. As computers are getting faster, systems are getting more and more complex, and design flaws are becoming an increasingly catastrophic problem (Hyman, 2002). So the second guideline is to anticipate failures—because they will happen.

In anticipation of failures at the infrastructure level, features that are transparent to software applications should be implemented to detect faults, to fail over to redundant components when faults are detected, and to recover from failures before they become catastrophic. To handle exceptions in the execution of specific software applications, application-specific features should be implemented. Another effect of increasing complexity is an increase in vulnerabilities—which serve as "opportunities" for malicious attack. Security features to detect, disable, and recover from malicious attacks, while preserving system stability and security, should be implemented.

Finally, safety-critical systems should be designed and built to fail in a safe state. Industries that deal with safety-critical systems, such as the aerospace, chemical, and nuclear power industries, routinely use software-safety methods to provide assurance that their systems will operate safely and, should a safety-critical component fail, it will not result in the loss of human life. Such methods include fault tree analysis, failure modes and effects analysis, state-machine hazard analysis, formal verification, and independent verification and validation.

Guideline 3: Anticipate Success

The systems planning process should anticipate business success—and the consequential need for larger networks, more systems, new applications, and additional integration. Modeling of use-case scenarios that anticipate hospital and clinic mergers, acquisitions, and a growing patient/customer base will enable the system designer to visualize the data flows, system loading, and network impact resulting from business growth and success. Such models can provide valuable input into planning for scalability and future integration.

Guideline 4: Hire Meticulous Managers

Managing and keeping complex networks and integrated systems available and responsive requires meticulous overseers—individuals who know that failures will occur and accept that failures are most likely to occur when they are least expected. Good system administrators meticulously monitor and manage system and network performance, using out-of-band tools that do not themselves affect performance. These managers use middleware to manage the workload across the network. They take emergency and disaster planning very seriously; they develop, maintain, and judiciously exercise plans and procedures for managing emergencies and recovering from disasters.

Guideline 5: Don't Be Adventurous

Imagine that a small start-up company called Cute Chutes has announced the availability of a new parachute unit that promises to revolutionize the sport of sky diving. The new product has an innovative release design developed in collaboration with the national space program, and it is constructed of a fabric (available in several popular colors) engineered in the textile department of the local university. The product's brochure urges the consumer to be adventurous and states that the company guarantees satisfaction or the purchaser's money will be cheerfully refunded. Would you buy this product?

Of course not! Then why do people in healthcare buy computer systems and software before these products are mature and proven? For dependability, one should use only proven methods, tools, technologies, and products that have been in production, under conditions, and at a scale similar to the intended environment. The enterprise with a requirement for dependable systems should not be the first (or second) to adopt a new technology.

Assessing the Healthcare Industry

Healthcare clearly has a need for dependable systems—both now and after the transformation, as the industry becomes increasingly dependent on IT in the delivery of patient care. This section provides an informal assessment of how well healthcare provider organizations follow the guidelines discussed above. This assessment is by no means "scientific," nor is it intended to represent "all" healthcare provider organizations. Rather it conveys observations of the healthcare industry as a whole and the opinions of a passionate advocate of dependable systems for healthcare. Figure 15.2 shows the results of this informal assessment as a "report card" for the provider community (Fig. 15.2).

Healthcare Architectures

For adherence to the first guideline "architect for dependability" the clinical care provider community gets a barely passing grade of "D." Healthcare organizations build—or perhaps "compose"—their systems from the top down rather than from the bottom up. The healthcare professionals select the user interfaces they like, and the IT team negotiates terms with the vendors who offer the systems that generate those interfaces. These systems are familiarly known as "departmental" systems because they generally are used only in one department, such as registration, laboratory, or pharmacy. EAI or "interface engines," are used to transfer data, most commonly from a clinical system to a billing system. As a result, healthcare systems are among the most complex—a loose collection of departmental systems that are unaware that each other exist. Creating further complexity are the mergers and consolidations of healthcare enterprises, each bringing into the merger its

HEALTH CARE INDUSTRY
Report Card

Year: 2004

Student Name: Clinical Care Provider Community

Subject: Information Technology Dependability

Guideline	Grade	Comments
Architect for Dependability	D	Builds systems top down instead of bottom up. Too complex.
Expect Failures	D	Assumes systems will work.
Expect Success	C	Assumes systems and networks are infinitely expandable and adaptable, but does not plan for system expansions and consolidations.
Hire Meticulous Managers	C	Sometimes, but doesn't give them adequate support.
Don't Be Adventurous	C	Yes and no.

☒ Complies with security regulations.		☒ Insists on sound science as the foundation of good medicine.
☒ Recognizes the importance of correct data.		☐ Insists on sound systems engineering as the foundation of dependable systems.
☐ Understands the role of security in system dependability, service availability, data integrity, and patient safety.		☐ Systems play well together.
☒ Optimistic attitude.		☐ Values information technology as core business asset.

Figure 15.2
An assessment of the healthcare provider community's adherence to guidelines for dependable systems reflects areas needing improvement.

own software applications, systems, and networks, as well as its own operational practices and procedures.

The Health Insurance Portability and Accountability Act (HIPAA) security regulation (DHHS, 2003) prescribes administrative, physical, and technical safeguards for protecting the confidentiality and integrity of health information and the availability of critical system services. The following eight required administrative safeguards represent important operational practices that clearly will contribute to system dependability:

1. Security management, including security analysis and risk management

2. Assigned security responsibility

3. Information access management, including the isolation of clearinghouse functions from other clinical functions

4. Security awareness and training

5. Security incident procedures, including response and reporting

6. Contingency planning, including data backup planning, disaster recovery planning, and planning for emergency mode operations

7. Evaluation

8. Business associate contracts that lock in the obligations of business partners in protecting health information to which they may have access

The five specified physical safeguards also contribute to system dependability by requiring that facilities, workstations, devices, and media be protected. Most of the required technical safeguards are widely viewed within the security community and security-aware industries as "minimal" security controls:

1. Access control, including unique user identification and an emergency access procedure

2. Audit controls

3. Data integrity protection

4. Person or entity authentication

5. Transmission security

As discussed above, security plays a critical role in achieving system dependability. However, security within clinical environments is very different from environments that seek to tightly restrict access to information, systems, and services. In a healthcare environment, access must be more liberally authorized than in many other security environments simply because access to information is a prerequisite to care. Indeed one might argue that the quality of medical and nursing care that can be delivered is directly correlated with the quantity and quality of patient information available to the caregiver. So operational needs dictate that healthcare environments be more "open" than other information-intensive environments, such as banking, law enforcement, or the military. Indeed, the HIPAA requirement for emergency access—that is, the ability to override security in an emergency situation—is unique to healthcare. Thus, the HIPAA security requirement for "information system activity review" is an important safeguard to counterbalance the necessity of authorizing many people access to patients' records. This requirement includes procedures to regularly review records of information system activity, such as audit logs, access reports, and security incident tracking reports.

While the HIPAA security standard is a tremendous contribution toward achieving dependable systems in healthcare, the current standard lacks fundamental system assurance requirements that are so important to system dependability. For example, the standard contains no technical requirements addressing strength of mechanism (i.e., the security feature's ability to withstand attack and to protect under a broad range of conditions), functional testing, or penetration testing. Nor does the standard contain any requirements for assurance or dependability metrics.

If healthcare enterprises fully recognized the important role security plays in system dependability, the fact that the HIPAA standard contains no assurance requirements may not be that important. Unfortunately, however, healthcare enterprises view security as a "compliance" issue and not a core business need. Data collected by the 2003 and 2004 Annual HIMSS Leadership Surveys sponsored by the Health Information Management and Systems Society (HIMSS) and Superior Consultant Company, Inc., confirm this fact. For both years, the survey participants most frequently identified upgrading security "to meet HIPAA requirements" as their top priority (HIMSS, 2004). Until the healthcare industry recognizes information security as a core business requirement, enterprise system dependability will not be achievable.

Anticipating Failures

For adherence to the second guideline "expect failures" the clinical care provider community gets another grade of "D." Medical technology and prescription drugs, as well as clinical treatment protocols, are required to undergo extensive validation before they can be used in clinical practice. So is it not reasonable to assume that clinical applications, computer systems, and networks used in clinical practice would be subjected to the same level of scrutiny and validation?

One certainly would not think a vendor could market and sell a software application to be used to record vital patient information or to order medications without that software first being thoroughly analyzed, tested, and "certified" by the Food and Drug Administration (FDA) or some other regulatory body. However, that is exactly what happens. Commercial, clinical software applications are not subject to FDA certification or any other type of certification.

The architectural complexity discussed above increases the opportunities for failures to occur. Further, medical applications that are hosted on PCs and personal data assistants (PDAs) have a higher likelihood of failure than applications hosted on server machines that are physically protected, managed by trained system administrators, and continuously monitored. PCs that connect to the enterprise network from outside (e.g., in the home), laptops with wireless modems, smart phones, and PDAs that synchronize with enterprise systems present risks to enterprise systems in that they can serve as convenient conduits for transporting malicious code into the enterprise and for transporting confidential patient information out.

Computers are increasingly being used in safety-critical clinical applications, and without careful and appropriate attention to software safety, we can reasonably expect that failures will contribute to the loss of human life. A widely cited example of what can occur when a software-controlled, safety-critical medical device fails is an incident involving a computer-controlled, radiation-therapy machine called the Therac-25. Many people consider this the worst safety incident in the history of medical accelerators.

Between June 1985 and January 1987, the Therac-25 massively overdosed six people, resulting in deaths and serious injuries. The manufacturer's initial response was a temporary "fix" distributed as a memo containing a warning not to use the up-arrow key for editing or any other purpose, along with instructions for removing the key cap and using electrical tape to fix switch contacts in an open position. A complete investigation of the Therac-25 accidents uncovered multiple problems, including management inadequacies, design and implementation flaws, and fundamental systems engineering failures. Among the failures identified were overconfidence in the software and overconfidence in risk assessment results (Leveson and Turner, 1993). The manufacturer of the Therac-25 did not "anticipate failures."

Since the Therac-25 incident, the FDA has improved its reporting system and augmented its procedures and guidelines to include software. Today the FDA requires failure modes and effects analysis for products with software components, which helps detect errors in software-controlled, medical devices that require FDA approval. However, few CIS product companies incorporate software safety design and assurance methods in their development environments. As specialized medical devices migrate to PC platforms, and safety-critical, clinical functions increasingly are relegated to information systems, special safety analyses and design procedures must be incorporated into safety-critical, software development projects.

Anticipating Success

With respect to the third guideline "expect success" the clinical care provider community has earned a mediocre grade of "C." Healthcare organizations definitely expect their software applications, computer systems, and networks to work. In fact, providers *assume* their systems will work as well as any other medical equipment—despite the fact that many of the software applications they use are running on the same kind of PCs that have failed them at home.

However, healthcare organizations do not foresee that their business success may increase their need for processing power and networking capability. Nor do they foresee mergers' and acquisitions' creating the need to consolidate their systems with those of another healthcare enterprise. The Boston CareGroup instance discussed earlier offers a good example of a hospital that did not anticipate its own success and the resultant need for its network to grow. In 1996, Beth Israel Hospital implemented a state-of-the-art network, and as Beth Israel merged with Deaconess Hospital and acquired additional clinical systems, including its PACS, the network was more and more heavily taxed.

So in November, 2002, the highly successful CareGroup was running its critical clinical applications on a vintage 1996 network that depended on Layer 2 switching technology instead of today's more flexible and resilient Layer 3 routing. A switched network uses something called a "spanning tree protocol" to figure out the shortest route to send network traffic to its destination, and when a researcher uploaded a multigigabyte image file to the PACS network, the spanning tree protocol was unable to handle it and went into a loop. The result was a dramatic, 6-day demonstration of what can happen when a healthcare organization fails to adequately anticipate and build the infrastructure necessary to support its success.

However, CareGroup learned a valuable lesson: that one must plan for success and the additional demands that success places on the system. Other healthcare organizations can be grateful for CareGroup's CIO's willingness to share the details of his experience so that they might benefit from the lessons learned (Berinato, 2003a).

IT Management

For the fourth guideline "hire meticulous managers" the clinical care provider community has been assigned a mediocre grade of "C." Many provider organizations truly do recognize the criticality of IT to their business success. These organizations have hired IT managers who appreciate the important role of IT in a healthcare environment and who recognize the need for dependable systems that can anticipate and recover from failures. IT managers who recognize the strong relationship between system dependability and the quality and safety of patient care implement fault-tolerant systems with strong security protection, middleware to manage workload, and tools to continuously monitor the health and performance of their applications, systems, and networks.

Healthcare organizations who view IT as a "support function" and costly (albeit necessary) business expense, frequently select IT managers who may understand the healthcare business, but may not understand the fragile nature of IT or the importance of Guideline 1—architecting for dependability. These IT environments tend to be loose composites of proprietary, departmental systems designed for specific business functions such as admission, discharge, and transfer (ADT), radiology, or pharmacy.

As an industry, healthcare's spending for IT lags far behind other industries. Over the past decade, healthcare has invested only 2% of its revenues in IT, compared to 10% for other information-intensive industries (Landro, 2003). Other industries spend $8,000 per worker per year for technology, compared to $1,000 per worker for healthcare (President Bush Touts Benefits of Health Care Information Technology, 2005). Thus, even IT managers who are conscientious, meticulous, and capable often are forced to operate within a meager budget.

Adventurous Technologies in Healthcare

The fifth and final guideline "don't be adventurous" is the most difficult to assess for healthcare. On the one hand, healthcare givers typically are not early adopters, but on the other hand, they seem to cast fate to the wind for technologies that catch their collective fancy. So a grade of "C" seems appropriate here.

Healthcare clinicians, including nurses, historically and typically are very resistant to change, largely because they are taught to be circumspect in considering new approaches, treatment protocols, and drug regimens. Before adopting any new idea, they investigate it, they talk about it among their colleagues, they watch someone else try it, and then perhaps, they may try it themselves.

For dependable IT, the healthcare practitioner's skepticism is a good thing! 24×7 operations demand proven methods, tools, technologies, and products—elements that have been in production, at scale, under similar conditions. Newness and change are anathema to stability. While well planned and carefully executed changes over time are desired and expected, healthcare provider organizations should not be overly eager to adopt new technologies for life-critical clinical systems.

Wireless networking and handheld computers can serve as a good example of technologies that are not yet mature enough for safety-critical applications. Yet, wireless information systems are one of the most frequently used technologies in healthcare. The HIMSS 2004 Technology Leadership Survey found that 72% of the surveyed healthcare organizations had wireless networks, and two of the leading technologies planned for adoption over the next 2 years were wireless appliances (47%) and handheld computers (55%) (HIMSS, 2004). This trend is supported by a recent survey on the use of mobile computing in nursing, which found that the nurses surveyed ($n > 100$) recognized the potential value of mobile computing in increasing productivity, efficiency, and patient safety (PDA, 2004).

While wireless networking and handheld computers clearly are central to the ability to provide pervasive care in the future, these technologies today represent significant threats to clinical environments. Wireless (IEEE 802.11) networks broadcast data, potentially providing a convenient "back door" onto enterprise networks, creating a threat to data integrity, information confidentiality, and service availability. Wireless technology experts and product vendors are working diligently toward comprehensive security solutions, but such solutions have not yet arrived. Further, handheld platforms typically have many of the same security vulnerabilities as the early PCs: weak authentication, no separation of execution domains, no (or weak) encryption support, and vulnerabilities to malicious code attacks directed at either the device itself or the enterprise network with which it synchronizes (Baker, 2003).

Summary and Conclusions

The healthcare industry is undergoing a dramatic transformation from today's inefficient, costly, manually intensive, crisis-driven model of care delivery to a more efficient, consumer-centric, science-based, model that proactively focuses on health management. IT is a key enabler for this transformation. As provider organizations become increasingly dependent on IT in the delivery of care, new risks emerge, and system dependability becomes essential for business success, quality care, and patient safety. Dependable systems are reliable; they are available when they are needed; they protect confidential information; they assure the integrity of data; they are responsive; and they are safe.

This chapter has described five guidelines for achieving dependable systems:

1. Architect for dependability

2. Anticipate failures

3. Anticipate success

4. Hire meticulous managers

5. Don't be adventurous

An informal assessment of the healthcare provider community suggests that thus far, the healthcare industry has exhibited little recognition of the importance of enterprise architecture and the strong interrelationship among information security, system dependability, and patient safety. However, this is not surprising for an industry just beginning to use IT for core business functions, such as clinical care.

The future looks much brighter than the current state. The mandate for the healthcare industry to conduct business more efficiently and to deliver a safer and a higher quality of care is being championed by industry consortia (e.g., The Leapfrog Group), the scientific community (e.g., the National Academy of Sciences), the federal government (e.g., HIPAA, Agency for Healthcare Research and Quality, Centers for Medicare and Medicaid Services), and industry regulators (e.g., Joint Commission on Accreditation of Hospital Organizations). The President's Health Information Technology Plan and the creation of a sub-cabinet-level position of National Health Information Technology Coordinator, along with the National Health Information Network (NHIN) initiative all point to the reality that healthcare is on the brink of radical change.

As business operations and priorities change, the role and status of IT within provider organizations will increase. The healthcare provider of tomorrow undoubtedly will consider IT a core business asset and system dependability a business imperative.

References

Ausman, D. (2004). Computer viruses affect hospitals, which learn to cope. *Health IT World*. September 18, 2003. Retrieved June 21, 2004, from *http://www.health-itworld.com/enewsarchive/e_article000183662.cfm*

Baker, D. B. (2003). "Wireless (in)security for healthcare." *Health IT Advisory Report* (Vol. 4, No. 4, pp. 10–23). Medical Records Institute.

Berinato, S. (2003a). All systems down. *CIO* (pp. 46–53).

Berinato, S. (2003b). A rash of IT failures. *CIO*. Retrieved June 21, 2004, from *http://www.cio.com/archive/061503/tl_health.html*.

Department of Health and Human Services (DHHS). (2003). Health insurance reform: Security standards, final rule. 45 CFR Parts 160, 162, and 164. *Federal Register*.

Health Information Management and Systems Society (HIMSS). (2004). *15th Annual HIMSS Leadership Survey*, sponsored by Superior Consultant Company, Inc. Final report: Healthcare CIO.

Hyman, G. (2002). *The Dark Side of Moore's Law*. Retrieved June 15, 2004, from *http://siliconvalley.internet.com/news/article.php/1442041*

International Council of Nurses (ICN). (2000). *The ICN Code of Ethics for Nurses*. Geneva, Switzerland. Retrieved July 9, 2004, from *http://www.icn.ch/icncode.pdf*

Landro, L. (2003). Wired patients. *The Wall Street Journal*.

Leveson, N. and Turner, C. S. (1993). An investigation of the Therac-25 accidents. *IEEE Computer* 26(7):18–41.

Moore, G. E. (1965). Cramming more components onto integrated circuits. *Electronics* 38(8). Retrieved June 21, 2004, from *ftp://download.intel.com/research/silicon/moorespaper.pdf*

PDAcortex. (2004). *Mobile Computing in Nursing Study*. Retrieved July 9, 2004, from *http://www.rnpalm.com/Mobile_Computing_Nursing_Study.htm*

System crashes. (2003). System crashes linked to Centrino, VPN client glitch. *Computerworld* (p. 10).

President Bush Touts Benefits of Health Care Information Technology. (2005). Washington, DC: The White House. Available at *http://www.whitehouse.gov/news/releases/2004/04/20040427-5.html*

CHAPTER **16**

Nursing Minimum Data Set Systems

Connie White Delaney

OBJECTIVES

1. Define the concept nursing minimum data set (NMDS).
2. Compare and contrast national NMDSs.
3. Analyze which of the defined/published NMDSs support the international nursing minimum data set (i-NMDS).
4. Apply the concept of "context" to the definition and use of NMDSs.

KEY WORDS

minimum data set
nursing

Introduction—Clinical Nursing Visibility from National to International Contexts

The impetus for access to and use of nursing data and information has never been stronger. Recognition of this growing need for nursing data has been powered by forces both internal and external to nursing (Institute of Medicine, 2000, 2001, 2004; Brooten et al., 2004; Maas and Delaney, 2004). Moreover, this growing need has been fueled by international as well as national factors. The identification of the NMDS visionary work begun in the United States in 1980s by Werley and Lang (1988), has indeed spurred activity extending to national efforts to develop similar data sets around the world. Moreover, these national efforts have supported an initiative to develop an international i-NMDS. This chapter provides a synthesis of historical, current, and future NMDS systems which can increase nursing data and information capacity to drive knowledge building for the discipline and profession and contribute to the standards supportive of the electronic health record (EHR).

NMDS Historical Summary

The NMDS identifies essential, common, and core data elements to be collected for all patients/clients receiving nursing care. The NMDS is a standardized approach

that facilitates the abstraction of these minimum, common, essential core data elements to describe nursing practice (Werley and Lang, 1988) from both paper and electronic records. It is intended for use in all settings where nurses provide care, spanning, for example, acute care, ambulatory centers, home healthcare, community practices, occupational health, and school health.

The NMDS was conceptualized through a small group work at the nursing information systems (NISs) conference held in 1977 at the University of Illinois College of Nursing (Newcomb, 1981). Werley and colleagues took the NMDS forward at the NMDS conference in 1985, held at the University of Wisconsin-Milwaukee School of Nursing. It was during this invitational conference that the NMDS was developed consensually through the efforts of 64 conference participants and formalized (Werley and Lang, 1988).

The NMDS includes three broad categories of elements: (a) nursing care, (b) patient or client demographics, and (c) service elements (see Table 16.1). Many of the NMDS elements are consistently collected in the majority of patient/client records across healthcare settings in the United States, especially the patient and service elements. The aim of the NMDS is not to be redundant of other data sets, but rather to identify what are the minimal data needed to be collected from records of patients receiving nursing care.

The NMDS was developed by building on the foundation established by the U.S. uniform hospital discharge

Table 16.1   The U.S. NMDS Data Elements

Nursing care elements
Nursing diagnosis
Nursing intervention
Nursing outcome
Intensity of nursing care

Patient or client demographic elements
Personal identification*
Date of birth*
Sex*
Race and ethnicity*
Residence*

Service elements
Unique facility or service agency number*
Unique health record number or patient or client*
Unique number of principle registered nurse provider
Episode admission or encounter date*
Discharge or termination date*
Disposition of patient or client*
Expected payer for most of this bill (anticipated financial guarantor for services)*

*Elements of the uniform hospital discharge data set (UHDDS)

data set (UHDDS). The number of new items—mainly the nursing care items—is relatively less. The nursing care elements of the NMDS (nursing diagnosis, nursing interventions, nursing outcome, and intensity of nursing care) were derived from the nursing process.

Eight benefits of the NMDS, when adopted and implemented nationally or internationally with a system of ongoing data collection, were identified. These benefits were:

1. Access to comparable, minimum nursing care, and resources data on local, regional, national, and international levels

2. Enhanced documentation of nursing care provided

3. Identification of trends related to patient or client problems and nursing care provided

4. Impetus to improved costing of nursing services

5. Improved data for quality assurance evaluation

6. Impetus to further development and refinement of NISs

7. Comparative research on nursing care, including research on nursing diagnoses, nursing interventions, nursing outcomes, intensity of nursing care, and referral for further nursing services

8. Contributions toward advancing nursing as a research-based discipline

Standards and Research Era—Twenty-First Century

Although the full benefits of the NMDS are still being realized, the NMDS work has influenced a number of advances. The NMDS influenced the work of the professional nurses association. In 1991, the American Nurses Association (ANA) recognized the NMDS as the minimum data elements to be included in any data set or patient record. The ANA consequently established the American Nurses' Association Steering Committee on Data Bases to Support Clinical Nursing Practice (since renamed the Committee on Nursing Information Infrastructure). This committee launched a recognition process for standardized nursing vocabularies needed to capture the NMDS data elements for nursing diagnoses, interventions, and outcomes in a patient record. To date 11 languages have been recognized by ANA (2004); in addition, two data sets have been recognized by ANA: the nursing management minimum data set (NMMDS) to complement the NMDS (see Table 16.2).

The NMDS serves as a key component of the standards developed by the Nursing Information & Data Set Evaluation Center (NIDSEC) (American Nurses Association, 1997). Established in 1996, NIDSEC develops and disseminates standards related to nomenclature, clinical associations, clinical data repositories, and system characteristics/decision support/contextual variables pertaining to data sets in information systems that support the documentation of nursing practice (NMDS). Further NIDSEC evaluates voluntarily submitted vendor data sets against these standards. The advancement of the NMDS has supported nurses' participation in developing computerized health information systems (HISs) (Androwich et al., 2003), utilization of data and information to support evidence-based practice (Pierce, 2000; Pravikoff, 2003; Tanner, 2000), and inclusion of information management as an essential component of the discipline. The American Association of Colleges of Nursing (AACN, 2003) White Paper on the Clinical Nurse Leader is one example of the recognition

Table 16.2 American Nurses Association Recognized Languages and Data Sets Supporting Nursing Practice

Languages	Data Sets
ABC codes	Nursing minimum data set (NMDS)
Clinical Care Classification (CCC) (formerly Home Health Care Classification)	Nursing management minimum data set (NMMDS)
International Classification for Nursing Practice (ICNP)	
Logical observation identifiers names and codes (LOINC)	
NANDA—nursing diagnoses, definitions, and classification	
Nursing Outcomes Classification (NOC)	
Nursing Interventions Classification (NIC) system	
Omaha System	
Patient care data set (PCDS)	
Perioperative nursing data set (PNDS)	
SNOMED CT	

of the essential core function of informatics expertise within practice (*http://www.aacn. nche.edu/NewNurse/ NewNurseWorkingPaperHL.pdf*).

Tools and methods to facilitate comparability of nursing data continue to evolve, including the International Classification for Nursing Practice (ICNP) and the International Standards Organization Reference Terminology Model for Nursing. Mapping of many of the recognized ANA languages into SNOMED CT (*http://www.snomed/snomedct/*), development of a validation method for this mapping (Lu et al., in preparation), and inclusion of the NMDS elements in SNOMED CT recognized nursing's contribution to healthcare as well. The NMDS has likewise been recognized by Health Level Seven (HL7) and validation of the inclusion of the NMDS elements within the HL7 information model has been completed (*http://www.hl7.org/*).

 ## National Nursing Minimum Data Sets

Established NMDSs

The early NMDS work in the United States spurred the development of NMDSs in numerous other countries. To date seven countries have identified NMDS systems, including Australia, Canada, Belgium, Iceland, The Netherlands, Switzerland, and Thailand (see Table 16.3). A perusal of these data sets reveals a definite consensus on the importance of the nursing care elements across all countries with identified NMDSs. There is variability as

to the level of granularity in the specification of these data sets. Some are very granular in specifying specific patient problems and specific interventions of interest, while other data sets maintain a high conceptual focus and emphasize empowering nursing to establish NMDSs that can address all nursing problems/interventions/outcomes per encounter. There is also support for collection of key characteristics related to the patient/client and the service. There is variation as to applicability of the data sets to settings other than acute care.

Emergent NMDSs

Several countries across most continents beyond North America are exploring development of NMDS systems. For example, in Europe, the World Health Organization (Ryan and Delaney, 1995) has been concerned with variables including nursing care, personal data, medical diagnosis, and service data. Many of these elements are similar to the U.S. NMDS. Work is ongoing in the United Kingdom, e.g., Scotland, to identify NMDSs to be congruent with the initiatives of the National Health Service. The Nordic countries likewise have much ongoing activity to identify NMDSs, e.g., Finland (Turtiainen et al., 2000), Denmark, and Sweden (Hansebo, 1999). France is pursing identification of a NMDS.

Moreover, Brazil is leading efforts in South America to identify a NMDS. Korea and Japan are focusing on development efforts as well. New Zealand has focused efforts on a diabetes-specific data set to date. In summary, it is clear that there is major work being accomplished

Table 16.3   National NMDS

Australia (Community Nursing Minimum Data Set [CNMDSA])[a]	Canada (Health Information: Nursing Components Data Set [HI: NC Data Set])[a]
Community nursing	**National scope across all settings**[b]
Purpose: compare performance of institutions, allocate resources, monitor and compare health status of the population, and deliver information	Purpose: deliver information about nursing care, and to demonstrate unique contribution of nurses to the public
NANDA	**NANDA**
Goals of nursing care	Nursing Interventions Classification (NIC)
Nursing interventions	Omaha System
Client dependency	Clinical Care Classification (CCC)
Nursing diagnosis	Nursing outcomes
Nursing resource utilization	
Patient demographics	**Patient demographics**
Birth date of client	Racial/ethnic
Sex of client	Unique geographical location
Ethnicity—country of birth	Unique lifetime identifier
Ethnicity—language spoken at home	Language
Location of client	Occupation
	Living arrangement
	Home environment, including physical structure
	Responsible caregiver on discharge
	Functional health status
	Burden on care provider
	Education level
	Literacy level
	Work environment
	Lifestyle data
	Income level
Medical diagnoses	Medical diagnoses
	Medical procedures
Resource utilization	Unique nurse identifier
Episode	Principal nurse provider
Agency/provider service	Mortality
Agency identifier	Physician, nurses, and consultant identifiers
Client identifier	Admit/discharge dates
Admission date	Length of stay
Referral source	
Discharge date	
Discharge destination (also a nursing element)	
Other support service	

Table 16.3   National NMDS (*Continued*)

NMDS Belgium Minimate Verpleegkundige Gegevens (MVG)/Resume Infirmier Minimum (RIM), Minimale Psychiatricsche Gegevens (MPG)[a,b,c,d]	NMDS in Iceland[e]
Use in general hospitals throughout the country, including psychiatric hospitals	Use across all healthcare settings
	Nursing diagnoses (NANDA)
	Nursing interventions (NIC)
Main diagnosis	Main medical diagnosis
Complications	Additional medical procedures and operation
Medical procedure and operations	Date of operation
	Responsible doctor for operation
Activities of daily living: (1) hygiene, (2) mobility, (3) elimination, (4) feeding assistance, (5) tube feeding, (6) mouth care, (7) dressing, (8) prevention of pressure sore, (9) intubation, (10) assessment, (11) training of activities of daily living, (12) crisis intervention, (13) reality orientation, (14) isolation, (15) taking vital signs, (16) physical parameters, (17) cast care, (18) taking blood samples, (19) medication management, (20) infusion care, and (21) wound care	Personal identifier
	Sex
	Residence
	Marital status
	Nationality
	Primary care doctor/district
Patient number	Principal nurse provider number
Year of birth	Provider nurse
Sex	Facility-agency
	Admission date
	Admission time
	Admission way
	Admission circumstance
	Admission reason
	Admit from
	Remitted by
	Discharge date
	Discharge time
	Discharge to
	Discharge destination
	Disposition of patient
	Date of ended effective medical treatment
	Date of arrival outpatients
	Days on day-unit
	Control after discharge
	Readmission

(*Continued*)

Table 16.3   National NMDS (*Continued*)

NMDS Belgium Minimate Verpleegkundige Gegevens (MVG)/Resume Infirmier Minimum (RIM), Minimale Psychiatricsche Gegevens (MPG)[a,b,c,d]	NMDS in Iceland[e]
Code of the hospital	
Code of the department	
Code of the nursing unit	
Day of admission	
Day of stay	
Day of discharge	
Nursing hours available on the nursing unit	
Number of nurses available	
Number of beds	
Nurse qualification mix	

The Netherlands (NMDSN)[f,g]	Switzerland (the Swiss Nursing Maximum Data Set)[h]
Aim for NMDSN: budget parameter for nursing	
Ten nursing processes: (1) assessment, (2) patient problems, (3) goals, (4) interventions, (5) daily reports, (6) flow chart, (7) forms to ascertain continuity of care, (8) risk for bedsore, (9) problems in vital signs, and (10) risk for falls	
Twenty-four nursing diagnoses/patient problems/ nursing phenomena:	
(1) problematic communication; (2) need for information, knowledge; (3) fear; (4) uncertainty about the future; (5) problems in contact with family; (6) insufficient insight in the health situation; (7) difficulty managing therapy; (8) lack of motivation to co-operate in treatment and care; (9) behavioral problems; (10) disorientation in time, place; (11) memory problem; (12) restlessness; (13) pain; (14) problems with rest/sleep; (15) difficulty with stressful situations; (16) pressure ulcer; (17) impairment in elimination; (18) fever; (19) breathing; (20) problems with food and fluids; (21) self-care limitation; (22) functional problem with activities of daily living; (23) high risk; and (24) impairment in vital functions	
Thirty-two nursing interventions/actions	
Four outcomes/results of nursing care: (1) patient falls, (2) satisfaction with care, (3) satisfaction with information, and (4) satisfaction with pain management	
Three complexity of care: (1) calculation of nursing intensity, (2) visual analogue scale on which nurses score the complexity of care, and (3) visual analogue scale on which nurses score the appropriateness of the amount of care that could be given	

Table 16.3 National NMDS (*Continued*)

The Netherlands (NMDSN)[f,g]	Switzerland (the Swiss Nursing Maximum Data Set)[h]
Patient characteristics: Sex Year of birth Admission date Discharge date Unique patient code Age	Semistandard languages: LEP, PRN, PLAISIR, RAI (Considering NANDA, NIC, NOC) Health status: nursing phenomena and results Interventions: treatment and nursing care, principal intervention, secondary interventions, frequency, contribution of social network, care times, individualized required care time, individualized given care time Action modalities: frequency, duration, presence/absence of activity, volume, number of contributors, constant presence, nurture of assistance, contribution of social network
Seven items described medical conditions: (1) admission medical diagnoses, (2) additional medical diagnoses, (3) complications, (4) predictability of the health situation (5) stability of the health situation, (6) life-threatening situations, and (7) the derived item multiple health problems	Name Date of birth Sex Town/city of residence nationally Civil status Professional status on admission Language used during care Interpreter Religion Type of insurance Payment of basic care Other source of payment Home care and assistance Type of dwelling Persons living at the same address Neonate: weight at birth, length, congenital deformity, and length of pregnancy
Healthcare settings: Hospital Ward Specialty Type of nursing delivery system Date of data collection	Nonnursing care and treatment: surgical operation, examinations, domiciliary assistance, other intra/extrainstitutional treatments or services, medication, pharmacotherapy Place: nature of location, services offered by each unit Unit infrastructure: number of beds per unit

(Continued)

Table 16.3   National NMDS (Continued)

The Netherlands (NMDSN)[f,g]	Switzerland (the Swiss Nursing Maximum Data Set)[h]
	Institution: identification
	Status
	Type of institution
	Professionals: Care personnel number/sex/
	Swiss or non-Swiss; professional training: number, diploma level

Thailand[i,j]
Nursing care elements:
Nursing problems
Nursing interventions
Nursing outcomes
Patient elements:
Patient first name and last name
Sex
Medical diagnosis
Health history of patient and family allergy
Address and phone number of patients
Referral
Laboratory tests
Patient's condition and medical instruments use before discharge
Discharge plan
Service elements:
Hospital number
Admission umber
Date of admission
Date of discharge/expiry
Health insurance

[a]From Ryan and Delaney (1995).
[b]Based on U.S. NMDS and Belgium data set
[c]From Sermeus (1992).
[d]From Evers et al. (2000).
[e]From Haraldsdottir (2001).
[f]From Goossen et al. (1998).
[g]From Goossen et al. (2001).
[h]From Berthou and Junger (2000).
[i]From Kunaviktikul et al. (2001).
[j]From Volrathongchai, Delaney, and Phuphaibul (2003).

across the globe to ensure that nursing essential data will be more comprehensively available in the future. There is varying capacity to capture variables related to the context of care.

Call for Standardized Contextual Data

Ample studies have demonstrated the significance of nurse staffing, patient/staff ratios, professional autonomy and control, organizational characteristics, unit internal environment, work delivery patterns, work group characteristics, external environment, staff work satisfaction, education of staff, multidisciplinary coordination/collaboration, and educational level on the quality and outcomes of patient care. For example, Aiken et al. (2003); Aiken et al. (2002); and Aiken, Smith, and Lake (1994) have maintained extensive research programs focused on examining the significance of these factors for quality of care. These studies have influenced the identification and use of NMDSs elements. Table 16.3 clearly indicates that several countries with established NMDSs have included some contextual data in the NMDSs. For example, Belgium calls for data related to number of beds and number of nurses available; Switzerland includes for specific workload data related to each nursing intervention. The U.S. NMDS addresses "intensity"; however, no current NMDS addresses the essential breadth of contextual variables.

The development within the United States of the NMMDS addresses this void. The 18 NMMDS elements are organized into three categories: environment, nursing care resources, and financial resources (see Table 16.4). The NMMDS is the minimum set of items of information with uniform definitions and categories concerning the specific dimension of the context of patient/client care delivery. It represents the essential data used to support the management and administration of nursing care delivery across all types of settings. The NMMDS most appropriately focuses on the nursing delivery unit/service/center of excellence level across these settings. The NMMDS supports numerous constructed variables as well as aggregation of data, e.g., unit level, institution, network, system. This minimum data set provides the structure for the collection of uniform information that influences quality of patient care, directly and indirectly. These data, in combination with actual patient data identified in the NMDS support clinical decision making; management decisions regarding the quantity, quality, and satisfaction of personnel; costs of patient care; clinical outcomes; and internal and external benchmarking.

Table 16.4   Nursing Management Minimum Data Set (NMMDS) Data Elements

Environment
Unit/cost center identifier
Type
Patient/client population
Volume
Accreditation
Organizational decision making power
Environmental complexity
Patient/client accessibility
Method of care delivery
Clinical decision making complexity
Nursing Care
Management demographic profile
Staffing
Staff demographic profile
Staff satisfaction
Financial Resources
Payer type
Reimbursement
Budget
Expense

NMDSs Relationship to International Nursing Minimum Data Set (i-NMDS)

Evolution of Concept

The i-NMDS includes the core, internationally relevant, essential, minimum data elements to be collected in the course for providing nursing care (Clark and Delaney, 2000). These data can provide information to describe, compare, and examine nursing practice around the globe. Work toward the i-NMDS is intended to build on the efforts already underway in individual countries. It is imperative that the national healthcare infrastructure supports the collection and reuse of nursing data. Consequently, partner countries participating in the development of the i-NMDS are encouraged to establish triads composed of (a) representative(s) of the National Nurses Association (preferably International Council of

Nurses [ICN] member), (b) International Medical Informatics Association Nursing Informatics Special Interest Group (IMIA NI-SIG) representative, and (c) informatics expert(s). Project teams provide coordination and communication of project work in each country.

The i-NMDS project is intended to build on and support data set work already underway in individual countries, as well as the work with another ICN initiative, the ICNP. Data collected in the i-NMDS pilot project will be cross-mapped and normalized to the ICNP. This i-NMDS work will assist in testing the i-NMDS and also advancing the ICNP as a unifying framework. Overall, the i-NMDS project focuses on coordinating ongoing international data collection and analyses of the i-NMDS to support the description, study, and improvement of nursing practice (Goossen et al., 2004).

Cosponsorship

The i-NMDS Research Center is lead by a steering committee of international representatives of countries with existing and emerging NMDSs as well as professional cosponsorship and areas of informatics expertise (*http://www.inmds.org*). The project is cosponsored by the ICN and the IMIA NI-SIG. Project work is also coordinated with international standards organizations and other stakeholders to assure harmonization of these efforts.

Purposes

The contribution of nursing care and nurses is essential to healthcare globally. The i-NMDS as a key data set will support:

- Describing the human phenomena, nursing interventions, care outcomes, and resource consumption related to nursing services
- Improving the performance of healthcare systems and the nurses working within these systems worldwide
- Enhancing the capacity of nursing and midwifery services
- Addressing the nursing shortage, inadequate working conditions, poor distribution and inappropriate utilization of nursing personnel, and the challenges as well as opportunities of global technological innovations
- Testing evidence-based practice improvements
- Empowering the public internationally

Data Elements

The i-NMDS elements are organized into three categories: setting, subjects of care, and nursing elements (Delaney et al., 2003). Setting variables include country characteristics as well as descriptors of the location of care, whether the setting is acute, ambulatory, home, and so on. Measures include care personnel characteristics, including numbers, full-time equivalents, education, gender, and so on. Subjects of care can include individuals, families, groups, or communities. Demographics of the subject (individuals, families, groups, and communities) are included, e.g., country of residence, disposition, age, gender, medical diagnosis are described. Last, nursing care elements include nursing diagnosis/subject of care problems, interventions, and outcomes. A measure of intensity of resource consumption will be developed. Nursing care data may be collected using standardized languages, e.g., Clinical Care Classification (CCC), Omaha, NANDA, NIC, NOC). All nursing care data will be normalized using the ICNP.

Issues

Continuing attention needs to focus on consistency with the i-NMDS as well as supporting development of NMDSs across all countries. Consensus has been established to support the development and adoption of NMDSs that support all core nursing data collection in information systems across all settings. However, congruent with the state-of-adoption, specific studies addressing critical areas of international import will be designed to support the inclusion of countries with the capacity to collect the data which is the focus of specific studies. Normalization of data definitions must occur. Normalization of data collection time periods is a difficult issue.

Future Directions

The power of NMDSs to describe nursing practice from an international perspective is daunting (Delaney, 1996; Delaney and Moorhead, 1995; Delaney et al., 2000; Delaney et al., 1998; Junger, Berthou, and Delaney, 2004; Karpiuk et al., 1997; Maas and Delaney, 2004; Mehmert and Delaney, 1991; Park et al., 2003; Rios-Iturrine et al., 1991; Saba, 1992a 1992b, 1997, in preparation). Knowing the human phenomena served by nursing, the interventions given and the outcomes realized are essential to improving outcomes, assuring patient/client safety, and providing wise stewardship of all resources, from human to financial. Information and knowledge are key to supporting an essential knowledge-driven professional service and improving healthcare through effective policy changes. Addressing the nursing shortage, inadequate working conditions, personnel satisfaction, all factors that research shows affect the quality of care, is dependent on nursing administration access to contextual as well as clinical data captured in the i-NMDS.

Access to the large data sets populated by the i-NMDS empowers nursing to capitalize on the emerging technologies of knowledge discovery, decision support, and advanced clinical information systems (Delaney, Reed, and Clarke, 2000; Delaney et al., 2000; Irwin and Saba, 2003). Hypotheses generation as well as pattern discoveries will revolutionize many aspects of nursing research. Moreover, these data and valid and reliable knowledge generation likewise can revolutionize education and educating knowledge workers.

 ## Case Scenario

There is a need to determine quality and outcomes of care for pain management in elders with fractured hip diagnoses both across settings of care within one healthcare system and within and across national healthcare system boundaries. The National Health Service in collaboration with the World Health Organization wishes to establish benchmarks for care. You are asked to file a report addressing the following:

1. What is the relationship between and among the number, education, certification, and experience of healthcare workers and the vacancy rate?

2. What is the relationship between and among the number, education, certification, and experience of healthcare workers and turnover rates?

3. What is the relationship between and among the number, education, certification, and experience of healthcare workers and the following outcomes:
   (a) Nosocomial infections
   (b) Discharge effectiveness (teaching/planning)
   (c) Patient/family satisfaction with care received
   (d) Length of stay appropriate to diagnosis
   (e) Morbidity/mortality
   (f) Nurse satisfaction

References

Aiken, L. H., Clarke, S. P., Cheung, R. B., Sloane, D. M., and Silber, J. H. (2002). Hospital nurse staffing and patient mortality, nurse burnout and job dissatisfaction. *Journal of the American Medical Association* 288(16):1987–1993.

Aiken, L. H., Clarke, S.P., Cheung, R. B., Sloane, D. M., and Silber, J. H. (2003). Educational levels of hospital nurses and surgical patient mortality. *Journal of the American Medical Association* 290(12): 1617–1623.

Aiken, L. H., Smith, H. L., and Lake, E. T. (1994). Lower Medicare mortality among a set of hospitals known for good nursing care. *Medical Care* 32(8):771–787.

American Association of Colleges of Nursing. (2003). *http://www.aacn.nche.edu/NewNurse/ NewNurseWorkingPaperHL.pdf*

American Nurses Association. (1997). *Nursing Information & Data Set Evaluation Center (NIDSECSM)*. Washington, DC: ANA.

American Nurses Association. (2004). *http://nursingworld.org/nidsec/prtlist.htm*

Androwich, I., Bickford, C., Button, P., Hunter, K., Murphy, J., and Sensmeier, J. (2003). *Clinical Information Systems: A Framework for Reaching the Vision*. Washington, DC: ANA.

Berthou, A. and Junger, A. (2000). *Nursing Data: Final Report Short Version 1998–2000 Period*. Retrieved date (April 1, 2002). Online *http://www.hospvd.ch/ public/ise/nursingdata*

Brooten, D., Youngblut, J. M., Kutcher, J., and Bobo, C. (2004). Quality and the nursing workforce: APNs, patient outcomes, and health care costs. *Nursing Outlook* 52:45–52.

Clark, J. and Delaney, C. (2000). Conceptualization and feasibility of an international nursing minimum data set (i-NMDS) [abstract]. In V. Saba, R. Carr, W. Sermeus, and P. Rocha (Eds.), *One Step Beyond: The Evolution of Technology & Nursing, Proceedings of the 7th International Congress on Nursing Informatics* (p. 865).

Committee on Quality of Health Care in America Institute of Medicine. (2000). *To Err Is Human*. Washington, DC: National Academy Press.

Committee on Quality of Health Care in America Institute of Medicine. (2001). *Crossing the Quality Chasm: A New Health System for the 21st Century*. Washington, DC: National Academy Press.

Committee on the Work Environment for Nurses & Patient Safety, Institute of Medicine. (2004). *Keeping Patients Safe*. Washington, DC: National Academy Press.

Delaney, C. (1996). Use of nursing informatics in advanced nursing practice roles for building healthier populations (clinical innovations). *Journal for Advanced Nursing Quarterly* 1(4):48–53.

Delaney, C., Goossen, W., Park, H., Junger, A., Oyri, K., Saba, V., and Coenen, A. (2003). Seeking international consensus on elements of the international nursing minimum data set (iNMDS) [abstract]. In H. Marin, E. Marques., E. Hovenga, and W. Goossen (Eds.), *Proceedings of the 8th International Congress in Nursing Informatics* (pp. 74–75).

Delaney, C., Herr, K., Maas, M., and Specht, J. (2000). Reliability of nursing diagnoses documented in a computerized nursing information system. *Nursing Diagnosis* 11(3):121–134.

Delaney, C., Mehmert, P., Prophet, C., and Crossley, J. (1998). Establishment of the research value of nursing minimum data sets [reprint]. In V. Saba (Ed.), *Nursing and Computers: An Anthology, 1987–1996*. New York: Springer.

Delaney, C. and Moorhead, S. (1995). The nursing minimum data set, standardized language & health care quality. *Journal of Nursing Care Quality* 10(1):16–30.

Delaney, C., Reed, D., and Clarke, M. (2000). Describing patient problems & nursing treatment patterns using nursing minimum data sets (NMDS & NMMDS) and UHDDS repositories [paper]. In J. M. Overhage (Ed.), *AMIA 2000 Converging Information, Technology, & Health Care* (pp. 176–179).

Delaney, C., Ruiz, M., Clarke, M., and Srinivasan, P. (2000). Knowledge discovery in databases: Data mining the NMDS [paper]. In V. Saba, R. Carr, W. Sermeus, and P. Rocha (Eds.), *One Step Beyond: The Evolution of Technology & Nursing, Proceedings of the 7th International Congress on Nursing Informatics* (pp. 61–65).

Goossen, W., Delaney, C., Semeus, W., Junger, A., Saba, V., Oyri, K., and Coenen, A. (2004). Preliminary results of a pilot of the international nursing minimum data set (i-NMDS) [abstract]. In *Proceedings of MedInfo 11th World Congress on Medical Informatics of the International Medical Informatics Association* (p. S103).

Goossen, W. T. F., Epping, P. M. M., Feuth, T., Dassen, T. W. N., and Hasman, A. (1998). A comparison of nursing minimum data sets. *Journal of the American Medical Informatics Association* 5(2):152–163.

Goossen, W. T. F., Epping, P. J. M. M., Feuth, T., van den Heuvel, W. J. A., Hasman, A., and Dassen, T. W. N. (2001). Using the nursing minimum data set for the Netherlands (NMDSN) to illustrate differences in patient populations and variations in nursing activities. *International Journal of Nursing Studies* 38:243–257.

Hansebo, G., Kihlgren, M., and Ljunggren, G. (1999). Review of nursing documentation in nursing wards-changes after intervention for individualized care. *Journal of Advanced Nursing* 29(6):1462–1473.

Irwin, R. G. and Saba, V. (2003). An electronic 3 care tracking system. In e-Health for all: Designing nursing agenda for the future. In H. Marin, E. Marques, E. Hovenga, and W. Goossen (Eds.), *Proceedings of the 8th International Congress in Nursing Informatics*.

Junger, A., Berthou, A., and Delaney, C. (2004). Modeling, the essential step to consolidate and integrate a national NMDS [paper]. *International Medical Informatics Conference*.

Karpiuk, K., Delaney, C., and Ryan, P. (1997). South Dakota statewide nursing minimum data set project. *Journal of Professional Nursing* 13(2):76–83.

Kunaviktikul, W., Anders, R. L., Srisuphan, W., Chontawan, R., Nuntasupawat, R., and Pumparporn, O. (2001). Development of quality of nursing care in Thailand. *Journal of Advanced Nursing* 36(6):776–784.

Lu, D. F., Eichmann, D., Konicek, D., Kanak, M., and Delaney, C. (in preparation). *SNOMED CT & Post-mapping Validation Methodology for Nursing Vocabularies*.

Maas, M. and Delaney, C. (2004). Nursing Process Outcome Linkage: An Assessment of Literature & Issues. *Medical Care* 42(2)(Suppl.):II-40-II-48.

Mehmert, P. and Delaney, C. (1991). Validating impaired physical immobility. *Nursing Diagnosis* 2(4):143–154.

Park, M. and Delaney, C. (2003). Enhanced nursing care profile of older patients with dementia using nursing minimum data set (NMDS) & uniform hospital discharge data set (UHDDS) in an acute care setting [paper]. In H. Marin, E. Marques., E. Hovenga, and W. Goossen (Eds.), *Proceedings of the 8th International Congress in Nursing Informatics* (pp. 490–494).

Pierce, S. (2000). Readiness for evidence-based practice: Information literacy needs of nursing faculty and students in a southern U.S. state. *Dissertation Abstracts International* 62(12B):5645. UMI No. 3035514.

Pravikoff, D., Pierce, S., and Tanner, A. (2003). Are nurses ready for evidence-based practice? *American Journal of Nursing* 103(5):95–96.

Rios-Iturrine, H., Delaney, C., Mehmert, P., Kruckeberg, T., and Chung, Y. (1991). Validation of defining characteristics of four nursing diagnoses using a computerized database. *Journal of Professional Nursing* 7(5):293–299.

Ryan, P. and Delaney, C. (1995). The nursing minimum data set: Research findings and future directions. In *Annual Review of Nursing Research* Vol. 13, pp. 169–194. New York, NY: Springer.

Saba, V. K. (1991). *Final Report: Develop and Demonstrate a Method for Classifying Home Health Patients to Predict Resource Requirements and to Measure Outcomes*. Washington, DC: HCFA (No. 17-C-98983/3: NTIS # PB92-177013/AS). Available at *http://www.sabacare.com*

Saba, V. K. (1992a). A classification of home health care nursing diagnoses and interventions. *Caring Magazine* 11(3):50–57.

Saba, V. K. (1992b). Home health care classification. *Caring Magazine* 11(5):58–60.

Saba, V. K. (1997). Why the Home Health Care Classification is a recognized nomenclature. *Computers in Nursing* 15(20):S67–S73.

Saba, V. K., O'Hare, A., Zuckerman, A. E., Boondas, J., Levine, E., and Oatway, D. M. (1991). A nursing intervention taxonomy for home health care. *Nursing and Health Care* 12(6):296–299.

Tanner, A. (2000). Readiness for evidence-based practice: Information literacy needs of nursing faculty and students in a southern U.S. state. *Dissertation Abstracts International* 62(12B):5647. UMI No. 3035515.

Turtiainen, A. M., Kinnunen, J., Sermeus, W., and Nyberg, T. (2000). The cross-cultural adaptation of Belgium Nursing Minimum Data Set to Finnish Nursing. *Journal of Nursing Management* 8, 281–290.

Volrathongchai, K., Delaney, C., and Phuphaibul, R. (2003). The development of NMDSs in Thailand. *Journal of Advanced Nursing* 43(6):1–7.

Werley, H. and Lang, N. (Eds.). (1988). *Identification of the nursing minimum data set (NMDS)*. New York: Springer.

PART **4**

Informatics Theory

CHAPTER 17

Theories, Models, and Frameworks

Carol J. Bickford

Kathleen M. Hunter

OBJECTIVES

1. Discuss the relationship between healthcare informatics and nursing informatics.
2. Discuss different definitions and models of nursing and healthcare informatics.
3. Discuss core concepts and the scope of practice of nursing informatics.
4. Describe nursing informatics as a distinct specialty.
5. Discuss key aspects of the electronic health record (EHR).
6. Discuss terminologies for nursing.
7. Identify available organizational resources.

KEY WORDS

informatics
electronic health record
competencies
terminologies

Abstract

Nursing informatics is an established and growing area of specialization in nursing. All nurses employ information technologies in their practice. Informatics nurses are key persons in the design, development, implementation, and evaluation of these technologies and in the development of the specialty's body of knowledge.

This chapter addresses the concepts, definitions, and interrelationships of nursing and healthcare informatics. The core concepts of nursing informatics are described and related to one another. The recognition of nursing informatics as a distinct nursing specialty, its scope of practice, and certification are discussed. Nursing informatics concepts and practices are described within the context of the electronic health record (EHR).

Introduction

Lifelong learning is based on the recognition of patterns and variances, builds on previous experiences and knowledge, and involves the use of analogies. Recognition of such learning principles proves invaluable for those exploring or already engaged in nursing informatics practice because the nurse in this specialty role is always learning and always teaching. Students often reflect significant diversity and may include information systems department staff, fellow nursing colleagues, other healthcare professionals, organizational leaders, students enrolled in healthcare professions educational programs, patients, community members, and others. Theories, models, frameworks, clearly stated definitions, and foundational documents can guide the nursing informatics learning activities for both students and faculty. By incorporating analogies based on clinical and other experiences, and by referencing previously learned foundational content and processes, the informatics nurse can assist the learner in understanding the relationships of data and information, computers and information sytem technologies, and communications and software applications to their work setting or personal life.

Foundational Documents Guide Nursing Informatics Practice

In 2001, the American Nurses Association (ANA) published the *Code of Ethics for Nurses with Interpretive Statements*, a complete revision of previous ethics provisions and interpretive statements that guide all nurses in practice, be it in the domains of direct patient care, education, administration, or research. Nurses working in the informatics specialty are professionally bound to follow these provisions. Terms such as decision-making, comprehension, information, knowledge, shared goals, disclosure, outcomes, privacy, confidentiality, disclosure, policies, protocols, evaluation, judgment, standards, and factual documentation abound throughout the explanatory language of the interpretive statements. Examine this guidance by reviewing the entire document posted for public access at *http://nursingworld.org/ethics/ecode.htm*.

In 2003, a second foundational professional document, *Nursing's Social Policy Statement, Second Edition*, provided a new definition of nursing:

> Nursing is the protection, promotion, and optimization of health and abilities, prevention of illness and injury, alleviation of suffering through the diagnosis and treatment of human response, and advocacy in the care of individuals, families, communities, and populations. (ANA, 2003, p. 6)

Again, informatics nurses must be cognizant of the statements and direction provided by this document to the nursing profession, its practitioners, and the public.

Nursing: Scope and Standards of Practice immediately followed in early 2004 and further reinforces the recognition of nursing as a cognitive profession (ANA, 2004). The measurement criteria explicate specific actions associated with each of the 15 standards and include data, information, and knowledge management activities as core work for all nurses. This cognitive work begins with the critical thinking and decision-making components of the nursing process that occur before nursing action begins.

The nursing process provides a delineated pathway and process for decision-making. First, assessment or data collection begins the nursing process. Diagnosis or problem definition, the second step, reflects the interpretation of the data and information gathered during assessment. Outcomes identification is the third step, followed by planning as the fourth step. Implementation of a plan is the fifth step. The final component of the nursing process is evaluation. The nursing process is most often presented as a linear process with evaluation listed as the last step; however, the nursing process really is iterative, includes numerous feedback loops, and incorporates evaluation activites throughout the sequencing. For example, evaluation of a plan's implementation may prompt further assessment, a new diagnosis or problem definition, and decision-making about new outcomes and related plans.

The collection of data about a client or about a management, education, or research situation is guided by a nurse's knowledge base built on formal and informal educational preparation, research, and previous experiences. In healthcare, as in most areas of our lives, data, information, and knowledge are growing at astronomical rates and demand increasing reliance on computer and information systems for collection, storage, organization and management, and dissemination. For example, in clinical nursing practice, consider the significant expansion in the amount and types of data that *must* be collected for legal, regulatory, quality, and other reasons; the data, information, and knowledge, like genetic profiles, related to specific client health conditions; and the information and knowledge about the healthcare environment, such as that associated with billing and reimbursement, health plan, and available formulary options. Collecting data in a systematic, thoughtful way, organizing data for efficient and accurate transformation into information, and documenting thinking and actions are critical to successful nursing practice. Nursing informatics is the nursing specialty that endeavors to make the collection, management, and dissemination of data, information, and knowledge easier for the practitioner, regardless of the domain and setting.

Definitions

Informatics and Healthcare Informatics

Informatics is a science that combines a domain science, computer science, information science, and cognitive science. Thus, it is a multidisciplinary science drawing from varied theories and knowledge applications. Healthcare informatics may be defined as the integration of healthcare sciences, computer science, information science, and cognitive science to assist in the management of healthcare information. Healthcare informatics is a subdiscipline of informatics. Imagine a large umbrella named informatics and imagine many persons under this umbrella. Each person represents a different domain science, one of which is healthcare informatics.

Because healthcare informatics is a relatively young addition to the informatics umbrella, you may see other terms that seem to be synonyms for this same area, such as health informatics or medical informatics. Medical informatics historically has been used in Europe as the preferred term for healthcare informatics. Medical informatics is now more clearly a subdomain of healthcare informatics and health informatics may mean informatics used in educating healthcare clients and/or the general public. As healthcare informatics evolves so will the clarity in definition of terms and scopes of practice.

Healthcare informatics addresses the study and management of healthcare information. Consider Fig. 17.1, where healthcare informatics is depicted as a large circle encompassing multiple healthcare-related disciplines. Note that the smaller circles inside the larger circle overlap. This represents the existence of areas of common knowledge and use among the disciplines. But each discipline also has specific knowledge and content areas that are unique to that discipline.

A similar model of overlapping discrete circles could depict the integrated content most often considered representative of the multiple and diverse aspects of healthcare informatics. Healthcare informatics again would be the largest encompassing circle surrounding smaller intersecting circles. These aspects include specific content areas such as information retrieval, ethics, security, decision support, patient care, system life cycle, evaluation, human-computer interaction (HCI), standards, telehealth, healthcare information systems, imaging, knowledge representation, EHRs, education, and information retrieval.

As shown in Fig. 17.1, nursing informatics is a subdomain of healthcare informatics. It shares common areas of science with other subdomains and therefore easily supports multidisciplinary education, practice, and research in healthcare informatics. Nursing informatics also has unique areas that address the special information needs for the discipline of nursing. Nurses work both collaboratively with other healthcare disciplines and independently when engaged in clinical nursing practice. Nursing informatics reflects this duality as well, moving in and out of integration and separation as situations and needs demand.

Nursing Informatics

In 1985, Kathryn Hannah proposed a definition that nursing informatics is the use of information technologies in relation to any nursing functions and actions of nurses (Hannah, 1985). In their classic article on the science of nursing informatics, Graves and Corcoran presented a more complex definition of nursing informatics. Nursing informatics is a combination of computer science, information science, and nursing science designed to assist in the management and processing of nursing data, information, and knowledge to support the practice of nursing and the delivery of nursing care (Graves and Corcoran, 1989).

The ANA modified the Graves and Corcoran definition with the development of the first scope of practice for nursing informatics. The ANA defined nursing informatics as the specialty that integrates nursing science, computer science, and information science in identifying, collecting, processing, and managing data and information to support nursing practice, administration, education, research, and the expansion of nursing knowledge (ANA, 1994). The explanation of the accompanying standards of practice for nursing informatics followed in 1995 with ANA's (1995) publication of the *Standards of Nursing Informatics Practice*.

In 2000, the ANA convened an expert panel to review and revise the scope and standards of nursing informatics practice. That group's work included an extensive examination of the evolving healthcare and nursing environments and culminated in the publication of the *Scope and Standards of Nursing Informatics*

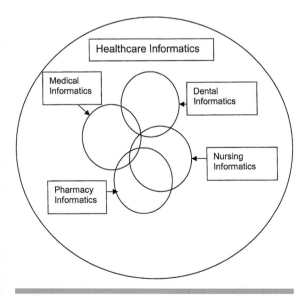

Figure 17.1
Healthcare informatics and subdomains of healthcare informatics.

Practice in 2001. This professional document includes an expanded definition of nursing informatics:

> Nursing informatics is a specialty that integrates nursing science, computer science, and information science to manage and communicate data, information, and knowledge in nursing practice. Nursing informatics facilitates the integration of data, information, and knowledge to support patients, nurses, and other providers in their decision-making in all roles and settings. This support is accomplished through the use of information structures, information processes, and information technology. (ANA, 2001b, p. vii)

The accompanying discussion of the scope of practice, informatics competencies, and standards of practice and associated measurement criteria provide more detail for a better understanding of this specialty. For a more rigorous review of nursing informatics definitions, see Staggers and Thompson's 2002 *JAMIA* article, "The Evolution of Definitions for Nursing Informatics: A Critical Analysis and Revised Definition." What is important to remember is that nursing informatics is a dynamic and evolving professional discipline.

Nursing Informatics as a Specialty

In early 1992, the ANA established nursing informatics as a distinct specialty in nursing with a distinct body of knowledge. Unique among the healthcare professions, this designation as a specialty provides official recognition that nursing informatics is indeed a part of nursing and that it has a distinct scope of practice. Following the recognition of nursing informatics as a specialty and the publication of the nursing informatics scope and standards, the American Nurses Credentialing Center (ANCC) established a certification examination and process in 1995 to recognize those nurses with basic informatics specialty competencies.

The scope of nursing informatics practice includes activities such as developing and evaluating applications, tools, processes, and strategies that assist registered nurses in managing data to support decision-making. This decision-making can encompass any and all of the following areas of nursing practice: client care, research, education, and administration. Information handling—the processes involved in managing data, information, and knowledge—includes naming, organizing, grouping, collecting, processing, analyzing, storing, retrieving, transforming and communicating data and information.

The core phenomena of nursing are the nurse, patient, health, and environment. Nursing informatics is interested in these core phenomena, decision-making, data,

information, and knowledge, as well as information structures and technologies. It is this special focus on the information of nursing that distinguishes nursing informatics from other nursing specialties.

As noted earlier in this chapter, nursing informatics is one component of the broader field of healthcare informatics. Nursing informatics intersects with other domains and disciplines concerned with the management of data, information, and knowledge. The boundaries and intersections are flexible and allow for the inevitable changes and growth that evolve over time.

Models for Nursing Informatics

Models are representations of some aspect of the real world. Models show particular perspectives of a selected aspect and may illustrate relationships. Models evolve as knowledge about the selected aspect changes and are dependent on the "world view" of those developing the model. It is important to remember that different models reflect different viewpoints and are not necessarily competitive; that is, there is no one "right" model.

Different scholars in nursing informatics have proposed different models. Some of these models are presented here to provide further perspectives on nursing informatics, to demonstrate how differently scholars and practitioners may view what seems to be the same thing, and to show that nursing informatics is an evolutionary, theoretical, and practical science. Again, remember that there is no one right model nor are any of the models presented here exhaustive of the possible perspectives of nursing informatics.

Graves and Corcoran's seminal work included a model of nursing informatics. Their model placed data, information, and knowledge in sequential boxes with one-way arrows pointing from data to information to knowledge. The management processing box is directly above, with arrows pointing in one direction from management processing to each of the three boxes (Graves and Corcoran, 1989). The model is a direct depiction of their definition of nursing informatics.

In 1986, Patricia Schwirian proposed a model of nursing informatics intended to stimulate and guide systematic research in this discipline (Schwirian, 1986). Her concern at that time was over the sparse volume of research literature in nursing informatics. The model provides a framework for identifying significant information needs, which in turn can foster research. There are four primary elements arranged in a pyramid with a triangular base. The four elements are the raw material (nursing-related information), the technology (a computing system), the users (nurses, students, and context), and the goal or objective toward which the preceding elements are directed. Bidirectional arrows connect the three base components of raw material, user, and computer system to form the pyramid's triangular base. The goal element is placed at the apex of the pyramid to show its importance. Similarly, all interactions between the three base elements and the goal are represented by bidirectional arrows (Schwirian, 1986).

Turley, writing in 1996, proposed another model in which the core components of informatics (cognitive science, information science, and computer science) are depicted as intersecting circles. Nursing science is a larger circle that completely encompasses the intersecting circles. Nursing informatics is the intersection between the discipline-specific science (nursing) and the area of informatics (Turley, 1996).

Data, Information, and Knowledge

Data, information, and knowledge are identified as current metastructures or overarching concepts for nursing informatics with specific definitions in the *Scope and Standards of Nursing Informatics Practice*. Data are "discrete entities that are described objectively without interpretation" and would include some value assigned to a variable. For example, a systolic blood pressure is a datum (ANA, 2001b, p. 6). Another datum may be a nursing intervention, a patient problem, or an outcome.

Information reflects interpretation, organization, or structuring of data (ANA, 2001b, p. 6). Information is the result of processing data. Data processing occurs when raw facts are transformed through the application of context to give those facts meaning or via the organization of data into a structure that connotes meaning (Graves and Corcoran, 1989).

Knowledge emerges from the transformation of information. "Knowledge is information that is synthesized so that relationships are identified and formalized" (ANA, 2001b, p. 6). Consider the continuity, the overlap reflected in the intersections, and the somewhat linear process with numerous bidirectional feedback loops in Fig. 17.2 (ANA, 2001b, p. 7). Note, however, that processing of information does not always result in the development of knowledge. Further, knowledge is necessary to the processing of data and information. Knowledge itself may be processed to generate decisions and new knowledge (Graves and Corcoran, 1989).

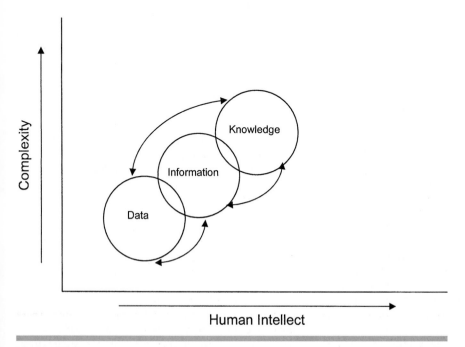

Figure 17.2
Transformation of data to knowledge.

Registered Nurses as Knowledge Workers

Knowledge work is the exercise of specialist knowledge and competencies (Blackleaf, 1995). The United States is becoming a nation of knowledge workers. Futurists predict that in the second millennium the primary domestic product of the United States will be knowledge and related knowledge services. Knowledge workers will be valued contributors to these products.

Registered nurses are consummate twenty-first century knowledge workers. Their skills in assessment, planning, critical thinking, and evaluation are transferable to many different settings but are most exquisitely employed in nursing practice. Knowledge work, of course, depends on access to data, information, and knowledge. Atomic level data are the foundation for the transforming processes by which knowledge work is accomplished. Atomic level data are raw, uninterpreted facts with values, and cannot be further subdivided. These data captured at the source in the course of clinical care are very useful in tracking the effectiveness of nursing decisions and are amenable to inclusion in electronic information systems as well as multiple forms of manipulation (Graves and Corcoran, 1989; Zielstorff et al., 1993). Analysis, combination, aggregation, and summarization are ways in which an information system can transform atomic level data to information and knowledge.

Competencies

Benner's (1982) work, built on the Dreyfus model of skill acquisition that describes the evolution of novice to expert, merits discussion for nursing informatics. This desired change in skills involves the evolution from a novice level to advanced beginner to competent to proficient to finally an expert level. Every nurse must continually exhibit the capability to acquire and then demonstrate specific skills beginning with the very first student experience. As students, most individuals can be described as novices having no experience with the situations and related content in those situations where they are expected to perform tasks. The advanced beginner can marginally demonstrate acceptable performance having built on lessons learned in their expanding experience base. Individuals at these levels often need oversight by teachers or experienced colleagues to help structure the learning experience and support appropriate and successful workplace decision-making and action.

Increased proficiency over time results in enhanced competencies reflecting mastery and the ability to cope with and manage many contingencies. Continued practice, combined with additional professional experience and knowledge, allows the nurse to evolve to the proficient level of appreciating the rules and maxims of practice and the nuances that are reflected in the absence of the normal picture. The expert has developed the capacity to intuitively understand the situation and immediately target the problem with minimal effort or problem solving.

Staggers, Gassert, and Curran recently published information about their research identifying the informatics competencies necessary for all nurses (Staggers, Gassert, and Curran, 2001). Their conceptual framework guiding the research included computer skills, informatics knowledge, and informatics skills as the informatics competencies (Staggers, Gassert, and Curran, 2002, p. 385). Their research, however, only identified informatics competencies for four levels of nurses: beginning nurse, experienced nurse, informatics specialist, and informatics innovator (Staggers, Gassert, and Curran, 2001). The comprehensive list of 304 competencies poses a significant challenge for professional development and academic faculties wishing to address each of the competencies when preparing curricula and then teaching educational programs for all skill levels.

Similar issues arise for the ANCC, which developed and maintains the nursing informatics certification examination. The ANCC content expert panel has oversight responsibility for the content of this examination and considers the current informatics environment and research when defining the test content outline. Currently, the topics addressed include human factors, system life cycle (system planning, analysis, design, implementation and testing, evaluation, maintenance, and support), information technology (hardware, software, communications, data representation, and security), information management and knowledge generation (data, information, knowledge), professional practice, trends, and issues (roles, trends and issues, ethics), and models and theories (foundations of nursing informatics, nursing and healthcare data sets, classification systems and nomenclatures, related theories and sciences). The detailed test content outline is available at *http://nursingworld.org/ancc/certification/cert/exams/TCOs/BSN27_Infor_TCO.html.*

The Healthcare Information and Management Systems Society (HIMSS) has recently established a certification program that may be of interest to informatics nurses. Certifications available include CPHIMS (Certified Professional in Healthcare Information & Management Systems), CHS (Certified in Healthcare Security), CHP

(Certification in Healthcare Privacy), and CHPS (Certified in Healthcare Privacy and Security). The content outlines for the examination and other administrative and application details are available at the HIMSS Web site at *http://www.himss.org/asp/prodevelopment_homepage.asp*.

Electronic Health Record

Today's healthcare environment is characterized by significant emphasis on establishing the EHR in all settings. Discussion of the associated database and data elements is critical in the implementation of the EHR. Data sets are comprised of data elements brought together for a specific reason. When values are assigned to the elements in a data set, the resulting data most often are stored in a database. Modern databases are used for storing data in a way that maintains the logical relationships among data elements, and are stored in a computer. Note, however, that the logical structure of a database is determined by the conceptual or theoretical views held by the database developers. That is, the same data elements may be organized and related in entirely different ways by different developers. Unfortunately, very often the healthcare organizations and final users have not been consulted in the database design phase, which then can result in major implementation and usability problems.

In healthcare and nursing, there are different types of databases, including bibliographic, payment claims, research, and the client record. Our focus in this chapter is on the client health record as a database. Any client health record, whether paper-based or computer-based, is a database made up of the myriad data elements for which data are gathered and which are used in health and healthcare decision-making by healthcare practitioners, providers, individuals, and families. A simple perspective is that the EHR is a client health record database supported by computer, electronic, and communications technologies.

The concept of the EHR emerged, initially, as a computer-based patient record or CPR and was given significant impetus by a 1991 report from the Institute of Medicine that advocated the adoption of the CPR as the primary source of client healthcare data and information (Dick and Steen, 1991; Dick, Steen, and Detmer, 1997). In this seminal work, the CPR was conceived as a longitudinal medical record receiving data from multiple worldwide sources, not simply an electronic copy of the traditional paper medical record.

Naturally, this concept and its definitions have evolved over time. Other terms for the CPR have been used, such as electronic medical record (EMR), electronic patient record (EPR), computerized patient record, or computerized medical record (CMR). Gradually, the informatics community has been adopting EHR as a name more in keeping with modern perspectives on comprehensive healthcare, health maintenance, and multidisciplinary practice.

American Society for Testing and Materials (ASTM) Standard E 1384-02a (ASTM, 2004, p. 31) defines the EHR as "any information related to the past, present, or future physical/mental health, or condition of an individual. The information resides in electronic system(s) used to capture, transmit, receive, store, retrieve, link, and manipulate multimedia data for the primary purpose of providing healthcare and health related services." An EHR encompasses the entire scope of health information in all media forms (Stetson, 1998). When implemented as part of an information system, the EHR is the primary source for information about a client; the place where client information is recorded or documented.

In 2001, the National Committee on Vital and Health Statistics (NCVHS) identified the patient medical record information (PMRI) as a model for the specific content necessary for the EHR, a component of the National Health Information Infrastructure (NHII). The healthcare provider, personal health, and population health dimensions are represented by intersecting circles. The personal health dimension includes the personal health record maintained and controlled by the individual or family, nonclinical information such as self-care trackers and directories of healthcare and public health service providers, and other supports to manage wellness and healthcare decision-making. The healthcare provider dimension promotes quality patient care, access to complete accurate patient data 24 hours per day 7 days per week, and includes provider notes, clinical orders decision support programs, and practice guidelines. The population health dimension includes information on the health of the population and the influences on that health. This information helps stakeholders identify and track health threats, assess population health, create and monitor programs and services, and conduct research (*http://www.ncvhs.hhs.gov/nhiilayo.pdf*).

There are many reasons for healthcare data and information documentation. These include compliance with law and regulations, adherence to the standards of accrediting agencies, communication with others providing healthcare to the client, conduct of research and clinical trials, provision of a basis for costing out services, and creation of claims for payment for services. For a clinical nurse, the status of the client and the recording of nursing care activities and decisions usually are priorities. This documentation of the nursing process and the delivery of nursing care allows nurses to accumulate the data to demonstrate nursing's impact on client health outcomes. In the modern healthcare environment, the availability of empirical evidence that one's discipline and practice positively affect an individual's or a community's health, is critical.

Without the EHR, it remains nearly impossible to extract nursing data from the paper health record in an efficient and affordable way. The logical structure of the database, that is, the EHR, along with the development of standardized terms for describing nursing practice, have made data collection a little easier. Informatics nurses serve an important role in designing, developing, implementing, monitoring, evaluating, and modifying

EHRs, so these records facilitate nurses' work, growth of the discipline, and nursing and health services research.

Progress toward this goal of the EHR has been hampered by the lack of attention to address workflow and the importance of clinical knowledge when designing the supporting information systems. Although it specifically references nursing, the organizing framework for clinical information systems in Fig. 17.3 is applicable to all healthcare disciplines participating in the EHR implementation activities (Androwich et al., 2003).

Terminologies

To convey important data and information to others, the communication must be understood by the listener and be interpreted as having meaning. This is best

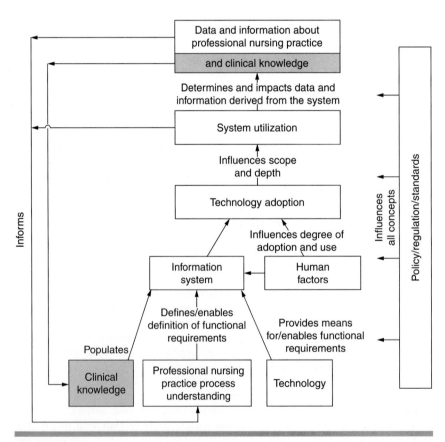

Figure 17.3
Organizing framework for clinical information systems: clinical knowledge as critical factor.

accomplished by using standard communication formats and terminologies, and recognized conventions for describing the concepts being presented. Concept representation involves the set of terms and relationships that describe the phenomena, processes, and practices of a discipline, such as nursing. Data elements, classifications, nomenclatures, vocabularies, and languages are some of the ways in which nursing concepts may be represented. Data elements are terms for which data are collected and for which values are assigned. A specific, purposeful group of data elements, representing a subset of concepts within a discipline, is a data set.

The nursing minimum data set (NMDS) developed through Dr. Harriet Werley's research is considered the foundational work for nursing languages and represents the first attempt to standardize the collection of essential nursing data. This data set contains 16 data elements divided into patient, service, and nursing care elements, and fosters the comparison of nursing data across time, settings, and populations (Werley and Lang, 1988). The four nursing care elements include nursing diagnosis, nursing intervention, nursing outcome, and intensity of nursing care. Patient or client demographic elements address personal identification, date of birth, gender, race, and residence. The seven service elements include unique facility or service agency number, unique health record number of patient or client, unique number of principal registered nurse provider, episode admission or encounter data, discharge or termination date, disposition of patient or client, and expected payer.

Most of these data elements, except for the nursing care elements and the unique identifier for the primary registered nurse, have long been captured in healthcare information systems. Werley and her colleagues envisioned collecting these data from everywhere nursing care is delivered, aggregating and storing these data in large databases, and using these data for policy analysis, evaluation of care, strategic planning, and nursing research. There are other data sets that contain nursing data elements, such as the minimum data set (MDS) developed for long-term care facilities (*http:// www.cms. hhs.gov/medicaid/mds20/default.asp?*) and outcome and assessment information set (OASIS), the home health data set that is used by home health agencies (*http:// www.cms.hhs.gov/ oasis/*).

Much of the early nursing terminologies research that helps describe nursing practice received initial federal funding support from the National Library of Medicine. The ANA further highlighted these efforts through establishment of a standardized data set recognition program based on defined review criteria. The ANA program

for recognition of terminologies that support nursing has evolved, in concert with the advancements in the research and terminology development efforts, to include new recognition criteria and differentiation of data sets, classification systems, and nomenclatures.

Nursing terminologies offer systematic, standardized ways of describing nursing practice and include data sets, taxonomies, nomenclatures, and classification systems. Nomenclatures are terms or labels for describing concepts in nursing such as diagnoses, interventions, and outcomes. Classifications are the ordering of entities, including nomenclatures, into groups or classes on the basis of their similarities (Gordon, 1998). Taxonomy is the study of classification, and simultaneously refers to the end product of a classification. It is often used interchangeably with classification (Gordon, 1998). Similarly, classification is an ordering of entities into groups according to a set of criteria as well as the end result of the ordering (Gordon, 1998). A nomenclature or vocabulary is a set of word labels for naming concepts. For example, SNOMED CT includes nursing diagnoses, interventions, and outcomes concepts within the hundreds of thousands of terms recently made available to the public through the National Library of Medicine.

Why are informatics nurses and nurse scholars so interested in terminologies? Nursing terminologies focus on the patient and care process, not reimbursement or mortality, and are increasingly important as EHRs become an integral component of healthcare services delivery. These terminologies are used to capture, store, and manipulate data in EHRs. Nursing is both blessed and challenged by the wealth of terminologies available for describing nursing practice and nurses' contributions to healthcare. This diversity offers practitioners choices in how to best describe their patient population and practice. A detailed presentation of each terminology recognized by the ANA as of 2004 is outside the scope of this chapter. Interested readers are referred to the terminology developers or custodians for more details (Table 17.1). What is important to remember is that each of the ANA-recognized terminologies was developed for specific purposes and does not yet provide the language to describe every segment of the nursing process.

NANDA

NANDA-I has evolved from an alphabetical listing in the mid-1980s to a conceptual system that guides the classification of nursing diagnoses in a taxonomy and includes definitions and defining characteristics. Currently NANDA-I includes 167 recognized diagnoses

Table 17.1   ANA-Recognized Terminologies

Terminology	Contact Information	ANA Recognition
NANDA-I:	E-mail: *info@nanda.org* Web site: *www.nanda.org*	1992
Nursing Interventions Classification (NIC)	Web site: *www.nursing.uiowa.edu/centers/cncce/*	1992
Clinical Care Classification (CCC) [Previously known as Home Health Care Classification (HHCC)]	Web site: *www.sabacare.com*	1992
Omaha System	E-mail: *martinks@tconl.com* Web site: *www.omahasystem.org*	1992
Nursing Outcomes Classification (NOC)	Web site: *www.nursing.uiowa.edu/centers/cncce/*	1997
Nursing management minimum data set (NMMDS)	E-mail: *connie-delaney@uiowa.edu* E-mail: *diane-huber@uiowa.edu*	1998
Patient care data set (PCDS)	E-mail: *judy.ozbolt@vanderbilt.edu*	1998
Perioperative nursing data set (PNDS)	E-mail: *pnds@aorn.org* Web site: *www.aorn.org*	1999
SNOMED CT	E-mail: *dkonice@cap.org* Web site: *www.snomed.org*	1999, 2003
Nursing minimum data set (NMDS)	E-mail: *connie-delaney@uiowa.edu*	1999
International Classification for Nursing Practice (ICNP)	E-mail: *coenena@uwm.edu* E-mail: *aamherdt@uwm.edu* Web site: *www.icn.ch/icnp.htm*	2000
ABC Codes	E-mail: *Melinna.Giannini@alternativelink.com* Web site: *alternativelink.org*	2000
Logical Observation Identifiers Names and Codes (LOINC)	E-mail: *susan.matney@ihc.com* Web site: *www.loinc.org*	2002

that are very different from the pathology and mortality focus of the ICD-9 CM terms used for medicine and third party payment claims.

Nursing Interventions Classification (NIC)

The fourth edition of NIC contains 514 nursing interventions that describe the treatments nurses perform, updated linkages with NANDA diagnoses, and core interventions identified for 44 specialty practice areas (including three new specialties). These terms differ from the surgically biased CPT-4 code set terms used by medicine and third party payment programs (Dochterman and Bulechek, 2004).

Nursing Outcomes Classification (NOC)

The latest edition of NOC has 330 research-based outcomes to provide standardization of expected patient, caregiver, family, and community outcomes for measuring the effect of nursing interventions. Each outcome

features a definition, a set of specific indicators, measures to facilitate clinical implementation, and references.

Clinical Care Classification (CCC) [Formerly Home Health Care Classification (HHCC)]

The CCC system is a research-based nomenclature designed to standardize the terminologies for documenting nursing care in all clinical care settings. The two interrelated terminologies: CCC if Nursing Diagnoses and Outcomes and the CCC of Nursing Interventions and Actions, classified by 21 Care Components, are designed to assess and document nursing care and also to classify and code care over time, across settings, population groups, and geographic locations.

Omaha System

The most recent revision of the Omaha System was released in November 2004. Originally developed for use in home health practice, the Omaha System is now used in all clinical settings. It includes an assessment component (Problem Classification Scheme), an intervention component (Intervention Scheme), and an outcomes component (Problem Rating Scale for Outcomes).

Perioperative Nursing Data Set (PNDS)

The PNDS provides a universal language for perioperative nursing practice and education and a framework to standardize documentation. The diagnostic component is based on NANDA, while the interventions are NIC terms and the outcomes are from NOC. The PNDS can be used in all perioperative settings and has been integrated into numerous commercial information systems for the operating room environment.

SNOMED CT

The SNOMED CT is a core clinical terminology containing over 357,000 healthcare concepts with unique meanings and formal logic-based definitions organized into multiple hierarchies. As of January 2004, the fully populated table with unique descriptions for each concept contains more than 957,000 descriptions. The July 2004 release contained HHCC Version 2, NANDA Taxonomy II, NIC Version 4, NOC Version 3, PNDS Version 2, and the Omaha System (1992). In 2004, the National Library of Medicine negotiated a long-term contract to place SNOMED CT in the public domain for low cost licensing through the National Library of Medicine. It is available in English, Spanish, and German language editions.

ABC Codes

The ABC codes provide a mechanism for coding integrative health interventions by clinician by state location for administrative billing and insurance claims. The data set includes complementary and alternative medicine interventions and codes that map all NIC, CCC, and Omaha System interventions.

Patient Care Data Set (PCDS)

The PCDS includes terms and codes for patient problems, therapeutic goals, and patient care orders. This data set was developed by Dr. Judith Ozbolt from research data from nine acute care hospitals throughout the United States.

Logical Observation Identifiers Names and Codes (LOINC)

The LOINC originated as a database of standardized laboratory terms for results reporting for chemistry, hematology, serology, microbiology, and toxicology. LOINC now includes about 32,000 terms, including a clinical portion with codes for observations at key stages of the nursing process, including assessments, goals, and outcomes. Such entries include vital signs, hemodynamic values, intake/output, ECG, obstetric ultrasound, cardiac echo, urologic imaging, gastroendoscopic procedures, pulmonary ventilator management, selected survey instruments, and other clinical observations.

International Classification for Nursing Practice (ICNP)

The ICNP is a combinatorial terminology for nursing practice developed by the international nursing community under sponsorship of the International Council of Nurses (ICN). The ICNP elements include nursing phenomena (nursing diagnosis), nursing actions (nursing interventions), and nursing outcomes. The ICNP facilitates cross-mapping of local terms and existing vocabularies and classifications.

Nursing Management Minimum Data Set (NMMDS)

The NMMDS includes terms to describe the context and environment of nursing practice, and includes terms for nursing delivery unit/service, patient/client population, care delivery method, personnel characteristics, and financial resources.

Organizations as Resources

Many organizations have emerged to provide information resources and value-added membership benefits that support those individuals interested in healthcare and nursing informatics. Clinical specialty and other professional organizations have also appreciated the evolving healthcare information management focus and have established organizational structures such as informatics sections, divisions, workgroups, or special interest groups. Some have incorporated informatics and information system technology initiatives in strategic plans with dedicated staffing and ongoing financial support. In many instances informal networking groups have evolved into international organizations with hundreds of members connected via the Web.

The ANA and its affiliates and several nursing specialty organizations have informatics committees and government affairs and lobby offices addressing information technology, EHRs, standards and other informatics issues. Other organizations are multidisciplinary in their membership composition. Some organizations restrict their membership to individuals, while others allow only other organizations to join.

The nature, purposes, and activities of the multiple informatics organizations have sufficient differences that there is bound to be at least one organization, if not more, for everyone interested in nursing informatics. Membership and active participation in such professional organizations demonstrate compliance with Provisions 8 and 9 of the *Code of Ethics for Nurses with Interpretive Statements* (ANA, 2001a) and Standard 15. Leadership described in *Nursing: Scope and Standards of Practice* (ANA, 2004).

Information about a few of these organizations is provided here. This is in no way an exhaustive presentation. To learn more about these organizations and others, consult the Internet, informatics colleagues, and the literature.

American Medical Informatics Association

The American Medical Informatics Association (AMIA) is an individual membership organization dedicated to the development and application of medical informatics in the support of patient care, teaching, research, and healthcare administration. (Note: AMIA believes that the term "medical informatics" represents all of the diverse interests, issues, and aspects of informatics in healthcare.) AMIA serves as an authoritative body in the field of medical informatics and frequently represents the United States in the informational arena of medical informatics in international forums and is the U.S. member of the International Medical Informatics Association (IMIA). The *Journal of the American Medical Informatics Association* (JAMIA), available online and in print copy, has emerged as one of the top healthcare infomatics resources.

Members include developers of many of the most significant clinical information systems in the United States, a large number of academically-based healthcare professionals devoted to the applications of computers in clinical care, and a representative number of users of healthcare information systems. Professionals who are members of AMIA include physicians, nurses, dentists, dietitians, educators, computer and information scientists, biomedical engineers, medical librarians, academic researchers, and others. Members may select membership

in special interest workgroups, including one for students. The Nursing Informatics Workgroup (NI-WG) has long been the most active AMIA workgroup and has established several competitive scholarships (*www.amia.org*).

Healthcare Information and Management Systems Society

The HIMSS represents a membership of over 14,000 individuals and 200 corporations interested in healthcare informatics, clinical systems, information systems, management engineering, and telecommunications. HIMSS members are responsible for developing many of today's key innovations in healthcare delivery and administration, including telehealth, CPRs or EHRs, community health information networks, and portable/wireless healthcare computing. HIMSS has special interest groups, local and state chapters, a fellows recognition program, and the recently established professional credentialing service offering four certifications: CPHIMS, CHS, CHP, and CHPS. HIMSS has assumed a leadership role in the healthcare information technology standards arena and holds the secretariate for International Organization for Standardization Technical Committee 215 (ISO TC-215) (*www.himss.org*).

National League for Nursing

The mission of the National League for Nursing (NLN) is to advance quality nursing education that prepares the nursing workforce to meet the needs of diverse populations in an ever-changing healthcare environment. Recent organizational restructuring consolidated numerous councils into four advisory councils with many integrated objectives related to information management and technology applications in the educational environment. The Educational Technology and Information Management Advisory Council (ETIMAC) was established to promote the effective use of technology in nursing education, both as a teaching tool and as an outcome for student and faculty learning, and to advance the integration of information management into educational practices and program outcomes. The NLN also addresses faculty development and educational research. Membership categories include individual, education agency, healthcare agency, and NLN agency/school of nursing members (*www.nln.org*).

Society for Health Systems

The Society for Health Systems (SHS) is a society of the Institute of Industrial Engineers. The SHS itself is an individual membership organization that exists to enhance the career development and continuing education of professionals who use industrial and management engineering expertise for productivity and quality improvement in the healthcare industry. Currently the 400 SHS members include management engineers, nurses, chief executive officers (CEOs), administrators, directors of continuous improvement, clinicians, physicians, and department managers (*www.shs.iienet.org*).

Association for Computing Machinery

The Association for Computing Machinery (ACM) was founded in 1947 and has become a major force in advancing the skills of information technology professionals and students worldwide. ACM's over 75,000 members have made possible the development of ACM's leading portal to computing literature and its authoritative publications, pioneering conferences, and twenty-first century leadership. Chapters and special interest groups serve individuals at the local level (*www.acm.org*).

ARMA International

ARMA International (ARMA) is a not-for-profit association serving more than 10,000 information management professionals in the United States, Canada, and over 30 other nations. ARMA International members include records and information managers, archivists, corporate librarians, imaging specialists, legal professionals, knowledge managers, consultants, educators, and healthcare professionals. The mission of ARMA International is to provide education, research, and networking opportunities to information professionals, to enable them to use their skills and experience to leverage the value of records, information, and knowledge as corporate assets and as contributors to organizational success. ARMA is responsible for developing and maintaining several American National Standards Institute (ANSI) standards. Chapters and industry-specific groups (ISG) provide local member support and numerous educational programs (*www.arma.org*).

American Society for Information Science and Technology

The American Society for Information Science and Technology (ASIS&T), established in 1937, describes itself as *the* society for information professionals leading the search for new and better theories, techniques, and technologies to improve access to information. The over 4,000 ASIS&T members include information specialists from such fields as computer science, linguistics, management, librarianship, engineering, law, healthcare, chemistry, and education, who share a common interest in improving the ways society stores, retrieves, analyzes, manages, archives, and disseminates information, coming together for mutual benefit. Local chapters and special interest groups provide professional support and educational programs on such topics as HCI, information architecture, information needs, and knowledge management (*www.asis.org*).

Many other organizations are available to the individual seeking colleagues with specific informatics interests, as well as tools, publications, and educational resources about diverse data, information, knowledge, and informatics topics. The explosion of the World Wide Web now makes those diverse resources continuously available from any world location.

Summary

Through the use of theories, models, frameworks, and definitions, some of the concepts of informatics, healthcare informatics, and nursing informatics were explained, and their relationships to each other were discussed. The core concepts of nursing informatics were presented and described in detail. The establishment of the specialty of nursing informatics was explained. The EHR was described and related to nursing informatics. The brief discussion of terminologies supporting nursing practice introduced several of the information management tools used by nurses to complete their work.

References

American Nurses Association. (1994). *The Scope of Practice for Nursing Informatics*. Washington, DC: American Nurses Publishing.

American Nurses Association. (1995). *Standards of Nursing Informatics Practice*. Washington, DC: American Nurses Publishing.

American Nurses Association. (2001a). *Code of Ethics for Nurses with Interpretive Statements*. Washington, DC: American Nurses Publishing.

American Nurses Association. (2001b). *Scope and Standards of Nursing Informatics Practice*. Washington, DC: American Nurses Publishing.

American Nurses Association. (2003). *Nursing's Social Policy Statement*, 2nd ed. Washington, DC: nursesbooks.org.

American Nurses Association. (2004). *Nursing: Scope and Standards of Practice*. Washington, DC: nursesbooks.org.

Androwich, I. M., Bickford, C. J., Button, P. S., Hunter, K.
M., Murphy, J., and Sensmeier, J. (2003). *Clinical
Information Systems: A Framework for Reaching the
Vision*. Washington, DC: American Nurses Publishing.

ASTM. (2004). *Annual Book of ASTM Standards 2004.*
West Conshohocken, PA: ASTM International.

Benner, P. (1982). From novice to expert. *American
Journal of Nursing* 82(3):402–407.

Blackleaf, F. (1995). Knowledge, knowledge work and
organizations: An overview and interpretation.
Organization Studies 16(6):1021–1046.

Dick, R. S. and Steen, E. B. (Eds.). (1991). *The Computer-
Based Patient Record: An Essential Technology for
Change*. Washington, DC: Institute of Medicine.

Dick, R. S., Steen, E. B., and Detmer, D. E. (Eds.). (1997).
*The Computer-Based Patient Record: An Essential
Technology for Change* (Rev.). Washington, DC:
Institute of Medicine.

Dochterman, J. M. and Bulechek, G. M. (Eds.). (2004).
Nursing Interventions Classification (NIC). St. Louis,
MO: Mosby.

Gordon, M. (1998). Nursing nomenclature and
classification system development. *Online Journal of
Issues in Nursing. http://www.nursingworld.org/ojin/
tpc7/tpc7_1.htm*

Graves, J. R. and Corcoran, S. (1989). The study of nursing
informatics. *IMAGE: Journal of Nursing Scholarship*
21(4):227–231.

Hannah, K. (Ed.). (1985). Current trends in nursing
informatics: Implications for curriculum planning. In
K. Hannah, E. J. Guillemin, and D. N. Conklin (Eds.),
Nursing Uses of Computer and Information Science.
Amsterdam: North-Holland.

Moorehead, S., Johnson, M., and Maas, M. (Eds.). (2004).
Nursing Outcomes Classification (NOC) (3rd ed.).
St. Louis, MO: Mosby.

NANDA International. (2003). *NANDA Nursing
Diagnoses: Definitions & Classification 2003–2004.*
Philadelphia, PA: NANDA International.

National Committee on Vital and Health Statistics.
(2001). *Information for Health: A Strategy for Building
the National Health Information Infrastructure*.
Washington, DC: U.S. Department of Helath and
Human Services. *http://www.ncvhs.hhs.gov/
nhiilayo.pdf*

Schwirian, P. M. (1986). The NI Pyramid-A model for
research in nursing informatics. *Computers in Nursing*
4(3):134–136.

Staggers, N., Gassert, C. A., and Curran, C. (2001).
Informatics competencies for nurses at four levels of
practice. *Journal of Nursing Education* 40(7):303–316.

Staggers, N., Gassert, C. A., and Curran, C. (2002). A
Delphi study to determine informatics competencies for
nurses at four levels of practice. *Nursing Research*
51(6):383–390.

Staggers, N. and Thompson, C. B. (2002). The evolution
of definitions for nursing informatics: A critical
analysis and revised definition. *Journal of the American
Medical Informatics Association* 9(3):255–261.

Stetson, N. (1998). The computer-based patient record: Its
role in the healthcare enterprise. *Journal of Healthcare
Information Management* 12(4):1–2.

Turley, J. (1996). Toward a model for nursing informatics.
IMAGE: Journal of Nursing Scholarship 28(4):
309–313.

Werley, H. and Lang, N. (Eds.). (1988). *Identification of
the Nursing Minimum Data Set*. New York: Springer.

Zielstorff, R., Hudgings, C., and Grobe, S. (1993). *Next-
Generation Nursing Information Systems: Essential
Characteristics for Professional Practice*. Washington,
DC: American Nurses Publishing.

18

Advanced Terminology Systems

Nicholas R. Hardiker

Suzanne Bakken

Amy Coenen

OBJECTIVES

1. Describe the need for advanced terminology systems.
2. Identify the components of advanced terminology systems.
3. Compare and contrast two approaches for representing nursing concepts within an advanced terminology system.

KEY WORDS

concept representation
terminology
vocabulary
standardized nursing language

The failure to achieve a single, integrated terminology with broad coverage of the healthcare domain has been characterized as the "vocabulary problem." Evolving criteria for healthcare terminologies for implementation in computer-based systems suggest that concept-oriented approaches are needed to support the data needs of today's complex, knowledge-driven healthcare and health management environment. This chapter focuses on providing the background necessary to understand recent approaches to solving the vocabulary problem. It also includes several illustrative examples of these approaches from the nursing domain.

Background and Definitions

The primary motivation for standardized terms in nursing is the need for valid, comparable data that can be used across information system applications to support clinical decision-making and the evaluation of processes and outcomes of care. Secondary uses of the data for purposes such as clinical research, development of practice-based nursing knowledge, and generation of healthcare policy are dependent on the initial collection and representation of the data. Given the importance of standardized

terminology, one might ask, "Why, despite the extensive work to date, is the vocabulary problem not yet solved?"

The Vocabulary Problem

Several reasons for the vocabulary problem have been posited in health and nursing informatics literature. First, the development of multiple specialized terminologies has resulted in areas of overlapping content, areas for which no content exists, and large numbers of codes and terms (Chute, Cohn, and Campbell, 1998; Cimino, 1998a). Second, existing terminologies are most often developed to provide sets of terms and definitions of concepts for human interpretation, with computer interpretation as only a secondary goal (Rossi Mori, Consorti, and Galeazzi, 1998). The latter is particularly true for nursing terminologies that have been designed for direct use by nurses in the course of clinical care (Johnson et al., 2003; Martin and Scheet, 1992; Saba and Zuckerman, 1992). Unfortunately, knowledge that is eminently understandable to humans is often confusing, ambiguous, or opaque to computers, and, consequently, current efforts have often resulted in terminologies that are inadequate in meeting the data needs of today's healthcare systems. This chapter focuses on providing the background necessary to understand recent concept-oriented approaches to solving the vocabulary problem. It also includes illustrative examples of these approaches from the nursing domain. Note that the word "terminology" is used throughout this chapter to refer to the set of terms representing a system of concepts.

Concept Orientation

An appreciation for the approaches discussed in this chapter has as a prerequisite an understanding of what it means for a terminology to be concept-oriented. The health informatics literature provides an evolving framework that enumerates the criteria (Table 18.1) that render healthcare terminologies suitable for implementation in computer-based systems. In particular, it is clear that such terminologies must be concept-oriented (with explicit semantics), rather than based on surface linguistics (Chute, Cohn, and Campbell, 1998; Cimino, 1998b; Cimino et al., 1989). Several studies have reported that existing nursing terminologies do not meet the criteria related to concept orientation (Henry and Mead, 1997; Henry et al., 1998).

In order to appreciate the significance of concept-oriented approaches, it is important to first understand the definitions of and relationships among things in the world (objects), our thoughts about things in the world (concepts), and the labels we use to represent and communicate our thoughts about things in the world (terms). These relationships are depicted by a model commonly called the semiotic triangle (Fig. 18.1) (Ogden and Richards, 1923). The International Organization

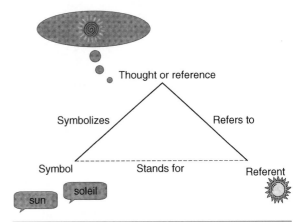

Figure 18.1

The semiotic triangle depicts the relationships among objects in the perceivable or conceivable world (referent), thoughts about things in the world, and the labels (symbols or terms) used to represent thoughts about things in the world.

for Standardization (ISO) international standard ISO 1087-1:2000 provides definitions for elements that correspond to each vertex of the triangle:

Concept (i.e., thought or reference): Unit of knowledge created by a unique combination of characteristics— a characteristic is an abstraction of a property of an object or of a set of objects.

Table 18.1   Evaluation Criteria Related to Concept-Oriented Approaches

Atomic-based—concepts must be separable into constituent components (Chute, Cohn, and Campbell, 1998)

Compositionality—ability to combine simple concepts into composed concepts, e.g., "pain" *and* "acute" = "acute pain" (Chute, Cohn, and Campbell, 1998)

Concept permanence—once a concept is defined it should not be deleted from a terminology (Cimino, 1998b)

Language independence—support for multiple linguistic expressions (Chute, Cohn, and Campbell, 1998)

Multiple hierarchy—accessibility of concepts through all reasonable hierarchical paths with consistency of views (Chute, Cohn, and Campbell, 1998; Cimino, 1998b; Cimino et al., 1989)

Nonambiguity—explicit definition for each term, e.g., "patient teaching related to medication adherence" defined as an *action* of "teaching", *recipient* of "patient", and *target* of "medication adherence" (Chute, Cohn, and Campbell, 1998; Cimino, 1998b; Cimino et al., 1989)

Nonredundancy—one preferred way of representing a concept or idea (Chute, Cohn, and Campbell, 1998; Cimino, 1998b; Cimino et al., 1989)

Synonymy—support for synonyms and consistent mapping of synonyms within and among terminologies (Chute, Cohn, and Campbell, 1998; Cimino, 1998b; Cimino et al., 1989)

Object (i.e., referent): Anything perceivable or conceivable.

Term (i.e., symbol): Verbal designation of a general concept in a specific subject field—a general concept corresponds to two or more objects which form a group by reason of common properties (International Organization for Standardization, 1990).

As specified by the criteria in Table 18.1 and illustrated in Fig. 18.1, a single concept may be associated with multiple terms (synonymy); however, a term should represent only one concept.

 ## Components of Advanced Terminology Systems

Within the context of the high-level information model provided by the Nursing Minimum Data Set (NMDS) (Werley and Lang, 1988), there has been extensive development and refinement of terminologies for describing patient problems, nursing interventions, and nursing-sensitive patient outcomes (Johnson, Maas, and Moorhead, 2000; Martin and Scheet, 1992; McCloskey and Bulechek, 2000; North American Nursing Diagnosis Association, 2003; Ozbolt, 1998; Saba, 2002) including the development of the International Classification for Nursing Practice (ICNP) (Coenen, 2003). These terminologies are described elsewhere in this text. The main component of more advanced terminology systems, however, is a concept-oriented terminology model or ontology representing a set of concepts and their interrelationships. The model is constructed using an ontology language that may be implemented using description logic within a software system or by a suite of software tools.

Terminology Model

A terminology model is a concept-based representation of a collection of domain-specific terms that is optimized for the management of terminological definitions. It encompasses both schemata and type definitions (Campbell et al., 1998; Sowa, 1984).

Schemata incorporate domain-specific knowledge about the typical constellations of entities, attributes, and events in the real world and, as such, reflect plausible combinations of concepts, e.g., "dyspnea" may be combined with "severe" to make "severe dyspnea". Schemata may be supported by either formal or informal composition rules (i.e., grammars).

Type definitions are obligatory conditions that state only the essential properties of a concept (Sowa, 1984), e.g., a nursing activity must have a *recipient*, an *action*, and a *target*.

There have been several published reports related to terminology models for nursing (Bakken, Cashen, and O'Brien, 1999; Hardiker and Rector, 1998; International Council of Nurses, 2001).

Representation Language

Terminology models may be formulated and elucidated in an ontology language (e.g., GALEN Representation and Integration Language [GRAIL]) (Rector et al., 1997), Knowledge Representation Specification Syntax (KRSS) (Campbell et al., 1998) or Web Ontology Language (OWL) (Rector, 2004). Ontology languages represent classes (also referred to as concepts, categories, or types) and their properties (also referred to as relations, slots, roles, or attributes). In this way, ontology languages are able to support, through explicit semantics, the formal definition of concepts in terms of their relationships with other concepts (Fig. 18.2); they also facilitate reasoning about those concepts, e.g., whether two concepts are equivalent or whether one concept, such as "pain", subsumes (is a generalization of) another, such as "acute pain".

Computer-Based Tools

A representation language may be implemented using description logic within a software system or by a suite of software tools. The functionality of these tools varies but may include among other things management and internal organization of the model, and reasoning on the model, such as automatic classification of composed

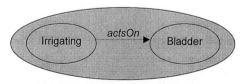

Figure 18.2

A simple graphical example of a formal representation of the nursing activity concept "Bladder Irrigation."

concepts based on their formal definition, e.g., "medication teaching" is a kind of "teaching".

In addition, the software may facilitate transformation of concept representations into canonical form (e.g., "cardiomegaly of the heart" is transformed to "cardiomegaly" since the location of the pathology is inherent in the concept itself), or support a set of sanctions (i.e., constraints) that test whether a proposed composed concept is sensible (e.g., "decubitus ulcer of the heart" and "impaired normal cognition" are not coherent terms). Other software support may be provided for knowledge engineering, operations management, and conflict detection and resolution.

The extent to which a terminology may be suitable for computer processing has been characterized in terms of "generations" (Rossi Mori, Consorti, and Galeazzi, 1998). First-generation terminology systems consist of a list of enumerated terms, possibly arranged as a single hierarchy. They serve a single purpose or a group of closely related purposes and allow minimal computer processing. Second-generation systems include an abstract terminology model or terminology model schema that describes the organization of the main categories used in a particular terminology or set of terminologies. The abstract terminology model is complemented by a thesaurus of elementary descriptors (i.e., terms) and templates or rules (i.e., grammar) for defining how categories may be combined. For example, "pain" and "severe" may be combined into "severe pain". Second-generation systems can be used for a range of purposes, but they allow only limited computer processing, e.g., automatic classification of composed concepts is not possible. Third-generation systems support sufficient formalisms to enable computer-based processing, i.e., they include a grammar that defines the rules for automated generation and classification of new concepts. Third-generation language systems are also referred to as formal concept representation systems (Ingenerf, 1995) or reference terminologies (Spackman, Campbell, and Cote, 1997).

Because they were designed primarily for direct manual use by nurses in the process of care or for classification purposes, the majority of existing nursing terminologies (e.g., NANDA, Nursing Interventions Classification [NIC]) can be characterized as first-generation systems. The *beta* 2 version of the ICNP is an example of a second-generation system (International Council of Nurses, 2001). Advanced terminology systems, i.e., third-generation terminology systems are the focus of the remainder of this chapter.

Advantages of Advanced Terminology Systems

Computer-based systems that support clinical uses such as electronic health records and decision support require more granular (i.e., less abstract) data than that typically contained in terminologies designed primarily for manual use or for the purpose of classification (Campbell et al., 1997; Chute et al., 1996; Cimino, 1998b; Cimino et al., 1989). Advanced concept-oriented terminology systems allow much greater granularity through controlled composition, while avoiding a combinatorial explosion of precoordinated terms.

In addition, as described previously in this chapter, advanced terminology systems facilitate two important facets of knowledge representation for computer-based systems that support clinical care: (a) describing concepts and (b) manipulating and reasoning about those concepts using computer-based tools. Advantages resulting from the first facet include (1) nonambiguous representation of concepts, (2) facilitation of data abstraction or de-abstraction without loss of original data (i.e., "lossless" data transformation), (3) nonambiguous mapping among terminologies, and (4) data reuse in different contexts. These advantages are particularly important for clinical uses of the terminology. Advantages gained from the second facet include automated classification of new concepts and an ability to support multiple inheritance of defining characteristics (e.g., "acute postoperative pain" is both a "pain" and a "postoperative symptom"). Both facets are vital to the maintenance of the terminology itself as well as to the ability to subsequently support the clinical utility of the terminology (Campbell et al., 1998; Rector et al., 1997).

Advanced Terminological Approaches in Nursing

Recently, there have been a number of initiatives that support the development of advanced concept-oriented terminology systems for the nursing domain. Following a brief description of three of these initiatives (ISO 18104:2003, the GALEN Project, and SNOMED), a nursing term is represented under GALEN and SNOMED approaches in order to illustrate similarities and differences between representations. A further illustrative example demonstrates one of the potential functions of an advanced terminology system for nursing, i.e., cross-mapping between existing terminologies.

ISO 18104:2003

An international standard (ISO 18104:2003) covering reference terminology models for nursing diagnoses (Fig. 18.3) and nursing actions (Fig. 18.4) was approved in 2003 (International Organization for Standardization, 2003). The standard was developed by a group of experts within ISO Technical Committee 215 (Health Informatics) Working Group 3 (Health Concept Representation) under the collaborative leadership of the International Medical Informatics Association—Nursing Special Interest Group (IMIA-NI) and the International Council of Nurses (ICN). The model built on work originating within the European Committee for Standardization (European Committee for Standardization, 2000).

The development of ISO 18104:2003 was motivated in part by a desire to harmonize the plethora of nursing terminologies in use around the world (Hardiker, 2004). Another major incentive was to integrate with other evolving terminology and information model standards—the development of ISO 18104:2003 was intended to be "consistent with the goals and objectives of other

specific health terminology models in order to provide a more unified reference health model." (International Organization for Standardization, 2003, p. 1). Potential uses identified for the terminology models include to (1) facilitate the representation of nursing diagnosis and nursing action concepts and their relationships in a manner suitable for computer processing, (2) provide a framework for the generation of compositional expressions from atomic concepts within a reference terminology, (3) facilitate the mapping among nursing diagnosis and nursing action concepts from various terminologies, (4) enable the systematic evaluation of terminologies and associated terminology models for purposes of harmonization, and (5) provide a language to describe the structure of nursing diagnosis and nursing action concepts in order to enable appropriate integration with information models (International Organization for Standardization, 2003). The standard is not intended to be of direct benefit to practicing nurses. It is intended to be of use to those that develop coding systems, terminologies, terminology models for other domains, health information models, information systems, software for natural langue processing, and markup standards for representation of healthcare documents.

ISO 18104:2003 has undergone substantial bench testing, both during its development and through more recent independent research (Hwang, Cimino, and Bakken, 2003; Moss, Coenen, and Mills, 2003). However, there is an outstanding need for further evaluation in terms of practical application and utility (Hardiker, Hoy, and Casey, 2000).

GALEN

A concept-oriented approach has been developed within the GALEN Program. GALEN can be used in a range of ways, from directly supporting clinical applications (Kirby and Rector, 1996) to supporting the authoring, maintenance, and quality assurance of other kinds of terminologies (Rogers et al., 1998).

GRAIL is an ontology language for representing concepts and their interrelationships—the source material for the construction of terminology models (Rector et al., 1997). Two integrated sets of tools are used in the development of a GRAIL model: a computer-based modeling environment and a terminology server. The modeling environment facilitates the collaborative formulation of models. It allows authoring of clinical knowledge at different levels of abstraction. The terminology server is

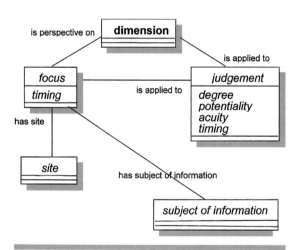

Figure 18.3

Reference terminology model for nursing diagnoses. (The terms and definitions taken from ISO 18104:2003 Health Informatics—Integration of a reference terminology for nursing, figures 1 and 2 [corresponding to Figs. 18.3 and 18.4 in this text] are reproduced with the permission of the International Organization for Standardization, ISO. The standard can be obtained from any ISO member and from the Web site of the ISO Central Secretariat at the following address: www.iso.org. Copyright remains with ISO.)

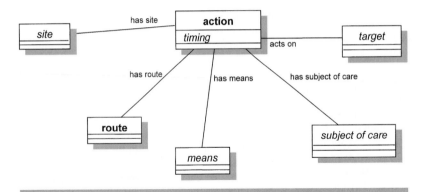

Figure 18.4

Reference terminology model for nursing actions.

(The terms and definitions taken from ISO 18104:2003 Health Informatics—Integration of a reference terminology for nursing, figures 1 and 2 [corresponding to Figs. 18.3 and 18.4 in this text] are reproduced with the permission of the International Organization for Standardization, ISO. The standard can be obtained from any ISO member and from the Web site of the ISO Central Secretariat at the following address: *www.iso.org*. Copyright remains with ISO.)

a software system that implements GRAIL. It performs a range of functions including (1) internally managing and representing the model, (2) testing the validity of combinations of concepts, (3) constructing valid composed concepts, (4) transforming composed concepts into canonical form, and (5) automatically classifying composed concepts into the hierarchy. The terminology server is also used to deliver the model for use by clinical applications and other kinds of authoring environments.

GALEN has been applied successfully in other areas of healthcare (Kirby and Rector, 1996). A major motivation for applying GALEN to nursing was the desire to meet the requirements of users of clinical applications (Heathfield et al., 1994). An additional factor was the need to provide a reusable and extensible model of nursing terminology. It is important to recognize that GALEN does not seek to replace existing nursing terminologies; rather, it seeks to contribute to the development of those terminologies, to supplement them, to allow comparisons among them, and to make them available for describing day-to-day nursing care.

For example, as part of another European project, TELENURSE, GALEN was applied to both the *alpha* and *beta* versions ICNP (Hardiker and Rector, 1998). The *beta* 2 version of ICNP is the first attempt in nursing to provide a formalized vocabulary of elementary concepts (International Council of Nurses, 2001);

however, the mechanism by which composed concepts are generated requires further specification. Within the TELENURSE project, GALEN provided a formalized mechanism for defining the syntax for sensible combinations of elementary ICNP concepts (Hardiker and Rector, 1998). In this experiment, the resulting GRAIL model of nursing terminology was shown to meet evolving evaluation criteria related to healthcare terminologies (Chute, Cohn, and Campbell, 1998; Cimino, 1998b). In so doing, it reinforces the view that advanced concept-oriented approaches can overcome many of the difficulties associated with existing nursing terminologies.

SNOMED RT

At the same time, an alternative concept-oriented approach was developed, through collaboration between the College of American Pathologists and Kaiser Permanente, based on SNOMED International. SNOMED Reference Terminology (RT) is a reference terminology optimized for clinical data retrieval and analysis (Spackman, Campbell, and Cote, 1997). Concepts and relationships in SNOMED RT are represented using modified KRSS rather than GRAIL (Campbell, et al., 1998). Concept definition and manipulation are supported through a set of tools with functionality such as (1) acronym resolution, word completion,

Table 18.2 Possible Representations of the Nursing Activity Concept "Bladder Irrigation", Using GRAIL and Modified KRSS

Generic Description Logic Representation	BladderIrrigation ≡ Irrigating ⊓ ∃ actsOn.Bladder
	Key
	≡ equivalentClass
	⊓ intersectionOf
	∃ someValuesFrom
GRAIL Representation	(Irrigating which actsOn Bladder) name "BladderIrrigation."
Modified KRSS Representation	(Define-concept BladderIrrigation (and Irrigating) (actsOn Bladder))

term completion, spelling correction, display of the authoritative form of the term entered by the user, and decomposition of unrecognized input (Metaphrase) (Tuttle et al., 1998), (2) automated classification (Ontylog), and (3) conflict management, detection, and resolution (Galapagos) (Campbell et al., 1998). More recently, along with U.K. Clinical Terms, SNOMED RT has been used as a foundation for a new terminology system, SNOMED Clinical Terms (CT), which has been developed collaboratively by the College of American Pathologists and the U.K. National Health Service (Wang, Sable, and Spackman, 2002). SNOMED CT possesses both reference terminology properties and user interface terms. A working group of the SNOMED International Editorial Board has led the integration of nursing concepts into SNOMED CT (Bakken et al., 2002).

Illustration of Representations Using GALEN and SNOMED RT Approaches

Table 18.2 illustrates the representation, using GRAIL and modified KRSS, of a single nursing activity. Although the two representations use different syntax, there are obvious similarities in how the concept "Bladder Irrigation" is defined.

Emerging Approaches

Outside the health domain, work in relation to the Semantic Web has resulted in an emerging "standard" (i.e., a W3C recommendation) ontology language, OWL (W3C, 2004). OWL is intended for use where applications, rather than humans, are to process information.

As such, it should be able to meet the requirements of advanced terminology systems that support contemporary healthcare. OWL builds on existing recommendations such as eXtensible Markup Language (XML) (surface syntax for structured documents), Resource Description Framework (RDF) (a data model for resources), and RDF Schema (a vocabulary for describing the properties and classes of resources) by providing additional vocabulary and a formal semantics. Software, both proprietary and open source, is available for (a) managing terminology models or ontologies developed in OWL (e.g., Protégé [Noy et al., 2003] with an OWL plug-in) and (b) reasoning on the model (e.g., Racer [Haarslev and Moller, 2001]). Although work within nursing (e.g., supporting the development of ICNP Version 1) and the wider health informatics community is still in its infancy, the results to date are promising.

An OWL representation (in XML) of the nursing activity concept "Bladder Irrigation" is provided in Table 18.3 for comparison with the GRAIL and KRSS representations in Table 18.2.

Advanced Terminology Systems in Practice

Figure 18.5 displays a potential mapping (to the right of the figure) between the NIC concept "Bladder Irrigation" (McCloskey and Bulechek, 2000) and the precoordinated Omaha System concept "Treatments and Procedures: Bladder Care" (Martin and Scheet, 1992). A computer-based reasoner can use the formal definitions of the corresponding composed concepts to infer a hierarchical relationship. The asserted properties for both concepts (in the center of the figure) are

Table 18.3   Possible OWL Representation (in XML) of the Nursing Activity Concept "Bladder Irrigation"

```
<owl:Class rdf:ID="BladderIrrigation">
  <owl:equivalentClass>
    <owl:Class>
      <owl:intersectionOf rdf:parseType="Collection">
        <owl:Class rdf:about="#Irrigating"/>
        <owl:Restriction>
          <owl:onProperty>
            <owl:FunctionalProperty rdf:about="#actsOn"/>
          </owl:onProperty>
          <owl:someValuesFrom>
            <owl:Class rdf:about="#Bladder"/>
          </owl:someValuesFrom>
        </owl:Restriction>
      </owl:intersectionOf>
    </owl:Class>
  </owl:equivalentClass>
</owl:Class>□
```

identical. The existing hierarchy (to the left of the figure) asserts that "Performing" subsumes "Irrigating". Thus, "BladderCare", which maps to the Omaha System concept "Treatments and Procedures: Bladder Care", is a generalization of "BladderIrrigation", which maps to the NIC concept "Bladder Irrigation", Hence, the NIC concept "Bladder Irrigation" potentially maps onto the Omaha System concept "Treatments and Procedures: Bladder Care" (but *not* vice versa).

Summary and Implications for Nursing

Several studies have supported the need for advanced concept-oriented terminology systems that (a) provide for nonambiguous concept definitions, (b) facilitate composition of complex concepts from more primitive concepts, and (c) support mapping among terminologies (Campbell et al., 1997; Chute et al., 1996; Henry et al., 1994). Because of the magnitude of resources and collaboration required, the development of advanced concept-oriented terminology systems is a fairly recent phenomenon and there is little documentation of the clinical impact of the approach. However, a number of benefits have been proposed: (1) facilitation of evidence-based practice (e.g., linking of clinical practice guidelines to appropriate patients during the patient-provider encounter); (2) matching of potential research subjects to research protocols for which they are potentially

eligible; (3) detection of and prevention of potential adverse drug effects; (4) linking online information resources; (5) increased reliability and validity of data for quality evaluation; and (6) data mining for purposes such as clinical research, health services research, or knowledge discovery.

The developers of nursing and healthcare terminologies and informatics scientists have made significant progress. From decades of nursing language research, there exists an extensive set of terms describing patient problems, nursing interventions and activities, and nursing-sensitive patient outcomes (Beyea, 2000; Coenen, 2003; Johnson, Maas, and Moorhead, 2000; Martin and Scheet, 1992; McCloskey and Bulechek, 2000; North American Nursing Diagnosis Association, 2003; Ozbolt, 1998; Saba, 2002). Through the efforts of nursing professionals, new terms have been integrated into large healthcare terminologies; terms, as demonstrated by nursing informatics research, which are useful for representing nursing-relevant concepts (Bakken et al., 2000; Bakken et al., 2002; Henry et al., 1994; Lange, 1996; Matney, Bakken, and Huff, 2003). Ontology languages supported by suites of software tools have been developed within the context of terminologies with broad coverage of the healthcare domain (Campbell et al., 1998). Applicability of these tools to the nursing domain has been demonstrated (Hardiker and Rector, 1998; Zingo, 1997). A major remaining challenge is the development of content. However, there is significant progress in that area as well;

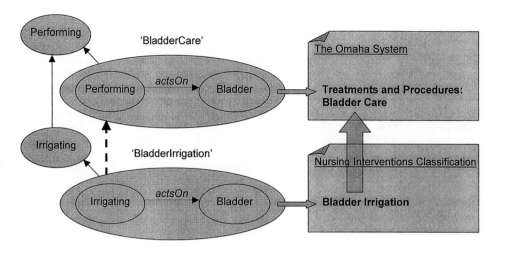

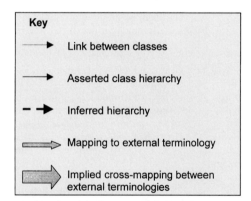

Figure 18.5
An illustration of a potential mapping using an advanced terminology system between nursing activity concepts from two existing terminology systems.

existing standardized nursing terminologies have shown themselves to be an excellent source.

A number of efforts within nursing (e.g., ICNP Version 1) and the larger healthcare arena (e.g., SNOMED CT) are aimed toward the achievement of advanced terminology systems that support semantic interoperability across healthcare information systems. In addition, other research has focused on examining how terminology models and advanced terminology systems relate to other types of models that support semantic interoperability, such as a domain model for nursing and the Health Level 7 Reference Information Model (RIM) (Goossen et al.,

2004). Such interoperability is a prerequisite to meeting the information demands of today's complex healthcare and health management environment.

References

Bakken, S., Cashen, M., and O'Brien, A. (1999). Evaluation of a type definition for representing nursing activities within a concept-based terminologic system. In N. Lorenzi (Ed.), *1999 American Medical Informatics Association Fall Symposium* (pp. 17–21). Philadelphia, PA: Hanley & Belfus Inc.

Bakken, S., Cimino, J. J., Haskell, R., Kukafka, R., Matsumoto, C., Chan, G. K., and Huff, S. M. (2000). Evaluation of the clinical LOINC (Logical Observation Identifiers, Names, and Codes) semantic structure as a terminology model for standardized assessment measures. *Journal of the American Medical Informatics Association* 7(6):529–538.

Bakken, S., Warren, J. J., Lundberg, C., Casey, A., Correia, C., Konicek, D., and Zingo, C. (2002). An evaluation of the usefulness of two terminology models for integrating nursing diagnosis concepts into SNOMED clinical terms. *International Journal of Medical Informatics* 68(1–3):71–77.

Beyea, S. (2000). Perioperative data elements: Interventions and outcomes. *Association of Operating Room Nurses Journal* 71(2):344–353.

Campbell, J., Carpenter, P., Sneiderman, C., Cohn, S., Chute, C., and Warren, J. (1997). Phase II evaluation of clinical coding schemes: Completeness, taxonomy, mapping, definitions, and clarity. *Journal of the American Medical Informatics Association* 4(3):238–251.

Campbell, K., Cohn, S., Chute, C., Shortliffe, E., and Rennels, G. (1998). Scalable methodologies for distributed development of logic-based convergent medical terminology. *Methods of Information in Medicine* 37(4–5):426–439.

Campbell, K. E., Oliver, D. E., Spackman, K., and Shortliffe, E. H. (1998). Representing thoughts, words, and things in the UMLS. *Journal of the American Medical Informatics Association* 5(5):421–431.

Chute, C., Cohn, S., and Campbell, J. (1998). A framework for comprehensive terminology systems in the United States: Development guidelines, criteria for selection, and public policy implications. ANSI Healthcare Informatics Standards Board Vocabulary Working Group and the Computer-based Patient Records Institute Working Group on Codes and Structures. *Journal of the American Medical Informatics Association* 5(6):503–510.

Chute, C. G., Cohn, S. P., Campbell, K. E., Oliver, D. E., and Campbell, J. R. (1996). The content coverage of clinical classifications. *Journal of the American Medical Informatics Association* 3(3):224–233.

Cimino, J. (1998a). The concepts of language and the language of concepts. *Methods of Information in Medicine* 37(4–5):311.

Cimino, J. (1998b). Desiderata for controlled medical vocabularies in the twenty-first century. *Methods of Information in Medicine* 37(4–5):394–403.

Cimino, J., Hripcsak, G., Johnson, S., and Clayton, P. (1989). Designing an introspective, multi-purpose, controlled medical vocabulary. In L. C.Kingsland, III (Ed.), *Symposium on Computer Applications in Medical Care* (pp. 513–518). Washington, DC: IEEE Computer Society Press.

Coenen, A. (2003). Building a unified nursing language: The ICNP. *International Nursing Review* 50(2):65–66.

European Committee for Standardization. (2000). *CEN ENV Health Informatics—Systems of Concepts to Support Nursing*. Brussels: CEN.

Goossen, W., Ozbolt, J., Coenen, A., Park, H., Mead, C., Ehnfors, M., and Marin, H. (2004). Development of a provisional domain model for the nursing process for use within the Health Level 7 reference information model. *Journal of the American Medical Informatics Association* 11(3):186–194.

Haarslev, V. and Moller, R. (2001). *Description of the RACER System and its Applications*. Paper presented at the International Workshop of Description Logics (DL–2001) 1–3 August 2001, Stanford, CA.

Hardiker, N. (2004). An international standard for nursing terminologies. In J. Bryant (Ed.), *Current Perspectives in Healthcare Computing* (pp. 212–219). Swindon, U.K.: Health Informatics Committee of the British Computer Society.

Hardiker, N., Hoy, D., and Casey, A. (2000). Standards for nursing terminology. *Journal of the American Medical Informatics Association* 7(6):523–528.

Hardiker, N. and Rector, A. (1998). Modeling nursing terminology using the GRAIL representation language. *Journal of the American Medical Informatics Association* 5(1):120–128.

Heathfield, H. A., Hardiker, N., Kirby, J., Tallis, R., and Gonsalkarale, M. (1994). The PEN and PAD Medical Record Model: Development of a nursing record for hospital-based care of the elderly. *Methods of Information in Medicine* 33:464–472.

Henry, S. B., Holzemer, W. L., Reilly, C. A., and Campbell, K. E. (1994). Terms used by nurses to describe patient problems: Can SNOMED III represent nursing concepts in the patient record? *Journal of the American Medical Informatics Association* 1(1):61–74.

Henry, S. B. and Mead, C. N. (1997). Nursing classification systems: Necessary but not sufficient for representing "what nurses do" for inclusion in computer-based patient record systems. *Journal of the American Medical Informatics Association* 4(3):222–232.

Henry, S. B., Warren, J. J., Lange, L., and Button, P. (1998). A review of major nursing vocabularies and the extent to which they have the characteristics required for implementation in computer-based systems. *Journal of the American Medical Informatics Association* 5(4):321–328.

Hwang, J. I., Cimino, J. J., and Bakken, S. (2003). Integrating nursing diagnostic concepts into the medical entities dictionary using the ISO Reference Terminology Model for Nursing Diagnosis. *Journal of the American Medical Informatics Association* 10(4):382–388.

Ingenerf, J. (1995). Taxonomic vocabularies in medicine: The intention of usage determines different established structures. In R. A. Greenes, H. E. Peterson, and D. J. Protti (Eds.), *MedInfo95* (pp. 136–139). Vancouver, BC: HealthCare Computing and Communications, Canada.

International Council of Nurses. (2001). *International Classification for Nursing Practice (beta 2 version)*. Geneva, Switzerland: International Council of Nurses.

International Organization for Standardization. (1990). *International Standard ISO 1087-1:2000 Terminology—Vocabulary—Part 1: Theory and Application*. Geneva, Switzerland: International Organization for Standardization.

International Organization for Standardization. (2003). *International Standard ISO 18104:2003 Health Informatics—Integration of a Reference Terminology Model for Nursing*. Geneva, Switzerland: International Organization for Standardization.

Johnson, M., Maas, M., and Moorhead, S. (Eds.) (2000). *Nursing Outcomes Classification (NOC)* (2nd ed.). St. Louis, MO: C.V. Mosby.

Johnson, M., McCloskey Dochterman, J. C., Maas, M., and Moorhead, S. A. (2003). *Nursing Diagnosis, Outcomes, and Interventions: NANDA, NOC, and NIC Linkages*. St. Louis, MO: C. V. Mosby.

Kirby, J. and Rector, A. L. (1996). The PEN and PAD data entry system: From prototype to practical system. In J. Cimino (Ed.), *1996 American Medical Informatics Association Fall Symposium* (pp. 709–713). Washington, DC: Hanley and Belfus.

Lange, L. (1996). Representation of everyday clinical nursing language in UMLS and SNOMED. In J. Cimino (Ed.), *1996 American Medical Informatics Association Fall Symposium* (pp. 140–144). Washington, DC: Hanley and Belfus.

Martin, K. S. and Scheet, N. J. (1992). *The Omaha System: Applications for community health nursing*. Philadelphia, PA: W. B. Saunders.

Matney, S., Bakken, S., and Huff, S. M. (2003). Representing nursing assessments in clinical information systems using the logical observation identifiers, names, and codes database. *Journal of Biomedical Informatics* 36(4–5):287–293.

McCloskey, J. C. and Bulechek, G. M. (2000). *Nursing Interventions Classification* (3rd ed.). St. Louis, MO: C. V. Mosby.

Moss, J., Coenen, A., and Mills, M. (2003). Evaluation of the draft international standard for a reference terminology model for nursing actions. *Journal of Biomedical Informatics* 36(4–5):271–278.

North American Nursing Diagnosis Association. (2003). *NANDA Nursing Diagnoses 2003–2004: Definitions and Classification*. Philadelphia, PA: North American Nursing Diagnosis Association.

Noy, N., Crubezy, M., Fergerson, R., Knublauch, H., Tu, S., Vendetti, J., and Musen, M. (2003). Protege-2000: An open-source ontology-development and knowledge-acquisition environment. In M. Musen, C. Friedman, and J. M. Teich (Eds.), *2003 American Medical Informatics Association Annual Fall Symposium* (p. 953).

Ogden, C. and Richards, I. (1923). *The Meaning of Meaning*. New York: Harcourt, Brace, and World.

Ozbolt, J. G. (1998). *Ozbolt's Patient Care Data Set, Version 4.0*. Nashville, TN: Vanderbilt University.

Rector, A.L. (2004). Defaults, context, and knowledge: Alternatives for OWL-indexed knowledge bases. *Pacific Symposium on Biocomputing* (pp. 226–237).

Rector, A. L., Bechhofer, S., Goble, C. A., Horrocks, I., Nowlan, W. A., and Solomon, W. D. (1997). The GRAIL concept modelling language for medical terminology. *Artificial Intelligence in Medicine* 9:139–171.

Rogers, J., Price, C., Rector, A., Solomon, W., and Smejko, N. (1998). Validating clinical terminological structures: Integration and cross-validation of Read Thesaurus and GALEN. In G. Chute (Ed.), *1998 American Medical Informatics Association Annual Fall Symposium* (pp. 845–849). Orlando, FL: Hanley and Belfus.

Rossi Mori, A., Consorti, F., and Galeazzi, E. (1998). Standards to support development of terminological systems for healthcare telematics. *Methods of Information in Medicine* 37(4–5):551–563.

Saba, V. (2002). Retrieved March 14, 2002, from the World Wide Web, *http://www.sabacare.com*

Saba, V. K. and Zuckerman, A. E. (1992). A new home health classification method. *Caring Magazine* 11(9):27–34.

Sowa, J. (1984). *Conceptual Structures*. Reading, MA: Addison-Wesley.

Spackman, K. A., Campbell, K. E., and Cote, R. A. (1997). SNOMED RT: A reference terminology for health care. In D. Masys (Ed.), *1997 American Medical Informatics Association Annual Fall Symposium* (pp. 640–644). Nashville, TN: Hanley and Belfus.

Tuttle, M., Keck, K. D., Cole, W. G., Erlbaum, M. S., Sherertz, D. D., C. G. Chute, Elkin, P. L., Atkin, G. E., Kahoi, B. H., Safran, C., Rind, D., and Law, V. (1998). Metaphrase: An aid to the clinical conceptualization and formalization of patient problems in healthcare enterprises. *Methods of Information in Medicine* 37(4–5):373–383.

W3C. (2004). *OWL Web Ontology Language Overview. W3C Recommendation 10 February 2004*. Retrieved June 16, 2004, from the World Wide Web: *http://www.w3.org/TR/owl-features/*

Wang, A., Sable, J. H., and Spackman, K. (2002). The SNOMED clinical terms development process: Refinement and analysis of content. In I. Kohane (Ed.), *2002 American Medical Informatics Association Fall Symposium* (pp. 845–849).

Werley, H. H. and Lang, N. M. (Eds.) (1988). *Identification of the Nursing Minimum Data Set*. New York: Springer.

Zingo, C. A. (1997). Strategies and tools for creating a common nursing terminology within a large health maintenance organization. In U. Gerdin, M. Tallberg, and P. Wainwright (Eds.), *NI97* (pp. 27–31). Stockholm, Sweden: IOS Press.

19

Implementing and Upgrading Clinical Information Systems

Marina Douglas
Marian Celli

OBJECTIVES

1. Describe the eight phases in developing, implementing, or upgrading a clinical information system (CIS).
2. Describe the personnel requirements for implementing or upgrading a CIS.
3. Describe the roles and responsibilities of nursing for implementing or upgrading a CIS.
4. Identify the various tools of the trade used in developing, implementing, and upgrading a CIS.
5. Describe the methods of evaluating a CIS.
6. Describe new challenges in implementing and upgrading CISs.

KEY WORDS

information systems
information technology
integrated system advances
information management systems
hospital information systems
clinical information system

What Is a Clinical Information System?

Nursing involvement in the design and implementation of a CIS is required at many levels. Nurses have been instrumental members of departmental teams in addition to their active involvement in nursing-focused projects. The nursing process used to deliver direct patient care (i.e., to observe, assess, plan, implement, and evaluate care) provides a strong parallel framework for nurses to succeed in the design and implementation of CIS projects (Douglas, 1995). The skills required to deliver direct patient care necessitate the ability to coordinate patient care involving multiple disciplines and departments. This provides nurses knowledge of the many aspects orchestrated for effective and efficient healthcare delivery.

The roles filled by nurses are at the heart of many development, implementation, and upgrading projects; these roles include being a member of departmental teams and serving as project team leaders, and experienced informatics nurses may be chosen to direct overall projects as project managers.

A CIS assists clinicians with data necessary for decision-making and problem solving. Clinical disciplines and specialty services share common user requirements as well as having specialized practice requirements. Just as multiple departments work in concert for optimum patient care delivery, the components of a CIS interact in much the same coordinated fashion.

If each discipline acted independently, the care of the patient would be fragmented, causing duplication of efforts and delays in treatment (Selker et al., 1989). A CIS must serve the organization and the patient in much the same way an efficient healthcare delivery system involves all appropriate departments in establishing healthcare delivery processes. The benefit of coordinated efforts to the patient and to the entire organization outweighs the singular advantage to any one discipline's or department's processes.

The nursing requirements of a CIS described in this chapter will focus on the requirements of nursing department of a healthcare facility providing direct patient care. As described, it is one department in a complex healthcare delivery system; to be effective, nursing must act in concert with the entire organization. The major CIS requirements for nursing are to (1) administer a nursing department, (2) assist the management of nursing practice, (3) assist nursing education, and (4) support nursing research (Zielstorff, 1985). The nursing component of a CIS can be designed as a stand-alone system, a subsystem of a larger system, or an integral part of the healthcare organization's overall information system (Simpson, 1993). It can be programmed for processing by a mainframe, minicomputer, or microcomputer, and it may share the same equipment other departmental systems in the facility use. The advantages of the nursing components (applications) being part of a subsystem or an integrated application are significant.

Because of increasingly complex technology and information requirements of healthcare, few hospitals and/or nursing departments have the resources to develop or create their own CIS or nursing computer applications. Some organizations have implemented CISs and maintained and even completed an evaluation of their nursing components. From the evaluation, new uses of the system have been demonstrated or suggested. To meet new legislation, new regulations, and new professional standards, CISs as young as 5 years need to be upgraded.

Regardless of the size or type of system, any CIS or single application design/implementation or upgrade must complete the eight phases of implementation listed below. The implementation of clinical information is a process introducing an application or information system to an organization, ensuring the full benefit and potential of the system are realized (Ritter and Glaser, 1994). The phases of implementation use a problem-solving, scientific approach. The problem solving begins with observation of the operations or problem in question. The second step requires an in-depth assessment of the issues. Developing and implementing a plan to resolve the problem are the third and fourth steps. The last step, evaluation, provides feedback on how well the solution resolves the problem. Countless iterations of the problem-solving approach are used during software implementation or

upgrading. Inherent in the implementation process is the need to recognize and manage change and its impact. "The ability to manage change often marks the difference between the success and failure of implementing a change initiative and moving an organization forward" (Ritter and Glaser, 1994, p. 168). Literature focusing on the workflow impact of a CIS and the cultural impact to an organization (Ash et al., 2000; Augustine, 2004; Kaplan, 1997; Lorenzi and Riley, 2000; Souton et al., 1997) is stressing the need to manage the change process (transition management) inherent in a CIS implementation if success is to be attained.

The eight phases of implementation are planning, system analysis, system design/system selection, development, testing, training, implementation, and evaluation (Fig. 19.1). The process of upgrading a CIS, entailing all eight phases of implementation, will be discussed.

Attempting to implement or upgrade a system without accomplishing the tasks associated with each phase generally results in system failure in one or more of the following areas:

- CIS does not meet the stated goal of the project.
- There is failure to gain end-user acceptance.
- Expenditures exceed budget.
- Anticipated benefits are unrealized.

The Planning Phase

The planning phase of the project begins once an organization has determined that an existing need or problem

---

EIGHT PHASES OF DESIGN, IMPLEMENTATION, and UPGRADING

Planning
System Analysis
System Design/System Selection
Development
Testing
Training
Implementation
Evaluation

Figure 19.1

Eight phases of designing, implementing, or upgrading a nursing information system.

may be filled or solved by the development or implementation of a CIS or application. Establishing the committee framework to research and make recommendations for the project is an important first step.

Clinical Information System Committee Structure and Project Staff The nursing administrator's involvement in the establishment of a CIS committee structure is paramount to the success of the project. The nursing administrator, in conjunction with the information system's management team, works to develop a committee structure and participation to best guarantee the success of the project. Assigning the appropriate resources, whether financial or personnel, is a critical success factor (Spillane et al., 1990; Protti and Peel, 1998; Schooler and Dotson, 2004).

Recent evaluations of both successful and less than successful implementations have stressed the need to anticipate the impact of the new system on the culture of the organization and to take active steps to mitigate the effects of change on the organization (Lorenzi and Riley, 2000; Peitzman, 2004). Transition management, as the process is sometimes called, is a series of ". . . deliberate, planned interventions undertaken to assure successful adaptation/assimilation of a desired outcome into an organization" (Douglas and Wright, 2003). The nursing administrator must direct both the assessment of the impact as well as be a visible leader in planning and leading the transition management efforts.

A three-tiered committee approach is recommended to accomplish the design, implementation, or upgrading of a complete CIS—a steering committee, a project team, and departmental teams.

Clinical Information System Steering Committee
Before a CIS is developed or selected, the organization must appoint a CIS steering committee. The CIS steering committee generally includes representatives from the following areas:

- Hospital administration/hospital finance
- Nursing administration
- Medical staff
- Information systems department at the director or manager level
- Major ancillary departments (laboratory, radiology, pharmacy, dietary, medical records/patient registration, patient accounting)
- Health information management (medical records)

- Legal affairs
- Outside consultants (as needed)
- Other appointed members (as needed)

The CIS steering committee is charged with providing oversight guidance to the selection and integration of a new CIS into the organization. The collective knowledge of the steering committee's members relative to the organization's operations provides global insight and administrative authority to resolve issues. This committee may need to meet frequently during the early planning phase and the implementation phases of the project, with less frequent meetings required during the middle stages (Fig. 19.2).

Project Team The project team is led by an appointed project manager and includes a designated team leader for each of the major departments affected by the system selection, implementation, or upgrade proposed. The objectives of the project team are to (1) understand the technology and technology restrictions, if any, of a proposed system, (2) understand the impact of intradepartmental decisions, (3) make decisions at the interdepartmental level for the overall good of the CIS within the organization, and (4) become the key resource for their application. A stated goal for the selection, implementation, or upgrading of a CIS is to improve patient care; gains made by one department at the expense of another department rarely work to improve overall patient care delivery. The project team's ability to evaluate multiple departments' information desires in light of the capabilities of the proposed system is important to the overall success of the project.

The project manager must be acutely familiar with the phases of implementation. Larger scale CIS implementations necessitate a project manager with significant implementation experience. The project manager is responsible for managing all aspects of the project. This management includes software application development, hardware, and networks, as well as oversight management of the interfacing and conversion tasks. The project manager must have good communication, facilitation, organizational, and motivational skills to be successful. A sound knowledge of healthcare delivery, hospital processes, and politics is important. The project manager must have full-time dedication to a large-scale design or implementation project (Fig. 19.3).

Departmental Teams The charge of the departmental teams is (1) to thoroughly understand the department's information needs, (2) to gain a full understanding of the

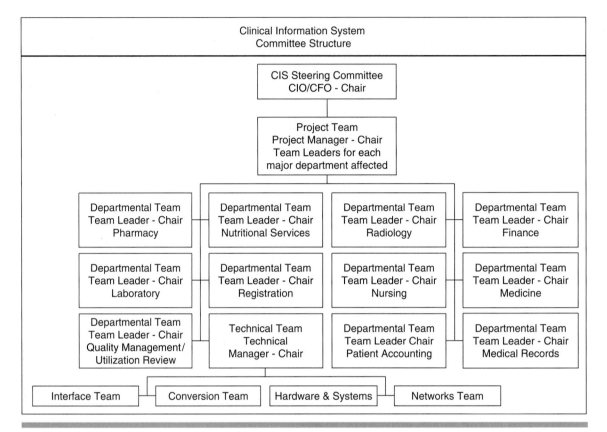

Figure 19.2
Commitee structure.

software's features and functions, (3) to merge the new system's capabilities with the department's operations, (4) to assist in the system testing effort, (5) to participate in developing and conducting end-user education, and (6) to provide a high level of support during the initial activation period of the new system. The team leaders must possess a sound knowledge of the hospital and departmental policies and procedures (both formal and informal), good organizational and communication skills, and must be adept at gaining consensus and resolving conflict. Successful implementations have provided decision-making authority at the level of project teams whenever possible.

A smaller scale project requires committee representation of a smaller scope. As an example, representation on the committees to implement an automated documentation project will have an emphasis on nursing members with less involvement from radiology, laboratory, and finance. Each of the major nursing subspecialty areas and ancillary departments scheduled to use the system for patient documentation is represented. A health information management representative and legal counsel assist the committee in planning for regulatory compliance. Physician involvement early in the planning process is recommended to ensure understanding of the information needs of the medical staff relative to patient documentation. The physician committee member assists in easing the medical staff's transition to the new documentation system. If the system will affect nursing interactions or communications with other departments, each of the major areas affected have committee representation and all areas/disciplines have involvement to ensure acceptance of the implementation plan at an early stage.

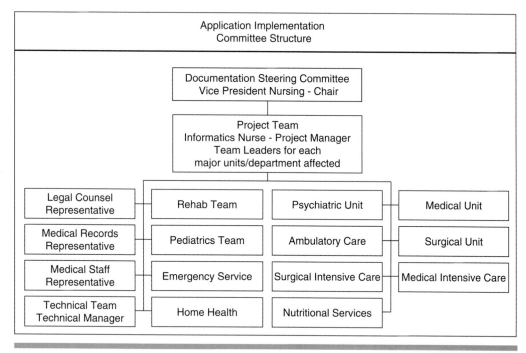

Figure 19.3
Application implementation committee structure.

Planning

During the planning phase, the information requirements necessary to solve the problem or accomplish the goal are assessed. The information needs for selecting, implementing, or upgrading a CIS, including their implications for nursing services, nursing practice, and quality care, must also be identified. In the American Society for Testing and Materials (ASTM) standards, the planning phase is referred to as the project definition. Commercial software developers and consultants rank this phase as the most critical factor in the selection of a system, even more important than the system itself (Zinn, 1989). Excellent planning is time-consuming and seemingly costly. It is estimated that the process can take up to 2 years to design and develop or to select and implement a new system (Ginsburg and Browning, 1989). This phase is critical whether a system is actually being developed or existing commercial systems are being evaluated for selection.

The planning phase involves the following steps:

- Definition of the problem and/or stated goal
- Feasibility study

- Documentation and negotiation of project scope agreement
- Allocation of resources

Definition of the Problem   Definition of the problem and/or stated goal precisely is essential and often not readily apparent. Not until the information requirements of the problem and/or stated goal and outcomes are precisely defined will the real characteristics of the problem be revealed (Fitzgerald et al., 1981).

For example:

- Unfair nurse staff assignments may relate to an invalid patient classification tool (inaccurate grouping of patients) rather than to workload measurements and/or acuity score.

- Duplicate health department reports may result in inappropriate statistics being collected instead of the collection of unique atomic-level data elements.

The project definition includes a description of how the system will be evaluated. Establishing the evaluation criteria early in the process supports the successful management philosophy of beginning with the end in mind (Convey, 1992). The results and improvements expected from implementing the system are described by realistic goals for the system. They might include increased processing capabilities, savings in processing time, decreased costs, or increased personnel productivity. When updating or expanding the CIS, the project definition includes the identification of equipment currently available, its age, the degree of amortization, and the need for hardware or operating system software upgrades prior to undertaking an upgrade project.

Feasibility Study   A feasibility study is a preliminary analysis to determine if the proposed problem can be solved by the implementation of a CIS or component application. The feasibility study not only clarifies the problem and/or stated goal but also helps to identify the information needs, objectives, and scope of the project. The feasibility study helps the CIS steering committee understand the real problem and/or goal by analyzing multiple parameters and by presenting possible solutions. It highlights whether the proposed solution will produce usable products and whether the proposed system's benefits outweigh the costs. Operational issues are reviewed to determine if the proposed solution will work in the intended environment. Technical issues are reviewed to ensure the proposed system can be built and/or will be compatible with the proposed and/or current technology. Legal and statutory regulations are reviewed to ensure compliance with local and federal law. The feasibility study includes a high-level description of the human resources required and how the selected system will be developed, utilized, and implemented. The feasibility study describes the management controls to be established for obtaining administrative, financial, and technical approvals to proceed with each phase of the project.

The feasibility study seeks to answer the following questions:

- What is the real problem to be solved and/or stated goal to be met?
- Where does the project fit into the overall strategic plan of the organization?
- What specific outcomes are expected from the project?
- What are the measurable criteria for determining project success from the above outcomes?
- What research and assumptions support the implementation project?

- What are the known limitations and risks to the project?
- What is the timing of the remaining phases of the project?
- Who will be committed to implementing the project?
- What are the estimated costs in both dollars and personnel time?
- What is the justification for the project, including the relationship between costs and benefits?

A feasibility study includes the following topic areas:

Statement of Objectives   The first step in conducting a feasibility study is to state the objectives for the proposed system. These objectives constitute the purpose(s) of the system. All objectives are outcome-oriented and are stated in measurable terms. The objectives identify the "end product" and what the CIS will do for the end users.

Environmental Assessment   The project is defined in terms of the support it provides to both the mission and the strategic plans of the organization. The project is evaluated relative to the organization's competition. The impact of legal, regulatory, and ethical considerations is reviewed.

Determination of Information Needs   This step, sometimes called a needs assessment, outlines the high-level information required by the users. Identifying the information needed helps clarify what users will expect from the system. Such knowledge is essential in designing the system's output, input, and processing requirements.

Determination of Scope   The scope of the proposed system establishes system constraints and outlines what the proposed system will and will not produce. Included in the scope are the criteria by which the success of the project will be judged.

Development of a Project Timeline   A project timeline is developed providing an overview of the key milestone events of the project. The projected length of time for each major phase of the project is established. Often called a project workplan, the major steps required for each phase are outlined in sufficient detail to provide the steering committee background on the proposed development or implementation process.

Recommendations   Committees may forget that not all projects are beneficial to the strategic mission of the organization, and a decision can be made not only to proceed, but also not to proceed, with a project. The viability of the project is based on the review of the multiple factors researched in the feasibility study. It is critical to consider whether more personnel or equipment is necessary rather than more computerization. In addition to identifying potential hardware and software improvements, the costs and proposed benefits are factored into the project's viability decision. In upgrading or considering expansion of a system, a concerted effort to maximize use of the current system and to make process improvements in the current management and coordination of existing systems should be undertaken before deciding to procure a new system(s).

If, based on the findings of the feasibility study, the project steering committee determines to continue with the project, a project scope agreement is prepared.

Documentation and Negotiation of a Project Scope Agreement

A project scope agreement is drafted by the project team and submitted to the project's steering committee for acceptance. The project scope agreement includes the scope of the project, the application level management requirements, the proposed activation strategy for implementing the CIS or application, and the technical management and personnel who will maintain the equipment. The agreement is based on the findings of the feasibility study.

The project scope agreement becomes the internal organizational contract for the project. It defines the short- and long-term goals, establishes the criteria for evaluating the success of the project, and expands the workplan to include further detail regarding the steps to be accomplished in the development or implementation of the CIS.

Allocation of Resources

The last step in the planning phase is determining what resources are required to successfully complete the project scope agreement. A firm commitment of resources for development of the entire CIS project scope agreement (including all phases of implementation) is needed before the system can fulfill its stated objectives. The following points should be considered when planning for resources:

- Present staffing workload
- Human resources (i.e., number of personnel, experience and abilities, and percentage of dedicated time to the project)

- Present cost of operation
- Relationship of implementation events with nonproject events (i.e., Joint Commission on Accreditation of Healthcare Organizations [JCAHO] reviews, state certification inspections, peak vacation and census times, union negotiations, and house staff turnover)
- Anticipated training costs
- Space availability
- Current and anticipated equipment requirements for the project team

Highly successful projects have spent the requisite amount of time to thoroughly complete the planning phase. Further, successful organizations have communicated senior management and administration's project expectations through dissemination of the project scope agreement to all departments in the organization.

The Key Role of the Nurse Administrator

Successful implementations of a CIS have been accomplished by many facilities; the active involvement of the nurse executive is considered a critical success factor of any CIS implementation or upgrade. Visionary nursing leaders who have implemented CISs and/or nursing components at their institutions have shared their recommendations and urge that a business plan be developed and incorporated into the process. The following features should be discussed in the business plan:

- An executive summary strongly supporting the power of timely and accurate information.
- An introduction, outlining the purpose and objectives of the proposed CIS and/or nursing application(s).
- An environmental assessment of the CIS and/or nursing components in use by similar hospitals.
- An analysis of the nursing department culture, infrastructure, policies, and information needs.
- An overview of the design and implementation plan describing the objectives, activation strategy to be used, a listing of equipment needs, staffing projections, time resources, potential costs, and evaluation methodologies for the CIS as a whole and the nursing component(s) in particular.
- A financial plan projecting staffing, budget, expenses, capital expenditures, and miscellaneous expenditures.

System Analysis Phase

The system analysis phase, the second phase of developing a CIS, is the fact-finding phase. All data requirements related to the problem defined in the project scope agreement are collected and analyzed to gain a sound understanding of the current system, how it is used, and what is needed from the new system. Process analysis is foundational to the actual system design, since it examines the objectives and project scope in terms of the end-user requirements, the flow of information in daily operation, and the processing of required data elements. Through the analysis effort, the individual data elements, interfaces, and decision points of the project are identified (Yourdon, 1989). Current costs and resources required for processing the data are compared with estimates for the cost of processing with the new system. If a system is being upgraded or expanded, the current equipment and functions are described. Careful evaluation is undertaken to ensure compatibility with the new system's requirements and to maximize the use of available equipment as long as possible. Depreciation costs of available equipment and projected budget expenditures are reviewed.

The importance of this phase should not be underestimated. Design changes made during the analysis stage often add minimal costs to the project; as the project progresses to the development and implementation phases, the cost of programmatic or design changes increases dramatically. According to one source, when a project is in the planning phase, the relative cost to make a design change or fix an error is one; in the analysis phase, the relative cost to fix the error/design change is three to six times that of the planning phase. The relative cost to fix an error or change a system design jumps to 40–1,000 times once the system is operational (Gause and Weinburg, 1989).

The system analysis phase consists of the following five steps:

- Data collection
- Data analysis
- Data review
- Benefits identification
- System proposal development

Data Collection

The collection of data reflecting the existing problem or goal is the first step in the system analysis phase. As a result of thorough data collection, refinements to the project scope agreement may occur. Added benefits to the organization may be realized through the small refinements. Larger project scope refinements should be carefully researched and evaluated (using the steps outlined in the feasibility study methodology) prior to requesting a major project scope change. Large or small, all changes must continue to support the goal(s) of the project and the strategic plan of the organization.

Two important documents are created as a result of data collection. The first is the creation of a workflow document for each major goal or problem to be resolved by the implementation of the new software or system; the second is a functional design document outlining how the new system will resolve the identified goals/problem.

Workflow Document The workflow document assimilates the data collected into logical sequencing of tasks and subtasks performed by the end users for each goal or problem area. Departmental standards of care, ordering patterns, procedures, operating manuals, reports (routine, regulatory, and year-end), and forms used in day-to-day operations are collected. Individual data elements required by clinicians in each department are identified and analyzed for continuity and duplication. The workflow document includes the following:

- A list of assumptions about the process or work effort
- A list of the major tasks performed by the user
- A list of the subtasks and steps the user accomplishes and outlines whether
  - The determination of optional or required status for each task
  - The frequency of the task being performed
  - The criticality and important factors of the tasks/subtasks
  - The order of the subtasks
  - The number and frequency of alternate scenarios available to the end user to accomplish a particular task

There are multiple sources of data for completing a workflow document. These include the following:

- Written documents, forms, and flow sheets
- Policy and procedure manuals
- Questionnaires
- Interviews
- Observations

Functional Design Document The functional design document is the overview statement of how the new system will work. It uses the workflow documents as its base, adding the critical documentation of the integration of each of the workflow documents to create a new system, implement a commercial software application, or upgrade a system. The functional design document, in this phase, outlines the human and machine procedures, the input points, the processing requirements, the output from the data entry, and the major reports to be generated from the new system. The functional design is a concise description of the functions required from the proposed computerized system and describes how the application will accomplish its task. From the functional design document, database structure will be determined.

When new software is being created, the functional design document provides the programmers with a view of screens, linkages, and alternate scenarios to accomplish a task. Initial programming efforts can begin once the functional design is accepted. In the instance where a commercially available system or application is being implemented, the functional design outlines how the end users will use the system's programs to accomplish their tasks. In some cases, commercial software provides multiple pathways to accomplish a single task; the functional specification may suggest deploying a limited number of available pathways.

Data Analysis

The analysis of the collected data is the second step in the system analysis phase. The analysis provides the data for development of an overview of the nursing problem and/or stated goal defined in the project scope agreement.

Several tools can be used in the development of the workflow and functional design documents. Some of the more common tools are:

- Data flowchart
- Grid chart
- Decision table
- Organizational chart
- Model

Data Review

The third step in the analysis phase is to review the data collected in the feasibility study, the workflow documents, and the functional specification and provide recommendations to the project steering committee for the new system. The review focuses on resolving the problems and/or attaining the goals defined in the feasibility study based on the best methods or pathways derived from the workflow documents and the functional design. Recommendations for streamlining workflow are suggested. The success of a CIS implementation project rests on the ability of the departmental and project teams to analyze the data and propose solutions benefiting the total organization without favoring certain departments at the expense of others. The benefits of a thorough structured analysis provide objective data to support these decisions. The careful analysis of end-user requirements and potential solutions has been proved to reduce the cost of design and implementation (Gause and Weinburg, 1989).

Benefits Identification

The overall anticipated benefits from the system are documented in the fourth step in the system analysis process. The benefits reflect the resolution of the identified problem, formulated and stated in quantifiable terms. The proposed benefits statements become the criteria for measuring the success of the project.

System Proposal Development

The final step in the system analysis stage is to create a system proposal document. The proposal is submitted to the project's steering committee for review and approval. It sets forth the problems and/or goals and the requirements for the new system's overall design. It outlines the standards, documentation, and procedures for management control of the project, and it defines the information required, the necessary resources, anticipated benefits, a detailed workplan, and projected costs for the new system. The system proposal furnishes the project steering committee with recommendations concerning the proposed CIS or application. The system proposal document answers four questions:

1. What are the major problems and/or goals under consideration?

2. How will the proposed CIS solution correct or eliminate the problems and/or accomplish the stated goals?

3. What are the anticipated costs?

4. How long will it take?

The system proposal describes the project in sufficient detail to provide a management level understanding of the system or application without miring in minutiae. Much of the information required in the system proposal is collected in the earlier phases of the analysis. It has been suggested that this proposal is best accepted when presented as a business proposal and championed by a member of the project's steering committee. The format of the final system proposal includes the following information:

1. A concise statement of the problem(s) and/or goal(s)
2. Background information related to the problem
3. Environmental factors related to the problem
   (a) Competition
   (b) Economics
   (c) Politics
   (d) Ethics
4. Anticipated benefits
5. Proposed solutions
6. Budgetary and resource requirements
7. Project timetable

Acceptance of the system proposal by the project steering committee provides the project senior management support. Following acceptance by the project steering committee, it is not unusual for major CIS proposals to be presented to the institution's governing board for their acceptance and approval and to receive funding. Often the requirement for board approval is dependent on the final cost estimates of the system. Acceptance of the proposal by the project steering committee and the governing board assures not only funding for the project but critical top-down management and administrative support for the project. The final system proposal is an internal contract between the CIS committees/teams (steering, project, and departmental) and the institution. When commercially available software is under consideration, the system proposal document assists the institution's legal team in formulating a contract with the software vendor as well as providing the basis for the development of a formal request for proposal (RFP) to potential vendors.

As noted earlier, the active support and involvement of the nursing executive in the development of the feasibility study are essential. The championing of the final system proposal greatly enhances the chances of acceptance of the system proposal.

The System Design Phase

In the system design phase, the design details of the system and the detailed plans for implementing the system are developed for both the functional and the technical components of the system. Acceptance of the system proposal by the steering committee heralds the beginning of the system design phase.

There are three major steps in the system design phase:

- Functional specifications
- Technical specifications
- Implementation planning

Functional Specifications

The functional specifications use the functional design document developed in the system analysis phase of a CIS and builds on the design by formulating a detailed description of ALL system inputs, outputs, and processing logic required to complete the scope of the project. It further refines what the proposed system will encompass and provides the framework for its operation.

Commercial software vendors generally provide a detailed functional specification document for their system or application in the form of manuals. The manuals, usually application-specific, include an introduction, a section for each pathway, and a technical section. From the provided documentation, the hospital's departmental and project teams produce the organization's functional specification by evaluating the available commercial software's functions with the workflow documents and making decisions on the pathways and functions to be used by the institution.

Data Manipulation and Output   There are several considerations for handling data manipulation and output (American Society for Testing and Materials, 1993). The detailed functional specifications are critical to the system's acceptance; each screen, data flow, and report the user can expect to see is analyzed. A significant level of detail with sketches, explanations, and/or examples is necessary (Hewlett-Packard, 1993). The examples incorporate real data into the explanations and drawings.

During this step, the departmental teams and users determine what the actual data will look like in its output form and gain consensus from the departmental teams for the proposed design. There is fluidity between the functional design, functional specification, and initial programming prototype efforts. The design team creating the new application often works closely with the programmers, making adjustments in the design and specification based on new perspectives, programming logic, and/or technologies. As the functional specification matures and major design decisions (e.g., selection of the underlying application technology and database structure) have occurred, a design "freeze point" is established. This indicates that the functional specification is complete and full programming efforts are established.

Once completed, the functional specification provides not only the road map for programming efforts, but the starting point for developing testing plans for verification of the software. It provides developers and the project teams of an implementation with the source for determining testing needs prior to releasing the application into a production, or "live," environment. The advantages of establishing testing plans in concert with the development of the functional specification include a more thorough test plan (pathways are not missed), and "what if" questions often spark the need to develop or allow alternate pathways for a function.

The following criteria are considered essential in selecting a CIS and can be used as a basis for evaluation. They include the following areas:

- Applications
- Use of industry standards to establish connectivity
- Overall system performance
- Evaluation features and pathways
- Ease of system use
- Configuration or programming performance
- Security
- Simplification of reports
- Database access
- Hardware and software reliability
- Connectivity
- System cost

Technical Specifications

In the system design phase, technical personnel work closely with the project and departmental teams to ensure the technical components of the proposed system work in concert with technology and end-user needs and to assist in the development of the implementation plan. As stated earlier, a dedicated technical manager is required. He or she is responsible for the coordination of efforts in four major areas. Each area requires that a detailed technical specification be developed. The project's technical manager and team leaders ensure that all of the components/applications of the CIS work in concert with all the other components. The four major areas include hardware, software, interfaces, and conversions.

Hardware   In the case of new software development, the technical project manager ensures the new software uses the best technology platform available. The ability to operate the new application on multiple hardware platforms is often desired. Technical specifications describing the recommended equipment are developed and tested in the development laboratory.

When commercial software is being implemented or upgraded, the technical project manager ensures that the physical environment for the new system conforms to the new system's technical specifications. This may include the need to build a new computer room, establish or upgrade a network, and procure the correct devices for the new system. The types of devices to be used (PCs vs. handheld vs. bedside devices) require dialog and testing with team leaders and department team members. The testing and deployment of the new equipment (terminals, printers, and/or handheld devices) are the responsibility of the technical manager. Ongoing maintenance for the new computer's central processing unit (CPU), operating system, and network is coordinated by the project's technical manager.

Application Software   The project's technical manager is responsible for establishing the technical specifications outlining the operational requirements for the new system. The specifications detail the procedures required to maintain the application software on a daily, weekly, and monthly basis. The specifications are compiled as the starting point for determining the operations schedule for the system and/or the institution. The operations plan includes detailed information related to when the system will be scheduled for routine maintenance, plans for operations during system failures, and acceptable periods during the week/month for the system to be unavailable to the users. Additional requirements for assuring data reliability and availability following planned and unplanned system downtime, as well as procedures outlining data recovery following a downtime are developed. "Change control" policies and procedures for identifying, tracking, testing, and applying software fixes are established.

Interface Systems   An interface system defines those programs and processes required to transmit data between two disparate systems. The project's technical manager coordinates all interfacing activities for the new application. While utilization of the industry's Health Level Seven (HL7) interface standards has greatly reduced the effort required to establish clinical interfaces by providing a standard specification for the transmission

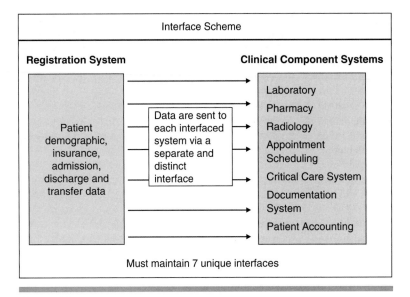

Figure 19.4
Interface scheme.

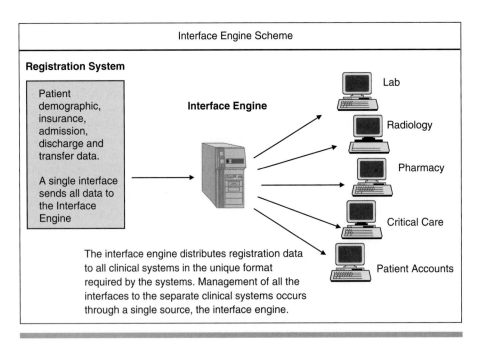

Figure 19.5
Interface engine.

of data, the number of clinical interfaces in a CIS has increased dramatically. It is not unusual for a CIS to interface with separate registration, patient billing, laboratory, radiology, and pharmacy systems. Recent interface methodology developments advocate the use of an interface engine decreasing the number of individual interfaces to be managed (Fig. 19.4). More complex environments may include interfaces to cardiac and fetal monitors and radio frequency-based portable devices and provide remote access into the hospital's clinical system for physicians and home care nursing staff (Fig. 19.5).

The interface specification details whether the interface will be one-way or bidirectional. A bidirectional interface implies that data are flowing both to and from a system. Conversely, a one-way interface may either send data to or receive data from a separate system but not do both.

The informatics nurse assists in development of the interface specification by assisting with the comparison of data elements in each system and helping to determine which data elements will be included in the interface.

Conversions The conversion of data from legacy systems to the new system is the fourth major area of coordination for the project's technical manager. Most hospitals currently use automated registration and billing systems; determining the conversion requirements and developing and testing the conversion programs are critical steps in implementing a new system or application.

While all steps are important in the implementation of a new system, the interface and conversion design and testing tasks are frequent areas that cause project delays for the implementation and/or upgrading of CISs. The importance of the project's technical manager and oversight management by the project manager in keeping these tasks on the established timetable and in ensuring that the departmental and project teams are informed of the interface and conversion plans should not be underestimated.

Implementation Planning

The last step in the system design phase is to establish a detailed implementation plan. The developed functional and technical specifications define a significant amount of form and substance for the new CIS. The next step is to assess the timeframes established in the final scope document with the development timeframes established during the system design phase and the interface and conversion requirements to establish a detailed workplan. The workplan identifies a responsible party and a beginning date and end date for each phase, step, task, and

subtask. This plan coordinates all tasks necessary to complete the development of new software, implement a new system, and/or upgrade a current system. Many software vendors and consultants provide an implementation workplan for their system or applications. The supplied workplans must be reviewed and revised to meet the individual needs and timetables of the institution's project.

Whether the project is software development or the implementation or upgrading of a system, the implementation workplan details the following:

- Personnel
- Timeframes
- Costs and budgets
- Facilities and equipment required
- Development or implementation tasks
- Operational considerations
- Human-computer interactions
- System test plan

These areas are detailed in an implementation workplan encompassing 14 steps. A successful implementation ensures all 14 steps are planned, executed, and tracked by the project manager and project team leaders (Fig. 19.6).

In the instance where commercially available software is being considered, completion of the design phase provides the steering committee and project team with

**Upgrade or Implementation Workplan
14 Steps for a Clinical System**

Project Planning/Administration
Hardware & Software Delivery
Application Administration
Application Verification
Team Leader Training
Conversion & Interface Planning
Building Databases (Files & Tables)
Policies and Procedures
Peripheral Device Identification
Functional Test
Integrated Test
End User Training
Live Operations
Post Implementation Evaluation

Figure 19.6
Fourteen steps for implementation/upgrading chart.

sufficient information to evaluate commercial system offerings. With the system design complete, the task of selecting a new system becomes more objective.

On the other hand, if the project steering committee decides to develop its own system programs, the project staff must proceed with the development phase of the system, which includes the following:

- Select hardware
- Develop software
- Test system
- Document system

Select Hardware   Selecting the correct hardware for the system depends on its design, application, and software requirements. Technical conditions may dictate selection of a mainframe, a minicomputer, a microcomputer, or a combination of the above. Computer hardware is obtained in several different ways. Mainframes and minicomputers may be purchased or leased from a hardware vendor for in-house use; however, when cost is a significant factor, timesharing computer processing with other facilities may be considered. Since microcomputers are small, they may be the most economical for some applications. Input, output, and processing media, including secondary storage, is selected, and all hardware must be installed and able to test the computer programs at the appropriate time.

Develop Software   When a new application or system is being created, the development phase becomes an iterative process of programming sections of the design established in the functional specification, testing the design with the informatics nurse and/or design team, evaluating options suggested as a result of testing, and refining/reevaluating the functional specification. The manager for the development project ensures the progress of the development and that timelines for completion of the project are met. Business aspects are detailed and managed. These may include determination of product packaging and marketing materials, establishment of product pricing, development of system/application documentation, and the establishment of a marketing plan.

The Testing Phase

The system, whether newly developed or commercially available, must be tested to ensure that all data are processed correctly and the desired outputs are generated.

Testing verifies that the computer programs are written correctly and ensures that when implemented in the production (live) environment, the system will function as planned. In the development scenario, the three levels of testing are often referred to as unit testing, alpha testing, and beta testing. Unit testing, described earlier, is conducted by the individual programmers as the programs are being coded. Systems are tested to determine if the programming protocols are used correctly and if the programs execute correctly. Alpha testing is accomplished by a testing (system assurance) group within the development organization. Alpha testing of a system or application, done in the development lab, focuses not only on the correct execution of the programs, but also on the integration of the programs with the entire application or system. Sample data mimicking true patient data are used whenever possible to test the integration of computer programs. Beta testing occurs at the first client site. Representatives of the development team assist the client in testing the programs for the first time in real-life situations.

When commercially available software is being implemented, three levels of testing are recommended. The first level is often called a functional test. During this round of testing, the departmental teams test and verify the databases (files and tables), ensuring that correct data have been entered into the files and tables. The expected departmental reports are reviewed to assure correctness and accuracy. Multiple iterations of the functional test often occur until the departmental team is confident of the system setup and profiles. The second level of testing, integrated systems testing, begins when all departments indicate the completion of their functional testing. During integrated testing, the total system is tested; this includes interfaces between systems as well as the interplay between applications within the same system. The integrated test must mimic the production (live) environment in terms of the volume of transactions, the number of users, the interfaced systems, and the procedures to be followed to carry out all functions of the system. It is at this point that testing of the organization-wide procedures to be instituted when the system is unavailable, downtime procedures, are thoroughly tested. Downtime procedures must be taught during end-user training. The final round of testing occurs during end-user training. As more users interact with the new system, previously unfound problems may surface. Evaluation of the severity of the newly discovered problems and the corrective action required is an ongoing process during implementation.

Document System

The preparation of documents to describe the system for all users is an ongoing activity, with development of the documentation occurring as the various system phases and steps are completed. Documentation should begin with the final system proposal. Several manuals are prepared: a user's manual, a reference manual, and an operator's maintenance manual. These manuals provide guides to the system components and outline how the entire system has been programmed or defined.

User's Manual

The user's manual highlights how to use the system and describes what outputs the system can produce. With commercially available software, the vendor's user's manual helps establish the organization's training manual.

Reference Manual

The reference manual is used by the project team members to understand how the system works. It describes what data are input, how the databases (files and tables) process the data, and the mechanisms used to generate outputs.

Operator's Maintenance Manual

This manual enables operators to keep the system up and running by providing the functional and technical specifications needed for the system. Manuals must be written in sufficient detail such that system users and operators understand how the system was developed, how it operates, and how it can be maintained, updated, and repaired.

 The Training Phase

It is essential to train the end users on how to use the system properly. A CIS will function only as well as its users understand its operation and the operations streamline the work. Two levels of training take place for the implementation of a system. The project team and selected members of the departmental team receive training from the developers or vendor. This training details the databases (files and tables), processing logic, and outputs of all the system's features and functions. End-user training, the second level of testing, takes place once the departmental and project teams have finished profiling the system to meet the functional and technical specifications developed and functional testing has been completed.

End-user training stresses how the user will complete his or her workflow using the new system.

All users of the new system or application must receive training. Training on a new system should occur no more than 6 weeks prior to the activation of the new system. When training occurs for more than 6 weeks before activation of the system, additional refresher training is often required by the end users.

Training takes place before and during the activation of a new system. After system implementation, refresher courses as well as new employee introductory training on the use of the new system are often provided by the institution. Training of the nursing department usually requires the development of a separate training plan. The large number of nursing staff members to be trained necessitates a significant amount of advance planning.

Training is most effective when hands-on, interactive instruction is provided. Training guides or manuals explain the system; however, retention of information is increased if the learners are able to interact with the new system in a manner simulating their workflow with the new system. Computer-assisted instruction (CAI) in a special training room or on the units can be used to provide hands-on experience. End-user training is offered with two perspectives. One perspective provides a general overview of the system, and the second perspective explains how the user will interact with the system to complete his or her daily work. While a user's/training manual is developed for the training sessions, most end users express the desire to have a pocket size reminder ("cheat sheet") outlining the key functions of the new system or application. Both the user's manual and the pocket reminders should be available for departmental use. When possible, a training environment on the computer system should be established for the organization. Establishing a training lab as well as providing access to the training environment from the departments and nursing units prior to the activation of the new system provides end users the opportunity to practice at times convenient to their work requirements and reinforces the training.

 The Implementation Phase

The implementation phase organizes all the steps into a detailed plan describing the series of events required to begin using the system or application in the production or live environment and details the necessary computer and software maintenance operations required to keep the system running. This phase ensures that once the system is installed in the live environment, the system and the delivery of healthcare in the organization will run smoothly. The schedule of operations begun in the design phase is documented in procedures manuals for the computer operators. The "go live" workplan includes a detailed description of the preparation steps required for all facets of the system, the timing requirements to accomplish the tasks, the defining elements indicating the completion of each critical task, and the party responsible for determining if the criteria to progress in the plan have been met. The activation of interfaces, the timing of the final conversion of data (if any) into the new system, and the activation activities for each of the nursing units and departments are detailed in this plan.

Four activation approaches are possible: (1) parallel, (2) pilot, (3) phased-in, and (4) big bang theory. In the parallel approach, the new system runs parallel with the existing system until users can adjust. In the pilot approach, a few departments or units try out the new system to see how it works and then help other units or departments to use it. In the phased-in approach, the system is implemented by one unit or department at a time. In the big bang approach, a cut-over date and time are established for the organization, the old system is stopped, and all units/departments begin processing on the newly installed system.

The timing of conversion activities and the activation of all interfaces require particular coordination between the technical staff and the project teams. The project's technical manager, in conjunction with the project manager, is responsible for assuring the development of thorough go live plans. A command center is established to coordinate all issues, concerns, and go live help desk functions. A sufficient number of phone lines and beepers are secured to support the move to the live production environment. Team members and trainers often serve as resources to the end users on a 24-hour basis for a period of time postimplementation. Sometimes called "super users," these team members are available in the departments and on the nursing units to proactively assist users during the first 1–2 weeks of productive use of the new system or application.

The coordination of all activities requires a cohesive team effort. Communication among the team members is as critical as keeping the end users informed of the sequence events, the expected time frames for each event, and the channels established for reporting and resolving issues.

The Evaluation Phase

The evaluation phase describes and assesses, in detail, the new system's performance. Using the criteria established in the planning and system design phases, the evaluation process summarizes the entire system, identifying both the strengths and weaknesses of the implementation process. An evaluation study often leads to system revisions and, ultimately, a better system.

During this phase, the system is evaluated to determine whether it has accomplished the stated objectives. A system evaluation involves a comparison of a working system with its functional requirements to determine how well the requirements are met, to determine possibilities for growth and improvement, and to preserve the lessons learned from the implementation project for future efforts.

To evaluate an implemented hospital information system, many principles are important for CISs. One authority suggests evaluating duplication of efforts and data entry, fragmentation, misplaced work, complexity, bottlenecks, review/approval process, error reporting (or the amount of reworking of content), movement, wait time, delays, setup, low importance outputs, and unimportant outputs (Young, 1981).

Evaluating the system is the final and ongoing step in implementation process. This evaluation component becomes a continuous phase in total quality management. The system is assessed to determine whether it continues to meet the needs of the users. The totally implemented system will require continuous evaluation to determine if upgrading is appropriate and/or what enhancements could be added to the current system. Formal evaluations generally take place not less than 6 months and routinely every 2–4 years after the system has been implemented. The formal evaluation should be conducted by an outside evaluation team to increase the objectivity level of the findings. Informal evaluations are done on a weekly basis.

Other approaches to evaluating the functional performance of a system exist. Investigating such functions as administrative control, medical/nursing orders, charting and documentation, and retrieval and management reports are used to assess system benefits. Each of these areas is evaluated through time observations, work sampling, operational audits, and surveys. System functional performance can be assessed by examining nurses' morale and nursing department operations (McCormick, 1983).

Documentation of care must be assessed if patient care benefits are to be evaluated. The following questions must be answered:

■ Does the system assist in improving the documentation of patient care in the patient record?

■ Does the system reduce patient care costs?

- Does the system prevent errors and save lives?

To evaluate nurses' morale requires appraising nurses' satisfaction with the system. The following questions may be considered useful:

- Does the system facilitate nurses' documentation of patient care?
- Does it reduce the time spent in such documentation?
- Is it easy to use?
- Is it readily accessible?
- Are the display "screens" easy to use?
- Do the displays capture patient care?
- Does the system enhance the work situation and contribute to work satisfaction?

To evaluate the departmental benefits requires determining if the CIS helps improve administrative activities. The following questions must be answered:

- Does the new system enhance the goals of the department?
- Does it improve department efficiency?
- Does it help reduce the range of administrative activities?
- Does it reduce clerical work?

Other criteria are necessary to evaluate technical performance; these include reliability, maintainability, use, response time, accessibility, availability, and flexibility to meet changing needs. These areas are examined from several different points—the technical performance of the software as well as hardware performance. The following questions must be answered:

- Is the system accurate and reliable?
- Is it easy to maintain at a reasonable cost?
- Is it flexible?
- Is the information consistent?
- Is the information timely?
- Is it responsive to users' needs?
- Do users find interaction with the system satisfactory?
- Are input devices accessible and generally available to users?

Cost-Benefit Analysis

A cost-benefit analysis is necessary to determine if the system is worth its price. The cost-benefit analysis relates system cost and benefits to system design, level of use, timeframe, and equipment costs. Each of these costs must be assessed in relation to benefits derived. Such an evaluation can help determine the future of the system.

Upgrading Clinical Information Systems

The upgrading of a system may be undertaken for a number of reasons. Software vendors often provide enhancements and upgrades to their system. New applications, features, and/or functions may be developed by the vendor and become available to the organization. Upgrading a system as a result of the addition of new subsystems and technology commonly occurs. To upgrade a system, the same phases and activities described for designing and implementing must occur; however, when upgrading, dovetailing the changes into the current system will require close evaluation. New technologies are an important consideration; the following new technologies may be considered:

- Bedside/point-of-care wireless devices
- Workstations
- Multimedia presentations
- Decision support
- Artificial intelligence
- Neural networks
- Integrated systems architecture
- Interfaced networks
- Open architecture

All of the above have been discussed within other chapters of this book, with the exception of the concepts of integrating, interfacing, or open architecture. These three important concepts are related to upgrading.

Workstations

The workstation becomes the mode to gain access to multiple applications. The user does not have to know or understand what type of hardware or software he or she is accessing, only that there is access to a broad array of information. The security and confidentiality issues raised by open architecture systems are being handled with the installation of security servers, registration centers to register use of information, and/or protocols requiring authorization.

According to Clayton et al. (1992), the advantages of updating using open architecture are modularity, rapid implementation, simultaneous existence of old and new systems running side by side, redundant pathways, and vendor and platform independence. The major disadvantage of open architecture is the lack of national standards dictating a common communication language between machines.

System Issues

As new technologies are evaluated and upgrading is considered, the design team or departmental team must reassess the original functional requirements. If the system has not been used to its limit, reserve capacity to expand the original functional requirements with the existing hardware may exist. As far as possible, the team needs to determine if a subsystem can be added to the working system. New functions might be required, necessitating the procurement of additional hardware.

Future Trends

The introduction of the computer-based patient record (CPR) has been recommended by the Institute of Medicine report. The report recommends that new system designs should expand to improve the fundamental resource in healthcare beyond the automating of patient records (Dick and Steen, 1991). Two key reports from the Institute of Medicine, To Err is Human: Building a Safer Health System (1999) and its sequel, Crossing the Chasm (2001) have been the imputus for national attention toward computerized order entry and computerized provider order entry as mechanisms needed to improve patient safety in the healthcare system. A significant number of works have been published on the impact of the implementation of computerized order entry on care providers and the delivery of patient care (Sengstack and Gugerty, 2004; Briggs, 2003; California Healthcare Foundation, American Hospital Association, Federation of American Hospitals and First Consulting Group, 2002; Bauer, 2004; Dambro et al., 1988; Aaarts, Doorewaard, and Berg, 2004). Efforts to improve long-term acceptance and assimilation of a CIS into everyday use must include

The CPR design will be more useful if it provides practical and accurate data, practitioner reminders and alerts, clinical decision support systems, links to bodies of medical knowledge, and other aids in expanding knowledge needed in clinical decision-making. Within this definition is the concept of broadening the CPR from more than an "automated patient record" to an

integral resource in the management of a lifelong healthcare record and in the extension of knowledge.

The fully configured workstations will require Active X or Web-enabled applications, accelerated processors, client/server architecture, graphical user interfaces (GUI), and large storage capabilities to retrieve and process data for case management, clinical pathways, and outcomes-of-care analysis. New user-oriented interfaces provide the user with high-powered workstations; graphical, object-oriented, and metaphoric interface; and relational databases that support ad hoc querying and multiprocessing.

 ## Summary

This chapter describes the process of designing, implementing, and/or upgrading a CIS in a patient healthcare facility. It outlines and describes the eight phases of the process—planning, system analysis, system design, system development, testing, training, implementation, and evaluation. The upgrading process uses all of the phases described.

The planning phase determines the problem scope and outlines the entire project to determine if the system is feasible and worth developing and/or implementing. The analysis phase assesses the problem being studied through extensive data gathering and analysis. The design phase produces detailed specifications of the proposed system. Development involves the actual preparation of the system. Testing is generally conducted on three levels for both the design and implementation of a commercially available system. Training includes the training of users in the use of the system for their everyday lives. Implementation outlines the detailed plans for moving the new system into the production or live environment. Evaluating the system determines the positive and negative results of the implementation effort and suggests ways to improve the system. Upgrading the system involves expansion or elaboration of initial functions by expanding capability or function or by adding entirely new applications. Upgrading projects requires that all implementation phases be completed to assure success.

References

American Society for Testing and Materials. (1993). Proposed standards (E622). *Standard Guide for Developing Computerized Systems*. Philadelphia, PA: ASTM International.

Ash, J., Anderson, J., Gorman, P., Zielstorff, R., Norcross, N., Pettit, J., and Yao, P. (2000). Managing change: Analysis of a hypothetical case. *Journal of the American Medical Informatics Association* 7(2):125–134.

Augustine, J. (2004). System redesign and IT implementation. *Advance for Health Information Executives* 8(1): 41–43.

Bauer, J. (2004). Why CPOE must become SOP. *Journal of Healthcare Information Management* 18(1):9–10.

Briggs, B. (2003). CPOE: Order from chaos. *Health Data Management*. Obtained from *www.HealthDataManagement.com* website archive.

California Healthcare Foundation. (2002). *Computerized Physician Order Entry: Cost Benefits and Challenges, A Case Study Approach* (pp. 28–36). Prepared by First Consulting Group, CA.

Clayton, P., Sideli, R., and Sengupta, S. (1992). Open architecture and integrated information at Columbia-Presbyterian Medical Center. *MD Computing* 9(5), 297–303.

Convey, S. (1992). *The Seven Healthy Habits of Highly Effective People: Restoring the Character Ethic* (pp. 95–144). New York: Fireside.

Dick, R. and Steen, E. (Eds.) (1991). *The Computer-Based Record: An Essential Technology for Health Care.* Washington, DC: National Academy Press.

Douglas, M. (1995). Butterflies, bonsai, and buonarroti: Images for the nurse analyst. In M. Ball, C. Hannah, S. Newbold, and J. Douglas (Eds.), *Nursing Informatics, Where Caring and Technology Meet 2000* (pp. 84–94). New York: Springer-Verlag.

Douglas, M. and Wright, B. (2003). Zoom–Zoom, turbo charging clinical implementations. *Presentation at Toward an Electronic Health Record—Europe, London, 2003.*

Fitzgerald, J., Fitzgerald, A., and Satllings, W. (1981). *Fundamentals of Systems Analysis* (2nd ed.). New York: Wiley.

Gause, D. and Weinberg, G. (1989). *Exploring Requirements: Quality before Design.* New York: Dorset House Publishing.

Ginsburg, D.A. and Browning, S.J. (1989). Selecting automated patient care systems. In V.K. Saba, K.A. Rider, and D.B. Pocklington (Eds.), *Nursing and Computers: An Anthology* (pp. 229–237). New York: Springer-Verlag.

Hewlett-Packard. (1993). *Choosing a Clinical Information System: A Blueprint for Your Success.* Waltham, MA: Hewlett-Packard.

Kaplan, B. (1997). Addressing organizational issues into the evaluation of medical systems. *Journal of the American Medical Informatics Association* 4(2):94–101.

Lorenzi, N. and Riley, R. (2000). Managing change. *Journal of the American Medical Informatics Association* 7(2):116–124.

Peitzman, L. (2004). Addressing physician resistance to technology. *Advance for Health Information Executives* 8(5):69–70.

Protti, D. and Peel, V. (1998). Critical success factors for evolving a hospital toward an electronic patient record system: A case study of two different sites. *Journal of Healthcare Information Management* 12(4):29–37.

Ritter, J. and Glaser, J. (1994). Implementing the patient care information system strategy. In E. Drazen, J. Metzger, J. Ritter, and M. Schneider (Eds.), *Patient Care Information Systems: Suggestful Design and Implementation* (pp. 163–164). New York: Springer-Verlag.

Schooler, R. and Dotson, T. (2004). Rolling out the CIS. *Advance for Health Information Executives* 8(2):63–70.

Selker, H., Beshansky, J., Pauker, S., and Kassirer, J. (1989). The epidemiology of delays in a teaching hospital. *Medical Care* 27:112–129.

Sengstack, P. and Gugerty, B. (2004). CPOE systems: Success factors and implementation issues. *Journal of Healthcare Information Management* 18(1):36–45.

Simpson, R. L. (1993). *The Nurse Executive's Guide to Directing and Managing Nurse Information Systems.* Ann Arbor, MI: The Center for Healthcare Information Management.

Spillane, J., McLaughlin, M., Ellis, K., et al. (1990). Direct physician order entry and integration potential pitfalls. In *Proceedings of the 14th Annual Society for Computer Applications in Medical Care* (pp. 774–778). Washington, DC: IEEE Computer Society Press.

Young, E.M. (Ed.) (1981). *Automated Hospital Information, Vol. 1: Guide to Planning, Selecting, Acquiring, Implementing and Managing an HIS.* Los Angeles, CA: Center Publications.

Yourdon, E. (1989). *Modern Structures Analysis.* Englewood Cliffs, NJ: Yourdon Press.

Zielstorff, R. (1985). Cost effectiveness of computerization in nursing practice and administration. *Journal of Nursing Administration* 15:22–26.

Zinn, T.K. (1989). Automated systems selection. *Health Care* 31:45–46.

Recommended Readings

American Nurses Association. (1994). *The Scope of Practice for Nursing Informatics.* Washington, DC: American Nurse Publishing.

American Nurses Association. (1995). *The Standards of Practice for Nursing Informatics.* Washington, DC: American Nurse Publishing.

Arnold, J. and Pearson, G. (1992). *Computers Applications in Nursing Education and Practice* (Pub. No. 14-2406). New York: National League for Nursing.

Axford, R. and Carter, B. (1996). Impact of clinical information systems on nursing practice: Nurses' perspective. *Computers in Nursing* 14(3):156–163.

Aydin, C., Rosen, P., Jewell, S., et al. (1995). Computers in the examining room: The patient's perspective. *American Medical Informatics Association Proceedings* (pp. 824–828).

Ball, M.J. and Collen, M.F. (Eds.) (1992). *Aspects of the Computer-Based Patient Record.* New York: Springer-Verlag.

Burnard, P. (1991). Computing: An aid to studying nursing. *Nursing Standard* 5(17):16–22.

Campbell, B. (1990). The clinical director's role in selecting a computer system. *Caring* 9(6):36–38.

Center for Healthcare Information Management (CHIM). (1991). *Guide to Making Effective H.I.S. Purchase Decisions.* Ann Arbor, MI: The Center for Healthcare Information Management.

Freudenheim, M. (2004). Many hospitals resist computerized patient care. *New York Times,* April 6, 2004.

Gillis, P.A., Booth, H., Graves, J.R., et al. (1994). Translating traditional principles of system development into a process for designing clinical information systems. *International Journal of Technology Assessment in Health Care* 10(2):235–248.

Holzemer, W.L. and Henry, S.B. (1992). Computer-supported versus manually-generated nursing care plans: A comparison of patient problems, nursing interventions and AIDS patients outcomes. *Computers in Nursing* 10(1):19–24.

Mills, M. (1994). Nurse-computer performance considerations for the nurse administrator. *Journal of Nursing Administration* 24(11):30–35.

Mohr, D., Capenter, P., Claus, P., et al. (1995). Implementing an EMR: Paper's last hurrah. *American Medical Informatics Association Proceedings* (pp. 157–161).

Protti, D. and Peel, V. (1998). Critical success factors for evolving a hospital toward an electronic patient record system: A case study of two different sites. *Journal of Healthcare Information Management* 12(4):29–37.

Ritter, J. and Glaser, J. (1994). Implementing the patient care information system strategy. In E. Drazen, J. Metzger, J. Ritter, and M. Schneider (Eds.), *Patient Care Information Systems: Successful Design and Implementation* (pp. 163–194). New York: Springer-Verlag.

Warnock-Matheron, A. and Plummer, C. (1988). Introducing nursing information systems in the clinical setting. In M. Ball, K. Hannah, U. Gerdin-Jelger, and H. Peterson. (Eds.), *Nursing Informatics: Where Caring and Technology Meet* (pp. 115–127). New York: Springer-Verlag.

Zielstorff, R., Grobe, S., and Hudgins, C. (1992). *Nursing Information Systems: Essential Characteristics for Professional Practice.* Kansas City, MO: American Nurses Association.

PART 5

Practice Application

CHAPTER 20

Practice Applications

Joyce E. Johnson
Molly Billingsley

OBJECTIVES

1. Review the history of informatics in healthcare and nursing.
2. Document the current definition of nursing informatics and its evolution.
3. Describe the national scope and standards of nursing informatics practice.
4. Delineate the informatics competencies for all nurses and those working as informatics specialists.
5. Identify the major applications of informatics within nursing practice.
6. Identify some future trends in computer use in nursing practice.

KEY WORDS

historical perspectives of documenting nursing practice
information systems for nursing practice
standards for nursing practice
care planning
outcomes management
discharge planning

 Historical Perspectives

More than 150 years ago, Florence Nightingale spoke about the critical importance of nursing informatics in patient care. "Decision making must be based upon the use of accurate data," she said (Ulrich, 1992, p. 68). The nursing pioneer also spoke of frustration from the difficulties of extracting such critical patient-related data from hospital records:

> In attempting to arrive at the truth, I have applied everywhere for information, but in scarcely an instance have I been able to obtain hospital records for any purposes of comparison. If they could be obtained they would enable us to decide many other questions besides the ones alluded to. They would show subscribers how their money was being spent, what amount of good was really being done with it, or whether the money was not doing mischief rather than good. (Nightingale, 1859, p. 187)

It was more than a century after Florence Nightingale's era that computers made their appearance on the hospital landscape. The first hospital information systems arrived in late 1950s to the mid-1960s, although these systems focused primarily on processing financial and administrative information. In 1965, the American Hospital Association conferences for hospital administrators signaled the emerging move toward more clinical adaptations of such systems in healthcare (Hannah, Ball, and Edwards, 1994, pp. 32–33). In the 1970s, the advent of the silicon chip allowed the focus to shift from one large supercomputer to smaller personal computers that could be adapted for many different applications throughout the hospital system. By the 1980s, the computer was being used for diverse hospital functions such as radiology, pharmacy, and laboratories. At this time, there emerged "a strong drive within healthcare to understand how clinicians would use the new tools to advance practice" (Zytkowski, 2003, p. 273).

Throughout the 1990s, expanded uses of computers evolved as nurses in keeping with the traditions begun 100 years before by Florence Nightingale, used computers to improve patient care and conduct research by analyzing patient trends, variability in practice, and outcomes of care. Nursing informatics at this time was characterized by concerns about accessibility, compatibility, and overall integration of informatics efforts within nursing practice and the entire healthcare system. That contemporary system of healthcare has been described by Carty (2001) as new terrain that is no longer confined to "hallowed halls of brick and mortar institutions." "Instead," said Carty, "it has become a point and click system with leveled boundaries that promotes unfettered public access to healthcare information and untraditional communication between providers and patients" (p. 11). It is in this new point and click system that contemporary nurses, in order to practice their profession, must build new competencies that reflect the digital era of healthcare. According to Zytkowski (2003), such competencies are needed because "nursing informatics is foundational to all areas of nursing practice" (p. 279). Snyder-Halpern and Chervany (2000) suggest that success with informatics is not only foundational but also key to survival in the modern day healthcare industry:

> The ability of healthcare delivery networks to effectively manage and leverage clinical information to meet strategic clinical goals is a cornerstone of their transformation and survival as integrated information-based clinical enterprises. (p. 591)

This chapter provides a critical look into how computer applications have been assimilated in nursing practice at the beginning of the new millennium. This time frame has been characterized as one in which "healthcare has shifted its focus from bringing individuals new technology to making the available technology work for clinicians" (Zytkowski, 2003, p. 273). The chapter specifically focuses on the degree to which technology has truly worked for nurses as they have collectively strived to assure that the voice of nursing—the unique language and contributions of nurses and the nursing process—is integrated into the field of healthcare informatics, and that computers are fully utilized in nursing practice to improve patient care.

Along with the most recent standards of nursing informatics practice which were set forth by the American Nurses Association (ANA) in 2001, the chapter also reviews the specific nature and extent of practice applications which involve computers, controversies surrounding nomenclature, the use of decision support systems, and nursing perspectives on the perceived value-added of using information systems in patient care. The chapter concludes with some thoughts about nursing informatics and the possible opportunities it continues to provide for the nursing profession to reexamine its language, its practice, and its contribution within the healthcare industry.

 ## Nursing Informatics: An Evolving Definition

One view of the changing nature of technology use in nursing practice can be seen through the evolving definition of nursing informatics. According to the ANA (ANA, 2001), since 1980, nursing informatics has been defined broadly either with a focus on the technologic aspects, on the concept of nurses interacting with technology to produce greater knowledge, or on the role of nurses who specialized in developing applications of technology to nursing practice. In 1989, Graves and Corcoran set forth what had become the most widely accepted definition of nursing informatics as a "combination of nursing science, information science, and computer science to manage and process nursing data, information, and knowledge to support the practice of nursing and the delivery of nursing care" (p. 227). This definition suggested that with the combination of three core sciences, nursing informatics was a unique and distinct specialty. The expanding role of the informatics nurse specialist was incorporated into a new definition published in 1992 by ANA's Council on Computer Applications in Nursing:

> A specialty that integrates nursing science, computer science, and information science in identifying collecting, processing and managing data and information to support nursing practice, administration, education, and research; and to expand nursing knowledge. The purpose of nursing informatics is to analyze information requirements; design, implement and evaluate information systems and data structures that support nursing, and identify and apply computer technologies to nursing. (ANA, 1992)

Two years later, the ANA again revised this definition by replacing specifics about the systems life cycle with a more general description of nursing informatics which suggested that:

> Nursing informatics supports the practice of nursing specialties in all sites and settings whether at the basic or advanced levels. The practice includes the development of applications, tools, processes and structures that assist nurses with management of data in taking care of patients or in supporting their practice of nursing. (ANA, 1994)

Although these definitions reflect various aspects of computer use in nursing, they did not acknowledge and incorporate what the ANA describes as the "phenomena of nursing"—the nurse, patient, health, and environment—in combination with the other critical elements which are relevant to nursing informatics:

Data, or the discrete entities that are described objectively *without* interpretation;

Information, or data that are interpreted, organized or structured;

Knowledge, or information that is synthesized so that relationships can be identified and formalized;

Nursing science, information science and computer science;

Decision-making, or the process of choosing among alternatives;

Information technology, which includes computer hardware, software, communication and network technologies derived primarily from computer science;

Information structures, which organize data, information, and knowledge for processing by computers; and,

Information management and communication. (ANA, 2001, pp. 6–11)

As depicted in Fig. 20.1, these diverse elements are involved in the dynamic process by which nurses use computers to make sound database and content-specific decisions about patient care. In anticipation of a new definition of nursing informatics for the twenty-first century, the ANA suggested that historical definitions underemphasized the role of the patient in informatics and participatory decision making, neglected the importance of both context and information communication, and focused too narrowly on data and information within nurses' decision-making (ANA, 2001, p. 17). Thus, the 2001 ANA Scope and Standards of Nursing Informatics offered the newest definition:

Nursing informatics is a specialty that integrates nursing science, computer science, and information science to manage and communicate data, information, and knowledge in nursing practice. Nursing informatics facilitates the integration of data, information and knowledge to support patients, nurses and other providers in their decision making in all roles and settings. This support is accomplished through the use of information structures, information processes and information technology. (p. 17)

The goal of nursing informatics, said the ANA, is to:

Improve the health of populations, communities, families, and individuals by optimizing information management and communication. This includes using

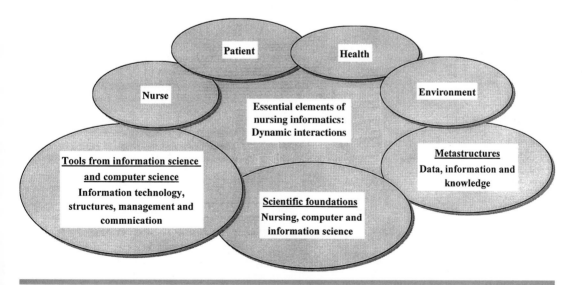

Figure 20.1
Essential elements of nursing informatics: dynamic interactions.
(Adapted from and reprinted with permission from American Nurses Association (ANA). (2001). *Scope and Standards of Practice for Nursing Informatics* (pp. 5–9). Washington, DC: American Nurses Publishing.)

technology in the direct provision of care; establishing administrative systems; managing and delivering educational experiences; supporting life-long learning, and supporting nursing research. (p. 17)

This description of nursing informatics reflects the key tenets of contemporary nursing informatics which, as identified by the ANA, include

clinical *and* non-clinical aspects of practice;
the importance of human factors (human-computer interaction, ergonomics and usability) in decision-making;
the focus on delivering the right information to the right person at the right time;
concerns about and commitment to ensuring the confidentiality and security of health care data and information and advocating privacy;
the central emphasis on the improvement of the quality of patient care, welfare of the health care consumer, and patient outcomes; and,
the importance of collaboration with other areas within healthcare informatics. (ANA, 2001, pp. 22–23)

What differentiates nursing informatics from the broader category of healthcare informatics? In 1997, the National Advisory Council on Nursing Education and Practice suggested that the general field of healthcare informatics included

identifying information to collect and process;
creating databases;
developing user-friendly data entry and retrieval screens;
educating users to work with and maximize available information resources;
installing and maintaining hospital information systems; and,
developing distance education and telehealth systems for information exchange.

Further, the council suggested that nursing augmented healthcare informatics by

bringing specific values and beliefs;
bringing a specific practice base that produces unique knowledge;
focusing attention on specific phenomenon; and
providing a unique language and word context.

A similar theme within the contemporary literature on nursing informatics was set forth by the ANA in the 2001 standards. The ANA stated, "Nursing informatics is a distinct area of specialty practice within nursing—it has a unique body of knowledge, formal preparation

within the specialty, and identifiable techniques and methods" (ANA, 2001, p. 22). Although nursing informatics shares many elements and commonalities with other informatics specialties, there are unique dimensions of informatics as used by nurses in practice today. According to the ANA:

The central issues of concern within nursing informatics are embedded within the discipline itself—data, information, and knowledge used for nurses' decision-making in any environment, in any nursing specialty. Although the boundaries between nursing informatics and other informatics specialties are not rigid, and the work of informatics nurse specialists typically occurs within interdisciplinary teams, informatics nurse specialists add a nursing *voice* to these interdisciplinary environments and often ensure that nurses' requirements are adequately addressed within these contexts. (ANA, 2001, p. 28)

According to Meadows (2002), that voice arises from nurses as they participate in a process of using clinical information systems to analyze data and information; exploring and understand the informational and cognitive foundations specific to nursing; "developing nursing wisdom"; and then applying this to affect patient care (p. 300). According to Abbott (2003), "the greatest struggle in nursing informatics is in the representation of nursing in a language that a computer can use. Nurses in general have not understood what is at stake with this 'nursing naming game' for computerized medical record systems. This lack of understanding has been costly to nursing as a whole" (p. 268).

This chapter reviews the controversy surrounding nursing nomenclature in information systems and examines more specifically how computers in the beginning of this new century have been assisting nurses to do the actual *work* of the nursing profession—delivering quality, cost-effective patient care, and advancing knowledge that improves such care at the bedside.

Standards for Practice

In 2001, an ANA workgroup reviewed and revised the existing scope and standards of nursing informatics practice. The new standards (ANA, 2001) built on the previous scope and standards of practice published by the ANA Task Force to Develop Measurement Criteria for Standards for Nursing Informatics (ANA, 1995). As described earlier, these new ANA standards have documented the evolving definition of nursing informatics that parallels the rapid evolution of informatics in healthcare. The new standards repeatedly emphasize the central role that information plays in the practice of nursing and the importance for *all* nurses, beyond those who specialize in nursing informatics, to develop their skills in managing and communicating information. The guidelines, however, clarify the different perspectives of nurses who are not nursing informatics specialists from those who are. As depicted in Fig. 20.2 these different perspectives present a contrast in emphasis. Nurses outside of nursing informatics are focused on the content of information while nurse specialists in informatics focus their concern on information systems, structure, applications, and the presentation of information for decision-making by nurses. Another major difference in emphasis lies in nurses' focus on using information technology and applications, rather than the focus of nursing informatics specialists who seek to optimize structures, applications, and technology for use in patient care settings.

Informatics Competencies: Beginning to Experienced

In the new 2001 standards of practice, the ANA makes a definitive statement about informatics competencies needed in nursing practice today. The ANA stated, "Informatics competencies are needed by all nurses whether or not they specialize in nursing informatics. As nursing settings become ubiquitous computing environments, all nurses must be both information and computer literate" (p. 24). The scope and depth of these competencies, as set forth by the ANA (2001), increase within each level of three major domains:

> Computer literacy skills: These are the basic computer skills needed to use a word processor; access a database; create a spreadsheet; communicate with e-mail; and interact with clinical documentation systems.

> Information literacy skills: These include the ability to recognize the need for information and the skill to access, evaluate and interpret information correctly. According to the Association of Colleges and Research Libraries (ACRL) (2000), information literacy includes determining the extent of information needed; accessing that information efficiently and effectively; evaluating the information and its sources critically; incorporating the information into one's own knowledge base; using information to accomplish a designated purpose; understanding the economic, legal, and social issues involved with the use of information; and ultimately using information in ethical and legal ways. (ACRL, 2000, p. 2)

> General informatics competencies: These basic skills are required for all nurses but are not sufficient for specialists: identifying, collecting and recording data relevant to the nursing care of patients; analyzing and interpreting patient and nursing information; using applications of informatics as an integral part of the nursing process; and implementing institutional and public policies regarding privacy, confidentiality and security of information. (ANA, 2001, p. 26)

Within the general nursing category, nurses who are the most experienced must be highly skilled in information management and communication. According to Staggers, Gassert, and Curran (2001), these nurses should be able to see relationships among data elements, make judgments based on trends and patterns within the data, use current informatics solutions, and also collaborate with the informatics nurse specialists. In addition, the authors suggest that experienced nurses must be able to use system applications to manage data, information, and knowledge within their particular specialty area; participate as a content expert to evaluate information and assist others in developing information structures and systems to support their area of practice; actively participate in efforts to improve information management and communication (e.g., the development and use of standardized nursing languages); promote the integrity and access to information related to confidentiality, legality, ethical, and security issues; and serve as a leader in incorporating innovations and informatics concepts into their area of specialty.

Although competencies in informatics are critical for all nurses in practice, Kerfoot (2000) made a strong case for positioning technical intelligence (IQ) as a core competency for leaders. Kerfoot described technical IQ as "not only knowing about specific functioning of technology, but also the interrelatedness between the technology, people, and systems that interact with this technology and how this translates into outcomes" (p. 29). Looking to the future, Kerfoot said:

> The success of the leader of the future will be measured by that person's ability to integrate the very complex issues of patient care and technology in a way that makes sense for patients, the organization, and the staff who will be working in a very complex environment. The leader's technical intelligence will be as important as other intelligences in the next 20 years. To be perplexed about technology will not be acceptable in the new millennium. The successful leader will understand the inter-relatedness between how technologies, computers, innovation, and the human condition interact. Leaders without this expertise will be as out of step as those who do not understand health care financial management. (p. 29–31)

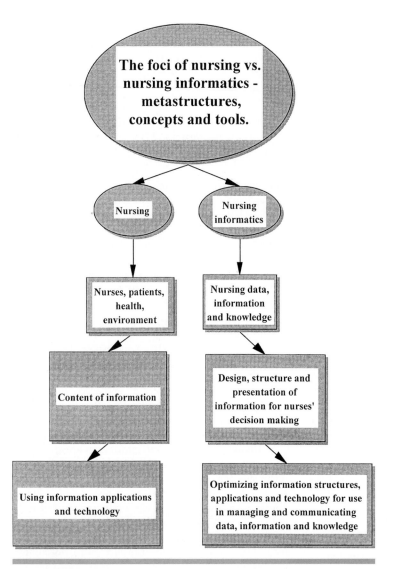

Figure 20.2
The foci of nursing vs. nursing informatics—metastructures, concepts
and tools.
(Reprinted with permission from American Nurses Association. *Scope and
Standards of Practice for Nursing Informatics* (p. 25). Washington, DC:
American Nurses Publishing, 2001.)

Problem Solving as an Organizing Framework

According to the ANA (2001), the informatics nurse specialist moves beyond the foundational competencies and into a practice specialty in which there are organized and recognized standards of practice and performance standards. As described in Fig. 20.3, these standards include six major areas that mirror the traditional nursing process (ANA, 2001, pp. 32–39). The ANA (2001) suggests that this "problem-solving framework supports all facets of informatics practice, including those without technology and all areas of nursing practice" (p. 32), and that the standards are overarching and "inherent in every aspect of practice" (p. 33).

The first standard assessment involves using data, information, and knowledge to clarify the presenting issue or problem. This process focuses on collecting data with different methodologies such as structured system and workflow analysis, and from a variety of sources such as stakeholders who are close to the problem. The second standard calls for identifying and evaluating possible solutions to information issues. This includes developing functional and technical specifications based on identified needs, designing new models for informatics solutions, considering costs and return on investment of informatics solutions, identifying measurable outcomes and terminal objectives, and advocating for informatics solutions with key stakeholders. The third standard includes all activities related to the identification of an appropriate informatics solution and planning for its application. It is at this stage that the informatics specialist skillfully matches the capabilities and limitations of hardware and software. This matching process involves many factors such as economic, technical, and human resources; established professional standards; selection criteria; critical success factors; vendor identification; and contract development.

Implementation is the fourth standard in which the informatics specialist acts as a process consultant and project manager for all interventions and activities related to the informatics application. This can involve a myriad of activities ranging from internal and external marketing, system testing, and training. Finally, the sixth standard sets forth criteria to be used as the efficiency and effectiveness of decisions, plans, activities, and applications are evaluated. This ongoing process serves as a means of not only evaluating the structure, process, and outcome of the informatics solution, but also the net effects of the informatics solution on nursing practice.

In addition to standards of practice, the 2001 ANA guidelines include standards that guide the work performance of nurses who specialize in informatics. This includes the process of assuring the quality and effectiveness of nursing informatics practice, approaches for performance appraisal, as well as guidelines for professional development, collegiality, collaboration, research, resource allocation, communication, and ethics (pp. 40–45). These performance standards, while designed for specialists in nursing informatics, provide a helpful resource for other nurses who wish to enhance their own competencies in this important and growing area of specialty within the nursing profession.

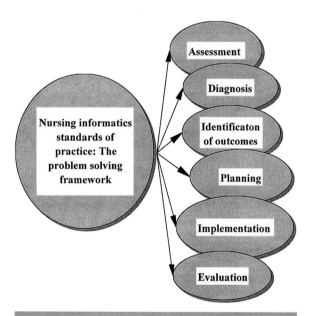

Figure 20.3

Nursing informatics standards of practice: the problem solving framework.

(Adapted from and reprinted with permission from American Nurses Association. (2001). *Scope and Standards of Practice for Nursing Informatics* (pp. 32–39). Washington, DC: American Nurses Publishing.)

Information Technology and the Actual Work of Nurses

At the beginning of the new century, much was written about the reality that information technology had become important in the delivery of contemporary healthcare. A federal report (U.S. Department of Health and Human Services, 2001) on proposed strategies to build a national health infrastructure emphasized the need for all healthcare providers to be skilled in using technology for decision-making, while other reports expressed concerns that the healthcare industry was lagging behind other industries in implementing information systems (Wong, Legnini, and Whitmore, 2000). At this time, the nursing literature was filled with individual voices from the profession and those of professional nursing organizations who echoed the importance of technology, emphasized its value in nursing practice and education, and expressed concerns about assuring that nurses and their unique perspectives were represented in the ongoing integration of information technology into patient care.

In her depiction of the future of the nursing profession in the twenty-first century, Saba (2001) left no doubt that computer technology needed to be part of professional nursing practice. This reality was confirmed by the ANA in 2001 when the revised *Scope and Standards of Nursing Informatics Practice* was published. But exactly how pervasive is information technology in nursing and in what ways are nurses in the twenty-first century using information technology in their work?

A Pattern of Underutilization

There are a number of approaches for exploring the use and importance of information technology in nursing practice applications. These include directly documenting the actual use of information technology tools and, more indirectly, through assessing specific information technology content areas taught in nursing schools. In a survey conducted by McNeil et al. (2003), the deans and directors of 266 baccalaureate and higher nursing programs were surveyed. A total of 172 (65%) of the respondents were nursing program administrators, directors, managers, or deans, while 74 (28%) were nurse educators. The survey was designed to determine the perceived current and future uses of information technology by practicing nurses, specific information technology knowledge and computing skills currently being taught in American nursing schools, and the extent to which faculty members were prepared to teach this knowledge and these skills (p. 342).

As depicted in Table 20.1, the results showed that the information technology tools most frequently used were remote monitoring devices, online consumer tools, and handheld computers, although these tools were used by only an estimated 50% of practicing nurses. The survey also showed that only 31% of the nurses were using decision support tools, i.e., software to mine data and applications that aid evidence-based decisions (p. 347) despite the recognized importance

Table 20.1 Perceptions of Current and Predicted Use of Information Technology Tools by Practicing Nurses (*n* = 266)

Tool	Nurses Who Currently Use Tool *n* (%)	Nurses Who Will Use Tool in Next 5 Years *n* (%)
Remote monitoring devices (i.e., machines that monitor a single function, such as electrocardiograms and temperature, pulse, and respiration)	152 (57)	87 (33)
Online consumer health (i.e., the ability to access and evaluate online healthcare resources)	140 (53)	100 (38)
Handheld computers that are used to document care or retrieve health information at the point of care	135 (51)	92 (35)
Mobile computers (i.e., wireless or other remote information processing technologies)	106 (40)	79 (30)
Telehealth tools (i.e., real-time video or audio for practitioner-patient encounters)	103 (39)	72 (27)
Telephony, which is a telephone that interfaces with a linked computer for collecting and transmitting health data	99 (38)	72 (27)
Decision support tools (i.e., software to mine data and applications that aid evidenced-based decisions)	81 (31)	74 (28)
Telecommunities (i.e., online support of patients and family members using computer links)	68 (26)	73 (27)
Robotics (i.e., managing healthcare using machine that integrate many functions and simulate encounters)	24 (9)	38 (14)

Source: Reprinted with permission, from McNeil et al. (2003). Nursing information technology knowledge, skills, and preparation of student nurses, nursing faculty, and clinicians: A U.S. survey. *Journal of Nursing Education* 42:347.

of these tools to evidence-based nursing practice (Bakken, 2001).

The survey also assessed the information technology content currently being taught in undergraduate and graduate nursing programs. The most frequently taught content at the undergraduate level included accessing electronic resources (50%), computer-based patient records (46%), and ethical use of information systems (46%), while at the graduate level, accessing electronic resources (38%), ethical use of information systems (36%), and evidence-based practice (34%) represented the top three content areas (p. 345). The findings show that information technology content included evidence-based practice in approximately 33% of the programs—a percentage that paralleled the reported use of decision support tools in actual practice. The three lowest reported information technology areas were the same for the graduate and undergraduate programs: Unified Medical Language Systems (17/11%), data/information system standards (14/6%), and the Nursing Information and Data Set Evaluation Center standards for information systems (12/5%) (p. 345).

McNeil and colleagues (2003) concluded that "there were many gaps in information technology taught at both levels" (p. 347), that most nursing programs rated their faculty as advanced beginners using Brenner's (1984) novice to expert framework (p. 346), and perhaps most importantly that "information technology competencies and tools use by most practicing nurses currently are not identified as expected outcomes of U.S. nursing program graduates" (p. 348). This pattern is also true in the United Kingdom, where Alpay and Russell (2002) have reported that "the absence of any agreed accredited IT training for practicing nurses has certainly contributed to the low level of IT literacy within this healthcare group" (p. 137). The underutilization of computers and the documented gap between education and practice further illustrates the need for more information technology training, more nurse informatics specialists, as well as nursing faculty with information technology expertise.

As depicted in Table 20.2, another study of current practice applications is the 2001 study by Dumas, Dietz, and Connolly of nurse practitioners' (NPs) use of computer technologies in practice. This research followed other studies of NPs which documented that patient care given by NPs and other nurses is enhanced with adequate use of current specialized information (National Center for Nursing Research, 1993), and a rural study in which NPs were able to document more consistent patient documentation, more efficient use of time for client data input, retrieval, and quality assurance (Yancey et al., 1998). In the 2001 study, 104 Californian NPs who were experienced nurses were surveyed about their use of computers, and the specific computer applications believed to most improve patient

Table 20.2   Nurse Practitioner Perceptions of Usefulness of Computer Applications for Improving Client Care

Computer Applications	Frequency (n = 104)	Mean (on a 5-Point Scale)	Standard Deviation
Obtaining client record information from other agencies and departments such as pharmacy and laboratories	77	4.56	0.90
Internet searches, e.g., MEDLINE and CINAHL	76	4.21	1.02
Entering electronic record information	69	4.16	1.13
Word processing	76	3.82	1.22
E-mail	81	3.77	1.30
Billing or accounting information	55	3.49	1.41
Spreadsheet	60	2.98	1.23
Presentation software	56	2.87	1.43
Desktop publishing	50	2.56	1.34

Source: Reprinted with permission, from Dumas, J., Dietz, E.O., and Connolly, P.M. (2001). NP use of computer technologies in practice. *Computers in Nursing* 19:39.

care. The NPs worked in a variety of practice settings including public clinics, private practice, HMOs, home care, nursing education, and other settings.

The survey results showed that within the three major practice areas, 94% used computers at their work site in the HMO setting, while the percentages in public clinics were 77% and in private practice, 71%. Less frequent use of computers was most often attributed to the unavailability of computers. The applications of computers in NP practice included obtaining records from other departments, entering client record information, conducting Internet searches, billing or accounting information, e-mail, word processing, spreadsheet, presentation software, and desktop publishing. The study showed that computer usage varied considerably by practice setting. For example, the two most frequently used applications in the three practice settings were e-mail and obtaining patient records, which were used by 87% of NPs in HMOs, by 40% in public clinics, and by only 11% of those in private practice. This pattern of highest use in HMOs and lowest in private practice pertained to entering electronic client record information and e-mail as well. Use of word processing, however, was highest in private settings (39.3%), as compared with 20% in public clinics and 10% in HMOs (Dumas, Dietz, and Connolly, 2001, pp. 36–38).

The researchers concluded that, "NPs underused computer applications that could improve client care in their practices" (Dumas, Dietz, and Connolly, 2001, p. 39). While some of the differences across practice settings were attributed to the lack of computer availability, greater emphasis on computer use by other office staff, and more extensive use of computers for administrative rather than clinical functions, the NP study suggested that further research was needed to better understand differences across practice settings and causes of underutilization.

These studies of computers in nursing practice suggest that while nurses perceive the many benefits from using computers in nursing practice, underutilization may be a norm in the beginning of the new century. As one American nursing leader (Hooper, 2003) suggested: "Nursing informatics is still new due to lack of awareness and exploding technology" (p. 4). This trend is consistent with recent findings from research in other countries (Alpay and Russell, 2002; Welling and Delnoij, 1997).

Alpay and Russel, for example, found patterns of underutilization of information technology in their study of British nurses who work in general practice areas. In this study, most nurses used information technology to maintain medical records in the practice, while only half

used technology to record appointments, manage skill mix and workload, input clinical codes, conduct online research, access health information, and write letters (p. 141). The researchers concluded that:

> The nurses had a high level of awareness of potential uses for IT and they had concerns about the lack of computer training to harness this potential. The ability to use IT was affected by the lack of practical knowledge in basic computer skills and lack of available knowledge about the adaptability of the software. Practicing nurses in other parts of Europe also face difficulties with their access to, use of and professional development in IT. (p. 141)

Underutilization has also been noted in other sectors of the healthcare industry as well (Major and Turner, 2003; Straub, 1997). Thus, it appears that the successful integration of automated information systems in healthcare is seen as both a goal to be attained and as a survival strategy in the regulated healthcare environment of today.

Nursing Documentation

Although this chapter is focused on specific practice applications, it would be incomplete without mention of the challenges, which lie in the area of nursing documentation, or the official recording of the essential applications of nursing practice. Nursing documentation in the patient record has become more complex as nursing practice has expanded to encompass care to critically ill and specialty patients, and as technologic advances have become standard of care in practice. In the beginning of the first decade of the new century, nursing documentation rests at an interesting and challenging intersection of history and technology.

In a 2001 report for the ANA, Coenen et al. cite pivotal points in recent history when ANA's emphasis on this critical issue was evident. In 1986, the ANA House of Delegates passed a resolution to promote the development of computerized nursing information systems (NISs) in nursing services (p. 240). In 1989, the Steering Committee on Databases to support Clinical Nursing Practice was established (McCormick et al., 1994). In 1993, the ANA House of Delegates passed another resolution to "develop nursing classifications specifically aimed at diagnosis, interventions, and nursing sensitive patient outcomes, and support activities directed toward the inclusion of nursing data elements in healthcare databases" (p. 240). In 1998, the Steering Committee on Databases to support Clinical Nursing Practice was renamed the Committee for Nursing Practice Information Infrastructure (CNPII) and charged with serving as the "primary authority for the ANA on nursing practice information infrastructure" (p. 214). This has involved "promoting relationships among data standards, the collection of data and the re-use of data for the ongoing development of practice standards and guidelines," which, said Coenen et al., are "essential to promoting nursing as an informed and valued partners in the health-care informatics and policy arena" (p. 240).

One view of the immense challenge of this task can be seen via the plethora of standardized languages now recognized by the ANA and outlined in Table 20.3.

These 13 standardized languages recognize and reflect elements of the nursing management minimum data set

Table 20.3   Recognized Terminologies that Support Nursing Practice

Resource	Recognition Date
NANDA—nursing diagnosis, definitions, and classifications	1992
NIC—Nursing Interventions Classifications system	1992
HHCC—Home Health	1992
OMAHA system	1992
NOC—Nursing Outcomes Classification	1997
NMMDS—nursing management minimum data set	1998
PCDS—patient care data set	1998
PNDS—peri operative data set	1999
SNOMED CT	1999
NMDS—nursing minimum data set	1999
ICNP—International Classification for Nursing Practice	2000
ABC codes	2000
LOINC—logical observation identifiers names and codes	2002

Note: The following 13 languages have been recognized by the American Nurses Association (ANA) as those classification systems that have been uniquely developed to document the entire process of clinical care for patients. For addresses and contact information for the above classification systems, refer to *www.nursingworld.org/nidsec*.
Source: Reprinted with permission, from ANA Recognized Terminologies that Support Nursing Practice—Revised November 14, 2003. Retrieved January 29, 2004, *http://www.nursingworlod.org/nidsec/class1st.htm*.

(Huber and Schumacher, 1997) and the nursing minimum data set (Werley and Lang, 1998) with their focus on administrative data, and the core principles and processes of the nursing process itself—nursing assessment, nursing diagnosis, outcomes identification, nursing interventions, and nursing outcomes.

The concerns expressed by Coenen et al. in 2001 focused on the "ongoing needs and issues to be addressed in the development of healthcare terminology standards" and the pressing needs in the nursing profession to "ensure that nursing practice data are captured in a manner suitable for use at the point of care and for reuse for purposes such as quality and cost management; clinical research, decision support, and healthcare policy development" (p. 245).Others such as Ballard (1997) have suggested that information technology provides a conduit for capitalizing on "nursing intelligence"—the information gathered by nurses in their nursing work.

Simpson (2003a) echoed the chorus of concerns from others in the nursing literature (ANA, 2001; Meadows, 2002; and Abbott, 2003) about the standardized structures for the computerized documentation of nursing when he said that:

> In the world of "prove it" health care, if something isn't coded, it doesn't exist. If nursing's contribution to patient outcomes can't be established, nursing becomes invisible once again. And in a fiscally tight market, invisibility can be expendability. Nursing must have a way to substantiate its role in the health care process and its essential nature to outcomes. Nursing needs a standardized language to describe its unique function. (p. 14)

Thus, while there are now 13 standardized languages at the turn of the century which speak what nurses do, the nursing profession appears to recognize that collecting nursing data, reusing data, capitalizing and leveraging such data, and understanding the relationships among types of date reflect the evolution of information technology in healthcare and the realities of nursing in the digital age.

Care Planning

The computer-based patient record facilitates the automation of the nursing care planning process. The benefits and the challenges of integrating computerized systems with care planning have been extensively reported in the literature during the last decade (Brazile and Hettinger, 1995; Axford and Carter, 1996; Adderley, Hyde, and Mauseth, 1997; Goossen, Epping, and Dassen, 1997; Yancey et al., 1998; McDonald et al., 1998; Allan and Englewright, 2000; Gohlinghorst et al., 2000). This research has focused on a wide range of topics related to the impact of computers on various aspects of nursing care such as contact time with patients, accuracy of documentation, charting time, transcription and medication errors, and communication between nurses and other healthcare professionals within a hospital. Summarized by Meadows (2002): "The ability to electronically record, integrate, and analyze data and information enables nurses to quickly move to the synthesis of nursing knowledge and the development of nursing wisdom, which they can then apply to patient care" (p. 300).

As described in Table 20.4 by Allan and Englewright (2000), today's care planning process may include a mix of individual patient data and data which can be used for decision-making such as facility standards of care, age-specific guidelines, care area standards of practice, specific patient problems identified by different disciplines, and physician orders (p. 93). An important feature is the requirement that caregivers must provide support for any exception to the standards of practice (p. 94). Ultimately, suggest Allan and Englewright, "managers were able to query the clinical record with questions about the provision and the results of care. The results from the system are useful to process improvement, performance evaluation, and strategic planning" (p. 95).

Decision-Making with Administrative Data

Although nursing leaders typically administer million dollar budgets and are held responsible for their unit's budget, they often:

> Lack the necessary information and decision support to manage their responsibilities effectively. Without day-to-day information on patient flow and acuity, resources use, staffing levels, costs and budgetary balance, they have little support for cost control and input into budgetary decision making. (Ruland, 2001, p. 187)

The desirability of cost containment in healthcare was the driving force behind the development of CLASSICA, a new Norwegian decision support system focused on financial management, resource allocation, activity planning, and budgetary monitoring and control. As reported by Ruland and depicted in Fig. 20.4, the core components of this system contain a wealth of data about patient flow and activity, staffing, the cost of nursing care at the nursing unit level, and relationships between costs and services. Capabilities include financial accounting options, trend analysis, as well as forecasting. The reports available included numbers and cost of extra hours and overtime, relationship between sickness leave and use of extra hours and overtime, unit's total cost for nursing care, cost per patient day, average cost per patient stay, total hours of absence/illness/education in terms of hours and costs, budget

Table 20.4   Care Planning Process

Data Source	Plan of Care	Documentation
On admission		
Location	Standards of care	Shift assessment
Age group	Standards of practice	Interventions
	Age-specific guidelines	Bundled interventions
		Age-related care
		Interventions
Initial assessment		
Nursing	Specific patient problems	
Therapies	Protocols	
Procedures areas		
Physician orders	Physician orders	Interventions

Source: Reprinted with permission, from Allan, J. and Englewright, J. (2000). Patient-centered documentation. *Journal of Nursing Administration* 30(2):93.

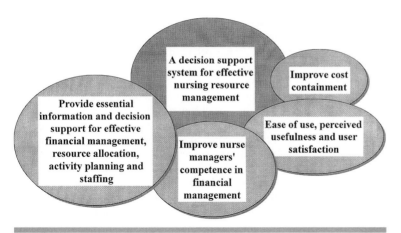

Figure 20.4
A decision support system for effective nursing resource management.
(Reprinted with permission from Ruland, C.M. (2001). Developing a decision support system to meet nurse managers' information needs for effective resource management. *Computers in Nursing* 19:188.)

balance, expense comparison year to year, ratio of float/agency nurses to regular staff, number of student nurses and nursing staff in orientation, nurse/patient ratio, and relationship between expenses, patient activity, staff level, and resources. Forecasting and simulation options include forecasting of expected deviation from budget at the end of the year based on expenditures so far this year; budget adjustments for the remaining part of the year to achieve budget balance, based on deviation from budget so far this year; and cost estimation of different staffing alternatives (Ruland, 2001, p. 191).

According to Ruland, the flexibility of an administrative system such as this enabled nurse managers to identify barriers to more effective resource management and to better understand the underlying factors in unsatisfactory resource management. This was facilitated by the integration of various types of financial, staffing, and activity measures. Ruland emphasized that the goal of improved resource management with a model like the CLASSICA system can only be realized when implementation of the system is paired with parallel financial management training for the nurse managers.

Decision-Making with Expert Systems

Broadly defined, the term clinical decision support system (CDSS) includes an array of computer-based applications that assist healthcare clinicians in the day-to-day work of patient care. These may include programs that involve artificial intelligence (AI); different types of knowledge such as uncertainty, heuristics, and fuzzy logic; expert systems; and decision support systems. Expert systems, also known as knowledge-based systems, process knowledge while conventional software process data. Expert systems have components that attempt to imitate human expertise by making inferences, which are defined by the Oxford Dictionary of Computing (1996) as *new* facts derived from a given set of facts. According to Power (2004), decision support systems have been in existence since 1965, when management decision systems first became available.

Generally, two types of AI—expert systems and machine learning—have been used to aid decision-making in nursing for more than a decade (Miller, 1994; Johnston et al., 1994; Cullen, 1998). These systems—which typically include a user interface, an inference engine, and a knowledge base—use knowledge and "thinking aloud" procedures to infer new information from what already is known about a problem, and to enhance understanding, reasoning, and decision-making. Expert systems solve problems by trial and error rather than using algorithms such as those used in convention programming. A successful expert system has the potential to capture and preserve expertise only if the procedural knowledge of experts can be articulated. Machine learning systems have been defined (Cullen, 1998) as a branch of AI concerned with construction of programs that learn from experience. Learning may take many different forms, such as learning from examples, by analogy, and by discovery to autonomous learning of concepts. Expert systems are similar to AI in that both technologies reproduce the human ability to select the relevant facts and draw logical conclusions.

In their recent review, Lyons and Richardson (2003) defined CDSS as a "tool used in health care to give data meaning, or to bundle data in clinically significant ways for application to patient care with minimum temporal delay" (p. 295). Some of these systems are freestanding and not connected to patient documentation systems. According to Lyons and Richardson (2003, p. 296), in today's healthcare environment many CDSS models are linked to information systems which carry vital patient data from a multitude of sources: laboratory, pharmacy, radiology, admit-discharge-transfer, computerized provider order entry, and the nursing electronic health record. The latter, according to Lyons and Richardson, "result in nearly simultaneous data retrieval, processing, and provider notification" (p. 295). A decision support or expert system can therefore guide, facilitate, and strengthen nursing decisions at the point of care or at the point of service. This might involve, suggest Lyons and Richardson, detection and prevention of untoward clinical events such as drug interactions, errors, or omissions, as well as trends in patient symptoms.

Nursing documentation systems that incorporate expert systems and AI offer nurses a valuable resource—the ability to improve clinical decision-making *at the point of care in real time.* This labor saving feature substitutes retrospective and labor-intensive analysis with trend analysis. This type of technology, sometimes referred to as push technology, can recognize predictive, discriminative, or explanatory patterns in individual patients and make comparisons across groups of patients. There are real savings in terms of nursing time and telephone time, as well as real benefits such as better patient monitoring, decision-making, and the capability of following a patient through the hospital system (Kuperman et al., 1999; Lyons and Richardson, 2003). Lyons and Richardson (2003) also state the obvious advantage of these systems:

> Nurses are human and therefore fallible. The CDSS can provide the best clinical data. It does not forget and does not misplace information. It is unresponsive to stress and does not get distracted. (p. 299)

Ultimately, the use of decision support systems yields direct benefits for patients—prevention of suffering, symptoms, and death—and for the entire healthcare industry in the form of reduced healthcare expenses from saved labor costs and fewer adverse events. For example, it has been estimated that adverse drug events cost an average of $2162 per event (Senst et al., 2001).

Lyons and Richardson (2003) point out that a CDSS may contain either synchronous or asynchronous alerting systems. Synchronous alerting occurs when an order is entered into a computerized order entry system. Order processing takes place under the watchful surveillance of an inference engine that acts when predetermined conditions are met. In this way clinicians can receive immediate feedback that can avoid duplicate testing or highlight additional testing which may be required. The obvious limitation of this type of system is that the patient's order must be entered into the computerized system. Asynchronous alerting, as the term suggests, provides clinicians with important but delayed feedback which is gleaned as the expert system combs through multiple databases. This type of system has advantages in that it can send messages via a number of modalities (cell phone, pager, personal data assistant [PDA], printer/fax, and computer terminal) to specific individual clinicians or multiple clinicians. An additional advantage of asynchronous alerting, suggest Lyons and Richardson, is its capacity to detect adverse events that occur over time.

Given the accelerated speed of innovation in information technology today, the expert systems that exist in our healthcare institutions at the beginning of the new century may face an early obsolescence. Kurzweil (1999) points out that the speed of computers, which doubled every 3 years at the beginning of the twentieth century and every 2–3 years in the 1950s and 1960s, now doubles in speed every 12 months. He predicts that computers will soon be able to read on their own, and understand and model what they have read by the next decade. Forecasters like Kurzweil believe that the changes in expert systems in the first two decades of the new century will be greater than all of those we experienced in the entire twentieth century.

Kosko (1999) has also suggested that innovations in what he calls "fuzzy thinking"—concepts without exact borders—and computer technology which mimics the organization of neural networks used by our brains as an operating platform will bring new and even more revolutionary systems to healthcare. These will include synchronous language translation systems and even more expert diagnostic systems.

The excitement about such new possibilities in expert systems is counterbalanced by a familiar warning from Lyons and Richardson. The voice of nursing cannot be included fully in the development and use of new age CDSSs until there are standards terms for diagnoses, interventions, and outcomes. Lyons and Richardson (2003) remind us that:

> The CDSS depends on computerized, standardized taxonomies. This is an opportunity for nurse informaticists and critical care nurses to collaborate and contribute to the design and testing process of computerized CDSSs, systems that have already proven beneficial to patient care. (p. 300)

Outcomes Management

A chapter on the use of computers in nursing practice today would be incomplete without a description of how informatics is being used to organize and implement systems for outcomes management. A look at outcomes management provides a powerful illustration of how nurses use informatics in daily practice to evaluate the relationship between patient goal attainment and nursing interventions. Since 1989, there has been an emphasis on outcomes management in healthcare as a result of new legislation and the efforts of the Joint Commission on Accreditation of Healthcare Organizations. Outcomes management is a simple premise with complex implications for healthcare providers. From a theoretical standpoint, outcomes are viewed as beneficial in healthcare while the implementation of appropriate nursing interventions are viewed as quality patient care (Larrabee, 1996; Mize, Bentley, and Hubbard, 1991). The outcomes

of healthcare, i.e., both the short- and long-term results of a treatment or clinical approach, should be monitored so that the nursing profession and the healthcare industry can determine and implement the best practices in healthcare (Aller, 1996; Wojner and Kite-Powell, 1997). Outcomes can include factors such as increased client satisfaction, decreased hospital admissions and ER visits, decreased costs and acuity of hospital stay, decreased morbidity and mortality, minimized hospital revenue loss, increased job satisfaction for nurses, and decreased job stress.

Nursing contributions to the expanding knowledge about outcomes management can be illustrated by reports in the literature that demonstrate the unique practice base of nurses and their contribution to outcomes assessment. Martin (1999) and Martin and Scheet (1995) have written extensively about the 20 year development of the Omaha system, with its problem classification scheme, intervention scheme, and problem rating scheme for outcomes. The outcomes capability of the system serves as a method for documentation and as a guide for nursing practice. As described in Table 20.5, the rating system was designed to measure problem-specific knowledge, behavior, and status throughout the time of service. Martin stated:

> When establishing the initial ratings for client problems, the nurse creates an independent data baseline, capturing the condition and circumstances of a client at a given point in time. This admission baseline is used to compare and contrast the client's condition

Table 20.5   Problem Rating Scale for Outcomes: The Omaha System

Concept	1	2	3	4	5
Knowledge: The ability of the client to remember and interpret information	No knowledge	Minimal knowledge	Basic knowledge	Adequate knowledge	Superior knowledge
Behavior: The observable responses, actions, or activities of the client fitting the purpose of the occasion	Not appropriate	Rarely appropriate	Inconsistently appropriate	Usually appropriate	Consistently appropriate
Status: The condition of the client in relation to objective and subjective defining characteristics	Extreme signs/ symptoms	Severe signs/ symptoms	Moderate signs/ symptoms	Minimal signs/ symptoms	No signs/ symptoms

Source: Reprinted with permission, from Martin, K.S and Scheet, N.J. (1995). The Omaha system: Nursing diagnoses, intervention and client outcomes. In *Nursing Data Systems: the Emerging Framework*. Washington, DC: American Nurses Publishing.

and circumstances with ratings completed at later intervals and at client dismissal. The comparison or change in ratings over time can be used to assess client progress in relation to nursing intervention and thus judge the effectiveness of the plan of care. (p. 2)

Data are used both for individual care planning and for aggregate analysis. Such analyses are used to interface with other components of an institution's informatics systems, and to evaluate the impact of patient care services, meet accreditation requirements, complete reports for third party payers, plan new programs, and ultimately advance progress in nursing.

A specific clinical example of nursing's key involvement in outcomes management was published in 1998 when Smith described a data-based system for simplifying data management for outcomes management of the mechanically ventilated patient population. According to Smith, an outcomes manager uses information obtained by outcomes measurement to monitor and trend data, and to determine the approaches for the clinical management of specific patient groups. In the past, the medical informatics infrastructure at this author's institution did not contain daily clinical data on this group of patients. Lack of such data made it difficult to identify trends and to identify areas for improvement in clinical practice. The author, a respiratory case manager, was then able to use the existing informatics systems at her institution, and adapt it for the monitoring, storing, and retrieving of data that could be used to determine best practices for patients who were being mechanically ventilated. This involved developing standardized criteria for such factors as reintubation rates and the starting and stopping points for weaning patients from the ventilation system. The data generated assisted the clinical staff in improving care protocols, quality improvement processes, and measurement tools.

In a 2000 study, Johnson and Nolan reviewed three systems that can be used for managing patient outcome data: traditional manual data entry, automated data entry scanning system, and a handheld device. Their findings suggest that in this period, when entire institutions are searching for integrated options for efficient and effective outcomes management, they may be wise to use interim approaches that integrate handheld devices with traditional data entry scanning systems.

In a more recent study, Larrabee and colleagues (2001) used a time series design to study the influence of a system-wide computerized NIS on document completeness of nursing assessment of patient outcomes, achievement of nursing outcomes, nursing interventions done, and routine assessments before and after implementation of a NIS in a 100-bed urban university hospital. Using retrospective chart review and a criterion referenced instrument at three time points (1 month before and 6 and 18 months after the implementation of the NIS), the researchers measured nursing assessments of patient outcomes, beneficence, or nurse goal achievement of desired patient outcomes, and nurse-patient perceived quality. The chart review used sections of the patient care plan as criteria for evaluating documentations of selected patient outcomes assessment, patient outcomes achieved, and nursing interventions done.

The study results showed that 6 months of experience using a NIS was not sufficient time for nurses to acquire documentation mastery. Over time, however, with continued use and regular and reeducation, documentation scores were shown to increase. The authors warned, however, that these results do not suggest that documentation of outcome assessment, goal achievement, interventions, and routine assessment is complete simply because a NIS is in place. The researchers concluded:

> The implication is that agencies should evaluate the completeness of chart documentation periodically after NIS implementation and use the information obtained to make ongoing improvements in their NIS or their nurses' use of the NIS. For greatest effectiveness, such improvements should address unit specific results. Demonstrated data validity is a pre-requisite to using patient record data to investigate the influence of nursing care quality on patient outcomes. (Larrabee et al., 2001, p. 63–64)

According to Simpson (2003b), "in order to effectively monitor outcomes, an organization must adapt one of the key tenets of CQI and TQM—make quality decisions up front—so there are quality outcome data at the end. Despite their limitations, information systems are still the best solutions for collecting, aggregating and creating information from data" (p. 355). Simpson concluded:

> With outcome measurement, nursing can become visible. The operative word here is "can"—without nursing specific taxonomies and nomenclatures, there can be no nursing-specific measures. Ands the result of that is continued invisibility. (p. 355)

Discharge Planning

The documentation of patient care usually begins with the admission assessment and ends with the discharge care plan. Discharge care planning systems provide for continuity of care from the home to the hospital and back to the community, another care facility, an outpatient department, or the home. A typical discharge plan includes five components:

- Summary of the admission assessment
- Summary of learning needs that the patient had at discharge
- Multidisciplinary plan including problems still unresolved and outcomes not met during hospitalization
- Medication and procedures that the patient must continue
- Summary of selected patient outcomes that a multidisciplinary team desired as minimal criteria for the patient to have achieved during hospitalization (Romano, McCormick, and McNeely, 1982).

Although the basic design of discharge plans has changed little from those used 30 years ago (Wessling, 1972), the extent and mode of communication about patient care throughout healthcare networks has changed dramatically. These networks, which represent the continuum of patient care, typically involve multiple healthcare providers, departments, and healthcare facilities. Healthcare professionals involved in the discharge planning process, for example, can include geographically dispersed and diverse professionals such as social workers, physicians, dieticians, occupational therapists, pharmacists, and physical therapists (Miller and Carlton, 1998).

Key to success and also central to much frustration in healthcare today is the ever-present issue of compatibility of the hardware and software infrastructure. Simpson (2003c) suggests that the increasing use of handhelds or PDAs in hospitals, medical groups, and other patient care organizations has done much to make the vision of patient-centered care a reality (p. 254). Lyons and Richardson (2003) have also emphasized that the ideal infrastructure allows communication with PDAs and many different modalities such as cell phone, pager, or fax machine. Closely coordinated communication among healthcare providers can result in up-to-date discharge plans that can be sent home with patients at the time of discharge, or to different institutions, or different wards within the same hospital.

Computerized discharge care plans also have the potential to be used for other purposes beyond direct patient care such as quality assurance, auditing, research, and coding at discharge for prospective payment. Thus, discharge planning in today's managed care environment,

like most of the critical activities involved in patient care, demands that nurses develop skills in using a variety of technologic applications such as e-mail, listservs, two-way video-conferencing, Web pages, electronic scheduling, electronic reminders, remote physiologic monitoring, and computer-based conferencing.

Healthcare Collaboration

Collaboration with other members of the healthcare team has always been a critical component of nursing. Advances in technology, however, have changed the ways in which members of interdisciplinary healthcare teams are and will be communicating with each other in the digital world of healthcare in new millennium. As Alpay and Russell (2002) have suggested, "the use of IT is part of the development and delivery of health services" (p. 136). In fact, predictions that collaboration and technology would become critical elements of the healthcare industry of the future (Miller and Carlton, 1998) have proven to be true as healthcare systems have grappled with the interdisciplinary challenges of implementing and expanding clinical information systems.

As primary caregivers at the bedside, nurses typically carry out the nursing process by interacting in person, writing, or telephone with a wide variety of healthcare professionals to share information and decision-making focused on improving patient care outcomes. Typically these interactions include sharing information, networking, consulting, and supporting. As Miller and Carlton suggested in 1998, this communication is communication in constant change sparked by the growing availability of telecommunication applications that allow both asynchronous and synchronous interaction.

Miller and Carlton's predictions that future healthcare practitioners such as nurses would be "active participants in collaboratively matching the wide range of telecommunications tools to the health care application need" have become the reality for many healthcare systems in the first years of the new century. For example, Miranda, Fields, and Lund (2001) have documented their 16-year experience implementing and expanding a four-phase point-of-care computer information system in their changing healthcare context in California. Begun in 1985 as a nursing documentation system in three intensive care units with 166 users for 35 beds with 49 computer workstations, this clinical information system at SharpHealthCare now has 2,584 interdisciplinary users for 384 beds with 477 workstations and plans for continued expansion. Miranda, Fields, and Lund have reiterated the advice of Henderson and Dean

(1996), who made a strong case against positioning the implementation of computer information systems in today's hospitals as a nursing task:

> The perception of the CIS as only a nursing tool plagued its use and support for many years. The primary lesson learned in this early phase was the importance of involving a wide range of potential users to create a CIS vision that could have capitalized on the flexibility of the CIS to meet the documentation needs of multiple disciplines. (p. 148)

Miranda, Fields, and Lund suggest that in their experience, making politically correct decisions—such as not mandating physicians to use the CIS—as well as failure to anticipate the "end users" reactions to collecting additional data and the additional time needed had strategically negative effects such as the parallel coexistence of a paper and electronic chart, diminished institutional capacity for sharing patient data electronically, and ultimately, an end product in which the desired computer information system did not encompass the entire patient stay and did not meet the data needs for both clinical documentation and research needs (pp. 149–150).

The experience documented by Miranda, Fields, and Lund opens a vivid window into the perils of not recognizing or advocating for healthcare collaboration at the initiation and during the implementation of a CIS. The creation of multidisciplinary task forces at SharpHealthCare, according to the authors, resulted in "consistent configuration across the three hospitals, group cohesiveness, respect among members, and better acceptance of the CIS" (p. 150). Thus, Miranda, Fields, and Lund recommended that when implementing a clinical information system, it is critical to "develop a broad support base for vertical and horizontal decisions in the organization by involving a cross-disciplinary team to select and implement the CIS" (p. 150). Thus, the experience at SharpHealthCare and other similar healthcare institutions reaffirms the essential role that interdisciplinary collaboration will play in the years ahead for assuring that technology as a tool is used to its best advantage for improving patient care.

Progress in Practice

The inevitable integration of computers into nursing practice has been accompanied by speculation, controversy, and research on the benefits, barriers, and real potential of NISs for improving clinical practice and giving nurses a voice in the development of healthcare

policy. Given growing concerns about a nursing shortage and previous estimates that nurses had been spending between 40 and 50% of their time on paperwork (McDaniel, 1997), there has been great interest in improving the speed and accuracy of nursing documentation, exploring approaches for using computer technology to enhance nursing care and healthcare delivery, and in conducting well-designed research studies on actual versus perceptions of the impact of computers on nursing practice. Table 20.6 describes a small sample of these studies.

Although related research on the practice applications of computers in nursing will certainly continue, there is general agreement that organization and use of data with computers have exerted a positive influence on the provision of patient care. The beginning of the new century appears to be a time of a deepening and shifting emphasis for informatics in nursing practice. In her review of contemporary nursing practice, Zytkowski (2003) provides us with a look at progress to date and what may lie ahead:

> Wireless communication, monitoring systems run with computerized backbones, and computerized ordering and documentation—all things unimaginable just a decade ago—are now fundamental to nursing practice. Nursing informatics is incorporated into all facets of nursing care and across all nursing specialties. Healthcare has shifted its focus from bringing individuals new technology to making technology work for these clinicians. This includes using information technology infrastructures currently in place to build Web-based services; enhance connectivity among specialties; link service areas; and enhance safeguards for protecting personal health information. (pp. 217–273)

Analysis of nursing research provides evidence of Kurzweil's predictions (1999) about the accelerating transformation in computer technology. In the 1990s, a major focus of informatics research in nursing was the comparison of nursing documentation at bedside terminals versus documentation at the nursing station (Herring and Rockman, 1990; Hendrickson and Kovner, 1990; Kahl, Ivancin, and Fuhrmann, 1991; Marr et al., 1993; Dillon et al., 1998). As these and other researchers (Bowles, 1997) studied factors such as ergonomic design, ease of use, elimination of redundant data, system support, availability and currency of data, and access to expert systems, there were some prescient voices in the nursing community who offered insights for the future

Table 20.6   Impact of Computerization on Nursing Practice: A Sample of Studies

Study	Year	Findings	Impact (+ or −)
Hendrickson and Kovner	1990	Time saved, less paperwork, fewer telephone calls, fewer errors; more complete documentation	+
Marr et al.	1993	No improvement in quality of documentation	−
Pabst, Scherubel, and Minnick	1996	No improvement in quality of documentation	−
McDaniel	1997	Identification of outliers, documentation of interventions	+
Kovner, Schuchman, and Mallard	1997	No time savings	−
Adderley, Hyde, and Mauseth	1997	Faster data entry, more consistent and more available data	+
Goossen, Epping, and Dassen	1997	Limited use and poor quality of systems	−
Yancey et al.	1998	More uniform reporting	+
Miranda, Fields, and Lund	2001	Consistent configuration across multiple sites, system used for both patient care and research	+
Larrabee et al.	2001	Improvement in blood pressure documentation, completeness of nurse assessment of patient outcomes, achievement of patient outcomes, and nursing interventions done	+
Dumas, Dietz, and Connolly	2001	Most useful applications were obtaining medical records, entering electronic client record information, communication with other healthcare agencies, pattern of under use	+
Flynn	2001	Improved utilization of ICU beds, increased accuracy of documentation	+

that have now become a reality. In 1995, for example, Patterson (1995) suggested that:

> The reports you get from a system are only as good as the data you put in, and the best place and time to record a supply used, a procedure administered, a pharmaceutical issued, is where and when it happens. (p. 16)

Patterson had also predicted in 1995 that nursing homes would be "going electric" because the managed care environment was requiring electronic billing and patient records.

Kasper (1996) and Kovner, Schuchman, and Mallard (1997) reported that community, home health, and rural care agencies were using handheld devices that could be easily carried to the point of care where patient data were recorded and transmitted to a central server.

In 1996, Kasper had noted that personal digital assistant (PDA) technology offered portability, accessibility, and accuracy with a *mobile medical record*, which provided instant access to current patient charts in a wide variety of practice settings. This allowed for patient records to be recorded instantly from remote settings and when nurses were at home and on call. With PDAs, nurses and other healthcare providers could complete a patient record, send a prescription to a pharmacy, order follow-up clinical procedures, collect billing information, and access vast amounts of medical information. At the time, some PDAs included built-in extensive pharmacy data and current ICD-9 codes that can assist in the billing process. Kasper reported that while few PDAs in the 1990s used software that was specific for nursing assessments of care plans, many were appropriate for clinical management, pharmacologic references, and patient history and physical examination data. In 2000, Ruland reported on the positive application of PDAs in documenting patient preferences.

The speed of advances in technology has allowed PDAs—with their wireless versatility and portability—to not only make bedside terminals obsolete, but also to change the healthcare landscape. These devices now can be found with nurses as they check vital signs; compare barcodes on medications and patient wristbands; review, enter, and transfer critical clinical data; and go about the daily delivery of patient care. According to Eandi (2001), Simpson (2003c), Zytkowski (2003), and Abbott (2003), PDAs keep nurses close to patients and the data needed to care for them. Hagland (2003) reports that many hospital-based organizations are now using handheld devices and most will implement handheld for clinical care within the next 2–3 years.

In 1995, Patterson suggested that wireless data communication in combination with pen-based computers would be the wave of the future as the healthcare industry attempted to broaden usage and lower the overall costs of point-of-care computing. Four years into the new decade, the nursing profession is still working toward a "computer in every hand" in the nursing profession and in healthcare. Yet, recent reports from the popular press (Kessler, 2004; Stone, 2004) suggest that the popularity of PDAs in the United States has waned in favor of smart phones, which carry full features and many of the same capabilities of PDAs. There are now predictions (Kessler, 2004; Stone, 2004) that in the future, the smart phone will equal the digital life of the twenty-first century. Such an advance would stimulate a new wave of adjustments for users and beneficiaries in society at large and in healthcare. Zytkowski (2003), Chastain (2003), Carty (2001), and other nursing leaders wisely advise us that although the future of computers in nursing practice looks bright, the exact course is difficult to predict.

Summary

Although the actual components of the nursing *process* have changed little over the years, the practice environment—with its technologic advances, regulatory constraints, changing patient needs, and shortage of nurses—certainly has. This chapter has described the use of the computers in the *work* of nurses within that twenty-first century practice environment. There are now new standards for practice in nursing informatics; a vast array of new, improved systems for nursing documentation systems, care planning, decision-making, and

outcomes management; and emerging technology that could drastically alter the digital landscape of the tomorrow's hospitals.

Yet, the excitement about advances in technology is tempered by concerns within the profession, as described earlier in this chapter, about patterns which show nurses' underutilization of technology and problems with standardization of computer languages. There is also concern about technology's focus on data collection per se rather than patient care (Ellis, 2000), and some voices which are focused on the potential negative effects of technology on the nurse-patient relationship (West, 2003; Baker, Reifsteck and Mann, 2003).

Simply maintaining the status quo with informatics in nursing practice is not a realistic option in the twenty-first century when the nursing shortage is of such concern. Nurses are key contributors to patient care and healthcare policy, and must be proactively engaged in all phases of information systems development. The presence of nursing in this process will assure that voice and work of nurses will be fully present in the digital world of healthcare today and tomorrow. If technology is the "tool of commonality" as Miller and Carlton (1998) suggested, then the nursing profession must use that tool to its fullest to advance patient care and nursing practice.

References

Abbott, P. (2003). Nursing informatics: A foundation for nursing professionals. *AACN Clinical Issues* 14:267–270.

Adderley, D., Hyde, C., and Mauseth, P. (1997). The computer age affects nursing. *Computers in Nursing* 15:43–36.

Allan, J. and Englewright, J. (2000). Patient centered documentation. *Journal of Nursing Administration* 30:90–95.

Aller, K. C. (1996). Information systems for outcomes movement. *Healthcare Information Manager* 10:37–53.

Alpay, L. and Russell, A. (2002). Information technology training in primary care: The nurses' voice. *Computer Informatics Nursing* 20:136–142.

American Nurses Association (ANA). (1992).Council on computer applications in nursing. Report on the Designation of Nursing Informatics as a Specialty. Congress of Nursing Practice unpublished report. Washington, DC: American Nurses Association.

American Nurses Association (ANA). (1994). *Scope and Standards of Practice for Nursing Informatics*. Washington, DC: American Nurses Publishing.

American Nurses Association (ANA). (1995). *Scope and Standards of Practice for Nursing Informatics*. Washington, DC: American Nurses Publishing.

American Nurses Association (ANA). (2001). *Scope and Standards of Practice for Nursing Informatics*. Washington, DC: American Nurses Publishing.

American Nurses Association (ANA). (2003). *ANA Recognized Terminologies that Support Nursing Practice*. Revised November 14, 2003. Retrieved January 29, 2004, from *http://www.nursingworlod. org/nidsec/class1st.htm*

Axford, R. and Carter, B. (1996). Impact of clinical information systems on nursing practice: Nurses' perspectives. *Computers in Nursing* 14:156–166.

Baker, L. H., Reifsteck, S. W., and Mann, W. R. (2003). Connected: Communication skills for nurses using the electronic medical record. *Nursing Economics* 21:85–88.

Bakken, S. (2001). An informatics infrastructure is essential for evidence-based practice. *Journal of the American Medical Informatics* 8:199–201.

Ballard, E. (1997). Important considerations about nursing intelligence and information systems. In U. Gerdin, M. Talberg, P. Wainwright (Eds.), *Nursing Informatics— The Impact of Nursing Knowledge on Health Care Informatics* (pp. 44–49). Amsterdam: IOS Press.

Bowles, K. W. (1997). The benefits and barriers of nursing information systems. *Computers in Nursing* 15:191–196.

Brazile, R. P. and Hettinger, B. J. (1995). A clinical information system for ambulatory care. *Computer Nurse* 13:151–158.

Brenner, P. (1984). *From Novice to Expert: Excellence and Power in Clinical Nursing Practice*. Menlo Park, CA: Addison-Wesley.

Carty, B. (2001). Nursing informatics: The future is now. *Journal of the New York State Nurses Association* 32:4–11.

Chastain, A. R. (2003). Nursing informatics: Past, present and future. *Tennessee Nurse* 66:8–10.

Coenen, A., McNeil, B., Bakken, S., Bickford, C., Warren, J. J., for the ANA Committee on Nursing Practice Information Infrastructure. (2001). Toward comparable nursing data: American Nurses Association. Criteria for data sets, classification systems and nomenclatures. *Computers in Nursing* 19:240–246.

Cullen, P. (1998). Gleaning patterns from practice: Intelligent systems in ambulatory care. *Nursing Economics* 16:133–136.

Dillon, T. W., McDowell, D., Salimian, F., and Conklin, D. (1998). Perceived ease of use and usefulness of bedside-computer systems. *Computers in Nursing* 16:151–156.

Dumas, J., Dietz, E. O., and Connolly, P. M. (2001). Nurse practitioner use of computer technologies in practice. *Computers in Nursing* 19:34–40.

Eandi, E. (2001). Handheld computers facilitate patient care and tracking. *Latitudes*. Retrieved 2/2/04, from *http: nlm.gov/psr/lat/v10n2/pda/html*.

Ellis, D. (2000). *Technology and the Future of Health Care: Preparing for the Next Thirty Years*. Chicago, IL: AHA Press.

Flynn, M. (2001). Nursing and informatics: Implications for critical care practice. *Critical Care* 21:8–16.

Gohlinghorst, S., Weir, C., Nutt, T., and McCarthy, C. (2000). Computer needs assessment based on nursing tasks. Paper Presented at 2000 Annual Conference of the American Medical Informatics Association, November 4–8, 2000, Los Angeles, CA.

Goossen, W. T., Epping, P. J., and Dassen, T. (1997). Criteria for nursing information systems as a component of the electronic patient record: An international Delphi study. *Computers in Nursing* 15:307–315.

Graves, J. and Corcoran, S. (1989). The study of nursing informatics. *Image—The Journal of Nursing Scholarship* 21:227–231.

Hagland, M. (2003). Handhelds and wireless. In "Nine tech trends." *Healthcare Informatics* 20:61, 80.

Hannah, K., Ball, M., and Edwards, M. (1994). History of health care computing. In K. Hannah and M. Ball. (Eds.), *Introduction to Nursing Informatics* (pp. 32–33). New York, NY: Springer-Verlag.

Henderson, R. D. and Deane, F. P. (1996). User expectations and perceptions of a patient management system. *Computers in Nursing* 14:188–193.

Hendrickson, G. and Kovner, C. T. (1990). Effects of computers on nursing resource use: Do computers save nurses time? *Computers in Nursing* 8:6–22.

Herring, D., and Rockman, R. (1990). A closer look at bedside terminals. *Nursing Management* 21: 554–561.

Hooper, W. (2003). The importance of nursing informatics. *Tennessee Nurse* 66:4.

Huber, D. G. and Schumacher, L. (1997). Nursing management minimum data set. *Journal of Nursing Administration* 27:42–48.

Johnson, C. and Nolan, M. T. (2000). A guide to choosing technology to support the measurement of patient outcomes. *Journal of Nursing Administration* 30: 21–26.

Johnston, M. E., Langton, K. B., Haynes, R. B., and Mathieu, A. (1994). Effects of computer-based clinical decision support systems on clinician performance and patient outcomes. *Annals of Internal Medicine* 120:135–142.

Kahl, K., Ivancin, L., and Fuhrmann, M. (1991). Identifying the savings potential of bedside terminals. *Nursing Economics* 9:391–400.

Kasper, C. (1996). Personal digital assistants and clinical practice. *Western Journal of Nursing Research* 18:717–721.

Kerfoot, K. (2000). Technical IQ—a survival skill for the new millennium. *Nursing Economics* 18:29–31.

Kessler, M. (2004). PDA sales slowing PDQ as cell phones add features. *USA Today*, 1B.

Kosko, B. (1999). *Fuzzy Future*. New York: Harmony Books.

Kovner, C., Schuchman, L., and Mallard, C. (1997). The application of pen-based computers technology to home health care. *Computers in Nursing* 15: 237–244.

Kuperman, G. J., Teiche, J. M., Tansijevic, et al. (1999). Improving response to critical laboratory results with automation: Results of a randomized controlled trial. *Journal of the American Medical Information Association* 6:512–522.

Kurzweil, R. (1999). *The Age of Spiritual Machines*. New York: Viking.

Larrabee, J. H., Boldreghini, S., Elder-Sorrells, K., Turner, Z. M., Wender, R. G., Hart, J. M., and Lenzi, P. S. (2001). Evaluation of documentation before and after implementation of a nursing information systems in an acute care hospital. *Computers in Nursing* 19:56–63.

Lyons, A. and Richardson, S. (2003). Clinical decision support in critical care nursing. *AACN Clinical Issues* 14:295–301.

Major, L. F. and Turner, M. G. (2003). Assessing the information requirements for behavioral health providers. *Journal of Healthcare Management* 48:323–333.

Marr, P., Duthie, E., Glassman, K., Janovas, D., Kelly, P., Graham, E., Kovner, C., Rienzi, A., Roberts, N., and Schick, D. (1993). Bedside terminals and quality of nursing documentation. *Computers in Nursing* 11:176–182.

Martin, K. S. (1999). The Omaha system. *On-line Journal of Nursing Informatics* 3:1–7.

Martin, K. S and Scheet, N. J. (1995). The Omaha system: Nursing diagnoses, intervention and client outcomes. In *Nursing Data Systems: The Emerging Framework*. Washington, DC: American Nurses Publishing.

McCormick, K. A., Lang, N., Zielstorff, R., Milholland, K. Saba, V., and Jacox, A. (1994). Toward classification schemes for nursing language: Recommendations of the American Nurses Association Steering Committee on Databases to Support Clinical Nursing Practice. *Journal of the American Medical Informatics Association* 1:421–426.

McDaniel, A. M. (1997). Developing and testing a prototype patient care database. *Computers in Nursing* 15:129–135.

McDonald, C. J. Overhage, J. M., Dexter, P. R., et al. (1998). Canopy computing: Using the web for clinical practice. *Journal of the American Medical Association* 280:1325–1329.

McNeil, B. J., Elfrink, V. L., Bickford, C. J., Pierce, S. T., Beyea, S. C., Averill, C., and Klappenbach, C. (2003). Nursing information technology knowledge, skills and preparation of student nurses, nursing faculty, and clinicians: A U.S. Survey. *Journal of Nursing Education* 42:347.

Meadows, G. (2002). Nursing informatics: An evolving specialty. *Nursing Economics* 20:300.

Miller, R. A. (1994). Medical diagnostic decision support systems—past, present, and future. *Journal of the American Medical Informatics Association* 1:8–27.

Miller, P. A. and Carlton, K. H. (1998). Technology as a tool for health care collaboration. *Computers in Nursing* 16:27–29.

Miranda, D., Fields, W., and Lund, K. (2001). Lessons learned during 15 years of clinical information system experience. *Computers in Nursing* 19:147–151.

Mize, C. P., Bentley, G., and Hubbard, S. (1991). Standards of care: Integrating nursing care plans and quality assurance activities. *AACN Clinical Issues in Critical Care News* 2:63–68.

National Advisory Council on Nurse Education and Practice (NACNEP). (1997). *A National Informatics Agenda for Nursing Education and Practice*. Rockville, MD: U. S. Department of Health and Human Services, Health Resources and Services Administration.

National Center for Nursing Research. (1993). Nursing informatics: Enhancing patient care: A report of the NCNR Priority Expert Panel on Nursing Informatics. NIH Publication No. 93-2419.

Nightingale, F. (1859). *Notes on Hospitals* (3rd ed.). London: John W. Parkers and Sons.

Oxford Dictionary of Computing. (1996, 4th ed.). Oxford, England: Oxford University Press.

Pabst, M. K., Scherubel, J. C., and Minnick, A. F. (1996). The impact of computerized documentation on nurses' use of time. *Computers in Nursing* 14:25–30.

Patterson, D. (1995). Bedside computing. *Nursing Homes* 44:16–18.

Power, D. J. (2004). *A Brief History of Decision Support Systems*. Available at *http://DSSResources.com/dsshistory/html*. Accessed June 2, 2004.

Ruland, C. M. (2001). Developing a decision support system to meet nurse managers' information needs for effective resource management. *Computers in Nursing* 19:187–193.

Saba, V. K. (2001). Nursing informatics: Yesterday, today and tomorrow. *International Review* 48:177–187.

Senst, B. L., Achusim, L. E., Genest, R. P., et al. (2001). Practical approach to determining costs and frequency of adverse drug events in a health care network. *American Journal of Health System Pharm* 57:1126–1132.

Simpson, R. L. (2003a). What's in a name? The taxonomy and nomenclature puzzle, part 1. *Nursing Management* 34:14.

Simpson, R. L. (2003b). The role of IT in health care quality assessment. *Nursing Administration Quarterly* 27:355.

Simpson, R. L. (2003c). The patients' point of view—IT matters. *Nursing Administration Quarterly* 27(3):54.

Smith, K. R. (1998). Outcomes management of mechanically ventilated patients: Utilizing informatics technology. *Critical Care Nursing Quarterly* 21:61–72.

Snyder-Halpern, R., and Chervany, N. (2000). A clinical information system strategic planning model for integrated health care delivery. *Journal of Nursing Administration* 30(12):583–591.

Staggers, N., Gassert, C. A., Curran, C. (2001). Informatics competencies for nurses at four levels of practice. *Journal of Nursing Education* 40:303–316.

Stone, B. (2004). Your next computer. *Newsweek* 51–54.

Straub, K. (1997). Behavioral health and the transition to integrated information systems. *Health Management Technology* 18:20–22, 24.

The Association of Colleges and Research Libraries (ACRL). (2000). *Information Literacy Standards Competency Standards for Higher Education*. San Antonio, TX: American Library Association.

Ulrich, B. (1992). Organizational structure. In W. Brotmiller (Ed.), *Leadership and Management According to Florence Nightingale* (p. 68). Norwalk, CN: Appleton & Lange.

U.S. Department of Health and Human Services. (2001). Information for health: A strategy for building the National Health Information Infrastructure. Report and Recommendations from the National Committee on Vital and Health Statistics. Washington, DC: Author.

Welling, N. and Delnoij, D. (1997). The practice nurse in British family practice—lessons from Dutch experiments. *Verpleegkunde* 1230:131–139.

Werley, H. H. and Lang, N. M. (Eds.) 1998. *Identification of the Nursing Minimum Data Set*. New York: Springer.

Wessling, E. (1972). Automating the nursing history and care plan. *Journal of Nursing Administration* 2:34–38.

West, E. A. (2003). Computers: Do they help or hinder patient care? *Nursing Forum* 38:29–31.

Wojner, A. W. and Kite-Powell, D. (1997). Outcomes manager: A role for the advanced practice nurse. *Critical Care Nursing Quarterly* 19:16–42.

Wong, H. J., Legnini, M., and Whitmore, H. (2000). The diffusion of decision support systems in healthcare; are we there yet? *Journal of Healthcare Management* 45:240–249.

Yancey, R., Given, B. A., White, N., DeVoss, D., and Coyle, B. (1998). Computerized documentation for a rural nursing intervention project. *Computers in Nursing* 16:275–284.

Zytkowski, M. E. (2003). Nursing informatics: The key to unlocking contemporary nursing practice. *AACN Clinical Issues* 14:271–281.

21

Critical Care Applications

Rosemary Kennedy
Ann Daddona

OBJECTIVES

1. Identify information technology applications in critical care.
2. Understand the basic components of arrhythmia monitors and physiologic monitors.
3. Describe how hemodynamic monitoring systems are used in critical care settings.
4. Understand the capabilities, purposes, types, benefits, and issues of critical care information systems (CCISs).
5. Describe the relationship between hemodynamic monitoring systems and CCISs.
6. Identify trends in monitoring and computerized information management.
7. Identify special-purpose applications available.

KEY WORDS

information systems
hospital information systems
critical care information systems
integrated information systems

Critical care nursing is the nursing specialty that deals with human responses to life-threatening problems (Lewis, 2004). Critical care is the multidisciplinary healthcare specialty that cares for patients with acute, life-threatening illness or injury. A critically ill patient is physically unstable with real or potential life-threatening health problems requiring continuous intensive assessment and interventions (American Association of Critical Care Nurses [AACN], 2003). Historically, critically ill patients were cared for in critical care units, but due to increased patient acuity and an aging population, critical care patients can be found in a variety of settings (Kidd, 2001). Implied in these definitions is a technologically intense environment geared to the monitoring and support needs of the critically ill patient (Bachman, 1995). Embedded in much of that technology are microprocessors, which permit gathering, processing, and storage of large volumes of clinical and financial data. In 1986, Saba and McCormick estimated that the volume of data collected by nurses in critical care settings on a daily basis was as high as 1,500 data points. Much of these data originate from the point-of-care medical devices found in the critical care environment. As the use of technology expands, the available information expands as well, making it increasingly difficult to access and manage the volume of data. The clinician in critical care integrates data from hemodynamic devices, mechanical ventilators, bedside testing devices, and observations from direct patient assessments to form a comprehensive picture of the patient's status and the effect of care. The data must be readily accessible at the point of care. The demand for cost-effective care continues to increase (Gardner, Bradshaw, and Hollingsworth, 1989). Resource shortages, both staff and time, increase the difficulty of data management. Information technology offers solutions to these difficulties through manipulation of large volumes of data and presenting them to the clinician in meaningful ways to guide quality and cost-effective decision-making. Effective and efficient integration of information drives improvement in patient care and hence is increasingly employed in critical care settings. Information technology is found in many patient care units in the critical care setting. The microprocessors that are embedded in many of the devices used with critical care patients facilitate downloading of the data that resides in the device to an information management system. Based on the sheer volume and complexity of the technology, the information management needs of the critically ill patient require different technology resources than those of other patient care areas. In this chapter, physiologic, arrhythmia, and hemodynamic monitors, and CCISs will be the focus of discussion. Descriptions of the specialized applications of information technology found in the critical care area and trends toward new applications will be included in the discussion.

Developments

Developers of automated approaches to information management in critical care settings have incorporated complex formulas into physiologic monitors, rapidly analyzed small samples of gas or fluids, maintained near-normal physiologic ranges with life-supporting equipment, and stored large volumes of data that would otherwise be disorganized, lost, inaccurate, or illegible. Information systems have been implemented to address alarms and clinical alerts that push significant patient data to the clinician at the point of care.

The advantages of these automated physiologic monitoring systems resemble the advantages of electronic nursing documentation: better control of patient observations to improve assessment, intervention, and evaluation of patient care. These systems focus heavily on collecting, storing, and displaying physiologic data. Usually, these systems are integrated into electronic patient documentation systems that address the nursing process and provide support for all facets of documentation such as assessments, medication charting, progress notes, and the interdisciplinary plan of care. The functions, purposes, and benefits of these nursing process capabilities are the same as noted elsewhere in this book.

Information Technology Capabilities and Applications in Critical Care Settings

Information technology in the critical care environment has several major capabilities:

- Process, store, and integrate physiologic and diagnostic information from various sources
- Present deviations from preset ranges by an alarm or an alert

- Accept and store patient care documentation in a lifetime clinical repository
- Trend data in a graphical presentation
- Provide clinical decision support through alerts, alarms, and protocols
- Provide access to vital patient information from any location, both inside and outside of the critical care setting
- Comparatively evaluate patients for outcomes analysis
- Present clinical data based on concept-oriented views (organize data by patient problem or by system).

There are several data-intense information systems that exist in the critical care environment from which data can be obtained and integrated in a meaningful way. The CCIS must include data from multiple sources, encompassing current and historical information. Information technology applications and functions typical in the critical care environment that will be described in this chapter include the following:

- Physiologic monitors, including arrhythmia and hemodynamic monitors
- Mechanical ventilators
- CCISs

Device Connectivity Infrastructure

Bedside monitoring devices are capable of sending information to software applications. In concept, the term Medical Information Bus (MIB) is used to classify the backbone of information exchange, allowing data to be moved from one point to another. This infrastructure is used to send the workload generated by the patient care devices (e.g., monitors, ventilators, infusion pumps) in the modern critical care setting. Most medical devices have small communication ports available that have the capability to transmit digital data to clinical software applications. Software developers design hardware and software interfaces to allow the devices to communicate and supply information to the clinical information system. Examples of messaging standards that are used to intercede informational workflows within the healthcare enterprise are Health Language Seven (HL7) standards and the Institute of Electrical and Electronics Engineers (IEEE) Medical Data Device Language (MDDL).

In late 1994, the IEEE's 1073 MIB won industry approval. This MIB standard provides a uniform model for the method of data captures and transport as well as the language used by various bedside devices, enabling them to communicate with a central information system (Data Trap, 1997). While emerging technology begins to adopt this standard, individual interfaces must still be developed for many devices. These interfaces decode the data output from the source device, translate the output into a format that is understood by the destination clinical information system, and transport the information in an orderly fashion from the source to the destination. Such interfaces are best developed with a cooperative effort between hardware and software vendors; however, it is possible for one vendor to reverse engineer an interface to be compatible with another vendor's product.

Physiologic Monitoring Systems

In the NASA programs of the 1960s, physiologic monitors were developed to oversee the vital signs of the astronauts. By the 1970s, these monitors had found their way into the hospital setting, where they replaced manual methods of gathering patient vital signs. These early monitors were large and cumbersome and had limited capabilities. In the 1980s, technology became cheaper, smaller, and significantly more powerful. These developments were used to improve overall patient monitoring capabilities (Wiggett, 1996). In the 1990s, the focus of development has shifted to integration of monitoring data into information systems. In fact, many monitoring vendors introduced clinical information systems into their standard product lines.

Most physiologic monitors consist of five basic parts as shown in Table 21.1. The sensor is the instrument that is coupled to the patient and transforms the physiologic signal (e.g., temperature, pressure, ionic current) into an electrical signal that can be detected by the monitor. Careful

Table 21.1   Basic Components of Physiologic Monitoring Equipment

---

Sensors (e.g., pressure transducer, ECG electrode)

Signal conditioners to amplify or filter the display device (e.g., amplifier, oscilloscope, paper recorder)

File to rank and order information (e.g., storage file, alarm signal)

Computer processor to analyze data and direct reports (e.g., paper reports, storage for graphic files, summary reports)

Evaluation or controlling component to regulate the equipment or alert the nurse (e.g., a notice on the display screen, alarm signal)

---

attention to the sensor's limitations is required, since signal errors can easily originate at this point. Physiologic signals are typically of very small amplitude and must be amplified, conditioned, and digitized by the device in preparation for processing by its embedded microprocessor. The microprocessor analyzes information, stores pertinent information in specific places, and controls the direction of reporting (e.g., a paper report, storage for graphic files, shift summary reports). The file holds the information (e.g., the storage files, signals, or alarms). The evaluation or the controlling component alerts the nursing personnel through a report, an alarm, or a visual notice (e.g., a notice on the display screen: "increase patient's oxygen or check for leaks"). Alternatively, the controlling component may regulate an external device as a result of its evaluation; e.g., drug delivery is altered via control of an infusion pump in response to a blood pressure change.

Today, most physiologic monitoring systems are available in conjunction with a clinical information system. Due to market demand, those same physiologic monitoring systems utilize open architectures, which render them capable of interfacing with clinical information systems from other vendors as long as an investment of labor and dollars is made to develop the interface. The attraction of purchasing a monitoring system that is a component of an integrated information system is that development of an interface between the monitoring system and the information system is not necessary. However, the strength of the individual monitoring and information system components must be weighed against the resources required to develop an interface when deciding to purchase an integrated system or to integrate dissimilar monitoring and information systems.

As the information from various sources is integrated into the clinical information system, the accuracy of each and every data element becomes more important. Errors that arise within the monitoring system can invade the information system, thus blurring the picture of the patient's status and making effective decisions about patient care more difficult. Regardless of the degree of sophistication of the monitoring technology, the information it processes is only as good as the input it receives. Faulty signals will continue to be processed and will result in an increase in nuisance alarms. The incidence of inaccurate information causing monitor alarms in the intensive care unit (ICU) setting was studied by Tsien and Fackler. They found that 86% of alarms were false positive alarms resulting from, in order of incidence, bad formats or connections, poor contact of sensors, electrocardiogram (ECG) wire movement, motion artifact, measurement during arterial line clamping or flushing, and probe disconnection (Tsien and Fackler, 1997). Considerable errors can be introduced to the monitoring system at the "front end" or patient side of the monitor, and hence the sensor and patient connections to the monitor demand particular attention. For example, pressure transducers must be zeroed properly to provide accurate pressure measurements, and ECG electrodes must be periodically changed with appropriate skin preparation in order to minimize motion artifact. As information from the monitoring system is integrated into the information system, the accuracy of the monitoring data becomes increasingly important (Belzberg et al., 1996).

Monitoring systems also store various data elements with a time stamp derived from the monitoring system's internal clock. These data elements are transported with their respective time stamps to the clinical information system. If the clocks of the monitoring system or other data sources and the clock of the clinical information system are different, the effectiveness of various interventions as integrated and recorded in the patient's record may be erroneously interpreted. Therefore, attention must be given to the synchronicity of information from a variety of sources.

Physiologic monitoring systems typically have a modular platform, allowing the selection of various monitoring capabilities to match the needs of a variety of clinical settings. A careful choice of physiologic parameters will allow a critical care unit to cost-effectively offer the appropriate monitoring capabilities for its patients without offering the costly capability to monitor every conceivable parameter at every bedside. Modular formats can also facilitate data collection during transport to various diagnostic locations using a smaller transport monitor from the same manufacturer as the bedside monitor. On return to the patient unit, that information can be downloaded into the bedside monitor for integration into the patient's record.

More specialized monitoring capabilities such as intracranial pressure or bispectral index monitoring are also available in modular format, but modular availability is usually developed sometime after the availability as a stand-alone monitor. Typically, the patent holder of the new monitoring technology will license its software development to monitoring manufacturers for incorporation into their monitoring system. An alternative approach is to work with the monitoring vendor to develop an interface with the stand-alone monitor such that information can be exchanged between the stand-alone monitor and the physiologic monitoring system. Once information from the stand-alone monitor is imported into the physiologic monitor, that information can be passed along by the physiologic monitor to the clinical information system.

The flexibility of the modular monitoring format allows the physiologic monitor to be built around the needs of the patient found in any care setting. In the critical care setting, physiologic monitors are usually built to incorporate both arrhythmia and hemodynamic monitoring capabilities.

Hemodynamic Monitors

Advanced hemodynamic monitoring systems allow for calculation of hemodynamic indices and limited data storage. Hemodynamic monitoring can be used to (Kenner, 1990; Gardner, Bradshaw, and Hollingsworth, 1989; Clochesy, 1989):

- Measure hemodynamic parameters
- Closely examine cardiovascular function
- Evaluate cardiac pump output and volume status
- Recognize patterns (arrhythmia analysis) and extract features
- Assess vascular system integrity
- Evaluate the patient's physiologic response to stimuli
- Continuously assess respiratory gases (capnography)
- Continuously evaluate blood gases and electrolytes
- Estimate cellular oxygenation
- Continuously evaluate glucose levels
- Store waveforms
- Automatically transmit selected data to a computerized patient database

Hemodynamic monitoring can be invasive or noninvasive. Invasive catheters are typically used to measure and monitor various pressures and cardiac output. Noninvasive monitoring methods are increasingly common and include pressure measurement using oscillometric techniques, oxygenation measurement using pulse oximetry technology, and measurement of cardiac output via Doppler. A screen from a bedside hemodynamic monitoring system is shown in Fig. 21.1.

Invasive hemodynamic monitoring techniques have traditionally involved use of the pulmonary artery catheter (PAC), which was originally designed for measurement of pulmonary artery and wedge pressures. Since its inception, design modifications have been made including incorporation of a thermistor, which facilitates measurement of cardiac output and incorporation of fiber-optic technology, which in turn facilitates measurement of mixed venous oxygen saturation (Headley, 1998). Use of the PAC has potential complications, such as infection, hemorrhage, and embolism.

With growing popularity of use, the PAC has come under recent and persistent criticism concerning its

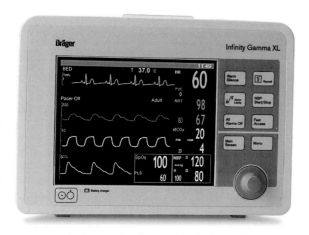

Figure 21.1
A bedside physiologic monitor: the universal clinical workstation.
(Courtesy of Draeger Medical Solutions.)

safety and appropriate use. This criticism prompted formation of the Pulmonary Artery Consensus Conference Organization (PACCO) with broad representation from professional nursing and medical societies. The PACCO determined that it is appropriate to use the PAC when either conventional hemodynamic therapies have not produced desirable results or hemodynamic therapies require the monitoring provided by the PAC. However, the PACCO supported further research on the impact of the PAC and found that clinical knowledge of the PAC, including clinical and technical aspects, probably warranted improvement (Ahrens, 1999a).

Intermittent measurement using thermodilution techniques has become the standard methodology for assessment of cardiac output; however, the accuracy of this technique is highly user-dependent for the following reasons (Headley, 1998; Burchell et al., 1997; Von Rueden and Turner, 1999):

- The bolus must be injected within 4 seconds
- The amount of the solution must be accurate
- The temperature of the injectate must be precisely measured and accurately maintained
- The catheter must be properly placed within the heart and pulmonary artery
- The computer must have the appropriate computation constant entered
- The bolus must be injected at the appropriate time in the respiratory cycle

The influence of these user-related issues is negated by using heating of a thermal filament embedded in the catheter to replace the injectate. The thermal filament is intermittently heated, thus sending pulses of heat energy into the right ventricle, which is then sensed by the thermistor in the pulmonary artery in much the same manner as in the traditional thermodilution technique. These measurements can be repeated at programmable intervals. The microprocessor keeps a running average of the last several minutes of values to obtain a continuously updated cardiac output measurement. Because of its more frequent measurements, this method may allow earlier detection and treatment of a change in cardiac output than conventional intermittent thermodilution. However, because this technique presents an averaged cardiac output, the response to acute changes may be considered to be slow (Headley, 1998; Mihm et al., 1998; Burchell et al., 1997).

An alternative means of measuring cardiac output noninvasively is provided by thoracic electrical bioimpedance. Four sensors are positioned on the sides of the neck and thorax. A low-amplitude, high-frequency signal is emitted by the sensors through the thorax. The amplitude of the signal detected by the sensors is proportional to the impedance of the path traveled by the electricity through the thorax. Because electricity follows the path of least resistance and because the path through the thorax is typically composed of fluid, the measured impedance provides information about the amount of fluid in the thoracic cavity. There are three compartments in the thorax that contain fluid, namely intravascular, intraalveolar, and interstitial. Since the aorta is the largest, most distensible, blood-filled vessel in the thoracic cavity, aortic blood flow contributes significantly to the measured impedance and hence is readily tracked via this method. As the heart beats and the blood within the thorax changes, the measured thoracic impedance will change. Monitoring these changes permits measurement of stroke volume; indices of contractility such as velocity and acceleration of blood flow, supraventricular rhythm, and index; and cardiac output and index. However, in conditions that increase the fluid in nonvascular compartments of the thorax, such as pulmonary edema and pleural effusion, measurements of cardiac output using the electrical bioimpedance method are less reliable. With these exceptions, satisfactory agreement with the thermodilution technique can be obtained using thoracic bioimpedance for cardiac output measurement (Shoemaker et al., 1994; Von Reuden and Turner, 1999; Lasater, 1998). Using bioimpedance as a factor integrated with analysis of the finger blood pressure waveform has also been demonstrated as a method of cardiac output measurement;

however, this method has not demonstrated sufficient agreement with established technique to be of clinical value (Hirschl et al., 1997).

A critical piece of hemodynamic information involves the availability of oxygen to bodily tissues. The gold standard for measurement of the blood's oxygen saturation is cooximetry, which is based on principles of spectrophotometry. Pulse oximetry is a noninvasive method of measuring arterial oxygen saturation that also uses spectrophotometry. The pulse oximeter uses two light-emitting diodes (LEDs), each of which emits light of different wavelengths. The light is emitted through a pulsatile arteriolar bed and then detected by a photosensor. Measurement of the amount of light detected at the photosensor and knowledge of the light absorption characteristics of oxyhemoglobin allow determination of the oxygen saturation. Because the blood volume in the arteriolar bed varies with the heartbeat, the amount of light absorbed will also vary with the pulse. This pulsatile nature allows the device to differentiate the amount of light absorbed by the venous blood and tissues from the amount of light absorbed by the arterial blood. The pulse oximeter is unable to distinguish between the various types of hemoglobin and hence the oxygen saturation is a functional saturation measurement that includes all types of hemoglobins including methemoglobin and carboxyhemoglobin.

The availability of a noninvasive oxygen saturation measurement device has resulted in widespread use of pulse oximetry in critical care environments. Unfortunately, the susceptibility of pulse oximetry to interference makes it the largest contributor to alarms in the ICU. Susceptibility to motion artifact is particularly problematic. Since the technology is dependent on its ability to differentiate blood content over a pulsatile cycle, any device such as a blood pressure cuff, tourniquet, or air splint that may cause venous pulsations will limit the sensor's ability to distinguish between arterial and venous blood. Since the technology is based on a measurement of light, any extraneous light source, including ambient light, may impact the accuracy of measurement (Ahrens and Tucker, 1999; Tsien and Fackler, 1997).

While pulse oximetry provides a measure of oxygen delivered to the tissue, mixed venous oxygen saturation (SvO_2) provides a measure of the amount of oxygen used by the patient. Normally, about 25% of the oxygen delivered is extracted for use. If more than 25% is extracted, then the body is compensating for an increased oxygen demand or a decreased oxygen delivery. Therefore, a drop in SvO_2 is a warning sign of a potential threat to tissue oxygenation. An increase in SvO_2 indicates that the tissue

is not receiving oxygen perhaps because of shunting of blood from vascular collapse or obstructions. (Ahrens, 1999b; Headley, 1998).

Hemodynamic monitoring can take place at the bedside or be conducted from a remote location via telemetry. As the volume of higher acuity patients that are serviced outside of the ICU increases, telemetry is more frequently utilized. Telemetry allows for the continuous monitoring of patients usually outside of the ICU. Physiologic data are sent by a transmitter to an antenna system that is distributed around the nursing unit or institution (usually in the ceiling) and displayed on the monitor screen at the telemetry station (Elder, 1991). The patient wears the transmitter, which is attached via surface electrodes for monitoring of ECG. The small size and weight of the transmitter enables the patient to be mobile as long as the patient remains in the area of antenna coverage. The radio frequency (RF) signal is received by a central monitor, processed, and then displayed at the central monitors as well as at specified remote sites. Transmitters can also be attached to portable devices, which in turn are connected to the patient. This approach enables telemetric monitoring of any parameter that can be monitored by the portable monitor. An example of this approach is shown in Fig. 21.2. Through utilization of an expansive antenna

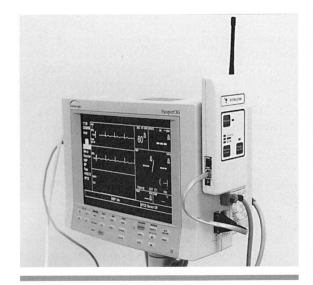

Figure 21.2
A transmitter couples to the output of a portable monitor.
(Courtesy of VitalCom, Inc., Tustin, CA and Datascope Patient Monitoring, Paramus, NJ.)

system, virtually any bed in the hospital can be monitored without purchasing monitoring hardware for every bed.

Through installation of an expansive antenna system, monitoring can be made available at virtually any bed without purchasing monitoring hardware for every bed. Use of this approach allows admission to the specialty area that best suits the patient's needs even when hemodynamic monitoring is necessary. However, it is important to remember that in that location, qualified staff members must be available to respond to alarms, attend to the patient, and make a complete assessment of the patient's cardiac condition. It is also important to remember that with telemetry, communication protocols between the central station and the bedside nurse are critically important. Pager systems that are linked to the telemetry system are now available to assist with this communication (Martin and Hendrickson, 1999).

Telemetry monitoring is susceptible to signal loss for a variety of reasons. The RF signal reception can be interrupted by obstacles in the environment including walls, furniture, and even the patient's own body. This signal loss is commonly referred to as "drop-out." Secondly, the RF signal can be interfered with by other extraneous RF signals of the same frequency. Medical telemetry is currently designated as a Part 15 or a Part 90 device by the Federal Communications Commission. According to the Part 15 and Part 90 rules, medical telemetry cannot interfere with licensed users, such as television and radio broadcasters and must endure any interference experienced from these licensed users. With the conversion to digital television as mandated by Congress, the refarming of the analog stations, and the expansion of private land mobile radio use, there is diminishing airspace left for telemetry use. The Federal Communications Commission is likely to designate some portion of the frequency spectrum for use by medical telemetry under a licensed by rule status. With this allocation, telemetry manufacturers are more likely to invest in the design of more robust products using more sophisticated modulation techniques. Only then will telemetry be more immune to signal loss and interference (American Hospital Association, 1999).

Computer-based hemodynamic monitoring offers the critical care nurse a wealth of information. However, the clinicians must keep in mind that the monitor and its information do not replace clinical judgment or necessarily imply quality patient care (Macy and James, 1971; Kenner, 1990). Conversely, the critical care nurse must learn to recognize the limitations of manual estimation of physiologic parameters and not use that estimation to diagnose a monitor malfunction. For example, manual calculation of mean arterial blood pressure is based only on two discrete

pressures, i.e., systolic and diastolic. The hemodynamic monitor calculates mean arterial pressure using a much larger sample of discrete pressures. Therefore, the manually calculated mean pressure is an estimate and the value calculated by the monitor is a derived measurement. The two values will not necessarily match.

Arrhythmia Monitors

Computerized monitoring and analysis of cardiac rhythm have proved reliable and effective in detecting potentially lethal heart rhythms (Widman, 1992). Standards for testing and reporting the performance of arrhythmia analysis systems have been developed by the American Heart Association. A key functional element is the system's ability to detect ventricular fibrillation and respond with an alarm. However, no standards currently specify the minimal accuracy of computerized detection systems (Mirvis et al., 1989). The basic components of arrhythmia monitors are shown in Table 21.2.

System Types There are two types of arrhythmia systems: detection surveillance and diagnostic or interpretive. In a detection system, the criteria for a normal ECG are programmed into the computer. The computer might survey the ECG for wave amplitude and duration and for the intervals between waves. The program may even include an alarm response if the R-R interval is either less than or equal to two-thirds of the average R-R interval. Each signal may then be analyzed to determine whether the QRS duration is greater than normal.

The next programmed search may be for the presence of a compensatory pause. (i.e., a prolonged R-R interval after a premature ventricular contraction [PVC]). The computer may then be programmed to store the number of PVCs per minute and sound an alarm or alert the nurse visually (e.g., a flashing red light) and audibly (a loud sound) when more than five PVCs occur within a minute. Detection systems can even store in memory the type of

Table 21.2 Basic Components of Arrhythmia Monitors

Sensor
Signal conditioner
Cardiograph
Pattern recognition
Rhythm analysis
Diagnosis
Written report

arrhythmia and time of occurrence, so that the patient's arrhythmia history can be plotted and compared to medication administration (Sorkin and Bloomfeld, 1982).

Arrhythmia systems can also be diagnostic; after the analog signals are digitized for processing, the program analyzes and diagnoses the ECG. The computer, after processing the ECG, generates an analysis report that is confirmed by a cardiologist, usually from another site. The computers that support these types of ECGs are usually dedicated systems (i.e., main memory is used only for ECG acquisition, analysis, and report generation). Diagnostic systems are usually capable of retrieving a patient's previous ECGs for comparison. Bedside monitoring capabilities are beginning to emerge that incorporate 12 lead ECG capabilities, the cornerstone of the diagnostic system.

Interpretive systems search the ECG complex for five parameters:

- Location of QRS complex
- Time from the beginning to the end of the QRS
- Comparison of amplitude, duration, and rate of QRS complex with all limb leads
- P and T waves
- Comparison of P and T waves with all limb leads

The findings are then compared to predetermined diagnostic specifications. Evaluation of these parameters is based on an arithmetic comparison of the patient's signal to a "normal" signal. Because the comparisons are arithmetic in nature, random signal noise can result in erroneous identification of arrhythmias. A purely arithmetic analysis will never replace the more discerning element of human review; therefore, arrhythmia monitors are merely another tool for use in the critical care environment, and will never replace the cognitive abilities of the caregiver.

Critical Care Information Systems

A CCIS is a system designed to collect, store, organize, retrieve, and manipulate all data related to care of the critically ill patient. It is focused on individual patients and the information directly related to the patients' care. The primary purpose of a CCIS is the organization of a patient's current and historical data for use by all care providers in patient care (Milholland and Cardona, 1983). The power of a modern CCIS is its ability to integrate information from a variety of sources and to manipulate that information in meaningful ways. The CCIS should include data and information from bedside devices; results from ancillary departments, medications, orders, physical assessment

findings gathered from the clinical team; and comprehensive plans of care to guide patient care. Integration of these data results in a more complete representation of the patient's status and can promote safaety, quality, and efficiency in patient care.

The hospital infrastructure of interfaces between medical devices and the CCIS allows the free flow of data between the critical care unit and other departments (McGrow, 2004). This provides a rich repository of patient information that can be integrated for use in outcomes management. The majority of information entered or integrated in the CCIS is clinical in nature. Within the CCIS, there are different views of information depending on the user and patient clinical condition.

Each patient's data can be accessed from any terminal or workstation. This capability can extend across units and departments or be restricted to a single unit. In some instances, an alarm on one patient can be "forwarded" to another patient location, as determined by the clinician.

CCISs offer many functions to facilitate the work of critical care nurses (Butler and Bender, 1999). The components of a CCIS include:

- Patient management
  - Admission, transfer, and discharge data can be directly entered or interfaced from the admissions department's information system, thus allowing compilation of unit statistics. Based on data elements entered, any variation of key statistics can be monitored. Service, length of stay, mortality, and readmit rates are examples of data that can be formatted into a report to assist in strategic planning.
  - Prognostic scoring systems can be integrated into the CCID to facilitate assessing the severity of illness for critically ill patients, such as the therapeutic interventions scoring system (TISS), the acute physiology and chronic health evaluation system (APACHE), the mortality predictor model (MPM), simplified acute physiology score (SAP), among others. These systems are useful in determining the likihood of survival (Rocker et al., 2004).
  - The CCIS can use the healthcare organization's system to schedule patient care activites, treatment, and diagnostic testing.

- Vital sign monitoring
  - Vital signs and other physiologic data can be automatically acquired from bedside instruments and incorporated into the clinical database. These data can be incorporated into

flow sheets with other data elements such as laboratory results, body system assessment findings, and problem lists. Any item entered via a flow sheet can be annotated. The annotations can be viewed via the flow sheet or as a set of notes, and they can be included with free-text notes entered separately.

- Interfaces to the monitoring system are available from vendors. The cardiohemodynamics flowsheet (Fig. 21.3) is an example of a flowsheet that collates vital sign data, performs

calculations, and summarizes critical therapies that may have influenced the patient information.

- Graphic displays of most data in the clinical database can be constructed. These displays may be preconfigured or may be developed dynamically as needed.
- Common groups of information can be displayed for easy viewing and trending.
- Monitor and device data can be interfaced to the CCIS flowsheet along with ventilator parameters.

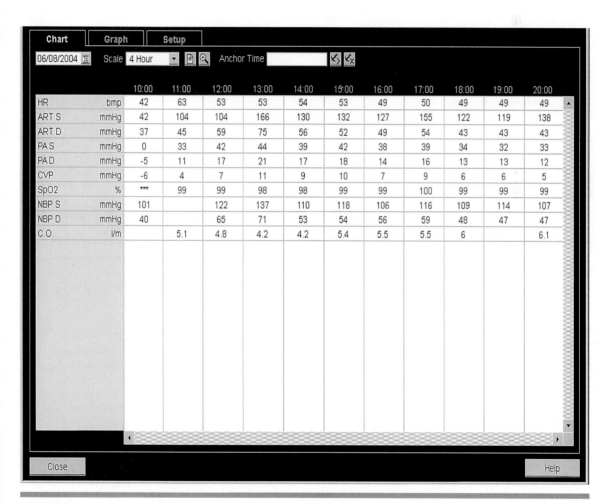

		Chart	Graph	Setup							

06/08/2004   Scale 4 Hour   Anchor Time

		10:00	11:00	12:00	13:00	14:00	15:00	16:00	17:00	18:00	19:00	20:00
HR	bmp	42	63	53	53	54	53	49	50	49	49	49
ART S	mmHg	42	104	104	166	130	132	127	155	122	119	138
ART D	mmHg	37	45	59	75	56	52	49	54	43	43	43
PA S	mmHg	0	33	42	44	39	42	38	39	34	32	33
PA D	mmHg	-5	11	17	21	17	18	14	16	13	13	12
CVP	mmHg	-6	4	7	11	9	10	7	9	6	6	5
SpO2	%	***	99	99	98	98	99	99	100	99	99	99
NBP S	mmHg	101		122	137	110	118	106	116	109	114	107
NBP D	mmHg	40		65	71	53	54	56	59	48	47	47
C.O.	l/m		5.1	4.8	4.2	4.2	5.4	5.5	5.5	6		6.1

Close

Help

Figure 21.3
A cardiohemodynamics chart.
(Courtesy of Siemens Medical Solutions.)

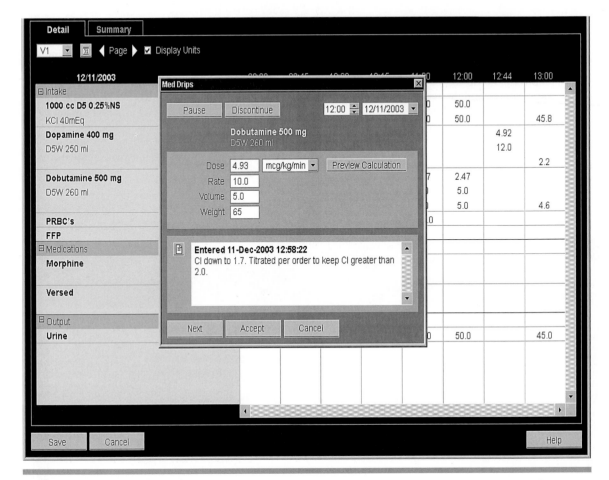

Figure 21.3 (Continued)

■ Diagnostic testing results
  ▪ Results can be displayed in flowsheets such as laboratory, radiology, and cardiology results.
  ▪ Clinicians can access picture archival information.

■ Clinical documentation to support the process of physical assessment findings
  ▪ Patient assessment flowsheets may be the cornerstones of the record, since they detail assessment findings that are regularly collected. As the critical care environment requires frequent assessments, these flowsheets may be configured to ease this extensive data collection. A shift assessment flowsheet can be created, for example, to capture more comprehensive baseline information, with a carry forward feature (data automatically "carries forward" from one time to the next) or mini assessment flowsheets used to record assessments not required as frequently. The use of drop-down menus in flowsheets such as these is particularly helpful in guiding the user to the most common choices based on evidence-based care guidelines. Structured lists of coded documentation choices are necessary for outcomes analysis.
  ▪ Flowsheets may also be organized by body system. A neurologic flowsheet (Fig. 21.4), for example, may record pupillary response, the

Chart	Setup								

Ventilator Type

		09/25/2003 09:07	09:28	09/29/2003 09:39	10/02/2003 12:44	13:28	13:30	13:32	13:34	10/03/2003 12:59
09/25/2003										
CMV FRAW	%	20	20	20	20	20	20	20	20	20
SIM FREQ	%	50	50	50	50	50	50	50	50	50
PEEP	cmH2O	0	0	0	0	0	0	0	0	0
RRv	breaths/m	20	20	20	20	20	20	20	20	20
i02	%	100	100	100	100	100	100	100	100	100
POP	cmH2O	60	60	60	60	60	60	60	60	60
MAP	cmH2O	20	20	20	20	20	20	20	20	20
Pause	cmH2O	60	60	60	60	60	60	60	60	60
TVi	ml	15	15	15	15	15	15	15	15	15
TVe	ml	15	15	15	15	15	15	15	15	15
MVi	l/m	3.0	3.0	3.0	3.0	3.0	3.0	3.0	3.0	3.0
MVe	l/m	0.3	0.3	0.3	0.3	0.3	0.3	0.3	0.3	0.3
Cdyn	ml/cmH2O									
Raw	cmH2O/l/s									
InspT%	%	75	75	75	75	75	75	75	75	75
etCO2*	mmHg	38	38	38						
iCO2*	mmHg	0	0	0						
I RISE %	%	60	60	60	60	60	60	60	60	60
INSP T%	%	30	30	30	30	30	30	30	30	30
Pause t %	%	40	40	40	40	40	40	40	40	40
RRc*	breaths/m	20	20	20						

Close   Help

Figure 21.3 (Continued)

Glasgow Coma Scale, sedation levels, pain ratings, motor strength, and intracranial and cerebral perfusion pressures, thus providing a comprehensive picture of a patient's neurologic status. Most systems allow annotations to the data elements so that qualifications or clarifications can be included. Noting that a patient has an endotracheal tube and cannot speak or to diminish intracranial pressures allows users to correctly interpret the data entered.

- All disciplines (nurses, physicians, respiratory therapists, and so forth), can document patient assessment findings into the CCIS.

Ability to document patient physical assessments for all disciplines. The findings entered by all clinicians can generate problem lists based on the physical assessment findings.

- Alerts automatically generated for patients at high risk for falls, pressure ulcers, and other factors.
- Automatic calculation of physiologic indices can be perfomed. As selected data are entered into the patient database manually or directly from bedside devices, customer-specified algorithms are employed to calculate the cardiovascular, respiratory, neurologic, and other indices.

	03/08/99 08:00	03/08/99 12:00	03/08/99 16:00	03/08/99 20:30	03/09/99 00:00	03/09/99 04:00	03/09/99 08:00
PUPILARY RESPONSE							
R Pupil Size	Small	Small	Small		Small		Normal
R Pupil Resp	Brisk	Brisk	Brisk		Brisk		Brisk
L Pupil Size	Small	Small	Small		Small		Normal
L Pupil Resp	Brisk	Brisk	Brisk		Brisk		Brisk
GLASCOW COMA SCALE							
Eyes Open	Speech	Speech	Spont		Speech		Spont
Best Verbal Resp	None	None	Confused		None		None
Verbal Response Qualifier	Trach/ET	Trach/ET	Trach/ET		Trach/ET		Trach/ET
Best Motor Resp	Obeys	Obeys	Obeys		Obeys		Localize
GCS Qualifier	None	None	None		None		MSO4 PCA
03/08 08:00 morphine gtt							
GCS	10	10	14		10		10
ASL	2 Sedate	2 Sedate	4 Rstlss		2 Sedate		2 Sedate
Pain Rating	5	0	5		3	11	11
03/08 08:00 pt admits to pain unable to use scale							
MOTOR STRENGTH							
R Arm Strength	VeryWeak	VeryWeak	VeryWeak		VeryWeak		Weak
L Arm Strength	VeryWeak	VeryWeak	VeryWeak		VeryWeak		Weak
R Leg Strength	VeryWeak	VeryWeak	VeryWeak		VeryWeak		Weak
L Leg Strength	VeryWeak	VeryWeak	VeryWeak		VeryWeak		Weak
MAP	93	97					

Figure 21.4

A neurologic chart.

(Courtesy of GE Marquette Medical Systems, Inc., Milwaukee, WI.)

- Automatic calculation capabilities have been extended to patient acuity, patient classification, productivity measures, and other indicators.
- Decision support
  - The CCIS can provide alerts and reminders to guide care in accordance with evidence-based guidelines. Prompts to guide the caregiver for required documentation can be integrated into the documentation process for all disciplines. Alerts on policies can facilitate adherence to protocols such as restraint management, pain management, and ventilator weaning.
  - Point-of-care access to knowledge bases that contain information on evidence-based guidelines of care, drug information, procedures, and policies can guide decision-making at the point of care where it has the most powerful impact in improving quality and safety.
  - Data from the CCIS can be integrated with patient information gathered outside of the critical care episode for outcomes analysis, performance improvement efforts, or to aid research.
- Medication management
  - The use of bar code scanning and an electronic medication administration record that is integrated into the CCIS can facilitate the medication administration process (Bates and Gawande, 2003).
  - Medication administration flowsheets incorporate the use of bar code technology, whereby the nurse scans the drug and the patient, while viewing medication administration data on a flowsheet, thus ensuring the five rights of medication administration (right drug, right patient, right dose, frequency, and route of administration). This supports patient safety and quality initiatives.
  - Calculation of intravenous medication dosage, intravenous flow rates, hyperalimentation, aminoglycoside dose, and total intake/output schedules are among the computations available. Depending on the system, these values may be part of the patient database or may be offered as an "off-line" calculator.
- Interdisciplinary plans of care
  - The CCIS supports multidisciplinary documentation and multidisciplinary planning of patient care (Muschlitz, 1998). Because each of the disciplines seeks different

information in often unique presentations, the ideal CCIS will allow the flexibility to meet these diversified needs (Cook, 1997).
  - Special flowsheets incorporating required treatments and interventions may be provided. In most instances, the nurse can document the care given and not given directly on this flow sheet (on the screen). At any time, the nurse can enter an explanatory note describing the patient's response or the reasons for not delivering a specific treatment or intervention.
  - Workflow management solutions that help orchestrate all of the numerous, simultaneous processes of caring for patients by pushing tasks to individual worklists, monitoring to ensure each tasks is completed and notification when tasks fail. These tools support nurses in critical processes such as medication administration, admission, patient rounding, discharge and transfer functions, to name a few. In addition, the use of communication support tools that contain a list of commonly called numbers with automatic call and recall can provide tremendous support to the entire clinical team.
- Provider order entry
  - Provider order entry plays a critical role in improving quality and safety. Electronic entry and communication of patient orders, combined with rules and alerts related to evidence-based care, can help clinicians improve communication, streamline processes, facilitate care, and can help all providers in managing quality.
  - Order set displays help to streamline the order entry process and also guide clinicians in adhering to evidence-based medical practices.
  - Integration of provider order entry with interdisciplinary plans of care that generate patient-focused worklists can help to guide the entire clinical team toward common goals.

CCISs solutions provided by vendors are usually flexible and allow for customization of the system functionality to fit the existing clinical practices and workflows at an individual institution. Because clinical input is essential to implementing and designing systems that reflect the reality of patient and caregiver needs, the clinician will be intimately involved in the development and implementation of the successful CCIS (Muschlitz, 1998). The degree of customization required will be largely dependent on the vendor's ability to provide clinically relevant data and flowsheet starter sets as well as the level of standardization previously completed by the healthcare organization. Therefore, in addition to evaluating a CCIS's flexibility, a CCIS vendor selection criterion might be their ability to provide evidence-based starter sets incorporating guidelines of care, assessment flowsheets with standardized scoring instruments, such as the Glasgow Coma Score and structured terminology that reflects nursing and clinical practice.

Considerable effort is being invested in the standardization of the language used in the CCIS and the electronic health record across the continuum of care, as previously discussed in other sections of this book.

It seems that the task of developing the clinical information system is never complete. As new technologies are introduced or new information needs arise, changes to the CCIS become necessary. As C. Peter Waegmann, the executive director of the Medical Records Institute says, "Getting to the electronic patient record is a journey" (Muschlitz, 1998). The human's inherent resistance to change and the seemingly unending task of implementing change relative to the CCIS makes the role of system champion imperative to its successful implementation. The system champion is responsible for overseeing and coordinating all aspects of system development and for avoiding or overcoming obstacles with the potential to stall its ongoing development and implementation. Only an evolving CCIS will meet tomorrow's needs.

As CCISs have matured, the functions they offer have expanded to encompass sophisticated data collection that also integrates the data with hospital information systems for longitudinal data access, after the patient leaves the ICU. In addition, the CCIS takes advantage of the functionality within the hospital information system for patient management functions related to admission, discharge, and transfer as well as provider order entry, results reporting, plans of care, and outcomes analysis.

Coordination and Scheduling of Patient Care Activities

The critical care flowsheet is a predominant display format for CCISs. As computer technology has advanced, the techniques for display of the flowsheet have been enhanced.

The goal of a CCIS is to have as much information integrated into the system as possible to obtain a comprehensive picture of the patient. As critically ill patients generate massive amounts of data, the challenge is to create logical "chunks" of information in the form of flowsheets.

Ultimately, all information pertaining to the patient should be contained in the electronic record. Access to comprehensive patient information collected across all care settings facilitates care delivery, safety, and quality.

Development of CCIS is a time-consuming process and requires user participation to ensure that the elements contained within the CCIS are appropriate for the organization and patient population(s). The selection of which CCIS function to implement and the order of implementation should also be considered carefully to facilitate a smooth transition to an automated record. The decision should be aligned with the goals and strategy of the critical care environment.

CCISs are most often used as bedside systems; i.e., there is usually access to the system at every bedside in a critical care unit as well as at the central station and various other locations. This, of course, will vary from hospital to hospital and is dependent on many factors, such as budget, space, and unit philosophy.

Personal computers (PCs) are almost universally employed in CCISs. These PCs are linked together by networks. The PCs perform data entry and screen management functions, and are frequently referred to as workstations. In addition, windows, structured lists, and icons can be used to make computer interaction easier and more meaningful to the clinical users.

Using PCs also allows access to the regular computer capabilities of the workstation. There is usually a method of exiting from the CCIS program and accessing the general computer functions of the workstation. This ability to leave the CCIS is controlled by the CCIS security system, and authorization to do so is determined by each organization. Once outside of the CCIS, the authorized user may have complete access to all computing features of the PC or may be restricted to a specific menu of software. Work processing, spreadsheets, and database management systems are some of the programs that could be available. In addition, if access to the full power of the computer is allowed, a user might write other programs to meet specific needs. As with central station monitors that allow the user to exit from the clinical applications, user organizations must consider the potential benefits and hazards of using this feature. Policies, procedures, and user education programs must be developed to address concerns and issues.

Although studies show that use of bedside documentation systems result in cost reductions based on reported full-time equivalent reductions, increased revenue, better bed use, documentation that supports patient charges, and identification of best practice patterns, there are other benefits to be reaped. Other benefits include improvement in nursing productivity, quality of nursing documentation, and bed management and a decrease in patient length of stay (Butler and Bender, 1999).

 Future Developments

As clinical information systems mature, their use in the patient care environment will become more pervasive. Adoption of a standard interface language will further promote the development of the clinical information systems. As the patient moves through the ambulatory, critical care and medical/surgical areas, patient caregivers will need easy access to secure information (Gartner, 2004). This necessitates thinking beyond the critical care environment in order to facilitate the integration of information between each of the patient care settings. Meaningful exchange of information will require standardized vocabularies in the various patient care settings. If this meaningful exchange can be achieved, a lifetime medical record for each patient becomes possible. A collection of these lifetime records in a clinical data repository enables trending for patient populations, comparison of an individual to that trend, and decision support for patient care strategies.

The development of clinical pathways and outcomes management are important in improving critical care performance. Outcomes are measurements made to determine the course of an illness and the effects of treatments on this course. CCISs can assist outcomes management by facilitating the identification and analysis of the relationships between clinical interventions and outcomes as well as between outcomes and cost. Three types of data are useful in supporting outcomes analysis: input variables, which stratify patients into comparable groups; interventions; and outcomes (Dolin, 1997). In order to measure clinical outcomes without bias, the performance of critical care areas must be evaluated in meaningful ways, and this may include data following discharge of the patient from the critical care area (Teres et al., 1998). This reinforces the need to use standard language between patient care settings.

CCISs have recently been discussed as tools to assist in diagnosis of patient conditions through use of neural networks. Neural networks are computer simulations of the brain that are capable of converting incoming activities into outgoing activities. The conversion includes weighting of the various inputs according to their strength of influence and then transformation of the inputs according to a predefined function (Hinton, 1992). If a set of diagnostic data could be defined as well as the relationships between those data points, the predictive ability of the neural network could be used to recognize patterns of symptoms, signs, and laboratory data diagnostic of a particular pathologic process. Before neural networks can be used in this manner, these definitions and relationships must be defined (Armoni, 1998; Buchman, 1995).

The evolution of computer hardware is extremely rapid. The swift growth of affordable memory permits storage of information that is processed and exchanged with increasing rapidity. This evolution supports previously unimaginable innovation in the area of patient care. An example of such an innovation is the use of voice recognition in controlling technology.

There is also a growing tendency to move information using wireless communications technologies (Muschlitz, 1998). As patient stays in the ICU become shorter and shorter, monitoring is going out of the ICU and into other clinical care areas. Using a wireless approach, it is possible to configure a portable bedside monitor to the patient's needs without buying a monitor for every bedside (Wiggett, 1996). Additionally, information that is collected at the bedside, e.g., admitting or registration data, can be transferred wirelessly to a remote database.

 Summary

Critical care nursing has been defined as a nursing specialty dealing with human responses to life-threatening problems. Critical care nursing can be practiced in any setting but is most often found in critical care units. The complexities of patient care in these settings have resulted in the development of technology to help nurses deliver that care. In this chapter, some of these technologies have been discussed. These include arrhythmia, hemodynamic, and physiologic monitoring systems; special-purpose systems; and CCISs. The basic functions of hemodynamic monitoring systems were described, as were the most common features that enhance their utilization. The trend toward noninvasive monitoring systems was discussed. Principal goals and purposes of CCISs, as well as a history of their development were presented. The most common CCIS information management features were presented. Modern CCISs incorporate PC technology into workstations that provide extensive computer power and many user-friendly functions. The monitor/device technology infrastructure allows multiple patient care devices to communicate with a CCIS. Technology continues to develop at a rapid rate, and the use of computers in critical care settings will continue to expand. Not only information systems, but also specific patient care devices, will proliferate and contribute to the information flood that has generated the need for the computer systems in the first place. Coping with technology overload is an essential skill for nurses. Learning the concepts and principles of CCIS applications presented in this chapter can be more important than focusing on a particular system or device. Understanding the basic elements will enable nurses to more easily adapt and adopt new equipment and systems.

References

Ahrens, T. (1999a). Hemodynamic monitoring. *Critical Care Nursing Clinics of North America* 11(1): 19–31.

Ahrens, T. (1999b). Continuous mixed venous (SvO$_2$) monitoring: Too expensive or indispensible? *Critical Care Nursing Clinics of North America* 11(1): 33–48.

Ahrens, T. and Tucker, K. (1999). Pulse oximetry. *Critical Care Nursing Clinics of North America* 11(1):87–98.

American Hospital Association. (1999). Report of the American Hospital Association Task Force on Medical Telemetry. Unpublished.

Armoni, A. (1998). Use of neural networks in medical diagnosis. *M.D. Computing* 15(2):100–104.

Bates, D. and Gawande, A. (2003). Patient safety: Improving safety with information technology. *New England Journal of Medicine* 348(25):2526–2534.

Belzberg, H., Murray, J., Shoemaker, W. C., et al. (1996). Use of large databases for resolving critical care problems. *New Horizons* 4(4):532–540.

Buchman, T. G. (1995). Computers in the intensive care unit: Promises yet to be fulfilled. *Journal for Intensive Care Medicine* 10(5):234–240.

Burchell, S. A., Yu, M., Takiguchi, S. A., Ohta, R. M., and Myers, S. A. (1997). Evaluation of a continuous cardiac output and mixed venous oxygen saturation catheter in critically ill surgical patients. *Critical Care Medicine* 25(3):388–391.

Butler, M. A. and Bender, A. D. (1999). Intensive care unit bedside documentation systems: Realizing cost savings and quality improvements. *Computers in Nursing* 17(1):32–38.

Clochesy, J. M. (1989). *Advanced Technology in Critical Care Nursing*. Rockville, MD: Aspen.

Cook, B. (1997). Computerized patient records—the off-the-shelf choice. *Healthcare Technology Management* 8(6):34–35.

Dolin, R. H., (1997). Outcome analysis: Considerations for an electronic health record. *M.D. Computing* 14(1):50–56.

Elder, A. (1991). Setting up and using a cardiac monitor. *Nursing* 91:21(3):58–63.

Gardner, R., Bradshaw, K., and Hollingsworth, K. (1989). Computerizing the intensive care unit: Current status and future direction. *Journal of Cardiovascular Nursing* 4(1):68–78.

Headley, J. M. (1998). Invasive hemodynamic monitoring: Applying advanced technologies. *Critical Care Nursing Quarterly* 21(2):73–84.

Hinton, G. E. (1992). How neural networks learn from experience. *Scientific American* 267(3):145–151.

Hirschl, M. M., Binder, M., Gwenchenberger, M., et al. (1997). Noninvasive assessment of cardiac output in critically ill patients by analysis of the finger blood pressure waveform. *Critical Care Medicine* 25(11):1909–1914.

Kenner, C. V. (1990). Hemodynamic monitoring. In B. Dorsey, C. Guzzetta, and C. Kenner (Eds.), *Essentials of Critical Care Nursing* (pp. 206–236). Philadelphia, PA: Lippincott.

Kidd, P. S. and Wagner, K. D., (2001). *High Acuity Nursing* (3rd ed.). Upper Saddle River, NJ: Prentice-Hall.

Lasater, M. (1998). The view within: The emerging technology of thoracic electrical bioimpedance. *Critical Care Nursing Quarterly* 21(3):97–101.

Lewis, S. M., Heitkemper, M. M., and Dirksen, S. R. (2004). *Medical-Surgical Nursing* (6th ed.). St. Louis, MO: Mosby.

Macy, J. and James, T. (1971). The value and limitations of computer monitoring in myocardial infarction. *Progress in Cardiovascular Diseases* 13: 495–505.

Martin, N. and Hendrickson, P. (1999). Telemetry monitoring in acute and critical care. *Critical Care Nursing Clinics of North America* 11(1):77–85.

McGrow, K. M., Roys, R., Maloney, R. C., and Xiao, Y. (2004). Using wireless technologies to improve information flow for interhospital transfers of critical care patients. *Critical Care Nurse.* 24:66–7.

Mihm, F. G., Geetinger, A., Hanson, C. W., et al. (1998). A multicenter evaluation of a new continuous cardiac output pulmonary artery catheter system. *Critical Care Medicine* 26(8):1346–1350.

Milholland, D. and Cardona, J. (1983). Computers at the bedside. *American Journal of Nursing* 83:1304–1307.

Mirvis, D., Benson, A., Goldberger, A., et al. (1989). Instrumentation and practice standards for electrocardiographic monitoring in special care units: A report for health professionals by a task force of the Council on Clinical Cardiology: American Heart Association. *Circulation* 79(2):464–471.

Muschlitz, L. (1998). Linda Reeder, HIMSS liaison and Intesys applications specialist. *Healthcare Technology Management* 9(4):32–34.

Rocker, G., Cook, D., Sjokvist, P., et al. (2004). Clinician predictions of intensive care unit mortality. *Critical Care Medicine* 32(5):1149–1154.

Shoemaker, W. C., Wo, C. C. J., Bishop, M. H., et al. (1994). Multicenter trial of a new thoracic electrical bioimpedance device for cardiac output estimation. *Critical Care Medicine* 22(12):1907–1912.

Sorkin, J. and Bloomfeld, D. (1982). Computers of critical care. *Heart and Lung* 11:287–293.

Teres, D., Higgins, T., Steinrub, J., et al. (1998). Defining a high-performance ICU system for the 21st century: A position paper. *Journal of Intensive Care Medicine* 13(4):195–205.

Tsien, C. L. and Fackler, J. C. (1997). Poor prognosis for existing monitors in the intensive care unit. *Critical Care Medicine* 25(4):614–619.

Von Reuden, K. T. and Turner, M. A. (1999). Advances in continuous, noninvasive hemodynamic surveillance: Impedance cardiography. *Critical Care Nursing Clinics of North America* 11(3):63–75.

Widman, L. (1992). The Einthoven system: Toward an improved cardiac arrhythmia monitor. In P. Clayton (Ed.), *Fifteenth Annual Symposium on Computer Applications in Medical Care* (pp. 441–445). New York: McGraw-Hill.

Wiggett, J. (1996). Off the wall with patient monitors. *Healthcare Technology Management* 7(11):24–25.

Bibliography

Kinney, M. R., Pacha, D. R., and Dunbar, S. B. (1988). *AACN's Clinical Reference for Critical Care* (2nd ed.). New York: McGraw-Hill.

Saba, V. K. and McCormick, K. A. (1996). *Essentials of Computers for Nurses* (2nd ed.). New York: McGraw-Hill.

Seyer, S. and Schroeder, L. (1997). Data trap. *Healthcare Technology Management* 8(6):24–27.

22

Community Health Applications

Cynthia M. Struk

Donna Ambler Peters

Virginia K. Saba

OBJECTIVES

1. Define the scope of community health nursing (CHN).
2. Describe vocabularies and classifications used for community health systems.
3. Discuss data sets and their use in community health nursing (CHN).
4. Discuss computer systems for community health.
5. Discuss use of telemedicine in community health.
6. Discuss future trends.

KEY WORDS

information systems
community health nursing (CHN)
public health
home health
home care
decision support

CHN is a synthesis of nursing practice and public health practice applied to promoting and preserving the health of populations (American Nurses Association, 1980). The scope is not limited to a particular age, diagnostic group, or practice setting. It requires a comprehensive understanding and knowledge of the framework of the community, its resources, and the sociocultural issues impacting people within the community. The focus is on the population as a whole even though nursing care may be directed toward families, individuals, or groups. The standards of CHN incorporate health promotion, health maintenance, health education, health management, coordination, and continuity of care using a holistic approach. CHN is practiced in public health departments, ambulatory care settings, group practices, outpatient clinics, freestanding community-based clinics, and in homes.

Computer systems and/or applications for CHN have been developed to support clinical practice but because of the broad scope of services there is a wide variance in applications. In addition, due to the multiple practice settings, applications are often targeted toward specific functional needs rather than clinical care or service delivery. Application examples may include population focused (tracking childhood immunization rates in a health department), continuity-of-care needs (patient hospital data available in an outpatient setting for specific diagnostic groups), and/or billing of services (point-of-care system for documenting home healthcare assessment to create a home health-related group [HHRG] for episodic payment). Since the underlying need for data varies in community health practice settings, the information system structures developed may offer functions for simple tracking of clinical data (vital signs, immunizations) to more complex applications related to portable medical data, billing, financial applications, statistical reporting, and decision support.

This chapter provides an overview of the development of CHN computer systems and/or applications as well as a description of the major types of community health, public health, and home health systems and/or applications.

Community Health Nursing System Development

CHN agencies have used computers since the late 1960s, when computers were introduced into the healthcare industry. Many of the early systems focused on regulatory compliance, billing applications, and statistical reporting related to community health, which encompasses public health and home health compliance. As healthcare services continued to evolve, community health services grew primarily due to consumer choice, cost control initiatives, and the increase in numbers of healthcare recipients with chronic illnesses. Concurrently the numbers of hospital beds were decreasing with an increase of services in community health settings (Elfrink and Martin, 1996).

The changing healthcare trends have been the impetus for increasingly sophisticated management information systems (MISs), which transformed data into information to measure outcomes, track client progress, exchange healthcare information among physicians, nurses, insurers, managed care companies, regulatory agencies, and public reporting, and analyze financial data. These systems supported clinical care delivery, electronic billing, and had the potential for multiple user access.

Further advancements led to four domains of concentration which directed unique MISs for practice: (1) public health that focused on population interventions and the outcomes related to epidemiologic and/or mortality/ morbidity trends; (2) home health that focused on skilled nursing care for individuals in the home and the outcomes related to care delivery for individuals or aggregated populations; (3) special population community practices (i.e., mental health) that focused on specific diagnostic care and/or treatment needs and the outcomes related to care delivery for individuals, diagnostic groups, and/or aggregated populations; and (4) outpatient care that focused on intermittent, episodic, or preventative care for individuals and the outcomes related to interventions for individuals and/or aggregate groups, inclusive of national health prevention standards. Concurrently, these MISs also offered clinical documentation capabilities at the point of care, provided billing functions, supported submission by computer of data for regulatory compliance, provided statistical reporting, and even developed decision support features.

Home Health

Medicare and Medicaid Legislation

With the enactment of the Medicare and Medicaid Legislation in 1965, reimbursement for home care services was allowed. Home healthcare is a very broad term used to describe the provision of preventive, therapeutic, restorative, and supportive healthcare in the home (Wieland, Ferrell, and Rubenstein, 1991). It is one part of the ongoing continuum of community health services.

This new legislation expanded the demand for home care services, increased the number of home health agencies (HHAs), and increased the information needs that created the driving force for computer systems. As a result, as early as 1969, several commercial vendors, service bureaus, and commercial companies developed billing and financial systems for HHAs. These data processing systems were primarily designed to satisfy the basic need for reporting to payers and regulatory bodies, processing the information required for billing, monitoring the certification requirements, and managing the home health services allowed by Medicare, Medicaid, and third-party payers. These systems captured patient demographics, visits, accounts payable, and journal entries for the purposes of producing standard reports, billing forms, regulatory documents (HCFA 485: Physician Plan of Treatment), visit summaries, and financial balances. Although valuable, they created organizational inefficiencies, because the basic software design did not share data among applications, and thus data had to be rekeyed when used for multiple purposes (Peters and McKeon, 1998; HCFA, 1980).

Balanced Budget Act

With the enactment of the Balanced Budget Act (BBA) of 1997, the need for information moved beyond billing information, statistical information, and the tracking of clinical data. Beginning, October 1, 2000, the Center for Medicare and Medicaid Services (CMS) instituted a prospective payment system (PPS) for Medicare home health beneficiaries as part of the BBA. The HHA relied on a 80-category case-mix adjuster to set payment rates based on 23 responses from questions from the outcome and assessment information set (OASIS) in the domains of clinical severity, functional status, and service utilization (CMS, 2003). The answers to these questions were weighted and scored, which were then equated to the relative intensity of care required by quantifying the dollar amount per 60-day episode. There were 80 possible iterations of scoring, which were entitled HHRG. These were similar to the hospital system of diagnostic related groups (DRG) that determined the level of reimbursement for hospitalized patients. This integrated payment system necessitated linkages between clinical, administrative, operations, and billing functions. In addition, it created a need for linkages among and between other home care providers, state regulatory bodies, and the fiscal intermediary responsible for paying Medicare reimbursement directly to the agency. OASIS information is also required to be transmitted to the state regularly with billing notification to CMS. Each agency is no longer able to provide care independently because a patient's 60-day episode of care is based with the agency that submits the initial request for anticipated payment (RAP) unless specific conditions are met for the transfer of care (HCFA, 2000). The interrelationship of these functions has created an even greater demand for information technology (IT) systems and/or applications in the home.

Outcome Measures Concurrently, a focus on quality initiatives further supported the need for IT. CMS began using the OASIS data set for the purpose of monitoring outcomes and adverse events based on risk-adjusted patient characteristics for all Medicare-certified HHAs. This has led to common home health outcome measures that are used for evaluating an individual agency's clinical practice based on regional and national benchmarks. These have also been publicly released to consumers for comparison among HHAs. The Joint Commission on Accreditation of Health Care Organizations (JCAHO) under their outcome-based quality improvement (OBQI) initiative has also supported the use of OASIS outcome measures as an important indicator of the quality and appropriateness of care (JCAHO, 2002).

◼ Public Health

The Institute of Medicine (IOM) defines public health as a "coordinated effort at the local, state, and federal levels whose mission is fulfilling society's interest in assuring conditions in which people can be healthy" (Institute of Medicine, 2004). Public health professionals focus on (1) preventing, identifying, investigating, and eliminating community health problems; (2) assuring that the community has access to competent personal healthcare services; and (3) educating and empowering individuals to adopt more healthy behaviors (National Institute of Health, 1996). The history and use of public health information systems have developed from this focus.

State and Local Health Departments

In the 1970s and early 1980s, many state/local official health departments developed statistical reporting systems for processing information on nursing personnel, programs, and services. Many of these reporting systems are still in use. They were primarily developed to manage the information requirements for the agency's CHN services. For example, one of the earliest systems, the Florida Client Information System funded by the Division of Nursing, Public Health Service, and DHHS, was developed to register eligible residents and to collect encounter information on those residents receiving CHN services. It was the first online statewide computerized community health system in the country (Florida Department of Health and Rehabilitation Services, 1983). The collection, analysis, use, and communication of health-related information has been called the "quintessential public health service," because all public health activities depend to some extent on the availability of accurate, comparable, and timely information (Lasker, 1995). Although, public health was an early adopter of computer technology, it has typically used information systems for categorical functions such as collecting electronic birth and death data, communicable disease reporting, immunization tracking, survey analysis, and incident and exposure tracking (NCHS, 1994).

Public Health Challenges

Currently, public health is facing many new challenges for information as a result of issues such as bioterrorism, health plans recognizing the need to evaluate prevention activities to improve the quality of life and reduce costs, healthcare providers recognizing the need to integrate public data into individual health records, and health departments needing to monitor the impact of community-wide interventions for improving the health of populations in communities.

For all venues of CHN, software developers responded by developing electronic IT systems instead of outdated data processing/computer systems. Their emphasis shifted from task support to providing both individual clinical information and population data as a strategic resource for community health practice. These IT systems allow for the following (Peters and McKeon, 1998):

◼ Relational databases that facilitate the retrieval of data for multiple purposes without rekeying

◼ Manipulation of data to create information and knowledge

- Point-of-care devices, computerized patient records (CPRs), and/or electronic health records (EHRs)
- Clinical repositories as a strategic resource for quality and practice
- Electronic interfacing systems to facilitate the sharing of data

The deployment of electronic IT systems will greatly increase the access to detailed information regarding community healthcare practice. As the richness of this information grows, healthcare providers, public health departments, patients, and others will want and need access to the information. This will drive the need for many new applications for integrated community information networks which can merge registries (vital statistics, immunizations), support local and federal initiatives for national public health information, provide linkage to healthcare providers (public clinics, private clinics, home health), and integrate data from key regulatory or public reporting systems.

A critical step in this process of generating more information for community health is the definition of a data set using a consistent health vocabulary or classification that will enable the sharing of information (Bruegel, 1998; Reichley, 1999). Aggregating clinical data sets of community health patients with like conditions provides the basis for standardizing and tracking processes and outcomes of care. Aggregating clinical data for all community health patients provides evidence to show the results of community health services in terms of value, quality, and cost-efficiency. A standardized language and/or nomenclature also allows for data to be used universally. Some of the projects involved in defining a community health data set, vocabulary, and/or classification system are described. The Public Health Data Standards Consortium was established to address these issues of standards and launched in 2003 to provide information about the consortium's committees and activities through its Web site (*http://phdatastandards.info*).

Data Sets

A uniform data set is a minimum set of items of information with uniform definition and categories, concerning the specific dimension of the service or practice setting that meets the essential information needs of multiple data users within the scope of the service or practice setting. Criteria that define a data set may include:

- Utility for multiple users
- Terms that can be defined and measured
- Common or shared language that is universally understood
- Relevance to national or local needs
- Uniformity with other applicable data sets
- Data can be coded for computer processing
- Data has portability to other applicable data sets
- Data can be structured in compliance with Health Insurance Portability and Accountability Act (HIPAA)
- Data can be collected easily and accurately through the functions of service delivery

Selected Data Sets

Several uniform data sets were developed by different organizations and governmental agencies for depicting their standardized vocabularies. The National League for Nursing developed one of the first prototypes for a basic minimum data set for CHN even though it is no longer being used (NLN, 1977). The nursing minimum data set (NMDS) developed by Werley and Lang (1988) was designed for all healthcare settings but focused primarily on the hospital setting. It consisted of 12 major elements, four of which are specific for nursing care: nursing diagnosis, intervention, outcome, and intensity. The remaining focus on the demographic and service elements. Other data sets that have impacted on CHN include the following.

Uniform Data Set for Home Care and Hospice

In 1993, the National Association of Home Care (NAHC) Resource Committee initiated a task force to develop a uniform data set for Home Care and Hospice. The need for a minimum data set was identified by NAHC as critical and was considered to be the first step toward achieving standardized, comparable home care and hospice data. The data set is organized into two major categories of organizational and individual level data elements. On an organizational level, the data set includes items that describe the organization, its services, its aggregate utilization, and its financial and personnel data. On the individual level, items include demographic, clinical, service, and utilization data for patients/clients (National Association of Home Care, 1994). In 1997, the NAHC Information Resources and Quality Assurance Committee added the OASIS data set to the uniform data set. The standardized data elements and definitions are available on their Web site (*www.nahc.org*). Figure 22.1 provides a sample of the clinical data elements and definitions. NAHC publishes the data elements and definitions so that entities involved in home care and hospice data collection can use these definitions when constructing surveys and questionnaires.

Outcome and Assessment Information Set (OASIS)

This is a group of items that represents the core items of a comprehensive assessment for an adult home health patient and forms the basis for measuring patient out-comes for purposes of OBQI (CMS, 2003). Most data items in the OASIS were derived as part of a CMS-funded national research program, co-funded by the Robert Wood Johnson Foundation to develop a system of outcome measures for home healthcare (Shaughnessy and Crisler, 1995). The core items were refined over time based on clinical and empirical research. The data set is comprised of 79 health and functional status patient assessment items that are discipline-neutral and when measured at two or more points in time serve as outcome measures (Fig. 22.2). They are not designed for mater-nity, pediatric, or hospice patients. These items are clini-cally more precise than most existing HHA assessment items, thereby maximizing the consistency of ratings among different clinicians collecting the same informa-tion. This allows for benchmarking data within and among HHAs. Agencies are required to integrate these assessment items into their existing assessment process and to collect them at defined time points in care delivery

---

CLINICAL ITEMS

54

Data Element Name: Medical Diagnosis
Definition: Any medical diagnoses that affect the care provided by the home care organization as defined by ICD-CM codes:
Principal: The diagnosis most responsible for the admission of the patient/client for home care service
Other: All other diagnoses that affect the care provided by the home care organization
Not applicable: If the home care services are not related to healthcare needs (e.g., homemaker)

55

Data Element Name: Surgical Procedures
Definition: Any surgical procedure that affects the care provided by the home care organization as defined by ICD-CM or CPT codes.

56

Data Element Name: Functional Status
Definition: Description of the individual's ability to perform activities of daily living and instrumental activities of daily living.
Comment: Need to decide on what measures to use. Some suggested sources are Katz, Uniform Needs Assessment, Long-Term Health Care Data Set, Nursing Home Resident Assessment Data Set, Outcome Assessment Item Set (OASIS), Functional Independence Measure (FIM), and Karnofsky Performance Scale.

57

Data Element Name: Patient/Client Problem
Definition: Clinical judgement made by professional healthcare personnel about a human response to an actual or potential health problem.
Comment: Possible approaches are Omaha system, Clinical Care Classifixation (CCC) previously Home Health Care Classification (HHCC), North America Nursing Diagnosis Association (NANDA).

Figure 22.1
Sample of hospice and home health data set definitions for clinical items.
(Courtesy of National Association of Home Health Care, 2004 *www.nahc.org*)

Severity rating

0—Asymptomatic, no treatment needed at this time
1—Symptoms well controlled with current therapy
2—Symptoms controlled with difficulty, affecting daily functioning: patient needs ongoing monitoring
3—Symptoms poorly controlled, patient needs frequent adjustment in treatment and dose monitoring
4—Symptoms poorly controlled, history of rehospitalizations

(M0230) Primary diagnosis	ICD-9-CM	Severity rating
a. _____	(_ _ _ _ . _ _ _)	☐ 0 ☐ 1 ☐ 2 ☐ 3 ☐ 4
(M0240) Other diagnoses	**ICD-9-CM**	**Severity rating**
b. _____	(■_ _ _ _ . _ _ _)	☐ 0 ☐ 1 ☐ 2 ☐ 3 ☐ 4
c. _____	(■_ _ _ _ . _ _ _)	☐ 0 ☐ 1 ☐ 2 ☐ 3 ☐ 4
d. _____	(■_ _ _ _ . _ _ _)	☐ 0 ☐ 1 ☐ 2 ☐ 3 ☐ 4
e. _____	(■_ _ _ _ . _ _ _)	☐ 0 ☐ 1 ☐ 2 ☐ 3 ☐ 4
f. _____	(■_ _ _ _ . _ _ _)	☐ 0 ☐ 1 ☐ 2 ☐ 3 ☐ 4

Effective 10/1/2003

(M0245) Payment diagnosis (optional): If a V-code was reported in M0230 in place of a case mix diagnosis, list the primary diagnosis and ICD-9-CM code, determined in accordance with OASIS requirements in effect before October 1, 2003-no V-codes, E-codes, or surgical codes allowed. ICD-9-CM sequencing requirements must be followed. Complete both lines (a) and (b) if the case mix diagnosis is a manifestation code or in other situations where multiple coding is indicated for the primary diagnosis; otherwise, complete line (a) only.

(M0245) Primary diagnosis	ICD-9-CM
a. _____	(_ _ _ _ . _ _ _)
(M0245) First secondary diagnosis	**ICD-9-CM**
b. _____	(_ _ _ _ . _ _ _)

(M0250) Therapies the patient receives **at home;** (Mark all that apply.)

☐ 1—Intravenous or infusion therapy (excludes TPN)
☐ 2—Parenteral nutrition (TPN or lipids)
☐ 3—Enteral nutrition (nasogastric, gastrostomy, jejunostomy, or any other artificial entry into the alimentary canal)
☐ 4—None of the above

(M0260) Overall prognosis: BEST description of patient's overall prognosis for **recovery from this episode of illness.**

☐ 0—Poor: Little or no recovery is expected and/or further decline is imminent
☐ 1—Good/fair: Partial to full recovery is expected
☐ UK—Unknown

(M0270) Rahabilitative prognosis: BEST description of patient's prognosis for **functional status.**

☐ 0—Guarded: Minimal improvement in functional status is expected; decline is possible
☐ 1—Good: Marked improvement in functional status is expected
☐ UK—Unknown

(M0280) Life expectancy: (Physician documentation is not required.)

☐ 0—Life expectancy is greater than 6 months
☐ 1—Life expectancy is 6 months or fewer

Figure 22.2
Sample of OASIS assessment form.
(Courtesy of 2002, Center for Health Services and Policy Research, Denver, CO OASIS-B1 SOC.)

which is minimally at admission to home healthcare and every 60 days. The data set was mandated by CMS in 1999 for all Medicare-certified agencies.

As of October 2000, the data set has also served as the basis for prospective payment. The answers to selected OASIS questions are weighted and compiled to create a case mix adjuster, which is mathematically formulated and based on patient risk-adjusted characteristics and the wage index in the metropolitan statistical area where the patient resides. It serves as a method to provide payment based on anticipated resource use for each 60-day episode of care.

Outcome-Based Quality Improvement   In early 2002, the OBQI framework was established (similar to a data set). It included two components: outcome analysis and outcome enhancement. The outcome analysis component begins with home care agencies transmitting the OASIS data to a central repository which then produces outcome, case mix, and adverse event reports on an annual basis. The all patients' outcome report provides a risk-adjusted comparison of agency performance measured in terms of patient outcomes that are relative to a national reference or benchmark sample. The 41 outcome measures include functional, physiologic, emotional/behavioral, cognitive, and healthcare utilization measures. The second component, outcome enhance-

ment, allows agencies to use the data for OBQI activities at the agency level and will assist the Medicare survey and certification process by providing specific information regarding the individual HHA's performance. As an extension of the OBQI initiative, selected outcome measures were made public in the fall of 2003 (Fig. 22.3). This is part of a four-prong effort to improve the quality of care for consumers by:

- Regulation and enforcement activities conducted by state survey agencies and CMS
- Improved consumer information on the quality of care provided by HHAs
- Continual community-based quality improvement programs for HHAs
- Collaboration and partnership to leverage knowledge and resources (CMS, 2003)

Health Plan Employer Data and Information Set (HEDIS)

HEDIS is a set of standardized performance measures designed to ensure that purchasers and consumers have the information for reliably comparing the performance of managed healthcare plans. The measures are related to many significant public health issues such as cancer,

Consumer Language	OASIS Outcome Measure
Patients who get better at getting dressed	Improvement in upper body dressing
Patients who get better at bathing	Improvement in bathing
Patients who stay the same (do not get worse) at bathing	Stabilization in bathing
Patients who get better getting to and from the toilet	Improvement in toileting
Patients who get better at walking or moving around	Improvement in ambulation/locomotion
Patients who get better at getting in and out of bed	Improvement in transferring
Patients who get better at taking their medicines correctly (by mouth)	Improvement in management of oral medications
Patients who are confused less often	Improvement in confusion frequency
Patients who have less pain when moving around	Improvement in pain interfering with activity
Patients who had to be admitted to the hospital	Acute care hospitalization
Patients who need urgent, unplanned medical care	Any emergent care provided

Figure 22.3
Home health quality measures consumer language.
(Courtesy of CMS, 2003.)

heart disease, smoking, asthma, and diabetes. There is also a standardized survey of consumers' experiences that evaluates plan performance related to customer service, access to care, and claims processing (NCQA, 2004). These measures cross many community health applications as they evaluate care along the continuum of practice from inpatient care through community-based care. Table 22.1 provides a summary table of measures and product lines.

Vocabulary Languages

Vocabularies are validated clinical reference languages, taxonomies, or terminologies that make healthcare knowledge more usable and accessible. The language, vocabulary, or taxonomy enables a consistent way of capturing, sharing, and aggregating health data across sites of care. The vocabulary serves as the vehicle to format messages that are exchanged between computer systems and the coding and classification scheme used within the messages. For data to flow between systems it is necessary for the messages to have agreement in syntax so that the individual data elements can be structured in a common way. There are several vocabularies in use for classifying and coding both medical and nursing vocabularies; however, the two most common nursing vocabularies or taxonomies in use for CHN include Clinical Care Classification (CCC) system (Saba, 2004) (previously known as the Home Health Care Classification [HHCC], Saba 1994a) and the Omaha System (Martin and Sheet, 1995).

Intensity Classifications

Classifications are broadly defined as the grouping or quantification of patients based on observable or inferred characteristics. These characteristics are then quantified as a measure of nursing effort and/or interventions needed for care delivery. Classification systems that focus on patient classification/intensity have been developed that provide information needed to measure care needs, predict resource use, and determine the requirements of home care. Classifying the intensity of patient needs for home care services depends on a great number of factors including physical well being, environment, level of independence, self-care ability, and the skill level of the patient and/or caretakers (Anderson, Pena, and Helms, 1998). Findings from Fortinsky and Madigan (1997) further support that patient outcomes and resource consumption are expected to vary accord-

ing to patients' admission characteristics and that changes in patients' clinical and functional health are expected to be influenced by the volume and intensity of home care services delivered. Home care needs are influenced by the actual health condition/diagnosis, environmental situation, support, and interventions required by the patient/caregiver to manage their disease condition. In home health, not all visits are equal; patients have different care needs and require different amounts of nursing care time.

HHAs have moved to episodic reimbursement for all Medicare patients and to some capitated models for non-Medicare patients based on disease condition or service. Therefore, patient needs have become critical for the HHA to be able to determine and/or predict the level of resources for an episode of care. Additionally, the resources used will also have an effect on the quality of care process and outcome for the individual patient and their caregivers.

Classification systems focusing on patient intensity developed for HHAs generally use different levels of care or client characteristics as the method for classifying patients. They are different from the acuity classification methods, based on workload measurements and developed for predicting nurse-staffing levels in hospitals. Generally, hospitals' methods predict hours of patient care required based on a list of patient care activities weighted by predetermined workload measures.

Clinical Care Classification System

The CCC system, previously known as the HHCC system is a standardized language/vocabulary consisting of two interrelated taxonomies—the CCC of Nursing Diagnoses and the CCC of Nursing Interventions—both of which are classified by 21 care components (Version 2.0). The CCC is designed to document, code, and classify for computer-processing patient care in any clinical setting by any healthcare provider using a standardized framework. Further they are used to electronically track and analyze patient care over time, across settings, population groups, and geographic locations (Saba and McCormick, 2001; Saba, 2004).

The CCC of Nursing Diagnoses (Version 2.0) consists of 182 (59 major and 123 subcategories) nursing diagnoses and/or patient problems which uses three modifiers: (a) improve patient's condition, (b) stabilize patient's condition, and/or (c) support the patient's deteriorating condition. These diagnostic modifiers depict 546 terms used to measure the actual outcomes of the nursing diagnoses and/or patient problems.

Table 22.1   HEDIS 2004 Summary Table of Measures and Product Lines

HEDIS 2004 Measures	Applicable To			
	Medicaid	Commercial	Medicare	PPO
Effectiveness of care				
Childhood immunization status	×	×		
Adolescent immunization status	×	×		
Appropriate treatment for children with upper respiratory infection	×	×		
Appropriate testing for children with pharyngitis	×	×		
Colorectal cancer screening		×	×	
Breast cancer screening	×	×	×	
Cervical cancer screening	×	×		
Chlamydia screening in women	×	×		
Osteoporosis management in women who had a fracture			×	
Controlling high blood pressure	×	×	×	
Beta-blocker treatment after a heart attack	×	×	×	
Cholesterol management after acute cardiovascular event	×	×	×	
Comprehensive diabetes care	×	×	×	
Use of appropriate medications for people with asthma	×	×		
Follow-up after hospitalization for mental illness	×	×	×	
Antidepressant medication management	×	×	×	
Medical assistance with smoking cessation	×	×	× (ASTQ only)	
Flu shots for adults age 50–64		×		
Flu shots for older adults			×	
Pneumonia vaccination status for older adults			×	
Medicare health outcomes survey			×	
Management of urinary incontinence in older adults			×	
Access/availability of care				
Adults access to preventive/ambulatory health services	×	×	×	
Children's and adolescents' access to primary care practitioners	×	×		
Prenatal and postpartum care	×	×		
Annual dental visit	×			
Initiation and engagement of alcohol and other drug dependence treatment	×	×	×	
Claims timeliness	×	×	×	×
Call answer timeliness	×	×	×	×
Call abandonment	×	×	×	×
Satisfaction with the experience of care				
CAHP 3.0H Adult Survey	×	×		
CAHP 3.0H Child Survey	×	×		×
ECHO 3.0H Survey for MBHOs		× (MBHO only)		

(*Continued*)

Table 22.1   HEDIS 2004 Summary Table of Measures and Product Lines (*Continued*)

HEDIS 2004 Measures	Applicable To			
	Medicaid	Commercial	Medicare	PPO
High plan stability				
Practitioner turnover	×	×	×	
Years in business/total membership	×	×	×	
Use of services				
Frequency of ongoing prenatal care	×			
Well-child visits in the first 15 months of life	×	×		
Well-child visits in the third, fourth, fifth and sixth years of life	×	×		
Adolescent well-care visit	×	×		
Frequency of selected procedures	×	×	×	
Inpatient utilization—general hospital/acute care	×	×	×	
Ambulatory care	×	×	×	
Inpatient utilization—nonacute care	×	×	×	
Discharge and average length of stay—maternity care	×	×		
Cesarean section rate	×	×		
Vaginal birth after cesarean rate (VBAC Rate)	×	×		
Births and average length of stay, newborns	×	×		
Mental health utilization—inpatient discharges and average length of stay	×	×	×	
Mental health utilization—percentage of members receiving services	×	×	×	
Chemical dependency utilization—inpatient discharges and average length of stay	×	×	×	
Chemical dependency utilization—percentage of members receiving services	×	×	×	
Identification of alcohol and other drug services	×	×	×	
Outpatient drug utilization	×	×	×	
Health plan descriptive information				
Board certification	×	×	×	
Total enrollment by percentage	×	×	×	
Enrollment by product line	×	×	×	
Unduplicated count of Medicaid members	×			
Diversity of Medicaid membership	×			
Weeks of pregnancy at time of enrollment in the MCO	×			

Source: Courtesy of HEDIS which is a registered trademark of the National committee for Quality Assurance (NCQA).

The CCC of Nursing Interventions (Version 2.0) consists of 198 (72 major and 126 subcategories) nursing interventions or services which use four modifiers (a) assess or monitor, (b) care or perform, (c) teach or instruct, and/or (d) manage or refer to depict the type of intervention actions. These action types modifiers depict 792 unique interventions used to treat the nursing diagnoses and/or patient problems.

These two taxonomies are classified according to 21 care components. A care component is a cluster of elements that represent four healthcare behaviors: health behavioral, functional, physiologic, and psychologic. The care components provide a holistic approach to patient care and are used to classify, link, code, analyze, and measure outcomes (Saba, 1994b, 1995). These are shown in Table 22.2.

The CCC uses the nursing process for its conceptual model with different labels for its six phases: (1) care components (assessment), (2) diagnoses/problems (diagnosis), (3) expected outcome (outcome identification), (4) nursing interventions (planning), (5) type action (implementation), and (6) actual outcome (evaluation). The six nursing process phases provide the framework for documenting clinical nursing practice. They include all major processes that nurses follow when caring for their patients and/or clients and are used as the basis of clinical decision-making. They reflect nursing responsibilities for all patients and fundamental to the standards that influence nursing practice (American Nurses Association, 1998; Saba, 1994a).

Background   The two CCC previously known as the HHCC taxonomies were empirically derived from a research study conducted by Saba and colleagues at Georgetown University, which collected data retrospectively from 8,967 random patient records sampled from 646 Medicare-certified community health agencies. The data that were collected included two sets of narrative statements representing approximately 40,000 patient problems and/or nursing diagnoses, and 72,000 nursing interventions or services provided during an episode of care (admission to discharge). They were electronically processed using key word sorts to develop the original CCC (Version 1.0) (Saba and Zuckerman, 1992; Saba 1994a). This version was found by researchers to be usable in any healthcare setting for documenting and coding patient care by all types of vendors of IT systems to document healthcare manually or electronically. As a result, a name change occurred and the original HHCC was changed to CCC Version 2.0 in 2004 (Saba, 2004).

The two CCC taxonomies are considered to be computer-based standards recognized by the American Nurses Association in 1992 as appropriate for documenting nursing practice. They have been registered as a Health Level Seven (HL7) language; integrated into LOINC (logical observation, identifiers, names, and codes), SNOMED CT (systematized nomenclature of human and veterinary medicine reference terminology), alternative medicine ABCcodes, and the metathesaurus of the UMLS (unified medical language system) of the National Library of Medicine (NLM). They are indexed in CINAHL (cumulative index of allied and health literature) and linked to ICNP (International Classification of Nursing Practice). They have been approved and evaluated by several standards organizations. Taxonomies have been translated in numerous languages such as Korean, Portuguese, German, Spanish, Slovanic, Dutch, Norwegian, and several others (Saba 2002). See Appendix A for CCC (Version 2.0)—CCC of Nursing

Table 22.2   Clinical Care Classification (CCC) 21 Care Components

Care Component
Activity
Bowel/Gastric
Cardiac
Cognitive
Coping
Fluid volume
Health behavior
Life cycle
Medication
Metabolic
Nutritional
Physical regulation
Role relationship
Respiratory
Safety
Self-care
Self-concept
Sensory
Skin integrity
Tissue perfusion
Urinary elimination

Diagnoses and CCC of Nursing Interventions classified by the 21 care components.

CCC Uses The two CCC taxonomies serve as a standardized language for nursing and other healthcare providers. They are being used by numerous vendors of IT systems to document healthcare manually or electronically. They are being used in all types of healthcare settings for documenting patient care and for implementing decision support and evidence-based practice modules. Many hospital IT developers are offering these taxonomies for documenting patient care and/or nursing practice in the EHR. They are being used in numerous research studies such as a study by Holzemer of AIDs patients with pneumonia. He determined that the 20 care components (Version 1.0) used to categorize all care terms were found to be 99% compliant (Holzemer et al., 1997). The CCC taxonomies are also being used in nursing education (Saba and Sparks, 1998). Bakken at Columbia University School of Nursing has developed a personal digital assistant (PDA) application for documenting patient care for the nursing and nurse practitioner students using selected sets of data elements in a clinical log including the CCC taxonomies. The data elements are downloaded via wireless communication into a database where they are aggregated across patients and students to allow students to benchmark their practice and enhance faculty and clinical preceptors to evaluate student performance (Bakken et al., 2004; Klein and Bakken, 2003).

Clinical Care Pathway An emerging use being offered by IT vendors for the CCC is as an application for a clinical care pathway (CCP) since such architecture already exists in many of the next generation IT systems. A CCP can provide the standardized framework for linking and tracking the care process.

In a CCP, the 21 care components are used to correlate the assessment data for a medical condition. For example, for each medical condition care requirement, a care component diagnosis and an expected outcome are identified based on the patient's assessment. Then, based on the expected outcome/goal, the nursing interventions and type actions are selected to treat the care component diagnosis. The CCP is used to identify the interventions and type actions needed for each encounter and/or visit for the episode of care or selected time periods. This process continues until the outcome/goal is met or not met for the identified care component diagnosis, whereas the interventions and type actions determine the amount of clinical care provided and time allocated

by a nurse or other healthcare provider for each encounter/visit. Together they form the basis for the acuity and cost of care. See an example of a CCC(c) sample clinical pathway/protocol for a pneumonia in Fig. 22.4 (Saba, 2004).

The CCC is used to improve quality, ensure safety, measure outcomes, and/or determine acuity and cost. It provides concept-oriented applications that establish a standardized vocabulary to describe, communicate, and evaluate nursing and interdisciplinary practice. It facilitates the electronic documentation at the point of care and the continual evaluation and improvement of services provided.

There are several major reasons why the CCC should be used to facilitate the electronic documentation of patient care at the point of care instead of traditional paper-based methods. They consist of discrete atomic-level terms (coded data). Data once collected and coded are used many times for many purposes making for more efficient aggregation, summarization, and analysis. The CCC taxonomies are coded and comply with the format of the International Classification of Diseases (ICD-10). Each term uses a five-digit alphanumeric code to link and cross-map the terms of the two taxonomies to each other and to other classifications. The coding structure makes it possible to assess, document, and track the care process during and between encounters/visits. They are flexible, adaptable, and expandable. Finally the two taxonomies are in the public domain and available to anyone for manual or electronic use without any cost but with permission (Saba 1991, 1997; Saba and Zuckerman, 1992). See Web Site *www.sabacare.com*.

Omaha System

The Omaha System is a research-based, comprehensive taxonomy designed to generate meaningful data following usual or routine documentation of client care (Martin and Sheet, 1995). It consists of three components: the problem classification scheme, intervention scheme, and problem rating scale for outcomes. The system provides a method for linking clinical data to demographic, financial, administrative, and staffing data.

The problem classification scheme is a vocabulary for CHN. It was developed in the 1970s by the Visiting Nurse Association (VNA) of Omaha. This vocabulary is consistent with the general and comprehensive practice of CHN (Simmons, 1980). Included in the system are 44 nursing problems that were arrived at empirically from the practice of the community health nurses employed by the visiting nurse agency. The problems are

Care component Nursing diagnosis Signs and symptoms	Care component Nursing diagnosis Expected outcome	Visit 1 Nursing interventions Type actions	Visit 2 Nursing interventions Type actions	Visit 3 Nursing interventions Type actions	Care component Nursing diagnosis Actual outcome
Q Sensory Q45.1 Acute pain alteration Pain when coughing, deep breathing.	Q Sensory Q45.1.1 Improve acute pain alteration	Q47.0.1 Assess pain control ▪ Location, intensity, and duration of pain Q47.0.3 Teach pain control ▪ Appropriate use of analgesics ▪ Splint with pillow when coughing ▪ Safe use of heat to control pain	Q47.0.1 Assess pain control ▪ Assess location, intensity, and duration of pain Q47.0.3 Teach pain control ▪ Return demonstrations		Q Sensory Q45.1.1 Acute pain alteration improved ▪ No pain when coughing
L Respiratory L26.2 Breathing pattern impairment Shortness of breath when walking more than 20 ft or climbing stairs; requires home oxygen therapy	L Respiratory L26.2.2 Stabilize breathing pattern impairment	L35.0.1 Assess oxygen therapy care ▪ Use of home oxygen L35.0.2 Perform oxygen therapy care ▪ Connect tubing to compressor and set liter flow at prescribed amount L35.0.3 Teach oxygen therapy care ▪ Correct set up of home oxygen equipment L36.1.3 Teach breathing exercises ▪ Pursed lip breathing L36.2.2 Perform chest physiotherapy ▪ Chest percussion	L35.0.1 Assess oxygen therapy care ▪ Use of home oxygen L35.0.2 Perform oxygen therapy care ▪ Change tubing and nasal cannula when tubing has been used for 1 week or when it becomes crusted or soiled L36.1.3 Teach breathing exercises ▪ Return demonstration: Pursed lip breathing L36.2.2 Perform chest Physiotherapy ▪ Chest percussion	L35.0.1 Assess oxygen therapy care ▪ Use of home oxygen L35.0.3 Manage oxygen therapy care ▪ Notify DME company before using the last tubing/cannula package	L Respiratory L26.2.2 Breathing pattern impairment stabilized ▪ No shortness 4 breath using home oxygen

Figure 22.4

CCC sample clinical pathway/protocol for pneumonia.

(Saba, V.K. (2004). *Clinical Care Classification (CCC) System*. Retrieved September 4, 2004, from *www.sabacare.com*.)

Care component Nursing diagnosis Signs and symptoms	Care component Nursing diagnosis Expected outcome	Visit 1 Nursing interventions Type actions	Visit 2 Nursing interventions Type actions	Visit 3 Nursing interventions Type actions	Care component Nursing diagnosis Actual outcome
H Medication **H21 Medication risk** Unable to take inhalant/mist medications unless administered by someone else	H Medication **H21.0.1 Improve medication risk**	**H24.4.1 Assess medication treatment** ■ Knowledge and use of metered dose inhaler (MDI) **H24.4.3 Teach medication treatment** ■ Assembly of MDI, method to dispense medication, and technique to inhale medication	**H24.4.1 Assess medication treatment** ■ Knowledge and use of metered dose inhaler (MDI) **H24.4.3 Teach medication treatment** ■ Return demonstration: Assembly of MDI, method to dispense medication, and technique to inhale medication ■ Side effects of inhaled medication, and actions to take if side effects occur		H Medication **H21.0.1 Medication risk improved** ■ Able to give MDI 69 self
N Safety **N33 Injury risk** Patient only able to complete small portions of tasks (related to management of equipment); caregiver requires considerable assistance but independently completes significant portions of task (related to management of equipment)	N Safety **N33.0.1 Improve injury risk**	**N42.2.1 Assess equipment safety** ■ Equipment location, condition **N42.2.3 Teach equipment safety** ■ Smoking precautions, use of prong outlet, and notification of DME company if alarm or warning light is noted **N42.2.4 Manage equipment safety** ■ Establish contact with DME company to ensure continuity of care and prevent duplication of services	**N42.2.1 Assess equipment safety** ■ Equipment location, condition **N42.2.3 Teach equipment safety** ■ Return demonstration: Smoking precautions, use of three prong outlet, and notification of DME company if alarm or warning light is noted ■ Inspection of electrical cord	**N42.2.1 Assess equipment safety** ■ Equipment location, condition	N Safety **N33.0.1 Injury risk stabilized** ■ Able to use equipment safely

Figure 22.4
(Continued)

organized by the four broad domains addressed by community health nurses: environmental, psychosocial, physiologic, and health-related behaviors. Each problem is described by a list of signs and symptoms. The problem may be referenced as health promotion, potential, or deficit/impairment/actual. The patient may be defined as an individual or family (Martin and Scheet, 1995).

The Omaha System also includes terms for interventions. The intervention scheme is an organized framework of community nursing activities designed to address specific nursing diagnoses using four broad categories of interventions: health teaching, treatments, case management, and surveillance. There is also a five-point Likert type outcome rating scale that measures the concepts of knowledge, behavior, and status for each identified nursing diagnosis.

Community Health Intensity Rating Scale

Another patient intensity classification system is the Community Health Intensity Rating Scale (CHIRS). The CHIRS is also predicated on the nursing process. The original CHIRS was a prototype classification tool that included 15 parameters that represented the same four home health domains as the Omaha System—environment, psychosocial, physiological, and health behaviors (Table 22.3).

Each of the 15 parameters included patient profiles to illustrate the extent of nursing input required for patient care for four levels of care contained within each parameter, for a total of 60 profiles. A profile was selected for each parameter, and then the rater implicitly integrated these into a categorical rating for the patient's resource requirements. These ratings were as follows: level 1, minimum requirements; level 2, moderate requirements; level 3, major requirements; and level 4, extreme requirements (Peters, 1988). Unfortunately, this format was challenging to apply in the workplace setting, so CHIRS has been reformatted into a comprehensive patient assessment form divided into the original 15 parameters. The responses for each of the assessment questions are weighted, producing a score for each parameter from 0 to 4 and a final intensity score between 15 and 60. Thus, a nurse can now get an intensity rating for a patient, while doing a comprehensive assessment at the same time.

The CHIRS concept of patient need incorporates not only the physiologic aspects of care, but also the context of patient need within a patient's support system (e.g., family, home environment, and community resources). All of these areas are especially important as home care

moves into managed care, where the goal of care is to educate and empower patients toward long-term independent management of their own health status and health problems. The CHIRS has been applied to several different community populations. These populations include maternal and child health (MCH), frail elderly, HIV/AIDS patients, patients using high technologies in the community, and substance-abusing homeless families. CHIRS is also being used in nursing education, and has been adapted for use in other countries. It has been translated into Turkish and has been found to be a reliable and valid tool for use in that country.

It has been adapted for school use as the School Health Intensity Rating Scale (SHIRS). The SHIRS is a four-level intensity rating scale for each of 15 parameters clustered in four domains: physiologic, psychosocial, environmental, and health behaviors (Table 22.4). The intensity ratings used to score each descriptor are severe dependency, significant services, moderate or limited services, and minimal or potential services needed. The SHIRS is being tested to enhance the school nurse's ability to make judgments about student healthcare needs across all parameters (Klahn, Hays, and Iverson, 1998).

Community Health Systems

"Community health systems" connotes those computerized IT systems specifically developed and designed for use by community health agencies, local and state health departments, community programs, and services. Community health systems address the broad areas of (1) healthcare programs, (2) agencies, and (3) settings. They support health promotion and disease-preventive programs, statistical information required by state/local health department programs, and funding information for federal block grants, categorical grants, or other grant programs. They also assist community health agencies in the decision-making processes for the management of nursing facilities. Community health systems are also used to evaluate the impact of noninstitutional nursing services on patients, families, and community health conditions. The following are some of the typically used systems in community health systems:

- Categorical systems
- Screening programs
- Client registration systems
- MISs
- Statistical reporting systems
- Special purpose systems

Table 22.3　Community Health Intensity Rating Scale Parameter Definitions

Environmental domain	
Finances	Available financial resources, including employment status of an individual/family reflecting the adequacy/availability of income related to financial obligations.
Physical environment/safety	Condition of client's home/neighborhood, including safety factors and availability of necessary facilities and transportation to those facilities.

Psychosocial domain	
Community networking	Individual family's knowledge and use of community resources/services, including their plan to deal with emergencies, and the availability and accessibility of the community resources.
Family system	Interpersonal relationships within the household (primary unit) and/or with relatives, friends, and significant others outside the household such as church members, social group members, and fellow employees. It includes the sufficiency of the family care-giving system.
Emotional/mental response	Mental status and the expression of feelings, including cheerfulness, grief, depression, anxiety, and coping behaviors that arise from an individual's/family's perception of self, considering their spiritual beliefs and cultural background, as it relates to current change.
Individual growth and development	Life development and maturation of cognitive, physical, and social tasks including ability to speak, read, and write as an individual moves from infancy to old age.

Psychosocial domain	
Sensory function	The body functions concerned with the use of senses to include vision, hearing, taste, touch, smell, proprioception, and an individual's perception of pain.
Respiratory/circulatory function	The body functions concerned with (1) the transfer of gases to meet ventilatory needs and (2) the supply of blood tissues via the cardiovascular system.
Neuromusculoskeletal function	The body functions concerned with the integration and direction of regulatory processes related to gross and fine body movements including level of consciousness, speech patterns, muscle strength, coordination, skeletal integrity, and degree of physical independence/mobility.
Reproductive/sexual function	The body functions concerned with menstruation, pregnancy, lactation, and sexual practices. Included are sexual organs and secondary sexual characteristics.
Digestion/elimination	The ability to ingest food and fluids, use nutrients, and excrete waste products from the body.
Structural integrity	The character and intactness of the body's protective mechanisms, including skin and/or the immunologic system.

Health behaviors domain	
Nutrition	An individual's/family's selection, preparation, and consumption of nutrients according to a prescribed diet that considers cultural and health factors.
Personal habits	An individual's/family's management of personal health habits. It includes sleep activity patterns, personal hygiene, and avoidance of harmful substances. It addresses client/family habits or preferences, not ability to perform activities of daily life.
Health management	An individual's/family's management of their own health status including a measure of their involvement, their technical abilities, and their ability to self-medicate.

Source: Modified, with permission, from Iyer and Camp (1999, p. 311).

Table 22.4   The School Intensity Rating Scale Domains and Parameters

Domain	Parameter
Environmental	Finances
	Physical environment and safety
Psychosocial	Community network
	Family system
	Emotional response
	Development
Physiological	Neuromuscular/skeletal
	Sensory function
	Respiration/circulation
	Reproductive/sexual
	Digestion/elimination
	Structural integrity
Health Behaviors	Nutrition
	Personal habits
	Descriptors: medications, special procedures, participatory involvement

Categorical Program Systems

Categorical program systems are designed to support data processing and tracking specific programs such as cancer detection, MCH immunization, or family planning. Other systems are designed to collect uniform longitudinal data for a specific disease condition, such as diabetes, that can be used for national databases for tracking incidence and prevalence of disease conditions. Categorical program systems generally count, track, and identify the health status of registered clients.

Screening Programs

Screening programs are used to detect individuals afflicted with a specific disease or predisposing health condition. Such programs generally use a computer system to collect important health information that may be mandated by federal, state, or local regulations. Results of screening tests are tracked so that data analysis can be used to measure the effectiveness of the screening program. A common application is tracking lead screening in high-risk pediatric populations.

Registration Systems

Client registration information systems (CISs) are designed to identify state/local residents/clients eligible for CHN services in clinics and homes. These systems generally consist of an online communication network, with terminals located in each of the local/district offices that are linked to a central computer facility used to collect, store, and process all data. The centralized registry can then be accessed from the local/district units prior to providing services.

Management Information Systems

Many state/local health departments have developed MISs, which focus on the management of statistical and operational needs of the agency and professionals. A client/personal management system is another type of MIS that provides the framework for collecting and reporting statistical as well as financial data needed for the management of health personal/client and programs. An example of an information system is the Ohio Department of Mental Health Multi-Agency Community Services Information System (MACSIS) which is designed to collect financial/reimbursement data, demographic data, and consumer outcomes for publicly funded clients (ODMH, 2004). The aggregate data are used for the management of consumer care both clinically and administratively, quality improvement, and public accountability.

Statistical Reporting Systems

Statistical reporting systems are community health computer applications that have been developed to collect and process statistical information primarily for state/local health departments such as epidemiologic data and immunization data. They emerged as the need for uniform information from all official state and local health departments became a national initiative.

Several state health departments have developed new systems for collecting community health statistics. They are implementing communication networks that link state and local community health agencies together. Many states, such as Michigan, Missouri, Florida, and Kentucky have implemented computer networks. They are primarily statistical reporting systems designed to collect and process online data required for federal, state, and local community health programs (NCHS, 1994).

Public Health Information Network   The Centers for Disease Control (CDC) also recognized that there are multiple systems in place that support communication for public health laboratories, the clinical community, and state and local health departments. Many of these systems operate in isolation and do not allow for early detection of public health issues and emergencies. The current development of a public health information network (PHIN) will enable consistent exchange of response, health, and disease tracking data between public health partners through defined data and vocabulary standards (CDC, 2004). The five key components include detection and monitoring, analysis, information resources and knowledge management, alerting and communications, and response.

National Electronic Disease Surveillance System

Additionally, the CDC has also supported the national electronic disease surveillance system (NEDSS) to promote the use of data and information system standards to advance the development of efficient and integrated surveillance systems at the federal, state, and local levels (CDC, 2004). The broad initiative is designed to (1) detect outbreaks rapidly and monitor the health of the nation, (2) facilitate the electronic transfer of appropriate information from clinical information systems in the healthcare system to public health departments, (3) reduce provider burden in the provision of information, and (4) enhance the timeliness and quality of information.

Special Purpose Systems

Special purpose systems have been developed to collect statistical data for administering a specific program (rather than an agency), regardless of what type of agency offers the program. Stand-alone systems are designed to collect and summarize management data on services in clinics, schools, and homes. These systems provide the statistics needed to obtain funds from federal, state, or local units for categorical programs and/or block grants. Programs such as maternal and infant (MI), children and youth (C/Y), children with medical handicaps, tuberculosis, drug abuse, or HIV have statistical reporting requirements that can be met by these systems.

Special study systems generally require a specially designed computer application. Studies that collect large volumes of data require computer processing using standard statistical software programs and/or specially designed computer-processing models. Generally, the data is collected for surveys, clinical trials, research studies, health policy, and other projects requiring volumes of data to resolve a problem. Many research studies collect information from federal databases to merge

with concurrently collected data. Other studies requiring special stand-alone systems are national surveys of nurses and/or CHN agencies.

One of the major obstacles in developing special study systems is the management of large databases that are complex and create time-consuming data entry tasks. The introduction of point of service online data entry terminals has replaced data collection forms, making it easier to develop special studies systems. With this approach, these systems can process the data as information is collected, improving the time for processing data, and generating information regarding research objectives.

School Health Systems   These are another type of special purpose systems. Computerized systems have emerged to improve data collection and monitor and evaluate health of school age students. These systems can be individual school-based or district-based allowing for collecting aggregate data about an educational district.

Commercial software options for school nursing take two basic forms. One form is to use a personal computer (PC)-based, stand-alone software product; the second form is to work with the health module that comes with the administrative software package used by the school district. The specialized PC-based software is more comprehensive, but using the health module of the school administrative package allows for integrating the health components with the financial, human resource, and broader student management modules, thus eliminating duplicate data entry (Hedberg, 1997b). Table 22.5 lists common capabilities of school nursing programs. Additional capabilities that vary among products include healthcare plans, student activity records, medication logs, appointment scheduling, and referral/tracking (Hedberg, 1997a).

The need to introduce computerized healthcare programs is becoming increasingly important in school nursing in order to provide an opportunity for collecting health-related data on the students and employees in the school and communicating that data in a meaningful way. These systems have many of the same issues as the computer-based patient record regarding data security and ensuring the privacy and confidentiality of the individual's (student) data.

Home Health Information Systems

Home health systems are designed to support home healthcare, hospice, and private duty programs provided by HHAs, such as VNAs, hospital-based programs,

Table 22.5   School Nursing Product Capabilities Common to All Software Packages

Product Capability	Capability Description
Individual student records	Individual files that contain each student's health record. Entering the student's name, a portion of the name, and/or an identifier can usually access this file.
Immunization records	The individual student record contains a special section for recording student immunizations. The programs that have this option allow for recording the date the immunization was given; some allow for dosage, lot number, and so forth.
Dental records	The individual student record contains a special section for the student's dental health records.
Other health screenings	The individual student record contains a special section for the student's other health screenings such as vision and hearing, heights and weights, and postural screening.
Family history	A section of the student health record that focuses on family history and/or diagnoses.
Multiple record diagnoses	Several diagnoses may be entered for one visit. Each diagnosis that is entered may be used to generate reports or lists.
Injury/incident reports	A section of the individual student record that focuses on incidents. In the case of injuries, this may include the type of injury, what the student was doing at the time of injury, and the place where the injury occurred.
Special emergency comment fields	This is a quick and easy-to-access file outside of the student record. The file contains emergency information such as the phone numbers of the student's parents and primary care physician and any student allergies.
Create reports and lists	This option allows the user to create a list or report based on individual student records such as those who have had chicken pox, injuries in specific areas of the school, or those behind in their immunizations.
Multiple school use	This function refers to situations in which one school nurse is servicing and collecting data on students from multiple school buildings using the same computer.
Daily log	The nurse's daily log keeps a record of the events for each day. This allows for easy review of trends or numbers of visits by a specific student without requiring a review of individual student records.
End-of-year processing	This function allows for the generation of annual reports as well as programming students to the next grade.

Source: Modified, with permission, from Hedberg, S. (1997b). A comparative analysis of PC-based school health software. *Journal of School Nursing* 13(1):30–38.

proprietary agencies, and other not-for-profit HHAs. Originally, home health systems were primarily designed to collect and process data in order to prepare the documents required by HCFA and third-party payers for the payment of home healthcare services. They have now evolved to include many applications including clinical service delivery, integrated financial functions, scheduling packages, decision support functions, payroll, personnel management, accounts payable, billing functions, general ledger, financial reporting, and statistical reporting capabilities.

Both the home healthcare industry and IT are changing rapidly due to some of the external driving forces including prospective payment, outcome measurement, electronic billing, disease management, and HIPAA legislation. The early community health computer systems were limited to time-sharing systems and stand-alone systems. The changing markets have brought together networked system products, client/server computing, and Internet applications.

Time-Sharing Systems

Time-sharing systems are computer-based systems developed by service bureaus/vendors that are shared by many HHAs. Generally the service bureaus purchase their own computer hardware with sufficient storage to share the data from many other HHAs and develop their own proprietary computer programs (software) to process the HHA data. The service bureaus design the computer screens and menus for collecting data, design the pathways, and processing of the data needed for preparing the billing and financial statements, OASIS reports, PPS reports, and other required reports. The bureaus develop manuals, provide training sessions, and support any other technological needs for their users.

The HHAs that use these service bureaus generally use PCs with fixed menus and screens designed to collect, store, and then transmit the data online via the Internet to the service bureau computer system. The users have real-time access to their patient information stored in their patient's designated database and in some cases can even generate special reports.

Stand-Alone Systems

Stand-alone systems on the other hand, are commercial systems developed for direct installation and implementation in an HHA. In this system, the commercial vendor generally develops the software for processing the data, maintains, updates, and supports all software programs as well as ensures that the software programs meet state and federal regulations. The vendor generally offers training courses to the HHAs on how to run the system. The major advantage of this option is that the agency owns its own computer hardware, software programs, and patient data and databases. The agency can then use the computer system for other applications such as word processing, Intranet communication, Internet resources, library access, and communicate to its staff via e-mail.

With the introduction of computer networks as a means of sharing and communicating data among users, the Internet is being used for both local area networks (LANs) and wide area networks (WANs) making it possible to link within an HHA, outside the HHA, and across large geographic areas. Networks allow the HHAs to share hardware and software for their individual computer system server while still using the network to communicate with each other's servers. Thus, the Intranet (worldwide network) has revolutionized the communication of data across all types of computer systems and servers that are connected to the Internet network.

Portability of Data

Portability of data is another important aspect of home health. Point-of-care technology uses a computer input device to input and retrieve clinical data at the point of care in the home. The data can then be transferred remotely to the main database through a client server. A server is a multiuser processor with shared memory that can provide common services to the user, such as shared communication and database access. This allows multi-

ple users access to the same information and supports the integration of clinical data to other functions within the database.

Point-of-Care Systems

Point-of-care systems also offer software-aided care planning and critical pathways allowing for care delivery based on evidence-based practice standards to reach a desired clinical outcome. This differs from the traditional care planning process by outlining a systematic plan for interventions and teaching through diagnostic categories. Laptop systems or personal digital assistants (PDAs) are designed to collect and transmit patient data. Many architectural designs using this new technology are being developed for nurses to chart visit details, patient care services, order supplies, and other functions related to service delivery. The clinician can query, collect, and retrieve data from the computer system. These systems generally use menu-driven Windows software, which prompts users through every step of the care delivery process. These systems may provide interaction with the clinician and can assist to provide logic and validity checks cuing the clinician to abnormal physiologic criteria, inconsistency within an assessment, and providing validation errors for required documents such as the OASIS assessment and/or Physician Plan of Treatment. Documentation is therefore more consistent, accurate, and accessible (Harrell, 1999). The HHA can aggregate clinical data from the point of care making it possible to identify trends in care, utilization, and outcomes. Data can also be used to generate information for managed care contracts, new business models, new services, and new organizational policies.

Reimbursable Models

Home health systems often integrate clinical, financial, and billing functions to support the Medicare episodic reimbursement model and fee-per-visit models still in use for private pay or managed care payers. The functions are primarily designed to furnish information essential for reimbursement of services provided to patients eligible for Medicare, Medicaid, and other third-party payers. These systems use a variety of input forms or data entry screens—admission data, assessment data, and plan of treatment data—to collect the required information. The data are needed to obtain approval for a patient to receive reimbursable services, as well as to obtain payment for visits and services provided by all types of disciplines. Services are billed for each specific patient, and payment is received based on the current Medicare regulations or private payer requirements. Revenue and cost data are periodically reconciled in order to determine the agency's position under the Medicare cost allocation system. These systems generally include the following applications: general ledger, accounts receivable, accounts payable, billing, reimbursement management, and cash management. Additionally, they generate financial reports related to the costs of delivering services inclusive of visits, supplies, personnel costs, and overhead expenses (mileage, administrative costs, and so forth).

Managed Care

The increase of managed care in the home health arena and the PPS for home care services has had an impact on the financial and billing systems. Most vendors have responded by expanding the back-end financial reporting capabilities and emphasizing reports that will help agencies identify the factors that impact delivery cost and profitability. Vendors are being more cautious about fundamental changes to the systems that can accommodate discounted fee-for-service billing, capitated reimbursement, and other scenarios different from the cost-reimbursement model (Bender, 1998; Williams, 1997).

An area that has experienced significant changes is electronic data interchange (EDI). EDI allows for data to move between payers and providers. Several states have implemented laws or instituted new programs that focused on cutting administrative healthcare costs by using EDI to transmit Medicare/Medicaid and other required claims data (Goedert, 1994).

Scheduling Systems

Scheduling systems are also being used to enhance HHA services. They are designed to schedule the clinicians providing services with the patients requiring the visit matching the clinician capacity with the required patient care. Some systems use graphical scheduling calendars and others provide road maps on how to travel to a location in the shortest distance. These systems can also track personnel by scheduling on and off duty time as well as generate payroll. Since these systems are interactive, schedules can be adjusted daily online, making edits and revisions to existing schedules more efficient. Schedules can be done for a month or more in advance, thus ensuring that patients receive the same staff for each home visit. This consistency in staff usually increases patient satisfaction. In general, scheduling systems reduce schedule conflicts, improve financial con-

trol, enhance productivity, reduce administrative costs, and decrease travel time. Scheduling systems may also use "the telephone," which allows the clinician to record the visit using phone technology and assists to verify clinician time in the home and may also be used to generate billing and payroll. The telephone systems are typically used for home care aides who may not have access to any other form of technology application for documenting care and/or service delivery.

In summary, information systems in home health must be able to capture and retrieve clinical and financial data that corresponds to the current functionality and operations of the agency (Struk, 2001). They are designed and structured to meet the information requirements of home care regulatory bodies, payers, accrediting bodies, state licensure and contractors with flexibility to meet business operations that may be unique to an individual agency. They support interrelationships between and among functions so that data is not repeated. Also, decision support should be a major consideration with alerts and triggers imbedded in the functionality of the products for both clinical and financial decisions. The portability of the database for point of care and remote operations is critical particularly for agencies using multiple sites or sharing data among facilities or providers.

Telemedicine

Telemedicine is being implemented to replace face-to-face home visits. It refers to the electronic transfer of medical information and services (voice, data, and video) from one site to another using telecommunication technologies (Kienzle, 1998). As home and community-based healthcare has evolved and technology has advanced, innovative home telemedicine systems are emerging. Technologies may include:

- Telemonitors with peripheral biometric attachments for remotely monitoring biophysical parameters
- Videophone with two-way audio-video connectivity which allows for the visualization of client activity
- In-home message devices with disease management education, advice, and vital sign monitoring
- Video cameras for monitoring all aspects of care delivery particularly focusing on wound management and home care aide supervision

- PCs with Internet connectivity for supervised communication
- Video conferencing that allows clinicians, physicians, and other healthcare providers to communicate about patient-specific care. This applicability is important for hospice care as interdisciplinary team conferences are a requirement of service delivery

Community Health Telemedicine Systems

Communication telemedicine systems link patients' homes to healthcare facilities and healthcare professionals, home care workers to their supervisors, and patients and families with community resources. Communication systems make it possible for patients to communicate with providers or other resources to get healthcare advice, avoid inconvenient and expensive visits to healthcare providers, and omit unnecessary visits to healthcare facilities.

Internet Applications

Using access to a computer terminal with Internet applications can be used by patients to (1) assist in self-diagnosis and preventive medicine, (2) reduce unnecessary outpatient visits, (3) provide self-directed triage, and (4) eliminate the "worried well" aspects of many patient-provider interactions. This leads to the following benefits:

- Improved patient and provider satisfaction
- Patient time savings in tracking and receiving information
- Reduced need to see a healthcare provider "face to face"
- Increased reliance on computer-based information
- Reduced information calls
- More cost-effective care

These terminals can also streamline administrative requirements such as obtaining physician orders and confirming appointments due to improved communications with the physicians and other healthcare professionals. Queries regarding immunizations for travel, flu vaccines, side effects of medications, nonprescription medications, and school and work health forms can increase early detection and reduce visits to health professional offices and hospitals.

Telemedicine Devices

HHAs are increasingly using devices that allow healthcare providers to communicate with patients in their homes. For example, the Texas Telemedicine Project in Austin, Texas is using two-way interactive video to connect specialists in major urban centers with health professionals in rural areas for diagnosis and consultation. Communication technology is used to transmit x-rays, electrocardiograms, and other clinical data for analysis by the specialists. Electronic healthcare allows rural professionals to "see" (via two-way interactive video) more clients without having to make "home visits," thus saving travel time and ultimately cost.

The home assisted nursing care network (HANC) is a system produced by HealthTech Services of Northbrook, IL. HANC is a programmed computer stationed in the patient's home. The unit is a voice-activated, 3.5-ft-tall robot with a video screen. A central nursing station is linked to the home system by telephone lines. HANC can walk patients through a dressing change, assess the condition of an intravenous (IV) site, or provide reminders for taking medications. HANC is FDA-approved and can be programmed in multiple languages (Warner, 1998).

The University of Iowa has used telemedicine to improve access to specialized services for both patients and providers. In 1994, they developed a telemedicine resource center, which is the administrative entity that oversees and coordinates the National Laboratory for the Study of Rural Telemedicine. The staff from the resource center provides support for project directors and other faculty and staff who are involved in delivery of health services to remote sites inclusive of technical support, on-site training, deployment of electronics and equipment to rural hospitals, and many other aspects of project support.

Community Health Network Systems

A community health network is an innovative ambulatory care system specially developed to provide services by computer. Computer terminals are placed in homes of "heavy users of healthcare," such as families with young children, pregnant women, disabled, and the elderly. The system allows the subscribers to telephone for assistance and guidance on services offered via the terminal. The system performs a triage of actions but not necessarily diagnoses. They include the following:

- Download the patient record from hospital to the home database.
- Enter a series of questions about symptoms using expert system logic until the pathways are concluded.
- Track self-care and, depending on the responses to questions, call or make an appointment with a clinician.
- Provide additional information on the condition if self-care is chosen to assist the client to resolve the problem.

Community health networks appear to increase client satisfaction, and it is anticipated that they will reduce telephone calls and unnecessary trips to the emergency room or physician offices for the "worried well." For example, ComputerLink was a project conducted by Case Western Reserve University (Cleveland, OH) that offered programs and services to support self-care in the home. They were primarily designed to support AIDS, as well as the caregivers of Alzheimer's disease patients living in their homes. ComputerLink ran within the Cleveland Free Net, a public access computer network. Computer terminals were placed in the homes of the patients using standard telephone lines to allow the patients and/or their caregivers to communicate with the Information Network Services staff at Case Western Reserve University. ComputerLink offered home care users information, communication, and decision support to enhance self-care and promote home-based treatment of their study patients. It served as a "support group without walls" (Brennan, 1993).

Home High-Tech Monitoring Systems

Home high-tech monitoring systems are using computers to link patients at home to healthcare facilities. Monitoring devices that transmit vital signs and other critical data are used in the home to conduct postsurgical checkups, for example. They allow healthcare providers to monitor the progress of their patients. Monitoring technology permits the transmission of healthcare information. Monitoring systems are being used not only for diagnosis and treatment but also for prevention.

Many HHAs are using telemonitoring for monitoring biophysical parameters that are remotely transmitted each time the user (patient) performs an assessment. The data is then reviewed by a nurse at a central monitoring station that is designed to alert the nurse to abnormal biophysical parameters for a particular patient. This allows for early intervention that could prevent complications and/or a hospital readmission (Lewis, 1999). Care Watch, a home telemonitoring program of the Visiting Nurse Health Care Partners of Ohio (VNAHPO) in Cleveland has used telemonitoring for its congestive heart failure patients leading to reduced hospitalization, reduced emergent care visits, and improved OASIS clinical outcomes when compared to the nonmonitored group (Jones, 2004).

Another monitoring device is a remote defibrillator that allows hospitals to diagnose and resuscitate a homebound patient who has suffered a cardiac arrest. A transtelephonic defibrillator device located in the home, called a briefcase, is linked to a hospital base unit. When a client feels that he or she is having a heart attack, a caregiver in the home opens the "briefcase," activates the transmitter, and places the electrode pads on the client's chest. An ECG is immediately transmitted to the hospital, and the interactive speakerphone is activated. If the hospital base unit determines that the client is having a heart attack, the device triggers an electronic shock to the patient to stimulate the heart.

Sophisticated telemetry devices such as digitized x-rays and ECG, electronic stethoscopes, and interactive video equipment are using telecommunications technology to enable specialists at a teaching hospital to examine patients in a remote clinic. The clinicians can examine patients, hear heartbeats, study x-rays and laboratory results, and perform other critical assessments with these devices. Two monitors are used to communicate between the two locations. One monitor is used to interact with the rural physician and patient, and the other is used to view the images close up from cameras attached to the biomedical devices.

Another type of monitoring device is alert systems that are widely used in home settings. Alert systems are primarily communication devices that allow the homebound to signal for help in an emergency. A one-way signaling device that is worn around the neck allows a patient, by pressing on a button, to signal for help to a friend, hospital emergency room coordinator, fire department, or other assistive facility. Another communication device being piloted is a two-way communication device that allows the healthcare provider in a hospital to communicate with.

Educational Technology Systems

Educational technology applications provide communication linkages, information access, and educational materials. These technologies meet the need for clients to reach beyond their environment to "see" and "hear," i.e., to experience, view, and visualize situations. These systems may also offer screening for compliance with health prevention standards and linkages to education.

Healthy Town is a unique program of the VNAHPO. It is a partnership with the Area Agencies on Aging (AAA) who serve seniors at neighborhood nutrition sites. It is founded on the federal initiative Healthy People 2010. It uses innovative computer screening technology to screen, refer, and link seniors with identified senior health risk issues such as safety and injury prevention, alcohol, drug and family abuse, anxiety and depression, and links seniors to follow-up for chronic illnesses (Stricklin, Jones, and Niles, 2000). The screening is done by the individual client using voice-interactive computerized technology. Screening risk can be identified individually but may also be aggregated by screening site so that the health needs of seniors are identified and service providers can develop appropriate on-site health programs or individually focused education which then supports state health policy and program funding (Fig. 22.5). A Web site has also been established to link both patients and providers to health promotion information accessible at *www.vnahealthytown.org*. Educational systems offer advanced learning applications. They use technological media to interact with and educate patients in the home and the community. The types of learning that can be communicated into the home are still being researched. However, the developed home teaching strategies using information technologies include active learning, personalization, individualization, cooperative learning, contextual learning, and sophisticated evaluation strategies.

Baby Care Link is a multifaceted telemedicine communication application of Beth Israel Deaconess Medical Center designed to provide individualized information to families of very low birth weight infants (Gray et al., 1998). The system is designed to interface with individualized Web pages and videoconferencing technology to enhance emotional support, provide education, provide information about services, and improve postdischarge care for these infants.

A critical component of home educational technologies is in bringing effective self-care and health promotion into the home or community setting. Home computers offer this information as an essential commodity. As new knowledge bases on treatments and alternate therapies as well as prevention and handling of chronic disabilities are developed, they will allow healthcare consumers to assume more responsibility for their self-care, wellness, and prevention of disease.

Patients using communication systems will have not only Internet access to clinical information about specific diseases on the World Wide Web (WWW), but also advice about an individual's health status and self-care, access to their own healthcare records, and evaluations of providers and therapies. Through interactive learning, communication, and Internet technologies in the home, patients will become active participants in healthcare decisions.

Home consultation is now available via computer-based stand-alone software programs that do not require a communication network. The use of computer-assisted instruction (CAI) and interactive video program tapes are available for the PC.

Databases systems are being developed, whereby consumers can be linked to a "smart database" with answers and healthcare advice for minor requirements such as a rash or a temperature. Once the two-way video networks are in place, clients will be able to consult with healthcare providers without making a physical visit to a clinician. Clinicians can then provide consultation, observe their patients, and feel connected. Visual and graphic interactive communications are far more effective in educating patients than pamphlets on topics such as nutrition. Clinicians can observe their patients and guide home health workers to use monitoring equipment, or view a specific part of the body, or teach a worker to conduct an examination for viewing. Additionally, the technology can enhance the use of electronic services to schedule healthcare appointments, automate insurance claims filing, and provide information on eligibility benefits and costs (Olsen, Jones, and Bezold, 1992).

Video-conferencing includes the transmission of a video image with a voice in real time and visual, interactive discussion between two or more parties in different locations (Little, 1992; Preston, Brown, and Hartley, 1992). Remote interactive video consultation has applications for both communication and rural access. It can reduce the need for patients to travel to specialists or for specialists to travel to rural hospitals (Fig. 22.6).

Once in place, the broadband networks can reach into the home through telephone or cable TV networks. They are able to offer video consultations and video instructions, support home care services for homebound patients, and allow clinicians to provide remote diagnostic evaluations and consultations.

Sample comprehensive health profile

Prevention needs:

Center health profile

Hearing screen
Take Rx meds
Mammogram (of females)
Take over counter meds
Alcohol risk
No regular doctor
Dental examination
Cannot care for self
Prostate examination (of males)
Eye examination

Chronic/disabling conditions

Smoking risk
Arthritis
Seat belt risk
Hypertension
No smoke alarm
Heart disease
Need blood pressure check
Diabetes

Mental health risk:
Lost someone close
Feel sad
Harm risk

Fall risk:
Blood pressure pills
Heart pills
Recent fall
Eye drops
Light headed
Use assistive device

Immunization risk:
TB screen
Tetanus
Pneumovax
Flu

Nutritional risk:
Wears false teeth
Eat three meals (no)
Weight loss
Weight gain
On special diet
Tooth/mouth problems
Need money for food

Figure 22.5
Healthy Town sample comprehensive health profile.
(Courtesy of Visiting Nurse Association Healthcare Partners of Ohio, 2002.)

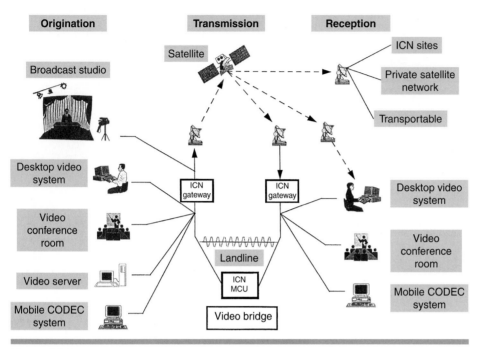

Figure 22.6
Video-conferencing model example.

Future Trends

Community health information networks will link multiple providers, patient information, and regulatory bodies on a single system allowing for integration of data, continuity of care, and the tracking of outcomes across service providers.

Decision support systems will become more sophisticated allowing community health agencies to easily use, analyze, and operate on large data sets. Information will be used to improve clinical practice, make better care delivery decisions, leverage financial resources, alert private and public providers to critical health trends, and allow for patients to make their own self-care decisions based on access to their own computerized record (Sheyte and Struk, 2003).

Geographic information system (GIS) technology which uses a computerized database for the capture, storage, analysis, and display of spatial information will become a powerful tool for public health applications. Mapping applications will be used for disease surveillance and control, allocation of resources, health plan-

ning, measurement of environmental data, and many other health-related concerns. Developments in spatial statistical computerized analysis are already in use for predicting health risk, exposure assessment, and other public health applications.

Summary

This chapter described the various computer applications found in community health. It presented an overview of the development of community health computer systems. Several of the development projects were discussed including vocabularies, data sets, classification systems, and OASIS.

An overview of the different types of community health systems was presented, including categorical systems, screening programs, client registration systems, MISs, statistical reporting systems, and special purpose systems. Applications for home health illustrated the importance of integrating various functions of service delivery into a MIS, integrating the clinical, financial, operational, and administrative functions.

The last section focused on home technology systems that include a wide range of home communication Internet systems, monitoring equipment, devices, alert systems, and educational technologies.

References

American Nurses Association. (1980). *A Conceptual Model of Community Health Nursing.* ANA Publication No. CH-10 2M 5/80. Kansas City, MO: American Nurses' Association.

American Nurses Association. (1998). *Standards of Clinical Nursing Practice.* Washington, DC: ANA.

Anderson, M. A., Pena, R. A., and Helms, L. B. (1998). Home care utilization by congestive heart failure patients: A pilot study. *Public Health Nursing* 15(2):146–62.

Bakken, S., Cook, S. S., Curtis, L., Desjardins, K., Hyun, S., Jenkins, M., John, R., Klein, W. T., Paguntalan, J., Roberts, W. D., and Soupios, M. (2004). Promoting patient safety through informatics-based nursing education. *International Journal of Medical Informatics* 7–8:581–589.

Bender, A. (1998). Management information systems: A required tool for survival. *Home Health Care Management and Practice* 10(2):37–42.

Brennan, P. P. (1993). ComputerLink: Computer networks and community health connections. *Nursing Dynamics* 2(1):9–15.

Bruegel, R. B. (1998). The increasing importance of patient empowerment and its potential effects on home health care information systems and technology. *Home Health Care Management and Practice* 10(2): 69–75.

Center for Disease Control and Prevention. (2004). *Overview of Public Health Information Network.* CDC [on-line]. Available at *www.cdc.gov*

Center for Medicare and Medicaid Services (CMS). (2003). *OASIS Data Set OASIS B-1 (10/2003)* [electronic version]. Baltimore, MD: CMS [on-line]. Available at *www.cms.hhs.gov/oasis*

Elfrink, V. and Martin, K. (1996). Educating for community nursing practice: Point of care technology. *Healthcare Information Management* 10(2): 81–89.

Florida Department of Health and Rehabilitation Services (1983). *HRS Manual: Systems Management: Client Information System: Personal Health.* Tallahassee, FL.

Fortinsky, R. H. and Madigan, E. A. (1997). Home care resource consumption and patient outcomes: What are the relationships? *Home Health Care Service Quarterly* 16(3):55–73.

Goedert, J. (1994). More states turn to EDI as a way to cut expenses. *Health Data Management* 2(7):54–55, 57–58.

Gray, J., Pompilio-Weitzner, G., Jones, P., Wang, Q., Coriat, M., and Safran, C. (1998). Baby care link: Development and implementation of a www based system for neonatal home telemedicine. *AMIA Symposium* (pp. 351–355).

Harrell, J. (1999). The future of point of care technology. *The Remington Report* 7(2):12–14.

Health Care Financing Administration. (1980). *Medicare: Provider Reimbursement Manual: Part II-Provider Cost Reporting Forms and Instructions.* Baltimore, MD: HCFA (1728), DHHS.

Health Care Financing Administration. (2000). Medicare program: Prospective payment for home health agencies. *Federal Register Rules and Regulations* 65(128):441128–441214.

Hedberg, S. (1997a). Administrative student information management software (AS/IMS) for school nurse record keeping and reporting. *Journal of School Nursing* 13(2):40–48.

Hedberg, S. (1997b). A comparative analysis of PC-based school health software. *Journal of School Nursing,* 13(1), 30–38.

Holzemer, W. L., Henry, S. B., Dawson, C., Sousa, K., Bain, C., and Hsieh, S. F. (1997). An evaluation of the utility of the Home Health Care Classification for categorizing patient problems and nursing interventions from the hospital setting. In U. Gerdin, M. Tallberg, P. Wainwright (Eds.), *NI'99 Nursing Informatics: The Impact of Nursing Knowledge on Health Care Informatics* (pp. 21–26). Stockholm, Sweden: IOS Press.

Institute of Medicine of the National Academies. (2004). *Public Health and Prevention* [on-line]. Available at *http://www.iom.edu/topic*

Joint Commission on Accreditation of Health Care Standards (JCAHO). (2002). ORYX requirement change. *JCAHO Homecare Bulletin* [on-line], Nov/Dec. Available at *www.jcaho.org*

Jones, S. (2004). 5 step plan for implementing a successful home telemonitoring program. Presentation: VNAA Annual Meeting.

Kienzle, M. (1998). *National Laboratory for the Study of Rural Telemedicine.* College of medicine, University of Iowa [online]. *www.telemed.medicine,uiowa. edu*

Klahn, J. K., Hays, B. J., and Iverson, C. J. (1998). The school health intensity rating scale: Establishing reliability for practice. *Journal of School Nursing* 14(4):23–28.

Klein, W. T. and Bakken, S. (2003). Design and implementation of a student clinical log database and knowledge base (pp. 617–622). In H. Marin, P. M. Eduardo, E. Hovenga, and W. Goosen (Eds.), *NI 2003: In Proceedings of the 6th International Congress in Nursing Informatics.* Rio de Janeiro, Brazil: E-papers Services Editorials, Ltd.

Lasker R. D. (1995). The quintessential role of information in public health. In *Data Needs in an Era of Health Reform. Proceedings of the 25th Public Health Conference on Records and Statistics and the National Committee on Vital and Health Statistics 45th Anniversary Symposium*, Washington, DC.

Lewis, A. (1999). Tough times for home care are better times for telemedicine. *The Remington Report* 7(2):4–6.

Little, A. D. (1992). *Telecommunications: Can It Help Solve America's Health Care Problems?* Cambridge, MA: A. D. Little.

Martin, K. S. and Scheet, N. J. (1995). *The Omaha System: Applications for Community Health Nursing* (2nd ed.). Philadelphia, PA: W. B. Saunders.

National Association of Home Care. (1994). *Progress Toward a Uniform Minimum Data Set for Home Care and Hospice*. Washington, DC: NAHC.

National Center for Health Statistics. (1994). *Subcommittee on State and Community Health Statistics: Minutes of Meeting*. Washington, DC: NCHS, National Committee on Vital and Health Statistics.

National Institute of Health. (1996). *Public Health Informatics: January 1980 through December 1995*. 471 Selected Citations/Prepared by Catherine Selden ... [et al.]. Bethesda, MD: U.S. Dept. of Health and Human Services, Public Health Service, National Institutes of Health, National Library of Medicine, Reference Section.

National League for Nursing. (1977). *Statistical Reporting in Home and Community Health Services* (Pub. No. 21-1652). New York: NLN.

NCQA. (2004). *Healthplan employer data and information set (HEDIS)* [on-line]. Available at *www.ncqa.org/programs/HEDIS*

Olsen, R., Jones, M. G., and Bezold, C. (1992). *21st Century Learning and Health Care in the Home: Creating a National Telecommunications Network*. Washington, DC: Consumer Interest Research Institute.

Peters, D. A. (1988). The development of a community health intensity rating scale. *Nursing Research* 37(4):202–207.

Peters, D. A. and McKeon, T. (1998). *Transforming Home Care: Quality, Cost, and Data Management*. Gaithersburg, MD: Aspen Publishers.

Preston, J., Brown, F., and Hartley, B. (1992). Using telemedicine to improve health care in distant areas. *Hospitals and Community Psychiatry* 43(1):25–32.

Reichley, M. (1999). Automation for the 21st century. *Success in Home Care* 12–16.

Saba, V. K. (1991). *Home Health Care Classification Project* (NTIS #PB92-177013/AS). Washington, DC: Georgetown University School of Nursing.

Saba, V. K. (1994a). *Home Health Care Classification (HHCC) of Nursing Diagnosis and Interventions* (Rev.). Washington, DC: Author.

Saba, V. K. (1994b). Twenty nursing diagnoses home health care components. In R. M. Carroll-Johnson and M. Paquette (Eds.), *Classification of Nursing Diagnosis: Proceedings of the Tenth Conference* (p. 301). Philadelphia, PA: J.B. Lippincott.

Saba, V. K. (1995). A new paradigm for computer-based nursing information systems: Twenty care components. In R. A. Greenes, H. E. Peterson, and D. J. Proti (Eds.), *Medinfo '95 Proceedings* (pp. 1404–1406). Edmonton, Canada: IMIA.

Saba, V. (2002). Nursing Classifications: Home Health Care Classification system (HHCC): An overview. *ONLINE Journal of Issues in Nursing*. Available at *http://nursingworld.org/ojin/tpc7/tpc7-htm*.

Saba, V. K. (2004). *Clinical Care Classification (CCC) System*. Retrieved September 40, 2004, from *www. Sabacare.com*

Saba, V. K. and McCormick, A., (2001). *Essentials of Computers for Nurses: Informatics in the New Millennium* (3rd ed.). New York: McGraw-Hill.

Saba, V. K. and Sparks, S. M. (1998). Twenty care components: An educational strategy to teach nursing science. In B. Cesnik, A. T. McCray, and J. R. Scherrer (Eds.), *Medinfo'98: Proceedings of the Ninth World Congress on Medical Informatics* (pp. 756–759). Amsterdam, The Netherlands: IOS Press.

Saba, V. K. and Zuckerman, A. E. (1992). A new home health care classification method. *Caring* 10(10):27–34.

Shaughnessy, P. W. and Crisler, K. S. (1995). *Outcome-based Quality Improvement*. Denver, CO: Colorado Center for Health Policy and Services Research.

Sheyte, R. and Struk, C. (2003). What is data decision support and why should I care? *Home Health Nurse* 21(10):652–654.

Simmons, D. A. (1980). *A Classification Scheme for Client Problems in Community Health Nursing* (DHHS Publication No. 80-16). Washington, DC: Government Printing Office.

Stricklin, M. L., Jones, S., and Niles, S. A. (2000). Home talk/healthy talk: Improving patient's health status with telephone technology. *Home Health Nurse* 18(1): 53–61.

Struk, C. (2001). Critical steps for integrating information technology in home care. *Home Health Nurse* 19(12): 758–765.

Warner, I. (1998). Telemedicine in home health care: The current status of practice. *Home Health Care Management and Practice* 10(2):62–68.

Wieland, D., Ferrell, B. A., and Rubenstein, L. Z. (1991). Geriatric home health care conceptual and demographic considerations. *Clinics in Geriatric Medicine* 7(4):645–664.

Williams, T. (1997). *Guide to Successful Automating Your Home Health Organization* (2nd ed.). Los Altos, CA: Home Health Business Resources.

23

Ambulatory Care Systems

Susan K. Newbold

OBJECTIVES

1. Understand information issues in ambulatory care including regulatory requirements.
2. Delineate the functions and benefits for information systems and sources for further information.
3. Describe the state of the art in using information systems in ambulatory care.
4. Describe future trends in ambulatory care information systems.
5. Define various roles for nurses in the ambulatory care arena.

KEY WORDS

ambulatory care information systems
ambulatory care physician order entry (ACPOE)
e-Prescribing
evidence-based medicine
regulatory requirements

On April 27, 2004, President George Bush announced a goal to establish electronic health records (EHRs) for all citizens within a 10-year time frame. He created the position of a national health information technology coordinator to develop a nationwide interoperable health information technology infrastructure. One responsibility for the national coordinator is to improve "the coordination of care and information among hospitals, laboratories, physician offices, and other ambulatory care providers through an effective infrastructure for the secure and authorized exchange of health care information" (White House Executive Order, 2004).

In July, then Health and Human Services Secretary Tommy G. Thompson, announced the "Decade of Healthcare Information Technology" and announced the publication of a report which reveals how vital it is to have automation in the physician's and ambulatory offices.

The report identifies four major goals, with strategic action areas for each (Decade, 2004):

■ Goal 1: Inform Clinical Practice. Bringing information tools to the point of care, especially by investing in EHR systems in physician offices and hospitals.

■ Goal 2: Interconnect clinicians. Building an interoperable health information infrastructure, so that records follow the patient and clinicians have access to critical health care information when treatment decisions are being made.

■ Goal 3: Personalize Care. Using health information technology to give consumers more access and involvement in health decisions.

■ Goal 4: Improve population health. Expanding capacity for public health monitoring, quality-of-care measurement, and bringing research advances more quickly into medical practice.

Where Ambulatory Clients are Being Treated

As a response to increasing costs of providing healthcare, the healthcare industry has moved away from the expensive inpatient, acute care environment to caring for clients in various ambulatory care settings. There are numerous organizations that fit within the umbrella of ambulatory healthcare. They include ambulatory clinics and surgery centers, single- and multispecialty group practices, diagnostic laboratories, health maintenance organizations, independent physician associations, birthing centers, and college and university health services. Other organizations that serve the ambulatory population are faculty medical practices, community health centers, prison health centers, Indian health centers, hospital-sponsored ambulatory health services, urgent and immediate care centers, office-based surgery centers and practices, pain management clinics, podiatry offices, networks, mobile clinics, nurse managed centers, and groups of ambulatory care organizations. Many single specialty providers offer care in settings such as birthing centers, cardiac catheterization centers, dental clinics, dialysis centers, endoscopy centers, imaging centers, infusion therapy services, laser centers, lithotripsy services, MRI centers, ophthalmology practices, oral and maxillofacial surgery centers, pain management centers, plastic surgery centers, podiatric clinics, radiation/oncology clinics, rehabilitation centers, sleep centers, urgent/emergency care centers, and women's health centers (JCAHO, 2004).

 ## Issues for Ambulatory Care

Issues surrounding those who work in ambulatory care are similar across the healthcare enterprise including increased accountability, the need for continuous and documented service improvements, pressures to control utilization, and the protection of confidential information. Effective reimbursement of services is paramount for continued operation.

Applications Necessary in the Ambulatory Environment

Ambulatory care information systems, usually computer-assisted, are designed to store, manipulate, and retrieve information for planning, organizing, directing, and controlling administrative and clinical activities associated with the provision and use of ambulatory care services and facilities. The applications needed in the ambulatory environment are similar to those required in the in-patient arena. Registration, billing, accounts receivable, accounts payable, patient and staff scheduling, and managed care functionality are the major application areas. The emphasis in the past has been on financial and administrative applications, but some organizations are now adding automated clinical applications. The benefits that can be achieved by using electronic records encompass the financial, administrative, and clinical areas.

 ## Financial Benefits

Financial benefits of the implementation of an automated information system include a cost-effective and timely bill submission process resulting in decreased days in accounts receivable and the reduction of rejected claims. In the financial arena, client benefits need to be verified and accurate insurance information obtained. A correct bill must be submitted to the proper payor. Larger ambulatory care organizations use electronic data interchange (EDI) to automate the exchange of data (typically between providers and payors) such as claims, submittals and remittances, and health plan eligibility information. Some organizations also provide integrated credit card payment applications so that patients may use credit cards, which are processed immediately. Payments when received, electronically or manually, must be posted to the proper account. If the payor or the client does not pay the bill within a predefined time period, a collections process must be instituted. The electronic or manual system must support adjudication which is the process of determining which payor pays which portion of the bill. The eligibility process needs to be conducted with each instance of service as clients may have changed insurance plans since the last contact with the healthcare organization. Claims submitted to the payor may be either electronic or paper. In the ideal electronic system, claims are edited prior to submission so that charges are paid and not rejected which necessitates further processing, costing time, and money.

Administrative Benefits

Administrative benefits of implementing an automated information system include a reduction in the size of the record room, reduced time spent finding and delivering charts, increase in the privacy of data, formats that are legible and comply with legal regulations, and the promotion of quality assurance and improved patient satisfaction. Additional administrative benefits for automated ambulatory care records are the ability for home access by physicians and nurse practitioners, alerts for incomplete data, and the integration of clinical data.

The patient scheduling system must link existing scheduling systems so that scheduled activities are coordinated across locations to schedule appointment times, providers, resources, and locations throughout the hospital or organization. The patient needs to be seen at the appropriate time with the proper personnel, equipment, supplies, and chart information.

The physicians and nurse practitioners must be credentialed in order to provide services. Credentialing is the exhaustive verification of the medical licenses and qualifications. Healthcare providers must be recredentialed on a regular basis. An automated system can enhance lookup and maintenance of this data.

 ## Clinical Benefits

Clinically, the automated healthcare record can provide a problem list, automated ambulatory care provider order entry (ACPOE), a medication record, vital signs, progress notes, results from the laboratory and radiology departments, flow sheets, growth charts, immunization records, medication allergies, profiles, alerts and reminders, and a follow-up system. Other applications for the clinical area can encompass a clinical decision support system, e-Prescribing, and evidence-based medicine.

A patient master index is the basis for collection of all patient-related data. If the ambulatory care organization is part of a greater healthcare enterprise, then this master patient index must be integrated into an enterprise-wide index. A master patient index is a central repository for patient/member information across the enterprise including sophisticated tools for querying, updating, and managing the index. It must be able to accommodate multiple patient identifiers so that different locations can maintain their current medical record identification system. The registration system collects patient demographics and insurance information.

Other functions of the ambulatory care environment can be enhanced by electronic information technology for data collection and management. Referrals are required by many health plans when a patient is to be seen (or referred) to another healthcare provider. Automatic transfer of these requests will aid patient care and payment of the bill. The multitude of contracts between the healthcare facility and the payor need to be documented and managed through a contract administration function. Reports must be included in any information technology application. Beyond standard reports, the user must be able to generate user-specified reports. Medical record location can be tracked automatically with an automated system.

Regulatory Requirements

Accounting for costs can be aided by information technology. Systems must support the resource based relative value scale (RBRVS) and the relative value unit (RVU). The RBRVS procedure fee pricing is a model designed by the Department of Health and Human Services (DHHS). In this system, each physician's current procedural terminology (CPT) code has a relative value associated with it. The payor will pay the physician on the basis of a monetary multiplier for the RVS value.

The ambulatory care arena, just like other healthcare sectors, requires data in order to manage care. The Health Care Portability and Accountability Act of 1996 requires six code sets. Behind the scenes, a database must be maintained of all the current coding schemes used for the ambulatory environment. These include Current Procedural Terminology, 4th Edition (CPT) (AMA, 2004), the Ninth Revision of the International Classification of Diseases (ICD-9-CM) (CMS, 2004), the Healthcare Common Procedure Coding System (HCPCS) (CMS, 2004), the National Drug Code (NDC), managed by the FDA (2004), and the Code on Dental Procedures and Nomenclature.

CPT codes describe medical procedures performed by physicians and other health providers. The codes were developed by the American Medical Association (AMA) to assist in the assignment of reimbursement amounts to providers by Medicare carriers. A growing number of managed care and other insurance companies, however, base their reimbursements on the values established by HCFA. The most recent version is CPT 2004, which contains 7,755 codes and descriptors (AMA, 2004).

The ICD-9-CM (CMS, 2004) is based on the official version of the World Health Organization's ICD-9 (2004). It is designed for the classification of morbidity and mortality information for statistical purposes, for the indexing of hospital records by disease and operations, and for data storage and retrieval. Diagnoses and procedures coded in ICD-9-CM determine the diagnosis-related group (DRG) that controls reimbursement by CMS programs and most other payors. The United States is currently using the ninth revision although other countries are using the tenth version (*http://www.cdc.gov/nchs/about/_otheract_/icd9_/abticd9._htm*).

The HCFA HPCS (2004) is a collection of codes that represent procedures, supplies, products, and services which may be provided to Medicare beneficiaries and to individuals enrolled in private health insurance programs. The codes are designed to promote uniform reporting and statistical data collection of medical procedures, supplies, products, and services.

The NDC system identifies pharmaceuticals in detail including the packaging. Its use is required by the FDA for reporting and it is used in many healthcare information systems to aid in reimbursement. At the end of 2001, there were over 1,313,786 NDC codes. The current edition of the NDC directory is limited to prescription drugs and a few selected over-the-counter products (FDA, 2004). The directory is available on the Internet at *www.fda.gov/cder/ndc/index.htm*.

Medicare's ambulatory payment classification (APC) system is a prospective payment system for hospital outpatient services. APCs were mandated by Congress as part of the Balanced Budget Act of 1997 (Public Law 105-32). All covered outpatient services are divided into 451 groups called APCs. Software is available to help ambulatory care organizations determine outpatient payment and verify payment received. It also makes it possible for outpatient managers to determine patterns, to predict cost of resource use, and to evaluate managed care and physician contracts.

There are a multitude of other federal, state, and local regulations including those from the Centers for Medicare and Medicaid Services (CMS) formerly known as the Health Care Financing Administration. Among these are the health plan employer data and information set (HEDIS) (National Committee for Quality Assurance, 2004). HEDIS is a standardized, comprehensive set of indicators used to measure the performance of a health plan. Another is outcome and assessment information set (OASIS) regulations for the home care industry. OASIS is a data set for use in home health agencies and is an initiative from the Health Care Financing Administration. The purpose is to provide a comprehensive assessment for an adult home care patient and measure patient outcomes for purposes of outcome-based quality improvement.

In the ambulatory care environment there is much emphasis on data at the individual patient level. Also, it is important to aggregate data to view patient care and payment trends.

Implementation Issues and Challenges

In 2004, there was a long way to go in implementing clinical EHRs in the ambulatory arena. Based on 7,808 ambulatory care facilities, in 2004 84% were *not* automated, 13% had software installed, and 3% had a contract signed but the software was not implemented (HIMSS, 2004). Only 7% planned to purchase software.

Doctors view improvements in tablet personal computers and wireless networks as assisting in the adoption of EHRs. Physicians are asking national policymakers to assist in the adoption of information technology in the clinical area by offering federal loans, grants, tax incentives, and matching funds.

The Role of the Nurse Using Informatics Concepts in the Ambulatory Arena

First and foremost, the nurse is a user of the data contained in automated systems. The objective is to take the data and put it together in meaningful ways, making information. An automated system can help in this management of data and the transformation from data to information to knowledge. Reports are generated that can be used in the better management of the health of the patient, managing the administrative aspects of the practice, generating financial information, or for conducting research. A nurse may be involved in the selection of an automated system based on a needs assessment of the environment. The ambulatory care nurse may be instrumental in the implementation of an automated system whether the emphasis be administration, financial, or clinical. All nurses must be mindful of the impact of the information system on the confidentiality and security of information.

Member Associations Involved in Ambulatory Care

As varied as the types of organizations that serve the ambulatory populations are, so are the organizations which serve the professionals that work in those organizations. Major ambulatory care organizations will be highlighted.

The American Academy of Ambulatory Care Nursing (AAACN) is a member organization specifically for nurses. The AAACN offers networking opportunities for the membership by geographic location through local networking groups and by specialty practice through special interest groups (SIGs). One SIG for informatics is working to develop an ambulatory care data set for nursing. The organization also represents ambulatory practice to other political advocacy organizations, to government and quasi-government agencies, and in the federal and state legislative arena. They offer education through publications, electronic media, and conferences. The headquarters are located at East Holly Avenue, Box 56 Pitman, NJ 08071-0056 856.256.2350 *.aaacn@ajj.com* (*http://www.aaacn.org/*)

The American Medical Informatics Association (AMIA) (*http://www.amia.org*) has physicians and nurses amongst their membership. Working groups include the Primary Care Informatics Working Group. The Spring 2005 meeting was dedicated to "Best Practices for ACPOE and Population Management with EHR." AMIA contact information is as follows: American Medical Informatics Association, 4915 St. Elmo Avenue, Suite 401, Bethesda, MD 20814, phone: 301-657-1291, fax: 301-657-1296.

The Medical Group Management Association (MGMA), founded in 1926 and based in Colorado, is a major organization in the United States representing physicians in group practice nationwide. About 11,500 healthcare organizations and 19,000 individuals are MGMA members, representing more than 237,000 physicians (*http://www.mgma.com*). The organization supports education, networking, job recruitment, research, and political action. Contact the MGMA: MGMA Headquarters, 104 Inverness Terrace East, Englewood, CO 80112-5306, phone: 303.799.1111; toll-free: 877.ASK.MGMA (275.6462), fax: 303.643.4439.

The Society for Ambulatory Care Professionals (*http://www.aha.org*) is associated with the American Hospital Association. It is an organization of management professionals across the continuum of healthcare services, including outpatient, ambulatory, and home healthcare in hospital and freestanding settings. They offer networking opportunities, education, publications, and legislative advocacy.

The Federated Ambulatory Surgery Association (FASA) is a nonprofit association representing the interests of ambulatory surgery centers in the United States. FASA represents the physicians, nurses, administrative staff, and owners industry before the media, Congress, state legislatures, and regulatory bodies. FASA publishes a bimonthly journal and other publications to inform its members and the public. Also FASA conducts educational programs on a variety of topics (*http://www. fasa.org/about.html*). Contact FASA at Federated Ambulatory Surgery Association, 700 N. Fairfax Street, #306, Alexandria, VA 22314, phone: 703-836-8808, fax: (703) 549-0976, e-mail: *FASA@fasa.org*.

The American Association of Ambulatory Surgery Centers (AAASC) is a member organization that promotes advocacy at the national level through relationships with the CMS and Congress, networking, and educational opportunities (*http://www.aaasc.org/*). See the following for more information: American Association of Ambulatory Surgery Centers, P.O. Box 5271, Johnson City, TN 37602-5271, phone: 423-915-1001, fax: 423-282-9712, e-mail: *info@ AAASC.org*.

The Association for Ambulatory Behavioral Healthcare is an international organization of ambulatory mental healthcare providers dedicated to the delivery of high-quality psychiatric and chemical dependency treatment within a continuum of care. This membership association

which started about 1975 is based in Fairfax, Virginia (*http://www.aabh.org/*). AABH, 11240 Waples Mill Rd., Suite 200, Fairfax VA 22030, phone: 703-934-0160, fax: 703-359-7562, e-mail: *info @aabh.org*.

American Health Information Management Association (AHIMA) with over 46,000 members is a membership organization of health information management professionals. The purpose is to foster the professional development of its members through education, certification, and lifelong learning thereby promoting quality information to benefit the public, the healthcare consumer, providers, and other users of clinical data in any healthcare setting (*http://www.ahima.org*). Many resources are available online and in hardcopy documents. See AHIMA, 233 N. Michigan Avenue, Suite 2150, Chicago, IL 60601-5800, phone: 312-233-1100, fax: 312-233-1090, e-mail: *info@ahima.org*.

HIMSS, the Healthcare Information Management Systems Society, has formed an Ambulatory Care Committee. The HIMSS Ambulatory Care Initiative was created in response to trends such as the aging population, the increasing prevalence of chronic diseases, and the development of minimally-invasive procedures that can be performed without hospitalization (*www. himss.org*). (HIMSS, 2005) 230 East Ohio Street, Suite 500, Chicago, IL 60611-3269, phone: 312/664-4467, fax: 312/664-6143.

There are local groups to support the ambulatory care information systems specialist professionals such as AIM—the Ambulatory Information Management association. It is a specialty organization of the California Health Information Association (CHIA).

Accreditation Organizations

Accrediting organizations validate standards of practice and promote quality care. A private, not-for-profit organization was formed in 1979 called the Accreditation Association for Ambulatory Health Care (AAAHC). Their mission is to develop standards and conduct a survey and accreditation program (*http://www.aaahc.org/accreditation/coop_agree_faq.shtml*).

COLA, headquartered in Columbia, Maryland, is a nonprofit, physician-directed, and national accrediting organization. The purpose of COLA is to promote excellence in medicine and patient care through programs of voluntary education, achievement, and accreditation (*http://www.cola.org*).

The National Committee for Quality Assurance (NCQA) is a private, not-for-profit organization dedicated to assessing and reporting on the quality of managed care plans. They are governed by a board of directors that includes employers, consumer and labor representatives, health plans, quality experts, policy makers, and representatives from organized medicine (*http://www. ncqa.org*).

The Joint Commission on Accreditation of Healthcare Organizations (*https://www.jcaho.org*) publishes Management of Information Standards for Ambulatory Care. Standards are updated yearly and recently new elements of performance were added to be consistent with HIPAA.

Journals and Conferences

Healthcare professionals who work in the ambulatory care arena need to keep up with regulatory and practice changes in the environment. Among the ways to obtain an education include journals and conferences, as well as membership in organizations.

The *Journal of Ambulatory Care Management* is a quarterly publication. Each issue focuses on one topic of interest related to ambulatory care. The *Ambulatory Pediatrics* is a publication of the Ambulatory Pediatric Association. The journal, started in 1999, is available both on the World Wide Web and in hardcopy for a fee. The *Journal for Healthcare Quality* is a publication started in 1979 by the National Association for Healthcare Quality. The articles in the journal are refereed.

Several conferences focus on information technology needs of the ambulatory care arena. One of the best known with the largest attendance is the MGMA, – Medical Group Management Association which provides a wide range of educational programs on topics that medical group practices need to be aware of.

AMIA –the American Medical Informatics Association (*www.amia.org*) meets twice yearly, primarily in the Washington, DC area. Over 3,000 attendees meet primarily to discuss hospital and clinic use of technology. In addition, TEPR, sponsored by the Medical Records Institute (*http://www.medrecinst.com/conferences/tepr/*) will have its 21st meeting in February 2005 with an expected 4,000 attendees.

Future Directions for the Adoption of Information Technology in Ambulatory Care

The goals set by President Bush and the appointment of Dr. David J. Brailer as the national coordinator will inject momentum into the adoption of automated systems into ambulatory care. There is a move to use computerized provider order entry (CPOE) systems in ambulatory care. The biggest area of impact is that of medication safety where it is thought that adverse drug events could be prevented. A major area of concern is who should pay for the implementation of these systems. Estimates for the use of electronic prescribing of medications is now between only 5 and 18% of physicians and other clinicians (eHealth Initiative, 2004).

Some ambulatory practices are using electronic mail, computer interviewing, voice recognition, handwriting recognition, smart card technology, wireless devices, and biometrics. Some seek the goal of a paperless record. Automating the physician's offices and ambulatory care practices is a primary step in the goal of EHRs for all citizens.

References

American Academy of Ambulatory Care Nursing. *http:// www.aaacn.org*

American Medical Association. (2004). *CPT® 2005 Professional Edition*. Chicago, IL: AMA.

American Medical Informatics Association. (AMIA). *http:// www.amia.org*.

Centers for Medicare and Medicaid Services. (2004). *ICD-9-CM*. Washington, DC. *www.cms.hhs.gov/ paymentsystems/icd9/*

Centers for Medicare and Medicaid Services. *www.cms.hhs.gov/medicare/hcpcs/*

The Decade of Health Information Technology: Delivering consumer-centric and information-rich health care. Department of Health and Human Services, July 21, *http://www.hhs.gov/news/press/2004pres/20040721a. html*eHealth Initiative. (2004). Electronic prescribing: Toward maximum value and rapid adoption. *Recommendations for Optimal Design and Implementation to Improve Care, Increase Efficiency and Reduce Costs in Ambulatory Care*. Washington, DC: DHHS.

FDA. (2004). *National Drug Code Directory*. Washington, DC. *http://www.fda.gov/cder/ndc/*

Health Care Portability and Accountability Act of 1996. *http://aspe.hhs.gov/admnsimp/index.shtml*.

Healthcare Information Management Systems Society. (2005). *www.himss.org* and the HIMSS Analytics Database Chicago, IL: HIMSS.

Johnston, D., Pan, E., Walker, J., Bates, D.W., and Middleton, B. (2004). *Patient Safety in the Physician's Office: Assessing the Value of Ambulatory CPOE*. California Healthcare Foundation.

Joint Commission on Accreditation of Healthcare Organizations. (2004). *http://www.jcaho.org/ accredited+organizations/ambulatory+care/*

National Committee for Quality Assurance. (2004). *HEDIS®*. Washington, DC: NCQA.

The Decade of Health Information Technology: Delivering consumer-centric and information-rich health care. Department of Health and Human Services, July 21, *http://www.hhs.gov/*

U.S. Department of Health and Human Services (DHHS). *aspe.os.dhhs.gov/admnsimp*

White House Executive Order. April 27, (2004), *http://www.whitehouse.gov/news/releases/2004/04/20040427-4.html*. Retrieved May 2005.

WHO. (2004). ICD-10. Geneva. *http://www.who.int/whosis/icd10/*

24

Internet Tools for Advanced Nursing Practice

Mary Ann Lavin
Michael Morgan

OBJECTIVES

1. Employ basic and advanced Internet search skills in retrieving information pertinent to advanced practice nursing.

2. Access a variety of clinical practice Internet-available tools, including bioterrorism information, organized within nursing process categories.

3. Integrate eClinicaLog and its informatics skills-building components into the educational development of advanced practice nurses.

KEY WORDS

Internet tools
search methods
clinical practice
nursing process
assessment
diagnosis
bioterrorism
standardized terminologies
NLINKS
PubMed
nursing treatment
outcomes
eClinicaLog

This chapter presents a variety of Web-based applications that help form the knowledge base of advanced nursing practice. Information relevant to clinical decision-making continues to expand, and its relevance will only increase as the electronic health record becomes a standard part of practice. Furthermore, Internet access per wireless personal digital assistants (PDAs) and notebooks, currently geographically limited due to requirements to stay with the geographic limits of a wireless local area network (WLAN) or physical proxim-

ity to high speed phone lines, is already being challenged by fixed wireless broadband technology (Fixed Wireless, *http://www.fixedwireless1.com/Overview%20of%20Fixed%20Wireless.htm* Spint is the commercial pioneer of fixed wireless broadband technology. It provides geographic mobility up to 35 miles. Both wireless and fixed wireless talk/Internet time is usually limited to about 5–6 hours with standby time up to 1 week.

Wireless applications permit Internet connectivity. Within some academic health science centers this allows for Web-based clinical decision support, patient and clinician e-mail communication, and point-of-care electronic health record data entry, data sharing, and messaging, including prescription writing.

The authors gratefully acknowledge the contributions of Matthew J. Euler, BSN, RN, Lieutenant, U.S. Army.

Wireless technology is electromagnetically safe. Bluetooth radio technology, on which wireless devices rely, was found to be safe and robust even within intensive care environments (Wallin and Wajntraub, 2004). Other issues surrounding wireless technology use are not minor (Delbanco and Sands, 2004; Newbold, 2004). Such considerations include:

- Secure portals and encryption, which are mandatory to safeguard patient privacy/confidentiality.

- Incorporation of a wide range of practice guidelines to frame clinician and patient expectations and responsibilities.

- Cost per clinician time considerations.

Whether access is mobile or not, the Internet is increasingly an important adjunct to safe practice. The number of practical tools available on the Internet increases each year. This may result in information overload, unless the user knows how to retrieve and structure available tools. Retrieval cannot solely depend on the book marking of Web pages. They change as Web editors and designers add new information and tools. As a result, the Web site you visited today may be changed or even unavailable tomorrow and, there may be no forwarding address.

Basic and advanced Internet search skills are needed to adapt to a frequently changing Internet environment and to retrieve the wealth of Internet information applicable to clinical practice in an efficient manner. To facilitate adaptation, this chapter

1. Describes basic and advanced Internet search methods

2. Structures the presentation of Internet-available clinical practice tools

3. Discusses the eClinicaLog and its applicability to advanced practice

Basic and Advanced Internet Search Methods

Regardless of the search engine used, certain search methodologies, if applied correctly, increase the efficiency of retrieval of needed information. The following search strategies proceed from basic to advanced. Clinical examples are provided to facilitate learning. The strategies are three: name precisely the information being sought, use search strings rather than single words, and enhance search strings by using boolean or natural language methods. Each of these strategies is described below.

- Name precisely the information being sought. The Internet is not a book. There is no need to go to a chapter on diabetes mellitus, then find the section on therapeutic management, and then locate the specific pages or paragraphs containing information on insulin dosing. If the search terms used are precisely chosen, the searcher goes directly to the desired information.

- Use a search string (one or more search terms) rather than a single word to increase the preciseness of a search. If information on insulin dosing is needed, then enter "insulin dosing" into the search box and not "insulin." This principle may appear simple, but many fail to apply the principle when searching the Internet. The end result is frustration over time wasted. If tempted to use a single term such as insulin, ask what is it about insulin I want to know? Insulin reactions? Insulin resistance? Insulin administration? Or, insulin dosing? Enter the precise search terms in a string, rather than a single term, e.g., insulin.

- Enhance search strings by boolean or natural language methods. Use the boolean terms: AND, OR, or NOT. The term "AND" is used when search terms or strings need to be added together. The term "OR" is used when equivalent terms or synonyms are used to capture the information required. The following is an example of how "AND" may be used to create a search string that precisely expresses the intent of the searcher. Suppose the searcher is looking for asthma death rates in children in 2002. Boolean terms may be used as follows.

asthma AND (death OR mortality) AND rates AND children AND 2002

The same search conducted in natural language follows.

asthma death or mortality rates in children in 2002

Both searches lead directly to the same hyperlink. Search efficiency is maximized and cost is minimized, where cost stands for search time used.

This section on search methods concludes with tips on evaluating the quality of government (gov), education (edu), organization (org), and commercial (com) domains.

When using Web sites for clinical decision support purposes, the clinician must understand differences among these domains and evaluate the credibility of the content retrieved. In general, clinical information obtained from governmental domains is likely to be less biased than information obtained from commercial sites. The credibility of content from educational Web sites varies and is likely to be directly related to the academic quality of the university the Web site represents. An organizational Web site is likely to present organizational interests and bias. There is a vast difference in quality among commercial Web sites. It is therefore incumbent on the clinician to evaluate the credibility of the information obtained.

Case 24.1 presents an exercise in evaluating credibility of information obtained on the topic of drug interactions associated with St. John's Wort. The above search methodology and quality considerations are applicable when the clinician is using a search engine, e.g., the National Library of Medicine's (NLM) PubMed, OVID, or commercial search engines, e.g., Google. They are also applicable when conducting a metasearch, i.e., a simultaneous search of multiple search engines or databases.

The term "metasearch" represents a process similar to parallel, federated, broadcast, or cross-database searches (National Information Standards Organization, *http://www.niso.org/committees/MetaSearch-info.html*). Examples of two metasearch providers are NLM Gateway (*http://gateway.nlm.nih.gov/gw/Cmd*) and a privately produced site Ithaki (*http://www.ithaki.net/indexu.htm*). There are also Internet sites that provide how-to information on adding a metasearch capability to a Web site. They include:

- Digital windmill (*http://digitalwindmill.com/*)
- eMetasearch (*http://emetasearch.com/*)

For additional information on Web searches, including metasearches, access the William H. Welch Medical Library Evidence Based Medicine Webpage and scroll down to "Meta-Search Engines) (Johns Hopkins Medical Institutions, Welch Medical Library, *http://www.welch.jhu.edu/internet/ebr.html#meta-analysis*).

Internet-Available Clinical Practice Tools

This section is divided into the most basic components of the nursing process: assessment, diagnosis, treatment, and outcomes evaluation. These components provide the outward structure for the development of a Clinical Information Database for Advanced Practice Nursing. The Internet sites selected are listed within this structure. Although the listing is not exhaustive, it does represent carefully selected examples of the types of clinical information available on the Internet. This structured approach to clinical information database development is clinically useful, helps clinicians organize their own knowledge databases, and facilitates ready access to needed information.

Assessment

Assessment refers to the systematic collection of data needed to arrive at one or more diagnoses. The tools included in this section include forms, miscellaneous screening tools, risk assessment instrument, and information of the manifestation of signs and symptoms. These tools represent a sampling of assessment content available on the Internet. Each category is described briefly.

Nursing assessment is the first step in the nursing process. The following site provides an example of a comprehensive nursing assessment form:

http://www.hospitalsoup.com/public/nursingassess2001.pdf

Craving, loss of control, physical dependence, and tolerance constitute four cardinal signs and symptoms of alcoholism. This Web site of the NIH National Institute on Alcohol Abuse and Alcoholism provides not only a reminder of signs and symptoms but also contain outstanding resource information:

http://www.niaaa.nih.gov

Domestic abuse assessment is an integral part of primary care practice. The following assessment tool, from the Vermont Department of Health, provides information on a professional approach to interviewing on the delicate topic and the essential questions to be asked. One additional tip is to have available directions to and the phone number of a safe house. Some domestic abuse counselors recommend that the information be given verbally, asking the patient to memorize it rather than placing the patient at added risk should the abusive partner find the written material and use it as an excuse for further abuse:

http://www.state.vt.us/health/abuse.htm

The following Web page is from the Connecticut Clearinghouse, a program of the Wheeler Clinic. It consists of multiple assessment and screening hyperlinks, useful in advanced nursing practice:

http://www.ctclearinghouse.org/

Risk assessment is an important part of clinical practice. The following Internet tools are health risk calculators that provide the evidence to support risk diagnoses.

Case 24.1 Drug Interactions Associated with St. John's Wort: A Comparison of the Information Obtained from Four Internet Domains

Government Domains Several government Web sites were selected: The Food and Drug Administration (*www.fda.gov*), the NLM PubMed database (*www.pubmed.gov*). The National Center for Complementary and Alternative Medicine (NCCAM) (*http://nccam.nih.gov/clinicaltrials/stjohnswort/*, retrieved on June 21, 2004). The site that provided the quickest access and the most concrete information on drug interactions was the FDA Web site with its warning letter to health professionals, dated February 10, 2000 (Food and Drug Administration, *http://www.fda.gov/ cder/drug/advisory/stjwort.htm*). To retrieve this letter, the search terms "St. John's Wort" or "St. John's Wort AND drug interactions" were entered into the FDA home page search box. The letter indicated that St. John's Wort lowers the plasma concentration and hence decreases the effectiveness of indinavir, a protease inhibitor. The letter postulated that the cause of the interaction is due to the metabolism of the two drugs. St. John's Wort induces the P450 metabolic pathway in the liver that indinavir relies on for its metabolism. Therefore, the metabolism (in this case, inactivation) of indinavir occurs more rapidly than normal. Consequently, its plasma concentration is thereby reduced. The FDA noted that similar interactions are likely to occur between St. John's Wort and other protease inhibitors metabolized by the same P450 subsystem.

The PubMed site provided additional information relevant to clinical decision-making. When the search terms "St. John's Wort AND P450" were used and results were limited to abstracts only, 46 citations were retrieved. St. John's Wort was found to reduce the plasma concentrations of:

Alprazolam (Markowitz et al., 2004)

Verapamil (Tannergren et al., 2004)

Alprazolam, amitriptyline, cyclosporine, digoxin, fexofenadine, indinavir, irinotecan, methadone, nevirapine, simvastatin, tacrolimus, theophylline, warfarin, phenprocoumon, and oral contraceptives (Izzo, 2004).

These interactions are secondary to the induction of P450 human isoenzymes, including CYP2C19 (Wang et al., 2004). CYP2C19 is responsible for the metabolism of drugs, e.g., proton pump inhibitors, phenytoin, diazepam, amitriptyline, and warfarin (Indiana University-Purdue University Indianapolis, School of Medicine, *http://medicine.iupui.edu/flockhart/table.htm*).

Other drug interactions with St. John's Wort were mentioned. It was found to:

Enhance *P*-glycoprotein efflux activity (Hennessy et al., 2002)

Induce serotonin syndrome when coadministered with selective serotonin reuptake inhibitors (Izzo, 2004)

A second search was conducted using the terms "cyclosporine AND St. John's Wort." This search led to several reports of organ rejection resulting from a cyclosporine and St. John's Wort drug interaction. Karliova, occurring when cyclosporine and St. John's Wort are taken in conjunction. These reactions included:

Acute rejection of a liver transplant (Karliova et al., 2000)

A sudden drop in the cyclosporine plasma concentration of a previously well-controlled, long-term kidney transplant patient (Mai et al., 2000)

Kidney and pancreas transplant organ rejection (Barone et al., 2001)

Acute rejection of organ transplants in two other patients (Ruschitzka et al., 2000).

On introducing the search terms "St. John's Wort AND P450" into its search box, the NCCAM reported the interaction effect of St. John's Wort with an "important" liver enzyme. The information, although useful, was written in language addressed to the lay consumer (Newsletter, *http://nccam.nih.gov/news/newsletter/previous/index.htm*). After inserting the same search string into the clinical trials page of NCCAM, several ongoing clinical trials were found to be investigating the effect of St. John's Wort on minor and major depression, oral contraceptives, herbal-opioid interactions, screening herbs for drug interactions, obsessive-compulsive disorders, and social phobia.

Educational Domains When the search phrase "P450 drug interactions" was entered into the Google search box, the first site listed in an edu domain was Indiana University, Purdue University Indianapolis P450 Drug Interactions Table (*http://medicine.iupui.edu/flockhart/table.htm*), where a P450 cytochromosal drug interaction table is provided. To use, enter "St. John's Wort" in the find box. Note that St. John's Wort is listed as a CY 3A4,5,7 inducer. Note the CY 3A4,5,7 substrates and inhibitors as well. As an inducer, St. John's Wort will lower the plasma concentration of all substrates and inhibitors within the same P450 isoenzyme subsystem.

Organizational Domains   Very little actual and no new information was found when the search string "St. John's Wort AND drug interactions AND organizations" was entered in Google. Of the first 10 sites listed, only one was an organizational site and when activated it linked to a commercial site alerting seniors to the drug interaction effects of St. John's Wort. Credibility was not the issue but rather the fact that organizations as such do not address drug interaction issues.

Commercial Domains   The credibility of commercial sites was mixed. Known sites were accessed first: medscape.com and rxlist.com. Medscape provided assessable, user friendly, and updated information. In the search box on the home page, enter the search terms, in this case "St. John's Wort" and then click on "drug information." When the drug information section

appears, click on "drug interactions." A comprehensive listing of the drug interactions appears. Another pharmacology reference site is rxlist.com. However, its St. John's Wort drug interaction page was last updated in 1999 and its use, therefore, was limited.

To obtain a listing of other commercial sites, a Google search was performed, using the search terms "St. John's Wort and P450." All, among the first 10 sites assessed, cited St. John's Wort drug interaction effects, the information was based on a few citations only, obtained from PubMed. It was obvious that the primary source, PubMed, provided more information in terms of quality and quantity of reports than any of the commercial sites.

Conclusions   Credible information on specific clinical topics is readily available on the Internet. The type and depth of information varies by domain and by the purpose of the web site within domains. For clinical decision support purposes, it is suggested that a database of sites be kept readily available for use. With this particular search, government and university sites provided the best available information.

- Body mass index calculator from the National Heart, Lung, and Blood Institutes of the National Institutes of Health (*http://nhlbisupport.com/bmi/bmicalc.htm*).

- Cancer risk tools are available on the Web pages of the Harvard Center for Cancer Prevention. Risks may be calculated for breast, prostate, lung (Case 24.2), colon, bladder, melanoma, uterine, kidney, pancreatic, ovarian, stomach, and cervical cancers (*http://www.yourcancerrisk.harvard.edu/*).

- Coronary heart disease risk calculator, a risk assessment tool for estimating 10-year risk of developing hard CHD (myocardial infarction and coronary death), based on age, gender, total cholesterol, high-density lipoprotein (HDL), smoker, blood pressure, and current medication for hypertension for the NIH National Heart, Lung, and Blood Institute (*http://hin.nhlbi.nih.gov/atpiii/calculator.asp?usertype=prof*).

- Health risk calculators from the University of Maryland Medicine for 24 health conditions, including asthma, depression, diabetes, pregnancy due date, HIV risk, nicotine dependency, teen suicide risk, and more (*http://www.umm.edu/healthcalculators/*).

The assessment of symptoms of illness and the education of patients regarding symptoms are major responsibilities of the advanced practice nurse. An outstanding resource for consumers and health professionals is the information available through the following NLM MEDLINE Plus Health Information hyperlink:

http://search.nlm.nih.gov/homepage/query?FUNCTION=search&PARAMETER=MEDLINE+Plus +AND+symptoms+AND+manifestations&DISAMBIGUATION=true&START=0&END=25& MAX=250&ASPECT=1

Assessment concludes with the listing of diagnoses, the next major category of Internet tools.

Diagnosis

Treatment is diagnostic-specific. Hence, diagnosis and treatment information categories are frequently not discreet. Practice guidelines often address assessment, diagnosis, and treatment. Disease directories often do the same. When developing the accompanying clinical information database, a diagnosis/treatment category was developed to respond to the overlap. Conceptually, however, it was thought best to divide the content sequentially. In the following section, the focus is on treatment; in this section, the focus is diagnosis.

Case 24.2

A 73-year-old male, retired insurance agent, who smoked between 14 and 25 cigarettes per day between the ages of 18 and 45 years, but never any cigars, asks you what his chances of developing lung cancer. How would you respond?

To answer this patient's question, the advanced practice nurse with the patient accesses the Harvard Center for Cancer Prevention.

Access http://www.yourcancerrisk.harvard.edu/ and click on cancer.

Then click, on "Lung Cancer," answer age and sex questions, and click next.

Answer question about any prior diagnosis of cancer and click next.

Answer questions about the number of vegetable and fruit servings per day and click next.

Answer questions about cigarette smoking history and click next.

Answer question about number of cigarettes smoked per day and click next.

Answer question about cigars smoked per day during the past year and click next.

Answer questions about city living and asbestos exposure and click next.

Answer question about chemical exposure and click next.

Answer question about exposure to various manufacturing processes and click next.

Answer question about diagnosis of lung cancer among immediate family members and click next.

Results　Based on the answers to these questions, this patient (who had no prior history of cancer, ate at least three fruits and vegetables daily, smoked between 14 and 25 cigarettes per day between 18 and 45 years, never smoked cigars, lived in a city his entire life, was never exposed to asbestos, carcinogenic chemicals or manufacturing process, and has no family history of lung cancer) has a below average risk of lung cancer, with the risk displayed graphically.

The etymology of the word "diagnosis" is based in its Greek roots. "Dia" means "through," and "gnosis" means "knowledge." Diagnosis is dependent on the knowledge base of the person diagnosing. Disease represents the knowledge base of physicians. Human responses to illness and health represent the knowledge base of nursing. A classification of functional health and disability terms represents a beginning step toward the elaboration of a unified health professional knowledge base. These knowledge bases are displayed within classification systems specifically

1. Medical classifications of diseases, e.g., the International Classification of Disease (ICD)-10-CM (World Health Organization [WHO], 1992) and the ICD-9 (American Medical Association, 2004)

2. Nursing classifications of human responses to illness and health, e.g., the NANDA Classification of Nursing Diagnoses (NANDA 2003–2004)

3. Functional health and disability, e.g., the International Classification of Functioning in Health and Disability (World Health Organization, 2002).

Classifications display in a systematic manner the array of diagnoses that represent the knowledge bases of the professions represented. Clinicians need to be aware of these classifications for data entry, aggregation, analysis, and reimbursement purposes. For clinical purposes, they need to know how to access information on the diagnoses themselves and how to contribute to their development. Clinicians today are faced with new threats to health, requiring rapid access to related information. These threats include emerging infections and bioterrorism events. Therefore, this section on diagnosis is divided into the following sections: new threats to health, disease/condition directories, examples of specific disease information, easy diagnosis tools, standardized diagnosis terminologies, and the unified medical language system (UMLS).

New Threats to Health　New threats to health include mass trauma, biologic and biochemical warfare agents, and emerging infectious diseases. Primary care and emergency department practitioners need readily accessible information to facilitate diagnosis. The CDC's

Emergency Preparedness and Response Web page is an excellent resource. Either click on "Emergency Preparedness and Response" within the left hand margin of *www.cdc.gov* or access the site directly at *http://www.bt.cdc.gov/*. Within the bioterrorism site, the following pages are available.

Mass Trauma Preparedness and Response   Mass trauma hyperlinks, featured on the CDC Emergency Preparedness and Response webpages include coping with a traumatic event, a primer for clinicians on dealing with explosions and blast injuries; fact sheets for injuries and mass trauma; possible research studies; and rapid assessment of injuries. The latter hyperlink contains a rapid assessment instrument available as an html, pdf, Word, and rich text file document. This instrument is especially useful in documenting the nature and scope of presenting injuries.

Bioterrorism Agents/Diseases   The CDC Emergency Preparedness and Response webpages present information on approximately 30 diseases e.g., anthrax, plague, smallpox, typhoid fever. When a particular hyperlink, e.g., smallpox, is activated, the information is available for everyone, specific groups (e.g., clinicians, health officials, responders), and diagnostic testing, infection control, and other specialized information for health professionals. Photographic images and/or video presentations facilitate clinical decision-making related to infectious agents that may be used for bioterrorism purposes.

Chemical Agents   The CDC Emergency Preparedness and Response webpages hyperlink information to more than 70 chemical agents. Some of the hyperlinks represent categories of agents, e.g., biotoxins, blister agents, and caustics (acids). When these categories are activated, listings of within category agents are provided. In addition to a toxicologic profile, most also include information on the clinical management of the toxins. Other hyperlinks represent single agents, e.g., ricin. When the ricin hyperlink is activated, the categories of information are basics for the public, information for clinicians, laboratory information, and information for first responders. Information for clinicians includes several topic categories: recognition, case management and surveillance, case definitions, toxic syndrome recognition, and a 2003 investigation of ricin at a postal facility.

Recent Outbreaks and Incidents   The Emergency Preparedness and Response page also includes informa-

tion on outbreaks, e.g., severe acute respiratory syndrome (SARS), West Nile virus, monkey pox, and mad cow disease; this site also includes information on incidents, e.g., wild fires, winter storms, and power outages. Detailed information is provided on each. For example, the West Nile virus hyperlink leads ultimately to a page that presents guidelines for clinicians, including disease diagnosis.

Other useful hyperlinks on CDC's Emergency Preparedness and Response page are those on radiation emergencies and natural disasters.

Bioterrorism Information Available through Academic Health Science Centers   Several academic health science centers have received federal funding to move biodefense research and education forward. These sites include the following.

- Agency of Healthcare Research and Quality in collaboration with the University of Alabama has a Web site devoted to bioterrorism education (*http://www.bioterrorism.uab.edu/*)
- George Mason University National Center for Biodefense (*http://www.gmu.edu/centers/biodefense/*)
- Saint Louis University Center for the Study of Bioterrorism and Emerging Infections (*http://bioterrorism.slu.edu/*)
- University of Pittsburgh Center for Biosecurity (*http://www.upmc-biosecurity.org/*)

Disease Diagnoses   The most familiar disease terminology is the ICD (World Health Organization, 1992). For use in the United States, WHO has authorized the Department of Health and Human Services National Center for Health Statistics to develop, in keeping with WHO ICD conventions, the ICD-10-CM, where CM refers to clinical modification. A prerelease version is available for review at the National Center for Health Statistics (*http://www.cdc.gov/nchs/about/otheract/icd9/abticd10.htm*) and preview books are available for sale at bookstores. Currently, ICD-9-CM is the classification still in use in the United States (American Medical Association, 2004).

Use of the ICD code allows for the aggregation of disease data across patient care settings. Because disease definitions are not static, codes are never finished products. Each year, the Centers for Medicaid and Medicare Services (CMS) Medicare Learning Network posts lists of new and revised ICD diagnosis codes and titles (*http://www.cms.hhs.gov/medlearn/icd9code.asp*).

There are several disease directories, with A–Z lists, that are Internet available. Examples include:

Centers for Disease Control and Prevention (CDC), Diseases and Conditions. The hyperlink is available in the left hand margin of the CDC homepage (*www.cdc.gov*) or may be accessed directly at *http://www.cdc.gov/node.do/id/0900f3ec8000e035*

A–Z list of cancers from the National Cancer Institute (*www.nci.nih.gov*)

The Karolinska Institute University Library in Sweden (*http://www.mic.ki.se/Diseases/*)

For disease definitions, online medical dictionaries are useful. One example is the On-Line Medical Dictionary published by the University of Newcastle upon Tyne Department of Oncology (*http://cancer-web.ncl.ac.uk/omd*). Its listing, which is not limited to oncology-related diseases, is a readily accessible, comprehensive dictionary.

While the above directories are appropriate for clinicians, there are also disease directories that target a lay audience and that provide outstanding health education information. Examples include the

National Institute of Diabetes, Digestive, and Kidney Diseases, National Digestive Diseases Information Clearinghouse (NDDIC) (*http:// digestive.niddk.nih.gov/ddiseases/a-z.asp*)

New York Online Access to Health (*www.noah-health.org*). The latter site has an A-Z Index, which is especially useful for providing laypersons with information on uncommon illness, for example: lupus erythematosus, Marfan's syndrome, Ehlers-Danlos syndrome.

Many Internet sites provide clinical information on tools useful in the diagnosis of specific diseases. For example, Brain Attack: Stroke Scales, National Institute of Neurological Disorders and Stroke (*http://www.stroke-site.org/stroke_scales/stroke_scales.html*).

Other sites are devoted to a group of diseases, related in some way. The new field of genomics fits this latter category. For information on genomics and disease prevention, access CDC, Genomics and Disease Prevention, *http://www.cdc.gov/genomics/default.htm*.

Human Response to Illness/Health Diagnoses

The Internet tools presented in this section are infrastructure tools, because much of the work that needs to be accomplished in the field of nursing diagnosis is at the infrastructure level. It is imperative that nurse informaticists continue to engage in this work, if the profession is to advance scientifically. It is equally imperative that advanced practice nurses enter, aggregate, and analyze data from nursing terminologies and subsets of other standardized healthcare terminologies (Keenan et al., 2003).

Terminologies designed for or listing nursing diagnoses include NANDA Diagnoses and Classification (NANDA–2005–2006, nanda.org), Home Health Care Classification (Saba, 2003, sabacare.com), The Omaha System (Martin, Elfrink, and Monson, 2001, omahasystem.org), and the perioperative nursing data set (*http://www.aorn.org/research/pnds.htm*). These classifications are recognized by the American Nurses Association, included in the UMLS of the NLM, and available through the standardized nomenclature of medical terminology—clinical terms (SNOMED CT). The latter is a terminology model approved as the U.S. standard for the entry and aggregation of electronic health record data (Lavin et al., 2004).

The nursing profession has yet to display its diagnoses, defining characteristics, and related factors in a manner as readily available to the clinician as the medical profession has displayed its array of diseases. The NLM's UMLS constitutes one exception. Clinicians, researchers, or educators may register with UMLS and access the diagnosis definitions and, in terms of the NANDA Classification of Nursing Diagnoses, access the defining characteristics and related factors, as well. To register with UMLS, access *http://www.nlm.nih.gov/research/umls/access.html*.

After UMLS registration, access the UMLS Knowledge Source Server (UMLSKS) to login. Once logged in, enter the nursing diagnosis search term, e.g., chronic pain, and click on "Metathesaurus Concept Search." There are three standardized definitions from which to choose: the CRISP Thesaurus, the Home Health Care Classification, and NANDA's Classification of Nursing Diagnoses. The latter provides NANDA's defining characteristics and related factors in addition to the definition.

Adjacent to Metathesaurus Concept Search are two other buttons: Semantic type and Specialist Lexical Search. Although the UMLS semantic type of chronic pain "is a" sign and symptom as it exists within disease terminology, the semantic type of chronic pain within nursing "is a" human response to illness/health diagnosis. In other words, the semantic types of disease and human response to illness/health terminologies are disjointed, in some cases. This difficulty makes adaptation of the UMLS for electronic health record purposes problematic. Resolution is possible by establishing a semantic type called "observation," as it is done in SNOMED CT. If chronic pain "is an observation," then it may be aggregated and analyzed as a sign or symptom in reference to disease and as a diagnosis in reference to illness/health human responses. When "chronic pain" is subjected to the Specialist Lexical Search, pain is referenced as a noun, but pain modified by the word chronic is appropriately excluded. Such modifiers are not essential to lexical searches.

To develop an array of nursing diagnoses that are evidence-based, an infrastructure is needed to facilitate the requisite literature searches reporting primary data results. Primary data refers to data collected at the point of patient contact, whether quantitative or qualitative (Lavin et al., 2005). A nursing diagnosis and primary data database that connects to PubMed (NLM, pubmed.gov) is available through the Network for Language in Nursing Knowledge Systems Research Center (*http://www.nlinks.org/research_main.phtml*); or, to retrieve citations on any single nursing diagnosis, follow these directions.

1. Access nlinks.org.

2. Click on Research Center.

3. Scroll down to the Nursing Diagnosis and Primary Data Database hyperlink and click on it.

4. A PubMed Web page will appear. In the search box is a nursing diagnosis and primary data filter. Do not alter the filter. Rather, place the cursor at the beginning of the filter.

5. Type in the nursing diagnosis of interest and use a Boolean AND to connect it to the filter already present in the search box.

6. Click on limits.

7. Limit the choices to "abstracts only" and, if desired, limit to "nursing journals" by click on "Subsets."

8. Click on "Go" to retrieve the abstracts of interest.

Save the search citations in PubMed's *My NCBI (Cubby)* directly (*http://www.ncbi.nlm.nih.gov/entrez/ login.fcgi?call=so.SignOn..Login&callpath=QueryExt. CubbyQuery..ShowAll&db=pubmed*). Scroll down the left hand margin on the PubMed Web page and click on "*My NCBI.*" NCBI is an acronym for the National Center for Biotechnology Information at the National Library of Medicine. Cubby refers to an electronic cubby hole, where personal searches may be stored. Register for *My NCBI* by entering the required ID and password registration information. Save and retrieve searches in your own *My NCBI (Cubby)* as needed.

Table 24.1 presents the results of NLINKS nursing diagnosis and primary data searches for two time periods. limited to abstracts only and the nursing journals

Table 24.1   Results of NLINKS Nursing Diagnosis and Primary Data Database Searches for the Years 1994 through 1998 and 1999 through 2003

Nursing Diagnosis	1994–1998	1999–2003
Knowledge deficit	6	3
Acute pain	73	92
Chronic pain	86	133
Self-care deficit	16	2
Anxiety	166	211

Note: Limited to abstracts only and nursing journal subset.

subset. Notice that primary data research on the diagnoses of deficient knowledge and self care have declined from the first to second time periods, while research abstracts on pain, chronic pain, and anxiety have increased. Other literature databases include MEDLINE (NLM, *www.pubmed.gov* click on Limits, then on Subsets, and then MEDLINE), PubMed's Clinical Queries Research Methodology Filters (NLM, *http://www.ncbi.nlm.nih.gov/entrez/query/static/clinical.html* or access in the left hand margin of the pubmed.gov homepage), and CINAHL (*http://www. cinahl.com*). Because each database relies on its own unique filter or filters, the results will be different even if the same search terms are used.

Methods of Contributing to Terminology Revision and Development   Like the ICD, standardized nursing terminology is in continual need of revision and development. Clinicians, informaticists, researchers, educators, and students may contribute to this process. Revision and new diagnosis submission forms and instructions are available at the NANDA Web site (*www.nanda.org*) and the Network for Language in Nursing Knowledge Systems Concept Analysis Center (*http://nlinks.org/cac_introduction.phtml*).

The International Classification of Functioning, Disability, and Health (ICF)   Standardized nursing diagnosis terminologies do not encompass the entire field. As a result, subsets from the ICD are used, especially in the provision of primary care services by advanced practice nurses. Another terminology of interest to nursing practice is the ICF. The ICF consists of four domains: body functions, body structures, activity and participation, and environmental factors. Of these, the body functions, activity and participation, and environmental factors contain subsets with terms applicable to or capable of being developed as nursing diagnosis.

An ICF browser is available at the Web site of the WHO (*http://www3.who.int/icf/onlinebrowser/icf.cfm*).

This browser includes a comments message box so that users may provide feedback on the domains and/or terms within domains. The ICF may also be accessed through the U.S. National Center for Health Statistics (*www.cdc.gov/nchs*) and clicking on "Disease Classifications" in the left hand margin.

The ICF is a classification of interest within the United States. Following an 18-month study, the U.S. National Committee for Vital and Health Statistics (NCVHS) enthusiastically approved the report "Classifying and Reporting Functional Status" in a letter of July 16, 2001 from the committee chair, John R. Lumpkin, MD, MPH, to the Department of Health and Human Services secretary, Tommy Thompson. The cover letter, report, and its appendices are available at *http://www.ncvhs.hhs.gov/010716rp.htm*. The Spring issue of the 2003 Centers for Medicare and Medicaid Services Health Care Financing Review, posted on the CMS Web site (*http://www.cms.hhs.gov/review/03spring/defaut.asp*) reported on conference proceedings on functional status. Several of the papers accessible at the site refer to ICF applications.

The ICF may assist nursing terminology developers in generating revised and new diagnose. It may also serve as a tool facilitating collaboration among leaders in the field of nursing diagnosis classifications. In a critical appraisal, Kearney and Pryor (2004) found it to be a useful conceptual framework for practice, education, and research. In a review, Lehman (2003) concluded that it provides a useful framework in researching health conditions, body structures and function, activity and participation, and environmental influences on patients with idiopathic intracranial hypertension. While recognizing its clinical applicability, Heerkens et al. (2003) noted that its lack of detail lends itself to development by multidisciplinary teams and publication as a clinical modifications manual, an ICF-CM. It is hoped that nursing terminology developers, informaticists, and clinicians become involved in this process and use the opportunity to contribute not only to a better ICF but to think creatively about the development of a more unified nursing diagnosis terminology as well.

Treatment

The term "treatment" is used here in lieu of interventions and nursing actions, because it expresses more precisely the broad clinical management focus of this section.

Nursing Treatment   Several Internet sites are available for those who desire more information on Saba's framework/structure examples. a NIC intervention example, Omaha System case studies, and PNDS examples and outcomes. They are:

- Home Health Care Classification (Saba, 2003, *www.sabacare.com*)
- Nursing Interventions Classification (NIC) (Dochterman and Bulechek, 2003, *http://www.nursing.uiowa.edu/centers/cncce/nic/index.htm*)
- Omaha System (Martin, Elfrink, and Monson, 2001, *http://www.omahasystem.org/*)
- Perioperative nursing data set (*http://www.aorn.org/research/pnds.htm*)

Calculators   Internet tools are available to facilitate calculations used in planning treatment. Examples include:

Martindale's Calculators Online Part I: Nutrition (*http://www.martindalecenter.com/Calculators1B_4_Nut.html*). In addition to folic acid, calcium, and calorie calculators, there is also a basal metabolism calculator especially applicable given interest in dieting and a surge in the proportion of the population who are overweight or obese. After entering age, sex, height, and weight variables, this calculator computes the number of daily calories required to maintain or lose weight and also provides the number of related grams of protein, fat, and carbohydrate (Cases 24.3 and 24.4).

Nursing calculators for drug administration purposes (Villanueva, *http://www.manuelsweb.com/nrs_calculators.htm*)

Medical calculators developed by Cornell University Medical College, Pediatric Critical Care Medicine (*http://www-users.med.cornell.edu/~spon/picu/calc/medcalc.htm*)

Drug Management   There is no shortage of information available on pharmacotherapeutics and the pharmacologic management of patients. The federal government provides a wealth of information.

1. Drug Enforcement Agency (*www.dea.gov*), excellent information on drugs and chemicals of concern (*http://www.deadiversion.usdoj.gov/drugs_concern/index.html*

Case 24.3

You have recently joined a primary care practice. One of your first patients, a 43-year-old, obese female secondary school teacher returns to the office for follow-up Type 2 diabetic management. She reports that her fasting blood sugars are between 230 and 255 mg/dL per finger stick. She indicates that she has been avoiding all sugars. For breakfast, she eats a dish of oatmeal with about one-half cup of milk and a little honey, a banana, and about 4 oz of orange juice. For lunch, she usually eats one or two slices of pizza or a pasta dish with the teachers at school along with a diet soda. Every now and then she will eat a small slice of cake, when it is a coworker's birthday. For supper, she will stop by a fast food restaurant for a hamburger and salad on the way home or eat part of a pot roast or stew she had prepared over the weekend. She eats graham crackers and milk at bedtime. Your diagnoses are Type 2 diabetes mellitus, obesity, and diabetic diet knowledge deficit. You would like to code all three, but you have been told by your nurse practitioner colleagues that there is no way to code nursing diagnoses for reimbursement purposes. What would you do?

The 2004 ICD-9th edition, as in previous editions, contains V-codes, which allow for the classification of factors influencing health status or contact with health services. The V-codes are numbered V-01-V83, but the V40-49 codes are designed for conditions affecting a person's health status. Nursing diagnoses, e.g., "risk" nursing diagnoses, deficient knowledge, and ineffective management of therapeutic regimen, may be coded with the ICD using V-codes, especially V49, other specified conditions influencing health status. These codes need to be explored for clinical application and reimbursement purposes. The following site provides free, online access to the codes (ICD-9, *http://icd9cm.chrisendres.com*).

Case 24.4

A 63-year-old woman asks what kind of diet she would need, to lose weight. Her height is 63.5 in. and her weight is 173 lb. What would you do?

> Access Martindale's Calculators Online Center Part I: I-N Nutrition (*http://www.martindalecenter.com/Calculators1B_4_Nut.html*)
>
> Scroll down and click on Basal Metabolism Calculators (*http://www.room42. com/nutrition/basal.shtml*).

Enter the patient's criteria

> Input weight is 173 in U.S. lb
>
> Input height is 63 in U.S. in.
>
> Input age is 63
>
> Input gender is female
>
>> Click on "calculate now."

The metabolism results that appear on the next Web page are:
1422.4 calories per day is the basal caloric rate. This is:

no more than 47.415 g of fat (30%) for the patient's basal caloric rate

53.341 g of protein (15%) for the patient's basal caloric rate

195.58 g of carbohydrate (55%) for the patient's basal caloric rate

1849.1 calories per day recommended for the patient's active caloric rate. This is:

no more than 61.639 g of fat (30%) for the patient's active caloric rate

69.344 g of protein (15%) for the patient's active caloric rate

254.26 g of carbohydrate (55%) for the patient's active caloric rate

No fewer than 1200 calories per day are recommended for a safe weight loss of 1 lb every 15 days. This is:

no more than 40 g of fat (30%) for weight loss rate

45 g of protein (15%) for your weight loss rate

165 g of carbohydrate (55%) for weight loss rate

2. Food and Drug Administration (*www.fda.gov*), with an outstanding search capability. Clinicians need to remember that herbal products, even though pharmacologically active, are listed under "Foods" and not under "Drugs." Within the FDA Web site, the following are especially useful pages.
   (a) Center for Drug Research and Evaluation (*http://www.fda.gov/cder/index.html*)
   (b) Medwatch: The FDA Safety Information and Adverse Event Reporting Program (*http://www.fda.gov/medwatch/index.html*)
   (c) Medwatch Adverse Event and Product Problem Forms (*http://www.fda.gov/medwatch/get-forms.htm*)
   (d) Vaccine Adverse Event Reporting System (*http://www.fda.gov/medwatch/safety/vaers1.pdf*)

3. NLM Clinical Alerts Database, may be accessed in the left hand margin of the *www.pubmed.gov* Web page or directly at *http://www.nlm.nih.gov/data-bases/alerts/clinical_alerts.html*

4. The National Institutes of Health (*www.nih.gov*) provide outstanding drug information. See especially the following.
   (a) National Institute on Alcohol Abuse and Alcoholism (*www.niaaa.nih.gov/*)
   (b) National Institute on Drug Abuse (*www.nida.nih.gov*)
   (c) National Center for Complementary and Alternative Medicine (*www.nccam.nih.gov*)

5. The CDC (*www.cdc.gov*) provide a wealth of information of vaccines as well as annually updated vaccine schedules for all age groups.
   (a) CDC Vaccines and Immunizations (*http://www.cdc.gov/node.do/id/0900f3ec8000e2f3*)
   (b) CDC National Immunization Program (*http://www.cdc.gov/nip/*)
   (c) More information on vaccines (*http://www.cdc.gov/nip/menus/vaccines.htm*)

6. University sites are excellent sources of information as well. Examples include:
   (a) Indiana University-Purdue University Indianapolis for its P450 drug interactions table (*http://medicine.iupui.edu/flockhart/table.htm*)
   (b) University of Missouri—Columbia, Pharmacy Services Department for its formulary (*http://www.muhealth.org/~formulary*)

7. There are also commercial sites that provide readily accessible manufacturer's information on drugs. These include:

(a) Medscape (*www.medscape.com*). Enter the drug name in the search box and click on "drug information."
(b) Rxlist (*www.rxlist.com*). In addition to providing manufacturer's information, this site provides for cost comparisons. Just click on "online pharmacy" in the right hand side of the tool bar. For example, 60 tablets of Tagamet 300 mg cost $66.14, whereas the generic cimetidine costs $16.57.

8. There are other commercial sites that provide excellent online clinical educational information. For example, clinicians and students can sharpen their clinical dosing skills at the Family Practice Notebook (*http://www.fpnotebook.com/END135.htm*) connects to AIDA, which is a free diabetes software program for purposes of teaching insulin dosing (*http://www.fpnotebook.com/END135.htm*).

Evidence-Based Practice Guidelines Government Sites Practice/treatment guidelines are available at several government sites.

1. CDC (www.cdc.gov)
   (a) Diseases and Conditions (*http://www.cdc.gov/node.do/id/0900f3ec8000e035*)
   (b) Sexually Transmitted Diseases Treatment Guidelines 2002 (*http://www.cdc.gov/std/treatment/*)
   (c) Tuberculosis Core Curriculum on Tuberculosis 2000 (*http://www.cdc.gov/nchstp/tb/pubs/corecurr/*)
   (d) Tuberculosis Treatment per American Thoracic Society, CDC, and Infectious Disease Society of American (CDC, Morbidity and Mortality Report, 2003, *http://www.cdc.gov/mmwr/PDF/rr/rr5211.pdf*)

2. National Guidelines Clearinghouse (*www.ngc.gov*). This site includes the practice guidelines for the major nursing and medical specialty organizations as well as those developed by Schools of Nursing and Schools of Medicine.

3. National Institutes of Health. Examples include:
   (a) Guidelines for the Diagnosis and Management of Asthma from the National Heart, Lung, and Blood Institute, *http://www.nhlbi.nih.gov/guidelines/asthma/asthgdln.htm* and 2002 update on selected topics *http://www.nhlbi.nih.gov/guidelines/asthma/index.htm*

(b) Detection, evaluation and treatment of high blood cholesterol in adults from the National Heart, Lung, and Blood Institute, *http://www.nhlbi.nih.gov/ guidelines/cholesterol/index.htm*, and recommendations regarding public screening of cholesterol measurements,

(c) Hypertension from the National Heart, Lung, and Blood Institute
   ▪ Blood pressure tables for children and adolescents, *http://www.nhlbi.nih.gov/ guidelines/ hypertension/child_tbl.htm*
   ▪ High blood pressure guidelines: Joint National Commission (JNC) 7, *http://www.nhlbi.nih.gov/ guidelines/hypertension/index.htm*

(d) Overweight and Obesity Clinical Guidelines from the National Heart, Lung, and Blood Institute, *http://www.nhlbi.nih.gov/guidelines/obesity/ ob_home.htm*

Practice and Treatment Guidelines: Professional Organization Sites

Many of the professional associations or societies include clinical practice guidelines or recommendations. They may be evidence-based or derived from expert opinion. Examples follow.

1. American Diabetes Association, Clinical Recommendations (*http://www.diabetes.org/for-health-professionals-and-scientists/cpr.jsp*)
2. American Cancer Society Guidelines for Screening, Surveillance, and Early Detection of Adenomatous Polyps and Colorectal Cancer (*http://www.diabetes.org/for-health-professionals-and-scientists/cpr.jsp*)
3. American Academy of Family Physicians, Clinical Recommendations (*http://www.aafp.org/x132.xml*)

Outcomes

Outcomes measurement is a tradition within nursing practice. When Florence Nightingale arrived in Crimea, she noted that soldiers, said to be dying from "wounds," were actually dying from "conditions," e.g., fever, diarrhea, fatigue, lack of clothing, and lack of shelter. When she initiated condition or diagnostic-specific nursing actions, death rates attributable to zymotic disease fell from 480.3 to 47.5 per 1,000 soldiers; deaths attributable to all other causes except wounds fell from 68.6 to 5.0 per 1,000 (Nightingale, 1859). Nightingale measured patient outcomes.

Many categories of patient outcomes are measured today. This section provides examples of outcome meas-ures within several categories. The categories are patient safety, nursing outcomes, nursing home and home healthcare setting outcomes, health plan outcomes, and the short form (SF) health survey.

This categorization of patient outcomes is not all-inclusive. It does not include listings of economic outcomes, e.g., costs/hospitalization, length of ICU stay, and length of hospital stay. A presentation of these economic variables lies beyond the scope of this section and has been addressed elsewhere (Stone, Curran, and Bakken, 2002; Lavin et al., 2004). It also tends to slight epidemiologic variables, e.g., infection rates and mortality rates, which Florence Nightingale relied on heavily. Such content is readily available in epidemiology texts. This section does present an array of outcome measures, tools, scales, or surveys that are used today and are Internet accessible. Many are available free on the Internet; others are available for purchase, with the purchasing information provided on the Internet. Because outcome data must be analyzed, this section concludes with information on Internet-available biostatistical analytical tools.

Patient Safety   Patient safety is an outcomes issue. There are several patient safety sites, which are of prime importance to advanced practice nurses. They include the following.

   ▪ Agency for Healthcare Research and Quality Web Morbidity and Mortality Rounds, an online forum for presentation and discussion of medical errors (*http://www.webmm.ahrq.gov/*)
   ▪ The patient safety page of Medscape.com, a free subscription service (*http://www.medscape.com/ pages/editorial/resourcecenters/public/patientsafety /rc-patientsafety.ov?src=hp24.rcbottom*)
   ▪ Institute for Healthcare Improvement (*http://www.ihi.org/ihi*)

Nursing Outcomes   The Internet sites presented within this section refer to standardized nursing terminologies that either present outcomes in a structured format or data sets that may be used for evaluative purposes.

   ▪ NOC is an acronym for the Nursing Outcomes Classification, a standardized nursing terminology. There are 330 outcomes listed in the third edition (Moorhead, Johnson, and Maas, 2003). Information of NOC may be obtained from the University of Iowa Center for Classification and Clinical Effectiveness (*http://www.nursing.uiowa.edu/centers/cncce*).

■ NMDS and i-NMDS are two related data sets. NMDS refers to the nursing minimum data set, dating back to the work of Werley, Lang, and Westgate (1986) and Werley and Lang (1988). The data set is now being managed by the U.S. Nursing Minimum Data Set Consortium (*http://www.nursing.uiowa.edu/sites/NI/research_frm.htm*). A position statement of the National Association of School Nurses promotes the use of a Nursing Minimum Data Set for School Nursing Practice (*http://www.nasn.org/positions/2004minimumdata.htm*). An international version, called i-NMDS, is being developed by the International Council of Nurses, as reported in the Nursing Matters fact sheet (*http://www.icn.ch/matters_i-NMDS_print.htm*), with the steering committee being chaired by Connie Delaney, PhD, RN, FAAN at the University of Iowa Nursing Informatics Center (*http://www.nursing.uiowa.edu/sites/ NI/research_frm.htm*).

Nursing Home and Home Healthcare Setting Outcomes
Related to nursing outcomes are those measures that evaluate the quality of care within nursing homes and home healthcare settings.

■ The minimum data set is a long-term care resident assessment instrument used by the Centers for Medicare and Medicaid (*www.cms.hhs.gov*). The MDS information site (*http://www.cms.hhs.gov/medicaid/mds20/*) provides historical questions, manual, forms, and technical specification hyperlinks. A complete listing of the version 2.0 MDS forms as pdf files are available at *http://www.cms.hhs.gov/quality/mds20/MDSAllForms.pdf*.

■ OASIS (outcomes assessment information set) measures are used to evaluate quality within home healthcare settings. A comparison of the OASIS measures and the consumer language used to describe the language may be found at the Centers for Medicare and Medicaid Web site (*http://www.cms.hhs.gov/quality/hhqi/HandOut1.pdf*). These measures rate improvement in performance of activities of daily living, mobility, cognition, and emergency prevention. The first phase of this Centers for Medicare and Medicaid quality initiative, begun in 2003, involved eight states: Florida, Massachusetts, Missouri, New Mexico, Oregon, South Carolina, Wisconsin, and West Virginia.

Health Plan Outcomes
The acronym HEDIS stands for health plan employer data and information set (*http://www.ncqa.org/Programs/HEDIS/index.htm*). It is a trademark name of the National Committee for Quality Assurance (NCQA). HEDIS measures (Case 24.5) are updated annually The 2005 listing may be found at (*http://www.ncqa.org/Programs/HEDIS/HEDIS%202005%20Summary.pdf*). Reports are issued annually and some states issue their reports online. The following are 2003 reports issued by Minnesota and Missouri. The reports are made in report card fashion and allow for quality and service comparisons among health plans.

Minnesota Department of Health HEDIS Reports may be found at *http://www.health.state.mn.us/divs/hpsc/mcs/hedishome.htm*. Their report card features allow for quality and service comparisons among health plans.

The Missouri Department of Health and Senior Services features a consumer's guide to commercial managed care plans. (*http://www.dhss.mo.gov/ManagedCare/Com_Bro_04.pdf*) and another consumer's guide to Medicaid Plus

---

Case 24.5   Finding HEDIS Measures

You are a nurse practitioner in a rural health clinic. You want to insure that your practice is in compliance with HEDIS measures. What would you do?

HEDIS measures are outcome measures designed for health plans but adaptable for use as quality measures within nurse practitioner clinics. Include HEDIS measures in your practice database, with measures derived from sites such as those listed in the text. HEDIS prod-ucts, including managed care organization standards, may be purchased from the National Quality (*http://www.ncqa.org*). You may also access a listing of the HEDIS measures as displayed in Web sites provided by the Minnesota Department of Health Managed Care Reports or the Missouri Department of Health Managed Care Guides (*http://www.dhss.mo.gov/ManagedCare/Com_Bro_04.pdf; http://www.dhss.mo.gov/ManagedCare/mcaid_04.pdf*).

managed care (*http://www.dhss.mo.gov/ManagedCare/mcaid_04.pdf*). Scroll down to find outcome-based report card results in each guide.

It is incumbent on the advanced practice nurses within primary care settings to know the HEDIS quality measures and evaluate the quality of their practices, accordingly.

Office Tools: Online Healthcare Record Audit and Patient Satisfaction Forms

Until the electronic health record is universal, the completeness of the health record or specific aspects of care need to be evaluated manually. The following links provide resources on auditing the health record and patient satisfaction. These measures are included together for two reasons. The first is that both the quality of the health care record and patient satisfaction reflect upon the quality of the care provided, a healthcare outcome. The second is that patient satisfaction variables provide clinicians with criteria to evaluate their own performance and that of the office in which they are practicing.

1. Heath care record audit criteria, adapted from the Santa Barbara Regional Health Authority (*http://www.sbrha.org/sections/ensuring_quality/provider_audit/pdf/Medical_Record_Review_Criteria.pdf*) (Table 24.2).

2. Patient Satisfaction Form (four-point scale), *http://www.geomedics.com/downloads/pss4.rtf*

3. Patient Satisfaction Form (five-point scale), *http://www.geomedics.com/downloads/pss5.rtf*

Short Form (SF) Health Survey

One of the long-lasting outcomes of the Medical Outcomes Study (Kravitz et al., 1992; Ware and Sherbourne, 1992) was the dissemination and use of the 36-item SF health survey (SF-36) and its subsequent versions and redactions. Another outcome was the formation of a nonprofit trust, called Medical Outcomes Trust (*http://www.outcomes-trust.org*) and SF-36.org (*http://www.sf-36.org*). After subscribing free at the SF-36 Web site, access information on SF-36 and its subsequent versions, SF-12 and SF-8. An SF-8 Internet demo is available. This survey tool is especially useful for population-based intervention studies or in cohort studies. Its eight items survey physical and mental health. Physical health items survey overall health, physical activity, interference with ability to work secondary to physical health problems, and pain. Mental health items survey overall energy, social activity, emotional problems, interference with ability to work secondary to emotional problems.

Table 24.2 General Health Care Record Audit Criteria Categories

Format of the healthcare record, e.g., client identification on each page, biographic and demographic data current, consistent organization of content

Documentation included in the record, e.g., allergies, status of advanced directives, emergency contacts, vaccine record, problem list, medication list

Coordination/continuity of care, e.g., diagnoses consistent with assessment data, presence of diagnostic-specific treatment plans, documentation of instructions for follow-up care, unresolved problems/issues addressed in subsequent visits, appropriate tracking recorded, outcomes evaluated as indicated (e.g., HbA1C, lipid levels)

Adult/pediatric preventive care, e.g., checklist of age-appropriate screenings preconception counseling, perinatal prevention activities recorded (e.g., prenatal assessment, visit documentation, WIC referral, HIV education, domestic violence assessment, home visits, postpartum assessment), breast and cervical cancer screening and treatment referrals, other cancer and treatment referrals, and other screenings and follow-up (e.g., weight, tobacco, diabetes mellitus, blood pressure, alcohol abuse, fall risk, car safety)

Source: Adapted from Santa Barbara Regional Authority Clinical Quality page (*http://www.sbrha.org/sections/ensuring_quality/clinical_pages/cp10_99.html, retrieved on April 28, 2005.*)

Outcomes Measurement: Internet-Available Biostatistical and Analytical Tools

Although the biostatistical measurement of outcome variables is not a routine part of clinical practice, it is likely to assume an important role when new programs or initiatives are begun. The following sites provide basic biostatistical tools available online including an AOL listing that includes free software and software packages available through the CDC.

1. Qualitative data creation, management, and analysis software (CDC, *http://www.cdc.gov/hiv/software/ez-text.htm*).

2. Qualitative database software (CDC, *http://www.cdc.gov/hiv/software/answr/howto.htm*)

3. Epidemiologic analysis software (CDC, *http://www.cdc.gov/epiinfo/*)

4. Chi-square calculator (Georgetown University, *http://www.georgetown.edu/faculty/ballc/webtools/web_chi.html*)

5. Student's *t*-test calculator (College of St. Benedict/St. John's University, *http://www.physics.csbsju.edu/stats/t-test.html*)

6. Extensive listing of free biostatistical software and biostatistical tests online (AOL, *http://members.aol.com/johnp71/javastat.html*)

eCLINICALOG (*http://www.eclinicalog.org*), A Web-Based Clinical Encounter Database

Healthcare settings are integrating clinical information systems into all aspects of care planning, delivery, and evaluation. To prepare clinicians to recognize and capitalize on the potential of this information to affect health outcomes, informatics needs to be integrated into the clinical course work. The eClinicaLog is part of an educational strategy, initially designed to build data entry, analysis, and synthesis skills in nurse practitioner students. As its versions have evolved, eClinicaLog has become relevant to undergraduate education as well.

Like other logs, eClinicaLog started out as a paper and pencil format. Nurse practitioner students used logs to track the number of patients seen in clinical practical and record basic demographic data, medical diagnoses, and medications prescribed. To facilitate student evaluation, some logs contained information regarding the extent of preceptor supervision during the encounter, the encounter length, and its complexity. The first version of what became the eClinicaLog was a spiral-bound, legal-sized, two-page grid of boxes that student filled in. This version lasted 1 year. It became apparent that a tracking system could do much more than serve as a ledger. Analysis of the paper version was time-consuming and frustrating. Items had to be counted and then entered into equations. Some items could not be analyzed, as students did not enter data in a standardized manner. Guiding principles were needed to guide the design of the next version.

After consulting the literature, especially the NMDS (Werley and Lang, 1988) as well as the National Organization of Nurse Practitioner Faculties' *Domains and Competencies of Nurse Practitioner Practice* (2000) and the AACN's *Essentials of Master's Education for Advanced Practice Nursing* (1995) a set of principles, or development parameters evolved. The next version addressed issues of retrievability, familiarity, availability; student acceptance, curricular congruence, and contribution to the discipline. Later versions incorporated HIPAA principles as well. Easily retrievable data are required for efficient analysis. This ruled out further use of paper-based collection instruments in favor of an electronic database. Students were amenable to the use of an electronic log, using the MS Access program. Within the Access format, the variables were arrayed as they were in the paper form. Subsequent student cohorts did not realize how much time this electronic format was saving them compared to the paper-based version and petitioned for an easier electronic format. The eClinicaLog migrated to a Web-based format.

Part of the notion of student buy-in was addressed when looking at curricular congruence. If students were to develop high-level skills—as opposed to being trained to be excellent data collectors—then there should be phases of skill development built into the curriculum that were tied to the clinical log exercise. Indeed, the topical outlines for the various theory courses also had to be revised to reinforce concepts that would be tested in the clinical arena. Even content thought to be clinically oriented was updated as the clinical log evolved to be more encompassing. In brief, inclusion of electronic and Web-based tools to facilitate student learning and curricular development is a bidirectional process.

The final development parameter, "contribution to the profession" was challenging and motivating. Previous versions of eClinicaLog were oriented to document the medical aspects of clinical encounters. Students frequently stated that they knew "all that nurse stuff' and wanted to focus on disease diagnosis and treatment. Yet, they were in a double bind: while adamantly insisting their practice was different from that of a physician assistant, nurse practitioner students were unable to articulate clearly their own discipline's concrete contribution to the clinical encounter. Unwittingly, the students were asking for ways to describe their practice. Standardized nursing terminology became this clinical log's contribution to the profession. NANDA, NOC, and NIC were chosen over other taxonomies due to familiarity (sometimes positive and sometimes negative) and the breadth of possibilities they presented. These terminologies provided a structure for students to explore the phenomena of concern for nursing (what we diagnose), what outcomes we expect to influence, and what interventions we employ to affect those outcomes.

The eClinicaLog consisted of three categories of variable: patient, program, and demographic. Since interprofessional collaboration is an important aspect of care delivery, it was important for nurse practitioner students to understand and use standardized terminologies from several disciplines. Within the patient category (subdivided into nursing, medical, pharmacy, and economic variables) several terminologies were employed. Nursing variables included NANDA, NOC, and NIC codes, included in SNOMED CT and registered with HL7. Medical variables included the ICD codes, CPT codes, and questions regarding laboratory/other diagnostic investigations performed, ordered, or interpreted. The pharmacy category relied on the American Hospital Formulary System terminology, which lends itself very well to tracking medications as specific drugs and within drug categories. Economic variables included the Level of Service codes from the CPT, including the wellness visit codes. Program variables included information on the date of service, preceptor, clinical site, patient encounter length, and extent of supervision. Demographic data, drawn from CMS descriptors, were limited to HIPAA approved fields and source of payment (insurance).

The learning process has been accelerated not only by having the clinical log available on the Web, but to have supportive information available on the Internet also. Students who buy nursing's diagnoses, outcomes, and interventions—NANDA, NOC, and NIC Linkages (Johnson et al., 2001)—have access to the Merlin system. There are numerous sites for looking up ICD codes. One free site is ICD-9 chrisendres.com (*http://icd9cm.chrisendres.com*) and a PDA version, the Stat ICD-9 Coder, is available at ICD-9 Coder (*http://www.statcoder.com/icd9.htm*). Students can use an active link to access all the acceptable ICD codes. Medication codes can be accessed via the University of Missouri—Columbia Health Care, Pharmacy Services Department (*http://www.muhealth.org/~formulary/*) and by subscription through STAT!Ref Electronic Media Library (*www.statref.com*).

The eClinicaLog is a useful pedagogic tool. It guides students through an informatics skill building and refinement process and assists professional development. Its successful use indicates that Internet applications are not just adjuvant educational tools but an integral part of the clinical learning process.

References

American Association of Colleges of Nursing. (1995). *The Essentials of Master's Education for Advanced Practice Nursing*. Washington, DC: Author.

Agency of Healthcare Research and Quality and University of Alabama, AHRQ's Bioterrorism and Emerging Infections Site. Retrieved July 8, 2004, from *http://www.bioterrorism.uab.edu*

Agency for Healthcare Research and Quality, Web Morbidity and Mortality Rounds. Retrieved July 8, 2004, from *http://www.webmm.ahrq.gov*

American Cancer Society Guidelines for Screening, Surveillance, and Early Detection of Adenomatous Polyps and Colorectal Cancer. Retrieved July 8, 2004, from *http://www.diabetes.org/for-health-professionals-and-scientists/cpr.jsp*

American Diabetes Association, Clinical Recommendations. Retrieved July 8, 2004, from *http://www.diabetes.org/for-health-professionals-and-scientists/cpr.jsp*

American Medical Association. (2004). *Physician ICD-9-CM: International Classification of Diseases, 2004.* Chicago, IL: American Medical Association.

America Online. *Web Pages that Perform Statistical Calculations*. Retrieved July 8, 2004, from *http://members.aol.com/johnp71/javastat.html*

Association of Perioperative Registered Nursing, Perioperative Nursing Data Set. Retrieved July 8, 2004, from *http://www.aorn.org/research/pnds.htm*

Barone, G. W., Gurley, B. J., Ketel, B. L., Lightfoot, M. L., and Abul-Ezz, S. R. (2001). Drug interaction between St. John's wort and cyclosporine. *Annals of Pharmacotherapeutics* 35(1):124–125.

Centers for Disease Control and Prevention. Retrieved July 8, 2004, from *www.cdc.gov*

Centers for Disease Control and Prevention, Diseases and Conditions. Retrieved July 8, 2004, from *http://www.cdc.gov/node.do/id/0900f3ec8000e035*

Centers for Disease Control and Prevention, Emergency Preparedness and Response. Retrieved July 8, 2004, from *http://www.bt.cdc.gov*

Centers for Disease Control and Prevention, Epidemiologic Analysis Software. Retrieved July 8, 2004, from *http://www.cdc.gov/epiinfo*

Centers for Disease Control, Genomics and Disease Prevention. Genomics Retrieved July 8, 2004, from Centers for Disease Control and Prevention, Genomics and Disease Prevention, *http://www.cdc.gov/genomics/default.htm*.

Centers for Disease Control and Prevention, National Immunization Program. Retrieved July 8, 2004, from *http://www.cdc.gov/nip*

Centers for Disease Control and Prevention, National Immunization Program, Vaccine Menus. Retrieved July 8, 2004, from *http://www.cdc.gov/nip/menus/vaccines.htm*

Centers for Disease Control and Prevention, Qualitative Data Creation, Management, and Analysis Software. Retrieved July 8, 2004, from *http://www.cdc.gov/hiv/software/ez-text.htm*

Centers for Disease Control and Prevention, Qualitative Database Software. Retrieved July 8, 2004, from *http://www.cdc.gov/hiv/software/answr/howto.htm*

Centers for Disease Control and Prevention, Sexually Transmitted Diseases Treatment Guidelines 2002. Retrieved July 8, 2004, from *http://www.cdc.gov/std/treatment*

Centers for Disease Control and Prevention, Tuberculosis Core Curriculum on Tuberculosis 2000. Retrieved July 8, 2004, from *http://www.cdc.gov/nchstp/tb/pubs/corecurr*

Centers for Disease Control and Prevention, Tuberculosis Treatment per American Thoracic Society, CDC, and Infectious Disease Society of American. Morbidity and Mortality Weekly Report, June 20, 2003, Volume 52, No. RR-11. Retrieved July 8, 2004, from *http://www.cdc.gov/mmwr/PDF/rr/rr5211.pdf*

Centers for Disease Control and Prevention, Vaccines and Immunizations. Retrieved July 8, 2004, from *http://www.cdc.gov/node.do/id/0900f3ec8000e2f3*

Centers for Medicare and Medicaid Services. Retrieved July 8, 2004, from *www.cms.hhs.gov*

Centers for Medicare and Medicaid Services, Comparison Table of Oasis Items Used in Oasis Measures and Publicly Reported Consumer Language in Home Health Compare. Retrieved July 16, 2004, from *http://www.cms.hhs.gov/quality/hhqi/HandOut1.pdf*

Centers for Medicare and Medicaid Services, Health Care Financing Review, Conference Proceedings Measuring Functional Status. Retrieved July 14, 2004, from *http://www.cms.hhs.gov/review/03spring/default.asp*

Centers for Medicare and Medicaid Services, MDS (Minimum Data Set) Information Site. Retrieved July 8, 2004, from *http://www.cms.hhs.gov/medicaid/mds20*

Centers for Medicare and Medicaid Services, MDS (Minimum Data Set) Forms (version 2.). Retrieved July 16, 2004, from *http://www.cms.hhs.gov/medicaid/mds20*

Centers for Medicaid and Medicare Services, New and revised ICD Diagnosis Codes and Titles. Retrieved July 8, 2004, from *http://www.cms.hhs.gov/medlearn/icd9code.asp*

Centers for Medicare and Medicaid Services, OASIS (Outcomes Assessment Information Set). Retrieved July 8, 2004, from *http://www.cms.hhs.gov/quality/hhqi/HandOut1.pdf*

Centers for Medicaid and Medicare Services, Medicare Learning Network. Retrieved July 8, 2004 *http://www.cms.hhs.gov/medlearn/icd9code.asp*

CINAHL. Retrieved July 8, 2004, from *http://www.cinahl.com.*

College of St. Benedict/St. John's University, Student's t test calculator, *http://www.physics.csbsju.edu/stats/t-test.html*

Cornell University Medical College, Pediatric Critical Care Medicine. Retrieved, from *http://www-users.med.cornell.edu/~spon/picu/calc/medcalc.htm*

Delbanco, T. and Sands, D. Z. (2004). Electrons in flight—e-mail between doctors and patients. *New England Journal of Medicine* 350(17):1705–1707.

Department of Health and Human Services, Indian Health Services, PCS Forms. Nursing Care Plan Form Parts I and II. Retrieved July 8, 2004, from *http://forms.psc.gov/forms/ihs/ps80.pdf and http://forms.psc.gov/forms/ihs/ps80-1.pdf*

Department of Health and Human Services, Indian Health Services, PCS Forms. Retrieved July 8, 2004, from *http://forms.psc.gov/forms/IHS/ihs.html*

Digital windmill. Retrieved July 8, 2004, from *http://digitalwindmill.com*

Dochterman, J. M. and Bulechek, G. (2003). *Nursing Interventions Classification (NIC).* St. Louis, MO: Mosby.

Drug Enforcement Agency. Retrieved July 8, 2004, from *www.dea.gov*

Drug Enforcement Agency, Drugs and Chemicals of Concern. Retrieved July 8, 2004, from *http://www.deadiversion.usdoj.gov/drugs_concern/index.html*

eCLINICALOG. Retrieved July 16, 2004, from *http://www.eclinicalog.org*

eMetasearch. Retrieved July 8, 2004, from *http://emetasearch.com*

EclinicaLog. Retrieved July 8, 2004, from *http://www.apnlog.wayne.edu*

eMetasearch. Retrieved July 8, 2004, from *http://emetasearch.com*

Family Practice Notebook. Retrieved July 8, 2004, from *http://www.fpnotebook.com/END135.htm*

Fixed Wireless. Retrieved July 8, 2004, from *http://www.fixedwireless1.com/Overview%20of%20Fixed%20Wireless.htm.*

Food and Drug Administration. Retrieved July 8, 2004, from *www.fda.gov*

Food and Drug Administration, Center for Drug Research and Evaluation (CDER). Retrieved July 8, 2004, from *http://www.fda.gov/cder/index.html*

Food and Drug Administration, FDA Public Health Advisory of February 10, 2000. *Risk of Drug Interactions with St John's Wort and Indinavir and other Drugs.* Retrieved July 8, 2004, from *http://www.fda.gov/cder/drug/advisory/stjwort.htm.*

Food and Drug Administration , Medwatch, Adverse Event and Product Problem Forms, Medwatch. Retrieved July 8, 2004, from *http://www.fda.gov/medwatch/getforms.htm*

Food and Drug Administration, Medwatch, FDA Safety Information and Adverse Event Reporting Program. Retrieved July 8, 2004, from *http://www.fda.gov/medwatch/index.html*

Food and Drug Administration, Medwatch, Vaccine Adverse Event Reporting System. Retrieved July 8, 2004, from *http://www.fda.gov/medwatch/safety/vaers1.pdf*

Geomedics—Business and Productivity Solutions for Healthcare Professionals, Patient Satisfaction Form (four point scale). Retrieved July 8, 2004, from *http://www.geomedics.com/downloads/pss4.rtf,*

Geomedics—Business and Productivity Solutions for Healthcare Professionals, Patient Satisfaction Form (five point scale). Retrieved July 8, 2004, from *http://www.geomedics.com/downloads/pss5.rtf*

George Mason University, National Center for Biodefense. Retrieved July 8, 2004, from *http://www.gmu.edu/centers/biodefense*

Georgetown University, Chi square calculator. Retrieved July 8, 2004, from *http://www.georgetown.edu/faculty/ballc/webtools/web_chi.html)*

Harvard Center for Cancer Prevention, Risks. Retrieved July 8, 2004, from *http://www.yourcancerrisk.harvard.edu*

Heerkens, Y., van der Brug, Y., Napel, H. T., and van Ravensberg (2003). Past and future use of the ICF (former ICIDH) by nursing and allied health professionals. *Disability and Rehabilitation* 25(11–12):620–627.

Hennessy, M., Kelleher, D., Spiers, J. P., Barry, M., Kavanagh, P., Back, D., Mulcahy, F., Feely, J. (2002). St. Johns wort increases expression of P-glycoprotein: Implications for drug interactions. *British Journal of Clinical Pharmacology* 53(1):75–82.

Home Health Care Classification (HHCC) System. Retrieved July 8, 2004, from *www.sabacare.com*

Hospital Soup. Retrieved July 8, 2004, from *http://www.hospitalsoup.com/public/nursingassess2001.pdf*

ICD-9 Coder, Stat ICD-9 Coder. Retrieved July 15, 2004, from *http://www.statcoder.com/icd9.htm*

ICD-9 chrisendres.com, sponsored by Practice Management Information Corporation (PMIC). Retrieved on July 15, 2004, from *http://icd9cm.chrisendres.com*

Indiana University-Purdue University Indianapolis P450 Drug Interactions Table. Retrieved July 8, 2004, from *http://medicine.iupui.edu/flockhart/table.htm*

Institute for Healthcare Improvement, *http://www.ihi.org/ihi*

International Council of Nurses, Nursing Matters: International Nursing Minimum Data Set. Retrieved July 8, 2004, from *http://www.icn.ch/matters_i-NMDS_print.htm*

Ithaki. Retrieved July 8, 2004, from *http://www.ithaki.net/indexu.htm*

Izzo, A. A. (2004). Drug interactions with St. John's Wort (Hypericum perforatum): A review of the clinical evidence. *International Journal of Clinical Pharmacology and Therapeutics* 42(3):139–148.

Johns Hopkins Medical Institutions, Welch Medical Library. Retrieved April 28, 2005 from *http://www.welch.jhu.edu/internet/ebr.html#metananalysis*

Johnson, M., Bulechek, G., Dochterman, J. M., and Maas, M. (2001). *Nursing Diagnoses, Outcomes, and Interventions: NANDA, NOC and NIC Linkages.* St. Louis, MO: Mosby.

Karliova, M., Treichel, U., Malago, M., Frilling, A., Gerken, G. and Broelsch, C. E. (2000). Interaction of Hypericum perforatum (St. John's wort) with cyclosporine A metabolism in a patient after liver transplantation. *Journal of Hepatology* 33(5):853–855.

Karolinksa Institute University Library, Diseases, Disorders, and Related Topics. Retrieved July 14, 2004, from

http://medwebplus.com/subject/Diseases_and_Conditions/Chronic_Disease/Directories

Kearney, P. M. and Pryor, J. (2004). The International Classification of Functioning, Disability and Health (ICF) and nursing. *Journal of Advanced Nursing* 46(2):162–170.

Keenan, G., Stocker, J., Barkauskas, V., Treder, M., and Heath, C. (2003). Toward collecting a standardized nursing data set across the continuum: Case of adult care nurse practitioner setting. *Outcomes Management* 7(3):113–120.

Kravitz, R. L., Greenfield, S., Rogers, W. H., Manning, W. G., Zubkoff, M., Nelson, E., Tarlov, A. R., and Ware, J. E. (1992). Differences in the mix of patients among medical specialties and systems of care: results from the Medical Outcomes Study. *Journal of the American Medical Association* 267(12):1617–1623.

Lavin, M. A., Avant, K., Craft-Rosenberg, M., Herdman, T. H., and Gebbie, K. A. (2004). Contexts for the study of the economic influence of nursing diagnoses on outcomes. International. *Journal of Terminologies and Classification* 15(2):39–47.

Lavin, M. A., Krieger, M.M., Meyer, G. A., Spasser, M. A., Cvitan, T., Reese, C., Carlson, J. H., Perry, A.G., and McNary, P. (2005). Development and testing of NLINKS evidence-based nursing (EBN) matrix and related databases. *Journal of the Medical Library Association* 93(1):104–115.

Lehman, C. A. (2003). Idiopathic intracranial hypertension within the ICF model: A review of the literature. *Journal of Neuroscience Nursing* 35(5):263–269.

Lumpkin, J. R. (2001). *Report of the National Committee for Vital and Health Statistics: Classifying and Reporting Functional Status* (*http://www.ncvhs.hhs.gov/010716rp.htm* and (*http://www.cms.hhs.gov/review/03spring/default.asp*).

Mai, I., Kruger, H., Budde, K., Johne, A., Brockmoller, J., Neumayer, H. H., and Roots, I. (2000). Hazardous pharmacokinetic interaction of Saint John's wort (Hypericum perforatum) with the immunosuppressant cyclosporine. *International Journal of Clinical Pharmacology and Therapeutics* 38(10):500–502.

Markowitz, J. S., Donovan, J. L., DeVane, C. L., Taylor, R. M., Ruan, Y., Wang, J. S., and Chavin, K. D. (2004). Effect of St. John's Wort on drug metabolism by induction of cytochrome p450 3A4 enzyme. *Obstetrical and Gynecological Survey* 59(5):358–359.

Martin, K. S., Elfrink, V. L., and Monson, K. A. (2001). Retrieved July 8, 2004, from The Omaha System, *www.omahasystem.org*

Martindale's Calculators Online Part I: Nutrition. Retrieved July 8, 2004, from *http://www.martindalecenter.com/Calculators1B_4_Nut.html* and *its Basal Metabolic Calculators from http://www.room42.com/nutrition/basal.shtml*

Medical Outcomes Trust. Retrieved July 16, 2004, from *http://www.outcomes-trust.org*

Medscape. (1994–2004). Retrieved July 8, 2004, from *www.medscape.com*

Medscape. (1994–2004). *Patient Safety Page.* Retrieved July 8, 2004, from *http://www.medscape.com/pages/editorial/resourcecenters/public/patientsafety/rc-patientsafety.ov?src=hp24.rcbottom*

MedWeb Plus, Diseases and Conditions. Retrieved July 14, from *http://medwebplus.com/subject/Diseases_and_Conditions/Chronic_Disease/Directories*

Minnesota Department of Health, HEDIS Reports. Retrieved July 8, 2004, from *http://www.health.state.mn.us/divs/hpsc/mcs/hedishome.htm*

Missouri Department of Health and Senior Services, 2004 Consumer's Guide: Commercial Managed Care in Missouri. Retrieved on May 2, 2005 from *http://www.dhss.mo.gov/ManagedCare/Com_Bro_04.pdf*

Missouri Department of Health and Senior Services, 2004 Consumer's Guide: MC+ Managed Care in Missouri. Retrieved on May 2, 2005 from *http://www.dhss.mo.gov/ManagedCare/mcaid_04.pdf*

Moorhead, S., Johnson, M., and Maas, M. (2004). *Nursing Outcomes Classification.* St. Louis, MO: Mosby.

NANDA. (2003–2004). *NANDA Diagnoses and Classification.* Philadelphia, PA: Author.

NANDA International. Retrieved July 8, 2004, from nanda.org

National Association of School Nurses, Position Statement on Nursing Minimum Data Set. Retrieved April 28, 2005, from *http://www.nasn.org/positions/2004minimumdata.htm*

National Cancer Institute, Cancer Treatment. Select from an A-Z listing. Retrieved July 8, 2004, from *www.nci.nih.gov*

National Center for Complementary and Alternative Medicine. Retrieved July 8, 2004, from *www.nccam.nih.gov*

National Center for Complementary and Alternative Medicine, Investigating the Science Behind Plants as Treatments. Retrieved July 8, 2004, from *http://nccam.nih.gov/news/newsletter/previous/index.htm*

National Committee for Quality Assurance (NCQA). Health Plan Employer Data and Information Set (HEDIS), 2005 listing. Retrieved July 8, 2004, from *http://www.ncqa.org/Programs/HEDIS/HEDIS%202005%20Summary.pdf*

National Guidelines Clearinghouse. Retrieved July 8, 2004, from www.ngc.gov

National Heart, Lung and Blood Institute, Blood pressure tables for children and adolescents. Retrieved July 8, 2004, from *http://www.nhlbi.nih.gov/guidelines/hypertension/child_tbl.htm*

National Heart, Lung and Blood Institute Body Mass Calculator. Retrieved July 8, 2004, from *http://nhlbisupport.com/bmi/bmicalc.htm*

National Heart, Lung, and Blood Institute, Coronary Heart Disease Risk Calculator. Retrieved July 8, 2004, from *http://hin.nhlbi.nih.gov/atpiii/calculator.asp?usertype=prof*

National Heart, Lung and Blood Institute, Detection, Evaluation, and Treatment of High Blood Cholesterol in Adults (Adult Treatment Panel III). Retrieved July 8, 2004, from *http://www.nhlbi.nih.gov/guidelines/cholesterol/index.htm*

National Heart, Lung and Blood Institute, Guidelines for the Diagnosis and Management of Asthma—Update on Selected Topics 2002. Retrieved July 8, 2004, from *http://www.nhlbi.nih.gov/guidelines/asthma/index.htm*

National Heart, Lung and Blood Institute, High blood pressure guidelines: Joint National Commission (JNC) 7. Retrieved July 8, 2004, from *http://www.nhlbi.nih.gov/guidelines/hypertension/index.htm*

National Heart, Lung and Blood Institute, National Asthma Education and Prevention Program Expert Panel Report 2: Guidelines for the Diagnosis and Management of Asthma. Retrieved July 8, 2004, from *http://www.nhlbi.nih.gov/guidelines/asthma/asthgdln.htm*

National Heart, Lung and Blood Institute, Overweight and Obesity Clinical Guidelines. Retrieved July 8, 2004, from *http://www.nhlbi.nih.gov/guidelines/obesity/ob_home.htm*

National Human Genome Research Institute, Specific Genetic Disorders. Retrieved July 8, 2004, from *http://www.nhgri.nih.gov/10001204*

National Human Genome Research Institute, Genetic, Rare and Orphan Disease Resources Online. Retrieved July 8, 2004, from *http://www.nhgri.nih.gov/10001200*

National Information Standards Organization. Retrieved July 8, 2004, from *http://www.niso.org/committees/MetaSearch-info.html*

National Information Standards Organization, *http://www.niso.org/committees/MetaSearch-info.html*

National Institute of Health (NIH). Retrieved on April 28, 2005 from *http://www.nih.gov*

National Institute of Diabetes, Digestive, and Kidney Diseases, National Digestive Diseases Information Clearinghouse (NDDIC). Retrieved on July 14, 2004, from *http://digestive.niddk.nih.gov/ddiseases/a-z.asp*

National Institute of Neurological Disorders and Stroke, Brain Attack: Stroke Scales. Retrieved July 8, 2004, from *http://www.stroke-site.org/stroke_scales/stroke_scales.html*

National Institute on Alcohol Abuse and Alcoholism. Retrieved July 8, 2004, from *www.niaaa.nih.gov/www*

National Institute on Drug Abuse. Retrieved July 8, 2004, from *www.nida.nih.gov*

National Library of Medicine, Clinical Alerts Database. Retrieved July 8, 2004, from *www.pubmed.gov* or *http://www.nlm.nih.gov/databases/alerts/clinical_alerts.html*

National Library of Medicine, Gateway. Retrieved July 8, 2004, from *http://gateway.nlm.nih.gov/gw/Cmd*

National Library of Medicine, MEDLINE. Retrieved July 8, 2004, from *www.pubmed.gov* (Click on "Limit." Click on MEDLINE from drop down "Subsets" menu).

National Library of Medicine MEDLINE Plus Health Information *http://search.nlm.nih.gov/homepage/query? FUNCTION=search&PARAMETER=MEDLINE+Plus+AND+symptoms+AND+manifestations&DISAMBIGUATION=true&START=0&END=25&MAX=250 &ASPECT=1*

National Library of Medicine, My NCBI (Cubby). Retrieved on April 28, 2005 from *www.pubmed.gov* (left hand margin) and from *http://www.ncbi.nlm.nih.gov/entrez/ login.fcgi?call=so.SignOn..Login&callpath=QueryExt. CubbyQuery..ShowAll&db=pubmed*

National Library of Medicine, PubMed. Retrieved July 8, 2004, from *www.pubmed.gov*

National Library of Medicine, PubMed's Clinical Queries Research Methodology Filters. Retrieved July 8, 2004, from *http://www.ncbi.nlm.nih.gov/entrez/query/static/ clinical.html*

National Library of Medicine, Unified Medical Language System. Retrieved July 8, 2004, from *http://www.nlm.nih.gov/research/umls/access.html*

National Organization of Nurse Practitioner Faculties. (2000). *Domains and Core Competencies of Nurse Practitioner Practice: Newly Revised*. Washington, DC: Author.

Network for Language in Nursing Knowledge Systems (NLINKS). Retrieved July 8, 2004, from *www.nlinks.org*

Network for Language in Nursing Knowledge Systems Concept Analysis Center (NLINKS). Retrieved July 14, 2004, from *http://nlinks.org/cac_introduction.phtml*

Network for Language in Nursing Knowledge Systems (NLINKS), Research Center. Retrieved July 8, 2004, from *http://www.nlinks.org/research_main.phtml*

Newbold, S. K. (2004). New uses for wireless technology. Nurse Practitioner 29(4):45–46.

New York Online Access to Health (NOAH). Retrieved on July 14, 2004, from *www.noah-health.org*

New York Online Access to Health (NOAH), Ehlers-Danlos Syndrome. Retrieved July 8, 2004, from *http://www.noah-health.org/english/illness/dermatology/ derm.html#ehlers*

New York Online Access to Health (NOAH), Lupus erythematosus. Retrieved July 8, 2004, from *http://www.noah-health.org/english/illness/arthritis/ lupus.html#Diagnosis*

New York Online Access to Health (NOAH), Marfan syndrome. Retrieved July 8, 2004, from *http://www.noahhealth.org/english/illness/genetic_ diseases/geneticdis.html#Marfan*

Nightingale, F. (1859). *A Contribution to the Sanitary History of the British Army During the Late War with Russia*. London: Harrison and Sons.

O'Connor, N. A., Hameister, A. D., and Kershaw, T. (2000). Developing a database to describe the practice patterns of adult nurse practitioner students. *Journal of Nursing Scholarship* 32(1):57–63.

RavenSearch. Retrieved July 8, 2004, from *http://www.ravensearch.net*

Ruschitzka, F., Meier, P. J., Turina, M., Luscher, T. F. and Noll, G. (2000). Acute heart transplant rejection due to Saint John's wort (comment). *Lancet* 355(9203): 548–549.

RxList. Retrieved July 8, 2004, from *www.rxlist.com*

Saba, V. K. (2003). *Home Health Care Classification (HHCC) System*. Retrieved July 8, 2004, from *www.sabacare.com*

Saint Louis University, Center for the Study of Bioterrorism and Emerging Infections. Retrieved July 8, 2004, from *http://bioterrorism.slu.edu*

Santa Barbara Regional Health Authority, Medical record audit criteria. Retrieved July 16, 2004, from *http://www.sbrha.org/sections/ensuring_quality/chart_ quality.html*

SF-36.org. Retrieved July 16, 2004, from *http://www.sf-36.org*

STAT!Ref Electronic Media Library. Retrieved July 16, from *www.statref.com*

Stone, P. W., Curran, C. R., and Bakken, S. (2002). Economic evidence for evidence-based practice. *Journal of Nursing Scholarship* 34(3):277–282.

Tannergren, C., Engman, H., Knutson, L., Hedeland, M., Bondesson, U., and Lennernas, H. (2004). St. John's wort decreases the bioavailability of R- and S-verapamil through induction of the first-pass metabolism. *Clinical Pharmacology and Therapeutics* 75(4):298–309.

University of Iowa Center for Classification and Clinical Effectiveness. Retrieved on July 16, 2004, from *http://www.nursing.uiowa.edu/centers/cncce*

University of Iowa Nursing Informatics Center. Retrieved on July 16, from *http://www.nursing.uiowa.edu/sites/ NI/research_frm.htm*

University of Maryland, Medicine Health Risk Calculator. Retrieved July 8, 2004, from *http://www.umm.edu/healthcalculators*

University of Missouri—Columbia, Pharmacy Services Department. Retrieved July 16, 2004, from *http://www.muhealth.org/~formulary*

University of Newcastle upon Tyne, Department of Oncology, On-Line Medical Dictionary. Retrieved July 14, 2004, from *http://cancerweb.ncl.ac.uk/omd*

University of Pittsburgh, Center for Biosecurity. Retrieved July 8, 2004, from *http://www.upmc-biosecurity.org*

USA Nursing Minimum Data Set Consortium. Retrieved on July 16, 2004, from *http://www.nursing.uiowa.edu/ sites/NI/research_frm.htm*

Vermont Department of Health, Clinician Reference Guide: Recognizing and Treating Victims of Domestic Abuse. Retrieved July 8, 2004, from *http://www.state.vt.us/health/abuse.htm*

Villanueva, M. Manuel's Web, Nursing Calculators. Retrieved July 8, 2004, from *http://www.manuelsweb.com/nrs_calculators.htm*

Wallin, M. K. and Wajntraub, S. (2004). Evaluation of Bluetooth as a replacement for cables in intensive care and surgery. *Anesthesia and Analgesia* 98(3):763–767.

Wang, L. S., Zhu, B., El-Aty, A. M., Zhou, G., Li, Z., Wu, J., Chen, G. L., Liu, J., Tang, Z. R., An, W., Li, Q., Wang, D., and Zhou, H. H. (2004). The influence of St John's Wort on CYP2C19 activity with respect to genotype. *Journal of Clinical Pharmacology* 44(6):577–581.

Ware, J. J. and Sherbourne, C. D. (1992). The MOS 36-item short-form health survey (SF-36). I. Conceptual framework and item selection. *Medical Care* 30:473–483.

Werley, H. H. and Lang, N. M. (1988). *Identification of the Nursing Minimum Data Set*. New York: Springer.

Werley, H. S., Lang, N. M., and Westlake, S. K. (1986). Brief summary of the nursing minimum data set conference. *Nursing Management* 17(7):42–45.

Wheeler Clinic Connecticut Clearinghouse. Retrieved July 8, 2004, from *http://www.ctclearinghouse.org/Vertical_Files/vf_assessment_screening.htm*

World Health Organization. (1992). *ICD-10 International Statistical Classification of Diseases and Related Health Problems, 1989 Revision*. Geneva: Author.

World Health Organization. (1992). *ICD-10-CM International Statistical Classification of Diseases and Related Health Problems, 1989 Revision*. Geneva: Author. [The Clinical Modifications version was developed in collaboration with the United States Department of Health and Human Services National Center for Health Statistics.]

World Health Organization. (2001). *International Classification of Functioning, Disability, and Health (ICF)*.Geneva: Author.

World Health Organization, International Classification of Functioning, Disability, and Health (ICF), Retrieved July 14, 2004, from *http://www3.who.int/icf/icftemplate.cfm*

World Health Organization, ICF Browser, Retrieved July 14, 2004, from *http://www3.who.int/icf/onlinebrowser/icf.cfm*

25

Informatics Solutions for Emergency Preparedness and Response

Elizabeth Weiner
Sally Phillips

OBJECTIVES

1. Describe current informatics solutions in emergency management and response.
2. Project areas of emergency management and response that would benefit from informatics assistance.

KEY WORDS

emergency management
emergency response
disaster management
bioterrorism
public health informatics

 Introduction

The events of September 11, 2001, catapulted the United States into the realization that the country was not adequately protected from terrorism. Then, within a short window of time, the anthrax outbreaks stressed the public health infrastructure to the point that bioterrorism arose as an additional deadly threat. As a result of these two events, the government of the United States responded at an unprecedented pace to better prepare and manage terrorist events.

Early response by the informatics community focused on contributions toward surveillance of threat detection; however, a broader assessment of possible informatics contributions unveiled that in addition to biosurveillance and bioagent detection, informatics could also contribute to increasing the efficiency in disaster response as well as providing a telepresence for remote medical caregivers (Teich et al., 2002).

The purpose of this chapter is to explore current and future roles of informatics in emergency preparedness and response. While it is recognized that terrorism has created a problem that is international in scope, this discussion will be limited to preparedness and response in the United States.

 Changes in the Federal System Affecting Emergency Preparedness and Response

A New Definition of Community

Community health has traditionally been defined in the United States as the provision of healthcare outside the hospital infrastructure. As such, the public health departments have been viewed as the major delivery system of healthcare. Unfortunately, over time the public health infrastructure has been deteriorating to the point that many of the rural health department settings did not even have fax machines to receive notices about potential public health threats. The anthrax scares made this situation most apparent, as all sorts of white powder mixtures were sent through the laboratory system of the state public health departments.

Federal funds were channeled through the Centers for Disease Control and Prevention (CDC) to the states in order to strengthen the public health infrastructure. At the same time, federal funds were directed to hospitals through the Health Resources and Services Administration (HRSA). Both funding agencies encouraged the development of systems that would intersect one another, and for the first time a concerted effort was made to promote a collaborative system that would best meet the needs of the nation's health.

Local agencies also began to work together. Reporting systems that had traditionally only been used within a hospital began to be used among several hospitals within a local region; however, these systems lacked standardization and thus led to a network of systems that could not communicate with one another.

Even the reporting of victims during a mass casualty event created challenges. After the attacks of September 11, thousands of family members circulated throughout the hospitals in the area in a futile attempt to locate their family members. There was no central place for them to access the information. Healthcare members in St. Louis wanted to make certain this did not happen to their community. As a result, they developed a bar code system to log and track their victims (Hamilton, 2003). In addition, PDAs were used by medics to log patients and belongings as well as notebook computers with wireless technology and networked desktop machines in command centers.

A report of the 2002 Coastal North Carolina Domestic Preparedness Training Exercise described the innovative use of telehealth technologies for terrorism response (Simmons et al., 2003). During this exercise, East Carolina University tested the in-place telehealth networks as well as deployable communications, networking, and data collection technologies such as satellite communication, local wireless networking, on-scene video, and clinical and environmental data acquisition and telemetry. Specific recommendations were shared based on their experience.

Unfortunately, not all communities have advanced to an electronic system of data management for healthcare professionals. For those small percentages of hospitals and clinics using electronic medical records, no standard exists for a reporting system (Snee and McCormick, 2004). The inability to access electronic health data creates barriers to continuity of care, quality of care, cost analysis, and vulnerabilities to exposures during bioterrorism events. It is anticipated that with the development of a national health information infrastructure (NHII) will come an improved public health information network (PHIN). At the same time, data sharing has to be carefully planned in order to stay in compliance with the Health Insurance Portability and Accountability Act (HIPAA).

Federal Responsibilities for Healthcare Providers

The U.S. Department of Health and Human Services (DHHS) is responsible for the education of healthcare

professionals in preparedness for emergencies, including potential terrorism (U.S. Department of Health and Human Services, 2004). Several specialized units exist under the auspices of DHHS. Three of the units focus on emergency planning and response: the CDC the Agency for Healthcare Research and Quality (AHRQ), and HRSA. Each of these agencies plays a critical role in emergency planning and response.

The organization of the new Department of Homeland Security (DHS) caused some confusion about whether education for emergency planning and response of healthcare professionals would remain within DHHS or move to other first responder training activities already instituted by the Federal Emergency Management Agency (FEMA). Typically, "first responders" have been identified as the police, fire, and emergency medical technicians who arrive first on the scene of an event. In a biologic threat, however, healthcare providers are likely to be the first to discover or detect a biologic pattern. As a result, the definition of first responder was recently expanded to include healthcare providers in Presidential Directive #8 (U.S. Department of Homeland Security, December 17, 2003). This allows for the healthcare community to be eligible for funding from the DHS.

New Visibility of CDC Promotes Informatics Solutions

The CDC is recognized as the lead federal agency for protecting the health and safety of people—at home and abroad, providing credible information to enhance health decisions, and promoting health through strong partnerships. CDC serves as the national focus for developing and applying disease prevention and control, environmental health, and health promotion and education activities designed to improve the health of the people of the United States (Centers for Disease Control and Prevention, 2004). As the lead federal agency for protecting the health and safety of people, CDC also compiles statistical information to guide actions and policies to improve the health of the nation. During and following the anthrax attacks, the CDC was suddenly in the national limelight, and Dr. Julie Gerberding (the director), called for changes that would strengthen the organization, particularly in the area of risk communication.

Funds from the Frist-Kennedy legislation were targeted to go to the states, but were channeled through the CDC. These funds were designed to upgrade the failing public health infrastructure, to improve emergency communication, and to educate healthcare professionals in emergency planning and response. Each state governor was asked to sign off on the plan created by their state officials. While the CDC made haste to get new federal funding to the states, they also realized that many of our nations' cities were at higher risk of bioterrorism attacks. As a result, funding for fiscal year 2005 was reduced to the states in order to channel funds to "high-risk" cities.

Several of the CDC initiatives require informatics support. The National Electronic Disease Surveillance System (NEDSS) is an initiative that promotes the use of data and information system standards to advance the development of efficient, integrated, and interoperable surveillance systems at federal, state, and local levels. It is a major component of the Public Health Information Network (PHIN). Table 25.1 describes the purposes of NEDSS (Centers for Disease Control and Prevention, NEDSS, 2004).

The health alert network (HAN) was begun in 1999 with 33 states and 3 city/county health departments (Centers for Disease Control, HAN, 2004). It was funded to develop capacity at the state and local levels for continuous, high-speed access to public health information, and to broadcast information in support of emergency communications. The HAN has now grown to all 50 states and 8 U.S. territories. Well over $300 million has been spent on information and communication infrastructure development at the state and local levels, thus making this system a vital component of the PHIN. The HAN homepage also provides directions to be followed in the event of an actual or threatened incident. Figure 25.1 illustrates the protocol to be followed in a bioterrorist event. Notice the communication links that are necessary for a successful notification procedure.

The CDC established the laboratory and response network (LRN) after President Clinton issued Presidential Decision Directive 39 in 1995, which outlined national antiterrorism policies and assigned specific missions to federal departments and agencies (Centers for Disease

Control, LRN, 2004). Its objective was to ensure an effective laboratory response to bioterrorism by helping to improve the nation's public health laboratory infrastructure, which had limited ability to respond to bioterrorism. Today, the LRN is charged with the task of maintaining an integrated network of state and local public health, federal, military, and international laboratories that can respond to both bioterrorism and chemical terrorism.

There is also an informatics component of the CDC, the Division of Public Health Surveillance and Informatics. Their purpose is to provide and improve access to and use of public health information (Centers for Disease Control, Division of Public Health Surveillance and Informatics, 2004). A wide variety of resources can be found on their Web site, including performance criteria for public health disease reporting systems, phone triage protocols, and guidance for public health alerts and advisories. Informatics tools such as knowledge representation, controlled vocabularies, heterogeneous databases, security and confidentiality, clinical decision support, data mining, and data visualization are now being applied with a new urgency to the task of early detection of intentional outbreaks of disease (Lober et al., 2002).

Role of AHRQ in Stimulating New Informatics Solutions

AHRQ's involvement in bioterrorism comes from the recognition that clinicians, hospitals, and healthcare systems have essential roles in public health infrastructure. In the fiscal year 2000, AHRQ received $5 million in support for bioterrorism research. Since that time, AHRQ received ongoing funding and has initiated many major projects, several of which focus on the use of informatics and other technologies and methods to improve linkages between personal healthcare systems, emergency response networks, and public health agencies.

Decision Support Systems Decision support systems and their role in disease management are an area of significant interest and importance. AHRQ's integrated delivery system research network (IDSRN) based at the Weill Medical College at Cornell University has collaborated with the New York City Department of Health and Mental Hygiene and Mayor's Office of Emergency Management to develop a computer simulation model for citywide response planning for mass prophylaxis and vaccination during bioterrorist attacks and other public health emergencies. Researchers at the Children's Hospital of Boston are building decision support models for information systems

Table 25.1 Purposes of the National Electronic Disease Surveillance System (NEDSS)

To detect outbreaks rapidly and to monitor the health of the nation

Facilitate the electronic transfer of appropriate information from clinical information systems in the healthcare system to public health departments

Reduce provider burden in the provision of information

Enhance both the timeliness and quality of information provided

Protocols:
Interim Recommended Notification Procedures for Local and State Public Health
Department Leaders in the Event of a Bioterrorist Incident

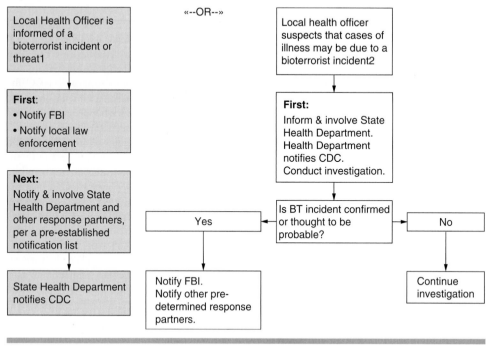

Figure 25.1
Procedures for dealing with bioterrorist event.
(*www.bt.cdc.gov/EmContact/Protocols.asp*)

of linked healthcare data, which would speed up reporting and enhance rapid dissemination of relevant information (AHRQ, 2004).

The University of California at San Francisco has reviewed and synthesized available evidence on the Information technology (IT) needs of first responder physicians in the event of bioterrorism or other public health emergencies. It has also examined the role of information technologies and decision support systems to assist in rapid diagnosis and management of disease resulting from an increased caseload. Findings were published by the AHRQ Publications Clearinghouse as well as by the National Library of Medicine Bookshelf (AHRQ, 2004).

Another project involving decision support systems is being undertaken at Boston Children's Hospital and Harvard University, in a joint study funded by AHRQ. This project seeks to develop a prototype database and Web site to facilitate clinician reporting of trends that

will be used to diagnose possible bioterrorist attacks. Four prototypes of decision support systems are being developed, so that clinicians can give "just-in-time" information and advice on appropriate responses. Such information systems would link together the public health infrastructure as well as the clinical care delivery system to speed up the reporting process and enhance dissemination of relevant information.

Syndromic Surveillance   IT systems can also aid intensively in syndromic surveillance. Syndromic surveillance is loosely defined as detection of a disease outbreak before the actual disease or mechanism of transmission is identified. The MPC Corporation, together with the University of Pittsburgh and Carnegie Mellon University, have undertaken a project to develop the "real-time outbreak and disease surveillance" (RODS) system. This system provides early warning of possible infectious disease outbreaks caused by bioterrorism or other public health emergencies. Additionally, the MPC Corporation is also working on a project which focuses on the use of information systems to track and plan for bioterrorist events, of which an important component is the prototype electronic bed-tracking tool. An assessment tool has been developed, which will aid public health officials in acquiring tools related to early warning surveillance systems and other IT systems addressing bioterrorism.

Helping Clinicians Respond   Provider training and education are also critical elements of a comprehensive plan for bioterrorism and public health preparedness in general. Researchers at the University of Alabama at Birmingham have developed continuing medical education training modules to teach healthcare professionals to identify various biologic agents, as many pathogens and conditions (such as smallpox) are rarely seen in the United States, which limits clinicians from being familiar with related infection. The six biologic agents covered on the Web site are anthrax, smallpox, botulinum toxin, tularemia, viral hemorrhagic fever, and the plague. These pathogens are classified at the Biosafety Level 4 (BSL-4) and are considered to be the most deadly agents. While these modules are meant for all healthcare professionals, there are specialized modules specifically for emergency room practitioners, radiologists, pathologists, and infection control specialists (University of Alabama Birmingham, 2004). The Research Triangle Institute (RTI), has also developed two prototype simulations to aid medical providers in responding to bioterrorist attacks and other public health emergencies.

The practice-based research network (PBRN) at the Children's Hospital Center in Cincinnati has developed a system to allow for electronic solicitation of data using handheld devices and wireless communications. This system has a primarily pediatric focus and allows real-time transmission of clinical impressions and symptoms, which will aid in bioterrorism surveillance.

Researchers at Vanderbilt University Medical Center have undertaken a study to determine the effectiveness and efficiency of learning programs to educate nurses volunteering in their local community Medical Reserve Corps. In this study, two types of learning programs will be compared, one with a traditional face-to-face format, while the other is an online version. Both programs are designed using the principles of the national How People Learn framework, and will also focus on defining user characteristics that predict selection of and effective completion of learning programs.

In 2004, AHRQ also hosted a series of Web conferences for state and local health system preparedness, further demonstrating how informatics can help providers learn about ways to improve response and preparedness in their respective healthcare systems (AHRQ news, 2004).

Role of HRSA in Promoting Informatics Educational Solutions

Two grant management programs exist under the management of HRSA related to bioterrorism: the Hospital Bioterrorism Preparedness Program and the Bioterrorism Training and Curriculum Development Program (BTCD). Because these grants were only awarded in 2003, much of the development continues to take place at the current time.

The purpose of the National Bioterrorism Hospital Preparedness Program is to aid state, territory, and selected entities in improving the capacity of the healthcare system, including hospitals, emergency departments, outpatient facilities, emergency medical services systems, and poison control centers, to respond to incidents requiring mass immunization, isolation, decontamination, diagnosis, and treatment, in the aftermath of terrorism or other public health emergencies (*http://www.hrsa.gov/bioterrorism/*). The BTCD program provides continuing education and curricular enhancement for practicing healthcare providers and current students. The developed materials are designed to equip a healthcare workforce to recognize indications of a terrorist event or other public health emergency, meet the acute care needs of patients, including pediatrics and other vulnerable populations in a safe and appropriate manner, rapidly and effectively alert the public health system of such an event at the community, state, and national level, and participate in a coordinated, multidisciplinary response to terrorist events (U.S. Department of Health Resources and Services Administration, 2004). The results of these programs should begin to be available during the fall of 2005.

Other Changes Affecting Emergency Preparedness and Response

Competency-Based Learning and Informatics Needs

Since the emergency department would most likely receive the first victims of a bioterrorism, chemical, or nuclear attack, it is no surprise that the first efforts to conduct a needs assessment and curricular review centered on those activities. The American College of Emergency Physicians (ACEP) formed a nuclear, biologic, and chemical task force to evaluate the status of bioterrorism training in the United States, identify barriers to this training, and offer recommendations for effective education (American College of Emergency Physicians—NBC Task Force, 2001). There were nursing representatives to the task force (Cheryl Peterson [American Nurses Association], Claudia Niersbach and Bettina Stopford [Emergency Nurses Association]). As a result, content needs were addressed for emergency nurses, emergency physicians, and emergency medical service providers. The U.S. DH HS Office of Emergency Preparedness sponsored the task force.

During their analysis, the task force focused on a thorough explanation of the problem that would result in specific recommendations. As a result, they produced a description of the target audiences/learners, an outline of the content that learners should be taught with specific objectives that indicate what learners must know and be able to do, clarification of barriers, and a review of existing educational materials.

Specific methods were used to adequately describe the targeted audiences including group interactions, interviews, review of materials, and agreement by the task force. The task force determined the relative similarities and differences among the groups in a number of areas. Based on the information gathered, a subject matter analysis was accomplished through interviews with task force members and other subject matter experts recommended by the task force. Additional detail was added after reviewing selected articles and other existing subject matter material. The content was organized into three proficiency categories—awareness, performance, and planning. Objectives for each of these categories were then developed.

A formal curriculum review was then undertaken. The focus of each review was to assess the current educational efforts regarding specific weapons of mass destruction (WMD) and to determine how to best integrate that content into the educational programs designed for each audience. The task force concluded, "from initial nurse education through the educational path selected to reach the emergency nursing specialty, emergency nurses are provided no course work specific to WMD incidents" (American College of Emergency Physicians—NBC Task Force, 2001).

The ACEP report was welcomed by the healthcare community as a starting point for mass casualty education. Critics were quick to point out that the findings of the report focused specifically on emergency departments and were not therefore generalizable to other audiences. In addition, the review focused on nuclear,

biologic, and chemical WMD rather than a broader view including explosive, incinerary, radiologic, or natural causes of events.

Concurrent to the development of the ACEP report was an initiative led by Kristine M. Gebbie, RN, DrPH, and funded by the CDC. Her focus was on assuring that the nation's public health workforce was ready to respond to emergencies. As a result, she published in 2001 the first version of competencies for all public health workers (Center for Health Policy, 2001). Some of the competencies were applicable to every worker; others were specific to workers in administrative, professional, technical, or support positions. Her work was recently expanded to encompass specific bioterrorism competencies and to include competencies for more job categories (Center for Health Policy, 2002). The document further reminds readers that "the application of any competency is always within the context of both agency and jurisdictional plans" (Center for Health Policy, 2002). The type of emergency and the emergency response plan for each jurisdiction also determines whether a public health agency is in the lead position, in a collaborative role, or in a secondary/supportive role. The same is true for other organizations that comprise an emergency response team. Gebbie (Center for Health Policy, 2004) went on to develop a "competency-to-curriculum toolkit" that is a resource for those planning a curriculum in emergency preparedness and response. She also listed specific informatics competencies for various job categories (Center for Health Policy, 2004, p. 38).

The International Nursing Coalition for Mass Casualty Education (INCMCE) is an international coalition consisting of organizational representatives of schools of nursing, nursing accrediting bodies, nursing specialty organizations, and governmental agencies interested in promoting mass casualty education for nurses. The vision of the organization is to be the point of influence for public policy that impacts the welfare of the public through nursing practice, education, research, and regulation for mass casualty incidents (MCI). Their mission is to assure a competent nurse workforce to respond to MCI. Their strategic plan has been developed in the priority areas of awareness, response, and research. One of the first activities was to develop a list of competencies for all nurses dealing with mass casualties. The completed competencies can be found on their Web site (International Nursing Coalition for Mass Casualty Education, 2004).

INCMCE members recognized that the assumption of limited curriculum content in nursing programs had never been validated, so a survey was prepared by a task force of INCMCE. In conjunction with the National

League for Nursing, this online curricular survey was sent to all deans and directors of nursing programs in the United States during the months of May and June 2003. The results of this survey not only provide baseline data in relation to what nursing programs are teaching at all levels in emergency response, but will be the source of annual data collection over the next 5 years (Weiner et al., 2004).

Over 300 schools of nursing representing 455 different nursing programs (from licensed practical nurses through doctorate) responded to the survey. Most striking was the finding that *75% of the respondents felt that faculty were not at all prepared or poorly prepared to teach disaster preparedness content.* Figure 25.2 describes the survey findings from the three academic years beginning with 2000–2001.

In 2000–2001, only 22% (N = 107) of the schools of nursing in the survey offered disaster preparedness content with natural disasters receiving the greatest emphasis (28% of programs). In 2001–2002, the percentage of nursing schools offering some disaster preparedness content rose to 39% with again an emphasis on natural disaster. However, disasters related to biologic and chemical agents began receiving more emphasis. It was not until this last academic year that content related to biologic agents occurred more frequently than content related to natural disasters and content related to chemical agents increased as well. It should be noted that content related to nuclear, radiologic, and explosive agents has lagged behind in all three academic years.

While biologic and chemical agents have received increasing emphasis in disaster preparedness content in nursing programs, the total contact hours over the 3 years *has not changed* significantly. The *average number of contact hours in disaster preparedness content is approximately 4 hours* (means ranged from 3.9 in year 2000–2001 to 4.2 in year 2002–2003). The majority of respondents were using Web sites (50%) and journal articles (45.8%) to provide content in disaster preparedness.

The Johns Hopkins University Evidence-based Practice Center was requested by the AHRQ during 2001 to summarize existing evidence on the effectiveness of training clinicians for public health events relevant to bioterrorism preparedness (Johns Hopkins Evidence-based Practice Center, 2002). The extensive literature and Web site search identified over 1,900 articles, although only 60 were found that described and evaluated an education intervention involving one of the key questions for the project. The majority of identified studies pertained to the training of clinicians for detection and management of an infectious disease outbreak. No literature was found that addressed the updating and reinforcing of clinician's training. No literature was found that addressed the training of clinicians to use Web or telephone-based central information sources. No literature was found on the topic of training clinicians to communicate with other healthcare professionals during a public health event. The authors concluded that there is a need for future research into the most effective way to train clinicians in areas that will improve their ability to respond to a bioterrorist attack or other public health event. In 2002, AHRQ awarded another contract to Hopkins to do further research. This work includes an update of the literature review on training practice for bioterrorism, with a new emphasis on disaster drills, and best practices to accomplish successful disaster drills. A tool was also developed for evaluating

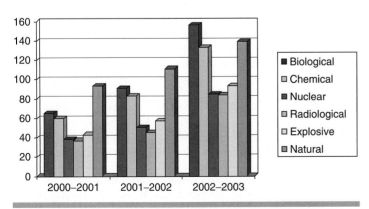

Figure 25.2
Focus of disaster preparedness content across three academic years.

such simulation exercises, and this tool was provided to the states through HRSA's National Hospital Bioterrorism Preparedness Program.

Informatics and the Emergency Operations Center

IT staff have long been familiar with emergency planning for disaster recovery related to their systems, but find themselves in a new role as part of a more comprehensive team approach to disasters and emergencies affecting the hospital. The incident management system (IMS) was first used by firefighters to control disaster scenes in a multijurisdictional and interdepartmental manner. The IMS calls for a hierarchical chain of command led by the incident manager or commander. Each job assignment is consistently followed by assigned personnel who refer to a specific job action sheet. The IMS has been adapted for hospital use and is called the Hospital Emergency Incident Command System (HEICS).

The Vanderbilt University Medical Center (VUMC) incorporated the HEICS system in 1999, in preparation for Y2K. As such, they adopted the organizational structure of an incident commander with eight direct reports: planning officer, operations officer, logistics officer, security officer, public information officer, liaison officer, safety officer, and finance officer. Using this organizational structure, the IT leader was "buried" four levels down under the command of the logistics officer.

Early initiations of HEICS at Vanderbilt occurred due to reasons not directly related to technology, but pointed out the importance of technology for an effective response. The testing of the bioterrorism subemergency plan pointed out that the IT leader was so low in the chain of command that critical information systems were not available when needed. A second incident involved a missing patient, and responders soon learned that the clinical workstations in the hospital emergency operations center did not include typical office products needed for effective communication. Mass communications were not easily generated through the HEOC workstations, as the Outlook accounts were not set up for individuals who had the authority to mass communicate throughout the VUMC. A third incident was created by the onslaught of the SQL Slammer worm that packet flooded the hospital network in a denial of service attack. In this situation (because of being caused by a technology problem), there was also an Information Management Emergency Operations Center (IMEOC) that was separate from the HEOC, but was also using principles of IMS. When the patient care online system became inaccessible, it was determined that a hospital-wide HEOC needed to be established. The effective management of this situation resulted in a revised organizational chart for HEICS, adding the positions of information management officer and physician officer to the first line of management. In addition, there was a job action sheet developed for the position of information management lead coordinator (Weiner, Chenoweth, and Hoffman, 2004).

As IT becomes more pervasive in the delivery of quality patient care, it takes on increased importance in managing a hospital through an internal or community emergency. For those emergencies caused by an IT threat, increased coordination is necessary between the HEOC and the IMEOC. During non-technology-related incidents, it is important to realize that other IT tools are needed to promote effective and efficient communication during times of crises. Furthermore, advanced modeling tools would be a helpful addition to the tool set, given that some data are known prior to an event (like when medications from the Strategic National Stockpile should arrive).

Informatics and Volunteerism

Healthcare volunteers are a necessary component of mass casualty events but also create challenges. How do you count volunteers so that they are only entered once? How do you educate them so that they can perform effectively when needed? How are liability issues dealt with? Are there certain tasks that lend themselves to volunteer effort? Some states (like Colorado and Texas) offer their nurses the opportunity to volunteer when they renew their nursing licensure. It is then possible for state-wide databases to be built, but these are only shared within the state system. Some states require a set number of hours of continuing education in emergency preparedness in order to renew licensure.

The federal government does have a system for organizing teams that are willing to travel to other regions of the country in the event of an emergency. These teams are called disaster medical assistance teams (DMATs). When DMATs are activated, members of the teams are federalized or made temporary workers of the federal government, which then assumes the liability for their services. Their licensure and certifications are then recognized by all states. The newer Medical Reserve Corps initiative (Medical Reserve Corps, 2004) was designed to assemble healthcare volunteers who are willing to respond at their local levels. This 2-year-old program is part of the larger Citizens Corps federal program. Another initiative sponsored by the American

Nurses Association is the National Nurses Response Team (NNRT) team. The NNRT will comprise 10 regionally-based teams of 200 registered nurses who could be called on to assist in chemoprophylaxis or vaccination (American Nurses Association, 2004). Their members will be enrolled in the National Disaster Medical System. The American Red Cross has a long history of volunteerism during disasters, and has education requirements for nurses depending on what roles they will play in disaster relief. Regardless of the group, nurses are urged to be a part of an organized group rather than simply showing up on the scene of a disaster and contributing to the confusion.

All of these initiatives require informatics solutions in order to function effectively. A national database of nurses who are willing to volunteer would allow for informed decisions and increased efficiency of services. Table 25.2 lists potential characteristics of a national volunteer nurses' database.

The National Health Information Infrastructure (NHII) in Fighting National Threats

Recent growth in the support for the NHII will help to support the standards that are currently lacking. David J. Brailer, MD, PhD, was appointed as the first national coordinator for Health Information Technology (Thompson and Brailer, 2004). The national coordinator was charged with directing health IT within DHHS and coordinating them with those of other relevant executive branch agencies. Public health monitoring, bioterror surveillance, research, and quality monitoring require data that depend on the widespread adoption of the principles of health IT (Thompson and Brailer, 2004).

Table 25.2   Characteristics of a National Volunteer Nurses' Database

Verification of licensure (can be multiple states)

Records of continuing education

Records of certifications

Organization(s) volunteering for (will need to decide how to only count individual once during an event)

Activation instructions

Prior emergency response experience (including dates of service)

Security clearance level

Summary

In summary, the challenges that bioterrorism and other emergency events bring to the informatics agenda are not unique. Many of the same hurdles that typically hamper healthcare information efforts are made exponentially worse because of the shortened timeline and sense of urgency. Healthcare workers are also faced with terroristic and natural threats that again draw attention to our need for better communication tools and data interfaces. We must continue to develop and refine informatics tools that meet the challenges of emergency planning and response. After all, the health of our nation depends on it.

References

AHRQ. Retrieved October 4, 2004, from *http://www. ahrq.gov/clinic/epcsums/bioitsum.htm*.

AHRQ news. Retrieved October 3, 2004, from *http:// www.ahrq.gov/news/ulp/biotconf.htm*.

AHRQ, Research. Retrieved October 4, 2004, from *http://www.ahrq.gov/research/biomodel.htm*.

American College of Emergency Physicians NBC Task Force. (2001). *Developing Objectives, Content, and Competencies for the Training of Emergency Medical Technicians, Emergency Physicians, and Emergency Nurses to Care for Causalities from Nuclear, Biological or Chemical (NBC) Incidents: Final Report.* Irving, TX: Author. Retrieved July 8, 2003, from *http://www. acep.org/library/pdf/NBCreport2.pdf*.

American Nurses Association. Retrieved September 15, 2004, *http://www.ana.org/news/disaster/response.htm*.

Center for Health Policy, Columbia University School of Nursing. (2001). *Emergency Preparedness: Core Competencies for All Public Health Workers.* New York, NY: Author. Retrieved December 13, 2002, from Columbia University, School of Nursing, Policy, *http://www.nursing.hs.columbia.edu/institute-centers/chphsr/compbroch.pdf*

Center for Health Policy, Columbia University School of Nursing. (2002). *Bioterrorism & Emergency Readiness: Competencies for All Public Health Workers: Preview Version III.* New York, NY: Author. Retrieved December 13, 2002, from *http://www.nursing. hs.columbia.edu/institute-centers/chphsr/btcomps.pdf*

Center for Health Policy Columbia University School of Nursing & Association of Teachers of Preventive Medicine. (2004). *Competency-to-Curriculum Toolkit: Developing Curricula for Public Health Workers.* Author.

Centers for Disease Control and Prevention. Retrieved October 1, 2004, from *http://www.cdc.gov/aboutcdc.htm*

Centers for Disease Control and Prevention. Retrieved September, 18, 2004, from *http://www.phppo.cdc. gov/han/*

Centers for Disease Control and Prevention, Division of Public Health Surveillance and Informatics. Retrieved September 20, 2004, from *http://www.cdc.gov/epo/dphsi/*

Centers for Disease Control and Prevention, LRN. Retrieved October 4, 2004, from *http://www.bt.cdc.gov/lrn/*

Centers for Disease Control and Prevention, NEDSS. Retrieved June 5, 2005, from *http://www.cdc.gov/nedss/*.

Hamilton, J. (2003). An internet-based bar code tracking system: Coordination of confusion at mass casualty incidents. *Disaster Management & Response* 1(1):25–30.

International Nursing Coalition for Mass Casualty Education. Retrieved October 1, 2004, from *http://www.incmce.org*

Johns Hopkins Evidence-based Practice Center. (2002). *Training of Clinicians for Public Health Events Relevant to Bioterrorism Preparedness* (AHRQ Publication no. 02-E011). Rockville, MD: Agency for Healthcare Research and Quality.

Lober, W. B., Karras, B. T., Wagner, M. M. Overhage, J. M., Davidson, A. J., Graser, H., et al. (2002). *Journal of the American Medical Informatics Association* 9:105–115.

Medical Reserve Corps. Retrieved October 5, 2004, from *http://www.citizencorps.gov/programs/medical.shtm*.

Simmons, S. C., Murphy, T. A., Blanarovicii, A., Workman, F., Rosenthal, D. A., and Carbone, M. (2003). Telehealth technologies and applications for terrorism response: A report of the 2002 Coastal North Carolina domestic preparedness training exercise. *Journal of the American Medical Informatics Association* 10:166–176.

Snee, N. L., and McCormick, K. A. (January/February, 2004). The case for integrating public health informatics networks. *IEEE Engineering in Medicine and Biology Magazine* 1–8.

Teich, J. M., Wagner, M. M., Mackenzie, C. F., and Schafer, K. O. (2002). The informatics response in disaster, terrorism, and war. *Journal of the American Medical Informatics Association* 9:97–104.

Thompson, R. and Brailer, D. J. (2004). *Progress Report: The Decade of Health Information Technology: Delivering Consumer Centric and Information Rich Healthcare*. Washington, DC: U.S. Department of Health and Human Services Office of the National Coordinator for Health Information Technology.

University of Alabama, Birmingham. Retrieved October 4, 2004, from *http://www.bioterrorism.uab.edu/*

U.S. Department of Health and Human Services. Retrieved October 7, 2004, from *http://www.hhs.gov/about/whatwedo.html/*

U.S. Department of Health Resources and Services Administration. Retrieved October 4, 2004, from *http://bhpr.hrsa.gov/grants/applications/03bioterror.htm*

U.S. Department of Homeland Security. Retrieved October 7, 2004, from *http://www.whitehouse.gov/news/releases/2003/12/20031217-6.html*, December 17, 2003.

Weiner, E., Chenoweth, K., and Hoffner, P. (2004). Elevating information technology in the hospital emergency operations center. In *Proceedings of MedInfo 2004*, San Francisco, CA, 1905.

Weiner, E., Irwin, M., Trangenstein, P., and Gordon, J. (2005). *Emergency Preparedness Curriculum in U.S. Nursing Schools. Accepted for publication in Nursing Education Perspectives*.

26

CHAPTER

Vendor Applications

Sheryl Taylor
Ann Farrell

OBJECTIVES

1. Review key trends, issues, obstacles, and opportunities facing the nursing profession with regard to adoption of healthcare information technology

2. Describe healthcare information technology vendors' responses to nursing demand for improved information systems.

3. Identify leading healthcare information technology vendors that provide organizationwide, hospital-centric information systems and address nursing applications in the context of a patient-centric, electronic medical record.

KEY WORDS

computerized medical record
electronic medical record
electronic health record
vendor
nursing philosophy
multidisciplinary systems
clinical terminology sets

Current Trends Toward Prime Vendors, EHRs, and Systems Integration

There are a wide variety of software products offered by an array of diverse vendors that nurses use to plan, document, manage, and evaluate patient care. "Niche" applications focus on a discrete set of nursing functions, e.g., care planning. "Departmental" systems address a more comprehensive set of functions for a single point of service, e.g., labor and delivery; or department, e.g., cardiology; or closely aligned group of departments, e.g., the perioperative suite. Departmental systems are more targeted and robust than comparable modules of EHR solutions since departmental systems focus on one or a few specialties and points of service. Thus, departmental systems continue to be sought by many organizations, particularly in academic medical centers and for high acuity, specialized care departments. Niche and departmental systems complement EHRs where they exist and share data with them via industry standard

data exchange technologies, e.g., Health Language Seven (HL7) and XML.

The current trend is to limit niche and departmental systems in order to create an EHR via well-integrated applications with a common database, tools, and technologies. Although the HCIT environment is by nature heterogeneous, healthcare organizations (HCOs) increasingly seek a primary clinical vendor who, to the degree possible, delivers a single system or suite of tightly coupled solutions that spans all points of service, automates core clinical processes of physicians and all care providers, and creates a multidisciplinary, longitudinal, and patient-centric record.

In addition to products that facilitate patient care, numerous vendors offer HCIT solutions that support quality management, staff scheduling, supply management, and other patient-care-related nursing activities. These applications and comparable capabilities within EHRs are increasing in importance as virtually every HCO faces quality of care, care management, and fiscal challenges on which nursing can have a significant positive impact, using IT as a tool.

New Technologies

New and emerging hardware and software technologies, e.g., handheld devices, are increasingly being incorporated in nursing applications. Key goals are to improve quality of care, mobility of caregivers, and collaboration among the care team. Currently, strong emphasis is being placed on delivering technology at the point of care via bedside terminals and wireless devices, e.g., personal digital assistants (PDAs), laptops, PCs, or computers on wheels (COWs). Even with automated systems, if all terminals are at the workstation, nurses waste enormous time and introduce the potential for error with duplicate charting in documenting care on paper notes and later entering them into the computer. Bedside terminal access can facilitate real-time charting, increase nursing time at the bedside, and eliminate "batch" end of shift charting. In addition, vendors are introducing a variety of enabling technologies, e.g., speech and handwriting recognition, that minimize nonproductive data entry time. It is unclear how seamlessly these new and emerging technologies can be integrated into nursing workflow and existing information systems, and thus whether they will gain widespread adoption by nurses in the near future.

Historical Perspective

Historically, nurse executives have not widely embraced IT as a strategic business tool. For a variety of reasons, nurses in the field have often lacked a deep understanding of the power of IT. With the ubiquity of technology in healthcare and everyday life, savvy nursing leaders increasingly view IT as viable means to address resource shortages, care delivery challenges, and fiscal pressures. A new breed of registered nurses (RNs) is entering the field with a greater appreciation for the value of technology as a means to improve patient care and job satisfaction.

With notable exceptions, the nursing profession has been largely underserved by HCIT vendors. This is surprising, given that nurses are by far the single largest user of clinical systems and key potential beneficiaries of information technology (IT). Contributing factors are cultural, gender-related, power-based, and economic in nature. Nurses are by far the largest and most well-respected healthcare professional group based on numerous national consumer surveys. Yet ironically, the nursing profession all too often lacks due respect in many settings, suffering triple biases as RNs in a MD-centric medical world, females (primarily) in male-dominated executive suites, and expense items in a revenue-constrained and cost conscious fiscal environment.

In most national and local healthcare debates, nursing has been essentially invisible. This is in part because nursing is the only profession that does not charge for services rendered. Unlike their professional counterparts, nursing care is bundled in room and bed charges like housekeeping services. In addition, because nursing lacks a standard nomenclature and nursing data are not codified, the direct correlation between nursing interventions and patient outcomes is difficult, if not impossible, to quantify. As such, the contribution of nursing to patient care has historically often been undervalued and nursing initiatives underfunded.

Current Situation

Today, the majority of nursing-related patient care applications are acquired as part of EHR decisions. Since nurse executives historically did not drive most EHR purchasing criteria or decisions, systems were all too often selected based on the priorities of more powerful constituents and occasional users, e.g., MDs. In these cases, nursing often does not fully embrace the system or take full advantage of its capabilities. Complicating the situation, in an effort to save time and money, some organizations overlay new clinical technologies on inefficient or poorly designed existing processes. This is a "dead on arrival" strategy that leads to user dissatisfaction and, frequently, "blaming" of the technology for the failures of the organization.

Perhaps not coincidentally, in the recent survey "Healthcare without Bounds: Mobile Computing in Nursing, June 2004" Gregg Malkary, managing director of Spyglass consulting, reports that an alarming percentage of nurse respondents perceived that nursing applications are not a high priority for their organization and, by and large, many current solutions are poorly designed, disjointed, and user-unfriendly for nurses. Commonly reported perceptions were:

- Nursing is an untapped and underserved resource in provider organizations.
- Workflow inefficiencies are not well addressed by existing solutions.
- Automation is not a high priority for nursing in their organizations.
- Vendors are out of sync with nursing needs.
- Some new tools and technologies have complicated rather than simplified nursing practice, at times decreasing productivity and introducing an element of increased risk to patients.

Root causes of poorly designed nursing applications include:

- Vendor product design processes driven by engineers, financial systems analysts, or MDs (non-nurses)

- Insufficient nursing representatives on vendor executive and development teams (majority of clinicians in sales and marketing)

- The HCIT industry's overall woeful lack of adequate requirements definition, functional specifications, and process analysis

- Early focus on automation of the paper chart without a full understanding of underlying nursing process, workflows, and ergonomic challenges

Automating the paper chart and existing workflows often exacerbates inefficiencies. With the advent of graphic user interfaces, some HCIT vendors simply "beautified" underlying chart forms, with minimal process improvement. With some clinical documentation systems, charting time has increased significantly, with little added value for the patient or clinician or return on investment (ROI) for the organization.

In recent years, there has been renewed national interest in exploiting IT as a tool to address mission critical issues facing virtually every HCO nationwide. Landmark Institute of Medicine reports: To Err is Human (1999) and Crossing the Chasm (2001), as well as efforts by the Leapfrog Group, a powerful consortium of employers, have focused nationwide attention on acute patient safety problems in U.S. hospitals.

In response to patient safety concerns, vendors and provider organizations have focused on two primary HCIT initiatives, i.e., computerized physician order entry (CPOE) and bar-code-enabled medication administration (BCMA). Based on 2004 Healthcare Information and Management Systems Society (HIMSS) survey data, these two initiatives dominate clinical system selection processes and are top IT priorities for HCOs today. Although market interest is high, adoption rates are relatively limited to date due to a variety of technology (hardware and software), workflow, and cultural issues and challenges.

While CPOE and BCMA drive most clinical system selections today, EHR vendors are delivering a broader, richer set of capabilities that enable more efficient, standardized clinical documentation, and interdisciplinary, evidence-based care. The role of well-designed, easy to use, online clinical documentation in facilitating safe and cost-effective care has long been undervalued. EHR vendors are increasingly aware of the need to deliver solutions that better support caregivers and managers in today's more holistic, collaborative, data intensive, and demanding patient care environment.

Purchase of an EMR product forces buyers to take a patient-centric, rather than departmental, view of clinical processes and systems. Nurses and all professional groups must consider not only their own requirements and preferences but also how new information systems will impact colleagues, patients, and the organization at large.

Nurses leveraging HCIT at facilities with well-implemented and well-supported clinical systems report significantly higher levels of job satisfaction than their counterparts using manual processes and paper records. The ability of nurses to clearly articulate and promote the value of HCIT for themselves, their patients, and their organizations could be a crucial factor in accelerating widespread adoption of advanced nursing applications.

Vendor Response

In response to market demand, HCIT vendors are delivering more robust and tightly integrated clinical solutions that better address the needs of all care providers for more coordinated, streamlined patient care delivery. While some vendors offer clearly superior nursing applications, no solution is perfect; each has different strengths and limitations.

Unlike with earlier systems that primarily automated the paper chart and basic patient care processes, vendors are now expected to deliver "next generation" clinical applications that:

- Support multi- and interdisciplinary care, i.e., nurses and allied health professionals, e.g., physical therapy (PT), respiratory therapy (RT), social services, and so forth, with all provider orders, care plans, and notes online and integrated in a common patient-centric patient record.

- Promote data integrity via data validity checks and embedded tools, e.g., intravenous (IV) dose/drip calculators.

- Provide ready access to internal standards, e.g., policies and procedures, and external knowledge bases, e.g., reference guides and drug databases.

- Enable evidence-based care via automation of integrated multidisciplinary clinical pathways and incorporation of decision support mechanisms, e.g., prompts and alerts.

- Collect work load management data as a byproduct of clinical documentation, including deriving prospective acuity data from orders and retrospective acuity data from clinical documentation.

- Support productivity management, staffing, and budgeting activities.

- Support process and outcomes monitoring, management, and continual improvement via standard reports and database mining.

- Support charge capture, supply management, and inventory reconciliation, e.g., replenishment of supplies and medications as a byproduct of clinical documentation.

- Support for medical (case, quality, risk, utilization, and infection control), disease, and population management.

Clearly, vendors and future nursing systems must address the critical (sometimes conflicting) needs of a broad base of nurse constituents, including executives, quality managers, and educators, while respecting the sensitivities and workload demands of the direct care providers.

EHR vendors' recognition of the vital role of nursing is evidenced by the number of appointments of nurse executives and growing investments in nursing and interdisciplinary system capabilities.

Table 26.1 reflects the perspectives of lead EHR vendor nursing executives regarding their organization's nursing vision and product differentiation.

All lead vendors can point to client success stories as well as failed implementations, each using the same underlying software. Although functionality and technology are important, more critical factors for system success are enthusiastic clinician champions and strong executive leaders who make IT part of organization's fiber and culture.

With strong clinical leadership and increasingly supportive systems, nursing now has an unparalleled opportunity to leverage IT for the well being of our patients and profession.

Vendor Comparison

For purposes of this chapter, side-by-side, feature function product comparisons will not be presented given the sheer number of vendors offering nursing solutions and time sensitive nature of the information.

Care Flow Diagram

The care flow diagram is a conceptual model that represents a patient-centric, interdisciplinary, inpatient-oriented view of a clinical information system that supports a fully integrated EHR. It includes care components, e.g., care planning and documentation that are automated in EHR systems as well as, in whole or part, in niche and departmental applications. This diagram reflects how core care components are interrelated and how clinical data are shared among multiple care providers. Each care component is displayed in relation to other components and the clinical process it supports (Fig. 26.1, shown on right).

The model assumes direct physician use of the EHR and represents a multidisciplinary team approach reflecting emerging care delivery models. Lead EHR vendors increasingly enable care delivery across the community and continuum of care, while also supporting traditional more episodic approaches to patient care. Although each vendor's vision, solution, and product differentiators are unique, the diagram is intended as a model for use as an education tool, framework for product evaluation, and benchmark for vendor comparison.

■ Key Clinical System Nursing and Multidisciplinary Care Components

For this section, readers should refer to the care flow diagram (Fig. 26.1) for a graphical representation of concepts presented.

Patient Access

The patient record is initiated in the admission, discharge, and transfer (ADT) system or administrative portion of the EHR. The collection of initial registration and admission data establishes a patient record and begins the clinical and financial encounter with the provider organization. As part of the scheduling and admitting processes, select patient demographic and clinical data are collected, stored, and available for retrieval by all authorized care providers. In many organizations data collected throughout each patient encounter are never archived, therefore a "birth to death" patient record is available online. In an EHR environment, nurses can access patient records for all encounters with the organization and compare clinical data across multiple episodes of care.

Every patient care process begins with a user sign-on to the information system, and location and selection of the patient from a list or roster. Patient lists are tailored to the individual provider, e.g., patients on the unit(s) that the nurse is assigned to support and that is customized based on individual preference .

While patients enter the hospital via scheduled admission, transfer from another facility, referral, walk in, and

Table 26.1 Vendors' Nursing Philosophy, Product Differentiation, and Vision for the Future

Cerner Corporation[a]

Philosophy for nursing

Cerner takes the paper out of healthcare by automating the workflow of the entire healthcare team with point-of-care solutions based on a common clinical data repository architecture. Clinical decision support tools provide safety nets with alerts and reminders to protect against errors. Best practice and evidence-based nursing knowledge are embedded in documentation and plans of care that come with our prebuilt clinical database as an organization's starter database. Cerner's CareNet Nursing solutions are designed to free nurses from non-nursing tasks, to remove inefficiencies and to allow nurses to do the things that only nurses can do.

Key differentiators

At Cerner, there is a nursing executive team with autonomy for solution development, business strategies, and the ability to represent nursing at the cabinet and board level. This results in nursing-centric solutions across the care continuum that support the practice, profession, and science of nursing. For example, our collaborative partnerships with academia/provider organizations to conduct evidence-based nursing practice research and two university-based schools of nursing to bring automation into the baccalaureate level of nursing curriculum.

Vision of the future

Most immediate is the extension of our current clinical systems to serve a community and health populations for a person's EHR that crosses geography and venues of care. Advancement in telephone/Web/voice documentation will support voice documentation at point-of-care, hand-free devices, and connection to the patient electronic chart over the phone with Web linkage. This is the near future. Technology embedded in uniforms that act as medical devices to scan the patient for vital signs, blood levels, and cardiac output will be a bit further out, but coming.

Department of Defense[b]

Philosophy for nursing

The Department of Defense (DoD) does not endorse any single nursing philosophy, but instead shapes published nursing philosophies around the vision and mission of the Military Health System (MHS). The vision of the MHS is to be a world-class health system that supports the military mission by fostering, protecting, sustaining, and restoring health. To achieve this vision, nursing professionals must focus their leadership, nursing skills, and selected nursing applications on providing health support for the full range of military operations and sustaining the health of all those entrusted to their care.

Key differentiators

The key distinction in DoD HCIT systems is the mandated requirements that apply to each clinical system that serves DoD beneficiaries. For example, any MHS clinical application must meet the executive order by the then President Clinton on 11/8/97: "... I am directing the DoD and VA to create a new Force Health Protection Program. Every soldier, sailor, airman and marine will have a comprehensive, life-long medical record of all illnesses and injuries they suffer, the care and inoculations they receive and their exposure to different hazards. These records will help us prevent illness and identify and cure those that occur ..."

Vision of the future

Our vision is to preserve the fighting strength by providing stellar nursing care services and exploiting the power of technology through access to data and knowledge. The DoD's worldwide readiness mission requires the delivery of nursing care in both deployable, hostile environments and peacetime environments. This global responsibility requires nursing professionals to blend nursing science, computer science, and information science in their practice of nursing and in their delivery of nursing care to active duty and retired members of the uniformed services, their families, veterans, and other selected DoD beneficiaries.

Veterans Health Administration[c]

Philosophy for nursing

Veterans Health Administration (VHA) office of nursing services believes that technology should be advanced to improve patient care and support the practice of nursing. Information systems should also offer veterans easy access to their health information and engage veterans to actively participate in managing their health.

(Continued)

Table 26.1 Vendors' Nursing Philosophy, Product Differentiation, and Vision for the Future (*Continued*)

Veterans Health Administration[c]

Philosophy for nursing

Nursing should benefit from technology that supports improving patient outcomes. Technology needs to serve all levels of nursing, creating seamless processes that support proactive practice in clinical, administrative, research, and education areas. New technology should have utility as well as efficiency. Nursing should provide input in every phase of technology design and implementation.

Key differentiators

The VA is recognized for leadership in employing technology to measure and improve patient care.

The VA EHR allows for increased accessibility of patient records and enables standardized, continuous documentation across disciplines, care settings, and overtime.

Bar code medication administration (BCMA) creates human/technical processes that minimize medication errors.

Clinical reminders, safety alerts (e.g., critical lab values), and nursing dashboards provide real-time decision support tools at the point of care.

Nurses have the opportunity to participate in designing and implementing innovative systems. For example, a VA nurse launched the idea for bar coding patient identification bands.

Vision of the future

Technology will be accessible, effective, easy to use, and available at the point of care. Technology will facilitate seamless processes that support nursing practice and patient care. Nurses have access to the latest hardware technology and are engaged in testing systems designed specifically to all age groups of nurses. Through design and implementation of a new generation of healthcare technologies, the VHA will remain in the forefront of healthcare informatics.

Eclipsys Corporation[d]

Philosophy for nursing

Eclipsys recognizes that nurses have always been at the center of patient care, from performing clinical assessments and administering complex treatment plans to counseling and educating patients and their families. With our advanced clinical solutions, Eclipsys supports nurses as care coordinators. With a view of patients' acuity scores and status and access to complete patient records, relevant orders and clinical documentation, nurses determine who has the most acute needs, what interventions are required, and how to efficiently use their time. In addition, nurse managers can manage appropriate nurse staffing levels. Eclipsys solutions help make healthcare safer for patients—and safer for nurses.

Key differentiators

Eclipsys' advanced clinical solutions improve workflow and help all members of the healthcare team catch errors and prevent complications. When all healthcare team members have access to evidence-based best practices, they can collectively work toward a common goal in partnership with the patient. Our solutions offer rich clinical content and the ability to manage patient acuity through an automated patient classification system. They put the right knowledge into the hands of the right person, at the right time and place, and on the right device. With relevant knowledge at their fingertips, clinicians and administrators can make the best possible decisions.

Vision of the future

Momentum is building in healthcare for the deployment of advanced clinical, financial, and management information systems that help improve patient safety, operational efficiency, and financial performance. Eclipsys' vision is to be a trusted value partner in a HCO's pursuit of superior clinical, financial, and operational outcomes. As the outcomes company, Eclipsys was founded with a simple mission: better healthcare through knowledge. Through the advanced clinical and financial solutions it offers today and the evolution of those tools to meet the changing needs of leading HCOs, Eclipsys strives to help nurses—and all healthcare professionals—reach their full potential.

IDX Systems Corporation[e]

Philosophy for nursing

Through technology, IDX creates innovative solutions for clinical excellence that improve outcomes, enhance satisfaction, and reduce costs. IDX Carecast nursing applications offer effective nursing tools that expedite excellent patient care. Our nursing applications integrate data and transform it into information that facilitates critical thinking, supports clinical judgment, and provides pertinent, real-time patient information, empowering nurses to deliver high-quality patient care now.

Table 26.1 Vendors' Nursing Philosophy, Product Differentiation, and Vision for the Future (*Continued*)

IDX Systems Corporation[e]

Key differentiators

IDX focuses on the needs of each customer and builds strong rapport with customer clinicians to meet business needs that support high-quality patient care. Nursing is viewed as a vital aspect of patient care delivery and products are evolved continually that support nurses across care settings. *Carecast* integrates clinical, financial, and administrative information on each patient on a single database, built on the foundation of the patient-centered, lifetime patient record that spans the continuum of care. *Carecast* is built on the principle of Advancing Fail-Safe Care: providing 99.9% uptime, sub-second response time, and clinical comprehensiveness.

Vision of the future

IDX's vision for the future is focused on patient safety and clinician satisfaction, including expansion of capabilities that support evidence-based practice and foster interdisciplinary collaboration.

McKesson Information Solutions[f]

Philosophy for nursing

McKesson knows how challenging it is for nurses to provide consistently safe, high-quality patient care, as patient loads increase, care becomes more complex and care processes are predominantly manual. Manual processes result in less than adequate collaboration and communication, inefficiency, and an absence of an interdisciplinary approach. Nurses face an avalanche of paperwork that affects the time available to care for patients. McKesson believes that the right information and technologies can streamline and improve the nursing process to help patients achieve the best outcomes in the safest possible way and support nurses better in caring for their patients.

Key differentiators

Only comprehensive medication safety solution, providing true closed-loop medication management. Over 60 live customer sites with BCMA.

Tight integration within Horizon Clinicals—sharing allergies, medical history, vital signs, orders, and documentation between all patient care settings.

Strong development history and customer base—more than 15 years of experience, 180+ customers, developed by nurses, for nurses—200+ nurses in development and customer service.

Leader in point-of-care, wireless technology using multiple device options.

Security of a Fortune 16 company with wide range of healthcare offerings, financial stability, ability to invest in R&D.

Vision of the future

Knowing the critical role that nursing plays in patient care and healthcare delivery, McKesson is committed to transforming the nurse's work environment through technology. Our goal is to continue developing technology solutions that eliminate inefficiencies, streamline work processes, and ensure patient safety, in order to support nursing in providing the safest, highest quality patient care. McKesson's strategy includes leveraging the success of proven Horizon Clinical products with unique new workflow capabilities, evidence-based knowledge, and tools to promote collaboration among all caregivers, to help support nurses in providing optimal care for every patient and their family.

Siemens Medical Solutions[g]

Philosophy for nursing

On the front lines of patient care, nurses are critical to quality and efficient healthcare. With a fierce nursing shortage,[h] mounting administrative burdens,[i] growing cost and quality pressures, Siemens is dedicated to improving care delivery and nursing practice, through nursing informatics, education, and research. To enhance the expertise of practicing nurses, Siemens develops tools that streamline workflow and allow nurses to concentrate on patients rather than documentation—helping healthcare facilities provide evidence-based care and attract and retain talented nurses. Integrating the knowledge of nursing into the global field of healthcare informatics ultimately assists populations in achieving optimum well-being.

(Continued)

Table 26.1   Vendors' Nursing Philosophy, Product Differentiation, and Vision for the Future (*Continued*)

Siemens Medical Solutions[g]

Key differentiators

Siemens provides information technology (IT) solutions that support nursing, enable high-quality evidence-based care and improve clinical and administrative workflow. Three fundamental differentiators for Siemens solutions are:

1. Innovative workflow-based solutions that support nurses in the management of information in an effective and meaningful way, improving collaboration among caregivers and standards of care

2. IT solutions that provide data content and knowledge to facilitate clinical decision-making, safety, and quality

3. Comprehensive IT that spans and integrates various clinical specialties, such as oncology, cardiology, diagnostic imaging, critical care, respiratory care, audiology, picture archiving and communication systems (PACS) and telecommunications.

Vision of the future

Technology advances quickly in today's world, and nursing informatics is no different. The vision for the future centers on using IT to create new knowledge, which will transform the standard of care. Today, HCOs can monitor performance by collecting metrics as a byproduct of IT. Tomorrow, systems will mine data for trends and patterns in order to create new knowledge about how to treat future cases. From a totally digital bedside to wireless patient monitoring to Web-enabled enterprisewide networking, Siemens is committed to driving a new paradigm in the role and quality of nursing for optimum healthcare delivery.

[a]Obtained from and published with permission of Cerner Corporation.
[b]Obtained from and published with permission of Department of Defense.
[c]Obtained from and published with permission of Veterans Health Administration.
[d]Obtained from and published with permission of Eclipsys Corporation.
[e]Obtained from and published with permission of IDX Systems Corporation.
[f]Obtained from and published with permission of McKesson Information Solutions.
[g]Obtained from and published with permission of Siemens Medical Solutions.
[h]According to the American Hospital Association, 89% of hospital chief executives report significant workforce shortages, with the job category most often reported being R.N. at 84%.
[i]Nearly 70% of nurses report the need to perform "non-nursing" functions, such as administrative tasks, as reported by ibid.

other sources, in many organizations 35–60% of hospital admissions originate in the emergency department (ED) and 20% of hospital net profits are yielded from the department (The Camden Group, 2003). This is a key motivator for acquiring ED IT capabilities that create efficiencies and enable cost savings. As a result, EDs, historically an IT "step child," are now more frequently acquiring ED departmental systems and being included in EHR selection processes where there is a desire to have a single integrated electronic record that spans the ED visit and entire inpatient stay.

Admission Assessments

Physicians perform history and physicals on patient admission. Similarly, nurses and allied health professionals perform initial patient assessments and intakes. EHR and niche nursing documentation systems have historically automated narrative notes by creating body systems-based forms, with items typically selected from lists of predefined data. Systems that simply replicate the paper record online with extensive free form, text-based charting offer little added value and no data analysis capability.

Many earlier generation electronic nursing assessments did not allow nursing data, e.g., height/weight and vital signs, to populate other caregiver records, resulting in significant duplicate data collection across disciplines. Well-designed applications offer more streamlined data entry via standard templates and checklists while eliminating unnecessary duplicate data entry among providers.

More advanced clinical systems support:

- Bringing forward select data from current and prior episodes of care in the EHR, for edit and reentry by the nurse (saving data entry time)

- Sharing of data among MD and the care team (avoiding duplicate requests for information and services)

- Automatic referrals based on entry of specific assessment data, e.g., height and weight triggers nutrition education dietary referral (improving quality of care)

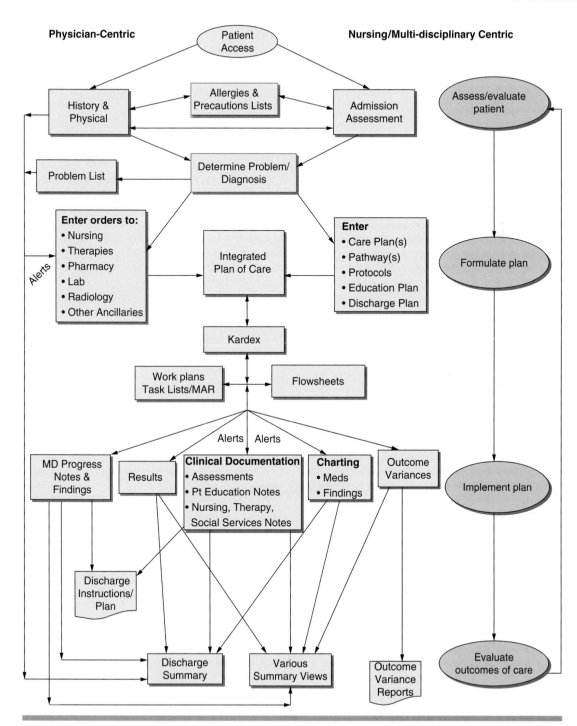

Figure 26.1
Care flow diagram.
(Copyright by Ann Farrell.)

■ Prompting of nurses for care plans and/or pathways based on initial diagnosis and nursing assessment data (promoting efficiencies and standard, evidence-based care)

■ Creation of separate allergies and precautions lists (promoting quality of care)

Diagnosis/Problem

The concept of a "nursing diagnosis" has been somewhat controversial since its inception. While the intent was to define nursing as a discrete discipline, there has been "push back" by those who maintain the record is patient-centric, with contributions from multiple physicians, nurses, and increasingly, allied health professionals.

A "problem list" is a common set of patient-specific problems that are maintained by the MD and care team. Any authorized care provider can add a problem to the problem list that is then tracked by the information system, with a status applied until the problem is resolved. While lead vendors can support the concept of nursing diagnoses and some HCOs embrace this concept, a current trend is for patients to have a single diagnosis and problem list based on the medical model, with inputs from diverse healthcare professionals.

Nursing and Multidisciplinary Orders and Plans of Care

Physicians can enter medical orders directly online (CPOE) or via authorized designees, e.g., RNs and clerks. In the manual system, physician orders are separate from orders of other care providers. Like physicians, nurses, and allied health professionals enter "orders," i.e., requests for services, individually and as part of order sets and plans of care. Nursing orders and care plans are typically entered into the system after an initial nursing assessment. In some systems, charting of specific data in the initial assessment prompts the nurse for associated plan(s) of care.

Nursing care plans are based on diagnoses, organization, and department standards of care and patient-specific nursing orders. The scope of nursing orders depends on national and state legal and regulatory requirements, professional practice standards and individual organization's policies.

Examples of nursing orders include activities of daily living (e.g., bed bath), treatments (e.g., wound care), and interventions (e.g., vital signs) that support established standards of care. Hospital protocols, e.g., blood administration policy can be integrated into nursing orders, e.g., blood administration procedures, and generated as auto-

matic byproducts of associated medical orders, e.g., administer 1 unit blood. In addition to treatment and procedure-related orders, multidisciplinary care plans should include education and discharge orders, which begin at the time of patient admission. Education and discharge planning are increasingly important aspects of care, given the increased acuity of hospital patients, decreased lengths of stay due in large part to reimbursement pressures and community-based multiprovider postdischarge care.

In early nursing applications, nurses built care plans "on the fly" by selecting appropriate interventions and expected outcomes from predefined checklists based on diagnoses and the individual patient's course of treatment. Even when automated, this process can be labor intensive and repetitive. Increasingly, hospitals are implementing clinical pathways for high-volume patients and those with more standardized care, e.g., cardiac, surgical, and orthopedic patients.

Clinical pathways, also known as care maps, are based on patient diagnosis. They provide a standard, evidence-based, time-driven plan of care, with predefined interventions to be performed and outcomes to be achieved in targeted time frames.

Clinical pathways are increasingly multidisciplinary so that care is coordinated within disciplines, e.g., nursing, and across the care team. With initiation of a multidisciplinary clinical pathway, the clinical system automatically generates, and where appropriate schedules all orders for all services to be provided to the patient.

Clearly, every patient cannot be managed using clinical pathways, e.g., patients with multiple or highly complex diagnoses. It was formerly believed that approximately 80% of patients can be managed with standard pathways tailored, as needed, to the individual patient and specific episode of care. Currently, due to the acuity level, severity of illness and co-morbidities of today's patient population, estimates for the percentage of patients that can be managed with clinical pathways is far lower than originally projected.

With the movement toward evidence-based medicine, care patterns incorporated in clinical pathways are analyzed over time for determination of the impact of prescribed interventions on clinical outcomes. In order to meet national best practice standards, pathways are typically based on research conducted by the government or in prestigious academic centers and specialty hospitals. Given scarce healthcare resources and focus on quality of care, treatment patterns and reimbursement are expected to be increasingly based on the proven effectiveness of specific interventions to achieve desired outcomes. Once clinical pathways are automated and utilized, they become the standard of care for the entire organization. Thus, as medical research rapidly progresses and new treatments are proven most effective, clinical pathways must be continually updated to reflect best practices.

Integrated Plans of Care

An integrated plan of care includes all orders for all services to be provided for a patient, including physician, nursing and multidisciplinary pathways, and orders and patient care plans. An integrated plan of care provides a single, patient-centric, rather than fragmented department-oriented, plan of care that can be accessed and used by the entire care team.

Kardex

A Kardex is a patient management tool used by nurses to collect, organize, and display summary patient information in one place. In a paper environment, the Kardex is a flip-file holding paper cards that contain patient data snapshots. Typically, a Kardex includes the patient name, medical record number, admission date, diagnosis, service, attending physician, primary nurse, patient age and date of birth, special needs/requests (e.g., prosthetics), allergies, medical alerts, and all currently active orders.

In an automated environment, the Kardex is more than just an online view of summary patient data. An electronic Kardex automatically gathers appropriate data already in the system via previously entered orders, plans of care, and clinical documentation. The Kardex can ideally be tailored to the needs and preferences of the individual organization, department, and work center. In advanced nursing systems, direct entry of data into the Kardex will update associated parts of the electronic record; conversely, charting updates automatically populate the Kardex. A Kardex is not a legal document and therefore it is not saved in the permanent patient record.

Workplans—Tasklists

EHRs support generation of work plans, known as task lists, as an automatic byproduct of orders and plans of care. These task lists help nurses organize, document, and manage patient care activities for individual or groups of assigned patients. Nurses can access task lists for an entire shift, or request them from the system as needed for a particular period of time. Completion of an activity or set of activities can be charted directly on the task list. Task lists can be generated for individual patients or groups of patients.

Two types of activities are presented on task lists, i.e., treatments/interventions and medications. Some organiza-

tions integrate these activities into a single, chronologic list of assigned medication and nonmedication related tasks. Most organizations prefer a task list for treatments and interventions and a separate medication task list, known as an electronic medication administration record (eMAR).

The eMAR contains all medication orders including one time, scheduled, unscheduled, and prn medications, IV additives, topical solutions, and any other pharmaceutical or homeopathic therapy. As soon as a medication order is entered, it automatically appears on the eMAR. The eMAR is accessible by authorized physicians, nurses, therapists, and pharmacists and offers clinicians a picture of the entire medication history, typically with 7-day views of data.

Nurses chart medications on the eMAR as "given" or "not given" and adjust schedules to accommodate held or missed doses. If a medication is not charted within a predefined time frame, the system can alert the nurse electronically on the information system via visual cues on the eMAR and, if desired, audible alerts via a pager or PDA.

Charting of medications on the eMAR can prompt the nurse for specific charting actions, e.g., pain assessment 30 minutes after administration of prn pain medication per Joint Commission of Healthcare Organization (JCAHO) requirements. Charting of a medication as given can automatically send a charge to the billing system and decrement the pharmacy inventory system or medication dispensing cabinet.

Current patient safety initiatives have prompted the adoption of bar coding technology to support medication administration. With bar code labels placed on patient armbands and medications, nurses can better support for the "five rights" of mediation administration, i.e., the right patient, drug, dose, route, and schedule.

BCMA requires charting at the point of care, via bedside terminals or wireless devices. Medication management is one of the most important aspects of an EMR given its role in patient care and patient safety. One of the most daunting challenges for HCIT vendors has been designing an electronic medication record that fully supports timely and accurate medication administration and enables efficient workflow and data interchanges among physicians, RNs, and pharmacists.

Results

Laboratory, imaging, and other ancillary department tests ordered by physicians, once completed, have results filed in the EHR database that are accessible to all authorized care providers. Lab values, radiology reports and, in some cases, x-ray images from picture archiving systems (PACS) can be retrieved, as needed, during the care process.

In more advanced systems, key lab result values are displayed automatically during the ordering process, e.g., a digitalis order automatically displays the last potassium level.

Most systems prompt users for orders of complementary tests or procedures where medically recommended, e.g., an order for Coumadin prompts for a partial thromboplastin time (PTT) and/or protime order, and display most recent lab values that impact medication dosage and treatment protocols.

In an EHR, results data can be viewed over time in tabular formats and graphed for display of trends. In most systems, multiple data types, including nursing interventions, can be displayed on the same graph, e.g., digitalis administration and potassium values.

Clinical Documentation

Physicians and all care providers document care in progress notes and ongoing assessments. In electronic systems, in addition to charting on the eMAR and task list, nurses document assessments in a number of online formats, including template-based notes, checklists, and flowsheets. Narrative notes are minimized in automated systems since they are difficult to read and data cannot be extracted for later analysis.

Clinical documentation is the major method by which diverse care providers collaborate across multiple points of service. When attempts are made to implement newer documentation models that promote efficiencies, e.g., charting by exception, some nurses resist, claiming these approaches "depersonalize" care and mask the "patient story." Nurse executives are discovering in early adopter sites that standardized charting will be more readily adopted by RNs if care can be personalized via patient-specific observations and comments. With education and system use, nurses see the value in efficient, structured data collection as long as documentation can be tailored to the individual patient and extracted information is shown to support quality of care and process improvements.

Given the enormous amount of time nurses spend in documenting care, 50% or more in some organizations, speed and efficiency of data entry is the top priority for clinical documentation across nursing constituents. However, while a primary goal is limiting the amount of charting time, patient care documentation must be legally defensible, regulatory-compliant, and clinically sound.

In the past, even when nursing care was automated, allied health departments often were either paper-based or had different departmental systems. Use of these disparate methods and systems often resulted in fragmented care and poor communications among the care team.

A confluence of factors is driving current heightened interest in standardized nursing and multiinterdisciplinary care and documentation including:

- A new organization model with a single clinical executive overseeing all clinical service providers (typically an RN)
- Increased recognition of potential value of improved clinical documentation and more collaborative team-oriented care delivery
- Patient demographics (e.g., aging population), the increased role of allied health professionals, and a growing focus on chronic disease management
- More IT savvy nurse and allied health clinical service directors
- Resource shortages, acute in nursing and allied health, and the need to recoup RN indirect care time
- Second and third generation IT systems—maturing technologies and applications

With an increasing number of critical care beds and monitored patients throughout the hospital, integration of monitored data in the patient record is increasingly important to HCOs. The effort to reenter electronic data collected by patient monitoring devices (e.g., cardiac monitors, ventilators, and IV pumps) into a departmental or EHR system is error prone, labor-intensive, and nonproductive. In more sophisticated systems, these data are integrated with the clinical system. Where an interface between the monitor and information system exists, data values from the monitoring device are displayed and verified by the nurse prior to entry into the EMR.

Discharge Summaries

The discharge summary is an increasingly important component of care with inpatient stays shortening and postdischarge care often provided by diverse providers in multiple venues of care across the community. Discharge summaries, now being addressed in the continuum of care record (CCR) initiative, support continuity of care goals by providing key patient data needed for transfer of care to the family and other facilities and providers in the community, e.g., the patient's primary care physician.

In addition to listing key patient demographic and clinical data, e.g., discharge diagnosis, key lab values, and current medication list, the discharge summary is accompanied by patient instructions and follow-up information and education forms. In an integrated EHR, discharge summary data are collected and updated throughout the patient stay and available for final review and completion prior to patient discharge or transfer to another facility or home.

Summary Reports

With the amount and density of patient data, key information is often difficult to extract and synthesize. Clinical systems offer a variety of "data snapshots" that provide customized views that facilitate rapid and timely evaluation of key relevant patient information. Patient summary reports are targeted for specific use and often designed to meet the needs and preferences of a medical specialty, e.g., cardiology or individual caregiver. Patient summaries can support rounding, initial patient assessment by consulting physicians, end of shift reporting by nurses, and other patient-care-related activities.

Outcomes Variance Reports

Virtually all HCOs are focused on improving patient safety and quality of care. For organizations to thrive, clinicians must be committed to continual performance improvement. In electronic systems, as a byproduct of patient care documentation, data are collected that continually measure key clinical processes and patient outcomes. For example, the interval of time between when a medication is ordered and administered is an important process measure for most HCOs. With the availability of this information, the organization and providers gain key insights regarding the timeliness of crucial therapeutic (e.g., antibiotics) and palliative (e.g., pain meds) interventions that impact quality of care and length of stay. Data analysis can pinpoint "lags" in process substeps, e.g., time from medication order to dispensing from pharmacy, that support root cause analysis of problems and targeting of process improvement efforts.

As standards of care and clinical pathways are more rapidly adopted, more rigorous analysis of care patterns can occur. Physicians are increasingly being asked to adopt clinical pathways, with the requirement to document the rationale for deviation from the standard in the information system. Unexplained variances are tracked by the system and available for management reporting. These variance reports can be used to identify practice "outliers," compare performance across providers, and

when appropriate, update the pathway to reflect more effective practices. High performing hospitals increasingly benchmark their outcomes by continually comparing their current performance to past performance, peers, best practices in industry, and (for nonclinical services) across industries, e.g., food service.

 ## Standard Terminology Provided with Clinical Applications

Expectation of the Marketplace

Despite the lack of a national consensus regarding one standard nursing terminology or data set, HCOs expect their EHR vendor to deliver a standards-based set of nursing content for charting and planning care. Implementation of an EHR system usually is a lengthy project; but the cost, time, and effort required can be decreased if a set of valid terminology is included with the software and customers can merely modify this set where necessary to meet their specific requirements. Without a "starter set" of standard terminology, the nursing and information systems departments must devote significant time and resources to selecting a nomenclature and configuring it "from scratch" into the tables and dictionaries of their EHR system.

Now that the federal government has recognized SNOMED (Systematized Nomenclature of Medicine) as the standard reference terminology, the expectation of HCOs has risen—they want the starter set of terminology provided with the EHR software to be one that "maps to" SNOMED. SNOMED facilitates sharing and aggregating healthcare information within and among HCOs. Facilities using terminologies that map to SNOMED are able to take advantage of these capabilities and ultimately participate in national and potentially international healthcare initiatives.

As most HCOs have adopted a multidisciplinary or even interdisciplinary approach to delivery of care, their expectation for predefined content extends beyond meeting the needs of nursing. Content to support clinical documentation for therapists, social services, and other members of the care team is being requested.

Current Status

Responding to this market demand, most of the major HCIT vendors now deliver at least a basic starter set of terminology. An increasing number of these vendors are including standards-based terminology with their clinical

Table 26.2   Clinical Terminology Sets and Related Applications Provided by Major HCIT Vendors

Cerner Corporation[a]

Data set

Cerner structures, deploys, and maintains clinical content as *Cerner Executable Knowledge* within *Cerner Millennium*. Cerner Knowledge Sources for nursing content include:

- H. Lee Moffitt—National Cancer Institute and Research Center—source of evidence-based content and standards for *Cerner Executable Knowledge* to support all stages of the care process for oncology, from screening to diagnosis and treatment
- The University of Iowa—*Cerner Executable Knowledge* automates University of Iowa nursing care standards such as gerontology, pain, wound healing, and informatics.
- The University of Wisconsin, Milwaukee—Cerner is codeveloping empirical and evidence-based nursing practices and protocols with the University of Wisconsin, Milwaukee focusing on care for clinical conditions in ambulatory and community health.

Clinical documentation application

Automated documentation practices—Includes embedded clinical "best practices knowledge" and "smart defaults"; from data gathered with the admission assessment, Discern Expert rules engine triggers alerts for nutrition consults, social service consults, restraint use, and aggressive nursing prevention of conditions, such as pressure ulcers and falls.

Plan of care application

CareNet *Power Plan*—Pathways system for automating

- Care plans, pathways, oncology protocols
- Nursing problems for most common components in medical, surgical, and critical care
- Patient safety measures (falls prevention, Foley catheter management, deep vein thrombosis prevention, venous/arterial catheter management, wound management, Warfarin management)

Power Plan integrates all functionality, including problem name based on standard SNOMED CT, for all disciplines, interventions, outcomes, and variance documentation from a single view to all care team members. Enables evidence-based protocols for all disciplines that cross the care continuum including the unique demands of oncology.

Department of Defense[b]

Data set

No one standard data set currently is used across all military treatment facilities with healthcare information applications. Based on mandated requirements for implementation of clinical applications, each facility has developed their own data sets.

Clinical documentation application

Nursing professionals working in military treatment facilities, use two DoD enterprise healthcare information applications to document care rendered to DoD beneficiaries:

- Composite Health Care System I and II (CHCS I and CHCS II)
- CliniComp's clinical information system (CIS)

Clinical documentation features of the healthcare information applications used in DoD facilities worldwide support history and physicals, nursing assessments, provider notes, nursing notes, and so forth.

The CHCS I/CHCS II is the DoD's enterprisewide medical and dental clinical information system that generates and maintains a comprehensive, lifelong, computerized patient record of all preventive care, and illness/injury treatment rendered to each authorized beneficiary. This application supports the commitment of the DoD to conduct population health management throughout the military health system (MHS).

The CIS is the application used for acute care, enabling care providers to have real-time access to complete inpatient documentation. The CIS integrates information from all care areas (including the CHCS I/CHCS II, departmental systems, ambulatory facilities, patient monitoring equipment, and nursing documentation) into a central repository for quick and easy access and analysis.

Table 26.2   Clinical Terminology Sets and Related Applications Provided by Major HCIT Vendors (*Continued*)

Department of Defense[b]

Plan of care application

Nursing professionals working in military treatment facilities, use two DoD enterprise healthcare information applications to generate and review the plan of care for DoD beneficiaries:

- Composite Health Care System I and II (CHCS I and CHCS II)
- CliniComp's clinical information system (CIS)

These applications support:

General order entry and retrieval	Specialty referrals
Pharmacy record and orders	Laboratory and radiology orders and results retrieval (narrative and images)

Veterans Health Administration[c]

Data set

A VA national task force currently is developing an enterprise reference terminology, which is anticipated to help with standardization of data between sites. A "clinical reminder" module uses national clinical guidelines for health maintenance schedules; reminders currently used by nurses include tobacco screening, seat belt education, weight and diet education, influenza immunization, pneumococcal immunization, and pain assessment. ICD-9 and CPT codes are used for diagnosis and treatment documentation. The Nursing Plan of Care module is site-configurable.

Clinical documentation application

Computerized Patient Record System (CPRS) is used throughout the VA for clinical documentation. CPRS is a fully integrated system that includes modules for vital signs/patient measurements, problem list, clinical reminders, encounter data, BCMA, and progress notes.

- **Progress Note module**—Supports documentation via free text or templates with embedded text. Templates can be created by informatics personnel for shared use or by each clinician and saved in a folder for personal use. Clinicians can copy and paste data (e.g., latest blood pressure, patient's age, latest blood glucose) from other documents in the medical record into their notes using "objects." Objects are hard-coded and are made available in a shared folder.

- **"Clinical Reminder" module**—Provides timely alerts for clinicians regarding health maintenance schedules for their patients and supports documentation of preventative measures based on national clinical guidelines. Documented encounter data include diagnosis, examinations, skin tests, health factors, immunizations, and patient education. Documentation of a clinical reminder note automatically populates the encounter information.

- **Commercial–Off-The-Shelf (COTS) application**—Used in critical care areas at several VA medical facilities, COTS provide various means of documenting patient care. One application currently has a progress note interface to the CPRS Progress Note module.

Plan-of-care application

Nursing Package, VISTA (Veterans Health Information Systems and Technology Architecture)—The VISTA plan-of-care module used by VA nurses is self-developed software that is site-configurable. This application is delivered with standard care plans that can be configured to meet the needs of each medical center at the care unit or specialty level. Care plans can be individualized for each patient. Interventions, goals, and outcomes can be updated online and an audit trail tracks these changes. All care plans entered for a patient are stored in the database and are available for future reference on subsequent admissions. Based on site-specific policy, these stored care plans can be copied forward and updated to meet the patient's needs for the current visit, or the nurse can enter a new care plan for each admission.

Eclipsys Corporation[d]

Data set

Eclipsys and the Clinical Practice Model Resource Center (CPMRC), an organization recently merged into Eclipsys, are working to deliver best practice guidelines. More than 180 clinical practice guidelines have been incorporated into Eclipsys' advanced clinical software solutions, which meets the professional standards of the Joint Commission on Accreditation of Healthcare Organizations (JCAHO) and the Magnet recommendations.

(*Continued*)

Table 26.2   Clinical Terminology Sets and Related Applications Provided by Major HCIT Vendors (*Continued*)

Eclipsys Corporation[d]

Eclipsys also has aligned with Wolters Kluwer Health, a multinational health information company, to expand the clinical content embedded within Eclipsys' solutions. Eclipsys has formed a strategic alliance with Clinician Support Technology, Inc., a provider of Internet-based technology, to provide HCOs, their patients, and families with specialty-specific content and communication in the areas of pediatrics and oncology.

Clinical documentation application

Sunrise Advanced Clinical Solutions Knowledge-Based Charting (KBC)—Eclipsys' advanced clinical solutions save nurses time and increase the quality of care by treating documentation as an *intervention* rather than a *task*. These documentation tools provide a complete patient story and address patient and staff safety by enabling both accurate and timely documentation. To meet the many regulatory requirements for patient charts, the advanced clinical solutions proactively provide clinicians with preconfigured, evidence-based content and tools to help prevent incomplete, inaccurate documentation, which also speeds and maximizes reimbursement.

Plan-of-care application

Sunrise Advanced Clinical Solutions Knowledge-Based Charting (KBC)—KBC includes over 180 clinical practice guides that contain evidence-based, diagnosis-specific knowledge, and reflect interdisciplinary scopes of practice. Patient data documented in KBC populates the patient record and is integrated into a specific plan of care. Redundant entry of information is eliminated and all clinicians have access to an accurate, individualized view of the patient they are treating. Information captured within the system as part of the care process becomes a blueprint from which individualized care can be designed. The system serves as a central communication tool that brings accurate information to each member of the interdisciplinary team real-time, helping him or her prepare and integrate their services.

IDX Systems Corporation[e]

Data set

Carecast is designed to support comprehensive clinical documentation, with expert rules capabilities that can be used to support nursing protocols, and with a focus on the needs of the interdisciplinary care team. IDX is refining use of standard nursing terminology for *Carecast*, including NANDA (North American Nursing Diagnosis Association), NIC (Nursing Intervention Classification), and NOC (Nursing Outcome Classification).

Clinical documentation application

Carecast Care Documentation—Provides clinician access to patient information and simplifies documentation activities; supports efficient, user-friendly documentation that fosters interdisciplinary collaboration. Combined displays provide options for filtering by discipline and sorting by date/time. Features include:

- Flowsheet charting—"Flowsheet Views" automatically creates patient flowsheets and graphs "on the fly"; displays data in a trended format, supporting faster nursing analysis.

- Charting and worklists—support efficient documentation of care needed and given

- Patient summary—single screen view of key patient data, supporting clearer, faster exchange of information at shift report, and throughout the shift

Plan-of-care application

Interdisciplinary Critical Pathways (includes patient plan)—Critical pathways contain orders and associated goals specifically related to the patient's needs, supporting interdisciplinary collaboration. Orders and goals may occur sequentially over limited phases/dates/times. Interdisciplinary Critical Pathways focuses on improving the quality of care delivered while decreasing the costs of care by managing the delivery of services and noting variances to the goals of the pathway. A critical pathway may be cross-continuum with phases that focus on the ambulatory, inpatient, and subacute episodes of disease, procedure, or problem management. It may incorporate evidence-based best practice guidelines as outcomes that may serve as benchmarks.

Table 26.2 Clinical Terminology Sets and Related Applications Provided by Major HCIT Vendors (*Continued*)

McKesson Information Solutions[f]

Data set

McKesson provides nursing clinical content and documentation data sets to support multiple specialty areas and disciplines including med-surg; critical care; pediatrics; respiratory care, occupational and speech therapy; nutrition services; case management; pastoral care; inpatient rehabilitation; and various other specialty areas. McKesson also provides documentation data sets to meet JCAHO standards, such as pain assessment (with associated alerts), restraint documentation, fall risk assessment, nutrition assessment, patient education, and age-specific requirements.

McKesson provides the following standard nursing terminologies:

- NANDA—incorporated in the Clinical Profile module, utilized for the problem list.
- NIC and NOC—incorporated into the structure of the–Plan of Care standard content.
- Braden Scale—incorporated into the skin assessment.
- PNDS (Peri-operative Nursing Data Set)—incorporated into Horizon Surgical Manager, McKesson's perioperative software solution.

All of the above meet the NIDSEC (Nursing Information and Data Set Evaluation Center) standards recognized by the American Nurses Association. Pathways Care Manager, the initial version of McKesson's current nursing documentation solution, was the first product to be recognized by the ANA's NIDSEC.

Clinical documentation application

Horizon Clinicals—includes several products and modules; primary clinical documentation modules used by nursing:

- **Horizon Expert Documentation** (previous version named Horizon Clinical Documentation): An advanced care documentation and assessment solution featuring an intelligent clinical documentation model that adapts to individual patient characteristics (such as age and gender) before displaying charting components. Includes a graphical user interface that integrates clinical data entry and review into a single view, while addressing workflow needs of the multidisciplinary care team. Clinicians are presented with information to support critical thinking and enable better decision-making.
- **Horizon Admin-Rx:** A point-of-care BCMA solution that is integrated with Horizon Expert Documentation, automating MAR documentation as well as providing streamlined access to view and document related events such as pain assessments, vital signs, responses to medications.
- **Clinical Profile:** Automates collecting and reviewing patient health history information such as family medical history, use of tobacco, immunization history, previous surgeries, medical and nursing problems, food/drug/environmental allergens, and medication history. Data is input once and confirmed or modified during subsequent encounters throughout a patient's lifetime.
- **Horizon Surgical Manager:** Horizon Surgical Manager offers real-time perioperative charting, physiologic recording, and anesthesia documentation at the point of care.

Plan-of-care application

Horizon Expert Documentation, Horizon Expert Orders and Horizon Order Management—Integrated Horizon Clinicals solutions that provide plan-of-care capabilities supporting collaboration and shared care within the interdisciplinary team. Nursing orders and protocols help drive standards and compliance as well as documentation and outcome management.

Guidelines—a critical pathways module that provides traditional critical path functions including phases and variance tracking.

Siemens Medical Solutions[g]

Data set

Siemens model solutions provide a starter set of structured terminology that integrates comprehensive clinical content needed to support business/clinical processes and delivery of evidence-based care. The documentation solutions include starter sets targeting evidence-based practice, along with tools that allow for client-defined adaptation of the applications to support safety and quality standards. The code sets provided by Siemens will evolve in accordance with industry standards and healthcare delivery needs.

(*Continued*)

Table 26.2   Clinical Terminology Sets and Related Applications Provided by Major HCIT Vendors (*Continued*)

Siemens Medical Solutions[g]

Data set

Example of starter codes and data sets include:

Assessment starter set

Critical care observations from various point-of-care monitoring devices

Critical care scoring tools

Interdisciplinary treatment plans

CCC (Clinical Care Classification) system

SNOMED CT

Standardized nursing vocabularies to describe the nursing process, document nursing care, and facilitate aggregation of data for comparisons (including ANA-recognized terminologies)

DRGs/APC/ICD/HCPCS/CPT4 code sets

Allergy and problem codes model rules

Operational and analytical reports

Workflow Starter Sets covering areas such as infection control, stroke management, antibiotic management, and health management, and other operational processes that benefit from workflow technology

Materials and supplies

Access to and integration with reputable knowledge content sources to facilitate best practice decision-making at the point of care.

Clinical documentation application

Clinical documentation—Supports clinical and administrative workflow and delivery of evidence-based care; composed of three fundamental components:

1. Access to comprehensive clinical information to support nurses in the management of information in an effective and meaningful way, improving collaboration among caregivers and standards of care

2. Automated documentation that provides data content and actionable knowledge to facilitate clinical decision-making, safety, and quality

3. Integrated documentation for seamless support of various specialties' care delivery models across the continuum of care, such as acute medical-surgical, critical care, oncology, home care, diagnostic imaging, and respiratory care

Supports the entire clinical team in documentation of patient problems, assessments, interventions and outcomes, and for capturing vital signs, allergies, intake and output, and progress notes. Templates display dynamically based on specific patient conditions. Charting functions are configurable to meet needs of the facility, regulatory requirements, and scope of practice. Automatically generated alerts and prompts display recommended actions to help ensure clinical documentation meets practice standards. Clinical documentation is a component of an integrated, adaptable system that provides online alerts and user-focused features to support the flow of patient information and resources throughout the health continuum.

Plan-of-care application

Inter-Disciplinary Treatment Plans—Enables communication and collaboration amongst all members of the clinical team utilizing best practice plans of care including individualized problems, goals, and interventions. Treatment plans support all aspects of care encompassing guidelines of care, order sets, and time sequenced clinical pathways and protocols. Clinicians can document the patient's progress against the plan of care. Interdisciplinary treatment plans generate worklists and calculate the acuity for each patient in order to facilitate workload management. Data collected in pathways communicate a comprehensive view of a patient's condition to all members of the clinical team. Fully integrated with **computerized provider order entry so** the clinical team has comprehensive view of all interventions and orders for each patient.

[a]Obtained from and published with permission of Cerner Corporation.
[b]Obtained from and published with permission of Department of Defense.
[c]Obtained from and published with permission of Veterans Health Administration.
[d]Obtained from and published with permission of Eclipsys Corporation.
[e]Obtained from and published with permission of IDX Systems Corporation.
[f]Obtained from and published with permission of McKesson Information Solutions.
[g]Obtained from and published with permission of Siemens Medical Solutions.

documentation application as well as evidence-based standards of care with their care planning and clinical pathways applications, and some are using standard terminologies that map to SNOMED. A survey of the major vendors, as well as federal agencies that have developed their own HCIT software, provided information about their current status regarding the terminologies they deliver and the clinical applications in which they are deployed (Table 26.2).

Summary

This chapter presented key trends, issues, obstacles, and opportunities facing the nursing profession with regard to utilization of HCIT. The focus was on leading HCIT vendors that provide organizationwide, hospital-centric information systems, and address nursing applications in context of a patient-centric EMR. The response of these vendors to the demand by nursing for improved information systems was discussed. In addition, the demand for delivery of standards-based nursing or clinical data sets with the software application and how leading vendors are responding to this demand were presented. HCIT vendors are making progress, although many challenges and gaps still exist. The role of nursing in patient care is essential and the time is right for nurses to lead the way in exploiting IT to the benefit of healthcare professionals and patients.

References

Institute of Medicine Reports. (2004). *To Err is Human (1999) and Crossing the Chasm (2001).* 15th Annual HIMSS Leadership Survey.

Malkary, G. (2004). *Healthcare without Bounds: Mobile Computing in Nursing.* Spyglass Consulting, spyglassconsulting.com

The Camden Group. (2003). *Hospital Emergency Departments in Crisis: Aggressive Planning is Needed* (Vol. VII, No. 1).

Further Information

Weaver, C. (May 2004). Vice President & Chief Nursing Officer, Cerner Corporation.

Williams, D. (May 2004). AN Deputy Director, Information Management Chief, E-Health Requirements and Operational Architecture, Department of Defense.

Rick, C. (June 2004). Chief Nursing Officer, Department of Veterans Affairs.

Cato, J (May 2004). Chief Nursing Officer, Eclipsys Corporation.

Sweeney, C. (May 2004). Senior Marketing Communications Specialist, IDX Systems Corporation.

Meadows, G. (May 2004). Director, Product Marketing Nursing Solutions, McKesson Information Solutions.

Kennedy, R. (May 2004). Chief Nursing Informatics Officer, Siemens Medical Solutions.

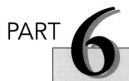

Administrative Applications

27

Administrative Applications of Information Technology for Nursing Managers

Roy L. Simpson
Charlotte Weaver

OBJECTIVES

1. Delineate nursing management's unique challenges, chances, and choices.
2. Provide an overview of implications and applications of information technology (IT) for nursing management.
3. Identify factors that determine system cost.
4. Discuss the need for nursing data standards.
5. Describe the benefits of administrative IT for nursing.
6. Delineate specific computer applications for nursing administration.
7. Examine the role of nursing management in system selection and implementation.

KEY WORDS

nursing administration
nursing management
nursing shortage
managing for patient safety
nurse manager's role in IT selection

 ## Nursing Management Today: Challenges, Chances, Choices

Ironically, the constituencies shaping healthcare—global leaders, healthcare CIOs and CEOs, vendors, and patients—are accidental jurists in the court of healthcare IT futures. They do not care about shaping tomorrow's healthcare; they just want their problems solved. But because they are such key players, their problems shape healthcare information technology solutions.

Nursing, which has traditionally steered clear of the process, must now trade in its IT blinders for binoculars, taking control of its own future by grappling with its present informational challenges. Three major issues have an administrative impact on the workplace, the profession, and the future of nursing managers and administrators. These issues are:

1. The nursing shortage
2. Increased demand for patient safety
3. The need for visibility

The Nursing Shortage

Within 10 years, 40% of working registered nurses (RNs) will be 50 years or older. As those RNs retire, the supply of working RNs will be 20% below requirements by the year 2020 (Buerhaus, Staiger, and Auerbach, 2000).

Three primary factors are contributing to the current shortage, including:

1. Steep population growth and an aging population, which are increasing the need for healthcare services: The U.S. population aged 65 and over is predicted to reach 82 million in 2050, a 137% increase over 1999. Between 2011 and 2030, the number of elderly could rise from 40.4 million (13% of the population) to 70.3 million (20% of the population) as "baby boomers" begin turning 65 (U.S. Census Bureau, 2000).

2. A diminishing pipeline of new students in nursing: Although enrollments in entry-level baccalaureate programs in nursing increased by 16.6% in 2003, this increase is not sufficient to meet the projected demand for nurses. Because the number of young RNs has decreased so dramatically over the past two decades, enrollments of young people in nursing programs would have to increase at least 40% annually to replace those expected to leave the workforce through retirement.

3. An aging nursing workforce: Forty percent of all RNs will be older than age 50 by the year 2010.

Unfortunately, there is no simple solution to the nursing shortage. Nursing must approach the problem from all angles, from finding ways to stem the tide of nurses leaving the profession, to attracting a new generation to it—all while not losing sight of patient care, safety, and satisfaction.

Increased Demand for Patient Safety

Patient safety is an international issue. In 2001, in Britain, there were more than 10,000 recorded medicine errors resulting in 1,100 deaths. The United States recorded 750,000 medical errors with a death rate of between 44,000 and 90,000. According to international statistics, one in every 300 errors will result in a serious, and possibly fatal, adverse effect.

Spurred into action by the impending nursing shortage and the rise in medical errors, the federal government, state legislatures, payer and provider groups, and accrediting organizations are authoring new policies and standards faster and more cooperatively than ever before. Consumers are now more discriminating and vocal about what they want, and health organizations are increasingly called on to be accountable for the results they achieve. We measure those results by outcomes.

In light of these startling numbers, managed care companies, the Joint Commission on Accreditation of Healthcare Organizations (JCAHO), and business coalitions like the Leapfrog Group increasingly require organizations to demonstrate their effectiveness and quality of patient care services. The pressure is not just external—outcomes measurement is a critical part of internal business requirements for both continuous quality and process improvement activities.

Standards focusing on the patient's well-being cut across all models of care, categories of disease and health conditions, and all types of providers. Simply stated, when healthcare organizations do the right things, they are most likely to have good outcomes, which translate into positives for patients, providers, and payers alike. But if quality is the goal, how do we get there?

Part of the challenge of measuring outcomes rests in defining exactly what an outcome is. Outcomes may be encounter-based or they may span the continuum of care. They could relate to an individual patient across several encounters or they might measure a system. Indeed, outcomes measurement can relate to any of the following areas:

1. Organizational performance
2. Clinical effectiveness
3. Patient satisfaction
4. Service quality
5. Appropriateness of care
6. Patient responses to treatments
7. Cost of services
8. Efficiency of services delivered (Simpson, 2003)

The Need for Visibility

In the world of "prove-it" healthcare, if it is not documented, it was not done. If nursing cannot establish its contribution to patient outcomes, nursing becomes invisible and in a fiscally tightened market, invisibility can mean expendability. Nursing must have a way to substantiate its role in the healthcare process and its vitality to outcomes.

Together, these three issues—the nursing shortage, the increased demand for patient safety, and the need for visibility—have created a wealth of opportunity for nursing in terms of IT. At the same time, they have created a challenge: When faced with limited time, personnel, and financial resources, should nursing pursue its mission to provide care or should it concentrate on mastering emerging technologies? The answer is both, given today's industrywide demands to increase the quality of care while decreasing its cost.

Nursing Management's Administrative Needs

In 2002, the American Healthcare Association (AHA) commissioned PricewaterhouseCoopers (PwC) to survey some of the American hospitals about their patient care and paperwork experiences (AHA, 2002). The results were disturbing:

1. In the emergency department, every hour of patient care requires 1 hour of paperwork.

2. For surgery and inpatient acute care, every hour of patient care requires 36 minutes of paperwork.

3. For skilled nursing care, every hour of patient care results in 30 minutes of paperwork.

4. For home healthcare, every hour of patient care results in 48 minutes of paperwork.

The rapid proliferation of nursing information systems compels nursing to face the vast challenge of learning and working within the age of technology. IT influences the manner in which nurses practice, how they are educated, and the methods of providing and documenting patient care (Rivers, Blake, and Lindgren, 2003). In addition, IT advances have become an integral link to staff development and continuing education, and nursing administrators now use informatics applications to assist with staffing, managing budgets, and disseminating information.

This chapter describes how computerized nursing systems—specifically administrative applications—can help nursing manage and use information to fulfill its unique data requirements, including:

- Clinical needs: Individual patient care, documentation, implementing services
- Business/strategic needs: Organizational performance, management, and support processes
- Quality management needs: Outcomes measurement and regulatory compliance
- Resource and personnel management needs: Scheduling, costing, and allocating nursing staff; managing productivity; continuing education/staff development

The chapter focuses on two levels of nursing administrators: nurse managers and nurse executives, which the American Nurses Credentialing Center defines as follows (ANCC, 2003):

1. *Nurse manager*: Nurses who hold an administrative position at the nurse manager level are responsible for:

- The proper allocation of available resources to provide efficient and effective nursing care.
- Providing input into executive-level decisions and collaborating with the nurse executive and others in organizational programming and committee work.
- Implementing the philosophy, goals, and standards of the healthcare organization
- Implementing clinical nursing services within their defined areas of responsibility.
- Planning, organizing, implementing, and controlling the care of individuals and aggregates across the spectrum of healthcare settings. This includes, but is not limited to, aspects of quality outcomes, staff development, care management, and research.

2. *Nurse executive*: The nurse executive is responsible for:

- Managing organized nursing services and the environment in which clinical nursing is practiced. Collaborating with other healthcare organization executives to make decisions about healthcare services and organizational priorities.
- Ensuring that standards of nursing practice are established and implemented, and are consistent with standards of professional organizations and regulatory agencies.
- Evaluating care delivery models and of services provided to individuals and aggregates.
- Fostering a climate for practice that enhances productivity, job satisfaction, and professional development.

Applications and Implications of Information Technology for Nursing Management

In the 1980s, nursing IT education—what little there was of it—taught the use of computers as tools for word processing, spreadsheet analysis, graphics production, and statistical applications (Klein, 2000). Today, however, rapidly changing technologies and dramatically expanding knowledge are influencing how nursing students acquire, apply, and evaluate new knowledge (Smalley, 2001). The American Association of College of Nursing's Nursing Education's Agenda for the 21st Century recognizes the importance of information skills, listing "information seeking, sorting, and selection" as third among nine essential cognitive curricula areas (AACN, 1999).

Definition of a Nursing Information System

In today's information age, nurses are expected to keep pace with rapidly advancing technology. Appropriate use of computers and information systems can help nurses make well-informed decisions regarding management and patient care issues (Klein, 2000).

Nurse managers and nurse executives must collect and analyze large amounts of data. This has become impossible to do effectively without automated clinical and administrative nursing information systems. But what is a nursing information system? For this chapter, we define nursing information system as:

> A software system that automates the nursing process from assessment to evaluation, including patient care documentation. It also includes a means to manage the data necessary for the delivery of patient care (e.g., patient classification, staffing, scheduling and costs).

To be effective, nursing information systems must be integrated into organizations' overall IT networks. For this reason, the nursing information system is typically a subsystem of the larger hospital information system. The nursing information system has both clinical and administrative functions that, ideally, are tightly integrated.

Ultimately, the data such systems provide help nursing administration fulfill its pivotal role to measure, monitor, and manage services by providing accurate answers to several key questions about nursing service:

1. **How often and when** are services provided?
2. What is the **cost** of services?
3. What **level of service** is required?
4. What **resources** are required to provide specific levels of service?
5. What is the **result** of services performed?

In addition to managing services, nursing administrators are also increasingly responsible for effective management of financial and patient care data to:

1. Demonstrate compliance with standards set by the JCAHO and other standard-setting organizations.
2. Document conformity to state and federal government regulations.
3. Manage credentialing.
4. Develop risk management programs to reduce organizational liabilities, identify legal risks, and minimize financial liability in legal matters.
5. Recruit and retain qualified staff.

6. Support the personnel, information, and technologic infrastructure necessary to further organizational goals.
7. Assure customer (patient) satisfaction.
8. Establish patterns of care, benchmarks, and outcomes necessary for evaluating past and forecasting future patient care quality.
9. Ensure effective and efficient use of facility, equipment, service, and financial resource utilization.
10. Determine case mix in terms of patient diagnosis, age, and other variables to optimize third-party payer reimbursement.
11. Assure follow-up care of chronic patients and assess efficiency of that care.
12. Satisfy data requirements of managed care contracts.
13. Demonstrate organizational efficiency, effectiveness, and performance to optimize competitive position.

Increasingly, nurse administrators must also focus on outcomes of care. While clinical systems collect the clinical data used to measure outcomes, administrative systems play a key role in interpreting that data.

 ## The "Real" Cost of Administrative Systems

To determine the true cost of automation, one must take three things into account:

1. Cost of the hardware and software: While hardware and software are often the only things considered when determining cost, they are, today, perhaps the least costly element given the constantly declining cost of technology. The administrative system that cost $4 million dollars in 1972 now costs less than $250,000. But today's $4 million system would be worth that much. The value of technology has caught up with its price.
2. Cost of education: A system is only effective if nurses use it and nurses cannot use a system unless they get the necessary training. Training costs can comprise everything from instruction fees to travel expenses and the cost for temporary staffing during training.
3. Intellectual resources: Nursing management should serve as advisors, directors, and influencers of the technology that nursing uses. In fact, in the selection

of patient care systems, the JCAHO now mandates nursing involvement and for good reason. This is the only way nursing can ensure that technology is applied to meeting nursing's information needs, advancing nursing practice, and realistically, ensuring nursing's continued viability (Simpson, 1999). Any system cost estimate should include the necessary resources for nursing management to be actively involved in system selection and evaluation.

To determine these costs, it is helpful to start with a model, either clinical or financial.

Healthcare organizations create, move, store, and retrieve billions of patient records every year. Although managed healthcare has increased healthcare's information requirements, advancing technology has increased the availability—and therefore the demand—that information be in electronic form. The only way for nursing management to effectively control this amount of information is through computerization.

Continued reliance on manual data collection is having and will continue to have serious implications, including:

- Increased administrative cost: National health expenditures are projected to total $2.2 trillion and reach 16.2% of gross domestic product (GDP) by 2008 (Health Care Financing Administration). Controlling administrative data and documenting practice to monitor quality and assess cost and value consumes as much as 20% of that total U.S. healthcare bill. This is at least twice and as much as 10 times what other countries—including those with national healthcare–expend.

- Compromised quality: At least 30% of the information required to make diagnosis and treatment decisions is unavailable at the time the decision needs to be made (Dick and Steen, 1991). Much of this information is nursing information. For example, inadequate documentation of medication administration has led to adverse drug events that add roughly $3 billion per year to hospital bills (Melmon, 1971).

The potential savings of automation are significant. Healthcare administrators can help reduce healthcare costs to a total of $36 billion per year through four applications of computers:

- Patient information management and transfer, $30 billion

- Electronic claims processing, $6 billion

- Electronic inventory management, $600 million

- Video conferencing for professional training, $200 million

Automation will allow nursing management—specifically—to reduce annual costs to hospitals by at least $12.7 billion. This will be accomplished by:

1. Reducing costs associated with adverse medical reactions.

2. Decreasing nursing clerical time.

3. Reducing costs associated with record maintenance.

4. Curtailing malpractice costs.

5. Hastening retrieval of valid and reliable information.

6. Easing aggregation of medical information for research.

7. Improving internal and external review of records (Little, 1992).

The Need for Nursing Data Standards

For some time, there have been standards motivating nursing to focus on effective and efficient administration. Established by the American Nurses Association (ANA) in 1988, these standards remain the prevailing measures by which professional nurses evaluate practice.

Several years after developing practice standards, ANA established the Nursing Information and Data Set Evaluation Center (NIDSEC) to create and disseminate standards for information systems. These standards were designed to ensure complete, accurate documentation of nursing practice and to serve as a guide by which to evaluate information systems. The ultimate goal of these standards is to expedite the evolution of large, accessible pools of patient data that reflect the true nature, cost, and effects of nursing practice.

The NIDSEC standards apply to four aspects of nursing data sets and the systems that contain them—nomenclature, clinical content, clinical data repository, and general system characteristics. Though most often applied in the selection of clinical systems, these standards could serve as an equally good model for evaluating administrative systems for nursing.

In addition, thanks to JCAHO initiatives that have shifted the orientation of healthcare information systems from monitoring processes to measuring outcomes, there is also a need for standards to facilitate:

- Combining data from different sources in new ways

- Linking clinical and administrative data

■ Evidence-based practice

■ Using external databases to monitor hospital performance (AONE and CHIM, 1993).

Specifically, the JCAHO's initiatives have created an additional need for standards to (Porter, 1994):

1. Support access to external comparison databases
2. Ensure data security and confidentiality
3. Promote the development of knowledge-based systems
4. Provide a link to physicians' information systems
5. Support continuous quality improvement projects
6. Ensure data integrity
7. Integrate with existing standards and procedures related to documentation requirements
8. Support needs assessments

Moreover, the lack of standards has become a key obstacle to the development of universal computer-based medical records, as recommended by the Institute of Medicine more than a decade ago.

There is a great deal of confusion in the standardization ranks, however. Making sense of it all starts with definitions of the foundational elements of a language—taxonomy and nomenclature:

1. Taxonomy is the classification of things into an ordered system based on natural relationships. In a larger sense, it comprises the science, laws, or principles of classification.
2. Nomenclature is a system of names; the names of the kinds and groups of things listed in a taxonomic classification. In healthcare, it is a system for naming things according to preestablished rules.

Confusion arises when "nomenclature" and "language" are used interchangeably with "taxonomy." Taxonomy is the process of deciding what constitutes a language and how it fits into a classification. Nomenclature, on the other hand, is a secondary process of deciding the correct name for procedures given a number of alternatives in the literature. If taxonomy is the "how," then nomenclature is the "what."

However, the practice of nursing does not lend itself easily to classification. How does one code caring? As a result, the ANA recognizes several different standardized nursing nomenclatures, each designed to address a specific area of nursing.

How Nursing Benefits from Information Technology

Nursing administrative systems fall into three basic categories of use:

1. Strategic
2. Operational
3. Tactical

In general, they help nursing:

1. Improve communication
2. Improve order entry
3. Improve continuity of care
4. Spend more time on patient care
5. Guide critical thinking
6. Tap into expert resources
7. Evaluate care

In addition, nurse administrators have identified several other specific benefits of using IT (AONE and CHIM, 1993) including:

1. Expanded use of nursing staff resources
2. Improved quality of patient care monitoring
3. Improved documentation
4. Improved communication
5. Improved planning
6. Increased standardization of nursing practice
7. Ability to define nursing practice and associated problems/issues
8. Ability to define methods to track patient care delivered, outcomes achieved, and revenue generated
9. Enhanced recruitment and retention
10. Improved evaluation of care provided
11. Support for the dynamic organization, capable of change.

While benefits come at the end of a successful system installation, the time to ensure their realization is at the beginning, during system implementation. As early as system selection and no later than initial planning, organizations should outline desired benefits, and then manage system implementation to those benefits via weekly updates, scorecards, and other evaluation/measurement methods.

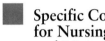

Specific Computer Applications for Nursing Administrators and Managers

Several administrative applications are available on computers for nurse administrators. Table 27.1 summarizes them.

Nurse Managers' Data Needs

In general, nursing managers use computer systems to collect data needed for planning, budgeting, and reporting, which ensure quality care. Their needs and the applications they use include:

1. Allocating available resources to provide efficient and effective nursing care and implementing clinical nursing services

Table 27.1 Computer Applications for Administrative Information Management

Applications for Nurse Managers	Applications for Nurse Executives
Nursing intensity	Forecasting and planning
Patient classification systems	Financial planning
Acuity systems	Hospital expansion
Staffing and scheduling systems	Preventive maintenance
Inventory	Planning systems
Budgeting and payroll	Quality assurance
Claims processing and reimbursement	Regulatory reporting
Patient billing	Consumer surveys
Unit activity reports	Evidence-based nursing
Utilization review	Personnel files
Shift summary reports	Risk pooling
Computer-based patient records (CPR)	Costing nursing care
Census	Case mix management
Poison control	
Allergy and drug reactions	
Error reports	
Incident reports	
Infection control	
Communication networks	
Training and education	

- Nursing intensity
- Patient classification systems
- Acuity systems
- Staffing and scheduling systems
- Inventory
- Budgeting and payroll
- Claims processing and reimbursement
- Patient billing

2. Providing input into executive-level decisions and collaborating with the nurse executive and others in organizational programming and committee work. Implementing the philosophy, goals, and standards of the healthcare organization.

- Unit activity reports
- Utilization review
- Shift summary reports

3. Planning, organizing, implementing, and controlling the care of individuals and aggregates across the spectrum of healthcare settings. This includes, but is not limited to, aspects of quality outcomes, staff development, care management, and research.

- Computer-based patient records (CPR)
- Census
- Poison control
- Allergy and drug reactions
- Error reports
- Incident reports
- Infection control
- Communication networks
- Training and education

Each of these applications has been described in the third edition (Simpson and McCormick, 2001). They remain essential as administrative applications but will not be described fully in this new edition. The reader is referred to the previous editions for classic descriptions of these applications.

Nurse Executives' Data Needs

Nurse executives' needs and the applications they use include:

1. Managing organized nursing services and the environment in which clinical nursing is practiced.

Collaborating with other healthcare organization executives to make decisions about healthcare services and organizational priorities.

- Forecasting and planning
- Financial planning
- Hospital expansion
- Preventive maintenance
- Planning systems

2. Ensuring that standards of nursing practice are established and implemented, and are consistent with standards of professional organizations and regulatory agencies. Fostering a climate for practice that enhances productivity, job satisfaction, and professional development.

- Quality assurance
- Regulatory reporting
- Consumer surveys
- Evidence-based practice

3. Evaluating care delivery models and of services provided to individuals and aggregates.

- Personnel files
- Risk pooling
- Costing nursing care
- Case mix

Each of these applications for nurse executives have been described in detail since 1986 and in the previous edition authored by Simpson and McCormick (2001).

Evidence-Based Nursing

An entire chapter is contained in this book that describes the methods toward achieving evidence-based nursing (EBN). In addition, several tools are described related to the computerization of evidence. From an administrative standpoint, the use of evidence in nursing will improve care and demonstrate effective and efficient care delivery. But what exactly is evidence-based practice or, more specifically, EBN? According to the University of Minnesota:

> Evidence Based Nursing is the process by which nurses make clinical decisions using the best available research evidence, their clinical expertise and patient preferences. Three areas of research competence are: interpreting and using research, evaluating practice and conducting research. (University of Minnesota, 2001)

In simple terms, EBN is caring grounded in investigation, intuition, and reaction (Simpson, 2004). Practice based on proof, professional experience, and response to patients. Nurses have always practiced based on the latter two—professional experience and response to patients. But the first one—proof-based practice—is only beginning to occur.

EBN improves care directly by putting actual knowledge—elements of practice that have been proven to work—in the hands of nurses. The globalization of healthcare, escalating healthcare costs, and the nursing shortage demand consistent practice based on effective, proven, and documented practice. Continuing challenges, such as the need to validate the importance of nursing, call for structured documentation of practice (Simpson, 2004).

What Nursing Administrators Need to Know about Selecting a System

By putting the patient at the center of the cost equation, managing care makes the *caregiver* a critical determinant of success. But caregivers can only be successful with the proper technological tools.

The key tasks of managed care—identifying best practices, coordinating caregiver team efforts, ensuring compliance with established clinical protocols and referral guidelines, and getting specialist feedback—are impossible without information systems support.

Increasingly, healthcare decision-makers understand this. CEOs view improved decision support for clinicians as one of the most pressing IT priorities. Other pressing IT needs for the integration of healthcare delivery systems include:

1. Networkwide information access
2. Networkwide master patient index
3. User-friendly system interfaces
4. Interface engines for system communications
5. Data repositories to facilitate data sharing
6. Specialized managed care software
7. Standards
8. Systems for data comparison
9. Software for longitudinal patient records
10. Standardization on "a limited number" of application vendors

Simply put, healthcare will not make the transition to a totally managed care environment without IT and

IT's influence will be seen primarily in three things:

1. *New-breed clinical information systems:* Managed care's need to monitor both the appropriateness and cost of care has led to a wave of new clinical applications. From workstation to bedside, these new systems integrate clinical and financial data, operate on the whole spectrum of hardware platforms using predominantly "open" operating systems, and put the patient at the center of the information gathering process. The result? Fusion of the best clinical practices into clinical care, and better documentation, which improves the quality of patient care by ensuring that the right information is collected and disseminated.

2. *Open systems:* Open architecture client/server systems are the only answer for true enterprisewide, integrated information transfer and access. A client/server-based system ensures access to critical information across both the enterprise and the continuum of care by integrating multiple care sites, multiple caregiver constituencies, and multiple episodes of care via local or wide area networks.

3. *Patient-centered care:* In the mid-1990s, the advent of managed care, followed closely by a drop in federal Medicaid reimbursements, set off an economic crisis that left one of every four hospitals in the red. So the hospitals followed the advice of healthcare consultants whose cost-cutting strategies invariably targeted hospitals' largest expense—nurse staffing—and set the foundation for the current and worsening nursing shortage. Thanks to such rampant, often injudicious cost cutting, clinicians are less able to separate the patient as person from the cost of his or her care. The result? Care delivery models based less on providing patient care than on getting paid for it. This scale is tipping back in favor of patients, however, thanks to the rise of consumerism and increasing concerns about patient safety, two areas in which IT can play a critical role.

Healthcare's increased focus on better quality, lower cost patient care means more organizations are turning to IT and clinical systems—and turning to nursing to help select them. Given this new responsibility, it is important for nursing to anticipate—and plan for—ongoing change and a difficult, time-consuming selection process. The normal time from deciding to purchase and installing is at least 2 years.

A key success factor in any implementation is the degree of administrative involvement. "C-level" (CEO, CFO, and CIO) buy-in and support ensures sufficient financing and, ultimately, successful implementation.

Nursing Administration's Role in IT Implementation

Times are tight and dollars are short in healthcare. With organizations questioning all expenditures, it is no surprise that they are increasingly asking "Why?" when it comes to nursing information systems. If nursing is to have the technology it needs, it better well have an answer to that question.

It is easy to understand how—with only a surface review—healthcare organizations might see nursing systems as possible candidates for cuts. Nursing's responsibility is to make sure that organizations understand the value of these systems and, despite what organizations may say about nursing systems, they can and do have value in the new healthcare equation. Indeed, although they require a significant initial outlay, they can often help an organization save money through gains in productivity, outcomes, and patient satisfaction.

Nursing systems can:

1. Maintain outcomes and demographic and health-related data to help organizations better manage what care they provide and to whom.

2. Eliminate routine manual documentation, optimizing human resources.

3. Improve accuracy and completeness to ensure timely reimbursement.

4. Support practice decisions aimed at providing higher quality care at a lower cost (Fitzgerald, 1996).

Advocacy for such systems does not occur at the bedside, however. Today, a nursing administrator's place is in the boardroom, or wherever the high-level systems decisions are made. If nursing is to have the systems it needs for continued viability, then nursing will have to make sure that organizations understand the contribution of nursing systems—and the work they support—to the bottom line. The survival and continued development of nursing informatics rests squarely on the shoulders of nursing.

The Future of Computerized Nursing Administrative Systems

Several critical trends—from globalization to the culture of change and the rise of the information age—will fuel development and deployment of future IT.

For nursing, technology is both a solution to short-term problems and the foundation of a long-term vision. In other words, technology is critical. Nursing can either embrace technology and bend it to the profession's purposes, or continue to wait in the wings, watching other industries and constituencies prosper and grow. Or, even worse, find itself replaced by the very technology it avoids in the name of patient care. Technology is the key to ensuring that nursing remains present and able to continue contributing to healthcare. Key emerging technologies include (Simpson, 2003):

1. Mobile technology (mHealth): As information and telecommunication infrastructures converge to create mobile health systems, and mobile technology improves in terms of availability, miniaturization, performance, and communication bandwidth, we can expect to see a host of cost-effective technologies that powerfully affect the way healthcare organizations deliver care.

2. Wireless local area networking and personal digital assistants (PDAs) are the foundation for mHealth. With wireless computing, caregivers access, update, and transmit critical patient and treatment information using radio signals. By providing and documenting care where they provide it, caregivers can eliminate the human error that happens in translation. In the next few years, we can expect to see rapid developments in the areas of wireless communications. This growth will rest on:

   ▧ Advances in Universal Mobile Telecommunications Service (UMTS), a third-generation (3G) broadband, packet-based transmission of text, digitized voice, video, and multimedia, that transmits at data rates up to 2 megabits per second (Mbps).

   ▧ Pervasive computing, which uses machines that are not personal computers, but very tiny (even invisible) apparatuses, either mobile or embedded in almost any type of object imaginable, including medical devices—all communicating through increasingly interconnected networks.

3. Picture archiving and communication systems (PACS) are a computerized way to replace conventional radiologic film. Users can acquire, store, transmit, and display images digitally, creating a "film-less" clinical environment. Although hundreds of PACS installations exist worldwide, most are small, linking, for example, the intensive care unit with the radiology department or networking a few workstations.

4. Single sign-on (SSO) is a session/user authentication process that allows a user to enter one name and password to access multiple applications. The SSO is requested at the session initiation and authenticates the user to access all the applications they have rights to on the server, eliminating future authentication prompts when the user switches applications during that particular session.

5. Thin-client computing uses low-cost, centrally managed computers with no CD-ROM players, disk drives, or expansion slots. These devices use a central system to store data, providing high levels of availability, reliability, and security.

6. Computerized provider order entry (CPOE) systems are designed to catch and prevent potential errors at the earliest possible point in the treatment process. With CPOE, the provider enters the order into a computer, then the system checks the order for incorrect dosages and/or drugs, drug-allergy interactions, drug-drug interactions, drug-food interactions, and other possible causes of error. The system monitors the treatment process to ensure that nurses administer the right drug to the right patient at the right time, issuing an alert if the patient's condition changes. For nursing, such technology removes the guesswork from medication administration, reducing stress levels, improving clinical effectiveness and productivity, and allowing nurses to focus on patient care rather than paperwork.

7. Virtual reality uses computers and multimedia peripherals to produce a simulated clinical setting of the future, better preparing today's students for everything from remote-controlled robotic surgery and nanotechnology, to voice-activation documentation and telehealth kiosks.

8. Electronic healthcare records (EHRs) are a critical way for nursing to document its contribution to healthcare.

For a summary of the implications of these emerging technologies, see Table 27.2 (Simpson, 2003).

▧ Summary

This chapter presented an update and the expanded responsibilities of today's nurse administrator. Because of increased pressures, this chapter also described the expanded systems that serve as tools for nursing services administration and nursing unit management. Because nursing administration has more obligations, there has been an increase in the number and depth of computer applications that facilitate efficient capture of financial data. Today's nurse administrator has moved into the role

Table 27.2   Emerging Technologies for Nursing

The Tech Trend	Requirements	Uses/Implications
■ Computerized physician order entry (CPOE)	■ ▭ Point-of-care devices ■ ▤ Speech recognition software ■ ▤ Relational databases ■ ▤ Clinical data repositories	■ ▭ Reduction in medical errors ■ ▤ Improved patient care ■ ▤ Streamlined documentation
■ Mobile technology (mHealth)	■ ▭ PDAs ■ ▤ WLANs ■ ▤ Tablet PCs ■ ▤ Smart phones	■ ▭ Notification/messaging ■ ▤ Internet access ■ ▤ Clinical decision support ■ ▤ Telemetry/patient care ■ ▤ Asset management ■ ▤ Information system access
■ Picture archiving and communication systems (PACS)	■ ▤ Workflow management systems ■ ▤ Middleware ■ ▤ High-resolution workstations ■ ▭▭ Flat panel displays ■ ▭▭ Physical imaging devices ■ ▭▤ High-speed networks ■ ▭▤ High volume archives	■ ▭▤ Streamlined intra and interdepartmental workflow ■ ▭▤ Instant access to patient data ■ ▭▤ Accelerated patient care
■ Single sign-on (SSO)	■ ▤ Smart cards ■ ▤ Biometrics	■ ▤ Security ■ ▤ Expanded access
■ Thin-client computing	■ ▭▤ Terminals ■ ▭▤ Cell phones ■ ▭▤ PDAs	■ ▤▭ Reduced support staff costs ■ ▤▭ Rapid and uniform deployment of applications ■ ▤▤ Improved access ■ ▤▤ Enhanced security

Source: Simpson, R.L. (2003). Today's challenges shape tomorrow's technology, part 2. *Nursing Management* 34(12):40–44.

of corporate executive officer with obligations to report to the institution, to society, and to national accrediting bodies. These responsibilities are also imposed by the professional practice of nursing. Today's nurse administrator needs more than a basic understanding of word processing and e-mail systems. Today's nurse administrator has a moral obligation to help improve healthcare costs by better managing nursing information.

■ References

American Association of Colleges of Nursing (AACN). (1999). *Position Statement: Nursing Education's Agenda for the 21st Century*. Online at *http://www.aacn.nche.edu/ Publications/positions/nrsgedag.htm*

American Association of Nurse Executives (The AONE) in Cooperation with the Center for Healthcare Information Management (CHIM). (1993). *Informatics: Issues and Strategies for the 21st Century Health Care Executive. Resource Book and Video Set*. Chicago, IL: American Hospital Association Services.

American Hospital Association. (2002). *Patients or Paperwork: The Regulatory Burden Facing America's Hospitals*. Online at *http://www.aha.org/aha/advocacy-grassroots/advocacy/advocacy/content/ FinalPaperworkReport.pdf*

ANCC, American Nurses Credentialing Center. (2003). Online at *http://www.nursingworld.org/ancc/certification/ cert/certs/admin.html*

Buerhaus, P. I., Staiger, D. O., and Auerbach, D. I. (2000). Implications of an aging registered nurse workforce.

Journal of the American Medical Association 283(22): 2948–2954.

Dick, R. S. and Steen, E. B. (Eds.) (1991). *The Computer-Based Patient Record: An Essential Technology for Health Care*. Washington, DC: National Academy Press.

Fitzgerald, J. M. *Application of computers in nursing: A position analysis*. The Nursing Resource Home page. *http://www.nursingnet.com/journal/Position.html*

Klein, J. A. (2000). *Nursing Informatics Education: Past, Present and Future*. Online at *http://nursingnetwork. com/education.htm*.

Little, A. D. (1992). *Telecommunication: Can it Help Solve America's Health Care Problems?* (Ref. No. 91810-98).

Melmon, K. (1971). Preventable drug reaction—causes and cure. *New England Journal of Medicine* 284(24): 1, 361.

Porter, S. (1994). Complying with JCAHO's IM Standards. *Healthcare Informatics* 11(7):62, 64, 66.

Rivers, F. H., Blake, C. R., and Lindgren, K. S. (2003). Information technology: Advancements in healthcare. *Online Journal of Nursing Informatics (OJNI)* 7(3). Online at *http://eaa-knowledge.com/ojni/ni/7_3/riversinfotech.htm*.

Simpson, R. L. (1999). Toward a new millennium: Outlook and obligations for 21st century healthcare technology. *Nursing Administration Quarterly* 24(1):94–97.

Simpson, R. L. (2003). Today's challenges shape tomorrow's technology, part 2. *Nursing Management* 34(12):40–44.

Simpson, R. L. (2004). Evidence-based nursing: Practice certainty for the uncertain world of healthcare. Presentation at the 10th Annual Japan Society of Nursing Diagnosis. Osaka, Japan.

Simpson, R. L. and McCormick, K. A. (2001). Administrative applications of information technology for nursing managers. In V. K. Saba and K. A. McCormick (Eds.), *Essentials of Computers for Nurses: Informatics for the New Millennium*. New York: McGraw-Hill.

Smalley, T. (2001). *Investigating Information Age Realities in the World of Work: Nursing informatics*. Online at *http://www.cabrillo.edu/~tsmalley/NrsgInformatics.html*

University of Minnesota's Evidence-Based Nursing Page. (2001). Available online at *http://evidence.ahc.umn.edu/ebn.htm#what%20is%20EBN*

U.S. Census Bureau. (2000). *U.S. Census Bureau News Release, Census Bureau Projects Doubling of Nation's Population by 2100*. Available online at *http://www.census.gov/Press-Release/www/2000/cb00-05.html*

28

Translation of Evidence into Nursing Practice: Evidence, Clinical Practice Guidelines, and Automated Implementation Tools

Kathleen A. McCormick

OBJECTIVES

1. Define clinical evidence and how it is used.
2. Define how evidence is translated into tools for clinical practice.
3. Discuss how guidelines are used and promote effective and efficient care.
4. Describe how to evaluate the quality of a guideline.
5. Discuss how specific implementation tools can be selected.
6. Identify two nursing roles relevant to guideline implementation.

KEY WORDS

evidence
clinical practice guidelines
implementation tools
computerized guidelines
performance measurement

Much of this chapter is based on the classic description of guidelines and computer implementation by McQueen and McCormick in 2001. However, this revised chapter contains a new major section which discusses scientific evidence and the development of clinical evidence-based guideline tools. The second section updates information on computerized tools to support guideline implementation. The first part provides fundamental information about evidence and evidence-based clinical tools. Guideline development methods, evaluation, and limitations are discussed. The second part deals with issues relevant to assessing the quality of evidence-based tools and implementation of tools to improve nursing practice.

Fundamentals of Clinical Practice

The current pace of change with healthcare knowledge and technology continues to accelerate. Computers and decision support systems provide tools for healthcare providers to manage this exponential increase in information so that the most effective treatment decisions can be made that will result in the optimal outcomes for the patient.

At the start of a new millennium, quality and cost issues drive the direction of change in healthcare. As policy makers, providers, researchers, and consumers simultaneously demand both high quality care and controlled health-related spending, population-based approaches to health promotion and disease management, such as evidence-based health, focus on twin goals: efficiency and effectiveness. Both are linchpins of quality. But tools are needed to make evidence-based health a reality. Computers can potentially house the most powerful tools available. As computers facilitate the organization of meaningful information about patients, providers, and organizations, the availability of this information makes it far easier to focus on efficiency and effectiveness.

We are heading toward diffuse information networks and infrastructures (Shortell et al., 1996). With these systems in place, providers will have the support needed for seamless translation of evidence into quality patient care and ongoing systemwide changes. Output will come from diverse, integrated quality tools (such as computerized guidelines with automated reminders) accessible within integrated clinical workstations. Once quality tools are automated and timely information is readily available across disciplines, continuous quality improvement (CQI), utilization management, and patient-centered care will be systematized (Institute of Medicine, 1992) and the delivery of effective and efficient care will be transparent. It will be built into what we do every day.

Information systems can provide the ability to access the needed information at the appropriate time and place. But the ability of these tools to improve and facilitate efficient and quality outcomes is limited to the quality of information that can be assessed within these systems.

Knowledge from clinical research increases daily. To provide the optimal care for their patients, nurses and other healthcare practitioners need to be aware of the massive amounts of information. Evidence-based practice (EBP) provides an approach to coping with the constantly changing knowledge base about what works best in healthcare. EBP is a systematic approach to clinical decision-making that uses the best evidence available in making decisions about patient care (Sackett et al., 2000).

EBP has three components: (1) a critical appraisal of the relevant research evidence, (2) the healthcare practitioner clinical expertise, and (3) the patient's values and preferences. The integration of these three sources of information provides the foundation for decisions about clinical practice. As with all interventions, an ongoing assessment of the relevant clinical outcomes that results from the implementation of evidence into practice should be made to provide additional information for future clinical decision-making (Fineout-Overholt, 2004).

The foundation of EBP is a systematic review of the research literature. This review gathers the evidence in a systematic way so that all relevant evidence is included

to prevent biases in the information derived from the studies. Many hierarchies of research designs have been developed usually with the randomized control trial (RCT). The RCT is considered the "gold standard" which indicates that it is the most appropriate design for evaluating the effectiveness of an intervention and less subject to potential bias than other study designs. One commonly used rating system is the Preventive Health Services Task Force Rating System (Woolf et al., 1996).

A systematic review needs clearly defined questions that indicate the population of interest and the relevant outcomes of the intervention. Often an evidence model/ analytic framework is developed to define the linkages between the intervention and the desired patient outcomes (Woolf, 2001). Once these have been developed, explicit rules are developed that will guide what studies will be included or excluded from the literature review. The search criteria and databases that are used are specified so that the search can be reproduced. The numbers of abstracts identified and reviewed are documented. The number of articles read and included or excluded is also noted. Most systematic reviews are based on computerized searches, but some include hand searches of certain publications to identify relevant literature and in some cases unpublished literature is scanned to address the issue of publication bias that results from journals being more likely to publish positive findings rather than studies of negative findings (Guyatt and Rennie, 2002).

Systematic reviews are based on the best evidence (Melnyk and Fineout-Overholt, 2002). In many cases RCTs are not available to answer clinical questions and in these cases other study types including observations studies are included. After the relevant articles have been identified, the quality of the individual studies is evaluated. Various methods are used to rate studies, such as the use of the study design hierarchy to rank studies of higher and lower quality and the use of rating scales that incorporate various domains. In addition, some systematic reviews also rate the strength and quality of the body of evidence found to answer a specific question. Results of studies may also be pooled using meta-analytic techniques to give a summary statistic that indicates the effect size of the intervention across multiple studies (Ciliska et al., 2001).

Systematic reviews require time and resources to perform. In addition to the publication of systematic reviews in the peer review literature, some databases of systematic reviews are available such as the Cochrane Database of Systematic Reviews and Evidence Reports published on the Agency for Healthcare Research and

Quality's (AHRQ) Web site at *http://www.ahrq.gov/clinic/epcindex.htm*. If an existing systematic review is not available, one can proceed with initiating a review of the literature to identify the best available evidence.

Systematic reviews state what the available research evidence shows. They do not make recommendations or prescribe an integrated course of clinical care for a given condition. The next step in evidence-based practice is the development of tools that may be used by the practitioner to assist in clinical decision-making.

Information from systematic reviews may also be used to develop tools that may be used at the organizational or system level to facilitate EBP. In this section the focus is only on tools that assist individual clinician decisions about the delivery of care.

Clinical practice guidelines are defined by the Institute of Medicine as "systematically developed statements to assist practitioner and patient decisions about appropriate healthcare or specific clinical circumstances" (Institute of Medicine, 1990). Evidence-based (scientifically grounded) clinical practice guidelines (also known simply as "guidelines" or "practice parameters") are gaining favor as instruments for promoting quality care.

EBP guidelines use the findings of the systematic review as the bases for the guideline recommendations. They provide documentation of the quality of evidence that supports the recommendations. In cases where systematic review findings are not available and recommendations are based on expert opinion or consensus of the guideline development panel, the guideline will indicate this. EBP guidelines integrate what is known from research with clinical expertise to provide information in clinically useful formats—thereby supporting informed decision-making for providers and patients (McCormick, 1998; McGlynn, 1996).

Guidelines provide a convenient way to present vast, complex data about outcomes, efficiency, effectiveness, patient preferences, policy, and costs as meaningful information (Cook et al., 1997) for clinical conditions. Guidelines are defined as quality tools because, when implemented effectively, they promote improved patient outcomes and reduce the outcome variations. These changes have been referred to in the third edition of this book, and documented over the past two decades (McQueen and McCormick, 2001).

A guideline is composed of multiple recommendations. Each recommendation links practice to supporting evidence for a specific intervention. For example, within a guideline about diabetes, there will be many individual recommendations concerning various aspects of prevention, diagnosis, and treatment. One recommendation might address foot assessment to prevent amputation, and another might involve patient education about glycemic control. In a quality guideline (evidence-based and developed using rigorous methods), the strength of the available evidence is explicitly stated for each recommendation so that clinicians and patients can judge for themselves (Eddy, 1990; Hadorn et al., 1996; Woolf et al., 1996).

Prior to using or computerizing a guideline, critical appraisal is needed (Sackett and Parkes, 1998). For many reasons, such as widespread gaps in the available evidence, many guidelines have limitations. These limitations need to be understood, and efforts should be made to minimize their effects (Anders et al., 1997). Again, this is especially important if computerization is being considered.

The first question to ask is "who developed this guideline?" Providers are more likely to use a guideline when they trust the credibility of the sponsor and do not suspect a serious political or financial agenda that would compromise objectivity (McQueen, 1998). The composition of the guideline panel is also significant. Although a multidisciplinary panel is sought, the appropriate makeup of the panel depends on the topic.

The scientific rigor of the development methods is key to the quality of the guideline (Sackett and Parkes, 1998; Woolf et al., 1996) and needs to be evaluated carefully. A central issue is whether or not the methods and the strength of evidence for each recommendation are plainly discussed so that providers can evaluate guideline credibility. A methods section will be part of a quality guideline and should clearly explain how the guideline was developed. It is particularly important to consider the data sources that were used, the inclusion/exclusion criteria used to select the data, and the currency of the information.

Evaluations of the methods used to analyze the data are critical. Who served as the methodologist? Were meta-analysis and other sophisticated statistical techniques used? Is the strength of the evidence explicitly stated? Strong evidence is not needed for each recommendation. Even in a quality, evidence-based guideline, the strength of the evidence will vary between recommendations, since there will typically be strong evidence for one intervention and missing or inconsistent evidence (uncertainty) for another. But the strength of the evidence for each recommendation should be presented clearly. The use of expert opinion should also be considered. While expert opinion may be necessary to fill in gaps in the evidence, over reliance on expert opinion raises issues of credibility.

Another guideline limitation is that patient preferences are often not adequately addressed (Bastian, 1996).

Patient participation in decision-making contributes to improved patient satisfaction and other positive outcomes (Deber, 1996; Hagen and Whylie, 1998). The needs of patients are especially important if the condition is a chronic and non-life-threatening condition, such as benign prostatic hyperplasia (Roberts, 1994). In these instances, the patient's preferences become the focus of the decision, and flexibility is needed to assure that personal choices are prioritized.

The absence of cost information is a common guideline limitation. Ideally, enough data about costs and outcomes are available so that the harms and benefits of different interventions can be easily compared and contrasted. Unfortunately, adequate cost information is rarely available or is outdated (Edinger and McCormick, 1998; Grady and Weis, 1995).

In summary, "guidelines are only as good as the evidence on which they are based" (Management Decision Research Center, 1998). Providers need to assess the quality of a guideline and evaluate whether or not it will contribute to improved patient outcomes. Key questions to ask are:

1. Who developed this guideline?
2. Is the guideline developed using an evidence-based approach (is it grounded in science and is evidence prioritized over expert opinion)?
3. Is the guideline current (when was it last updated)?
4. Is it presented in a flexible format? (Are patient preferences taken into account? Is there a capability for shared decision-making with patients, and is individual clinical judgment possible?)
5. Are the benefits and harms presented to support sound decision-making?
6. Are costs considered? Is this important for this specific topic?

Since guidelines are not directives, flexibility and discretion in application are needed. A guideline can be used as is, adapted for use based on local circumstances, and/or used as a basis for developing algorithms, critical paths, and other ("spin-off") quality tools (Anders et al., 1997; Gates, 1995). Not all guideline recommendations fit every clinical circumstance or every patient. In addition, the provider must generally trust that compliance will ultimately improve outcomes, or the guideline should not be used. This is especially important when deciding to computerize a guideline. Computerizing quality tools, such as guidelines, is resource-intensive

and should not be started until credibility of the guideline content has been established.

 # Implementation

What is Implementation?

Implementation is defined as applying textual information to real situations. Successful implementation implies compliance and the ability to manage change. Because real situations are fluid, implementation is a dynamic process that is by nature complex and multifaceted (McQueen and McCormick, 2001).

Implementation is the *active* employment of a guideline to promote effective and efficient care in order to improve patient outcomes. Although much additional study is needed, reports of guideline implementation have risen sharply over the past decades. The use of guidelines has been studied and described in a wide variety of settings. Many studies were previously described by McQueen and McCormick (2001) in the third edition.

Effect of Guidelines

Much is still being learned about the effect of guidelines on the outcomes of clinical practice. Since the early studies by Grimshaw and Russell (1993), published evaluations of guideline effectiveness report statistically significant improvements in professional performance and significant improvement in patient outcomes. They have the potential to improve the quality of care delivered and the outcomes of that care. The ability of guidelines to improve the quality of care depends on what evidence is incorporated with the guideline and the implementation of that guideline into practice.

Evaluation of Guidelines

Evaluation of the effects of clinical practice guideline use by practitioners focuses now on the computerization of guidelines. Due to the myriad of complex factors that impact outcomes, there is a lack of conclusive evidence about what works and does not work when using guidelines in real situations. Little is also known about how to manage diversity across settings. Instead, publications relevant to guideline implementation cover a diverse range of topics, and the meaning of the cumulative literature is elusive. Effective implementation of guidelines has been associated with quality improvements, and others report a positive association between guideline use and patient outcomes (McQueen and McCormick, 2001).

The nature of implementation studies is shifting. Early investigations of guideline implementation typically focused on strategies designed to change physician practice. Donabedian's (1980) measurement of treatment structures, processes, and outcomes was the theoretical basis for many studies, but processes—not outcomes—were typically the focus. The processes studied included provider processes, such as "buy-in," as well as patient/provider-influenced factors, such as compliance.

Although processes are still studied, reports of appropriateness from Brook (1996), McGlynn and Asch (1998), and others at RAND heightened awareness of the need to also focus on *outcomes*. During the 1990s, it became obvious that the amount of work needed to improve outcomes had been consistently underestimated (Forrest et al., 1996). For example, the effort required to implement guidelines and other quality tools effectively—let alone efficiently—is now the focus of many studies. But the field is still young in nursing research. Issues relevant to the translation of evidence into nursing practice (including the use of guidelines as a tool for this purpose) are only starting to be adequately addressed.

Putting Nursing Guidelines into Practice: Finding WHAT Works

The lessons learned from nursing care plans are applicable: guidelines that sit on a shelf will collect dust and not contribute to improved outcomes. Quality improvement using guidelines and other quality tools is most likely achieved and sustained over a long period when there is ongoing commitment from leaders to manage change proactively. Strong leadership promotes an active, multipronged, and theory-based approach (McQueen and McCormick, 2001). Long gone are notions that distributing a guideline to providers ("throwing it over the wall") will ultimately improve the health of a patient or make a provider's job easier.

Guideline implementation has long been recognized as a social process that is best promoted when users have time to gain awareness of the guideline content, develop a favorable attitude, and make a choice to adopt (Rubinstein et al., 2000). The ability to manage change is at the center of this process. After initial, active/multipronged/theory-based dissemination and implementation efforts are completed reinforcement and confirmation are needed indefinitely in order to sustain any quality improvements. But these social

processes are strengthened when implementation decisions are grounded in science and mandated by organizational leaders and guideline champions (Gates, 1995; Rubenstein et al., 2000).

Also during the last decade, awareness of the significance of social factors grew, and increased attention was paid to the organizational barriers and facilitating factors associated with the use of guidelines (McQueen and McCormick, 2001). The need for strong collaborative teamwork has been a common theme across organizational studies. Some studies consider general organizational factors, while others focus on specific disciplines or settings.

Since the early nineties, no single implementation strategy has been found to work consistently across settings. For this reason, increased attention has been directed toward organizational strategies designed to promote best practices rather than trying to change providers. Organizational strategies are typically tailored to match implementation goals to real world circumstances. Kaluzny et al. (1995) emphasized the importance of implementing guidelines in stages, providing "small wins," and building on existing governing mechanisms already in place within the institution. Goldberg et al. (1998) conducted a clinical trial to determine the effectiveness of academic detailing (AD)—a form of individualized, targeted education (Soumerai, 1990)—and CQI on increasing guideline compliance. Positive results were found when AD and CQI were used together. From these and other studies, evidence has accumulated regarding effectiveness of strategies and tools, but far more nursing research is needed. Ultimately, whatever strategies and tools are chosen to facilitate guideline implementation, a systematic approach is beneficial

Computers as a Tool to Facilitate Evidence-Based Practice and Guideline Implementation

This section presents new information for providers seeking computerized tools to promote guideline implementation. Since the third edition (McQueen and McCormick, 2001), there has been movement into developing, implementing, evaluating, and determining outcomes from computerizing guidelines. There have been numerous publications on guideline implementation models including GLIF, sharable active guideline environment (SAGE), and GEM. These will be described further in this chapter. In addition, another model has been evaluated in work related to guidelines at the Sowerby Centre for Health Informatics at Newcastle

(SCHIN). This model has been called clinical practice guideline architecture (CPGA) and it is being analyzed as a component model for incorporation into Health Level Seven (HL7) (Jenders and Sailors, 2004). According to Jenders and Sailors, there has even been convergence on a standard for representing clinical guidelines in HL7 in order to make guidelines more sharable. They reported that it was necessary to describe a terminology representation for guidelines when representing guidelines in HL7. This guideline expression language is called GELLO. As more professionals have delved into implementing guidelines, the evolving roles for nurses have changed and will also be discussed later in this chapter.

Computers and Guidelines

At their best, automated tools are the most powerful resource available to facilitate guideline implementation. For many reasons, computers are potentially an ideal match for guidelines: (1) computers permit centralized storage and retrieval of guidelines; (2) computers facilitate communication between different providers or between providers and patients; (3) computers enhance the speed, timeliness and presentation of feedback and other reports; (4) computers expand the accessibility of guidelines and related decision analysis tools; (5) computers make decision analysis infinitely easier and more powerful; and (6) computers provide a means for integrating guidelines with clinical information about effectiveness and outcomes. In short, computers make it easier for providers and patients to access, use, and communicate guideline-related information. This promotes sound decision-making and facilitates change.

Evidence to support the benefits of using computers as a guideline implementation tool has been growing. Shiffman et al. (1999a,b) stress the importance of implementation strategies that promote workflow integration and describe an information services model designed to maximize such integration. The authors provide a checklist for those using computers as an implementation tool and also describe a model for evaluating computerized guideline implementation tools. In a systematic review of 25 studies (including nine randomized controlled trials) published between 1992 and January 1998, the authors found that guideline compliance improved in 14 out of 18 systems and that documentation improved in four out of four studies. Shiffman and colleagues identified numerous diverse factors (such as the provision of a wide array of information management services) that potentially influence the success or failure of computer-

ized guideline systems. In a more recent publication, Shiffman and Michel (2004) provide a standardized approach for representing guideline documents using eXtensible Markup Language (XML). This model, called guideline elements model (GEM) adheres to the Conference on Guideline Standardization (COGS) standardized checklist for promoting guideline quality and facilitating information technology (IT) implementation (*http://ycmi.med.yale.edu/GEM*).

Research relevant to the intersection of guideline implementation and informatics becomes increasingly technical as issues relevant to technology transfer are prioritized. For example, work relevant to unified language and coding is proliferating. Extensive work is currently under way by InterMed that studies the cognitive processes relevant to computerized guideline encoding. The InterMed collaboration is a partnership between Columbia, Harvard, Stanford, and McGill universities. Investigators from these diverse institutions collaborate in the development and testing of software, tools, and system components that facilitate and support the standardized implementation and sharing of guidelines (Patel et al., 1998). To pursue their goals, InterMed collaborators developed a standardized, common language to represent guidelines. This language is called the guideline interchange format (GLIF) and has been studied as a vehicle for disseminating guideline text (Ohno-Machado et al., 1998).

The advantages of using a common format such as GLIF have been previously described to (Patel et al., 1998):

- Support multidisciplinary teams developing guidelines
- Reduce the duplication efforts in guideline development
- Provide feedback mechanisms to update guidelines concurrent with advances in medical and nursing knowledge

Recently, an innovative methodology to update guideline content was described by Scott-Wright et al. (2004). In the GLIF model, guideline content was created in a hierarchical and modular manner, thus allowing updates and revisions using axiomatic design theory (AD).

Other systems have been developed to allow local variation of guidelines. Fridsma et al. (1996) proposed a simple prompted diskette that allows the user to convert guideline recommendations into locally useful applications. Lobach (1995) described a model of local adaptation using five national guidelines implemented at Duke University.

In a more recent study of the use of national standardized guidelines for regional localization, Mattison et. al. (2004) discussed issues in implementing national guidelines into a large managed care delivery system—Kaiser Permanente. They developed guiding principles for managing local variation in specific data recommended by national guidelines.

In summary, computers can be used as quality implementation tools in a variety of ways depending on creativity, resources, and the organizational culture present (Harvey and Kitson, 1996). The technological sophistication of automated tools crosses a spectrum. Some computerized guideline tools, such as those using artificial intelligence, are complex, while others, such as the dissemination of text using the Internet or an Intranet, are relatively simple and easily created. Regardless of the level of sophistication, opportunities to use computers as tools to improve patient outcomes are still under development and are being evaluated.

As recommended by Mittman et al. (1999) and others, a *theory-based* approach to considering tools helps to assure that implementation decisions are rational and grounded in science. Evidence summarized in McQueen and McCormick in 2001 suggested that an *active* and *multipronged* approach is also beneficial. An active approach has also been shown to discourage use of only passive dissemination and implementation methods—such as merely handing out a guideline to providers and assuming that it will be read and followed. A multipronged approach means that several diverse guideline implementation tools will be used simultaneously and supported by leaders from the top down (e.g., by policies issued by leaders) and from the bottom up (e.g., by staff at all levels and across disciplines serving as champions and guideline promoters). The goals of this combined approach are (1) rational choices and (2) change management. Discussions of several computerized tools to consider are listed below. Using a theory-based, active, and multipronged approach, nurses should consider which of the following tools best-fit local needs.

In a recent article by McQueen et al. (2004), the Veterans Health Administration (VHA) Quality Enhancement Research Initiative (QUERI) is described after 6 years of design and implementation. The article describes the model and information systems infrastructure needed to demonstrate continuous quality measurement and improvement policies and practices. In a complementary article, Hynes et al. (2004) describes the information systems needed to support the QUERI process and the components needed in the Veterans Health Information System and Technology Architecture (VistA).

In an effort to develop a knowledge representation framework for interoperable sharing of guidelines, the IT community developed a national project funded by National Institute of Standards and Technology (NIST) called SAGE (Campbell et al., 2003). This provides a guideline model and a public domain workbench model (Protégé-2000) knowledge authoring tools, with standards such as standardized nomenclature of medical terminology—clinical terms (SNOMED-CT), logical observation identifiers, names, and codes (LOINC), and HL7 to employ open system interface. This collaboratory has a Web site and useful tools for persons interested in using guidelines imbedded into information systems. The Web site is *http://www.sageproject.net/ guidelines/guidelines. htm*. Evaluation of the experience with SAGE has demonstrated the complexity of accomplishing such a task (Parker et al., 2004).

SAGE has been integrated into a clinical information system called IDX Systems Corporation with cooperation from research at the University of Nebraska, Mayo Clinic—Rochester, Intermountain Health Care, Apelon, Inc., and Stanford University (Ram et al. 2004). In addition, the guideline had been encoded based on standard medical terminologies (SNOMED CT and LOINC) and HL7 data types. It is a real-time model of the integration of a clinical practice guideline (immunization guideline) into an electronic health record (EHR). In progress is a new application on a different clinical information system using a different clinical practice guidelines (ADA Diabetes guideline) in order to determine interoperability and sharability.

Decision Support Systems

Decision analysis offers a way to link the probability of a clinical course to the likelihood of specific outcomes. The results of clinical decisions can then be predicted, and the probability of alternative strategies can be quantified. Decision models, data, and complex analyses are required. There are many ways in which these systems can be applied to guideline implementation. For example, providers could learn about, test, and improve a new guideline using a decision support system. But there are potential limitations. Invalid or conflicting evidence is sometimes used in analyses. In addition, coding is complex, and lack of expertise and resources currently prohibit widespread use. But this is changing as applications become more powerful and integrated systems are capable of capturing performance information and linking it concurrently with outcomes.

Problems with adherence to guidelines, even when implemented in decision support systems, have also been recently described (Chan et al., 2004). In another study, Tu et al. (2004) describe modeling guidelines into clinical workflow. They use the SAGE guideline coding methodology and find problems with sharability and terminology. Without standard clinical vocabularies with reference terminology features, true interoperability of decision support technology for guidelines is lacking.

Computerized Reminder Systems

Many common reminder systems are not automated. Laminated cards, posters, preprinted forms within charts, and pocket guides are all reminders familiar to most providers. Automated reminders are infinitely more powerful, especially when they cannot be ignored or turned off easily. Whatever their form, reminders are most useful when used in "real time" (at the point of patient contact). Both automated and paper reminders are ideal for health promotion and preventive care. For example, a computer can be programmed to analyze a patient's age, risk factors, and other data to generate a screening reminder at the appropriate time. Although they are still being studied, automated reminders may be the most promising guideline implementation tools now available—particularly when the reminders are integrated within decision support programs or other integrated systems during real time.

When information is fed back to providers and facilities, quantitative performance data are linked to social processes such as peer influence. For example, data collected about the interventions of a group of providers can be linked to outcomes and fed back. In some instances, benchmarks are used; other times, provider performance is compared to colleague performance. As accountability is increasingly demanded of all professions, nurses can expect wider use of feedback and performance profiling. Since computers can readily be programmed to feed back the vast quantity of clinical and administrative data now being collected by many organizations, these applications should proliferate. Audit and feedback of information are generally most useful when provided at the time of the patient encounter or soon after and when the feedback is stimulating and interactive. Delayed or disconnected feedback is less useful or counterproductive, and over auditing may contribute to inappropriate use (Robinson et al., 1996).

An innovative use of interactive voice response (IVR) technology in assisting consumers who are in a smoking cessation program has been described by nurses at Indiana University (McDaniel et al., 2004). By using telephone prompts and educational messages, they have demonstrated adherence to a smoking cessation clinical practice guideline and achieved smoking relapse prevention.

Online Access to Guidelines

Online communication provides a convenient, cost-effective vehicle for information dissemination and exchange. Online tools are more powerful when integrated within an overall communication strategy and targeted to the specific information needs of each stakeholder. Soon it will be hard to imagine guideline implementation without the World Wide Web. In 2001, McSweeney et al. listed several sources for the nurse practitioner to access and evaluate clinical practice guidelines.

The U.S. government has provided valuable access to guidelines on the Internet since the early 1990s. The National Library of Medicine (NLM) and the AHRQ have full text and abstracted versions of guidelines available. The latest access to guidelines is a cosponsored U.S. Guideline Clearinghouse that involves the government and private sector resources. Table 28.1 provides the key URLs to access valuable guideline content online.

Patients search online guideline-derived patient brochures and discuss guideline recommendations with online providers. Patients and providers easily download guideline text, rural clinics gain access to the latest update of a guideline, and facilities within large organizations use the Intranet to exchange information about compliance. As the "digital age" promotes Web applications, their influence on clinical decision-making and outcomes will expand rapidly but remain difficult to measure. Zielstorff (1998) has studied the issue and obstacles associated with online practice guidelines and provides specific suggestions for overcoming barriers, including better accommodation of imprecise knowledge in clinical algorithms using fuzzy logic. Dugas (1998) reported the use of Intranet-based information systems specifically for nurses. Additional research on this topic continues to be needed.

Table 28.1 A listing of URLs in the United States to Obtain Full Texts of Clinical Practice Guidelines Online

http://www.ahcpr.gov
http://www.ngc.gov

Automated Flow Sheets as Part of an Electronic Patient Record

As the level of integration described by Shortell et al. (1996) becomes a reality, EHR are gaining popularity as a way to combine stored data repositories with information management tools. For example, computerized records provide a practical way to use guidelines to support creation of clinical protocols (Bazzoli, 1995). This allows knowledge to be represented in various formats so that it is available to facilitate accurate and timely decisions. Tang et al. (1999) also reports use of EHR for evaluating interventions designed to improve guideline compliance. As EHR evolves, mechanisms for recording data will improve so that the frequency of events within specified time periods can be more easily analyzed. These data can then be linked to a variety of computerized tools relevant to guidelines. For example, automated flow sheets used to collect patient information relevant to guideline compliance should become more sophisticated. Flow sheets could then be easily transferred from portable computers and used by providers at the bedside or linked to patient education information.

Computers Used to Facilitate Academic Detailing

AD is an acronym used to describe customized "educational outreach." Individual providers are targeted for education. Computers can supplement AD in a variety of ways. For example, computer-assisted instruction or videodisc technology can be used to convey information about a guideline and allow the provider to explore this information safely prior to applying it to real patients. Unlike conferences or workshops, which are often passive, computerized AD provides focused, individualized education that can be highly interactive. The stimulating and engaging nature of computer-facilitated AD promotes success.

Choosing Computerized Tools

Although a theory-based, active, multipronged approach aids in the initial consideration of appropriate tools, the unique needs of each healthcare setting also guide implementation decisions about tools. Once a systematic approach has been used to consider various options, multidisciplinary guideline implementation teams can identify strategies to guide their selection of specific tools for a guideline implementation tool kit. The team will also need to address how tools can best be combined

with each other and integrated into systemwide quality improvement initiatives (Kinney and Gift, 1997).

Numerous strategies directly linked to informatics are available to facilitate guideline implementation. Duff and Casey (1998) describe strategies for using informatics to promote access, communication, and evaluation of guidelines. Shiffman et al. (1999a) stress the importance of implementation strategies that promote workflow integration and describe an information services model designed to maximize such integration. The authors provide a checklist for those using computers as an implementation tool and also describe a model for evaluating computerized guideline implementation tools.

The Department of Veterans Affairs (VA) taxonomy (Management Decision Research Center, 1998) can guide selection of tools for a guideline implementation tool kit. Computerized tools from all four categories can be considered: knowledge-based, attitude-based, behavior-based, and maintenance-based tools.

Knowledge-based tools will sometimes be the top priority depending on the culture. For example, computers can be used to provide diabetes guideline text to providers or patients or to forward algorithms to providers showing the logic of the guideline. Providers may also want to consider attitude-based tools. For example, professional organizations or specialty groups associated with diabetes to convey their endorsement of the guideline to providers and patients can use computers. When seeking behavior-based tools, administrative systems can be used to determine staffing needs after a guideline is implemented, or to calculate the resource changes associated with guideline implementation. For example, perhaps implementation of the diabetes guideline leads to increased patient education. Additional staff time may be needed and there may be financial implications. Computers can track this information over time. Perhaps computers contribute most to systemwide quality improvement when used as maintenance-based tools. Used in this capacity, computerized reminder systems, computerized standing orders, and automated audit/feedback systems can be integrated to assure that the quality improvement gains (such as decreased amputation rates) associated with guideline implementation are sustained over time. Maintenance is an important, sometimes neglected, priority when implementing guidelines.

Once the tools have been selected and the tool kit is being used to facilitate implementation, the work is just starting. Change management principles suggest that use must be encouraged over time and that each tool be evaluated. Information about what works in a specific environment is gained through iterative processes. Barriers to implementation as well as facilitating factors are revealed as each tool is used in various situations; adjustments are then made accordingly. Cumulative information from the evaluation is also fed back to providers and facilities on an ongoing basis. As information is gained over time, a culture of critical thinking and organizational learning is fostered, and guideline use becomes part of the daily routine.

Nursing Role in Using Automated Tools

As computer applications in quality improvement expand, so do nursing roles. These roles increasingly appear in published literature, and it is obvious that many new roles are evolving. Many guideline-related studies focused on nursing and the use of specific guidelines (McQueen and McCormick, 2001). Publications have covered a diverse range of topics: the integration of IT with outcomes management, coding and taxonomy issues relevant to outcomes including standardized language and other issues tied to the nursing minimum data set, and the development of nurse-sensitive outcome measures.

An issue of specific relevance to nursing relates to the composition of guideline development panels and the critical appraisal of guidelines. There is currently no national professional or academic group with overall responsibility for assessing nursing content within guidelines or for suggesting appropriate representation of nurses on multidisciplinary panels. Guideline developers do not readily know where to turn when seeking nurse's involvement.

Summary and Conclusions

As quality and cost issues drive the explosive pace of change in modern healthcare organizations, issues related to the provision of effective and efficient care come into focus. Clinical practice guidelines are fast becoming a primary quality improvement tool for promoting efficiency and effectiveness. But not all guidelines are created equal. Since providers are held accountable for their decisions, it is important to know how to evaluate a guideline, adapt it to an individual patient, and promote its use throughout the organization. An active, multipronged, and theory-based approach combined with judgment about the needs of the specific organization can be helpful when seeking tools to leverage guideline use. Computerized tools should be considered carefully because they are potentially so powerful. Computerized tools come in many forms, including decision support systems and automated reminders. The tools can be used together or

in isolation, but their use should be evaluated over time and contain mechanisms for revision and updating as the evidence base for practice evolves.

References

Anders, R. L., Tomai, J. S., Clute, R. M., and Olson, T. (1997). Development of a scientifically valid coordinated care path. *Journal of Nursing Administration* 27(5):45–52.

Bastian, H. (1996). Raising the standard: Practice guidelines and consumer participation. *International Journal for Quality in Health Care* 85(5):485–490.

Bazzoli, F. (1995). Clinical protocols: The next automation frontier. Computerized records will play a key role in the implementation of clinical guidelines. *Health Data Management* 3(2):30–32, 34–46.

Brook, R. H. (1996). Practice guidelines: To be or not to be? *The Lancet* 348(9033):1005–1006.

Campbell, J. R., Tu, S. W., Mansfield, J. G., Boyer, J. I., McClay, J., Parker, C., Ram, P., Scheitel, S. M., and McDonald, K. (2003). The SAGE guideline model: a knowledge representation framework for encoding interoperable clinical practice guidelines. Stanford Medical Informatics Report SMI-2003-0962. *http://smi-web.stanford.edu/pubs/SMI_abstracts/SMI-2003-0962.html*

Chan, A. S., Coleman, R. W., Martins, S. B., Advani, A., Musen, M. A., Bosworth, H. B., Oddone, E. Z., Shlipak, M. G., Hoffman, B. B., and Goldstein, M. D. (2004). Evaluating provider adherence in a trial of a guideline-based decision support system for hypertension. In M. Fieschi, et al. (Eds.), *MEDINFO* (pp. 125–129). Amsterdam: IOS press.

Ciliska, D., Cullum, N., Marks, S. (2001). Evaluation of systemic reviews of treatment or prevention interventions. *Evidence Based Nursing* 4(4):100–104.

Cook, D. J., Mulrow, C. D., and Haynes, R. B. (1997). Systematic reviews: Synthesis of best evidence for clinical decisions. *Annals of Internal Medicine* 126:364–371.

Deber, R. B. (1996). Shared decision making in the real world. *Journal of General Internal Medicine* 11:377–378.

Donabedian, A. (1980). *Explorations in quality assessment and monitoring. Volume 1: The definition of quality and approaches to its assessment.* Ann Arbor: Health Administration Press.

Duff, L. and Casey, A. (1998). Implementing clinical guidelines: How can informatics help? *Journal of the American Medical Informatics Association* 5(3):225–226.

Dugas, M. (1998). An intranet-based information system for nurses. *MD Computing* 15(3):158–161.

Eddy, D. M. (1990). Guidelines for policy statements: The explicit approach. *Journal of the American Medical Association* 263:3077–3084.

Edinger, S. and McCormick, K. A. (1998). Databases—their use in developing clinical practice guidelines and estimating the cost impact of guideline implementation. *Journal of the American Health Informatics Association* 67(4):52–60.

Fineout-Overholt, E., and Melnyk, B. M. (2004). Evaluation of studies of prognosis. *Evidence Based Nursing* 7(1):4–8.

Forrest, D., Hoskins, A., and Hussey, R. (1996). Clinical guidelines and their implementation. *Postgraduate Medical Journal* 72:19–22.

Fridsma, D. B., Gennari, H. J., and Musen, M. A. (1996). Making generic guidelines specific. *Proceedings of the American Medical Informatics Association Annual Fall Symposium* (pp. 597–561).

Gates, P. E. (1995). Think globally, act locally: An approach to implementation of clinical practice guidelines. *Joint Commission Journal on Quality Improvement* 21(2):71–85.

Goldberg, H. I., Wagner, E. H., Fihn, S. D., et al. (1998). A randomized controlled trial of CQI teams and academic detailing: Can they alter compliance with guidelines? *Joint Commission on Quality Improvement* 24(3):130–142.

Grady, M. I. and Weis, K. A. (Eds.). (1995). *Cost Analysis Methodology for Clinical Practice Guidelines.* Rockville, MD: U. S. Department of Health and Human Services, Agency for Health Care Policy and Research, AHCPR Publication No. 95-0001.

Grimshaw, J. M. and Russell, J. T. (1993). Effect of clinical guidelines on medical practice: A systematic review of rigorous evaluations. *The Lancet* 342: 1317–1322.

Guyatt, G. and Rennie, D. (2002). Users' Guide to the Medical Literature. Chicago, IL: AMA Press.

Hadorn, D. C., Baker, D., Hodges, J. S., and Hicks, N. (1996). Rating the quality of evidence for clinical practice guidelines. *Journal of Clinical Epidemiology* 49(7):749–754.

Hagen, N. A. and Whylie, B. (1998). Putting clinical practice guidelines into the hands of cancer patients [editorial]. *Canadian Medical Association Journal* 158(3):347–348.

Harvey, G. and Kitson, A. (1996). Achieving improvement through quality: An evaluation of key factors in the implementation process. *Journal of Advanced Nursing* 24:185–195.

Hynes, D. M., Perrin, R. A., Rappaport, S., Stevens, J. M., and Demakis, J.G. (2004). Informatics resources to support health care quality improvement in the veterans health administration. *Journal of the American Medical Informatics Association* 11:344–350.

Institute of Medicine. (1990). In Field, M. J. and Lohr, K. N. (Eds.). *Clinical Practice Guidelines: Directions for a New Program.* Washington, DC: National Academy Press.

Institute of Medicine. (1992). Field, M. J. and Lohr, K. N. (Eds.). *Guidelines for Clinical Practice: From Development to Use.* Washington, DC: National Academy Press.

Jenders, R. A. and Sailors, R. M. (2004). Convergence on a standard for representing clinical guidelines: Work in Health Level Seven. In M. Fieschi, et al. (Eds.), *MEDINFO* (pp. 130–134). Amsterdam: IOS Press.

Kaluzny, A. D., Konrad, T. R., and McLaughlin, C. P. (1995). Organizational strategies for implementing clinical guidelines. *Joint Commission Journal on Quality Improvement* 21(7):347–351.

Kinney, C. F. and Gift, R. G. (1997). Building a framework for multiple improvement initiatives. *Joint Commission Journal of Quality Improvement* 20(4):181–191.

Lobach, D. F. (1995). A model for adapting clinical practice guidelines for electronic implementation in primary care. *Proceedings of the 19th Annual Symposium on Computer Applications in Medical Care* (pp. 581–585).

Management Decision Research Center. (1998). *Clinical Practice Guidelines.* Boston: VA Health Services Research and Development Service, in collaboration with the Association for Health Services Research.

Mattison, J. E., Dolin, R. H., and Laberge, D. (2004). Managing the tensions between national standardization vs. regional localization of clinical content and templates. In M. Fieschi, et al. (Eds.), *MEDINFO* (pp. 1081–1085). Amsterdam: IOS Press.

McCormick, K. A. (1998). New tools—new models to integrate outcomes into quality measurement. *Seminars in Nursing Management* 6(3):119–125.

McDaniel, A. M., Wewers, M. E., Hudson, D. (2004). An integrated smoking relapse prevention system. In M. Fieschi, et al. (Eds.), *MEDINFO* (pp. 1749). Amsterdam: IOS Press.

McGlynn, E. A. (1996). Setting the context for measuring patient outcomes. *New Directions in Mental Health Services* 71:19–32.

McGlynn, E. A. and Asch, S. M. (1998). Developing a clinical performance measure. *American Journal of Preventive Medicine* 14(Suppl. 3):14–21.

McQueen, M. L. (1998). *Interests in Evidence: Politicians' Involvement in Developing Evidence-Based Policies.* Ann Arbor, MI: UMI Services of The Bell and Howell Publishing Company.

McQueen, L. and McCormick, K. A. (2001). Translating evidence into practice: Guidelines and automated implementation tools. In V. K. Saba and K. A. McCormick (Eds.), *Essentials of Computers for Nurses: Informatics for the New Millennium* (3rd ed.). New York: McGraw-Hill.

McQueen, L., Mittman, B. S., and Demakis, J. G. (2004). Overview of the Veterans Health Administration (VHA) Quality Enhancement Research Initiative (QUERI). *Journal of the American Medical Informatics Association* 11:339–343.

McSweeney, M., Speis, M., Cann, C. J. (2001). Finding and evaluating clinical practice guidelines. *The Nurse Practitioner* 26(9):30–49.

Melnyk, B. M. and Fineout-Overholt, E. (2002). Key Steps in evidence-based practice: Asking compelling clinical questions and searching for the best evidence. *Pediatric Nursing* 28(3)262–263.

Mittman, B. S., Pugh, J. A. Rubenstein, L. V., and Charns, M. P. (1999). Making ongoing improvement a reality. *Presentation at the Second Annual Meeting for the Quality Enhancement Review Initiative.* Reston, VA: Department of Veterans Affairs, Health Service Research and Development.

Ohno-Machado, L., Gennari, H. J., Murphy, S. N., et al. (1998). The guideline interchange format: A model for representing guidelines. *Journal of the American Medical Informatics Association* 5(4):357–372.

Parker, C. G., Rocha, R. A., Campbell, J. R., Tu, S. W., and Huff, S. M. (2004). Detailed clinical models for sharable, executable guidelines. In M. Fieschi, et al. (Eds.), *MEDINFO 2004* (pp. 145–148). Amsterdam: IOS Press.

Patel, V. L., Allen, V. G., Arocha, J. F., and Shortliffe, E. H. (1998). Representing clinical guidelines in GLIF: Individual and collaborative expertise. *Journal of the American Medical Informatics Association* 5(5):467–483.

Ram, P., Berg, D., Tu, S., Mansfield, G., Ye, Q., Abarbanel, R., Beard, N. (2004). Executing clinical practice guidelines using the SAGE execution engine. In M. Fieschi, et al. (Eds.), *MEDINFO 2004* (pp. 251–255). Amsterdam: IOS Press.

Roberts, R. G. (1994). New guidelines based on symptoms and patient preferences. *Geriatrics* 49(7):24–31.

Robinson, M. B., Thompson, E., and Black, N.A. (1996). Evaluation of the effectiveness of guidelines, audit and feedback: Improving the use of intravenous thrombolysis in patients with suspected acute myocardial infarction. *International Journal of Quality in Health Care* 8(3):211–222.

Rubenstein, L. V., Mittman, B. S., Yano, E. M., and Mulrow, C. D. (2000). From understanding health care provider behavior to improving health care: The QUERI framework for quality improvement. *Medical Care* 38(Suppl. 6):129–141.

Sackett, D. L. and Parkes, J. (1998). Teaching critical appraisal: No quick fixes [editorial]. *Canadian Medical Association Journal* 158(2):203–204.

Sackett, D. L., Straus, S. E., Richardson, W. S., Rosenberg, W., and Hayes, R. B. (2000). *Evidence-Based Medicine: How to Practice and Teach EBM.* London: Churchill Livingstone.

Scott-Wright, A. O., Fischer, R. P., Denekamp, Y., and Boxwala, A. A. (2004). A methodology for modular representation of guidelines. In M. Fieschi, et al. (Eds.), *MEDINFO 2004* (pp. 149–153). Amsterdam: IOS Press.

Shiffman, R. N., Brandt, C. A., Liaw, Y., and Corb, G. J. (1999a). A design model for computer-based guideline implementation based on information management services. *Journal of the American Medical Informatics Association* 6(2):99–103.

Shiffman, R. N., Liaw, Y., Brandt, C. A., and Corb, G. J. (1999b). Computer-based guideline implementation systems: A systematic review of functionality and effectiveness. *Journal of the American Medical Informatics Association* 6(2):104–114.

Shiffman, R. N. and Michel, G. (2004). Toward improved guideline quality: Using the COGS statement with GEM. In M. Fieschi, et al. (Eds.), *MEDINFO 2004* (pp. 159–163). Amsterdam: IOS Press.

Shortell, S. M., Gillies, R. R., Anderson, D. A., et al. (1996). *Remaking Health Care in America.* San Francisco, CA: Jossey-Bass Publishers.

Soumerai, S. B. and Avorn, J. (1990). Principles of educational outreach ('academic detailing') to improve clinical decision-making. *Journal of the American Medical Association* 263(4):549–556.Tang, P. C., LaRosa, M. P., Newcomb, C., and Gorden, S. M. (1999). Measuring the effects of reminders on outpatient influenza immunizations at the point of clinical opportunity. *Journal of the American Medical Informatics Association* 6(2):115–121.

Tu, S. W., Musen, M. A., Shankar, R., Campbell, J., Hrabak, K, et al. (2004). Modeling guidelines for integration into clinical workflow. In M. Fieschi, et al. (Eds.), *MEDINFO 2004* (pp. 125–129). Amsterdam: IOS Press.

Woolf, S. H., DiGuiseppi, C. G., Atkins, D., and Kamerow, D. B. (1996). Developing evidence-based clinical practice guidelines: Lessons learned by the U. S. Preventive Service Task Force. *Annual Review of Public Health* 17:511–538.

Woolf, S. H. (2001). Evidence-based medicine: A historical and international overview. In *Proceedings of the Royal College of Physicians Edinburgh* (Vol. 9, Suppl. 31, pp. 39–41).

Zielstorff, R. D. (1998). Online practice guidelines: Issues, obstacles, and future prospects. *Journal of the American Medical Informatics Association* 5(3):227–236.

29

Data Mining and Knowledge Discovery

Patricia A. Abbott

Sun-Mi Lee

OBJECTIVES

1. Describe the uses of data mining.
2. Describe knowledge discovery in datasets and how they are applied in large data collections.
3. Discuss the uses of Bayesian networks.
4. Articulate the differences between quality of the data and the tools or methods used in analyzing them.

KEY WORDS

data mining
knowledge discovery
decision making

 Introduction

Decision-making in healthcare is a knowledge-intensive activity that may surpass the ability of the human cognitive processing. The impact of disease processes, care processes, and environmental influences all combine to present a continually shifting target for decision-makers in healthcare. In their seminal work from the seventies, Pauker et al. (1976) assert that clinicians make clinical decisions on "guesses" of initial hypotheses, which are based on minimal amounts of data. The difficulties inherent in clinical decision-making are now further compounded by the rapid proliferation of massive and distributed healthcare data warehouses that are unwieldy for purposes of analysis. Factors that contribute to patient outcomes can be related to specific patient characteristics; external forces such as facility ownership, reimbursement patterns, and regulatory agencies; and internal forces such as case-mix and staffing ratios. These data points are captured and stored in a variety of systems, both internal and external to the agency and/or enterprise.

The standards used to structure these data are in disarray and are often not transportable or interpretable by outside systems. Correlations and patterns that may emerge when integrated are trapped in these disparate data silos, termed by McCormick (1981) two decades ago as "data cemeteries." The challenge facing information technologists is how to unlock the information trapped in these massive and fragmented sets to determine causation or look for predictors of untoward outcomes and then to incorporate such findings into systems that support decision-makers. The webs of causality in healthcare are exceedingly complex and often covert, requiring new approaches to discovery and application.

The purpose of this chapter is to introduce and detail a method known as knowledge discovery in datasets (KDD) and to discuss its applicability for use in large collections of data. Several approaches are discussed, with special attention given to a very promising approach using Bayesian networks (BNs) to mine healthcare data.

The term data mining is often misperceived. Commonly associated with "fishing" and "dredging," many in the past have chosen to avoid exploration of this technique. Such approaches are now becoming more mainstream, yet nursing remains mired in misconception. It is important to emphasize that the *tools* of KDD are totally independent from the *data* on which they operate. Therefore, KDD utility is domain-independent and can be used in any large collection of data. The value of KDD as an approach is often confused with the character of the data, which in healthcare has a tendency to be noisy or dirty. One should never confuse the validity of the tools and approaches of KDD with the characteristics of the data. The use of data mining approaches should be approached with the same level of rigor as any scientific method; reliability, validity, and reproducibility are paramount. Arguments supporting the use of KDD are offered in this chapter.

Innovative Approaches to Information Management in Healthcare

The move toward integrated health systems and the tracking of data from cradle to grave has highlighted the need for a method by which the vast amounts of data being collected can be analyzed and visualized. The need for automated and intelligent database analysis is receiving increasing levels of attention as healthcare enterprises and payers struggle to make sense of the data that tremendous amounts of resources are being spent to capture. The problem arises in the intensive multidimensionality, fragmentation, and distribution of healthcare data that can overload human cognitive capacity as well as traditional methods of aggregation and analysis.

The question becomes, therefore, how can we begin to harness the data that are being collected, how can we turn the data into information, and how can we use the information to generate new knowledge? Discovery-based approaches such as KDD—sometimes referred to as "data mining"—may be one method of working with massive, distributed, and multidimensional healthcare data.

Knowledge Discovery in Large Data Sets

KDD is defined by Abbott (2000) as the "melding of human expertise with statistical and machine learning techniques to identify features, patterns, and underlying rules in large collections of healthcare data." Fayyad et al. (1989, p. 6) define KDD as the "non-trivial process of identifying valid, novel, potentially useful, and ultimately understandable patterns in data." According to Goodwin et al. (1997, p. 22) data mining and KDD in healthcare uses a "combination of artificial intelligence (AI) and computer science techniques to help build knowledge in complex healthcare domains." In essence, KDD can be viewed as extracting high-level knowledge from low-level data (Fayyad et al., 1989). KDD uses discovery-based approaches in which pattern recognition and matching, classification or clustering schemas, and other algorithms are used to detect key relationships in the data.

The techniques used in KDD and data mining are not new, having been discovered in the field of AI research in the 1980s. The finance and banking industry have a strong history in the use of KDD approaches. Data mining has been used extensively in business to predict future customer markets and current customer behavior (Wasserman, 2001). Future customer characteristics are predicted based on past behavior and strategies are implemented based on the projected future characteristics (Saarenvita, 1999). For example, "market-basket analysis" is a type of KDD where large databases containing customer buying patterns are examined for purchases that cluster together. A market-basket analysis may demonstrate that the purchase of a man's suit is closely linked with the purchase of a new shirt and tie. The business manager would then use this information prospectively to enhance the probability of the sale of a new shirt and tie by offering an incentive to the customer to purchase the additional pieces at the same time as the new suit. Other common applications of KDD include predicting loan default by identifying factors that contribute to this negative outcome and applying them prospectively in loan approval systems.

Aside from the logistic issues when working with very large collections of data, substantial work is needed to influence a movement beyond traditional and comfortable approaches to analysis of healthcare data. This is not to imply that the gold standard approaches to analysis are no longer of value; however, one size does not and cannot fit all. In light of the challenges of terabytes of data and market-driven, rapid competition for resources and customer bases, innovative approaches to data analysis in healthcare warrant further attention. Munhall (1997, p. 203) asserts that

> Manuals and methods are the antithesis of creative thought. They mobilize behavioral assumptions and prescribe consistency of presentation and forbid wandering to a different form of rhetoric and discourse that is 'out of the box.' . . . unless he or she already knows that living knowledge and discovery lies outside the box.

The push is on for innovative discovery-based approaches to data analysis; we must begin to look for the living discovery and knowledge outside the comfort range of traditional approaches.

Differentiation of Verification versus Discovery Approaches

How are traditional approaches different from KDD? Current statistical models based on regression offer the possibility of in-depth analysis but may require unrealistic assumptions about the distribution and interdependence of data or errors. Traditional analysis supports a *verification-based approach* to hypothesis testing. A specific hypothesis is made, variables suspected to be contributors to the phenomenon of study are isolated, and analytic tools are used to either refute or prove the original postulate. This requires that the investigator have a detailed understanding of all (obvious and nonobvious) elements that could affect the outcome and then complete complex iterative queries of the data to further refine the analysis.

The effectiveness of this approach can be limited by a variety of issues including the knowledge base of the investigator, the ability of the investigator to detect trends in the data and to pose proper questions, the ability to compose the complex queries required, the character and quality of multivariate data, and the ability to work with constrained or artificially imposed constructs. Most statistical models focus on the values that are expected—those elements that appear as the unexpected (outliers) are those that invalidate the model.

In contrast, KDD is based on *discovery-driven approaches* to hypothesis testing, where the unexpected is valued. This technique can be used to sift through large repositories to "discover" trends, predictive patterns, or correlations in data; confirm hypotheses; and highlight exceptions. KDD is particularly valuable for use in nonlinear, combinatorially explosive, and non-monotonic problems.

The two primary goals of KDD lie within prediction and description. Description in KDD deals with the discovery of patterns interpretable by humans, which are used to describe the data. Prediction focuses on using variables within the data set to predict future or unknown values of other variables of interest. In working with large healthcare data sets, the discovery of interpretable patterns that illuminate the phenomenon under study in concert with the discovery of information that can be used to predict such phenomena could be incorporated into automated systems, leveraging the value of the data that we are spending thousands of dollars to collect.

It is important to emphasize that KDD as a *process* is different from (but complementary to) the frequently applied term of "data mining." KDD focuses on the overall process of discovering useful knowledge from data and is composed of several steps (Fig. 29.1), while data mining generally refers solely to the use of algorithms for extracting patterns from the data. KDD is interactive and iterative, involving the application of the algorithms to extract the patterns and then a concerted effort to *interpret* the patterns that have been presented. It could be said then that the application of the techniques without a matching strong understanding of the

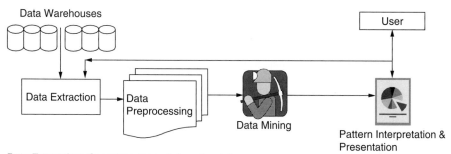

Data Extraction: Searching for and choosing data
Data Preprocessing: Choosing variables, dealing with noise and multidimensionality
Data Mining: Analysis of data using association, clustering, modeling, classification, etc.
Pattern Interpretation & Presentation: Interpretation, evaluation, and presentation of patterns

Figure 29.1
KDD process.
(Source: Abbott, P. (2000). Knowledge discovery in large datasets: A primer for data mining applications in healthcare. In M. Ball, K. Hannah, S. Newbold, and J. Douglas (Eds.), *Nursing Informatics: Where Caring and Technology Meet* (3rd ed.). New York: Springer-Verlag.)

problem domain is not evidence of the application of KDD as a process. Work with data mining algorithms, however, is one of the most active research areas in KDD.

Background of Knowledge Discovery in Large Data Sets

Analyzing large data sets in the quest to find "nuggets" of useful and interesting patterns of information has been labeled with many different titles. The terms, such as knowledge extraction, data mining, data pattern processing, data archaeology, and information discovery, can be found in much of the literature. The term knowledge discovery in databases (KDD) was coined in 1989 to "refer to the broad process of finding knowledge in data, and to emphasize the 'high-level' application of particular data mining methods" (Fayyad et al., 1989). These authors assert that the term data mining has traditionally been used by the management information systems (MIS) community, while AI and machine learning researchers have adopted KDD.

As noted earlier, the use of KDD in the truest form is the application of the techniques of KDD to discover useful knowledge from data. This is in contrast to the term data mining, which refers to the application of algorithms to extract patterns without the further use of the additional steps critical to KDD (such as interpreting the results and the requisite understanding of the problem domain). The additional steps of KDD are what differentiate the technique from data mining in the singular sense. The application of data mining techniques without a firm understanding of the problem domain has been labeled as "fishing" or "dredging" in the statistical literature (Keppel, 1991). These terms refer to the improper discovery of erroneous patterns that may be elicited and presented without understanding the spurious nature of the results and the consequential negative impact on statistical conclusion validity.

Broad outlines of the nine steps in KDD are presented here, based on the work of Fayyad et al. (1989). This practical overview demonstrates the interactive and iterative nature of the KDD process.

The initial step of KDD involves obtaining an in-depth understanding of the application domain via experience and examination of prior knowledge generated in the domain. It also involves in-depth work with the end-user to obtain an understanding of the needs and/or goals of the persons that the application of KDD will serve. The secondary step involves creating a target data set, which involves selecting the warehouse or data

set on which KDD is to be tested. At this point, the data subselection process has not begun. The third step involves subselection, preprocessing, and cleaning of the data to examine the impact of outliers and noise on the data set. It is during this step that decisions related to missing or "dirty" data are made. Wreden (1997, p. 47) refers to this step as "Purgatory before Nirvana." Brachman and Anand (1996) make the point that caution in "scrubbing" away anomalies in the data is warranted, since these could be crucial indicators of interesting domain phenomena.

The fourth step involves feature or dimension reduction. As is often the case, the number of variables that are gleaned in the second step are highly dimensional, and frequently there are certain dimensions that can be used to identify the factor structure and then model for the set of variables (Stevens, 1996). The use of dimensionality reduction or transformation methods is applied in this phase. Brachman and Anand (1996) label this reduction as parameter restriction and suggest it as a way to deal with massively overwhelming amounts of data. These authors state that not all variables will have utility in an analysis and believe that parameter shrinkage makes a model more robust. A commonly used approach is called a principal components analysis (PCA).

The fifth step involves choosing the data mining task. The selection of the data mining approach is based on a goal of the KDD process such as summarization, dependency modeling, classification, regression, or others (Fayyad et al., 1996). Each of these approaches has strengths and weaknesses, and the decision of what method to use is dependent on the task at hand and the inclination of the modeler. Brachman and Anand (1996) assert that the choice of approach can be determined as data sets are being investigated, a point that emphasizes the intertwining of data analysis and model creation in the KDD approach. These authors frame the model selection process in a "human-centered" approach, asserting that when completing the knowledge engineering that is required for model selection "background knowledge of the domain expert is crucial" (Brachman and Anand, 1996, p. 47). This factor contributes to the growing popularity of BNs. The BN's ability to incorporate human expertise into the modeling process is very powerful.

Subsequent to step five is the selection of the data mining algorithm, once again based on the overall goal of the KDD process. The selection of the best method to search for patterns in data is made. In addition, considerations of the needs of the end-user are included here, for example, making the determination if the system is to be used to explain or predict.

The seventh step involves the actual data mining, which is the active investigation of the transformed data set for interesting patterns, frequently via the use of data mining tools such as neural networks (NNs) or BNs. The final two steps involve the interpretation of the output of the data mining and finally the incorporation and/or dissemination of the knowledge out to the users. Generally, output involves the analysis of results and can be represented in many different formats such as reports of goodness of fit, outliers, scatterplots, graphical representations, and alarming (or monitoring) functions. The type of output (called "visualization") and dissemination is once again based on the needs of the user and the type of problem. The final step also involves reconciling new findings with previously known facts, a point of particular importance in clinical situations.

Data Mining Tools   In the healthcare/medical domain, commonly used data mining tools for knowledge discovery include NNs, BNs, decision trees, and classification and regression trees (CART). NN are known as connectionist, meaning that they parallel distributed processing models or AI and are designed to mimic the parallel processing ability of the human brain (Rumelhart, Hinton, and Williams, 1986). Decision trees create a binary tree structure until no more relevant branches can be derived, using a repeating series of branches that describes associations between attributes and a target variable. CART is used to build classification and regression trees for predicting categorical predictor variables (classification) and continuous dependent variables (regression). The use of BNss in KDD is gaining popularity due to its ability to handle uncertainty and to allow the inclusion of human expertise into the model building—very important traits when analyzing healthcare data (Lee and Abbott, 2003).

 The Use of Bayesian Networks in Healthcare KDD

BNs have emerged in recent years as a powerful data mining technique for handling uncertainty in complex domains and a fundamental technique for pattern recognition and classification (Heckerman, 1996; Pearl, 1988). The BN represents the joint probability distribution and domain (or expert) knowledge in a compact and understandable way. The BN provides a graphical diagram offering a comprehensive method of representing relationships among nodes (variables). The BN is based on the assumption that the classification of patterns is expressed in probabilistic terms between predic-

tors and outcome variables (Luttrell, 1994). As they are based on probability theory, BNs inherit many of the efficient methods and strong results of mathematical statistics (Sox et al., 1988).

BNs have been shown to have high performance of prediction in the medical domain. In particular, Bayesian approaches have been successfully applied to the diagnoses of pneumonia and breast cancer (Aronsky and Haug, 2000; Burnside, Rubin, and Shachter, 2000), classification of cytologic findings (Hamilton et al., 1995; Montironi et al., 1995), prediction of patient compliance to medication (Korrapati, Mukherjee, and Chalam, 2000), prediction of clinician compliance to medical practice guidelines (Abston et al., 1997), prognosis of head injuries (Sakellaropoulos and Nikiforidis, 1999), determination of the obesity risk factors (Bunn et al., 1999), and pattern recognition in narrative clinical reports (Wilcox and Hripcsak, 1999). The use of BN in nursing research, however, is almost nonexistent.

Explaining Bayesian Networks

The BN is a state-of-the-art representation of probabilistic knowledge. The BN illustrated in Fig. 29.2 is drawn from a well-known example from literature (Jirousek and Kushmerick, 1997; Lauritzen and Spiegelhalter, 1988). As mentioned earlier, BNs represent knowledge qualitatively through a graphical diagram (BN structure) with nodes (representing variables) and edges (arrows representing relationships). Quantitatively, the degree of dependency is expressed by probabilistic terms (parameters).

The network in Fig. 29.2 is defined by a graph, with the five nodes in the domain capturing the prior and conditional probabilities among nodes, shown adjacent to each node. Each root node (nodes without parents: X_1 [smoker] and X_2 [family history of cancer]) has a prior probability distribution only, and the nonroot nodes (child nodes with parents nodes: X_3 [bronchitis], X_4 [lung cancer], and X_5 [x-ray]) have conditional probability distributions quantifying the parent-child probabilistic relationships. The network in Fig. 29.2 can be interpreted to show that for instance, smoking can causally influence whether lung cancer is present, which can in turn causally influence whether a patient has a positive x-ray finding indicating lung cancer.

Note: A BN is expressed by prior and posterior (conditional) probabilities. In a situation where no other information (evidence) is available, the probability of an event occurring is a prior probability. Prior probability, for example, $P(X_3)$, is used only when no other information is available. The prior probability

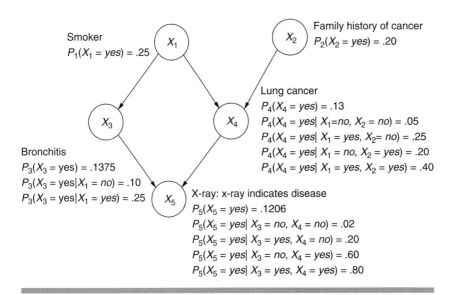

Figure 29.2
Typical Bayesian network.

becomes a posterior or conditional probability once the evidence is obtained. When clinicians have new information X_1, they can use the conditional probability of X_3 given X_1 instead of $P(X_3)$, which can be denoted as $P(X_3|X_1)$, meaning "the probability of X_3, given X_1" (Jensen, 1996).

Data Mining with Bayesian Networks

When BNs are used as data mining algorithms within the KDD process, the modeling process of BNs consists primarily of two learning phases. The first is the structural learning phase, which serves to construct a directed acyclic graph (a BN structure) that encodes dependence and independence relationships among variables. The second is the parameter learning phase, which assesses the prior and local conditional (posterior) probabilities, the so-called parameters, which in turn quantify the dependence relations defined by the BN structure.

Structural Learning Phase A potentially useful consequence of the network structure learning is that a hidden or unknown structure in the domain, frequently missed by investigators using conventional statistical methods, is identified (Spirtes, Glymour, and Scheine, 2000). There are two different approaches in finding a proper structure: search-and-score-based and constraint-based algorithms.

A search-and-score-based algorithm searches for a best model structure using a scoring metric, which reflects the goodness of fit of the structure to the data. Examples of systems that implement a search-and-score-based algorithm include the Bayesian knowledge discoverer (Ramoni and Sebastiani, 1997; BayesiaLab, 2003).

A constraint-based algorithm searches for a best possible structure by finding all of the possible conditional independence and dependence within a statistical test (e.g., Chi-square test). The systems that implement this algorithm include HUGIN (Jensen et al., 2002), BN PowerConstructor and BN PowerPredictor (Cheng, Bell, and Liu, 1997; Cheng, 1998; Cheng, 2000), and TETRAD (Spirtes et al., 2000). Constraint-based approaches allow the researcher to specify the relationships between variables using domain knowledge (personal expertise) in learning a structure. The use of constraints in the learning phase enables the investigators to feed the learning algorithm with existing and well-established structural knowledge of the domain. In other words, the specification of dependence or independence among pairs of variables can be manipulated by the investigator, based on the investigator's personal knowledge base and experience.

This use of human expertise is useful in guiding the learning algorithm toward the best possible model. In this step, researchers can incorporate domain knowledge obtained by a theoretical research framework, literature, or observational experience. This is one aspect of the BN approach which makes it so powerful and desirable to users.

Parameter Learning Phase   Once a satisfactory dependence structure is obtained, the next step is to estimate conditional probability relationships given BN structure and the data. The parameters can be assigned by expert knowledge, or learned from data by inducing a learning algorithm. The combination of both methods may strengthen the performance of a model. If a database includes complete data (no missing variables), the estimation of parameters is simple and can, given the link of the Bayesian structure, be done by simply calculating (counting and dividing) the prior or conditional probabilities; however, missing data commonly exists in the real world, especially in the healthcare domain. This requires the use of parameter estimation methods that address missing data.

The most commonly used parameter, learning algorithm, is the expectation-maximization (EM) algorithm (Lauritzen, 1995). This approach is useful for estimating the parameters of the conditional probability distributions in the case of missing data. The EM algorithm is an iterative algorithm that, given a Bayesian structure and a database of cases, determines a local maximum estimate of the parameters by assuming the pattern of missing data is uninformative (missing at random or missing completely at random). Maximum a posterior (MAP) is estimated in this situation when initial knowledge about the parameters is assigned; maximum likelihood (ML) is not. The software programs, such as HUGIN and Netica, provide the parameter learning algorithms. A full description and examples of the use of BN algorithms are beyond the scope of this chapter. A primer on the basics of BNs for nurse researchers can be found elsewhere (Lee and Abbott, 2003).

The use of BNs by nurse researchers is projected to gain momentum. One of the most attractive advantages of BNs to nurse researchers is the ability to use domain knowledge and personal expertise in the process of model building. In addition, the presentation of data and relationships in a graphical format and the ability to directly manipulate the structure based on personal knowledge and expertise is powerful. The BN approach is also known to be more robust to errors in the researcher's prior knowledge and uses rigorous methodology for dealing with missing data.

BNs can be used in various ways in nursing research. For instance, the structural learning method used by BNs can assist researchers in identifying the contributing factors (expected and nonexpected) relating to a specific patient outcome. Those identified contributing factors can be used to build a model to predict patients' outcomes, which allow for modification of nursing actions to improve quality of care. Knowledge discovery, using either the Bayesian approach or others mentioned earlier in this chapter, may be useful in discovering new patterns, contributors, and evidence of the nursing contribution to patient outcomes.

 Summary

As healthcare moves into a highly automated future where massive data warehouses are the norm, innovative discovery-based approaches will become increasingly important. This will require adoption of techniques different from the familiar traditional statistical approaches so common to data analysis in healthcare today. Healthcare may find itself in a position similar to other industries, where the importance of prediction may begin to rival that of explanation.

Management of patient outcomes requires a linkage and analysis of cost data, resource data, and clinical data, creating massive data repositories. Significant challenges present themselves due to the distribution, complexity, size, fragmentation, and frequently erroneous nature of healthcare data; however, when these components are merged, there is much to be discovered. What exists in the data that we do not know yet? How can we discover this knowledge and harness it to improve the quality of care? How can we handle huge sample sizes where the assumptions required of traditional approaches cannot be made? These questions will require that we begin to use new and innovative approaches to harness and analyze healthcare databases.

 References

Abbott, P. (2000). Knowledge discovery in large datasets: A primer for data mining applications in healthcare. In M. Ball, K. Hannah, S. Newbold, and J. Douglas (Eds.), *Nursing Informatics: Where Caring and Technology Meet* (3rd ed.). New York: Springer-Verlag.

Abston, K. C., Pryor, T. A., Haug, P. J., and Anderson, J. L. (1997). Inducing practice guidelines from a hospital database. In *Proceedings/AMIA Annual Fall Symposium* (pp. 168–172).

Aronsky, D. and Haug, P. J. (2000). Automatic identification of patients eligible for a pneumonia guideline. In *Proceedings/AMIA Annual Symposium* (pp. 12–16).

BayesiaLab [computer software]. (2003). Version 1.3.1. France: Bayesia SA.

Brachman R. and Anand, T. (1996). The process of knowledge discovery in databases. In U. Fayyad, G. Piatetesky-Shapiro, and P. Smyth (Eds.), *Advances in Knowledge Discovery and Data Mining* (pp. 37–57). Cambridge, MA: MIT Press.

Bunn, C. C., Du, M., Niu, K., Johnson, T. R., Poston, W. S. C., and Foreyt, J.P. (1999). Predicting the risk of obesity using a Bayesian network. In *Proceedings/ AMIA Annual Symposium* (p. 1035).

Burnside, E., Rubin, D., and Shachter, R. (2000). A Bayesian network for mammography. In *Proceedings/ AMIA Annual Symposium* (pp. 106–110).

Cheng, J. (1998). *BN PowerConstructor* [on-line]. *http://www.cs.ualberta.ca/~jcheng/bnpc.htm*.

Cheng, J. (2000). *BN PowerPredictor* [on-line]. *http://www.cs.ualberta.ca/~jcheng/bnpp.htm*.

Cheng, J., Bell, D. A., and Liu, W. (1997). An algorithm for Bayesian belief network construction from data. In *Proceeding of AI & STAT* (pp. 83–90).

Fayyad, U., Piatetesky-Shapiro, G., and Smyth, P. (1996). From data mining to knowledge discovery. In U. Fayyad, G. Piatetesky-Shapiro, and P. Smyth (Eds.), *Advances in Knowledge Discovery and Data Mining* (pp. 1–36). Cambridge, MA: MIT Press.

Goodwin, L., Schlitz, K., and Jasion, B. (1997). Data mining for improved patient outcomes. *Tarheel Nurse* 59(4):21–22.

Hamilton, P. W., Montironi, R., Abmayr, W., Bibbo, M., Anderson, N., Thompson, D., et al. (1995). Clinical applications of Bayesian belief networks in pathology. *Pathologica* 87:237–245.

Heckerman, D. E. (1996). Bayesian networks for knowledge discovery. In U.M. Fayyad, G. Piatetsky-Shapiro, P. Smyth, and R. Uthurusamy (Eds.), *Advances in Knowledge Discovery and Data Mining* (pp. 273–305). Menlo Park, CA: MIT Press.

Jensen, F. V., Kjaerulff, U. B., Lang, M., and Madsen, A. L. (2002). HUGIN-The tool for Bayesian networks and influence diagrams. In *Proceedings of the First European Workshop on Probabilistic Graphical Models* (pp. 212–221).

Jirousek, R. and Kushmerick, N. (1997). Constructing probabilistic models. *International Journal of Medical Informatics* 45:9–18.

Keppel, G. (1991). *Design and Analysis: A Researchers Handbook* (3rd ed.). Upper Saddle River, NJ: Prentice Hall.

Korrapati, R., Mukherjee, S., and Chalam, K. V. (2000). A Bayesian framework to determine patient compliance in glaucoma cases. In *Proceedings/AMIA Annual Fall Symposium* (p. 1050).

Lauritzen, S. L. (1995). The EM algorithm for graphical association models with missing data. *Computational Statistics and Data Analysis* 19:191–201.

Lauritzen, S. L. and Spiegelhalter, D. J. (1988). Local computations with probabilities on graphical structures and their application to expert systems. *Journal of the Royal Statistical Society Series B* 50:157–194.

Lee, S.-M. and Abbott, P. (2003). Bayesian networks for knowledge discovery in large datasets: Basics for nurse researchers. *Journal of Biomedical Informatics* 36:389–399.

Luttrell, S. P. (1994). Partitioned mixture distribution: An adaptive Bayesian network for low-level image processing. *IEE Proceedings on Vision, Image and Signal Processing* 141:251–260.

McCormick, K. (1981). Nursing research using computerized data bases. In H. Heffernan (Ed.), In *Proceedings of the 5th Annual Symposium on Computer Applications in Medical Care*. Silver Spring, MD: IEEE Computer Society Press.

Montironi, R., Bartels, P. H., Thompson, D., Scarpelli, M., and Hamilton, P. W. (1995). Prostatic intraepithelial neoplasia (PIN). Performance of Bayesian belief network for diagnosis and grading. *Journal of Pathology* 177:153–162.

Munhall, P. (1997). Out of the box. *Image: Journal of Nursing Scholarship* 29(3):203.

Pauker, S., Gorry, G., Kassier, J., and Schwartz, W. (1976). Toward the simulation of clinical cognition: Taking a present illness by computer. *The American Journal of Medicine* (60)[7]:981–996.

Pearl, J. (1988). *Probabilistic Reasoning in Intelligent Systems: Networks of Plausible Inference*. San Francisco, CA: Morgan Kaufmann Publishers.

Ramoni, M. and Sebastiani, P. (1997). *Learning Bayesian networks from incomplete databases* (Rep. No. KMI-TR-43). Milton Keynes, U.K.: Knowledge Media Institute.

Rumelhart, D. E., Hinton, G. E., and Williams, R. J. (1986). Learning internal representation by error propagation. In D. E. Rumelhart and J. L. McClelland (Eds.), *Parallel Distributed Processing*. Cambridge, MA: MIT Press.

Saarenvita, G. (1999). Data modeling for direct mail: A lesson in predictive modeling. *DB2* 4(1):40.

Sakellaropoulos, G. C. and Nikiforidis, G. C. (1999). Development of a Bayesian network for the prognosis of head injuries using graphical model selection techniques. *Methods of Information in Medicine* 38:37–42.

Sox, H. C., Blatt, M.A., Higgins, M. C., and Marton, K. I. (1988). *Medical Decision Making*. Boston, MA: Butterworths.

Spirtes, P., Glymour, C., and Scheine, R. (2000). *Causation, Prediction, and Search*. (2nd ed.). Cambridge, MA: MIT Press.

Stevens, J. (1996). *Applied Multivariate Statistics for the Social Sciences*. (3rd edition). Mahwah, NJ: Lawrence Erlbaum Associates.

Wasserman, M. (2000). Data mining. *Regional Review* Quarter 3, Vol. 10, No. 3. Accessed August 17, 2004: *http://www.bos.frb.org/economic/nerr/rr2000/q3/ mining.htm*

Wilcox, A. and Hripcsak, G. (1999). Classification algorithms applied to narrative reports. In *Proceedings/AMIA Annual Symposium* (pp. 455–459).

Wreden, N. (Feb. 17, 1997). The mother lode: Data mining digs deep for business intelligence. *Communications Week* 43–47.

PART 7

Consumer's Use of Informatics

CHAPTER 30

Consumer and Patient Use of Computers for Health

Rita D. Zielstorff

OBJECTIVES

1. Review the types of computer applications used by patients and consumers related to health.
2. Discuss several issues related to patient and consumer applications in health, and promising developments for dealing with these issues.
3. Explain the nurse informatician's role in patient and consumer computing.
4. List some areas for research related to patient and consumer computing.
5. Provide a list of resources for further learning.

KEY WORDS

consumer computing
patient computing
Internet-based health applications
computer information systems
consumer health informatics
nursing informatics

Introduction

Consumerism has seen a dramatic rise in the United States over the past decade. More recently, this movement has expanded into the arena of health. Consumers of health services (patients, families, and family caregivers) are educating themselves on all aspects of health, wellness, and disease. Armed with this education, they are demanding a greater say in decisions that affect them and the persons they care about. The traditional role of the patient as the object of care, acquiescent to decisions made by the experts, is being challenged (Solucient, 2003; Ferguson, 2002c). Today, patients and families expect to be partners in care, evaluating with their caregivers the implications of diagnostic tests and the ramifications of treatment modalities, including cost and effectiveness (Solucient, 2003; Oster et al., 2000; Fox and Rainie, 2000).

The Health Insurance Portability and Accountability Act (HIPAA) Privacy Rule grants specific rights to patients and family members regarding their health information. For example, patients must be made aware when their record is shared outside of prespecified boundaries, and patients must be granted the ability to view their medical record, and to correct information if that is warranted (USDHHS, 2003).

The Internet has been a boon to healthcare consumerism. A Google search on any health topic will typically return thousands of pages, varying greatly in relevance and quality, but nonetheless usually useful to the health information seeker (Fox and Fallows, 2003). Caregivers routinely report the phenomenon of patients arriving for a visit with a ream of printouts related to their diagnosis or treatment, asking the physician or nurse to comment on the material's relevance to their particular case (Ferguson, 2002d).

Static content pages are only one type of health-related resources on the Web. Links to diagnosis-specific support groups, the ability to communicate with family, friends, and healthcare providers about one's health, and a variety of interactive resources for record-keeping, monitoring, and decision-making are also available. In this chapter, we will provide an overview of these applications, discuss several issues related to consumer use of computers for health, and review current developments for dealing with these issues. In addition, we will provide a rationale for nurses' involvement in this arena, list special considerations in designing computer applications for patients and consumers, and discuss some areas for research related to patient and consumer computing for health.

 ## Application Areas: Consumer Use of Computers for Health

Information Seeking

Information seeking about health matters is a common use of computers by patients and consumers. According to a 2002 HarrisInteractive survey, approximately two-thirds of the adult U.S. population has access to the Internet, of these, about 80% had used the computer recently for health-related matters (Harris Interactive, 2002a,b).

In a different survey, the Pew Internet & American Life project found that the number of persons who have used the Internet to seek health information grew by 59% between March 2000 and December 2002. The researchers report that 73 million persons, or two-thirds of the online population, had used the Internet to get health-related information (Madden, 2003). Information seekers declared that they use the Internet because it is fast, anonymous, and always available. By searching multiple sites and looking for commonality in the content, they are able to discern the accuracy of the information. The topics most frequently searched on, according to another Pew report, are diseases, treatments, and diet or nutritional information (Fox and Fallows, 2003).

Sponsorship of static content sites varies widely. Healthcare organizations may offer their communities a public Web site that includes health articles developed by their own professional experts, or licensed from vendors. A well-known example is the Mayo Clinic, whose public site, *mayoclinic.com*, provides a wealth of health information and tools. For-profit entities such as pharmaceutical firms, drugstore chains, and durable medical equipment vendors frequently sponsor public sites. An example is *diabetes.com* sponsored by GlaxoSmithKline. Professional societies and foundations frequently sponsor public sites devoted to educating consumers about health matters that are their particular focus. Examples are *americanheart.org*, sponsored by the American Heart Association, and *lungusa.org*, sponsored by the American Lung Association. Some vendors develop health Web site appli-

cations and license them to other entities, allowing branding or co-branding by the licensing organization. Two of these companies are Healthvision, Inc. and HealthGate Data Corp.

The U.S. government has developed several resources for consumers seeking health information. These include *healthfinder.gov*, a collection of vetted links to health-related Web sites that is sponsored by the Office of Disease Prevention and Health Promotion of the U.S. Department of Health and Human Services; *medlineplus.gov*, a consumer-friendly site developed by the National Library of Medicine and the National Institutes of Health; and *medicare.gov*, devoted to information specific to the Medicare program and to health topics for seniors, sponsored by the Centers for Medicare and Medicaid Services (CMS) of the U.S. Department of Health and Human Services.

Communication and Support

Electronic mail continues to be the "killer app" of the Internet. Many e-mail users find it particularly useful for health-related matters. They may communicate informally with friends and family about health. They may use e-mail to keep family informed about the health status of one of the family. They may engage in online support groups whose focus is on a particular disease or condition or they may communicate directly with their healthcare providers about their own or a family member's condition (Fox and Fallows, 2003).

Online support groups can provide an indispensable, even life-saving resource to patients and families. Interested persons can find an online support group for almost any condition, ranging from Alzheimer's disease to Zellweger syndrome. Again, the sponsorship varies, from healthcare organizations providing local groups for their patients, to national organizations and foundations, to privately sponsored groups, to grant-funded research projects. Participation in the group can also vary. Some groups are monitored by health professionals such as medical social workers, nurses, or physicians. Others are unmonitored. For suffering patients and families, the knowledge that others are facing similar situations, and have found ways to cope, can be a source of hope and consolation (Brennan, 1995; Fox and Fallows, 2003; Gustafson et al., 2001; Ferguson, 2002a). In addition, members of the group sometimes share information about latest research, treatments, and clinical trials that may not be common knowledge (Ferguson, 2002a). For those who are homebound, the online group may be a lifeline. Technical aids such as screen readers for the visually impaired can even assist those who have physical disabilities to use the computer for online support.

Direct communication with one's healthcare provider is high on the list of desired resources for most patients and families. A survey by HarrisInteractive found that 90% of Internet users would like to be able to communicate with their doctor or doctor's staff (HarrisInteractive, 2002). More than half of these would switch doctors or health plans to get the service, and more than one-third would even be willing to pay for it. The most frequently cited reasons for wishing this type of communication are to (a) get health reminders, (b) get personalized information after the doctor's visit, (c) ask questions when a visit is not necessary, (d) make appointments, (e) renew prescriptions, and (f) get lab results (HarrisInteractive, 2000, 2002). Couchman and colleagues found similar results among their patients in Houston who had access to the Internet (Couchman, Forjuoh, and Rascoe, 2001).

The number of providers offering this type of service is much less than the demand. A recent survey by Manhattan Research (2004) found that about 20% of physicians currently offer online communication with their patients. Generally the reasons for reluctance to offer the service include (a) liability, (b) reimbursement, (c) confidentiality and security, and (d) impact on office workflow (MacDonald, 2003; Manhattan Research, 2004; Patt et al., 2003; Wilson, 2003). Those who do offer it note increased patient satisfaction and increased sense of partnership with patients who participate (Patt et al., 2003). In some arrangements, patients communicate with staff for issues such as appointment requests and prescription renewal requests. In others, patients are able to send nonurgent clinical questions to nursing staff or directly to the physician. Generally the practice absorbs the cost of the technology supporting the service, although some health plans may charge a subscription fee for clinical messaging (MacDonald, 2003).

The technology for providing the service ranges from simply giving patients the provider's e-mail address, to registering them with a username and password to use a secure Web site. The Web site may be administered by the practice, or by the provider group or network, or the clinician may subscribe to a vendor-provided service. For example, Medem, an organization formed by several physician professional associations, offers secure patient messaging to member physicians and their staffs for a nominal monthly subscription fee. The fee can be waived if the physician agrees to allow "sponsor" ads to appear on the physician's home page. The physician is able to set up the site using online tools. (For details, visit *http://www.medem.com.*)

Further along the spectrum are "e-visits," structured interactions that enable patients to describe a problem in some detail (usually with the help of a topic-specific questionnaire), and receive advice from the healthcare provider, thus avoiding the time and expense of an in-person visit. An independent study sponsored by RelayHealth, a vendor of this type of application, found in a pilot study that patients who had access to the online visit service spent on average $1.87 less per member per month on office visits, yielding savings on the part of the insurer of $1.54 per member per month (RelayHealth, 2002). The majority of physicians and patients were satisfied with the service, and indicated that they would like to continue using the service after the pilot period (RelayHealth, 2002). First Health, a managed care company, will reimburse providers at a rate of $25 each for up to 24 consultations per year, believing that the service not only serves patient satisfaction, but could potentially reduce costs (Smith, 2002).

The California HealthCare Foundation recently released a comprehensive report on the subject of patient-provider communication and the technological solutions available for meeting the need. The report compares the solutions with respect to complexity of infrastructure; degree of integration with systems in the office; degree of structure in the messaging, cost, security of information, and potential for reimbursement (MacDonald, 2003). The report contains interviews with healthcare providers where the solutions are implemented, providing a real-world glimpse of the issues and benefits of these applications. A number of organizations have published guidelines for clinicians thinking of offering the service to minimize the risks (see Federation of State Medical Boards, 2002; Kane and Sands, 1998; Medem, 2002; SCPIE, 2002).

Personal Health Records

Even though patients' medical records are more available to them now, thanks to the HIPAA privacy rule, many consumers are daunted by the size, complexity, illegibility, and sheer number of institutionally-based medical records that accumulate over a person's lifetime. As an alternative, many keep their own personal health records, both for themselves and for their family members. The structure of computer-based personal health records varies widely, from those that simply collect text under major headings such as allergies, problems, drugs, procedures, and so forth, to those that encode users' entries with ICD9 and CPT codes, or even with the broad range of terms found in the National Library of Medicine's Unified Medical Language System.

Consumers can buy a personal health record application in any software store, loading the program onto their own computer, and storing their record there. One example is RecordSmart, supplied by MyHealth123, another is Health-Minder, which can be downloaded from *www.health-minder.com*. Alternatively, consumers can subscribe to a Web site where their record will be held securely. Insurers and health plans frequently offer an online personal health record application as a member benefit. Many healthcare organizations offer the service on their community Web sites. A number of these applications include interactive health management tools such as health risk assessments, smoking cessation programs, fitness trackers, pregnancy centers, calorie intake monitors, and any number of calculators. WebMD's Personal Health Manager, available through sponsoring organizations that offer it on their Web site, even includes the ability for the user to subscribe to a wireless messaging service. Reminders can be sent to the user's Web-enabled phone to take medication, record blood pressure, and so forth. Built-in alerts can advise the user to call the physician if recorded values are outside the acceptable range.

Different from comprehensive medical record-keeping applications, a number of sites allow the consumer to keep a record of personal disease-specific information. For example, MyDiabetes.com and MyAsthma.com allow the patient to record parameters specific to those diseases, providing graphs, decision aids, and a wealth of related materials geared to supporting the patient who has those conditions.

A number of issues arise when the personal health record is stored in a place other than the user's own computer. Security of access to the data must be assured as well as privacy. Will the data be shared with anyone other than the user? Are policies for data sharing clearly described and accessible to the user? Can the user opt out of data sharing or e-marketing of goods and services based on the data entered in the record? If the user terminates his or her relationship with the vendor, can a paper or electronic version of the accumulated record be provided, and will the data be subsequently purged? If the vendor goes out of business, will the user be notified, and what will happen with the information that is stored on the vendor's servers?

Several organizations have developed standards and guidelines relating to the consumer's relationship with vendors who supply personal health record systems over the Internet. They include URAC (*www.urac.com*), Hi-Ethics (*www.hi-ethics.org*), and ASTM International (Standard E2211.02, available at *www.astm.org*).

Bridging the gap between the professional's record and the personal health record is the shared patient record, one in which both professional and patient contribute information. Two examples: Caregroup's PatientSite is a Web-based application that permits patients to view their medical record, and to record information online in a separate section of the record (see *http://www.caregroup.org/patientsite.asp*). Palo Alto Medical Foundation provides an application called PAMFOnline that permits secure communication with the physician's staff (and with the physician or nurse for a nominal subscription fee); patients can view components of their medical record and obtain their health summary. They can make notes on the record for their own personal use (see *https://mychart.sutterhealth.org/pamf/default.asp*). Tang and colleagues find that the service improves patient access to health information, improves communication with physicians and staff, promotes patient satisfaction, and improves office efficiency (Tang et al., 2003).

The effects of providing the patient with access to their online medical record have not been widely evaluated, since the application is so new. In a small study at Columbia University, Cimino and colleagues concluded that "use of the system enhanced the patients' understanding of their conditions and improved their communication with their physicians," with no reported adverse effects (Cimino, Patel, and Kushniruk, 2002).

Decision Support

A broad range of decision-support applications is available to the interested consumer. Some incorporate multimedia presentations of patients who have the condition that is the subject of the search (for example, *www.dipex.org* has videos on several cancer subjects as well has heart conditions, epilepsy, and others). Others incorporate statistics-based presentations on alternatives in areas such as treatment of early-stage prostate cancer or hormone replacement therapy (for example, see the Health Decision Guides at *www.mayoclinic.com*). Some of these programs offer prognostic information based on personal information entered (for example, see the Health Decision Guide on adjuvant therapy for breast cancer at *www.mayoclinic.com*).

Some applications are straightforward decision trees that offer advice for follow-up depending on the information entered (for example, the Healthwise Knowledgebase, available for free from many hospital community Web sites, offers a "Check Your Symptoms" section for many health topics, including fever in children). Several sites allow users to enter the names of medications they are taking to obtain drug-drug interactions (one example is at *www.drugdigest.org*). Brennan and colleagues provided decision-support tools to caregivers of Alzheimer's patients in an application that included an array of support functions (Brennan, 1995). The Comprehensive Health Enhancement Support System (CHESS) system also includes an array of support functions that includes decision-support tools, though it is not primarily a decision-support application (Gustafson et al., 2002).

Some sites provide sophisticated risk assessment tools that use the consumer's input to summarize health risks, then suggest individualized changes in lifestyle that may influence these risks (for example, the Personal Health Manager tools available to registered users of WebMD can take a variety of health risk assessments, both general and topic-specific). There are smoking cessation programs available that survey the user about readiness to change, then offer action steps appropriate to the user (one example is at *www.lungusa.org*).

Schwitzer provided a review of five decision-support applications, and noted that none of them offered all four of what he considers to be key Web-enabled features: (a) outcomes probability data tailored to the individual user, (b) multimedia presentations of patient interviews, (c) an interactive support network, and (d) free access over the Internet (Schwitzer, 2002). Use of the computer for decision support among patients and consumers is covered in more depth in another chapter in this book.

Disease Management

Technological support for joint patient-provider collaboration in disease management is a promising application area, though not yet widespread. Patients or family caregivers are enrolled in a program and participate using one of a number of technologies. They may log on to an Internet portal to record parameters such as blood pressure, blood sugar, or peak flow; periodically complete a disease-focused questionnaire that captures broader data about mental and physical function or use a device that captures physical parameters such as weight or blood sugar and connect it to a telephone or computer, causing the information to be relayed to nurses whose responsibility is to monitor the incoming data. Interactive voice response systems have been used successfully to monitor patients with conditions such as obsessive-compulsive disease, hypertension, asthma, and others. Values outside the desired range may prompt a phone call requesting the patient to alter their regimen or come in for a visit (Adams et al., 2003).

There have been reports of reduced hospitalizations and reduced incidence of complications of chronic disease by employing these technologies. At this time, these programs are used mainly by insurers and health plans, who see cost benefits by aggressively managing populations of patients with specific chronic conditions. For example, one Kentucky-based health plan found 37% reduction in incidence of heart attacks and 26% reduction in costs by employing an online disease-management program that coordinates several aspects of care (Anonymous, 2003).

In a large government-funded randomized control trial at Columbia University named IDEATel (Informatics for Diabetes Education and Telemedicine), researchers will assess the effects of a comprehensive home-based telemedicine program with underserved rural and inner-city patients with diabetes (Shea et al., 2002). Live videoconferencing with nurses, use of devices to record and electronically transmit fingerstick glucose and blood pressure, and access to a project Web site are the technologies that are being used with the intervention group. Variables such as costs, outcomes, and patient satisfaction will be assessed.

In a more consumer-driven mode, some Web sites offer the user a disease self-management program, providing educational materials, tools, links to additional resources, and the ability to record disease-specific parameters. One such example for diabetics is *www. diabetes-self-mgmt.com*.

 ## Issues in Consumer Computing for Health

Variability in Quality of Information Available to Consumers

Because there are no quality controls on the content of health information available on the Internet, health professionals have been concerned about the influence of unreliable information on consumer and patient behavior. Research shows, however, that the fears may be unfounded. Ferguson observed that although both health professionals and patients are concerned with the quality of information available on the World Wide Web, patients are less so. They claim that the Web is no more a dangerous medium than is print information, or even verbal information dispensed by well-meaning but occasionally incorrect healthcare professionals (Ferguson, 2002c,d). Researchers for the Pew Internet and American Life project found that consumers used a variety of tactics to discern the veracity of materials. The most common one was to see whether the same information appeared on more than one site. If so, the information was deemed to be reliable (Fox and Fallow, 2003).

Guidelines have been published to assist both the developer of health-related materials, and the health information seeker. The Health On the Net Foundation (HON) has developed a set of principles and corresponding guidelines for developers of health information published on the Web. Those who follow the guidelines are encouraged to place the HON code seal on their Web pages. The eight principles are authority, complementarity, confidentiality, attribution, justifiability, transparency of authorship, transparency of sponsorship, and honesty in advertising and editorial policy (Health On the Net Foundation, 1997).

A number of organizations have developed guidelines for health information seekers to use when evaluating the quality of materials they read. For example, The Consumer and Patient Health Information Section of the Medical Library Association evaluates Web sites based on the following criteria: credibility, sponsorship/authorship, content, audience, currency, disclosure, purpose, links, design, interactivity, and disclaimers. Its list of top ten health Web sites is at *http://www.mlanet.org/resources/medspeak/topten.html*. Links to sites that offer guidelines for evaluating health materials are gathered in a special section of the National Library of Medicine's MedlinePlus site: *http://www.nlm.nih.gov/medlineplus/evaluatinghealthinformation.html*.

Some organizations now certify health sites, offering the consumer another level of confidence with the credibility of the site. URAC applies a rigorous set of 50 standards when evaluating a site. The standards cover such areas as privacy and security, disclosure, how content is developed and revised, and how the site chooses to link to other sites. There are also standards about policies, procedures, and quality oversight processes. The URAC seal on a Web site assures the user of the site's compliance with these standards. Further information can be found at *http://Webapps.urac.org/Websiteaccreditation/default.htm*.

Lack of Security in Internet-based Transactions

As stated earlier, there is a great demand from consumers to communicate with their healthcare providers online. Clinicians sometimes offer their patients the ability to communicate with them via open Internet e-mail. This poses several problems, however. For one thing, it is not uncommon for families to share a single e-mail address. Messages sent to a patient may be read by family members, resulting in possible violation of privacy. Also, open Internet transactions are subject to interception, resulting again in possible violation of privacy. The HIPAA privacy rule strongly encourages providers and organizations to use more secure means of communications with patients and consumers (USDHHS, 2003).

The preferred approach is to offer the patient or family caregiver a secure method of communication. This may be accomplished by using a message encrypting service, or by offering the patient a password-protected secure site, where all transactions are encrypted. This requires that the patient's computer have the capability for 128-bit encryption, but the software is easily downloadable for free. For a tutorial on security, privacy and confidentiality issues on the Internet, see Kelly and McKenzie (2002).

Uneven Accessibility Across Age, Ethnic, and Socioeconomic Groups: The Digital Divide

From the time that statistics were first gathered about Internet usage, it was apparent that Internet users were not representative of the population at large. Surveys consistently show that Internet users are better educated, wealthier, younger, urban, and largely White (Harris Interactive, 2003, 2004). Although the demographics of Internet users are slowly changing, there persists what has become known as the Digital Divide (Lenhart et al., 2003). This is a matter of concern to health providers and public health officials, because poorer, minority, and older populations have more health problems, and are the very ones who could benefit from Internet-based healthcare applications.

Healthy People 2010, the U.S. government's agenda for population health in the current decade, has as one of its overarching goals the elimination of health disparities among different segments of the population (USDHHS, 2000). In the focus area of health communication, one specific objective is to "Increase the proportion of households with access to the Internet at home." Recognizing that unequal access to technology poses a number of social and public health consequences among underserved populations, the U.S. government has initiated several programs to overcome the Digital Divide. The National Cancer Institute has funded pilot programs that enhance access to health information, cancer information, decision-support tools, and computer training for underserved populations (Kreps, 2002). The National Library of Medicine has funded several initiatives that are described in the online proceedings of the American Medical Informatics Association's 2003 Spring Congress (available at *http://www.amia.org/meetings/archive/s03/info.html*).

This is a small sample of the many initiatives underway that are intended to remedy the existing disparity in access to online applications and content.

Educational and Cultural Barriers

Even among those who have access to the Internet, factors such as literacy, language preference, and cultural background can be barriers to use of the Internet for health.

The 1992 Adult Literacy Survey (the most recent one performed) found that up to 47% of adults were functionally or marginally illiterate, and that up to 66% of adults age 60 or over had inadequate or marginal literacy skills (Kirsch et al., 1993). It is generally accepted that persons with low literacy will also have low health literacy, because so much of medical terminology is dense and complex. A recent report from the Institute of Medicine estimates that nearly half of the American adult population has low health literacy (IOM, 2004). Yet most Web-accessible material related to health is written at high-school level or greater. Lazarus and Mora found that of 1,000 Internet sites reviewed, only 10 were appropriate for limited literacy adults (Lazarus and Mora, 2000). Croft and Peterson found that asthma-related patient education material in 90 Web sites required an average reading level of 10th grade, and that only nine of them contained multilingual patient education material (Croft and Peterson, 2002).

Solutions to the problem of reaching low-literate populations include (a) better writing techniques (HSPH), (b) greater use of visuals and interactivity (Lazarus and Mora 2000; Croft and Peterson 2002), and (c) adherence to empirically derived usability principles (Spool et al., 1999; USDHHS, 2004).

Some vendors have developed consumer-friendly terminologies that map to medical terminologies to assist consumers with finding, understanding, and recording health-related material. For example, Intelligent Medical Objects, Inc. has developed a Personal Health Terminology (PHT) that contains synonyms for the most commonly used ICD9 and CPT codes (Intelligent Medical Objects, 2000). Wellmed Inc. has developed the Consumer Health Thesaurus, a large thesaurus of consumer terms that maps to terms in the Unified Medical Language System (UMLS) (Marshall, 2000). Apelon, Inc. a supplier of healthcare terminology software and services has developed a Distributed Terminology System (DTS) whose knowledge base includes a Consumer Health Vocabulary (CHV). The CHV contains over 15,000 commonly used words and phrases that include medical conditions, symptoms, tests, and procedures (Apelon, 2003).

This writer has advocated for the development of a consumer-friendly nomenclature that ideally would be included in the UMLS and available in the public domain (Zielstorff, 2003). Tse and Soergel provide a cogent discussion of the challenges such an effort would pose. These include (a) constantly evolving lay expressions for health matters, (b) much local variation, and (c) imperfect lay understanding of medical concepts (Tse and Soergel, 2003). Developers of MedlinePlus assert that a special nomenclature may not be needed, and that a terminology server using special algorithms can assist users with common misspellings and other support measures to find appropriate information (McCray et al., 2000).

Physical and Cognitive Disabilities

Fox and Fallows found in 2002 that only 38% of persons with disabilities went online, compared with 58% of all Americans. Of those, 20% said their disability makes using the Internet difficult (Fox and Fallows, 2002, p. 21). Yet the Internet has enormous potential to assist the homebound and disabled. Zeng and Parmanto found that of 103 consumer health information Web sites, none complied completely with Web accessibility guidelines. For example, text equivalents for all nontext objects on a page should be embedded in the code, so that it is accessible to automated screen readers that are used by the blind (W3C, 1999).

Elderly users are even more specialized in their needs. In a review of design considerations for elderly users, Demiris and colleagues point out that diminished visual acuity and color discrimination, memory deficits, and increased need for processing time impose specific requirements on the design of applications. In addition, a large proportion of the elderly are inexperienced using computers, so the applications must be especially easy to use (Demiris, Finkelstein, and Speedie, 2001). The American Association of Retired Persons found that common "Web words" like "URL," "visit [a site]," and "link" are not understood by Web-naïve elderly persons (Chisnell, Lee, and Redish, 2004).

Impact on Relationship with Healthcare Providers

Just as computers have revolutionized consumers' and patients' abilities to care for themselves, so have they affected patient-clinician relationships. The knowledgeable patient is no longer so dependent on the clinician's advice, and, in fact, may challenge it. The empowered patient wishes to collaborate in the clinician's care, and wants to be treated respectfully as a full-fledged partner in achieving mutually agreed-on goals (Brennan, 1999). Some clinicians welcome the new partnership, believing that better-quality, lower-cost care will result (Zablocki, 1998; Kaplan and Brennan, 2001). Others have a more difficult time adjusting to the power shift, and would rather not deal with patients who will not accept their recommendations at face value. Ferguson calls this disconnect "The Gap," and believes that providers who cannot accommodate to the new paradigm will lose patients to those who can (Ferguson, 2002b). Dickerson and Brennan (2002) provide a theoretical discussion of the Internet's role in changing the traditional model of provider-patient relationship, shifting from the gatekeeper model to one that is more egalitarian.

Another area that threatens many healthcare professionals is the notion of patients as independent copractitioners. Online support groups provide consolation, comfort, hope, and empathetic human contact—hallmarks of the care that any good nurse would provide. Furthermore, these are available 24 hours a day and on demand, something that no individual professional could do. In addition, support groups may provide cutting-edge knowledge of disease processes, treatments, and clinical trials of which even the patients' providers may not be aware. Patients within the group may bring their background expertise to the knowledge that is shared, helping to evaluate it for validity (Ferguson, 2002a).

Kaplan and Brennan (2001) advocate for a new, three-way partnership among patient, provider, and technology. This partnership should be centered on the patient/consumer, not on the provider or institution. The authors advocate that health informaticians develop tools to support this new relationship.

The Nurse Informatician's Role in Consumer and Patient Computing

Scope and Standards of Nursing Informatics Practice   It seems obvious that a technology that so impacts patients' and consumers' health decisions should be a central focus of nurse informaticians. The most recent edition of the American Nurses Association Scope and Practice of Nursing Informatics Practice (ANA, 2001) makes this explicit. The new definition of the field states that:

> Nursing informatics facilitates the integration of data, information, and knowledge to support *patients*, nurses and other providers in their decision-making in all roles and settings [emphasis added]. [p. vii]

In addition, the revised Scope and Standards make several references to patients' use of technology for managing their health, and the role of nursing informatics specialists in supporting that function. For example, the patient is now included as a focus of education about effective and ethical uses of technology (p. 19), and the patient's use of information tools and resources for health information is included as a focus for nursing informatics research (p. 20).

Areas of Nursing Expertise that can be Applied to Consumer/Patient Computing   Informaticians who are nurses bring unique skills to the arena of consumer informatics by virtue of their professional education in nursing. Among these skills:

- *Deep expertise in patient education:* A core competency of nursing professionals is patient education. Nurse informaticians can combine their expertise in patient education with their informatics skills to design content and applications that are effective for imparting knowledge and skills needed to maintain health and manage acute and chronic conditions. It is well within the nursing informatics skill set to design content that is interactive, effective, and sensitive to patients' literacy, language, and cultural needs.

- *Cultural diversity in the workforce and a strong ethic of cultural sensitivity:* The nursing workforce itself is more ethnically and culturally diverse than most professions. Cultural sensitivity is highly valued in nursing education and practice. This background serves nurse informaticians well in producing applications and materials that are culturally appropriate.

- *Strong background in both patient- and community-focused research:* Nurses have a long tradition of patient-focused research, a strength that can be applied to the many areas of consumer and patient computing that are begging for research. At the same time, nurses are very comfortable in the areas of implementing and evaluating interventions targeted at populations, by virtue of their expertise in community health.

- *Strong heritage of patient advocacy and patient empowerment:* While nurses are not immune to feeling threatened by the empowered patient, it is also true that nurses have always had as a central goal to assist each patient to achieve as much self-sufficiency as possible (ANA, 2003).

Encouraging and enabling the patient to use technology to achieve that self-sufficiency is a natural extension of nursing care.

Special Considerations in Designing Applications for Patients and Consumers

Nurse informaticians who have designed or implemented applications for health professionals to use should be aware of the special considerations required in applications for consumers and patients. They may need to seek further education to gain the skills and knowledge needed to design, implement, and evaluate these systems. These special considerations include:

■ *Lay versus professional nomenclature:* Professional nomenclature is so ingrained in most clinicians that they often are not even aware that they are using language that is foreign to the patient or consumer. Interactive applications, forms, and static content designed for patients and consumers must be scoured for professional terms. Lay terms must be substituted whenever possible. When professional terms must be used, a definition or an equivalent lay term in parentheses should be supplied. Though it does not incorporate a formal consumer nomenclature, the UMLS has many consumer-friendly synonyms for medical terms. The UMLS Metathesaurus can be browsed online by applying for a free license at *http://umlsks.nlm.nih.gov/kss/ servlet/Turbine/template/admin,user,KSS_login.vm.*

■ *General literacy and health literacy:* It is a myth that materials written at an 8th grade level will not be appropriate for more highly educated people. All readers, no matter what their educational level, appreciate material that is written clearly and in plain language (National Cancer Institute, 1994). There are many books, courses, and other resources to assist the health educator or system designer to develop materials that are accessible and understandable to most readers. Comprehensive bibliographies and references on this topic are available in the IOM report and in Healthy People 2010.

As with general literacy, applications and content must be designed to be effective when the user has limited health literacy. The Harvard School of Public Health's National Center for the Study of Adult Learning and Literacy Web site (*www.hsph.hardard.edu/healthliteracy//index.htlm*) has a wealth of resources, including an annotated bibliography and a page that lists resources for designing Web pages that are readable, easy to use, and accessible to persons with disabilities.

■ *Computer literacy and the digital divide:* Using a computer for a health-related application (such as participating in a support network or recording physiologic parameters from home) may be a person's introduction to the use of the technology. Nurses who have implemented health-related systems to persons who are not computer literate realize the importance of system design that emphasizes ease of use and easily available help functions. Some designers feel that if a user must access help information, they have failed in achieving usability. Web site usability poses a different set of requirements from desktop applications, so the nurse who is expert in one may not necessarily be expert in the other. There are many books available on user interface design and usability principles and methods of testing. These include Brinck et al. (2001), Nielsen (1993 and 2000), Krug (2000), and Spool et al. (1999). Shneiderman (2003) advocates for "universal usability," with principles that foster a better user experience for all persons, regardless of age, educational status, or physical impairments. Those interested in periodic newsletters delivered online can subscribe for free to Jakob Nielsen's Alertbox by visiting *www.useit.com* and to Jared Spool's usability articles by signing up at *http://www.uie.com/uietips.htm.*

The U.S. Department of Health and Human Services sponsors a highly useful site named Usability.gov that lists, among other things, research-based guidelines for usability (*www.usability.gov*). While some designers think that usability is largely a matter of taste and opinion, the guidelines compiled on this site are rated for relative importance in overall success of the Web site, and for strength of evidence.

■ *Special needs of the elderly:* Good resources for learning more about the needs of elderly users can be found at *www.aarp.org/olderwiserwired*. The National Institute on Aging and the National Library of Medicine have jointly published "Making Your Website Senior Friendly," a checklist with research-based guidelines that can be downloaded from *http://usability.gov/checklist.pdf*. The Center for Medicare Education has published a document entitled "Creating Senior-Friendly Web Sites" which can be downloaded from *www.medicareed.org/content/CMEPubDocs/V1N4.pdf*. Demiris and colleagues (2001) offer many practical suggestions for designing Web sites that take into account the limitations of older users.

■ *Accessibility to persons with disabilities:* The World Wide Web Consortium's Web Accessibility Initiative (W3C/WAI) is an international effort to establish guidelines and promote technologies to increase accessibility of the World Wide Web to persons with physical and cognitive impairments. To see the guidelines and a prioritized checklist for assessing compliance with the guidelines, visit *http://www.w3.org/WAI*. The federal government has mandated accessibility for all government-sponsored Web sites under Section 508 of the Rehabilitation Act Amendments of 1998. The standards are available at *www.access-board.gov/sec508/508standards.htm*. Designers wishing to use an automated tool to assess compliance of their Web pages with W3C/WAI guidelines and Section 508 standards can visit *www.cast.org/bobby* to assess one page at a time for free, or to purchase software that will evaluate an entire site.

■ *User-centered design:* While nurse informaticians undoubtedly learn the importance of user-centered design during their education, nowhere is this more important than in designing applications for patients and consumers. The patient's and consumer's view of the world will be highly influenced by age, by health and computer literacy, by health status, by socioeconomic status, and by language and culture. Focus groups, iterative testing and validation with target users, and a multidisciplinary approach that may include representatives of the target population, are central to the process. Chambers and colleagues describe an exemplary process that involved elderly users from five European countries to design a multimedia telehealth application for elderly caregivers (Chambers et al., 2003).

Some Research Areas Related to Consumer and Patient Computing

It is difficult to read any article, report, or book about consumers' use of computers for health without finding the phrase "more research is needed." The "e-health revolution" is a relatively new phenomenon, and every area described in this chapter could be a focus for in-depth research. Some fine examples are the work of Brennan and colleagues (1995, 2001), Gustafson et al. (2001), Kaufman, Starren, and Patel (2003), Cimino, Patel, and Kushniruk (2002) and while much good work is in progress, the surface has barely been scratched.

Ferguson (2002c) refers to the "terra incognita of online consumer health." He recommends, among other topics, investigating the dynamics of online support communities, how their members operate, what benefits they provide to participants, and how these communities sometimes contribute to formal medical research. He also advocates ethnographic examination of patient-doctor online communication, examining the evolution of the patient-doctor relationship over a period of time. Some research has been done in the area of content of patients' electronic communications, but many questions remain. For example, beyond patient satisfaction, does use of online communication contribute to patient outcomes, safety, or to patient cooperation with treatment regimen?

Gustafson (2004) advocates for various levels of evaluation studies of e-health systems based on the type of service offered. Services for patients who are in serious crisis situations demand higher standards of acceptability, usability, and veracity, and should be evaluated for such before implementation. Cost evaluations are infrequently carried out, but claims of replacing traditional forms of service with less expensive alternatives must be substantiated. Systems developed for underserved populations must be evaluated for usability, effectiveness, and impact.

Schwitzer (2002) believes that there has been inadequate evaluation of the merits of one type of decision support over another in multimedia decision-support applications. Are streaming video stories more effective than tailored prognostic information? Are moderated discussion groups more effective than unmoderated ones? These and many more questions remain unanswered to date.

Greenberg, D'Andrea, and Lorence (2004) advocate research into search technologies to help consumers to search more effectively and to evaluate the quality of what they find. Among other priorities are methods that would allow searches to learn from user behavior.

Kaplan and Brennan, summarizing the proceedings of the Spring 2000 Congress of the American Medical Informatics Association, noted three particular areas of research: (1) defining whether the user is a patient, consumer, or client, and whether the definitions make a difference, and whether the term might change with circumstances; (2) determining how the roles of the patient/consumer/client and healthcare providers are changing, and with what implications; and (3) examining what the term empowerment means, and what effect it might have on care (Kaplan and Brennan, 2001).

Additional areas for research (among many more that could be mentioned) include:

- Development and evaluation of technologies to automatically translate health content and medical record data to meet the user's native language and educational level

- Effect of the empowered patient on patient-nurse dynamics

- Effectiveness of various outreach methods to reach less educated, less wealthy, and more culturally diverse populations

- Needs of underserved, less literate populations with respect to computer applications for health

- Contribution of automatic push of health-related materials based on user's expressed interests and recorded health problems to patient behavior and outcomes

- Contribution of consumer-friendly terminology to retrieval of health information online

- Unmet needs of patients and consumers with respect to online services

- Contribution of access to online medical record to patient-provider communication, and to accuracy and completeness of medical record

- Effects of highly tailored prognostic information based on user's individual profile on patient decision-making

- Influence of e-health technology on educational interventions in patient care

- Ethical considerations in all aspects of e-health, including disclosure, informed consent, and providing full access to the medical record

- Differences in effects of synchronous versus asynchronous communication with patient (e.g., videocalls vs. secure messaging)

Conclusion

Clearly, the field of consumer health informatics, though young, is broad and multifaceted. It does not belong to any one discipline, but draws on the expertise of a variety of health, science, social, and technical fields. Armed with the additional knowledge of the special considerations in designing, implementing, and evaluating applications aimed at patients and consumers, nurse informaticians have much to contribute to the field.

References

American Nurses Association. (2001). *Scope and Standards of Nursing Informatics Practice.* Washington, DC: American Nurses Publishing.

American Nurses Association. (2003). *Nursing's Social Policy Statement* (2nd ed.). Washington DC: American Nurses Association. Pub. #03NSPS.

Anonymous. (2003). *Qmed, Inc. and CHA Health Achieve 37.1% Reduction in Heart Attack Incidence.* Press Release, January 7, 2003. Retrieved July 30, 2004, from *http://www.biospace.com/news_story.cfm?StoryID= 11302920&full=1*

Brennan, P. F. (1995). The effects of a special computer network on caregivers of persons with Alzheimer's disease. *Nursing Research* 44(3):166–172.

Brennan, P. F. (1999). Health informatics and community health: Support for patients as collaborators in care. *Methods of Information in Medicine* 38(4–5):274–278.

Brennan, P. F., Moore, S. M., Bjornsdottir, G., et al. (2001). HeartCare: An Internet-based information and support system for patient home recovery after coronary artery bypass graft (CABG) surgery. *Journal of Advanced Nursing* 35(5):699–708.

Brinck, T., Gergle, D., and Wood, S. D. (2001). *Usability for the Web: Designing Web Sites that Work.* San Francisco, CA: Morgan Kaufmann Publishers.

Chambers, M. G., Connor, S. L., McGonigle, M., and Diver M. G. (2003). Multimedia software to help caregivers cope. *Journal of the American Medical Informatics Association* 10(5):504–511.

Chisnell, D., Lee, A., and Redish, J. (2004). *Designing Web Sites for Older Users: Comparing AARP's Studies to Earlier Findings.* Retrieved July 29, 2004, from *http://www.aarp.org/olderwiserwired/oww-features/ Articles/a2004-03-03-comparison-studies.html*

Cimino, J. J., Patel, V. L., and Kushniruk, A. W. (2002). The patient clinical information system (PatCIS): technical solutions for and experience with giving patients access to the electronic medical records. *International Journal of Medical Informatics* 68(1–3):113–127.

Couchman, G. R., Forjuoh, S. N., and Rascoe, T. G. (2001). E-mail communications in family practice: What do patients expect? *Journal of Family Practice* 50(5):414–418.

Croft, D. R. and Peterson, M. W. (2002). An evaluation of the quality and content of asthma education on the World Wide Web. *Chest* 121(4):1301–1307.

Demiris, G., Finkelstein, S. M., and Speedie, S. M. (2001). Considerations for the design of a Web based clinical monitoring and educational system for elderly patients. *Journal of the American Medical Informatics Association* 8(5):468–472.

Dickerson, S. S. and Brennan, P. F. (2002). The internet as a catalyst for shifting power in provider-patient relationships. *Nursing Outlook* 50(5):195–203.

Federation of State Medical Boards. (2002). *Model Guidelines for the Appropriate Use of the Internet in Medical Practice.* Dallas, TX: Author. Retrieved July 28, 2004, from *http://www.fsmb.org.*

Ferguson, T. (2002a). God bless my CML support group. The Ferguson Report, No. 8, January 2002. Retrieved July 15, 2004, from *http://www.fergusonreport.com/articles/fr00803.htm*

Ferguson, T. (2002b). "The Gap" between Health Professionals' and Patients' views of online health. The Ferguson Report, No. 8, January. Retrieved July 15, 2004 from *http://www.fergusonreport.com/archives.idx008.htm*

Ferguson, T. (2002c). *The Robert Wood Johnson Online Health Project: What Kinds of Online Health Research are Really Needed?* Retrieved July 19, 2004, from *http://fergusonreport.com/articles/fr00802.htm*

Ferguson, T. (2002d). From patients to end users [editorial]. *British Medical Journal (BMJ)* 324:555–556.

Fox, S. and Fallows, D. (2003). *Internet Health Resources.* Washington DC: Pew Internet & American Life Project. Retrieved June 20, 2004, from *http:// www.pewinternet.org/pdfs/PIP_Health_Report_July_2003.pdf.*

Fox, S. and Rainie, L. (2000). *The Online Health Care Revolution: How the Web Helps Americans Take Better Care of Themselves.* Washington, DC: Pew Internet & American Life Project. Retrieved July 15, 2004, from *http://www.pewinternet.org/pdfs/ PIP_Health_Report.pdf*

Greenber, L., D'Andrea, G., and Lorence, D. (2004). Setting the public agenda for online health search: A white paper and action agenda. *Journal of Medical Internet Research* 6(2):e18.

Gustafson, D. H. (2004). Evaluation of Ehealth systems and services: We need to move beyond Hits and Testimonials [editorial]. *British Medical Journal* 328(7449):1150.

Gustafson, D. H., Hawkins, R. P., Boberg, E. W., et al. (2002). Chess: 10 years of research and development in consumer health informatics for broad populations, including the underserved. *International Journal of Medical Informatics* 65(3):169–177.

Gustafson, D. H., Hawkins, R., Pingree, S., et al. (2001). Effect of computer support on younger women with breast cancer. *Journal of General Internal Medicine* 16(7):435–445.

Harris Interactive. (2002a). *Cyberchondriacs Update. Health Care News.* Retrieved July 20, 2004, from *http://www.harrisinteractive.com/harris_poll/index.asp?PID=299*

Harris Interactive. (2002b). *Internet Penetration at 66% of Adults (137 Million) Nationwide. Health Care News.* Retrieved July 20, 2004, from *http://www. harrisinteractive.com/harris_poll/index.asp?PID=295*

Harris Interactive. (2003). Those with Internet access continue to grow but at a slower rate. *Health Care News.* Retrieved July 20, 2004, from *http://www. harrisinteractive.com/harris_poll/index.asp?PID=356*

Harris Interactive. (2004). More than one-third of Internet users now have broadband. *Health Care News.* Retrieved July 20, 2004, from *http://www.harrisinteractive.com/ harris_poll/index.asp?PID=432*

Institute of Medicine. (2004). *Health Literacy: A Prescription to End Confusion.* Washington, DC: Institute of Medicine.

Intelligent Medical Objects, Inc. (2000). *Product Description: Personal Health Terminology™ (PHT).* Retrieved June 20, 2004, from *http://www2.e-imo.com/ Products.asp.*

Kane, B. and Sands, D. Z. (1998). Guidelines for the clinical use of electronic mail with patients. *Journal of the American Medical Informatics Association* 5(1), pp. 104–111. Retrieved July 30, 2004, from *http://www.amia.org/ pubs/fpubl.html*

Kaplan, B. and Brennan, P. F. (2001). Consumer informatics supporting patients as co-producers of quality. *Journal of the American Medical Informatics Association* 8(4):309–316.

Kaufman, D. R., Starren, J., and Patel, V. L. (2003). A cognitive framework for understanding barriers to the productive use of a diabetes home telemedicine system. In M. Musen, C. P. Friedman, J. M. Teich (Eds.), *Proceedings of 2003 AMIA Symposium* (pp. 356–360).

Kelly, G. and McKenzie, B. (2002). Security, privacy, and confidentiality issues on the Internet. *Journal of Medical Internet Research* 4(2):e12. Retrieved on July 30, 2004, from *http://www.jmir.org/2002/2/e12/.*

Kirsch, I. S., Jungeblut, A., Jenkins, L., and Kolstad, A. (1993). *Executive Summary of Adult Literacy in America: A First Look at the Results of the National Adult Literacy Survey.* Washington, DC: US Department of Education. Retrieved July 10, 2004, from *http:// www.nces.ed.gov/naal/resources/execsumm.asp*

Kreps, G. L. (2002). Enhancing access to relevant health information. In R. Carveth, S. B. Kretchmer, D. Schuler (Eds.), *Shaping the Network Society: Patterns for Partici-pation, Action and Change* (pp. 149–152). Palo Alto, CA: CPSR. Retrieved June 25, 2004, from *http://www. amia.org/meetings/archive/s03/presentations/Access.pdf*

Krug, S. (2000). *Don't Make Me Think: A Common Sense Guide to Web Usability.* Indianapolis, IN: New Riders Publishing.

Lazarus, W. and Mora, F. (2000). *Online Content for Low-Income and Underserved Americans: The Digital Divide's New Frontier.* Santa Monica, CA: The Children's Partnership. Retrieved June 20, 2004, from *http://wdr.doleta.gov/research/rlib_doc.cfm?docn=6007.*

Lenhart, A., Horrigan, J., Rainie, L., et al. (2003). The *Ever-Shifting Internet Population: A New Look at Internet Access and the Digital Divide*. Washington DC: Pew Internet & American Life Project. Retrieved June 20, 2004, from *http://www.pewinternet.org/pdfs/ PIP_Shifting_Net_Pop_Report.pdf*

MacDonald, K. (2003). *Online Patient-Provider Communication Tools: An Overview*. Oakland, CA: California HealthCare Foundation. Retrieved on July 30, 2004, from *http://www.chcf.org/topics/view.cfm?item ID= 21600.*

Madden, M. (2003). *The Changing Picture of Who's Online and What They Do*. Washington, DC: Pew Internet & American Life Project. Retrieved June 20, 2004, from *http://www.pewinternet.org/pdfs/PIP_Online_Pursuits_ Final.PDF.*

Manhattan Research. (2004). *Taking the Pulse(r) v4.0: Physicians and Emerging Information Technologies.* New York, NY: Manhattan Research.

McCray, A. T., Dorfman, E., Ripple, A., et al. (2000). Usability issues in developing a Web-based consumer health site. In *Proceedings 2000 AMIA Symposium* (pp. 556–560).

Medem. (2002). *ERisk Working Group for Healthcare: Guidelines for Online Communication*. San Francisco, CA: Author. Retrieved July 15, 2004, from *http://www.medem.com/phy/phy_eriskguidelines.cfm*

National Cancer Institute. (1994). *Clear & Simple: Developing Effective Print Materials for Low-Literate Readers*. NIH Pub. No. 95-3594.

Nielsen, J. (1993). *Usability Engineering*. San Diego, CA: Academic Press.

Nielsen, J. (2000). *Designing Web Usability*. Indianapolis, IN: New Riders Publishing.

Oster, N., Thomas, L., Joseff, D., and Love, S. (2000). Making informed medical decisions; where to look and how to use what you find. Cambridge, MA: O'Reilly.

Patt, M. R., Houston, T. K., Jenckes, M. W., Sands, D. Z., and Ford, D. E. (2003). Doctors who are using e-mail with their patients: A qualitative exploration. *Journal of Medical Internet Research* 5(2):e9. Retrieved on July 29, from *http://www.jmir.org/2003/2/e9/.*

Schwitzer, G. (2002). A review of features in Internet consumer health decision-support tools. *Journal of Medical Internet Research* 4(2):e11. Retrieved on July 29, from *http://www.jmir.org/2002/2/e11/.*

SCPIE. (2002). New guidelines minimize risk in doctor-patient online communications. *Safe Practice* 8(6) 1–2. Retrieved July 30, 2004, from *http://www.scpie.com/ publications/safe_practice/200212.pdf*

Shea, S., Starren, J., Weinstock, R. S., et al. (2002). Columbia University's Informatics for Diabetes Education and Telemedicine (IDEATel) Project: Rationale and Design. *Journal of the American Medical Informatics Association* 9(1):49–62.

Shneiderman, B. (2003). *Leonardo's Laptop: Human Needs and the New Computing Technologies.* Cambridge, MA: MIT Press.

Smith, S. P. (2002). Internet visits: A new approach to chronic disease management. *Journal of Medical Practice Management* 17(6):330–332.

Solucient. (2003). *National Trends in Health Care Consumerism: A White Paper Report*. Retrieved July 20, 2004, from *http://www.solucient.com/forms/ nationaltrends.shtml.*

Spool, J., Scanlon, T., Schroeder, W., et al. (1999). *Web Site Usability: A Designer's Guide*. San Francisco, CA: Morgan Kaufmann Publishers.

Tang, P. C., Black, W., Buchanan, J., et al. (2003). PAMFOnline: Integrating ehealth with an electronic medical record system. In M. Musen, C. P. Friedman, J. M. Teich (Eds.), *Proceedings of 2003 AMIA Symposium* (pp. 644–648).

Tse, T. and Soergel, D. (2003). Exploring medical expressions used by consumers and the media: An emerging view of consumer health vocabularies. In M. Musen, C. P. Friedman, J. M. Teich (Eds.), *Proceedings of 2003 AMIA Symposium* (pp. 674–678).

U.S. Department of Health and Human Services. (2000). *Health People 2010* (2nd ed.). Washington, DC: U.S. Government Printing Office.

U.S. Department of Health and Human Services. (2003). *Summary of the HIPAA Privacy Rule*. Retrieved June 20, 2004, from *http://www.hhs.gov/ocr/ privacysummary.pdf.*

U.S. Department of Health and Human Services. (2004). *Usability.gov*. Retrieved on July 17, 2004, from *http://www.usability.gov/index.html*

W3C. (1999). *Web Content Accessibility Guidelines 1.0. World Wide Web Consortium (W3C) Web Accessibility Initiative (WAI)*. Retrieved August 3, 2004, from *http://www.w3.org/TR/WCAG10/*

Wilson, E. V. (2003). Asynchronous health care communication. *Commun ACM* 46(6):79–84.

Zielstorff, R. D. (2003). Controlled vocabularies for consumer health. *Journal of Biomedical Informatics* 36(4/5):326–333.

▮ Recommended Readings

Reports, Surveys

California HealthCare Foundation—iHealth & Technology: *http://www.chcf.org/topics/index. cfm?topic=CL108*

HarrisInteractive. *www.harrisinteractive.com*

Pew Internet and American Life Project. *www.pewinternet.org*. Search for "internet for health" or "demographics."

Principles, Guidelines, Standards

Hi-Ethics—Health Internet Ethics. *www.hiethics.org*
HON—Health On the Net Foundation. *www.hon.ch*
Medem. *www.medem.org*
URAC Health Web Site Accreditation Program. *http://Webapps.urac.org/Websiteaccreditation/ default.htm*
W3C—World Wide Web Consortium Web Accessibility Initiative. *www.w3c.org/wai*

Tools for Consumers to Evaluate Health Information on the Web

Health on the Net Foundation. *http://www.hon.ch*
MedlinePlus—Evaluating Health Information. *http://www.nlm.nih.gov/medlineplus/ evaluatinghealthinformation.html*
Medical Library Association. A User's Guide to Finding and Evaluating Health Information on the Web. *http://www.nlm.nih.gov/medlineplus/ evaluatinghealthinformation.html*

Publications on Consumer Health Informatics

Ferguson, T. (2002). From patients to end users. [editorial]. *BMJ* 324:555–556.

Ferguson T. *Ten Rules for Online Health Professionals.* Available at *www.fergusonreport.com/articles/ fr049905.htm.* Accessed Feb. 4, 2004.

Kaplan, B., Brennan, P. F. (2001). Consumer informatics supporting patients as co-producers of quality. *Journal of the American Medical Informatics Association* 8(4):309–316.

Rice, R. E. and Katz, J. E. (Eds.). (2001). *The Internet and Health Communication: Experiences and Expectations.* Thousand Oaks, CA: Sage.

Slack, W. and Nader, R. (2001). *Cybermedicine: How Computing Empowers Doctors and Patients for Better Care.* San Francisco, CA: Jossey-Bass.

CHAPTER 31

Decision Support for Consumers

Patricia Flatley Brennan

Shirley M. Moore

David M. Haight

Gail R. Casper

OBJECTIVES

1. Identify the challenges that patients face in understanding health risks, treatment options, and QOL issues when making medical decisions and the role that decision support technologies can play in empowering them as active participants in the management of their care.

2. Critically appraise patient-centered medical decision support tools differentiating experimental and theoretical applicability and effectiveness by specific characteristics of medical decision contexts.

3. Synthesize appropriate subsets of decision support methodologies, tools, and resources that can be effectively applied to specific decision contexts and identifying barriers to their adoption and appropriate utilization.

KEY WORDS

consumer health
decision support
decision theory

 Introduction

Quality healthcare demands that patients assume increasingly central and active roles in personal health promotion and disease management. Patients who are more informed and knowledgeable about clinical and quality of life (QOL) aspects of their disease and its treatment are more likely to have increased satisfaction with their care process and treatment outcomes. There has also been a significant increase in consumerism in health-related contexts driving patients to actively seek out information about treatments. Consumers are direct targets of advertising campaigns by pharmaceutical

companies and pieces focused on stimulating consumers' desire for screening for cancer and genetic defects are increasingly being published and televised in the mass media. A study of the effect of direct to consumer drug advertising determined that 19% of the participants requested a prescription and an additional 35% asked their physician for additional information about a drug after seeing an advertisement (Wilkes, Bell, and Kravitz, 2000). Enabling patients to be effective participants in the management of their health states and disease treatment requires that they have both the information and an understanding of their health risks, treatment options, and associated QOL issues.

The kinds of decisions that patients face and that they must make range from the one-time treatment choices that accompany a sudden acute disease to the ongoing health management process common to chronic diseases and to the daily affirmations of actions and attitudes

Supported in part by grants from the National Institutes of Health (NR 2001, AG 8614, LM 6543). Portions of the material were first presented at the NI'97 meeting and published in JAMIA.

that enable and empower a commitment to a healthy lifestyle. The application of computer technologies, including telecommunications systems, the Internet and the World Wide Web (WWW), and multimedia information display, has been shown to enable patients, their family caregivers, and concerned others to become active, informed participants in the management of the healthcare process.

The previous 10 years have witnessed an explosion of computer-based applications designed to help patients make better decisions about the health services they need and the health behaviors they seek to adopt. Some of these tools employ models from decision theory to guide patients in understanding and performing a structured analysis of the options they face and the values they wish to employ as they make these choices. Other approaches employ an expert decision-making model, where the computer tool is used to provide information, advice, and coaching based on the experiences of other patients who have had similar health problems or the expertise of clinicians who diagnose and treat those problems. A third approach uses general-purpose computer tools, including the WWW, to allow consumers to autonomously collect health-related information that can be used to help them understand diseases and their treatments or to reflect on their behaviors and sense of self, and incorporate incremental choices into adopting a more healthy lifestyle. Still other approaches to computer-based decision support work to provide patients with tools that let them view their clinical records and link these records with current literature databases.

This chapter will explore the many aspects of health-related patient decision-making, with particular emphasis on examining how computer technology can enhance patients' ability to gather, analyze, and understand information key to their empowerment as active participants in the management of both their health and interactions with the healthcare system.

Health-Related Decision-Making

Health-related decision-making is challenging for patients for several key reasons. First, decision-making itself is a complex, perceptual, cognitive, and social process. The talents and limits of humans as decision makers, particularly in the face of substantial uncertainty, are well known and well described in the work of the human information processing theorists (Tversky and Kahneman, 1972). Essentially, information processing is a complex challenge, and humans employ simplifying mental mechanisms as coping strategies to help them sort significant from insignificant facts, to organize and interpret complex observations, to facilitate recall and synthesis of known knowledge with new facts, and to apply judgments under conditions where consequences and outcomes are uncertain. Stressors, such as anxiety, time pressures, and lack of knowledge, lead these efficient processes to deteriorate in such a way as to lead to suboptimal or even incorrect decision processes. Lay persons facing health crises simultaneously experience many stressors, thus, their information processing skills are taxed repeatedly.

Second, health-related decision-making is complicated because the substance of the problems and choices is itself complex and exceeds the knowledge and education of most laypersons. At the very point that patients face a threat to their integrity as persons they are challenged to manage and attempt to understand large amounts of new and complex information, much of which they may not have the knowledge base to effectively process. So, with diminished information processing skills, the individual must attempt to comprehend and interpret new and unfamiliar facts and relate them to their own system of values and beliefs. Even those persons who are not in a health crisis may have difficulty locating and evaluating the quality and relevance of health information. Facts from authoritative sources mix with hearsay from unreliable mass media or personal interactions, resulting in an unsound basis for making health-related decisions such as following primary prevention recommendations or carrying out healthy lifestyle choices.

Finally, health-related decision-making is complex because it generally involves more than a single person. Two key groups must be considered: the family members of the person facing a health crisis or in need of health information and the healthcare delivery team. Family members hold values, beliefs, and attitudes that implicitly or explicitly influence the health choices of an individual. The healthcare industry holds clinical care standards, values, and attitudes about patients' responsibilities for their care and organizational or personal traditions that may interfere with the person's right to self-determination and self-care.

Healthcare decision-making is challenging because it involves uncertainty, taxes human information processing capabilities, deals with subject matter that is unfamiliar to the involved person, and there are multiple constituencies that must be served.

Shared Decision-Making and Informed Choice

The emphasis on involving patients in healthcare decision-making has greatly increased with the widespread acceptance of shared decision-making approaches, which advocates that patients are best able to determine which values should govern their care. Traditionally, clinicians have assumed responsibility for judging the appropriateness of the clinical treatments and their associated outcomes in the frame of reference of both their own values and those of the patient. Shared decision-making is also known as relationship or collaborative decision-making which empowers patients to choose among the options available to them in consultation with their clinician(s) using their personal values to frame the choice among alternatives. In a study of women with breast carcinoma, 89% preferred an active or shared role in decision-making (Mitchell, McConnahie, and Sullivan, 2003). In another study of women with breast cancer, 22% wanted to make the decision on their cancer treatment, 44% wanted to make the decision collaboratively with their clinicians, and 34% wished to defer the decision to the judgment of their clinicians, while only 42% of patients believed that they had experienced the level of control of the decision that they preferred (Woloshin et al., 2001). To accommodate this range of preferred involvement, clinical providers must adapt through flexible and effective communications mechanisms (Schwartz, McDowell, and Yueh, 2004).

Related to shared decision-making is the concept of evidence-informed choice. Informed consent has been an established practice that involves the patient acknowledging that they have received adequate information to assent to the care that is recommended by the clinician. Informed consent is a passive process that simply requires that a patient has knowledge of the treatments and the probable outcomes (O'Connor and Jacobsen, 2003). Evidence-informed choice sets a much more rigorous standard that requires that patients both receive and understand information that enables them to evaluate risks and benefits of alternative options, examine how they value the benefits versus the risks, and then use that information collaboratively with their clinicians to decide on the optimal course of action consistent with the joint values of clinicians and patients (Ledley and Lusted, 1999). There are strong legal and ethical motivations for driving the clinician/patient relationship as far in the direction of informed choice as possible. The following is an excerpt from a malpractice case decided by the New Jersey State Court:

> Accordingly, the doctor must discuss all medically reasonable courses of treatment, including non-treatment, and the probable risks and outcomes of each alternative. By not discussing these alternatives, the doctor breaches the patient's right to make an informed choice and effectively makes the choice for the patient. The doctor has a duty to explain, in words the patient can understand, all material medical information and risks. (NJ State Court Malpractice ruling)

A study of patients with breast cancer found that one-third of the time patients and surgeons disagreed as to whether alternative treatments were discussed before surgery (Keating et al., 2003). Decision support technology is a key tool to enable a higher level of understanding and evaluation of alternatives available to the patient and thus serves as a key to achieving informed choice by insuring that information regarding courses of treatment is comprehensively and uniformly communicated.

A major determinant of choice and decision-making is the context provided by the values held by an individual; therefore, in this discussion of health-related decision-making we now turn attention to the concept of patient preferences.

Patient Preferences

Attention to patient preferences as an input into health-care decision-making is rooted in the application of decision theory to understand personal choice. von Neumann and Morgenstern (1964) first proposed that the personal values and attitudes that drive individual choice could be understood through mathematical formulations. These formulations are based on an economic analysis model where numerical rating of a health state corresponds to its relative desirability. Following on their work, Ledley and Lusted (1999) introduced the concepts of mathematical reasoning to medical decision-making, with particular attention to decision-making under uncertainty. Raiffa (1968) explicated decision analytic strategies that brought the treatment of personal preference and uncertainty into a form accessible in an interpersonal interview. Recently, the work of Pauker and McNeil (1981) and associates (Sonnenberg and Pauker, 1986; Pauker, Pauker, and MacNeil, 1981) demonstrated the feasibility of using decision analysis to better understand treatment choices that are complicated by multiple uncertainties and personal values. These works offer a theoretical foundation for building health informatics tools that aid in the assessment of patient preferences.

The two main branches of decision theory: decision analysis and normative decision theory, both help make patient preferences accessible for clinical decision-making. Decision analysis helps in choosing one course of action from several when the most desired strategy depends, in part, on the knowledge of the costs, benefits, and probabilities of the resolution of the outcomes of that strategy.

Multiattribute utility theory (MAUT) provides the mechanisms for quantifying the subjective value of health states and therefore can be very useful to patients who must make healthcare decisions (Ledley and Lusted, 1999; Keeney and Raiffa, 1976). In MAUT, a utility is a numerical representation of the value, desirability, or preference for a health state. MAUT defines preferences as the ordering of entities over a value space where the ordering corresponds to the relative preference for the entity (Keeney and Raiffa, 1976). The entities about which one developed preferences are discrete objects, such as cars or job candidates or in healthcare parlance, specific health outcomes and the order of the preference value for an entity is a surrogate for the relative preference of the entity itself. Entities were viewed as multidimensional with the value space describing the n-dimensional intersection of a specific set of entities specified simultaneously on all dimensions. The set of possible values in each of the dimensions and the relative weights of each defined the ordering of the preference structure. MAUT provides a way to establish a quantitative expression of an individual's values with respect to a given set of alternatives, with preference for a given health outcome being expressed as a score on the weighted sum of the entities and their relative weights. A utility function computes a score for each treatment alternative that explicitly incorporates the probability of the outcome of each treatment and a quantitative estimate of the desirability of the outcomes following each treatment.

MAUT is based on compensatory rules that allow for assessing tradeoffs among entities in such a way that a high value for one entity is compensated for by a low value in another entity. The method of incorporating both desirability and probability results in a value that reflects both risk and cost/reward. The highest weighted score thus calculated would be the choice preferred by a rational decision maker under this decision model.

The work of Pauker and colleagues provided the operational strategies to move decision analysis into the clinical arena. Pauker's group employed decision analysis to aid patients and clinicians in the challenges of selecting treatment courses when the choice of an intervention depended on two key unknowns: the extent to which a patient preferred the outcomes likely to follow the treatment and the probabilities that those outcomes would occur. Importantly, they devised the strategies to elicit from patients their quantitative estimates of the desirability of various outcome states. In a series of studies, this group explored preferences for cancer treatment (Sonnenberg and Pauker, 1986), prenatal testing (Pauker, Pauker, and McNeil, 1981), and surgical intervention for cardiac disease (Sonnenberg and Pauker, 1986). The treatment with the highest resulting utility value became, by definition in this model, the patient's preference. This use of preference as a synonym for the most desired action is consistent with, but not identical to, its use within normative decision theory, where an individual's preference for an entity was its utility, a composite of how well that entity performed on each important dimension.

Decision analysis is then combined with MAUT to provide a framework for structuring a choice among a sequence of uncertain alternatives. In most cases, instead of a preference for a single alternative, preference for a treatment involves analyzing a sequence of interdependent alternatives. Many complex medical conditions require a stepwise decision process with the evaluation of alternatives at the next treatment step being dependent on the health outcome of the previous treatment step. For example, a breast cancer patient on initial diagnosis may elect to have a lumpectomy after applying decision theory encompassing all possible future health states. At some later time there may be a recurrence of the cancer and then the decision process must begin anew given the new preferences and future health state probabilities that arise with the newly ascertained health state.

Decision theory provides mechanisms for analyzing and ranking a sequence of health states under uncertainty to derive a numerical measure to each possible path's[s2] utility. Decision theory rests on the assumption that rational decision makers will prefer the immediate decision alternative that has the highest expected utility for the entire sequence of possibilities.

The expected utility is based on a set of probabilities for each outcome. Determining the correct probabilities can be very difficult as can be expected for a large set of patients given some aggregated estimate of probability of outcomes drawn from an appropriate patient population. Very often this data on probability of outcomes for a given treatment is extracted from clinical trials or other experimental or experiential studies. This leads to the difficult problem of applying the group derived outcome and probability data to a unique patient (Feinstein and Horwitz, 1997). Decision support systems are beginning to be deployed that assess outcome probabilities based on some set of the attributes of the patient such as age, pathology, and health history leading to preference assessments that are more specific to the individual (Whelan et al., 2003). In general, as the discrimination in the attributes that characterize the group from which the probability measure is derived increases, the precision of the probability as applied to a unique patient increases.

Most informatics tools designed to elicit patient preferences are grounded in these decision theoretic conceptualizations (Lenert and Soetikno, 1997). In this context, the preference statement denotes the extent to which given health states are desirable according to some implicit or explicit valuing scheme. Other uses of the term patient preference also exist.

Alternate Meanings of the Term "Preferences"

The distinction between preferences as formalization of values, vis-à-vis a set of healthcare entities and preferences as the identified option chosen from the set of healthcare-related entities becomes important when one examines how computers could be of assistance in eliciting patient preferences. Different kinds of computer programs and utilities support decision-making; some consider preference as an input to a decision while others view preference as the final choice resulting from a decision. Clarifying the exact referent of preferences is a necessary precursor to the design of computer systems to support the use of patient preferences in healthcare. Donabedian's three-part quality model (Donabedian, 1968) provides a useful heuristic for sorting out the various referents about which individuals may develop preferences. Individuals may establish preferences about structural aspects of healthcare, such as belonging to a health maintenance organization (Sainfort and Booske, 1996) or their preferences for information or decision-making (Deber, Kraetschmer, and Irvine, 1996). Preferences for treatment options, such as surgical versus medical interventions, represent the individual's appraisal about process aspects of healthcare. A third referent for preference is the outcomes of health actions.

Some use the term "preference" to represent an individual's final choice of one option from many possible treatment options. For example, the man coping with an enlarged prostate may be said to have a "preference for surgery" if, after considering watchful waiting, medications, or surgical treatment, he finally decides on the surgical intervention as his final choice of treatment (Barry et al., 1995). However, this perspective introduces confusion in that the same term is used to refer to the general concept (valuing of individual options for treatment) as well as a specific instance (most desired treatment).

Moore and Kramer (1998) used the term "preferences" to identify those features of cardiac rehabilitation programs deemed most desirable by patients. In this case, the preferences express the desirability of the features of a program, not the program (entity) itself. Henry and Holzemer (1995) identified preferences as "patient-specific inputs to the care process." Under this definition, preferences are atomic judgments that can be integrated with other components of the patient assessment and subsequently used to select treatment strategies.

Challenges to Using Patient Preferences for Health-Related Decision-Making

Although the value of understanding and using patient preferences in healthcare decision-making is well-recognized (O'Connor et al., 1999; Eraker, Kirschtk, and Becker, 1984), actually doing so can present a daunting challenge to patients (Gerteis et al., 1993). Imagining what a future health state could be like and determining the desirability of that future state is a complex cognitive task. Additionally, many patients lack experience with thinking about abstract concepts such as values, preferences, and risks. When patients are asked to evaluate complex situations with potentially adverse consequences under the stressful circumstance of the clinical encounter their cognitive ability is taxed to an even greater degree. Skilled interpersonal interaction can lead to an accurate assessment of an individual's preferences but the fragmented, time-limited nature of contemporary health encounters leaves little opportunity to conduct the intense, interpersonal exploration needed to elicit and use patient preferences (Sonnenberg and Pauker, 1986; Pauker and McNeil, 1981).

The determination of preferences is subject to a number of biases that result in departures from assessments that would normally be expected from rational, fully informed patients. Framing effects are the most pervasive potential form of bias in preference elicitation. Patients' assessment of the desirability of a health state or their attitude toward risk can vary substantially depending on the frame (positive or negative) in which the information is presented. In a classic study, one-half of the participants were asked for their preference given a set of survival probabilities (positive frame) and the other one-half were given the complementary set of mortality probabilities (negative frame) that conveyed the identical outcome prediction. Those who were basing their decision on survival data preferred the treatment in question less often than those who were basing their preference on mortality data. A study on the use of multimedia testimonials in which a patient describes his or her experience with a health state or with a treatment decision process found that a mismatch between the race or gender of the patient in the video presentation and the viewing patient affected the preference for the predicted health states (Fortin et al., 2001). Another study showed that the ratio of positive to negative testimonials affected the preference for angioplasty or bypass surgery (Ubel, Jepson, and Baron, 2001).

Furthermore, under traditional models of care which are still in common practice, patients and clinicians both presume clinician preeminence in decision-making, and frequently patients prefer to defer to the judgment of the clinician. However, the scientific and clinical knowledge of clinicians does not always provide adequate direction for treatment of complex illnesses, and despite increasing utilization of a shared decision-making model it may be difficult for many patients to engage reluctant physicians in a collaborative model (Elwyn et al., 1999; Gerteis et al., 1993).

Preference assessment is an iterative, cognitive process designed to help a person understand and clarify personal values, healthcare situations, treatment options and likely outcomes, and to elicit statements of preference. Benefiting from behavioral decision-making research, an interactive analysis process is used to help an individual focus on key components of a decision problem. Preference assessment can be accomplished by a skilled interviewer using probes and reflection. Recently, Ruland (1998) demonstrated that staff nurses can be trained to effectively elicit patient priorities regarding the focus of care, and that such elicitation can lead to improved satisfaction with care. Interactive computer systems can be used to either supplement or supplant the human analyst or interviewer.

Computer technology can assist in meeting the challenges inherent in accessing and employing patient preferences in healthcare practices. Computer packages that focus on elicitation and values clarification may serve to help patients think about complex, abstract issues, such as the desirability of future states (Barry et al., 1995). Multimedia displays use sound, pictures, and full-motion video to help patients envision future health states with greater clarity. When delivered via the WWW, these programs facilitate patients' exploration of preferences in the privacy of

their homes or away from anxiety-producing health encounters (Lenert and Soetikno, 1997). The use of carefully developed, automated preference elicitation methods can eliminate the possibility of bias or variability that can be introduced by a human interviewer and the preferences obtained through automated means can be more precise through the use of interactive feedback methods such as graphical displays (Lenert, Sherbourne, and Reyna, 2001).

Additionally, computer technology can store and communicate assessment data gleaned through a human- or computer-directed analysis. Such use of computer technology reduces the demand for repetition of analysis or communication on the part of the patient and helps to insure that data collected is transmitted in a timely fashion to involved clinicians. The information elicited on preferences must be available to the clinicians to improve the outcome of the course of treatment as measured by the perspective of the patient. The inclusion of preference information in the patient's electronic health record (EHR) allows for the consideration of the patient's preferences at each stage of his or her treatment but vocabulary standards for encoding and storing these preferences in an EHR is an immature field, most decision support system (DSS) applications currently are stand alone, and their output is not integrated into the care provider's information system (Ruland and Bakken, 2001).

Typically, the patient is the direct user of these computer technology preference applications, but the results of the preference assessment are used collaboratively in a shared decision process with his or her clinician. The process by which the patient's preferences are incorporated into the clinician-patient relationship and dialogue requires a merging or reconciliation between the patient's, clinician's, and healthcare organization's possibly conflicting values. In a study of patient's preferences for anticoagulation therapy, 61% of the patients preferred to be treated, which is much smaller than the proportion that was indicated by applying the accepted clinical guidelines. Of the patients who preferred treatment, only 47% would have been treated according to consensus clinical guidelines, while of those who preferred not being treated, 87% would have been treated according to those same guidelines (Protheroe et al., 2000).

These discrepancies between patient's preferences and clinical guidelines indicate that the inclusion of preferences into clinical practice may require substantial cultural and organizational shifts. While it is clear that decisional authority remains with the patient in all cases, there may be conflicts between the right of the patient to make important decisions and the imperative of clinicians to strongly recommend a course of action when the consensus guidelines indicate a clear and unambiguous course of action (Whitney, 2003). What happens when patients choose an alternative that is not supported by the evidence? In these cases adhering to the ideals of the shared decision process can pose significant challenges to the care provider. Achieving congruence between a patient's preferred and actual role in the decision-making process contributes to the level of satisfaction with the treatment process (Janz et al., 2004).

Reviewed next are prototype, experimental systems that aid in the assessment of patient preferences and in using those preferences for making health-related decisions.

Computer Technology and Patient Decision-Making

Assessing Utilities of Health Outcomes

The Stanford Center for the Study of Patient Preference (the Center) was a pioneer in the use of computers and the Internet for low-cost elicitation of patient preferences for health states. Initially, computerized surveys and instructional programs available on the WWW walked the patient through classic decision analytic methods to help them clarify their preferences. Subsequently, patients approached a rating task through programs that elicit preferences for specific health states (Lenert and Soetikno, 1997; Goldstein et al., 1994). These preference assessments used visual analog scales (VAS), pair-wise comparisons (PWC), standard gamble (SG), and time trade-off (TT) methods to measure patient utilities (Keating et al., 2003).

The SG method asks the patient to determine the indifference point where living in specified health state is perceived to be equivalently preferable to a specific probability of death, which provides a preference ordering where alternatives that are equivalent to a higher probability of death are preferred. The VAS method uses a visual representation of a linear scale with one end representing the best possible health state and the other representing the worst possible health state. Patients are asked to place the health state being evaluated in the position that best describes their preferences relative to the extremes, yielding an ordering of alternatives based on the visual analog scale. PWC asks patients to evaluate their preferences for each possible heath state or treatment in a pair-wise fashion, which then determines a preference ordering for all alternatives.

The TT method asks the patient to determine the number of years that life in perfect health would be equally preferable to a longer period in the health state in question. The resulting ratio represents the preference for the poorer health state.

The result of the preference elicitation using one of the described methods yields a preference ordering of health states or treatments which can then be used as inputs to the MAUT function to determine the overall preference for a set of alternatives and their health outcomes. Through tools developed by the Center, data can be collected on an appropriately-equipped computer connected to the Internet. Patient preference data are then checked and stored rapidly and confidentially, ready for analysis.

Cognitive processes involved in the assessment can be quite demanding. For example, the SG and the TT methods deal with abstractions and expressions of preferences for life and death, and varying degrees of impairment and health conditions. Despite the complexity of the activity, the Center demonstrated that computer elicitation of preferences using VAS and SG produces consistent and reliable results and that this means of preference elicitation is well accepted by most patients. However, the assessment of alternatives typically requires the use of some mathematical concepts, thus the validity of utility assessments has been shown to be dependent on the numeracy of the patient. The need for information to be presented in a manner most appropriate for individual cultural and literacy factors also has been demonstrated (Schwartz et al., 2004; Woloshin et al., 2001; Lenert et al., 2001).

Investigators using the services of the Center were able to download their patients' responses over the WWW. In addition to the Internet-based assessments, stand-alone multimedia preference determination of the elicitation software incorporated health state descriptions (iMPACT3) have been tested by the same group (Lenert, Sturley, and Watson, 2002). Multimedia descriptions of health states that patients have not yet experienced have been shown to improve patients' understanding of these states' impact on QOL and to improve patients' abilities to rate preferences. Multimedia presentations have been used in some Center studies to describe the effects of antipsychotic drugs and Gaucher disease (Goldstein et al., 1994).

Envisioning Treatment Options

The technology-based Shared Decision-Making Program (SDP) was developed within a framework grounded in the idea that rational treatment decision-making considers both what the patient wants and what the clinician views as appropriate. The SDP was designed for use in the clinic setting to aid patients facing complex treatment choices (Liao et al., 1996; Kasper, Mulley, and Wennberg, 1992). The SDP for benign prostatic hyperplasia (BPH) has been clinically tested and evaluated since 1989, and the foundation for Informed Medical Decision-Making has gone on to develop similar programs for other medical conditions such as low back pain, mild hypertension, breast cancer, and recently, ischemic heart disease (Longo, 1993). In the SDP designed for BPH, following diagnosis and introduction to the program, patients receive an informational brochure and complete a questionnaire about demographics, current symptoms, feelings about symptoms, and health outcome preferences. Self-reported and other data are entered into the program, which then tailor estimates of risks and benefits to specific patient situations. In addition to verbal and graphic display of patient-specific probabilities, SDP presents videotaped interviews with individuals facing similar problems. For example, in the BPH program, a taped interview with two physician-patients who chose either prostatectomy or watchful waiting is shown so that an understanding of the possible outcomes is made more real. This "core" segment lasts 22 minutes. In the "elective" segment that follows, the patient may view additional offerings on acute retention, sexual dysfunction, incontinence, and emerging treatments. The elective segments can add to 25 minutes of material. Printed summaries for the patient and clinician are made available (Barry et al., 1995).

A prospective randomized trial to evaluate the impact of SDP for BPH on subsequent treatment decisions was recently carried out in Washington state. After a 1-year follow-up, SDP subjects had significantly better scores than control subjects on BPH knowledge, satisfaction with the process of decision-making, general health perceptions, and physical functioning. The distribution of treatment decisions did not differ between groups. No difference was also found on satisfaction with the decisions themselves, BPH severity, social functioning, and preference for decision-making participation (Glanz, Lewis, and Rimer, 1997).

Facilitating Data Management

At Dana-Farber Cancer Institute, reports of health-related quality of life (HRQOL) are obtained from cancer patients each time they go to the breast cancer outpatient clinic. Patrick and Erikson (1993) define HRQOL as "the value assigned to the duration of life as modified by the social opportunities, perceptions,

functional states, and impairments that are influenced by disease, injuries, treatments, or policy." Patients' assignation of a value to their current QOL, vis-`a-vis their preference for a health state, can be quantified on a continuum from 0 to 1. The longitudinal elicitation of patients' perceptions of the effects of both the cancer and the treatment on their QOL presents the clinician with multiple opportunities to improve patient care. The clinician receives self-reported information that can instigate further discussion with patients about their preferences during the visit. These elicited data also act as feedback to the clinician about the outcomes of care since the last visit. At each point of contact, there is patient-reported information that can provide the basis for customizing patient care plans. In addition, the pen-based application used for the assessment has proven acceptable to patients, minimizes data entry, generates reports, is integrated with the institution's Oracle database, and works on a handheld computer called Newton MessagePad (Le, Kohane and Weeks, 1995).

Linking Preferences with Treatment Decisions

The Department of Family Practice at the Medical College of Virginia, Virginia Commonwealth University, designed HealthTouch, a computerized health information system for health promotion and disease prevention for use in primary care (Williams, Boles, and Johnson, 1995). Evaluated in a randomized clinical trial involving 29 primary care practices, HealthTouch was intended to supplement clinician involvement in patient-focused preventive services. As factors that contribute to variation in health and prevention outcomes, patient preferences regarding diet management, exercise routines, weight control strategies, and other practices served as the basis for the customized computer recommendations for prevention. The preference assessment in HealthTouch is semantic in nature and does not rely on an explicit decision theoretic model.

Patients used a touch screen to answer 20–25 questions on personal and family history and patient preferences that affect lifestyle. The system then generated patient-specific intervention criteria and education materials as well as clinicians chart reminders, reports, and order forms that facilitated both prescribing interventions and documenting the interaction with the patient. The clinicians were able to modify the recommendations, to further document patient preference to accept or decline implementation of the recommended activity, and to order the interventions or screenings, if appropriate.

HealthTouch was incorporated into clinic practices in two ways: actively, by staff directing the patients to complete the survey and passively, by placing the computers in the waiting area and allowing use based on patient choice. Regardless of the circumstances, follow-up surveys revealed that 77% of the patients who used HealthTouch received copies of their personalized health promotion recommendations and of these patients, 93% read the reports. Patients who were actively asked to complete the questionnaire were more likely to have had their practitioner discuss the report with them and to have completed suggested interventions than were patients who completed the survey at their own initiative. Nearly 9 out of 10 patients reported being very satisfied with HealthTouch and saw it as a personally valuable tool for their health (Williams et al., 1995).

Efficacy of Decision Aids

Decision aids for providing information regarding treatment options and health states leading to the elicitation of patient preferences have been developed to provide assistance to patients who are facing complex healthcare decisions. As described earlier, patients may have preferences for the structural, process, or outcomes dimensions of healthcare. Clinicians and health providers generally place a high value on achieving optimal clinical outcomes. While the value systems of the patients and clinicians may sometimes conflict, the goal is for decision aids to support and enhance patients' ability to choose a course of treatment that is consistent with their values along each of these three dimensions while simultaneously yielding optimal clinical outcomes. Measures of efficacy should therefore evaluate the degree to which the decision aids positively impact all of these outcomes. The Ottawa Health Research Institute (OHRI) has developed a set of evaluation measures and instruments that can be used by implementers of DSS to asses their systems performance along the dimensions of choice predisposition, decisional conflict, regret, acceptability, knowledge, realistic expectations, values, preparation for decision-making, and decision self-efficacy (*http://decisionaid.ohri.ca/eval.html*).

A systematic review of 17 studies of interventions that provided patient decision support for treatment or screening of health-related issues was performed by members of OHRI. The studies they analyzed included only randomized control trials (RCT) that helped to provide patients make "specific and deliberative choices among options by providing information on the options and outcomes relevant to a patient's health" (O'Connor et al., 1999). The restriction to RCTs enabled comparisons against a control group selected from the same pool of patients who did not receive the intervention. It was determined that decision aids improved patients' knowledge of outcomes and options, increased their comfort level with the decision-making process, and increased the level of participation in the decision process without an increase in anxiety. Decision aids have no effect on the retrospective satisfaction with the treatment decisions made. There was a variable effect on the actual patient decisions with little or no effect on the chosen course of treatment for major surgical procedures and a somewhat larger effect on the choices for treatments that were more minor in nature. The decision aids that provided more detailed information and allowed for a finer granularity of preference assessment improved both decision comfort level and knowledge.

OHRI also has performed a less rigorous review of approximately 130 decision aids involving a literature search and a summative analysis on each. The results from this review mirror the study cited previously with the conclusions including improvement in the knowledge and realistic expectations, lower decisional conflict, enhanced informed choice, and improved congruence between a patient's values and the choice of treatments (O'Connor et al., 2004).

A range of studies of decision aids for specific diseases has shown results that are similar to the systematic review (Janz et al., 2004; Sculpher et al., 2004; Whelan et al., 2003) and one showed an increase in social support for the patient (Lenert and Kaplan, 2000) with another showing decreased costs of treatment (Kennedy, et al., 2002). At this point, there are no studies that show conclusive improvements in clinical outcomes for those patients who used decision aids when compared to those who did not, which is consistent with their focus on improving the congruence with the values and preferences of patients, which are distinct from the health providers' values on clinical outcomes.

Points of Decision Support System Intervention

DSSs have been introduced at several types of intervention points. The most commonly deployed systems are those that are used when a patient has entered an acute phase of a disease. In these cases, DSS are narrowly targeted to providing the patient with a level of information adequate to allow them to make informed choices and participate in the shared decision process.

This intervention point characterizes most of DSS discussed up to this point in this chapter.

An emerging application of computer-based DSS is in the area of chronic disease management. The success of the management of chronic disease is characterized by the need to timely monitor patients' status and their compliance with the treatment protocols over an extended period of time. Patients may require access to information and their clinician throughout the course of their illness so that they can understand their health states and move toward self-management of their disease. The computer-based DSS can function as an intelligent disease management agent, which can be used to remotely acquire and transmit health indicators such as heart rate and weight and can be used to prompt patients when it is time to take their medicine or perform physical therapy activities.

The need for patients to make decisions regarding screening for diseases or for genetic defects is becoming increasingly common as the number and range of diagnostic tests available continue to multiply (Entwistle, 2004). Screening tests are used to identify latent diseases. There is a vast range of implications of the results of a screening test as the sensitivity and specificity as well as the efficacy of treatment that are associated with a particular screening test vary widely. There is the potential for harm, in that psychologic health may be affected by increased stress and the treatment options in the case of a false or misleading result may cause harm to the physical health of the patient. DSS has been demonstrated to be effective at assisting patients with assessment of the individual risks of having the latent disease along with understanding of the implications of the result of the test as viewed through the patient's values.

Effective behavior change is needed in diverse areas such as weight control, good nutrition, smoking cessation, or substance abuse treatment. In addition, behavior modification methods are important in increasing compliance with medication in conditions such as hypertension, asthma, diabetes, and human immunodeficiency virus-acquired immunodeficiency syndrome (HIV-AIDS). Computer-based DSSs have great potential to provide the information and reinforcement that is required to achieve changes in the chain of decisions that define an undesirable behavior.

Acute Disease Decision Support Systems

DSSs that are employed in the support of acute disease states typically are narrowly focused on supporting the patient by providing for their informational and preference determination needs regarding a single episode of treatment choices. The degree of comprehensiveness of the DSS is tailored to meet the specific characteristics of the disease with regard to the level of decision that the patient is going to be called on to participate in. Generally these disease states with these types of characteristics require increasing levels of information presentation and decision support (Kassirer, 1994).

- Alternatives differ greatly in their outcomes, complications, or side effects.
- Alternatives require trading off long-term and short-term outcomes.
- A choice or choices may result in a small chance of a grave outcome.
- There are only small differences in the outcomes of treatment alternatives.

Commonly, the disease has been diagnosed by a specialist with whom the patient may only have a newly formed relationship. In this case, the clinician-patient relationship that is a prerequisite for the shared decision process does not exist. It is particularly important, in this case, for the DSS to provide a structured method of the joint examination of the patient's preferences that result and that the DSS include mechanisms for determining and conveying to the clinician the level of participation and control in the decision process that the patient prefers.

The Comprehensive Health Enhancement Support System (CHESS) is a health promotion and support network application that operates as a module-based computer system for in-home or healthcare setting use (Gustafson et al., 1994). People with major illnesses or health concerns can access information, decision support, social support, skill training, and a referral resource. Several of the CHESS services help patients to clarify their values in preparation to make decisions that are consistent with their preferences.

Decision aid, based on an additive multiattribute utility model, can be used for condition-specific treatment decisions. The process involves the patient in understanding available options, in choosing possible decision criteria, in assigning weights to the criteria based on preference, and in assignation of a utility score to each criterion-option pair. Descriptions of suggested options and criteria or a personal story of someone who chose that option are offered. The program can also accommodate user-preferred options if the expert-generated lists do not contain the desired one. User-weighted decision criteria are shown in bar graph form, displaying the relative importance of all criteria. Likert-type utility scoring of criterion-option pairs is also graphically displayed in conjunction with summaries of how well each option satisfies its paired criterion. The system can predict the decision the user will make. When used as a conflict analysis aid, CHESS will compare the different weights and utilities and identify areas in which compromise is possible (Boberg et al., 1997).

Chronic Disease Management Decision Support Systems

Chronic diseases such as multiple sclerosis (MS), HIV/AIDS, amyotrophic lateral sclerosis (ALS), asthma, cancer, and hypertension are present at significant and growing rates in many of the countries around the world. Computer-based DSSs have the capability to enable the patient to better monitor and treat these diseases resulting in increased lifespan and QOL. There have been a relatively large number of clinical trials that employ computers as key mechanisms for management of chronic diseases and they have been shown to improve outcomes (Montgomery and Fahey, 1998), enhance treatment compliance, and increase shared decision-making. The primary difference between DSS that support chronic diseases from those that support singular treatment acute diseases is their extension to handle symptom management (Ruland et al., 2003).

The primary components of a chronic disease DSS are assessment, information, and communication. The assessment component is used to measure the patient's health state along the key dimensions of physical condition, functional status, and behavioral tendencies. These systems allow the patient to determine these levels through self-assessment exercises in the privacy of their own residence. These assessments are then available for use by the patient or when transmitted via the Internet by the clinician. The availability of these periodic, timely self-assessments is the basis for monitoring the health state and alerting the patient or clinician when a significant change has occurred. These assessments are also used as the basis for evaluating the health state of the patient relative to their preferences for health states, thereby allowing for the adjustment of their treatment to better align their preferences and outcomes. The assessments also can be used to drive the accessing or delivery of information that is specific to their current health state and symptoms and to focus shared decision process discussions with their clinicians. Critical pathways describe the specific process and sequence of care that can be used to project the expected course of the illness and the associated symptoms and treatments.

Chronic care management can take advantage of critical pathway information by tracking the level of correspondence between the actual and expected pathways and adjusting the future projections based on current health state and treatment plan.

The information component is used to provide information and guidance that is customized to the current health state of the patient. For example, if patients indicate that they are experiencing a particular symptom, the DSS can provide a structured set of documents that inform them about the symptom and recommended therapies or treatments that will address it. The information provided is constantly updated in response to new data acquired by the system.

The communication component provides an integrated mechanism for communicating with the clinician. E-mail interfaces are provided that allow patients to send their health status along with any questions or comments that they have to their clinician and thus serve as a portal into the healthcare provider. Many systems such as CHESS provide for a forum where the patient can network with other patients to provide and receive emotional and therapeutic support.

Most of the computerized decision-making tools described so far in this chapter exist as freestanding programs. While this approach to decision support is valuable, it can also lead to artificial separation of the decision support tool from the patient's day-to-day health information management. In the ComputerLink project an attempt was made to provide a range of integrated electronic services. ComputerLink provided participants with access to an integrated set of computer utilities targeting the needs of homebound patients and their family caregivers: coping with social isolation, managing novel and unexpected problems, and fulfilling unpredictable needs for health information (Flatley-Brennan, 1998; Brennan, 1994). Participants in the research projects used Wyse30 computer terminals based in their homes and linked via plain, ordinary telephone systems to a computer network.

The ComputerLinks each provided three services. The Electronic Encyclopedia consisted of information screens designed to enhance self-management, promote effective home-based treatment of patients, and promote patient/caregiver understanding of illness-specific issues. The Communication service included several public/private options: (1) an unrestricted public bulletin board, which allowed users to post by name or anonymously anything that was on their minds for open, ongoing discussion; (2) private electronic mail, through which users could send and receive their own private electronic mail, including messages from the nurse responding to their personal healthcare inquiries; (3) a question/answer area, in which answers to questions posed anonymously by users were posted by the nurse moderators. The third service, Decision Support, helped ComputerLink users make choices about which personal decisions were necessary, how they could best express these decisions, and how they could best generate insights for such decisions.

The effects of the ComputerLink interventions were evaluated in a field experiment. One study involved 60 persons living with AIDS (PLWAs). Sixty PLWAs participated in a 6-month field evaluation. Each group was randomly halved, with one group receiving typical home care and the other using ComputerLink. There were approximately 15,000 logons to both ComputerLinks, averaging 10–13 minutes per logon. Participants' use of the DSS provides some insight into how and why lay persons would use computer support tools.

Several approaches were used to measure the impact of the DSS. Participants responded to a 15-item survey assessing decision-making confidence and related a recent decision situation, recounting the alternatives chosen and the rationale for their choice. This strategy to obtain information about decision-making skill followed that suggested by von Winterfeldt and Edwards (1986) and others, who recommended that appraisal of the effects of a DSS target those dimensions of the decision problem likely to be amenable to ComputerLink influence. In MAU modeling, the perceived benefit arises from an increased ability to generate alternatives (Humphreys and McFadden, 1980) and an improved ability to understand their rationale (Fisher, 1979). Because decision situations familiar to the subject were used as a data source, this strategy avoided the biases engendered by posing hypothetical situations to the respondent. The strategy does, however, suffer from the bias of recency and saliency (Tversky and Kahneman, 1972); therefore, subjects were instructed to consider only decisions faced within the past 2 weeks. In addition, the effect of the substantive aspects of the decision problem on the number of alternatives generated could not be controlled.

A PLWA choosing to analyze a decision problem using the ComputerLink would first make modem access to ComputerLink from the home-based computer terminal, and then select the option "Make a Decision" from the opening menu. English-language prompts guide the analysis, sometimes incorporating words and phrases into subsequent questions typed by the PLWA in response to earlier items. First, the PLWA responded to a request to label the decision problem. This step is believed to help focus the user to the problem at hand. By permitting the PLWA to employ his or her own words for problem definition, the ComputerLink supported the analysis of problems as viewed by the individual. Next, the ComputerLink screens prompted the PLWA to list the alternatives under consideration, followed by the factors or characteristics deemed by the PLWA as important to the problem. By responding to a sequence of screens, one for each factor, the PLWA then designated on a visual analog scale each of the options under consideration met the factor or characteristic presented on the screen. The length of this line in millimeters became the single-attribute score. To assess the relative importance of each factor to solving the decision problem, subjects completed a weighting scheme suggested by von Winterfeldt and Edwards (1986), in which they assigned 10 to the least important factor, and then assigned a multiple of 10 to indicate how much more important than the index factor was each additional factor. To construct a recommendation, each alternative received a score computed as the weighted sum of each single-attribute score times the weight of the attribute. The final screen presented a list, in rank order, of the alternatives under consideration. Interested subjects could call for detail screens that provided explanations of the computations.

The 29 PLWAs involved in the computer network experience used the decision support tool 195 times over the course of the experiment, each session lasting less than 10 minutes. Subjects used the ComputerLink for a wide range of decision problems. Labels provided by the PLWA of their decisions were classified by their manifest content as either relating to "day-to-day choices" or "health management."

It is impossible to separate out the effects of one part of the computer network intervention on global measures of impact. However, there is evidence of the effect of the overall ComputerLink use, which on some occasions involved use of the ComputerLink on decision-making-related outcomes.

No evidence was seen, however, to suggest that access to the ComputerLink improved decision-making skill (t test of difference in the number of alternatives generated = 0.237, 46 df, $P > 0.05$). PLWAs with access to the DSS generated a mean total of 4.5 alternatives solutions to two decision problems before the experiment, and 5.4 following the experiment. Control subjects showed a mean gain of 0.7 in decision skill scores. Thus, the effect of using a computer network incorporating a decision support function appears to be an increase in decision-making confidence but no change in decision-making skill.

Many of the decision topics analyzed by PLWAs using the ComputerLink addressed issues faced by PLWAs in their day-to-day living. Twelve of the analyzed decisions were directly related to health issues; most of these dealt with choices about treatment or illness management. Topics included "quit smoking," "decide whether or not to go to an analyst," and "bone marrow transplant." Only one decision suggested that the PLWA may have used the ComputerLink to help resolve an emergent health crisis; this person indicated that his decision was to "Decide To Call a Doctor" (upper case characters provided by PLWA). Other decisions analyzed using this system reflected daily living concerns. It is possible that the decision support tool provided in the ComputerLink was better suited to the one-time, exotic decisions and less well suited to the day-to-day choice challenges faced by individuals. We now turn to other uses of computer tools for decision-making, including data management, future state visioning, and health behavior change support.

 ## Decision-Making to Promote Health Behavior Change

Several models of health behavior change provide insight into individuals' decision-making and motivation about changing health and lifestyle habits. More than a dozen theoretical models have been proposed for how to bring about change in health behaviors and lifestyles. According to Glanz and colleagues (Glanz et al., 1997), these proposed changes fall into three broad categories: individual change, interpersonal change, and community change. Four theories for individual change are the health belief model (Janz and Becker, 1984; Rosenstock, 1960), stages of change model (Prochaska, 1984), reasoned action (Fishbein, 1967), and stress and coping model of change (Lerman and Glanz, 1997). These theories focus on the individual and imply that change or the lack of it can be explained by individual characteristics. Three theories of interpersonal health behavior are social cognitive theory (Bandura, 1997), social support theory (Israel and Rounds, 1987; Cassel, 1976), and patient provider communication (Roter and Hall, 1997). These focus on the interaction of two or a group of individuals and how these interactions can promote change. Four theories of community or group intervention models are community organization (Garvin and Cox, 1995), diffusion of innovations (Rogers, 1983), organizations change (Kaluzny and Hernandez, 1998), and communication theory (Bryant and Zillman, 1994; Gerbner, 1983). These models are helpful for leaders who want to make changes in organizations. In addition, other scientists have combined several existing theories into more broad set of models for behavior change (Petraitis, Flay, and Miller, 1995; Stokols, 1992; Ewart, 1989).

However, most behavior change models assume that individuals are aware of their alternatives, know their own values, and process information quickly and efficiently to choose what is in their best interest. Widespread data suggest that these models posit a degree of decision-making about everyday aspects of our lives that is just not that systematic (Nisbett and Ross, 1980). One conceptualization is that people attempting health behavior changes do not decide about single behaviors; they follow that which is implied by their habits from a web of prior decisions (Alemi et al., 2000). In this view, lasting change is a function of multiple decisions over a long time. During that time, a series of interrelated and dependent decisions are made. These decisions lead to actions that are both affected by and alter the state of the world and the rewards the decision-maker receives. When actions are repeated frequently over time, habits are formed. Decisions are linked to many prior large and small choices, and affect future options. It is necessary to go beyond the immediate decision about a single act to see how prior choices concerning a number of related behaviors affect current events. In this conceptualization, habits emerge from a series of linked decisions as opposed to a single decision. There is a shift away from a focus on will power and self-discipline to a focus on problem solving.

To change habits, it is not enough to change a single act. All related decisions and reinforcements also must be examined and modified. Successful change requires careful study of reinforcements and an understanding of linkages among decisions so that all decisions support the same action. For example, the decision to reduce fat intake does not make sense when people continue shopping the same way as before. To maintain new habits, behaviors and decisions that promote the needed change should be coupled with or incorporated into existing routines so that they occur without thought and effort. An avalanche of related small and large decisions is made to make one habit change. This could be seen as analogous to a personal pyramid scheme in which the choice of continuing with an unwanted habit is no longer possible.

It is proposed that to change the system that maintains a habit one must (1) identify and examine the linkages among decisions, (2) measure and receive feedback about behaviors, (3) propose and try out new activities to improve these habits, and (4) build these decisions and behaviors into everyday routines that continue over a long period of time (Alemi et al., 2000). In this context, willpower and discipline are organized and enhanced by changing the system of linked decisions. The conscious decision is not in changing the behavior, but in changing the system that produces the behavior.

Initiatives in the design of computers to aid the decision-making process to date primarily have focused on the construction of tools with a discrete application, such as breast cancer treatment or hormone replacement therapy. The use of computers to assist decision-making for more general purposes, such as making health behavior and lifestyle changes, may require computer tools that focus on the process of decision-making more than the specific content of any one decision. Under the directed access of a clinician, a client could learn to examine a series of decisions about their health behaviors and the linkages among them. This approach to making health behavior change is being refined in a project in which interdisciplinary clinical teams work with an electronic community of individuals to change cardiac risk factors (Moore, in press). As part of an interdisciplinary course in quality improvement, clinical teams: (1) develop a therapeutic relationship with clients over a computer network, (2) assess clients' current health patterns regarding diet and exercise compliance with heart-healthy lifestyle guidelines, (3) coach clients to make self-improvements in health behaviors, and (4) track and trend data related to diet and exercise behavior over the project period. Using a self-improvement Web site created by the authors (*www.csuohio.edu/hca/hca615/improve.htm*), interdisciplinary clinical teams apply several theories of health behavior change, including the health belief model, reasoned action, self-efficacy enhancement, stage of change, and relapse prevention. Clients are electronically "coached" using strategies of goal setting, benefits/barriers assessment, problem-solving skills, diary keeping, social support, buddy system, contracting, tailored messages, relapse analysis, and feedback. Clinicians successfully conduct learning needs assessments with clients, implement strategies to change behaviors, and evaluate client outcomes using online methods. In this project 95% of the 15 clients using this approach have made their desired health behavior changes. They reported feelings of connectedness to their care provider (electronic coach) and stated that the emphasis on making small changes and receiving frequent data and feedback about the changing trends in their behavior were particularly important to making the behavior change.

Although computer interactions between clinicians and clients are not required to apply this approach to health behavior change, computers offer the ability to efficiently provide information to increase understanding, provide timely feedback, track and display behavior data in ways that are easily understood by clients, and offer an ongoing (almost daily) presence in someone's life. Although the role of computers to provide social support to users is controversial, it appears that directed support or coaching from a clinician may work because it brings new information and feedback to the problem (Cassel, 1976; Cobb, 1976). Kessler and McLeod (1985) suggest that support works because it reduces stress and provides a sense of belonging and happiness. Sarason, Pierce, and Sarason (1990) argue that support works because individuals worry less about where help might come from and spend more time facing their problems. In addition to professional support, this approach encourages (demands) that clients participate in understanding and changing the web of decisions that comprise their behavior pattern. Data show that participation in decision-making enhances implementation chances (Roter and Hall, 1997). Also, early and frequent feedback may be an important reinforcement for maintaining a behavior or abandoning a behavior. Data about behaviors help an individual to understand. Data are needed to discipline our intuitions and prevent us from making false claims and attributions. Lasting change requires changes in understanding, not changes in attitude.

Some challenges to using an electronic care delivery system to support decision-making for health behavior change include obtaining patient hardware for electronic communications needed for Internet access and obtaining sufficient software to graphically display patient data to support behavior change. Clinicians also must increase their learning about combining and applying knowledge from the disciplines of health behavior change and computer science. For example, what is the ideal "client load" that can be reasonably managed electronically by a clinician or team, how much electronic client contact should be done individually or in groups, to what extent should clients' families be involved, and what is the correct balance between the amount of work done with clients online and using other forms of communication, i.e., telephone, written, or face-to-face. Importantly, experience also has shown that electronic delivery of care to clients is a good way to foster interdisciplinary approaches to care. This approach broadens clinician exposure to different views of patient problems and interventions from multiple disciplines.

Decision Support in Screening for Latent Health Conditions

The advent of a wide variety of new medical technologies has enabled the screening for the presence of latent diseases or health problems ranging from genetic testing for mutations for such diseases like BRCA-1/BRCA-2 for breast cancer susceptibility, evaluating metabolic markers such as the prostate-specific antigen (PSA) antigen test for identifying potential for the presence of prostate cancer and amniocentesis which allows for the screening of fetuses for a variety of health conditions including genetic diseases such as Huntington and Down syndromes. Patient decision-making in the context of the application of screening tests has a different set of characteristics than those applied in acute, chronic disease management, or behavioral modification situations. Screening tests may have effects on a patient's life that are far broader than just their state of health and carry a different set of side effects including the potential for individual and familial psychologic harm (Richards and Williams, 2004) as well as for affecting a person's ability to obtain insurance (Low, King, and Wilkie, 1998) and employment. Certain screening tests involve invasive procedures that can result in harming physical health such as those for colorectal which can cause intestinal perforation (Dolan and Fisina, 2002) or amniocentesis which can cause miscarriage. These negative effects can occur irrespective of the actual outcome of the test and as a result the decision to undergo testing in and of itself requires adequate information and counseling to facilitate an informed choice by patients which reflects their personal value set. In the event the patient chooses to undergo screening, an additional layer of decision-making requiring decision support is undertaken to determine what clinical course of treatment is to be followed in the context of the test results.

This additional level of decision-making can be similar to that found in the acute or chronic disease phases if the test indicates the presence of a disease in the patient who has been tested. There are, however, screening test outcomes such as testing positive for being a Huntington gene carrier that does not require any immediate health-related decision-making for the benefit of the carrier but instead requires decision-making relating to lifestyle or life choice, in this case that decision would involve whether to have children given the knowledge of being a carrier. These types of decisions are quite different from those typically found in the clinical setting and require different approaches to information presentation and decision analysis.

As discussed earlier, patients find the assessment of probabilities in the context of healthcare decision-making to be a challenging and stressful task. Decisions regarding screening invoke an additional layer of uncertainty that involves the correctness of the test results, which is their sensitivity and specificity. Sensitivity is the ability of a test to determine which patients have a disease and specificity is the ability of a test to determine which patients do not

have a disease. All medical testing involves a degree of probabilistic uncertainty, which gives rise to both false positive and false negative results, resulting in some portion of patients who have the disease but are told that they do not and others that do not have the disease but are told that they do.

In the context of screening tests for diseases, a false positive can lead to substantial psychologic harm and can expose the patient to further invasive procedures that can increase health risks, and false negatives can lead to an increase in malpractice claims (Patrick and Erikson, 1993). A false negative can have tragic implications as the disease goes untreated. The decision process involved in evaluating screening decisions involves a complex combination of probabilities. The addition of probabilities for false positives and false negatives results in a situation where the risk assessment capacity of patients is quickly overwhelmed. There are no significant studies to date that examine the effect of the inclusion of the specificity and sensitivity information in DSSs and this information is typically not presented to patients for their consideration in decision-making.

Patients who were made aware of the potential adverse side effects of the colorectal screening tests through use of a structured multicriteria decision aid which assessed their values as they related to the screening context chose to undergo the screening procedure at a substantially reduced rate (18%) versus those who were given only traditional educational materials (37%) (Dolan and Fisina, 2002). This decrease in preference for screening tests following a combination of education and preference assessment has been repeated in the context of several different diseases. The PSA test that measures an antigen, which is associated with prostate cancer, is an example of the complexity of the decision process that screening tests can require. Prostate cancer is the second leading cause of cancer death in men and is often curable when detected at an early stage. PSA screening in asymptomatic men may reveal slow growing cancers which will never affect health and there is no clinical trial data that mortality due to prostate cancer is reduced through screening. The treatment for prostate cancer carries the risk of erectile dysfunction and incontinence potentially leading to health and QOL issues. The large amount of uncertainty in the specificity of the test combined with the uncertainty of the benefits of early detection lead to a decision process that is highly dependent on the patient's preferences for outcome of treatment (Volk et al., 1997).

In two separate studies a combination of an educational videotape with a utility preference assessment and the utility preference elicitation of both husband

and wife were used to determine the preference for PSA screening (Volk, Cass, and Spann, 1999). In the first study, the preference for screening was reduced by 17% in the group that received education and the utility assessment indicating that a combination of comprehensive education and risks leads to decisions that were aligned with the values of the patient.

In the second study, the time TT method was used to elicit patients, wives, couples, and physician-expert surrogates' utilities for complications of prostate cancer treatment which directly assesses how much time in a state of perfect health is judged to be equivalent to a period with the complication that is being evaluated. The preferences in this study differed clearly between the husband's and wife's utility for life expectancy and complications. Husbands had much lower utility for complications than did wives who were generally unwilling to trade-off lack of complications for reduced life expectancy. This indicates that men are more likely to adopt a "watchful waiting" choice where the PSA test is not taken but are vigilant for other symptoms that may make the choice to undergo a PSA screen more preferable.

The differences for preferences in screening are not unique to prostate cancer and given the effect of both the disease and the treatments on the intimate aspects of a couple's relationship, this study points out the value in employing DSS tools in combination with educational materials to the familial unit affected by a screening decision. Screening decisions that would fall in the same category and thus would benefit from this type of DSS application may include diseases that affect or include reproduction such as genetic profiling and screening for breast cancer.

The screening context is a complex milieu of risks, probabilities, and consequences that interact in different ways for the groups that receive one of the four possible outcomes: true positive, true negative, false positive, and false negative. There is clearly a very different set of consequences for each of the above categories and it is plausible to posit that a different set of educational information and differing decision support methodologies are appropriate for each of the subgroups. Aside from the difficulty in determining those differing needs, the primary problem is that a priori it is not possible to distinguish which group a patient falls into and thus the only information available to guide the application of DSS would be some measure of risk that is specific and measurable to the individual.

In a study evaluating the knowledge about prenatal screening for Down syndrome, the association between attitudes, knowledge, and uptake (decision to have screening test done), it was determined that the level of knowledge is not related to the rate at which screening is chosen nor is knowledge related to the attitudes toward screening (Austoker, 1999).

The contrast between this study and the studies on PSA testing indicates that the application of DSS techniques may be most appropriate in situations where uncertainty levels of disease presence and treatment outcomes are high and individual preferences for outcomes vary widely among patients. In cases where uncertainty of outcome is low or where the attitudes toward outcome are fairly uniform among patients, the use of DSSs will tend to provide education that is valuable in affecting the emotional responses to test outcomes through improving understanding but will not alter screening decision characteristics.

Summary: Decision-Making and Choice in Healthcare

Decision-making and choice in healthcare is shaped by three important trends: recognition of both the value and limits of science as a guide for care, a philosophy of care management that emphasizes standards and coordination, and a growing importance of the patient as a key participant in selecting and implementing clinical treatment. Each of these trends supports the need for explicit consideration of patient preferences as a guide to choosing healthcare practices. Yet, each poses specific barriers to the use of patient preferences. Scientific advances that can be made explicit and stated in a logical fashion may overshadow the more elusive, difficult to characterize, patient values. Managed care models may establish clinical care practices that leave little time for the intense, interpersonal process necessary to elicit a coherent understanding of patients' values and preferences. Patients themselves may hold personal attitudes that interfere with their ability or desire to explore these intimate parts of the self, to uncover and make explicit personal preferences, and choose care in accord with those preferences.

In summary, computer technology can solve some, but not all, of the challenges inherent in employing patient preferences in healthcare practices. As new computer tools are developed to support health-related decisions, clarity about the models of decision-making being employed and their match to the type of decisions being addressed is crucial. Given the wide range and vastly different characteristics of various types of health decisions, computer tools of both general purpose and specific purpose and requiring both directed and nondirected access are most likely needed. Computer packages that focus on elicitation and values clarification may serve to help patients think hard about complex, abstract issues such as preferences for life support or health outcomes. Computer networks can insure the rapid, efficient transmission of patient preferences from the point of elicitation to the point of care and may facilitate patients' exploration of preferences in the privacy of their homes or away from an anxiety-producing health encounter. Computer algorithms, built and integrated into a computer-based patient record, have the ability to insure that care is in accord with patient preferences by producing alerts when care deviates from explicit patient preferences. The WWW, CD-ROMs, and other computer tools can deliver informational interventions tailored to the needs, interests, and display requirements of individuals.

References

Alemi, F., Neuhauser, D., Ardito, S., Headrick, L., Moore, S., Hekelman, F., and Norman, L. (2000). Continuous self improvement: Systems thinking in a personal context, results. *Joint Commission Journal of Quality Improvement* 26(2):74–86.

Austoker, J. (1999). Gaining informed consent for screening is difficult but many misconceptions need to be undone. *British Medical Journal* 319:722–723.

Bandura, A. (1997). *Social Learning Theory*. Englewood Cliffs, NJ: Prentice Hall.

Barry, M. J., Fowler , F. J., Mulley, A. G., Henderson, J. V., and Wennberg, J. E. (1995). Patient reactions to a program designed to facilitate patient participation in treatment decisions for benign prostatic hyperplasia. *Medical Care* 33(8):772–773.

Boberg, E. W., Gustafson, D. H., Hawkins, R. P., Bricker, E., Pingree, S., McTavish, F., et al. (1997). CHESS: The comprehensive health enhancement support system. In P. F. Brennan, S. J. Schneider, and E. Tornquist (Eds.), *Information Networks for Community Health*. New York, NY: Springer-Verlag.

Brennan, P. F. (1994). Use of a computer network by persons living with AIDS. *International Journal of Technology Assessment in Health Care* 10:253.

Brennan, P. F. (1998) Improving health care by understanding patient preferences: The role of computer technology. *Journal of the American Medical Informatics Association* 5(3):257–262.

Bryant, J. and Zillman, D. (Eds.). (1994). *Media Effects: Advances in Theory and Research*. Hillsdale, NJ: Erlbaum.

Cassel, J. (1976). The contribution of social environment to host resistance. *American Journal of Epidemiology* 104:107–123.

Cobb, S. (1976). Social support as a moderator of life stress. *Psychosomatic Medicine* 38:300–314.

Deber, R. B., Kraetschmer, N., and Irvine, J. (1996). What role do patients wish to play in treatment decision-making? *Archives of Internal Medicine* 156(13):1414–1420.

Dolan, J. and Fisina, S. (2002). Randomized control trial of a patient decision aid for colorectal cancer screening. *Medical Decision Making* 22(2):125–139.

Donabedian, A. (1968). Promoting quality through the evaluation of patient care. *Medical Care* 6: 181–202.

Elwyn, G., Edwards, A., Gwyn, R., and Grol, R. (1999). Towards a feasible model for shared decision making: Focus group study with general practice registrars. *British Medical Journal* 319:753–756.

Entwistle, V. E. (2004). The potential contribution of decision aids to screening programs. *Health Expectations* 4:109–115.

Eraker, S. A., Kirschtk, J. P., and Becker, M. H. (1984). Understanding and improving patient compliance. *Annals of Internal Medicine* 100:258–268.

Ewart, C. K. (1989). A social problem-solving approach to behavior change in coronary heart disease. In S. A. Shumaker, E. B. Schron, and J. K. Ockene (Eds.), *The Handbook of Health Behavior Change* (pp. 153–190). New York, NY: Springer.

Feinstein, A. R. and Horwitz, R. I. (1997). Problems in the "evidence" of "evidence based medicine." *American Journal of Medicine* 103(6):529–535.

Fishbein, M. (Ed.) (1967). *Readings in Attitude Theory and Measurement*. New York, NY: Wiley.

Fisher, G. (1979). Utility models for multiple objective decision making: Do they really represent human judgment? *Decision Science* 10:451.

Flatley-Brennan, P. (1998). Computer network home care demonstration: A randomized trial in persons living with AIDS. *Computers in Biology & Medicine* 28(5):489–508.

Fortin, J. M., Hirota, L. K., Bond, B. E., O'Connor, A. M., and Col, N. F. (2001). Identifying patient preferences for communicating risk estimates: A descriptive pilot study. *BMC Medical Informatics and Decision Making* 1(2):2.

Garvin, C. D. and Cox, F. M. (1995). A history of community organization since civil war with special reference to oppressed communities. In J. L. Erlich and J. E.Tropman (Eds.), *Strategies of Community Organization* (5th ed.). Itasca, IL: Peacock.

Gerbner, G. (1983). Field definitions: Communication theory. In *1984–85 US Directory of Graduate Programs* (9th ed.). Princeton, NJ: Educational Testing Services.

Gerteis, M., Edgman-Levitan, S., Daley, J., and Delbanco, T.L. (1993). *Through the Patient's Eyes*. San Francisco, CA: Jossey-Bass.

Glanz, K., Lewis, F. M., Rimer, B. K. (Eds.) (1997). *Health Behavior and Health Education: Theory, Research and Practice.* San Francisco, CA: Jossey-Bass.

Goldstein, M. K., Clarke, A. E., Michelson, D., Garber, A. M., Bergen, M. R., and Lenert, L.A. (1994). Developing and testing a multimedia presentation of a health-state description. *Medical Decision-Making* 14:337.

Gustafson, D. H., Hawkins, R., Boberg, E. W., Bricker, E., Pingree, S., and Chan, C. L. (1994). The use and impact of a computer-based support system for people living with AIDS and HIV infection. *Proceedings/the ... Annual Symposium on Computer Application [sic] in Medical Care.* 1:604–608.

Henry, S. B. and Holzemer, W. L. (1995). A comparison of problem lists generated by physicians, nurses, and patients: Implications for CPR systems. *Proceedings of the Annual Symposium on Computer Applications in Medical Care* (pp. 382–386).

Humphreys, P. and McFadden, W. (1980). Experiences with MAUD: Aiding decision structuring vs. bootstrapping the decision maker. *Acta Psychological* 45:51.

Israel, B. A. and Rounds, K. A. (1987). Social networks and social support: A synthesis for health educators. *Advances in health education and promotion* 2:311–351.

Janz, N. K. and Becker, M. H. (1984). The health belief model: A decade later. *Health Education Quarterly* 11:1–47.

Janz, N., Wren, P., Copeland, L., Lowery, J., Goldfarb, S., and Wilkins, E. (2004). Patient-physician concordance: Preferences, perceptions and factors influencing the breast cancer surgical decision. *Journal of Clinical Oncology* 22(15):3091–3098.

Kaluzny, A. D. and Hernandez, S. R. (1998). Organizational change and innovation. In S.M. Shortell and A. D. Kaluzny (Eds.), *Health Care Management: A Text in Organization Theory and Behavior* (2nd ed.). New York, NY: Wiley.

Kasper, J. F., Mulley, A. G., and Wennberg, J. E. (1992). Developing shared decision-making programs to improve the quality of health care. *Quality Review Bulletin* 18(6):183–190.

Kassirer, J. P. (1994). Incorporating patients' preferences into medical decisions. *New England Journal of Medicine* 330:1895–1896.

Keating, N. L., Weeks, J. C., Borbas, C., and Guadagnoli, E. (2003). Treatment of early stage breast cancer: Do surgeons and patients agree regarding whether treatment alternatives were discussed? *Breast Cancer Research and Treatment* 79(2):225–231.

Keeney, R. and Raiffa, H. (1976). *Decisions with Multiple Objectives.* New York, NY: Wiley.

Kennedy, A., Sculpher, M. J., Coulter, A., Dwyer, N., Rees, M., Horsely, S., Cowley, D., Kidson, C., Kirwin, C.,

Naish, C., and Stirrat, G. (2002). Effects of decision aids for menorrhagia on treatment choices, health outcomes and costs. *Journal of the American Medical Association* 288(21):3701–3703.

Kessler, R. C. and McLeod, J. D. (1985). Social support and mental health in community samples. In S. Cohen and S. L. Syme (Eds.), Social *Support and Health.* Orlando, FL: Academic Press.

Le, P. P., Kohane, I. S., and Weeks, J. C. (1995). Using a pen-based computer to collect the health-related quality of life and utilities information. *Proceedings Annual Symposium Computer Applications in Medical Care* (pp. 839–843).

Ledley, R. S. and Lusted L. B. (1999). Reasoning foundations of medical diagnosis. *Science* 130:9–21.

Lenert, L. A. and Kaplan, R. M. (2000). Validity and interpretation of preference-based measures of health-related quality of life. *Medical Care* 38(Suppl. 9):138–150.

Lenert, L. A., Sherbourne, C. D., and Reyna, V. (2001). Utility elicitation using single item questions compared to a computerized interview. *Medical Decision Making* 21(2):97–104.

Lenert, L. A. and Soetikno, R. M. (1997). Automated computer interviews to elicit utilities: Potential applications in the treatment of deep venous thrombosis. *Journal of the American Medical Informatics Association* 4(1):49–56.

Lenert, L. A., Sturley ,A., and Watson, ME. (2002). iMPACT3: Internet based development and administration of utility elicitation protocols. *Medical Decision Making* 22(6):464–474.

Lerman, C. and Glanz, K. (1997). Stress, coping and health behavior. In K. Glanz, F. M. Lewis, and B. K., Rimer (Eds.), *Health Behavior and Health Education: Theory, Research and Practice.* San Francisco, CA: Jossey-Bass.

Liao, L., Jollis, J. G., DeLong, E. R., Peterson, E. D., Morris, K. G., Mark, D. B. (1996). Impact of an interactive video on decision-making of patients with ischemic heart disease. *Journal of General Internal Medicine* 11:373.

Longo, D. R. (1993). Patient practice variation: A call for research. *Medical Care* 31(5):YS82–YS83.

Low, L., King, S., and Wilkie, T. (1998). Genetic discrimination in life insurance: Empirical evidence from a cross sectional survey of genetic support groups in the United Kingdom. *British Medical Journal* 16(1):20–35.

Mitchell, E., McConnahie, A., and Sullivan, F. (2003). Consultation computer use to improve management of chronic disease in general practice: A before and after study. *Informatics in Primary Care* 11(2):61–68.

Montgomery, A. A. and Fahey, T. (1998). A systematic review of the use of computers in the management of hypertension. *Journal of Epidemiology and Community Health* 52:520–525.

Moore, S. M. (in press). Expanding information for clients: Using continuous improvement techniques to achieve health behavior change. *Quality Management in Health Care*.

Moore, S. M. and Kramer, F. M. (1998). Women's and men's preferences for cardiac rehabilitation program features. *Journal of Cardiopulmonary Rehabilitation* 16(3):163–168.

Nisbett, R. and Ross, L. (1980). *Human inference: Strategies and shortcomings of social judgment*. Englewood Cliffs, NJ: Prentice Hall.

O'Connor, A. and Jacobsen, M. J. (2003). Workbook on developing and evaluating patient decision aids. Available at *http://decisionaid.ohri.ca/docs/Resources/Develop_DA.pdf*

O'Connor, A., Rostom, A., Fiset, V., et al. (1999). Decision aids for patients facing health treatment or screening decisions: A systematic review. *British Medical Journal* 319:731–734.

O'Connor, A. M., Stacey, D., Entwistle, V., Llewellyn-Thomas, H., Rovner, D., and Holmes-Rovner, M. (2004). Decision aids for people facing health treatment or screening decisions [Cochrane review]. *Cochrane Database of Systematic Reviews*. 2(2):CD001431.

Patrick, D. L. and Erikson, P. (1993). *Health Status and Health Policy: Quality of Life in Health Care Evaluation and Resource Allocation*. New York: Oxford University Press.

Pauker, S. G. and McNeil, B. J. (1981). Impact of patient preferences on the selection of therapy. *Journal of Chronic Diseases* 34:77–86.

Pauker, S. G., Pauker, S. P., and McNeil, B. J. (1981). The effect of private attitudes on public policy: Prenatal screening for neural tube defects as a prototype. *Medical Decision Making* 1(2):103–114.

Petraitis, J., Flay, B., and Miller, T. (1995). Reviewing theories of adolescent substance use: Organizing pieces in the puzzle. *Psychological Bulletin* 117(1):67–86.

Prochaska, J. O. (1984). *Systems of Psychotherapy: A Transactional Analysis* (2nd ed.). Pacific Grove, CA: Brooks-Cole (originally published 1979).

Protheroe, J., Fahey, T., Montgomery, A. A., and Peters, T. J. (2000). The impact of patients' preferences on the treatment of atrial fibrillation: Observational study of patient based decision analysis. *British Medical Journal* 320:1380–1384.

Raiffa, H. (1968). *Decision Analysis: Introductory Lectures on Choice Under Uncertainty*. Reading, MA: Addison-Wesley.

Richards, F. and Williams, K. (2004). Impact on couple relationships of predictive testing for Huntington Disease: A longitudinal study. *American Journal of Medical Genetics* 126A:161–169.

Rogers, E. M. (1983). *Diffusion of Innovations* (3rd ed.). New York, NY: Free Press.

Rosenstock, I. M. (1960). What research on motivation suggests for public health. *American Journal of Public Health* 50:295–301.

Roter, D. L. and Hall, J. A. (1997). Patient provider communication. In K. Glanz, F.M. Lewis, and B.K. Rimer (Eds.), *Health Behavior and Health Education: Theory, Research and Practice*. San Francisco, CA: Jossey-Bass.

Ruland, C. M. (1998). Improving patient outcomes by including patient preferences in nursing care. *Proceedings/AMIA Annual Symposium* (pp. 448–452).

Ruland, C. M. and Bakken, S. (2001). Representing patient preference-related concepts for inclusion in electronic health records. *Journal of Biomedical Informatics* 34:415–422.

Ruland, C. M., White, T., Stevens, M., Fanicullo, G., and Khilani, S. M. (2003). Effects of a computerized system to support shared decision making in symptom management of cancer patients. *Journal of the American Medical Informatics Association* 10(6):573–579.

Sainfort, F. and Booske, B. C. (1996). Role of information in consumer selection of health plans. *Health Care Financing Review* 18(1):31–54.

Sarason, B. R., Pierce, G. R., and Sarason, I. G. (1990). Social support: The sense of acceptance and the role of relationships. In B. R. Sarason, I. G. Sarason, and G. R. Pierce (Eds.), *Social Support: An Interactional View* (pp. 97–128). New York, NY: Wiley.

Saunders, G. and Courtney, J. (1985). A field study of the organizational factors influencing DSS success. *MIS Quarterly* 9(1):7.

Schwartz, S. R., McDowell, J., and Yueh, B. (2004). Numeracy and the shortcomings of utility assessment in head and neck cancer patients. *Head and Neck* 26(5):401–407.

Sculpher, M., Bryan, S., Fry, P., Winter, P., Payne, H., and Emberton, M. (2004). Patients' preferences for the management of non-metastatic prostate cancer: Discrete choice experiment. *British Medical Journal* 328:382–384.

Sonnenberg, F. A. and Pauker, S. G. (1986). Elective pericardiectomy for tuberculous pericarditis: Should the snappers be snipped? *Medical Decision Making* April–June:110–123.

Stokols, D. (1992). Establishing and maintaining healthy environments: Towards a social ecology of health promotion. *American Psychologist* 47(1):6–22.

Tversky, A. and Kahneman, D. (1972). Judgment under uncertainty: Heuristics and biases. *Science* 185:124–131.

Ubel, P. A., Jepson, C., and Baron, J. (2001). The inclusion of patient testimonials in decision aids: Effects on treatment choices. *Medical Decision Making* 21(1):60–68.

Volk, R., Cantor, S., Spann, S., Cass, A., Cardenas, M., and Warren, M. (1997). Preferences of husbands and wives for prostate cancer screening. *Archive of Family Medicine* 6:72–76.

Volk, R., Cass, A., and Spann, S. (1999). A randomized control trial of shared decision making for prostate cancer screening. *Archive of Family Medicine* 8:333–340.

von Neumann, J. and Morgenstern, O. (1964). *Theory of Games and Economic Behavior*. New York, NY: Addison-Wesley.

von Winterfeldt, D. and Edwards, W. (1986). *Decision Analysis and Behavioral Research*. Cambridge, MA: Cambridge University Press.

Whelan, T., Sawka, C., Levine, M., Gafni, A., Reyno, L., Willan, A., Julian, J., Dent, S., Abu-Zahra, H., Chouinard, E., Tozer, R., Pritchard, K., and Bodendorfer, H. (2003). Helping patients make informed choices: A randomized trial of a decision aid for adjuvant chemotherapy in lymph node-negative breast cancer. *Journal of the National Cancer Institute* 95(8):581–587.

Whitney, S. N. (2003). A new model of medical decisions: Exploring the limits of shared decision making. *Medical Decision Making* 23(4):275–280.

Wilkes, M. S., Bell, R. A., and Kravitz, R. L. (2000). Direct-To-Consumer prescription drug advertising: Trends, impacts and implications. *Health Affairs* 19(2):110–117.

Williams, R. B., Boles, M., Johnson, R. E. (1995). Patient use of a personal computer for prevention in primary care practice. *Patient Education Counseling* 3:283–292.

Woloshin, S., Schwartz, L. M., Moncur, M., Gabriel, S. G., and Tosteson, A. (2001). Assessing values for health: Numeracy matters. *Medical Decision Making* 380–388. New York, NY: Wiley.

PART 8

Educational Applications

32

The Nursing Curriculum in the Information Age

Barbara Carty
Iris Ong

OBJECTIVES

1. Identify how technology is reshaping higher education and the nursing curriculum.
2. Identify resources needed to move the nursing curriculum into the information age.
3. Describe strategies to integrate information and computer technology into the nursing curriculum.
4. Describe a nursing informatics curriculum.

KEY WORDS

cognition
curriculum
computer literacy
faculty development
informatics
information technology
interactive learning

This chapter presents nursing education within the context of rapidly evolving and deploying of information technology within education. Curriculum implications including faculty development, Web-enhanced and interactive learning, cognition, electronic communications, and informatics are summarized. Models are presented and strategies suggested for meeting the educational challenges of the information age.

Nursing is an information-intensive profession, and nursing education relies heavily on the acquisition of information to educate students in their professional programs. Thus, the acceleration of technological development and availability of information will have profound effects on how students learn, how nursing is taught, and how care is delivered. The National Academy of Sciences in a report issued in 2002, "Preparing for the Revolution: Information Technology and the Future of the Research University" makes a clear mandate that education will be dramatically changed by the rapid proliferation and

deployment of digital technology. No longer will education be constrained by department and discipline boundaries, but rather information technology will change how universities are organized, financed, and governed.

In a very short period of time, higher education in general, and nursing education in particular, has moved from the delivery of educational content via isolated networked computer-assisted instruction (CAI) to the development of dynamic Web-based interactive delivery sytems that integrate voice, video, and text. The acquisition of educational materials and information now involves sophisticated communication and information systems that students can access from home, classroom, and clinical settings. Wireless technology, considered the fourth generation of computing, is just beginning to make inroads into both education and healthcare delivery systems. Access to data, information, and learning materials can be "on-demand" anywhere, anytime. In 2003, it is projected that American colleges are expected to spend more than \$5.2 billion on information technolgy; this is a 5% increase over 2001–2002 (Olsen, 2003).

Not only must educators in nursing programs be concerned with the overall rapid changes in technology and its application, faculty have to be equally aware and knowledgeable about various methods of content delivery and how student outcomes are effected by the use of information technology in both communication and learning.

Additionally, informatics, a discipline in its early stages, has become intricately related with the delivery of information in education and practice. Research indicates that the concept of informatics needs to be articulated in curricula in the context of cognition and information processing, including information science as well as the technology that supports these functions (Patel and Kaufman, 1998; Ribbons, 1998a; Patel, 2001; Carty, 2001). In short, when curriculum and nursing education are examined, it needs to be done through the lens of information technology and information science. This is the future vision of education.

Informatics as applied to healthcare and education has changed dramatically in the past decade. Propelled by the advances in information and computer technology, we are now poised for yet another paradigm shift in the information era of the twenty-first century. The experience we have had with computers and information technology over the past decade allows us to incorporate new information, develop innovative models, and apply research findings to the field of informatics as it relates to nursing education and practice.

In the past, literature on educational applications related to the use of computers to enhance and promote education. There is currently a paradigm shift in society generally, and informatics specifically, that emphasizes the communication and collaborative components of information technology rather than the computing aspects (Carty and Rosenfeld, 1998; Connors et al., 2002). Nursing literature supports that the teaching of computer literacy or skills alone will not prepare nurses for the knowledge and integrative competencies they will need for the adequate managing of information in their profession (Staggers, Gassert, and Curran, 2002; Chastain, 2002; McNeil et al., 2003).

This chapter will present the rapidly evolving changes taking place in the development and delivery of education material in nursing education and will focus on the processes of information management and technology as they apply to the nursing curriculum. Education will be discussed within the context of information technology

and information science and specifically relate to:

1. Information management and the educational environment
2. Faculty development
3. Cognition and interactive learning
4. Nursing informatics and the curriculum

Information Management

The management of information is and will continue to become one of the most daunting challenges for faculty, students, and nurses. Maintaining currency with the technology as well as with the dramatic changes within the education system as a result of digital technology will occupy the energies of faculty and administrators. Initiatives such as Internet2 (available at *http://www.internet2.edu/about/aboutinternet2.html*) will have a lasting impact on the culture and intellectual activities of the university. The creation of collaborative information technology intensive ventures among publishing, business, and education will result in a "knowledge and learning" industry that will alter the way faculty deliver content, students access learning materials, and administrators finance higher education (National Academy of Sciences, 2002). Mirroring the urgency in higher education to promote information management and technology is the American Association of Colleges of Nursing (AACN) Agenda for the 21st Century (1999) to support and foster the development of information and healthcare technologies among both faculty and students. A number of other efforts both within and outside of nursing support the necessity for nurses and students to be able to process, manage, and access information in education and nursing practice (Ribbons, 1998b; Young, 2002). These demands will only increase as our society becomes more dependent on information and technology continues to move to seamless interactive systems that incorporate cognition and decision support into the ebb and flow of education and practice.

Studies indicate that in many ways nursing education programs have neither incorporated information technology nor developed strategic plans that promote faculty development, financing, and support for information management in a comprehensive and measurable way (Carty and Rosenfeld, 1998; McNeil et al., 2003). Of primary importance for the successful integration of information management in education is an organizational infrastructure that supports resources both human and technical, promotes faculty development, and incorporates informatics into the curriculum.

Educational Environment

A discussion of the process of education in the context of information technology and information management necessitates inclusion of the educational environment to promote the delivery of curriculum content. Studies demonstrate that the majority of nursing schools have technology in place to deliver learning materials. However, there are marked differences as to the level of faculty involvement in teaching and facilitating information technology. McNeil et al., (2003) reported that the majority of nurse educators surveyed, were at a novice or advanced beginner level in the use of such applications as bibliographic retrieval and graphic software presentations. Chastain (2002) found 18.7% of faculty surveyed ($N = 79$) did not include information technology in the curriculum. So while there may be the availability of technology for delivery of learning materials, there is a pressing need for integration of information technology into nursing curricula.

Students as well as faculty need to learn how to access information, integrate it, and apply it in the learning environment as well as the practice environment. The use of appropriate technology for course delivery and assessment and management of healthcare information must be fostered in an environment of collaboration among departments and institutions to assure adequate distribution of resources, quality assurance, and professional recognition (Winter, 2001; National Academy of Sciences, 2002).

A successful plan for the integration of information technology into the education process requires the presence of an environment that engenders and sustains (1) a supportive infrastructure, (2) the availability of centralized technology resources, (3) collaborative, interdisciplinary courses, and (4) alliances among education, business, and government. Such a model, which crosses department lines and assures adequate resources to all members of the educational community, can effectively and efficiently prepare faculty and students to manage information for education and practice.

Supportive Infrastructure

The educational and curriculum goals of nursing education are forced by the nature of information technology to operate within an infrastructure that shares and supports access to available technology and technological innovations. Such an environment embraces (1) adequate technical support, including personnel; (2) an educational resource/technology planning committee; and (3) allocation of financial resources. Administrators and faculty in education should assure their consumers that planning and resources in information technology will be integral to the governance and delivery structure of the institution. One of the first steps in assuring organizational recognition for information technology is a study of the computer and information learning needs within the organizational structure. An assessment of resources as well as learning needs of both faculty and students will provide data to support informed decision-making for both computer technology and information management planning.

Financial resources and budget allocations have been one of the most difficult challenges for educators to reconcile in planning for technological resources. In one of the only studies that examined available financial resources for technology in schools of nursing throughout the country (Carty and Rosenfeld, 1998), financial resources ranged from no monies to as high as $156,000 annually, the mean being only $7,000, the most frequently allocated amount was $1,000. In addition, only one-third of schools reported monies allocated for personnel, with the mean reported as $8,000. In a more recent nationwide study of schools and the status of technology application, 75% of 672 schools reported having "a champion information technology user" (McNeil et al., 2003, p. 348). These findings continue to demonstrate how academic nursing education departments need to legitimize and demand resources to maintain currency in the information age of education. Schools of nursing also need to examine their strategies and formulate innovative methods to assure that existing resources are made available to both faculty and students.

Centralized Resources

With the availability of interconnectivity and both Internet and Intranet capability, schools are in a position to develop and share resources with other departments and divisions in an academic setting. Centralized resources are a natural extension of the information superhighway and the Internet II initiative of the government. The evolution of the Web-based platform not only allows for the transfer of information, but also the sharing of data, group discussions, access to educational programs, and the facilitation of research. Wide area networks (WANs) within schools of nursing promote immediate access to large shared databases and the pooling of resources. As academic settings expand their connectivity and Internet capability, nursing programs should have a seat at the table and contribute to the planning and allocation of resources. Representation on interdisciplinary strategic planning committees for technology implementation is essential as universities restructure and chief information officers (CIOs) form teams to develop long-range plans and goals. Similarly, technical support can be jointly supported by a number of departments, and nursing students can be encouraged to collaborate with students from other disciplines, including business and computer science. Such collaborative methods can decrease operational costs and provide for access to a large array of digital information including library databases, educational software, and research resources. The advent of learning platforms such as Blackboard and Web CT are promoting centralized resources for the authoring and delivery of content. These platforms have become commonplace and robust in the past 5 years and many faculty have had to reengineer and learn how to integrate the technology into their pedagogy.

Collaboration

Rogers (1996, p. 29) maintains that the rapid advances in technology will continue to "create financial and infrastructure needs that university campuses will be forced to address: new equipment, more user training, and new courses." The development of collaborative models in which faculty formulate interdisciplinary courses, share resources, and promote student interaction can be an exciting paradigm of the future. Hairston (1996) states that "for tomorrow's successful college and university, it will matter much less that departments exist, but far more that faculty, students, and all others interrelate." These themes have been reiterated more recently on a national level. ". . . university strategies (should) include the development of sufficient in-house expertise among faculty and staff to track technological trends and assess various courses of action; the opportunity for experimentation; and the ability to form alliances with other academic institutions" (NAS, 2002, p. 3).

The development of interdisciplinary courses and the cross-fertilization of experiences can benefit both faculty and students as they acquire skills in computer literacy and knowledge of information management. Various course models (Carty, 2000) have recently been

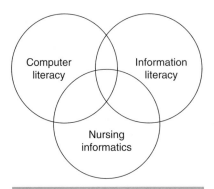

Figure 32.1
Relationships and interrelationships of computer literacy, information literacy, and nursing informatics. (Reproduced, with permission, from Nelson, R. (2000). Core informatics: Content for an undergraduate curriculum. In Carty (Ed.), *Nursing Informatics Education for Practice*. New York: Springer.)

proposed by educators as successful strategies to enhance education, maximize resources, and promote innovative learning. Nelson (2000) describes a computer and information literacy model for preparing healthcare practitioners for the future (Fig. 32.1). The model emphasizes the concept of computer and infromation literacy in an undergraduate program and reinforces collaboration among faculty in a college setting. Indeed, both faculty development and student learning are dependent on interdisciplinary collaboration and the use of information and communications technology.

Clearly, in a number of college settings, a major revolution is taking place in which technological innovations are being incorporated into the infrastructure and instructional operations. The collaborative paradigm in healthcare practice in which nurses work with information specialists, system designers, and technical experts should be emulated in the education setting.

Faculty Development

For faculty development programs to be successful at integrating information technology into the curriculum, they must be sensitive to both faculty interests and time limitations. Faculty values and pedagogic methods can be used to improve student learning, research projects, and clinical practice, so it is important that these aspects of faculty development be considered. In addition to the many demands placed on faculty, we are currently faced with a severe faculty shortage, an aging faculty, and rapid deployment of information technology within academic settings (AACN, 2003; Chastain, 2002). Research indicates that individuals move through several phases as they integrate the use of computers and instructional technology (Harris, 1995; Hilz 2002). This suggests that technical aspects should be taught before moving on to instructional applications of information technology. Table 32.1 lists categories and examples of content for faculty development programs designed to integrate information technology into the curriculum.

Barriers to Faculty Development

Integration of information technology into the curriculum forces major changes within an organization and its individuals. As with any change, driving and restraining forces exist that impact on the integration of innovation. Attention to the change process is crucial if information technology is to be successfully integrated into nursing curricula. In 1998, Cravener developed a faculty development paradigm for integrating information technology into nursing education. Underlying this paradigm is the principle that adoption of information technology for teaching and scholarship is an innovation issue requiring application of change theory so that

faculty's affective responses to change are understood and the desired outcome of change in faculty teaching behaviors are achieved. Subsequent surveys have supported that faculty may be reluctant or are not equipped to develop the knowledge and skills needed to teach information technology and integrate into the curriculum (Chastain, 2002; McNeil et al., 2003).

Faculty development programs that focus on enhancing faculty skills with the use of information technologies will be most successful if known areas of resistance to change are specifically addressed during the planning and implementation phases of program development. Resistance to the integration of technology comes from the anxieties and fears that people have when faced with major personal and institutional changes. From a faculty perspective, issues commonly associated with resistance to change and some strategies to overcome these barriers include institutional cultures, affective responses to the challenge of learning new instructional strategies, competing demands on faculty time, and perceived validity of computer-mediated teaching and learning. McNeil et al. (2003) found in their study that a gap exists in the ". . . knowledge needed by nursing faculty to prepare nurses to be skilled in information technologies and its use to manage clinical information in daily practice" (p. 347). The study also indicated that there are "many gaps in information technology taught in both graduate and undergraduate nursing programs" (p. 347).

Traditionally, institutions of higher learning have been authority- and knowledge-centered. The availability of e-learning and the ubiquitous use of technology have

Table 32.1   Content for Faculty Development Programs to Integrate Information Technology into the Curriculum

Computer Literacy Skills	Information Literacy Skills	Technical Skills	Knowledge for Teaching Information Technology Strategies
Computer systems for delivering healthcare	Electronic mail and Internet/WWW access	Campus and distance course delivery skills such as Internet skills, videoconferencing, multimedia, Blackboard, and Web CT access.	Cognitive theories and information science. Evidence-based practice skills and knowledge
Software packages such as word processing, spreadsheet applications, database, and computer-based testing systems	Library database access Understanding the impact of automation on healthcare delivery Evaluating the quality of information on the Internet		

created a shift to a more lateral structure where faculty serves as facilitators of learning. This new role can be considered a threat to faculty; combined with a perceived inability to control the teaching process, this can place much stress on faculty. Integration of information technology can also create fear of loss of employment. Faculty strategies need to be redesigned and faculty-student relationships reconsidered in light of the new technology (Ryan, Hodson Carlton, and Ali, 2004).

Affective Responses   Integrating information technology can create a potential threat to faculty self-concept in a variety of ways. Proposing that an educator needs to learn new media for teaching implies that the old way is not optimal. Faculty development programs should emphasize that new technologies are neither good nor bad, but merely a means for solving new problems. An educator's beginner role with instructional technology and/or Internet communications contrasts with his or her normal view of the self as a scholar and discipline expert. Development of technical skills needs to be taught in a nonthreatening manner. The availability and ease of use of e-learning platforms such as Blackboard and Web-CT have fostered the development of technical skills among faculty. They also challenge faculty to create innovative and interactive methods to deliver learning materials and measure student outcomes.

Competing Demands   Integration of information technology into the curriculum is a time-intensive process. A realistic assessment of this time variable and the impact of information technology on faculty workload need to be addressed to prevent faculty disillusionment with the process. Faculty participation in information technology training sessions should be recognized as valid continuing professional education programs by their department chair, and integration of information technology into the curriculum should be part of the tenure and posttenure review criteria.

Nursing faculty in particular may feel that computers disrupt interpersonal relationships with students and patients that are central to building caring and therapeutic relationships. Forces promoting the integration of information technology that can be used to encourage its adoption include new social and economic conditions, technology supports of excellence, risk-taking faculty, and change agents.

As the need for adult lifelong learning gradually spreads through educational systems, the introduction of Web-based instruction provides opportunities to enroll new populations of adult students. Uses of technology to support high-quality teaching and learning can serve as strong selling points during faculty development programs. Reinforcing the fundamental rationale for academic use of Web-based resources, potential advantage for individual faculty, the institution, and students, is crucial to the success of any faculty development program.

Rogers' (1983) theory on innovation-diffusion still has relevance as we attempt to integrate new knowledge and skills into our pedagogy. Hilz (2000) illustrates how one may adopt aspects of Rogers' theory into both clinical and classroom environments while valuing the motivations and perceptions of individuals. Faculty development programs that anticipate potential reactions to change and innovation and value individual differences will be the most sucessful. To keep pace with rapidly changing technological innovations, ongoing faculty development programs for the integration of information technology should be provided. Additionally, adequate resources in the form of hardware, software, and technical support need to be available immediately and on an ongoing basis to decrease faculty frustration while they integrate technology. Faculty development programs need to occur not only on an institutional level but also on the national level.

Cognition and Information Technology

In a discussion of cognition and information technology, it is essential to emphasize both the content taught and the delivery method. With the complex clinical practice environment of the next millennium, it is anticipated that nurses will face escalating information management challenges as well as require psychomotor skills to use ever-changing technology in their nursing practice. As the AACN has stated in *Position Statement: Nursing Education Agenda for the 21st Century* (Rev. 1999), nursing education must encompass the requirements for entry into practice and, to the greatest extent possible, anticipate the requirements for nursing practice in the future. This challenges nursing education to prepare practitioners who have not only appropriate computer literacy skills but also cognitive skills for the effective use of information technologies. Nelson (2000) describes the need for both computer and information literacy in nursing curricula. Computer literacy is the ability to perform computer operations at a skill level high enough to meet the demands of society. In healthcare environments, it involves the computer systems that are used to deliver healthcare and the common microcomputer software packages. Information literacy is the ability to use the tools of automation in the process of accessing, evaluating, and using information. This includes understanding the impact of automation on healthcare. The acquisition of specific information technology skills and knowledge has been supported by a number of authors (Staggers, Gassert, and Curran, 2002; Connors et al., 2002; Mc Neil et al., 2003).

More recently, in addition to the skills for information technology, cognition has been introduced as an important aspect in both the delivery and acquisition of the content of information technology. Turkle (2004) suggests that the tools we use to think "change the way we think" (p. B26). As the tools of information technology become more pervasive we are subtly changing how knowledge is acquired and integrated. Not only must we master the tools of technology, but we must also be cognizant of how users and technology interact, the human-computer interaction. Understanding learning styles and the roles that memory, reasoning, and problem-solving play in learning with interactive technology is essential to developing and implementing sucessful strategies.

The foundational cognitive skills of information acquisition, assessment, management, and use are necessary for effective problem-solving and clinical decision-making. Information technology is a tool that can facilitate or hinder the development of learning and awareness of the cognitive constraints that users impose on systems can promote the optimal development and use of learning systems. Using knowledge domain software, as seen in CAI, supports context-specific knowledge reproduction while tools such as word processing, spreadsheets, and e-mail promote knowledge construction or learning outcomes to apply knowledge across a wide variety of content and context domains. These broader-based learning outcomes occur as a result of cognitive residue (Ribbons, 1998a). Cognitive residue is the skills, understanding, and attitudes that remain with the individual as a result of human-computer interaction. Cognitive tools should foster the development of higher order thinking skills required for the effective acquisition, management, and use of healthcare information. There is very little research related to cognitive tools and metacognition in relation to computers and information technology in the nursing literature.

More recently emphasis has been placed on cognition and its role in the development and application of clinical systems (Patel, Arocha, and Kaufman, 2001; Zhang, Patel, and Johnson 2002). In healthcare, computer systems play a unique role because users will interact more with sophisticated systems that will advise, prompt, and alter knowledge in the process of supporting patient care. So an understanding of how users are affected by computer interaction both within education and the practice setting is essential to consider and examine in the information age of healthcare delivery. Patel et al. (2001) maintain that medical (clinical) cognition is essential to understanding how to design and develop systems for clinical applications. The application of cognitive theory is also necessary in comprehending how memory, partcicularly long- and short-term memory, is affected by clinicians' use of clinical systems. The incorporation of the use and application of clinical systems into student learning experiences to promote the understanding of complex clinical situations and improve cognitive understanding of clinical processes should become a major focus in nursing education. Innovative approaches include partnering with vendors to develop prototypes for clinical education (Connors et al., 2002) and incorporating cognition and learning into curricula. Future research directions for the application of computers as cognitive tools in education and healthcare settings are promising areas of research.

Nursing Education and the World Wide Web (WWW)

Nursing education is being reconceptualized by the increasing use of online instruction. The number of traditional college-age students has decreased while the nontraditional part-time student who works and has family obligations has become the norm for most programs (Sullivan, 1997; Halstead, 2000). Although the initial development of Web-based courses appears to be primarily an administrative-driven initiative, the trend is also being sustained by faculty, many of whom find the online learning environment dynamic and well suited to their individual teaching style (Christianson, Tiene, and Luft 2002).

Issues associated with online instructions have been described by several authors to include preplanning strategies, preparation of materials, incorporation of interactivity, and other pedagogic considerations (Byun, 2000; Landis, 2000; Liaw, Huang 2000).

Design and interactivity are important in developing interactive components of Web-based or Web-enhanced courses to ensure effective learning environments. Thurmond (2003) defines four types of interactions in relation to Web-enhanced course: learner-content, learner-learner, learner-instructor, and learner-interface. In learner-content interactions, the student studies the course content and participates in course activities. Strategies to enhance interaction with an online course include online discussions that may be in forms of synchronous chat, threaded weekly discussions, or e-mail.

With learner-learner interactions, students interact with each other to provide an exchange of ideas with different perspectives, which may reinforce understanding of what is being taught in course. Promoting this type of interaction may be achieved through collaborative group work/ projects. The third type of interaction, learner-instructor, is the most common. This type of interaction is used by students to reinforce understanding of course content and clarify nebulous points. Faculty may use several activities to achieve this within an online environment. Examples of these activities may be posting syallabus, responding quickly to student questions using email or online discussions, and addressing students personally. The last type of interaction, learner-interface, deals with how students interact with technology medium used in the course. Issues with access, compounded with lack of computer experience create frustration for the student. Strategies to promote a more satisfying learner-interface interaction would include posting of minimal hardware computer requirements and computer skills. Review of navigation and overview of the online course is recommended in the beginning of the course during a face-to-face session. Research also supports that hybrid courses or a combination of face-to-face and online interactions may be the best approach for some students (Kozlowski, 2002).

With the proliferation of e-learning platforms such as Blackboard and Web-CT, universities have evolved into Web-enhanced environments that support multimedia delivery and supplement face-to-face traditional teaching methods.

Multimedia

Multimedia, with its ability to deliver text, full color graphics, sound, video, and animation, provides an excellent example of how learning can be enhanced by computer-based systems. The most important characteristic of multimedia is its ability to deliver an effective and flexible method of instructional material that attracts the learner's interest, maintains attention, and accommodates a diversity of learning styles. In more recent years mutlimedia has been adapted to the WWW environment with its capability for video streaming and its ability to accomodate interactive power point presentations. Technology allows faculty to design and develop multimedia software that includes case studies and tutorial applications (Mills, 2000; Wilkie et al., 2001; Ross and Touvinen, 2001). Ribbons (1998c) suggests a variety of practical guidelines for the development of interactive multimedia applications in nursing education. In order for multimedia to be

an effective teaching tool, it is essential that the application be based on firm pedagogic principles.

CD-ROM/DVD

CD-ROMs (compact disk-read only memory) as teaching-learning tools for clinical nursing education incorporate multimedia capability, portability, and large storage capacity. Authoring software is available and allows for individuals to create programs to meet individual learning needs. The multimedia capability of CD-ROM technology allows for an interactive on-screen situation that mimics reality with graphics, sound, and movement. The technology and materials needed to record CD-ROMs are now commonly available for personal computer production. CD-RW disks usually hold 74 minutes (650 MB) of data, although some can hold up to 80 minutes (700 MB). Within the next decade, the DVD storage medium will supplant the CD-ROM. Both are written and read by optical means on a photosensitive disc that stores data as 1-μm-wide dots of light and dark. The dots are read by a laser, converted to an electrical signal, and then to audio or visual display for playback. Unlike the CD, there are several storage capacities for a DVD, currently ranging from single-sided, single layered 4.7 GB to double-sided, double layered 17 GB.

A CD player will only read an audio CD disc while a CD-ROM is able to read media of audio CD, CD-R, CD-ROM, and Photo CDs. A CD-R drive will be able to read CD-ROM and CD-R with writing once on CD-R disks. A CD-RW drive will be able to read CD-R disks and CD-RW disks with writing/rewriting abilities to CD-RW disks. A DVD-RAM drive will be able to read all CD formats and DVD-ROMs and will reads/ writes to DVD disks.

Interactive CD-ROM Programs/ Simulation Software

Self study modules/interactive CD-ROM programs and simulation software are computer-assisted learning programs designed to achieve greater mastery of content and learning than is possible with didactic instruction. This is achieved by allowing the learner to interact with the computer at his or her own pace and as many times as needed to master content. Most programs are text-based and include illustrations with audio and visual graphics of a procedure. Multiple topics are available to meet the range of professional learners. Available programs include drill and practice, tutorials, and simulations. Drill and practice routines allow the student to practice previously learned material through answering multiple choice questions. The program may score and track the student's progress and provides feedback. Tutorials or remedial instructions are computer-assisted learning software that provides didactic information and includes drill exercises to provide the learner with feedback about her or his mastery level of content. Simulations are case studies and/or models designed to provide opportunities to deal with realistic clinical or administrative problems. Clinical simulations provide the learner with opportunities to develop clinical decision-making skills in a nonthreatening environment.

Computer-assisted learning programs can be cost-effective and user-friendly, and the content can be customized to meet learner needs. For a computer-assisted learning program to be an effective educational tool, it must be designed in a stimulating and motivating way. It is essential that the educational strategy be clear and the program be appropriate to course objectives and the level of the student. There are several strategies that can be used to develop, review, and evaluate the usefulness of multimedia programs (Ross and Touvinen, 2001).

Testing System

Since April 1994, the National Council Licensure Examination for Registered Nurses (NCLEX-RN) has been an online, computer-based test administered in selected locations in every state and United States territory. Although computer literacy is not essential for taking the test, student familiarity and comfort with computer adaptive testing prior to taking the licensure examination are helpful to decrease anxiety levels and improve computer literacy. In response to this need, testing systems and software programs have been designed by developers and faculty to promote computer-based testing (CBT) in schools. The first published report of computerized testing in nursing education found that students taking examinations on computer performed "as least as well as, and in some cases better than" those given paper and pencil tests. The study further concluded that computerized testing was not detrimental to grades or to learning for the limited number of students who participated in the study (Bloom and Trice, 1997). In a more recent study, experience with CBT helped to decrease anxiety but did not improve NCLEX performance (Reisling, 2003). Concerns related to CBT include test security, use of honor codes, and positive student reactions to the choices accompanying computer testing.

Reported benefits of computerized testing for faculty include a reduced amount of time invested in the development, administration, and scoring of tests; the ability to generate a variety of question types; the establishment of test banks with varying degrees of psychometric properties; the ability to import questions from textbook computerized test banks; and prompt processing of grades and analysis of questions through access to students' answer files. Students report that feedback on questions during or immediately after the test promotes their learning. Other student benefits reported include immediate reports on their grades and scheduling of testing dates and times spread over several days to fit their academic and personal needs. Students feel that exposure to computers for evaluative purposes prepares them for taking the licensing examination on the computer. In an updated review of test development software (Kirkpatrick et al., 2000), the authors conclude that online testing is prevalent with many applications now in a Web-based format. The availability of Web-based formats such as Blackboard allow faculty to develop test banks, promote item analysis, and produce group and individual reports.

The production of commercial packages for online testing has become a big business with companies developing testing for licensure, school admissions, and competency evaluation.

Electronic Communications

The Internet with the WWW as a platform offers access to a host of information and communication resources for students and educators. Multiple benefits include the ability to exchange e-mail messages, transfer computer files, connect to and use distant information services and databases, participate in and obtain information from special interest group mailing lists, and obtain electronic journals. Today electronic communications are pervasive as we access communications from laptops, cell phones, PDAs and Internet cafes. Computer-mediated communication has become as commonplace as the stationary telephone once was. The literature includes many examples of the benefits of electronic communications in both nursing practice and education (Wright, 1996; Torrance, Lasome, and Agazio, 2002). Probably the most revolutionary aspect of electronic commmunication will be in the realm of patient-provider communication (Kane and Sands 1997; Mayer, et al., 2002). To prepare students for the practice environment in which they will be working, experience in using these applications during their educational program is essential.

E-mail

E-mail remains the primary and most prominent use of the Internet. E-mail can be used for computer-mediated communication (CMC) between faculty and students, to facilitate group work, and to distribute lecture notes and tutorial information. Many benefits of electronic communication have been reported by both faculty and students. These benefits include increased control over the learning environment, satisfaction in having mastered technical skills, the timeliness and convenience of personal communication with their instructor, and student belief that their responses were more thoughtful/reflective because of the delay imposed by writing. Students who describe themselves as reluctant to share opinions in a traditional face-to-face situation or unable to think quickly in a classroom setting are more comfortable and better able to reflect in an online environment (Kozlowski, 2004). Cravener and Michael (1998) conducted a study designed to investigate the extent to which campus-based students who were not inclined to participate in classroom discussions would use CMC for that purpose and to determine which individual differences among students appeared to be associated with student selection of class discussion or CMC. The study findings support the belief that students who used class and office time to talk about education-related concerns were the same individuals who used CMCs. For campus-based students who communicated frequently with faculty, the educational advantage of CMC was related to expansion of time for access to faculty. Todd (1998) used e-mail in an undergraduate child health nursing course to promote critical thinking by requiring students to respond to 10 critical thinking questions posted by the faculty. As a result of the electronic dialogue, misconceptions were clarified and students with learning disabilities participated more readily than in a traditional classroom discussion.

Blogs/Listservs/Forums/Newsgroups

Weblogs sometimes called blogs or a newspage began as personal journals that were frequently updated and published on the Web. They were intended largely for general public consumption as "Web diaries," reflecting the author's personality. Topics tended to include philosophical musings, commentaries about the Internet, social issues, and links to other sites that the author favored. The essential characteristics are its journal form, with entries on a daily basis and informal style. Weblogs also provide a feature allowing users to post comments to Weblog entries so long as the proper netiquette is observed. Blogs are used in education to share ideas with colleagues, eliciting feedback using the comments function. Opportunities to create like-minded persons questioning, interacting, and sharing on a blog is superceding the more traditional text-based e-mail and listservs that have been prominent in the last two decades (Glogoff, 2003).

Over the past decade, listservs have been developed and provide information and discussions on an enormous range of topics from patient support groups to nursing and healthcare to research and clinical practice. A user subscribes to the group by sending an e-mail to a listserv. These mailing lists give the user direct access to hundreds of like-minded clinicians and academics throughout the world. Listservs can be used in nursing courses to facilitate faculty and student communication and interaction. They provide a forum for class content and related topics of discussion on both a national and international level.

Newsgroups work by posting messages, much like putting a message on a bulletin board. The most common newsgroup network is Usenet. Newsgroups can be set up to run on a LAN, acting very much like an electronic bulletin board to be used for facilitating an electronic tutorial or a virtual classroom. Electronic tutorials can be used for sharing information and may facilitate critical thinking and questioning.

Synchronous Technologies

Electronic meeting software is a collection of software tools to automate and improve the quality of group process and team building. A form of this technology is called chat or instant messenger. It can be used to support a variety of processes in higher education including strategic planning, research collaboration, student program evaluation, and classroom instruction. A meeting support software system consists of a suite of decision support tools. Several advantages of electronic meetings over traditional meetings have been identified. The ability to work in the same area or at remote sites allows for greater control of personal time. The ability of all members to express ideas at the same time, speaking in parallel, increases participation and idea building. An increased awareness of and value for different perspectives is promoted through expression of ideas in a nonjudgmental environment (O'Brien and Renner, 1998). A study of the effectiveness of group system software for teaching a nursing management course indicated that examination scores and frequency of class participation were higher for the study group than the control group of students who experienced the same course using lecture. Student evaluations revealed that they believed the process enhanced application and understanding. Negative aspects of this methodology were increased preparation time for faculty and students' lack of tolerance when technical difficulties were encountered (Ayoub et al., 1998). E-learning platforms such as Blackboard and Web-CT allow for synchronous chats that can be moderated and promote valuable exchanges of ideas among faculty and students.

Nursing Informatics and the Curriculum

In 2000, the American Nurses Association (ANA) revised the definition of nursing informatics proposing, "Nursing Informatics is a specialty that integrates nursing science, computer science, and information science to manage and communicate data, information, and knowledge in nursing practice. Nursing informatics facilitates the integration of data, information, and knowledge to support patients, nurses, and other providers in their decision-making in all roles and settings. This support is accomplished through the use of information structures and information technology" (p. 17).

The position of the ANA was a direct outcome of the national endorsement of automating healthcare information, the establishment of the computer-based patient record, and the development of standards to facilitate the transmission of healthcare information across settings.

Prior to the ANA recognition, Graves and Corcoran-Perry (1989) defined nursing informatics as the "combination of computer science, information science, and nursing science, designed to assist in the management and processing of nursing data, information, and knowledge to support the practice of nursing and the delivery of nursing care."

Competencies in informatics include but are not limited to computer literacy, information literacy, the ability to use informatics strategies and system applications to manage data, information, and knowledge (ANA, 2001).

The emphasis on automated healthcare systems has created within the professions an imperative to identify, develop, and design data and information that reflects discipline specific as well as interdisciplinary domains. Nursing informatics is an area of practice that is being propelled by the advances of information technology in healthcare and the rapid evolution of the automated patient care record. Professional opportunities and roles are evolving at a rapid rate, and gradually more graduate

informatics programs are being developed (CIN, 2003). Not only has the specialty been recognized but also a subspecialty within the realm of nurse practitioners has been proposed (Curran, 2003). This would indicate an increase over the number of schools Carty and Rosenfeld (1998) found to be implementing informatics content in the curriculum. In 1997, the National Advisory Council on Nurse Education and Practice issued a report to the secretary of the Department of Health and Human Services on "A National Informatics Agenda for Education and Practice." Among the many issues addressed in the report was the call for nursing informatics education including:

- Identification of core informatics content for students and practicing nurses
- Advanced informatics preparation for nurses
- Faculty preparation in informatics

It is essential, therefore, that nursing education continue to address the learning needs of students and prepare them to practice in this millennium of healthcare. Mastery of information technology and managing health information are essential areas of curriculum content for all undergraduate and graduate nursing programs.

Nursing Education Informatics Models

In the past, emphasis has been on acquiring basic computer skills and knowledge of generic applications such as word processing and spread sheets. The focus now is on mastering information technology and information management as it applies to nursing information and knowledge (Staggers, Gassert, and Curran, 2002; Curran, 2003). The rapid advances in information technology, the availability of information in flexible, retrievable formats, and the need for faculty, students, and nurses to manage large amounts of data and information have driven this shift. The change in education and informatics has been from computer literacy to information literacy and management (Nelson, 2000).

A number of models have been presented for educators to emulate in designing curriculum for the inclusion of nursing informatics. Travis and Brennan (1998) propose a model that emphasizes the inclusion of information science as essential in the undergraduate curriculum (Fig. 32.2).

Focusing on the three concepts of information, technology, and clinical care processes, the authors support the incremental progression of informatics in the undergraduate curriculum. Such a model provides for both the theoretical and practical components of informatics

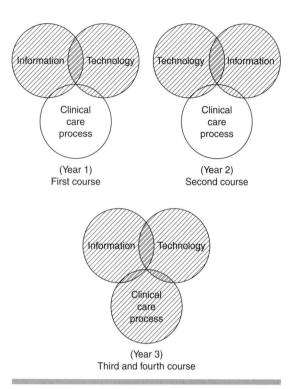

(Year 1)
First course

(Year 2)
Second course

(Year 3)
Third and fourth course

Figure 32.2
Travis and Brennan model.
(Reproduced, with permission, from Travis, L. and Brennan, P. (1998). Information science for the future: An innovative nursing informatics curriculum. *Journal of Nursing Education* 37:162–168.)

and emphasizes the smooth integration into course sequencing. Mastering the basics of information technology in the first and second year, students progress to the actual application of information technology to the science of nursing in the third year. The correlation between information technology and patient care is reinforced in the clinical environment. A final project concludes the students' understanding of the information of nursing by requiring the completion of a project in a selected area of nursing informatics that has practice implications.

Another approach to integrating nursing informatics into the curriculum has been proposed by Riley and Saba (Riley, 1996). In the Nursing Informatics Education Model (NIEM) (Fig. 32.3), the domains of computer science, information science, and nursing science are integrated throughout the curriculum in a progressive

leveling to ensure the development of nursing informatics competencies. In the Riley and Saba model, undergraduate students master computer literacy and progress to information management and its application to the clinical setting.

The challenge remains to design and develop strategies for integration into the undergraduate curriculum. Informatics competencies ranging from beginner to expert (Staggers, Gassert, and Curran, 2002) support the notion that informatics can and should be integrated throughout the nursing curriculum.

Nursing informatics at the graduate level has a vital role in both education and practice. Currently there are 18 graduate programs offering a specialty in nursing informatics (*http://www.amia.org/working/ni/education/cat1.html*). In addition, a number of schools offer graduate nursing informatics specialization courses. As nursing informatics attempts to define its role in the education and healthcare arena, there is discussion on the nature of the discipline. Some proponents see it as more of an interdisciplinary focus, while others propose a nursing focus (Mays et al., 2001). Current research efforts to support the domain of nursing, by developing nursing taxonomies, language, and classification systems, and designing clinical systems that reflect patient outcomes and effective nursing interventions, champion the recognition of an area of informatics specific to nursing. The presence of data warehouses and large clinical data repositories are auguring a new era for informatics. Carty (2000) proposes an informatics model in graduate informatics that expands on the Grave and Corcoran-Perry model of data, information, and knowledge. The model proposes an interpretation of data, information, and knowledge that is complex and nonlinear (Fig. 32.4). The model reflects three important developments in informatics: (1) the ability to transform and model knowledge in complex, interactive systems; (2) the advances that have been made in researching and developing standardized nursing terminology taxonomies; and (3) the availability of large clinical data sets and data repositories. As proposed and developed in the New York University graduate informatics curriculum, the concept of data, information, and knowledge can be taught at the undergraduate level. The more advanced concepts of information and knowledge representation are presented at the graduate level. The knowledge discovery content is introduced at the master's level, but is more thoroughly presented at the research and doctoral level, as students model large data sets and propose knowledge discovery through large dataset (KDD) projects.

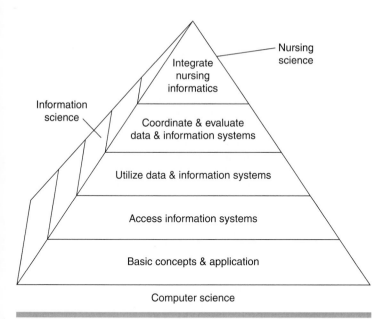

Figure 32.3
Nursing Informatics Education Model (NIEM).
(Reproduced, with permission, from Riley and Saba.)

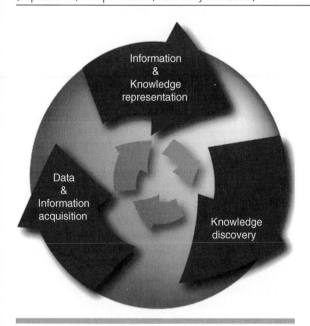

Figure 32.4
Nursing Informatics Graduate Education Model.
(Reproduced, with permission, from Carty, B. (2000). Nursing informatics: Graduate education. In Carty (Ed.), *Nursing Informatics: Education for Practice*. New York: Springer.)

Nursing Informatics Education: Domain-Specific and Interdisciplinary

It has been suggested that nursing informatics has a specific nursing focus, but there are acknowledged areas of interdisciplinary and collaborative foci that need to be explored and studied. Turley (1996) proposes a model for nursing informatics that incorporates other disciplines including cognitive science that has implications for education. This model supports a multidisciplinary approach and encompasses computer science, information science, and cognitive science within the domain of nursing science. The intersection of the information, cognitive, and computer sciences underpins informatics (Fig. 32.5). The Turley model gives credence to the importance of cognition in the application of information technology and management in nursing education.

In addition to Turley, several others have supported the inclusion of the science of cognition within a model of informatics (Patel and Kaufman, 1998; Ribbons, 1998; Patel, Arocha, and Kaufman, 2001). The paradigm shift from emphasis on technology to the cognitive or human computer-interaction has important implications for nursing education. How do students learn with technology, and how does technology affect the learner?

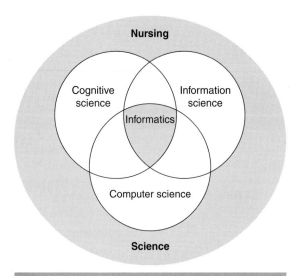

Figure 32.5
Turley model.
(Reproduced, with permission, from Turley, J. (1996).
Toward a model of nursing informatics. *Image: Journal of
Nursing Scholarship* 28(4):309–313.)

These are fertile areas for the emerging field of informatics and pose exciting research initiatives for educators.

Another interdisciplinary focus of informatics specifically relates to the collaborative nature of the discipline (National Advisory Council on Nurse Education and Practice, 1997; Gassert, 1998; Willson et al., 2000). Nurse informatics specialists work with programmers, information management teams, and system designers. Many nurse educators collaborate with other departments including computer scientists, education design specialists, and system analysts. This trend will continue as the need to manage and deliver information becomes the essential component of education and healthcare.

As computer hardware and software become more powerful and sophisticated, the ability to manage data and information and represent knowledge will affect how students learn in an educational environment and clinicians practice in a healthcare environment. The incorporation of decision support systems into clinical systems and the ability to access knowledge sources and research repositories will provide users with sophisticated knowledge systems that will have the potential to improve care. The communication and collaborative capability of information technology will have the effect of producing seamless, interactive systems that will sup-

port knowledge representation, facilitate human interaction, and provide new avenues for research in both practice and education.

Current and past literatures reveal enormous efforts by nurse informaticians to develop, design, and research nursing-specific as well as interdisciplinary areas of patient care data. Specialists in nursing informatics will continue to expand their work with interdisciplinary teams to develop sophisticated programs for decision support, interactive multimedia healthcare, and telehealth delivery systems. At the same time, there will remain the necessity to educate nursing informatics specialists to contribute to the ever-expanding field of healthcare informatics. It will be these specialists who will be able to cross the interdisciplinary boundaries and advance nursing knowledge and promote the domain of nursing within systems. This new area in nursing will grow as our society essentially relies on information systems to deliver, research, and teach healthcare.

References

AACN. (Rev. 1999). *American Association of Colleges of Nursing Agenda for the 21st Century.* Available at *http://www.aacn.nche.edu/publications/positions/nrsgedag.htm*

AACN. (2003). *American Association of Colleges of Nursing: Faculty Shortages in Baccalaureate and Graduate Nursing Programs: Scope of the Problem and Strategies for Expanding the Supply.* Available at *http://www.aacn.nche.edu/publications.htm*

American Nurses Association. (2001). *The Scope of Practice of Nursing Informatics and the Standards of Practice and Professional Performance for the Informatics Nurse Specialist.* Washington, DC: ANA Publishing.

Ayoub, J., Vanderboom, C., Knight, M., et al. (1998). A study of the effectiveness of an interactive computer classroom. *Computers in Nursing* 16:333–338.

Bloom, K. C. and Trice, L. B. (1997). The efficacy of individualized computerized testing in nursing education. *Computers in Nursing* 2:82–84.

Byun, H., Hallett, K., and Essex, C. (2000). Supporting instructors in the creation of online distance education courses: Lessons learned. *Ed Tech* 40(5):57–60.

Carty, B. (2000). Nursing informatics: Graduate education. In Carty B (Ed.), *Nursing Informatics: Education for Practice.* New York: Springer.

Carty, B. (2001). Informatics: The future is now. *Journal of the New York State Nurses Association* 1(32):11–14.

Carty, B. and Rosenfeld, P. (1998). From computer technology to information technology: Findings from a national study of nursing education. *Computers in Nursing* 16:259–265.

Chastain, R. (2002). Are faculty members ready to integrate information technology into the curriculum? *Nursing Education Perspective* 23(4):187–190.

Christianson, L., Tiene, D., and Luft, P. (2002). Web based teaching in undergraduate nursing. *Nurse Educator* 27(6):276–282.

CIN. (2003). Computers in Nursing, Special Report. Education and networking in nursing informatics. 5(21):275–286.

Connors, H., Weaver, C., Warren, J., and Miller, K. (2002). An academic-business partnership for advancing clinical informatics. *Nursing Education Perspectives* 23(5):228–233.

Cravener, P. (1998). A psychosocial systems approach to faculty development programs. *http://horizon.unc.edu/TS/development/1998-11.asp*

Cravener, P. and Michael, W. (1998). Students use of adjunctive CMC. In *Proceedings of the 5th Annual National Distance Education Conference.* *http://www.cravener.net/articles/austin1.html*

Curran, C. (2003). Informatics competencies for nurse practitioners. *AACN Clinical Issues* 3(14):320–330.

Gassert, C. (1998). The challenge of meeting patients' needs with a national nursing agenda. *Journal of Medical Informatics Association* 5:263–268.

Glogoff, S. (2003). *Blogging in an Online Course: A Report on Student Satisfaction among First-time Bloggers [PDF] E-Learn 2003.* Phoenix, AZ. Retrieved May 14, 2004, from *http://www.ltc.arizona.edu/blogginginonlineworldpdf.pdf*

Graves, J. and Corcoran-Perry, S. (1989). The study of nursing informatics. *Image: Journal of Nursing Scholarship* 21(4):227–230.

Hairston E. (1996). A picaresque journey. *Change* March/April:32–37.

Halstead, J. and Coudret, N. (2000). Implementing Web-based instruction in a school of nursing: Implications for faculty and students. *Journal of Professional Nursing* 16(5):273–281.

Harris, J. (1995). Curricularly infused telecomputing: A structured approach to activity design. *Computers in the Schools* 11:49–59.

Hilz, L. (2000). The informatics nurse specialist as change agent: Application of innovation-diffusion theory. *Computers in Nursing* 18(6):272–279.

Internet2. Available at *http://www.internet2.edu/about/aboutinternet2.html*

Kane, B. and Sands, D. (1997). Guidelines for the clinical use of electronic mail with patients. *Journal of American Medical Informatics Association* 1(5):104–111.

Kirkpatrick, J., Billings, D., Hodson-Carlton, K., Cummings, R., Dorner, J., Jeffries, P., Robinson, L., Rowles, C., Schafer, K., Sebrey, K., Siktberg, L., Smolen, R., and Taylor, S. (2000). Computerized test development software: A comparative review updated. *Computers in Nursing* 18(2):72–86.

Kozlowski, D. (2002). Using online learning in a traditional face-to-face environment. *Computers in Nursing* 20(1):23–30.

Kozlowski, D. (2004). Factors for consideration in the development and implementation of an online RN-BSN course. *Computers in Nursing* 22(1):34–43.

Landis, M. (2000). Faculty strategies for distance teaching. *Ed Tech* 40(6):55–57.

Liaw, S. and Huang, H. (2000). Enhancing interactivity in Web-based instruction: A review of the literature. *Ed Tech* 40(3):41–45.

Mayer, C., Stern, D., Dobiack, K., Cox, D., and Katz, S. (2002). Bridging the electronic divide: Patient provider perceptions on e-mail communication in primary health care. *American Journal of Managed Healthcare* 8(5):427–433.

Mays, D., Brennan, P., Ozbolt, J., Corn, M., and Shorttliffe, E. (2000). Are medical informatics and nursing informatics distinct disciplines? *Journal of Medical Informatics Association* 7(3):304–312.

McNeil, B., Elfrink, V., Bickford, C., Pierce, S., Beyers, S., Averill, C., and Klappenbach, C. (2003). Nursing information technology knowledge, skills, and prepapation of student nurses, nursing faculty, and clinicians: A U.S. survey. *Journal of Nursing Education* 42(8):341–349.

Mills, A. (2000). Creating web-based, multimedia, and interactive courses for distance learning. *Computers in Nursing* 18(3):125–131.

National Academy of Sciences. (2002). Preparing for the revolution: Information technology and the future of the research university. Washington, DC: National Academy Press.

National Advisory Council on Nurse Education and Practice. (1997). *A National Informatics Agenda for Nursing Education.* Rockville, MD: Department of Health and Human Services.

Nelson, R. (2000). Core informatics: Content for an undergraduate curriculum. In Carty B (Ed.), *Nursing Informatics Education for Practice.* New York: Springer.

Olsen, F. (2003). Colleges expect to increase spending on information technology by 5%. *Chronicle of Higher Education* 49:31a.

Patel, V., Arocha, J., and Kaufman, D. (2001). A primer on aspects for medical informatics. *Journal of Medical Informatics Association* 8(4):324–343.

Patel, V. and Kaufman, D. (1998). Medical informatics and the science of cognition. *Journal of American Medical Informatics Association* 5:493–501.

Reisling, D. (2003). The relationship between computer testing during a nursing program and NCLEX performance. *Computers in Nursing* 21(6):326–329.

Ribbons, R. (1998a). The use of computers as cognitive tools to facilitate higher order thinking skills in nurse education. *Computers in Nursing* 16:223–228.

Ribbons, R. (1998b). Practical applications in nurse education. *Nurse Education Today* 18:413–418.

Ribbons, R. (1998c). Guidelines for developing interactive multimedia applications in nurse education. *Computers in Nursing* 16:109–114.

Riley, J. B. (1996). Education applications. In Saba, V. and McCormick, K. *Essentials of Computers for Nurses*, 2d ed. (pp. 527–573). New York: McGraw-Hill.

Rogers, E. M. (1983). *Diffusions of Innovations* (3rd ed.). New York: The Free Press.

Rogers, E. and Green, K. (1996). The coming ubiquity of information technology. *Change* 2:24–31.

Ross, G. and Touvinen, J. (2001). Deep versus surface learning with multimedia in nursing education. *Computers in Nursing* 19(5):213–233.

Ryan, M., Hodson Carlton, K., and Ali, N. (2004). Reflections on the role of faculty in distance learning and changing pedagogies. *Nursing Education Perspectives* 2(25):73–80.

Saba, V. and McCormick, K. (1996). *Essentials of Computers for Nurses*. New York: McGraw-Hill.

Staggers, N., Gassert, C., and Curran, C. (2002). A delphi study to determine informatics competencies for nurses at four levels of practice. *Nursing Research* 51(5):383–390.

Sullivan E. (1997). A changing higher education environment. *: Journal of Professional Nursing* 13(3):143–148.

Thurmond, V. (2003). Defining interactions & strategies to enhance interactions in Web based courses. *Nurse Educator* 28(5):237–241.

Todd, N. (1998). Using e-mail in an undergraduate nursing course to increase critical thinking skills. *Computers in Nursing* 16:115–118.

Torrance, R., Lansone, C., and Agazio, J. (2002). Ethics and computer mediated communication. *Computers in Nursing* 32(6):346–353.

Travis, L. and Brennan, P. (1998). Information science for the future: An innovative nursing informatics curriculum. *Journal of Nursing Education* 37:162–168.

Turkle, S. (2004). How computers change the way we think. *The Chronicle of Higher Education* 50(21):30.

Turley, J. (1996). Toward a model of nursing informatics. *Image: Journal of Nursing Scholarship* 28(4): 309–313.

Wilkie, D., Judge, D., Kay, M., Wells, M., and Berkley, I. (2001). Excellence in teaching end-of-life care: A new multimedia toolkit for nurse educators. *Computers in Nursing* 22(5):226–230.

Willson, D., Bjornstad, G., Lussier, J., Matney, S., Miller, S., Nelson, N., Neiswanter, M., Pinto, K., and Thompson, C. (2000). Nursing informatics: Career opportunities. In Carty B (Ed.), *Nursing Informatics: Education for Practice*. New York: Springer.

Winter, J. (2001). Built environment: Appropriate technology for learning. Available at *http://www.uwe.ac.uk/fbe/beatl/summary_report.pdf*

Wright, K. B. (1996). The internet and nursing: A vital link. *MEDSURG Nursing* 5:209–211.

Young, J. (2002). The 24 hour professor. *The Chronicle of Higher Education* 48(38).

Zhang, J., Patel, V., and Johnson, T. (2002). Is the solution medical or cognitive? *Journal American Medical Association* 9(Suppl. 6):15.

33

Accessible, Effective Distance Education Anytime, Anyplace

Patricia E. Allen

Jean Arnold

Myrna L. Armstrong

OBJECTIVES

1. Explore the past and present perspectives of distance education.

2. Compare and contrast important interactive electronic tools to support learning at a distance.

3. Examine essential strategies and support required for the distance education learner and faculty.

4. Recognize further nursing research needed to propel future trends in distance education.

KEY WORDS

distance education
distance learning
faculty workload
distance education research
interactive learning
Internet or Web courses
educational platforms
faculty development

Programs for distance learning are exploding, especially Internet courses. The advertisement "new distance learning programs for working professionals" certainly has appeal, capturing the attention of many people seeking to fit further education into their busy schedules. The military has allotted a record 6-year appropriation of $600 million for solider training using distant education methodologies (as cited in Thurmond, 2002). Even businesses and investors are looking at distance education such as the World Bank's announcement of their $20 million contribution since 1997 to 16 distance learning centers in developing countries. Yet, many questions are frequently asked: Are these courses for "real"? Can I actually acquire a degree in my home or workplace without driving long distances and sitting in tedious lecture classes? And for us in nursing, do they really have application to nursing, especially for the clinical work I want to do? This progressive movement toward another way of providing both academic and continuing nursing education (CNE) is not only due to the development and use of technologies (video, audio, and computer equipment) that can be used for distance education, but also the market-driven demands of educational reform and creative, visionary faculty. Thus, the outcome is an empowerment of the nursing student and working professional to have numerous important educational choices. Often these decisions are based on accessibility and the amount of time needed to complete the course or program. Web sites are now available dedicated to find online nursing programs, such as allnursingschools.com.

While distance education has been available in this country since before the turn of the nineteenth century, many methodology changes, especially in synchronous and asynchronous technologies have occurred. Following a brief review of the historic approaches to distance education up to the present day, this chapter will focus on today's high-quality, cost-effective, learner-centered approach to distance education, examining it from both the student and faculty perspectives. This will include the importance of applicable educational principles needed to promote interactivity, active learning, and effective learner support, as well as some of the major academic and pedagogic issues impacting faculty developing creative courses. Additionally, this chapter will include the following:

- A definition of distance education
- An examination of various educational platforms
- Strategies and support for the learner
- Faculty support for course development and delivery
- Legal, ethical, and copyright issues
- Future trends and associated research questions

Currently, the 25-year and older age group is still the major group participating in distance education courses with more women than men enrolling in courses delivered at a distance (Neal, 1999; Thompson, 1998). Minority student enrollment is unclear. Some believe distance education offers a less threatening alternative because their mainstream educational settings were unsatisfactory nor can they leave their community or employment for further education; others still believe they prefer traditional classrooms. What is known, according to the National Center for Education Statistics (2004), is that the number of course enrollments in distance education has increased from 1.7 to 3.1 million between 1997–1998 and 2000–2001. Now, an "overall growth rate of almost 20% is expected in number of students studying online" (Allen and Seaman, 2003, p. 23).

There are still some traditional students who do not pay attention to distance education and there are still some faculty who avoid the concept by raising questions of quality rather than exploring the educational principles used in distance education. Yet overall distance education has moved on, capturing new types of educational experiences and innovative kinds of pedagogy, transforming education for both the students and faculty (Shomaker and Fairbanks, 1997). In essence, what has been learned is that good distance education theory and good education

theory are actually the same; the education just transcends the barriers of time and space (Dede, 1990; Mahan and Armstrong, 2003; Schlosser and Anderson, 1994).

 ## What is Distance Education?

Distance education differs from the traditional classroom in two essential elements. The majority of a course or program of study, whether with teachers and students or with students and students, is separated by (1) physical distance and (2) often time, thus the term "education—anytime, anywhere."

 ## Effectiveness of Distance Education

Educational outcomes are similar for both the on-campus and distance education students. Students usually drop out for personal and family crises rather than the educational modality (Pym, 1992). Distance education students, regardless of the delivery methods, receive the same grades or do better than those students receiving traditional instruction. Overall, student evaluations are good to very good following distance education activities. One factor commonly identified by students as a tremendous value in distance education is a collection of learners at a location that promotes the sharing of ideas, partners to debate the issues, and educational camaraderie (Armstrong, 2003; Shomaker and Fairbanks, 1997).

 ## Perspectives of Distance: The Past and Present

In the past, schools and educators needed an excuse to develop and conduct education at a distance. Documentation of need frequently had to be substantiated (Clark, 1993). Regulatory agencies had to approve off-campus or extension sites when the sites were separated from the originating school or when geographical barriers existed; some states even defined the number of miles for approval. Distance education, depending on the school's technological resources, could also mean that the faculty drove "the distance" to the off-campus site.

Today, the term "distance" education is associated with learner accessibility, whether learning is experienced locally or globally, at-home, a dormitory, or in the workplace, regardless of a rural or urban setting, across state lines, and even internationally.

The Evolution of Distance Education

Distance education has experienced bumps and surges of acceptance with the evolving presence of print, audio, television, and the various computer-interactive technologies. Distance education courses started out focusing on vocational training, but now many different disciplines have capitalized on distance education as an option of instruction (Neal, 1999).

Correspondence and Radio Courses

Although it can be said that today's distance education is new, the earliest form began in the nineteenth century as correspondence courses in Sweden. In the United States, support for this educational movement was from the Boston-based Society to Encourage Studies at Home in 1873. In 1885, the University of Wisconsin became the leader in distance education by developing "short courses" and farmer's institutes. By 1891, a commercial school for correspondence studies had developed in Pennsylvania. In 1900, enrollment figure was 224,000 and by 1920, enrollments had risen to more than 2,000,000 (Schlosser and Anderson, 1994). Unfortunately, dropout rates averaged around 65%. Radio, in 1919, was the first technology used for distance education.

Telephone, Television, and Satellite Courses

The ongoing changes in distance education have been termed as moving from plain old telephone service (POTS) to pretty amazing new stuff (PANS) (Zetzman, 1995). Audio conferencing used telephone handsets, speaker phones, and an audio bridge to connect multiple phone lines. This provided the first two-way interaction within distance education for physicians and nurses in Wisconsin.

Next came television for motion and visuals so that complex and abstract concepts could be illustrated through visual simulation. Yet, this additional technological idea for distance education did not become practical, feasible, and finally a reality until the 1950s (Mahan and Armstrong, 2003; Neal, 1999; Schlosser and Anderson, 1994). In 1971, the Open University of the United Kingdom began offering full degree programs through the innovative use of media. The popularity of this concept was astounding. By 1984, over 69,000 students had completed requirements for their Bachelor of Arts degree (Schlosser and Anderson, 1994).

Satellite technology for distance education in the United States was implemented in the early 1980s. These methodologies began to offer distance students greater transparency of the technology which enhanced the educational experience. Some interactive technologies such as cable, compressed video, and videoteleconferencing continue to be used supplementally for simulated face-to-face contact and simultaneous two-way interaction.

Computer Technology and the Internet

Computer technology came slowly to the forefront of distance education, and then its use exploded. In the late 1970s, computer-based education (CBE), computer-assisted instruction (CAI), and computer-managed instruction, were implemented cautiously, like so many other types of technologies used for distance education to supplement traditional classroom courses. Now, more and more faculty and student nursing education are moving toward Internet, a powerful worldwide "network of networks" connecting people globally (Billings, 1996b). This electronic education is incorporating multimedia, animations, graphics, print, audio, and video to the Internet technology (Ribbons, 1998).

With the emergence of online learning, a variety of mechanisms for course delivery have evolved. For some nursing classes, the traditional face-to-face course has become **Web-enhanced** extending the classroom by incorporating some of the electronic tools. In a Web-enhanced course, the instructor may use online modules, electronically provide required handouts or printed materials, and may use a few synchronous or asynchronous chats to extend the learning experience for the student enrolled in a traditional face-to-face course. This methodology emphasizes the advantages of traditional learning, yet capitalizes on convenient and accessible tools to supplement added communication beyond the classroom walls.

Hybrid course formats have also emerged in the era of online learning. This format allows instruction to be delivered using the best of both teaching methodologies for a mixture of up to 50% of the learning online and 50% of the learning in the classroom. The focus of hybrid courses is to blend the instructional methodologies to allow for efficient use of classroom time and facilities and encourage anywhere, any time learning with online formats such as Web-CT or Blackboard (see Educational Electronic Platform section) (Boener, 2003). The difference between a hybrid course format and Web-enhanced courses is in the amount of technology use.

Finally, Web-based or online courses have emerged with the total instruction using a variety of electronic communication tools. The online course incorporates all learning materials with the use of e-mail, synchronous chats, asynchronous chats, discussion or message boards, module completion, course management, and presentations delivered with audio and/or video streaming. Here, the fax and telephone become supplemental tools for further communication.

Educational Consortiums

Numerous consortia are present across the United States with state or multistate memberships to promote distance education. In 2003, the U.S. Department of Education reported that 60% of schools participating in electronic learning belonged to distance education consortium, such as the virtual college universities (VCU) consortia, Western Cooperative for Educational Telecommunications (WCET), and State Higher Education Executive Officers Consortium (SHEEO) (as cited in Western Cooperative Educational Telecommunications, 2004a).

The WCET will be further described due to its early origin and voluminous contribution to the field. It is a multistate organization that was founded by the Western Commission for Higher Education in 1989. This "virtual university" is sponsored by 15 states and one U.S. territory and the Committee on Institutional Cooperation made up of 12 large universities, so this consortia represents the higher education community, nonprofit organizations, schools, and corporations. The primary goal of this organization is to address telecommunication concerns relevant to the new distributed learning environments, especially when these environments are experienced by off-campus students (Western Cooperative Educational Telecommunications, 2004a). One of WCET endeavors is the founding of EduTools which provides comparisons, reviews, analysis, and automated decision-making tools for course management, student services, and e-learning policies (EduTools, 2004; Western Cooperative Educational Telecommunications, 2004b). Detailed information, updated review of educational products, and a purchase decision guide are available on their Web site (EduTools, 2004). One of these electronic products is educational platforms that assist the delivery of Internet courses.

Educational Electronic Platforms

An educational platform is an electronic product that assists the delivery of Internet courses. As colleges are faced with decisions regarding which educational platform to use for facilitation of online instruction, EduTools

has done a thorough assessment. Table 33.1 presents some of the major characteristics of the five common educational platforms used for distance education including Angel, Blackboard, eCollege AU+, First Class, and Web-CT Campus Edition.

A major consideration is what type of **hardware** and **software** is needed. Both students and instructors need to have access to the educational platforms with home-based personal computers and software. All five educational platforms run on IBM compatible personal computers. The most dominant browser requirement is Microsoft Internet Explorer and or Netscape. Macintosh browser is available for Angel and eCollege AU+.

Access to students is based on **authentication** requirements. Ease of authentication is defined as the use of a user and password login. The communication characteristics are also central to distance education. These include discussion capabilities, file exchange, e-mail capability, and real-time chats.

Access to students is based on **e-mail capability** by both the learner and instructor. Internal e-mail capability (within the educational platform) is only available for a few of the products such as First Class and Web-CT; otherwise students are required to have their own external e-mail address.

The **group work feature** is defined as the educational platform's capability to allow the instructor to assign students to groups with discussion forums and presentation folder or file exchange. All five educational platforms have this feature but group e-mail is also available for Blackboard, Angel, and eCollege AU+.

The educational platform table defines the **file exchange** feature as allowing the student and instructor to upload files to a digital group box. This option decreases the virus problems that can be associated with e-mail attachments. Four of the five described educational platforms have this feature with First Class being the exception.

Progress review, assessment capabilities, and online grading features are valued by the instructor and learner in distance education due to their convenience and feedback. Assessment features include automated testing with scoring and online grading. These characteristics are available for four of the five educational platforms with the First Class educational platform being the exception.

Student tracking is a feature that provides instructor with reports and statistics regarding student usage. An example is accessing of course content and discussion forums. Since participation in online discussion is an expected behavior, the ability to have student statistics is a means and time saver to evaluate this behavior.

Table 33.1 Characteristics of Five Educational Platforms Commonly Used for Nursing Distance Education

Characteristics	Angel	Blackboard	eCollege AU+	First Class	Web-CT Campus Edition
Developer Web site	Cyberlearninglabs	Blackboard	eCollege	Centrinity	Web-CT
Hardware	IBM & MAC	IBM & PDA	IBM & MAC	IBM & MAC	IBM
Discussion by date and thread	Y	Y	Y	Y	Y
File exchange	Y	Y	Y	N	Y
Internal e-mail	N	N	N	Y	Y
Real-time chats	Y	Y	Y	Y	Y
Progress review	Y	Y	Y	N	Y
Automated testing and scoring	Y	Y	Y	N	Y
Grade book	Y	Y	Y	N	Y
Group work	Y	Y	Y	Y	Y
Software version	6.0	6.0	Same version for all	7.0	4.1
Browser requirement	Internet Explorer (IE) & Netscape	IE & Netscape	IE, Netscape & MAC	No information	IE & Netscape
Student orientation/ help	Y	Y	Y	Limited	Y
Instructor help	Y	Limited	Y	N	Y
Course templates	Y	Y	Y	N	Y
Student tracking	Y	Y	Y	N	Y
Product demo	N	Y	Free trial	Tour	Tour
Instructional standards compliance	Y	Y	Limited to self-testing	N	Limited to self-testing and self-reports
Student home page	Y	Y	N	Y	Y
User and password login	Y	Y	Y	Y	Y

Note: Y = yes and N = no. This table was developed from an at-home instructor's perspective using the following criteria: (1) reviewed by EduTools, (2) longevity, (3) company profile, (4) comparable characteristics, and (5) usage in higher education. First Class and College AU+ were developed in 1990, Web-CT and Blackboard in 1997, and Angel in 2000.

The **help capability** was examined from both a student and instructor perspective with the goal to have adequate support provided by the vendor. For this table, instructor help was defined as the use of an online course manual and availability of online courses and user groups. All five educational platforms offered some form of help, some providing more details than others.

Course templates are critical to the instructor because it allows the user to categorize course information. This is the infrastructure of the educational platform that provides course building blocks. There was no description of course templates for First Class in the reviews by EduTools or at the vendor's Web site. Both Angel and Web-CT and Blackboard include a content editor. Common templates include course content, course units, syllabus, and discussion. **Announcement capability** is available in Angel, Blackboard, and eCollege AU+. Other course template features are described in details at the EduTools Web site.

The Distance Nursing University of the Twenty-First Century

Nurses know that knowledge is power. Power to control their nursing practice and access to educational opportunities is a vital way to maintain their professional practice, to meet the challenges of healthcare changes, and to effectively participate in the health team (Bachman and Panzarine, 1998; McGonigle and Mastrian, 1998). Yet, the ability to "keep up" will be intensified as dollars for travel and conferences continue to disappear, while the demands of rotating shifts, marketing for future opportunities, and family commitments continue (Dawes, 1998; Carlton, 1997). Accessibility to distance education can assist these problems.

Nursing education, especially for the registered nurse (RN), has a long history of using various modalities to deliver RN-BSN (bachelor of science in nursing), as well as CNE while graduate programs are evolving. The use of distance education has been an effective way to increase RN retention at healthcare facilities, build professional commitment, and promote quality care, while the nurse stays in her community (Armstrong, 2003). Additionally, there tends to be a higher enrollment and completion rate of minority students in distance education programs, because after they have their basic nursing education, they do not leave the community to take further courses due to family and work demands (Shomaker and Fairbanks, 1997). A recent survey by the National League for Nursing of 162 nursing schools found all of the respondents currently had or planned to have a distance learning component added to the course delivery methods (as cited in Ali et al., 2004).

Augmenting existing technological skills while pursuing new informational skills will help nurses remain competitive in the healthcare market. Thus, when nurses take on this lifelong learning commitment, distance education should become a tremendous mechanism for nurses to become "adept users and information connoisseurs ... discriminating users of the cyberspacial arena that spans the informational gambit from junkyard to gold mine" (McGonigle and Mastrian, 1998).

Another recent technological advance in the healthcare environment and distance education is personal digital assistants (PDAs) used by both faculty and students. PDAs are used for storing and retrieving clinical assessment data, drug information, language translation, calculations, identification of normal laboratory values, pediatric developmental milestones, medical sign language, medical terms, anatomy, acuity of illness scales, growth charts, and immunization guidelines. The PDA

can be uploaded with a wide variety of software and allows for beaming of programs between users. This technological advance is a tool for use in decreasing medical errors in today's nursing practice arena. Another feature is that students, with their fully loaded wireless PDA, are no longer required to carry heavy textbooks to the clinical setting for resource material (White et al., 2005).

Strategies and Support for the Distance Education Learner

Principles and Evaluation Criteria

Any quality education should be based on learning objectives and educational outcomes. Distance education courses and programs are no different (Massoud, 1999). They need to adhere to the same national accreditation and educational standards of the originating school (Hanna et al., 1998; Milstead and Nelson, 1998).

A self-assessment quiz for aspiring distance education learners can be found (*http://www.wgu.edu/*) with accompanying rationale for the potential student's responses. It is important to determine if course credits can be transferred to other universities. Students should seek information about the course design, expectations, and method of interaction between faculty and student and between students. Additionally, students should determine what arrangements are needed for technology troubleshooting, registration, student services, literary sources, and textbook acquisition (Milstead and Nelson, 1998). Samples of criteria that the student (and faculty) can use for evaluating effective distance education programs are available from the Western Cooperative for Educational Telecommunications (*http://www.wiche.edu*). To foster and support higher quality education programs, they have developed "Principles of Good Practice for Electronically Offered Academic Degree and Certificate Programs." The Southern Association of Colleges and Schools (*http://www.sacs.org/*) also has evaluation criteria.

The Role of Faculty Will Change

While the nursing content will remain the same as in the traditional classroom, providing education via distance will mean some methodological changes when delivering the educational materials. Because the Internet has been described as the "library card to the world" (Smith, 1997), the faculty role will change to more of a facilitator of learning rather than an imparter of all the information (Aucoin and Armstrong, 2003; Bachman and Panzarine, 1998; Billings, 1997). With information so accessible, the emphasis will go beyond just locating the information to a role of filtering the information. To facilitate learning, "the faculty's role will be to teach the student how to swim because they will be drowning in data" (Aucoin and Armstrong, 2003; Dede, 1990).

Importance of Orientation

Students seem to pass through a series of steps toward self-directed learning, almost like experiencing a sense of loss. Using Kubler-Ross's patterns of grieving (denial, anger, bargaining, depression, and acceptance), Cravener (1997) cites examples of students' grief as they move toward the resolution of a new learning role. Thus, the design and format of the orientation must foster relationships among the distance learners, providing the support and direction to enable them to make the transition from the traditional classroom to self-directed learning. Additionally, they need to know (and feel) that their online faculty care and want to assist them achieve success in their academic work. The creation of either video or written user tutorials or specific Web pages dedicated to quick reference topics can overcome initial student unfamiliarity with such topics as the use of e-mail, network software and file transfer (Carlton, 1997; Cravener, 1999; Milstead and Nelson, 1998; Ribbons, 1998). Designated coaching time from the technology team for individual learners on the system is extremely valuable and proactive; this can be initiated during their orientation time (Craig, 1994).

Importance of Communication and Flexibility

Internet education may be partially or fully text-based, so the ability to carry on a dialogue/discussion/interchange, whether in a synchronous or asynchronous mode, is vital to the connectivity of the student's experiences with the faculty and fellow students. Strategically placed questions in the text will be helpful in extracting major concepts; computer-based conferencing tools such as chat sessions and/or bulletin boards can provide further opportunity to explore important concepts with synchronous or asynchronous feedback (Milstead and Nelson, 1998; Carlton et al., 1998). The knowledge and the willingness to learn how to use the equipment for communication, the accessibility of the equipment, the required computer capabilities, as well as the commitment to be an active participate in the interchange format will be valuable tools for student success (Plank, 1998; Sparks and Rizzolo, 1998). Otherwise, the education experience reverts to passive learning, similar to the old correspondence course model (Sherry, 1996).

Both faculty and students will spend more time writing, actively promoting learning, and building knowledge

by interaction (Cravener, 1999). Interestingly, developers of computer-based courses describe the increased amount of communication as richer in depth and content as well as exciting because it seems to better meet the needs of all the learners online (Carlton et al., 1998; Achterberg, 1996). This results from using computerized communication tools; they become "an equalizer because the message is sent with no signs of race, gender, physical appearance, shyness, or external socioeconomic and status cues, which may be especially attractive to students not comfortable in the traditional classroom" (Armstrong, 2003, p. 419; Craig, 1994). Messages are also documented, so a running tabulation of responses can be recorded. Since writing is often improved with further writing, the interaction becomes an excellent method to encourage "an organized and fluent thought pattern, an application of learning, and an analysis of relationships" (Larson and Dunkin, 1997). This in turn assists both the faculty and student's evaluation of the learning process. Peer critique may also be part of the course interaction, leading to further collegiality, networking, and perhaps even mentoring (Billings, 1996b; Larson and Dunkin, 1997).

Yet, expected and frustrating obstacles can develop when working with any type of technology, especially at the initiation of the course (Milstead and Nelson, 1998; Todd, 1998). Flexibility should remain the watchword as both faculty and students will experience technological problems with the lack of reliable access to Internet-connected hardware, ever-threatening virus, difficult interfaces, and sometimes frustrating technical support during the course (Achterberg, 1996; Bachman and Panzarine, 1998; Billings, 1996b; Craig, 1994; Cravener, 1999).

Student Development of Self-Directed Learning Skills

Computer-based course faculty agree that successful distance education students become "more assertive, independent, and organized, than in a traditional classroom setting" (Achterberg, 1996; Craig, 1994; Cravener, 1999; Milstead and Nelson, 1998). RN students in Craig's study (1994) cite the ability to "time-shift," or study when able to, as an important advantage to developing this independence as well as an increasing proficiency with computers. Thus, support is provided for the development of self-directed learning skills such as active listening, working independently in the absence of a live instructor, and time skill management. Students inquiring about new learning experiences and possessing diligence and a positive attitude will be supported (Billings, 1997).

Strategies and Support for the Distance Education Faculty

Nursing programs are now delivering total programs online without the boundaries of regions or states or even countries dictating enrollments. The community of learners without walls presents many new and exciting challenges for faculty and administrators as well as program competition, which is a new arena for nurse educators. Online delivery has allowed faculty to rethink the critical components of the topic area for learning and to develop new and exciting ways for students to obtain knowledge. Creativity in teaching is the key to online delivery and faculty commitment to change should be ongoing.

Faculty Presence in Distance Education Programs

There is a change in status of who is providing distance education instruction. In many total online programs, many distance educators are not identified as faculty. In some cases, the faculty are invisible at the institution, unlike a traditional university site, where the faculty listing appears at the college's Web site. Instead they may have a title of facilitator, mentor, instructor, or guide. This occurs because many are not full-time faculty at the institution offering the course or the institution does not have full-time faculty. Adjunct faculty now constitute 37% of distance education personnel; this figure represents a 34% increase since 1998 (Sistek-Chandler, 2000). Educational changes for faculty will evolve around a redistribution of communication, online course management, and faculty workload.

Communication with Learners

Online faculty will find themselves needing to be available for student contact beyond the classroom setting guidelines of appointed office hours whether it be by accessed online chat office hours, e-mail, fax, or cell phone. Faculty response is no longer between 9 a.m. and 5 p.m. and this accessibility to faculty allows the learner to query the faculty member, whether they are presenting in Madrid, or while the student is on vacation at the beach.

Additionally, faculty will have to rethink their classroom habits and practices that have been taken for granted (Billings, 1996a). For example, what kind of interaction can be planned with students when there are no face-to-face classroom entry and exit rituals, nor the usual verbal or nonverbal clues such as intonation of audio presentation when teaching (Clark, 1993)?

Considerable thought must be given to the communication process in distance education as the "communication is judged by the words on the computer screen and the ideas expressed" (Milstead and Nelson, 1998). Recommendations to liven up the discussions and reduce the stiffness of entirely word-based material include using words (chuckle, chuckle), "emoticons," or Internet shorthand that helps the user express feelings (such as smiley faces [] or [:-)), and colloquialisms ("Go for it, keep cooking") (Bachman and Panzarine, 1998).

Communication with an Instructional Team

For online course development, content knowledge is no longer the only faculty responsibility. Rather, content knowledge goes hand in hand with blending of instructional design strategies and faculty knowledge of the capabilities of the course online learning format being utilized by the educational platform. Experts to help faculty include instructional designers and technical partners associated with the computing telecommunications systems. They are essential to help faculty pull courses together for distance education delivery and will provide great assistance to altering teaching methods and modifying instructional materials (Billings, 1997).

Online Course Development

Teaching strategies that encourage active involvement and critical thinking with the course content are very important (Billings, 1996b; Carlton et al., 1998; Todd, 1998). Critical thinking assignments such as case scenarios for problem solving followed by discussion boards for reflection and data sharing work extremely well in online course delivery for distance education (Ali et al., 2004). But, the opportunity for problem solving and then reflection is key for the development of critical thinking skills.

Whether a novice or experienced online educator, a distance education yardstick is available for use. Examples include:

1. "The Best Practices for Electronically Offered Degree and Certificate Program" is an excellent reference developed by eight regional accrediting commissions and includes institutional context and commitment, curriculum and instruction, faculty support, student support, and evaluation and assessment information (Perroots, n.d.). This is a simplified version of a basic assessment inventory used during accreditation visits.

2. "Guiding Principles for Faculty in Distance Learning is from The University of Idaho's Department of Engineering Outreach. It offers 13 guides regarding distance education and the content areas of these guides range from glossary, instruction development strategies, research and evaluation, technology, and copyright in distance Education (Willis, n.d.).

3. The Indiana Higher Education Telecommunication system guide focuses on the instructor's perspective of teaching and learning. This resource provides information about principles and subprinciples related to faculty benchmarks, course design, and issues. Faculty principles include course design, program design, faculty development, course evaluation, assessment of student outcomes, copyright ownership, and delivery methods (Indiana Higher Education Telecommunication System, n.d.).

To assist the reader in developing and maintaining online teaching skills Table 33.2 uses an alphabet format to share techniques, methods, and responsibilities of the rewarding and effective role of an online distance educator.

Assistance in Course Development Curriculum has been bundled for online access on many topics for student or healthcare providers seeking continuing education credit. One example of this, as well as online assessment of knowledge, is created by Healthstream, an organization that provides competency validation at the touch of the student's fingertips (*http://www.cmecourses.com/gateway/cscatalog.cfm?method=CourseInfo&iCourseID=8708&SID=&PID=46*). Additionally, nursing textbooks routinely have an established URL for additional student resources. The following is an example of the many Web resources that are available to provide nursing online course delivery such as for a health assessment course.

■ Delivery of an Online Health Assessment Course

A health assessment course is commonly included in a baccalaureate nursing program. The student is expected to take a health history and perform a physical examination on a client, whether a peer or paid actor. Traditional campus-based courses consists of a didactic and laboratory component with lectures about each human body system followed by practice of the physical examination associated with each body system. The performance requirement is considered an essential component for successful completion of the course. With the distance education learner, the nurse educator is faced with the dilemma of how to evaluate these behaviors. A sampling of a distance education health assessment course is described in Table 33.3.

Five of these courses are available online. Four colleges offer these courses, which include Canyon College, The Ohio State University, Southwest Missouri State University, and Thomas Edison State College. The health assessment Web site offers the sale of its Nursing Education Health Assessment Physical Examination products to single or multiusers. The Ohio State University mentions the use of this product in its course. The target audience for these courses are nurses or nursing students with some clinical experience, who are seeking a baccalaureate degree or continuing education units. Readers should seek further clarification whether these courses are open to the public.

Instructors will have to rethink how to address the psychomotor component of health assessment. Each of these six health assessment courses require adjunct materials that are compact disks, and/or textbooks, and/or or videotapes. Three of the health assessment courses use the Blackboard educational platform for course delivery. The physical examination component was assessed by written examination, a "comprehensive head to toe examination, and case studies." An actual performance of a physical examination on a client was not mentioned in any of the course descriptions.

Faculty Workload

An increase in faculty workload can be expected. This topic in distance education remains the most controversial factor for faculty assigned to distance education. Several schools are proactive with faculty recognition in this type of delivery medium, others are not. With the increase of faculty workload, the instructional costs, especially during the initial phases, will increase. "Design and development of online degree programs can cost between $15,000 to $20,000 per credit hour," according to Boettcher (2004, p. 4). Yet, it is often not the content that is changed, but the learning and incorporation of creative, sophisticated, and complex instructional tools to provide the content that increases the instructional mileu. With the emrgence of online courses, faculty enhance their instructional design and computer technology skills that increase their faculty workload time for course preparation and delivery, yet the end result is an intense, rich learning environment for the learner.

Assignment Time for Course Preparation At least one semester of preliminary course planning is important

Table 33.2   Distance Educator Role Alphabet

Availability: Faculty start their day by checking in with students by e-mail to determine if someone has an individual question, then reads postings in the discussion forums and their other assignments. Often this process is repeated twice or three times a day. Separate discussions regarding specific assignments are recommended to address student concerns as they occur.

Background: Start your course with a short autobiography and request one from each learner to know something about your student's educational and work experiences.

Breaks: Give student breaks for the opportunity to discuss their concerns in an open discussion and so each student can read the other student's questions.

Concern and counseling: Communicate your concern for the learners' welfare through frequent contacts; counsel learners individually by e-mail and telephone as needed.

Design: Design your course prior to its onset; provide detail in lessons that foster independent learning.

Empathy: Be alert for student concerns. For example, students were requested to discuss their presentation assignment in a "show and tell" session. One student stated "I am anxious about sharing my presentation with other students." An empathetic response could be "it is your option to share whatever you want about your presentation, whether it be a description of the presentation and/or your feelings about creating one."

Engage: Engage in discussions so your presence is felt. Online learners need to know you are there. Three times per week on different days is a recommendation based on experience teaching in three different online college curriculums. Faculty notification of their absence from a discussion for any expended period is also recommended. A better option is to have a substitute instructor or backup staff member during your absence.

Encourage: Encourage by stating, "hang in there" or "you are on target." Support phrases may be the key to keeping the learners online instead of disappearing into cyberspace.

Empower: "Make students responsible for summarizing the week's discussion, taking the lead of a discussion, or teaching others a concept. This approach will empower them and save you time." (University of Colorado, n.d., p. 1).

Feedback: Online learners appear to desire more feedback than traditional face-to-face students especially in the early phases of their distance education experience. A response to a learner's inquiry cannot come soon enough. This is a critical element to successful distance education. Feedback sheets for each assignment, based on the criteria, also enhance learning. Individual feedback is ideal. Group feedback regarding a given assignment is not as effective, because learners think it applies to someone else.

Facilitate learning: For active participation, challenge the learner to think by asking stimulating questions in the discussion arena. Expand their thoughts through further examples and questions. Ask the learner to provide substantive comments that build on other responses and are based on references from the literature.

Good comments: Praise students when they make a qualitative response in a discussion or prepare a good paper. Online learners can easily misconstrue your text-based feedback. Remember to provide constructive feedback that includes the good points of their writing and give advice regarding how to improve their weak areas.

Hindsight: Be an online instructor that learns from your experiences such as a summary of student comments on course evaluations. Further detailed assignment directions were incorporated from feedback of online learners.

Interaction: Moore describes three types of interactions important for successful distance education: (1) learner-content interaction, (2) learner-instructor interaction, and (3) learner-learner interaction (as cited in Smith, Ferguson, and Cavis, 2001). An example is the creation of learner materials that require the learner actions, pose a discussion question based on a Web site, require the learners to discuss these questions in small groups, and then send a draft summary of their responses to the instructor. The instructor in turn monitors the small group discussion, provides feedback, and then requires submission of final small group summaries in the class discussion.

Insight: Students do learn from interactions. Comment about their insights when they occur in discussions and overall at the end of a given discussion.

Jump in: When students are moving off the topic in a chat, bring them back to the issue on hand.

Knowledge: "Tap learners' knowledge. Create activities where students integrate new ideas with existing knowledge. Provide them with a frame of reference within the online environment" (University of Colorado, n.d., p. 1).

Learn: Learn with the learners—you **do** learn from the learners! When you receive a student example of a concept, provide feedback regarding their contribution.

Manage: Both faculty and students should use a calendar to manage due dates for course assignments.

(Continued)

Table 33.2   Distance Educator Role Alphabet (*Continued*)

Model: Role model effective pedagogic behavior in discussions.

Measurement: Identify criteria for each assignment and share them with the learners. Supply feedback to students on completed assignments using the criteria.

Notice: Send individual e-mails to inform learners that you are noticing their performance whether it be on track or not. Make announcements to learners regarding course activities as needed.

Obligation: Remind learners of their obligation to be an active participant in online courses and to complete their share of group work on time.

Objectives: Create lesson plans and assignments that have clear objectives.

Post: Role model and remind learners to make meaningful postings.

Personalize: Personalize your comments to learners; use first names in discussions.

Photos: Use photos of yourself and ask students to do so but remember that students should sign releases for the recording of their images if they use their pictures on the Web; students seem to sense your presence more if they have a photo. When the writer met a group of students at a site visit, their comment was "I would know you anywhere."

Participation: "the use of various learning options can stimulate learner participation and interaction. Small group discussion, debates, polling activities, dyadic learning partnership exchanges, and one-on-one messages recognizing students postings are some of the activities to use when encouraging participation" (Berge, 1995, p. 3).

Query: For the learner who is not participating send an e-mail to query the learner, hopefully to stimulate further discussion.

Reminders: Reminders for due dates and assignment criteria help learners stay on track and remind them of your ongoing presence.

Support: Provide words of encouragement and praise in written feedback of discussions and assignments.

Sharing: Online education is about sharing what you know and learn from each other.

Statistics: Educational platforms provide course statistics that paint a picture of your learners' activities online.

Threads: Add threads to discussion as needed to organize discussions; "Use the threaded discussions to provide motivation, support, and feedback for discussion—thank students, summarize responses, bring the discussions back on track, but allow students to discuss amongst themselves." (University of Colorado, n.d., p. 1).

Undertaking: Recognize that distance education is a large undertaking in time and energy resulting in a heavier workload.

Vary amount of contribution: "if there is a participant who appears overly outspoken, ask that person (privately) to wait a few responses before contributing. Similarly, ask less outspoken individual to participate more actively" (Berge, 1995, p. 6).

Victory: Acknowledge when success is achieved by a learner.

Ventilate: Allow learners to express their feelings regarding your comments about their performance in discussion or on assignments. It may take time but it is necessary to insure a positive learning experience.

Willingness: Convey your willingness to listen by providing your e-mail and phone number; also arrange a designated time for office hours.

X-ray vision skills are needed to read between the lines of online talk and the lack of face-to-face contact.

Yardstick: Yardstick provides benchmarks that learners recognize as your expectations; give the "whole nine yards" in terms of detail.

Zero hour: Let student know when the due date is and stick to your timetable.

Zeal: Communicate with zeal

---

to alter teaching methods and modify instructional materials for distance education (Milstead and Nelson, 1998). While the time in design/development has decreased from 18 hours per hour to 10 hours per hour of instruction, because the usual campus infrastructure now for distance education is usually in place, it is still the "transformational design and the building of technology habits that takes the time now" (Boettcher, 2004, p. 3). Proactive faculty development and ongoing institutional support can smooth out some of the frustrations. Trying to get the

Table 33.3   Health Assessment Distance Education Courses

Delivery Method	Distance Education Method	Source	Web Site
Compact disk option	Independent	Vendor	*www.healthassessment.com*
Online college course using compact disk	Independent or used as continuing education course	Ohio State University	*www.ohsu.edu/son/ce*
Online college course using Blackboard educational platform	Time-based course with four scheduled required meetings with comprehensive head-to-toe examination	Southwest Missouri State University	*www.ecollege.smsu.edu*
Online college course	Time-based course for 8 weeks with two examinations and required questions	Canyon College	*www.canyoncollege.edu*
Online college course using Blackboard educational platform	Time-based for 12 weeks with asynchronous discussions, papers and case study, teaching plan	Thomas Edison State College	*www.tesc.edu*
Online college course using evolve interactive learning system	Classroom or online using combination of discussions and textbooks	Elsevier publisher in partnership with Blackboard Company	*www.evolve.elsevier.com/Home*

Source: Padgett Coehlo, D. *Nursing Health Assessment Physical Examination CD Learning Package*. Retrieved June 1, 2004, from *health assessment.com*

Southwestern Missouri State University. *Health Assessment*. Retrieved June 1, 2004, from *http://www.eschool.smsu.edu*

online course to the desired level of efficacy will also take a good portion of time, some believe at least three semesters are needed (Achterberg, 1996; Billings, 1996a; Clark, 1998). Faculty workload during those three semesters should be adjusted for that learning curve. Achterberg (1996) describes tripling the time (when comparing a traditional classroom setting) to implement an electronic delivered course, yet on completing the course, she was ready to design more distance education because of the satisfaction of reaching so many students and stimulating a more "learner-centered system." Billings (2002) and Carlton et al. (1998) describe similar responses.

The Apple Classrooms of Tomorrow (Sherry, 1996) describe their perceptions of faculty response to distance education:

> It may take at least two years to change [the] focus from being anxious about themselves and equipment malfunctions, . . . to anticipating problems and developing alternate strategies, exploring software more aggressively, sharing ideas more freely, increasing student motivation and interest, and using technology to their advantage. Educational change takes time, a great deal of support, peer networking, and guidance. In general, teachers tend to focus on the increased workload and drawbacks associated with an innovation before the benefits of change emerge and the innovation takes hold.

Online Course Management   Two factors important in this discussion are faculty effort and student-faculty ratios. The three seasoned nurse educator/authors of this chapter concur that the faculty effort to provide instruction in an effective and interactive manner to produce a student-friendly Web-based course will take at least twice as much time than traditional classroom instruction. More intense and frequent student interaction time is the main reason.

As to student-faculty ratio, the mode tends to be one faculty to 20–25 online students per section to deliver the intense interactive communication exchange that is required of distance education students (Vilic, 2004). Public institutions of higher learning tend to peak about 34 students at the undergraduate level and 32 at the graduate level, whereas private institutions average lower course caps of 22 and 21. Although many schools of nursing allow for faculty time for this new method of delivery, the adherence to this "best practice educational principle" is difficult for faculty colleagues that can have over a 100 face-to-face students in traditional classrooms, especially now with the nursing shortage and the intense push for more nurses. Yet, the focus should always be on the course and program goals, as well as the institutional characteristics (Vilic, 2004). Regardless of the time commitment, "adequate operational and administrative infrastructure to support the distance education teaching endeavors" is vital (Clark, 1993; Bachman and Panzarine, 1998).

Legal, Ethical, and Copyright Issues

The faculty are accountable for any kind of educational endeavor, including that for distance learning (Menix, 1998). Legal concerns relate to established laws associated with telecommunication technologies, whereas the ethical concerns relate to the rights and wrongs stemming from the values and beliefs of the various users of the distance education systems. Three major areas that are of concern regarding legal issues include copyright protection, interstate commerce, and intellectual property. Additionally, there are cyberethical issues such as "privacy, confidentiality, censorship, freedom of speech, and an ever-increasing concern for control of personal information" (Bachman and Panzarine, 1998).

Intellectual property should be explored from two perspectives: faculty ownership of distance education products and the need to obtain permission for the various pieces of intellectual property of others (Billings, 2002). While no new federal mandates except the Copyright Act of 1976 exist to address multimedia educational concerns, the Consortium of College and University Media Centers has published the *Fair Use Guidelines for Educational Multimedia* (Dalziel, 1996). Faculty may own the materials they have developed for use in their distance education programs, but it is always good to have a memo of understanding documenting the specific use of the materials as well as the accrued benefits (Billings, 1996b). For any type of written and nonprint materials, permission should always be obtained from the copyright holders, followed by the appropriate recognition of their work (Menix, 1998).

The bottom line of this section is that faculty should know their employer's policy pertaining to intellectual property rights. Over the last several years, universities, government, and private organizations have noted the need to clearly delineate their policies in this area. For example, Texas Tech University has an established universitywide committee providing advisory opinions to the Provost on matters related to patentable discoveries and inventions, and/or copyrightable material, which had been developed by University employees. Extensive resources on intellectual property law and rights can be found at the following sites:

- The Copyright Management Center at Indiana University Purdue University at Indianapolis (*http://copyright.iupui.edu/*).

- Office of Technology Transfer and Intellectual Property at Texas Tech University (*http://www. depts.ttu.edu/transferandintellectualproperty/faq. html*)

- Legislative initiatives regulating intellectual property and copyright are found in the Technology, Education and Copyright (TEACH) Act (*http://www.arl.org/info/frn/copy/TEACH.html*)

- The World Trade Organization has an international perspective on intellectual property rights (*http://www.wto.org/english/tratop_e/trips_e/intel1_e.htm*)

- The Berkley Digital Library at Sunsite is an excellent resource for national perspectives on intellectual property (*http://sunsite.berkeley.edu/Copyright/*).

Further Research for Distance Education

Most of the research associated with distance education in the past has focused on comparing traditional and distance education instruction. Now, a more holistic evaluation of student issues is being sought. Some of these issues include the following.

Professional Socialization

Students comment that after completion of their online academic program they think and perceive the profession differently. These changes were always thought only to take place with face-to-face role modeling and mentoring. Yet, how can that change still be accomplished with the use of distance education (Milstead and Nelson, 1998; Reinert and Fryback, 1997) suggest that "sensitive indicators must be developed to determine when, how, and what socialization actually does occur."

Faculty and Student Interaction As Well As Critical Thinking

How much interaction is important during distance education, both between student and faculty and between students (Abrahamson, 1998)? With interactive video, Threlkeld and Brzoska (1994) found that adults tend to value the logistical elements of learning (rapid test return, feedback on writing assignments, and so forth) more importantly than discussing the issues, whereas high school students report greater emphasis on course design and interaction. Data from interactive video instruction may provide different findings than Internet courses. Additionally, what types of questions enhance critical thinking, what type of feedback is most beneficial, and at what time in the instruction is questioning most important (Armstrong, 2003)?

Gender and Environment Issues

With the large numbers of women in nursing using distance education for academic and continuing education, is gender a variable (Craig, 1994; Green, 1999; Koch, 1998; Pym, 1992)? Nurses expect support from family, friends, employers, and coworkers when they return to school, yet this may or may not be the case. According to Koch (1998), "some faculty claim that women and men behave and learn differently with distance education, in course satisfaction, academic performance, and retention." Also, are there learning differences between RN students from rural areas and urban areas? Gender differences in those locations should also be explored (Barker, 1985).

 ## Future Trends

Just as many graduate and nurse practitioner programs initially resisted online education, which is now basic, accelerated second degree, and doctoral education in nursing are slowly becoming the next horizon for distance learning. The consumer drive will push to meet this need for online education creating an avenue of reality. Also, transfer of credit and similarities in state nursing program curriculum will emerge as costs rise and the need to reduce duplication of resources emerges. Could standardization in nursing programs allow students to move from one state institution to another without leaving their home?

 ## Summary

Forging ahead in the cyber world has benefited both those taking the journey and those persons remaining behind to provide support and encouragement. The fallout or benefits have supported the technology explosion in nursing education where no faculty member is without a desktop, laptop, and PDA. Classrooms have gone wireless and laptops now have wireless cards. Online library access has become the norm with many traditional, as well as distance students, completing degrees without ever entering the on-campus library building, rather searching and retrieving all information from their dorm room. The notion of anywhere, anytime learning is truly now a reality in nursing education.

References

Abrahamson, C. E. (1998). Issues in interactive communication in distance education. *College Student Journal* 32(1):33–42.

Achterberg, C. (1996). Tips for teaching a course by e-mail. *Journal of Nutrition Education* 28(6):303–307.

Ali, N. S., Hodson-Carlton, K., and Ryan, M. (2004). Students' perceptions of online learning: Implications for teaching. *Nurse Educator* 29(3):111–115.

Allen, E. I. and Seaman, J. (2003). Sizing the opportunity: The Quality and extent of online education in the United States, 2002 and 2003. Needham and Wellesley, MA: The Sloan consortium.

Armstrong, M. L. (2003). Distance education: Using technology to learn. In V. A. Saba and K. A. McCormick (Eds.), *Essentials of Computers for Nurses: Informatics for the New Millennium* (3rd ed., pp. 413–425). New York: McGraw-Hill.

Aucoin, J. and Armstrong, M. L. (2003). Faculty development: A cornerstone of distance education. In M. L. Armstrong and S. Frueh (Eds.), *Telecommunications for Nurses: Providing Successful Distance Education and Telehealth* (pp. 55–69). New York: Springer.

Bachman, J. A. and Panzarine, S. (1998). Enabling student nurses to use the information superhighway. *Journal of Nursing Education* 37(4):155–161.

Barker, B. O. (1985). Understanding rural adult learners: Characteristics and challenges. *Lifelong Learning* 9(2):4–7.

Berge, Z. L. (1995). Facilitating computer conferencing: Recommendations from the field: The role of the online instructor/facilitator. *Educational Technology* 35(1):22–30. Retrieved June 2, 2004, from *http://www.emoderators.com/moderators/teach_online.html*

Billings, D. M. (1996a). Distance education in nursing. *Computers in Nursing* 14(4):211–212.

Billings, D. M. (1996b). Distance education in nursing: Adapting courses for distance education. *Computers in Nursing* 14(5):262, 263, 266.

Billings, D. M. (1997). Issues in teaching and learning at a distance: Changing roles and responsibilities of administrators, faculty, and students. *Computers in Nursing* 15(2):69–70.

Billings, D. (2002). Conversations in: E-learning. New York: Springer.

Boener, G. L. (2003). Delivering equitable online education: Online vs. hybrid course formats. Target Global Campus.

Boettcher, J. V. (2004). *Online Course Development: What Does it Cost?* Retrieved July 7, 2004, from *http://www.syllabus.com/article.asp?id=9676*.

Carlton, K. H. (1997). Refining continuing education delivery. *Computers in Nursing* 15(1):17–18, 22.

Carlton, K. H., Ryan, M. E., and Siktberg, L. L. (1998). Designing courses for the Internet: A conceptual approach. *Nurse Educator* 23(3):45–50.

Clark, C. (1993). Teaching and learning at a distance. In D. M. Billings and J. A. Halstead, (Eds.), *Teaching in Nursing: A Guide for Faculty* (pp. 331–346). Philadelphia, PA: W.B. Saunders.

Clark, D. (1998). Course redesign: Incorporating an Internet web site into an existing nursing class. *Computers in Nursing* 16(4):219–222.

Craig, C. E. (1994). Distance learning through computer conferences. *Nurse Educator* 19(2):10–14.

Cravener, P. A. (1997). Promoting active learning in large lecture classes. *Nurse Educator* 22(3):21–26.

Cravener, P. A. (1999). Faculty experiences with providing online courses. *Computers in Nursing* 17(1):42–47.

Dalziel, C. (1996). *Fair Use Guidelines for Educational Multimedia. http://www. libraries, psu.edu/mtss. fairuse/dalziel.html*

Dawes, B. S. (1998). Can distance learning provide a twenty-first century hallmark? *AORN Journal* 68(2):170, 172, 174.

Dede, C. J. (1990). The evolution of distance learning: Technology-mediated interactive learning. *Journal of Research in Computing in Education* 22(3):247–264.

EduTools. (2004). *EduTools Product Comparison.* Retrieved May 27, 2004, from *http://www.edutools.* and *http://edutools.info/course/product*

Green, M. (1999). *Streaming Video and Streaming Media. http://www.whatis.com/streamvd.html.*

Hanna, K. P., Wolford, N. R., and James S. G. (1998). Distance education and accreditation. *AANA* 66(2):113–116.

Indiana Higher eEducation Telecommunication system. (n.d.). *Guiding Principles for Faculty in Distance Learning.* Retrieved May 30, 2004, from *www.ihets. org/progserv/education/distance/guiding principles*

Koch, J. V. (1998). How women actually perform in distance education. *Chronical of Higher Education* A60.

Larson, O. M. and Dunkin, J. W. (1997). Writing in the interactive classroom. *Journal of Nursing Education* 36(6):298–301.

Mahan, K. and Armstrong, M. L. (2003). Distance education: What was, what's here, and preparation for the future. In M. L. Armstrong (Ed.), *Telecommunications for Nursing: Providing Successful Distance Education and Telehealth* (pp. 19–37). New York: Springer.

Massoud, L. (1999). *So You Want to Be a Distance Learning Instructor.* Flint, MI: Mott Community College.

McGonigle, D. and Mastrian, K. (1998). Learning along the way: Cyberspacial quests. *Nursing Outlook* 46:81–86.

Menix, K. D. (1998). Ethics and legal perspectives in distance education and telehealth. In M. L. Armstrong (Ed.), *Telecommunications for Health Professionals: Providing Successful Distance Education and Telehealth* (pp. 245–263). New York: Springer.

Milstead, J. A. and Nelson, R. (1998). Preparation for an online asynchronous university doctoral course: Lessons learned. *Computers in Nursing* 16(5): 247–258.

National Center for Education Statistics. (2004). *Highlights from the Condition of Education 2004.* U.S. Department of Education. Retrieved, from *http://nces.ed.gov//programs/coe/highlights/index.asp*

Neal, E. (1999). Distance education: Prospects and problems. *Phi Kappa Phi Journal* 79(1):40–43.

Perroots, S. D. (n.d.). *Best Practices for Electronically Offered Degree and Certificate Program.* Retrieved May 24, 2003, from *http://elearn.wvu.edu/zpolicies/ edpcheklist*

Plank, R. K. (1998). Nursing on-line for continuing education credit. *Journal of Continuing Education in Nursing* 29(4):165–172.

Pym, F. R. (1992). Women and distance education: A nursing perspective. *Journal of Advanced Nursing* 17:383–389.

Reinert, B. R. and Fryback, P. B. (1997). Distance learning and nursing education. *Journal of Nursing Education* 36(9):421–427.

Ribbons, R. M. (1998). Guidelines for developing interactive multimedia: Applications in nurse education. *Computers in Nursing* 16(2):109–114.

Schlosser, C. A. and Anderson, M. L. (1994). *Distance Education: Review of the Literature.* Washington DC: Association for Educational Communications & Technology.

Sherry, L. (1996). *Issues in Distance Learning. http//::www.cudenver.edu/~lsherry/pubs/issues.html.*

Shomaker, D. and Fairbanks, J. (1997). Evaluation of a RN-to-BSN distance education program via satellite for nurses in rural health care. *Journal of Nursing Education* 36(7):328–330.

Sistek-Chandler , C. (2000). Webifying courses: Online educational platforms. *Converge Magazine.* Retrieved May 24, 2004, from *http://.convergmag.com*

Smith, R. P. (1997). The Internet for continuing education. *MD Computing* 14:414–416.

Smith, G. G., Ferguson, D., and Cavis, M. (2001). Teaching college courses online vs. face-to-face. *The Journal.* Retrieved June 2, 2004, from *www.thejournal. com/magazine/vault/A3407.cfrm*

Sparks, S. M. and Rizzolo, M. A. (1998). World Wide Web search tools. *Image: Journal of Nursing Scholarship* 30(2):167–171.

Thompson, M. M. (1998). Distance learners in higher education. In C. C. Gibson (Ed.), *Distance Learners in Higher Education: Institutional Responses for Quality Outcomes* (pp. 10–18). Madison, WI: Atwood Publishing.

Threlkeld, R. and Brzoska, K. (1994). Research in distance education. In B. Willis (Ed.), *Distance Education: Strategies and Tools* (pp. 41–66). Englewood Cliffs, NJ: Educational Technology Publications.

Thurmond, V. A. (2002). Considering theory in assessing quality of web-based courses. *Nurse Educator* 27(1):20–24.

Todd, N. A. (1998). Using E-mail in an undergraduate nursing course to increase critical thinking skills. *Computers in Nursing* 16(2):115–118.

University of Colorado. (n.d.) Faculty development: Tips for online teaching. Retrieved June 2, 2004, from *http://www.cuonline.edu/faculty/teaching_tips.shtml*

Vilic, B. (2004). Online course caps: A survey. *Syllabus July 1, 2004.* Retrieved July 22, 2004, from *http://www.syllabus.com/article.asp?id=9679*

Western Cooperative for Educational Telecommunications. (2004a). *About WCET.* Retrieved May 26, 2004, from *http://www.wcet.info*

Western Cooperative for Educational Telecommunications. (2004b). *EduTools.* Retrieved on May 26, 2004, from *http://www/eduTools.info*

White, A., Allen, P., Goodwin, L., Breckinridge, D., Dowell, J., and Garvy, R. (in press). Infusing PDA technology into an accelerated baccalaureate nursing program. *Nurse Educator.*

Willis, B. (n.d.). *Distance Education at a Glance.* University of Idaho. Retrieved May 16, 2004, from *www.uidaho.edu/eo/distglan.html*

Zetzman, M. R. (1995). Telemedicine, POTS, and PANS technology, and rural health care in Texas. *Texas Journal of Rural Health*, 14:1–4.

34

Innovations in Telehealth

Diane J. Skiba
Amy J. Barton
Marilyn M. Nielsen

OBJECTIVES

1. Explore how telehealth innovations will transform healthcare, education, and research.
2. Examine the challenges and issues of these transformations.

KEY WORDS

information systems
telemedicine
telehealth
e-health
m-health
Internet

"The future of humanity is inextricably linked to technology," says John L. Petersen (2004), president of the Arlington Institute. "The future of the globe pivots on the kinds of tools we do or do not create in the coming years. Enlightened people with old tools will be significantly limited in what they can do to change the planetary footprint. We have to learn how to utilize new breakthrough technologies to solve our biggest, intractable problems—and not kill ourselves in the process." (Peterson, 2004)

Scientific advances in computing and communications technologies are transforming the way we live, work, and interact with each other. These technologies have transformed and will continue to transform the delivery of healthcare and learning in our society. These transformations will affect the practice of both healthcare and education. Telehealth applications will become commonplace and individuals will be able to participate in learning opportunities regardless of geographic location, age, physical limitation, or personal schedule (President's Information Technology Advisory Committee, 1999). In the mid-1990s, Kassirer (1995) predicted that the rapid growth of computer-based electronic communication coupled with patient empowerment and patient comfort with the electronic retrieval of

information would have a profound influence on the delivery of healthcare. Forkner-Dunn (2003) described the next generation of healthcare delivery as an Internet-based patient self-care model and concurred with Kassirer's perceptions that electronic communications will ultimately trigger widespread social and healthcare delivery transformations. Forkner-Dunn (2003) stated so aptly,

"The eHealth care train has not only left the station but it is rapidly moving down the track carrying ten of millions of e-patients and many possibilities for transforming patient self-management, improving health outcomes and enhancing the patient-clinician relationship. (p. 6)

This chapter highlights the transformations in healthcare and education within the context of advances in computing and communications technologies. The goals of this chapter are twofold: to explore how telehealth innovations will transform healthcare, education, and research and to present the challenges and issues as a result of these potential transformations. The chapter covers such topics as the concept of telehealth, the progression of telehealth applications, future innovations in advanced practice, education, and research, and the challenges and issues as a consequence of these transformations.

The Concept of Telehealth

Providing healthcare and education at a distance is not a new phenomenon. Distance education, the provision of learning opportunities at a distance, can be traced to the nineteenth century soon after the introduction of the postal service (Phipps and Merisotis, 1999). Correspondence courses were commonplace. This trend continued into the twentieth century with the arrival of new media such as radio and television. Similarly, telemedicine efforts can be traced to the late 1950s (Grisby and Sanders, 1998) with initial efforts focused on providing healthcare consultation to rural or remote environments (Bloch, 1999).

In order to understand the concept of telehealth, it is important to first define the term "telecommunications." According to the Institute of Medicine (IOM, 1996), "it is the use of wire, radio, optical or other electromagnetic channels to transmit and receive signals for voice, data and video communications." In the world of telecommunications, the media are telephone, video, and computer systems, and the methods of transmissions are phone lines, fiber optics, satellites, and microwave systems (Witherspoon, Johnston, and Wasem, 1994).

The IOM (1996) broadly defined telemedicine "as the use of electronic information and communication technologies to provide and support health care when distance separates the participants." Telemedicine has a variety of applications, some of which are often not thought of as telemedicine, since they are so commonplace. One such example is emergency calls to 911 that make use of "plain old telephone" technology (Institute of Medicine, 1996). Telephone triage, such as services like Ask a Nurse, is also another example that is often overlooked. More recent applications include remote telesurgery. Almost every specialty in medicine has some form of a telemedicine application (Grisby and Sanders, 1998).

In nursing, the American Nurses Association (ANA) (1997) wanted a more inclusive term and proceeded to define telehealth as "delivery of health care services or activities with time and distance barriers removed and using technologies such as telephones, computers, or interactive video transmissions." This organization considers telehealth as an umbrella term that encompasses telemedicine, telenursing, teleradiology, and telepsychiatry. Accordingly, telenursing is considered a form of telehealth where nursing practice is delivered via telecommunications. Perhaps the broadest definition is provided in *Mosby's Medical and Nursing Dictionary*

(1998). Telehealth is defined as:

> use of telecommunication technologies to provide health care services and access to medical and surgical information for training and educating health care professionals and consumers, to increase awareness and educate the public about health related issues and to facilitate medical research across distances. (Mosby, 1998)

A similar definition is provided by Bloch (1999), "telehealth is a broad term that can refer to educating health professionals and consumers, disseminating information on public health, performing research, and administering health services."

Loane and Wootten (2002) suggested that telehealth is not a technology but rather a technique for the remote delivery of healthcare. The *2001 Report to the Congress on Telehealth (2002)* defined it as "the use of telecommunication and information technologies (IT) to provide health care services at a distance, to include diagnosis, treatment, public health, consumer health information and health professions education." Brantley, Laney-Cummings, and Spivack (2004) expanded the defintion to include "a comprehensive system for integrating various applications—clinical health care delivery, management of medical information, education, and administrative services—within a common infrastructure." This report (Brantley et al., 2004) stated that "any examination of the nation's healthcare system should also acknowledge the convergence that combines such healthcare technologies as medical devices, healthcare informatics, IT for healthcare, telehealth and healthcare over the Internet (e-health)."

Thus, using the broadest definition of telehealth as a foundation, this chapter will explore the past, present, and future innovations as they apply to healthcare delivery, education, and research.

Progression of Telehealth Applications

For the last century, telehealth applications have evolved from simple communications to sophisticated pervasive and ubiquitous systems in the home that make use of wireless, wearable, robotic, and multisensorial technologies. In the past, trends in telehealth applications were grouped according to the various media: voice, data, and video. But with the convergence of these technologies, newer technologies merge across these media. Despite, these newer technologies, voice applications remain a mainstay of telehealth applications, since the telephone offers many advantages. According to Witherspoon et al. (1994), the telephone has the following advantages: relatively low cost for installation, low cost per use, minimal training for use, and ubiquity. Universal phone service was established as a public policy goal in the 1930s. Telephone service is enhanced to provide the following: conferencing, voice mail, facsimiles, computer communications, and videophones. Cell phone and other wireless technologies have generated a new movement called mobile health or m-health.

Voice technologies are now being supplanted with other medical devices to assess, monitor, and interact with patients, especially chronically ill patients in their homes. The Health Buddy device is one such example. Health Buddy, from Health Hero Network, is an appliance that attaches to a phone and prompts patients with a series of questions. On completion of questions, the appliance remotely transfers the data to a health professional's desktop. This appliance can also connect glucose meters, weight scales, blood pressure cuffs, and other medical devices so additional patient data are sent to the healthcare professionals. The Health Buddy system has been used with a variety of patients including coronary artery bypass graft (Zimmerman et al., 2004), chronic heart failure (LaFramboise et al., 2003), diabetes (Cherry et al., 2002), and asthma (Guendelman et al., 2002). E-Health or health over the Internet continues to be the area where there is the largest projected growth.

Without a doubt, the Internet and its accompanying data communications applications are transforming the way healthcare is delivered. The predecessor to many e-health applications was data communication applications developed by consumers or early healthcare pioneers. Data communications applications can be classified according to whether the applications were developed by the consumer or by healthcare professionals. These applications evolved from simple electronic bulletin board systems running on the FidoNet network (Sparks, 1992) to more elaborate multimedia systems designed to provide patient care in the home. For almost any diagnosis, there was an electronic support group that consumers could access. As an outgrowth of these electronic support groups, community-computing systems were established in many communities across the United States. These networks allowed communities to design computer networks to support their needs, including healthcare information. The first community network was the Cleveland Free Net that was used as a basis for the pioneering work done by Brennan et al. (1991a). Another community network, the Denver Free-Net also maintained electronic support groups and

healthcare information designed by consumer and healthcare professionals (Skiba and Mirque, 1994).

With the introduction of the World Wide Web (WWW), electronic support groups expanded to offer other healthcare services such as e-mail communication with providers, decision support tools, and customized discharge planning. Consumer demand for e-mail has continued to place demands on healthcare professionals. Early e-mail practices (Fridsma et al., 1994; Widman and Tong, 1997; Borowitz and Wyatt, 1998; Diepgen and Eysenbach, 1998) and corresponding guidelines (Kane and Sands, 1998; Spielberg, 1998) provided a solid foundation for the increasing demand for electronic communications between consumers and providers. Recent studies conducted by the Pew Internet and American Life studies indicated that over 50% of the U.S. population have accessed the Web for healthcare information either for themselves or for a family member or friend (Fox and Fallows, 2003). Given the tremendous increase in the usage, it is not surprising that consumers used e-mail to communicate with their healthcare providers. A recent editorial (Ferguson and Frydman, 2004) described the first generation of e-patients. They noted two observations e-patients have "better health information and services and have different, not necessarily better, relationships with their doctors" (Ferguson and Frydman, 2004).

Healthcare professionals and healthcare institutions have been actively creating Web-based applications for the direct delivery of healthcare. Pioneering work by Brennan et al. (1991a,b) served as a catalyst for the development of computer-mediated systems to provide healthcare for persons living with AIDS and caretakers of Alzheimer's disease patients. In both instances, Brennan and colleagues used a community-computing network, ComputerLink, to provide support services (contact with a nurse, informational resources, electronic support groups, and access to a decision-making tool) into the homes of patients and their caretakers. Results of these experiments (Brennan and Ripich, 1994; Brennan et al., 1995) demonstrated the value and effectiveness of computer-mediated support systems. As a continuation of this work, Brennan et al. (2001) designed HeartCare that created individual Web pages for cardiac artery bypass graft patients on discharge. The delivery of this healthcare recovery series via the Web will also provide direct communication via e-mail with the patient's healthcare provider.

The last type of telehealth applications incorporates video as a part of the application. The use of video within nursing applications is emerging as broadband capacity becomes available for consumers. For the past 30 years, medicine and psychiatry were the primary users of video applications. Store and forward radiology, dermatology, and pathology images were primary transmissions in medicine. There were also real-time patient visits for medical consults and telepsychiatry. A pioneering effort in nursing is the BabyCare Link project developed at the Beth Israel Deaconess Medical Center in Boston. This Web-based system connects families to their infants in the neonatal intensive care unit (Gray et al., 1998, 2000). The system allows parents to have updated information about the condition of their infant, such as weight gain and view images of their infant.

In more recent years, video applications have moved from the hospital to the home environment. The growth in managed care and demand management strategies has increased the interest in using video technologies with chronically ill patients. Videophones, desktop video systems, and televisions are common methods used in the home care market. In addition, Kinsella (1998) reports that video visits are augmented with vital sign devices with telecommunication capabilities such as blood pressure cuffs and glucometers. As video applications move to the home market, there is more potential for use by the nursing profession.

There have been several projects in nursing demonstrating the use of video applications in the home. Schlachta and Pursley-Crotteau (1997) pioneered an experimental program, Electronic Housecall, where chronically ill patients received healthcare through a personalized two-way interactive video system using a cable television network. Kaiser Permanente in Sacramento established a program, Tele-Home Health, to deliver care to a group of patients with advanced medical problems (Johnson, Wheeler, and Deuser, 1997). This project used a videophone augmented with an electronic stethoscope. A recent systematic review of telehealth interventions (Hersh et al., 2001) revealed that 25 studies met the criteria for inclusion and demonstrated various applications across different disease populations. "The strongest evidence for the efficacy of clinical outcomes were from home-based applications in the area of chronic disease management, hypertension and AIDS" (Hersh et al., 2001).

In summary, there has been a tremendous growth in the use of telehealth applications in nursing. Nursing applications have evolved over time and will continue to increase as we enter the next decade of healthcare. The rapid growth in home healthcare and managed care strategies serve as a catalyst for continued explorations in telehealth applications. These applications are transforming the way nursing care is delivered to patients.

Technological Innovations

Technological advances are providing healthcare with many opportunities to transform the business. This is particularly true in the area of telehealth. In the twentieth century, healthcare was in the infancy stage of telehealth. As the twenty-first century unfolds, technological innovations will advance the ability of nurses to participate in telehealth applications. What follows is a brief overview of technological advances for the next decade.

Applications for Advanced Practice: Transforming the Practice of Healthcare

Healthcare is undergoing evolution due to major societal changes and the need to provide access to quality and cost-effective care. Patients as "health consumers" are becoming more health conscious and more active in managing their own health. Telehealth applications are changing as well as moving into a *third generation*. Advances are occurring in digital imaging, remote wireless monitoring, videoconferencing, robotics and remote control, simulation and training, and diagnostics (Lymberis and Olsson, 2003; Brantley, Laney-Cummings, and Spivack, 2004).

Nursing practice must progress with these technologies that promote patient-centered care, access, evidence-based practice, and patient safety (Brantley, Laney-Cummings and Spivack, 2004; Institute of Medicine, 2001). As telehealth solutions are applied to healthcare situations, nurses must think about how these technologies will impact patient care, and understand the functional capability of the application within the healthcare delivery system (Constantelou and Karounou, 2004).

Nurses are actively involved with telehealth technologies: personal digital assistants (PDAs) are used at the bedside to enhance the safe delivery of care with access to clinical resources, drug databases, and medication calculation functions (Rempher, Lasome, and Lasome, 2003); diabetics use PDAs as electronic diaries to log food intake, glucose levels, medications, and activity (Kerkenbush and Lasome, 2003); home healthcare nurses document stages of wound healing with a digital camcorder (Demarest and Acoraci, 2004; Chetney and Sauls, 2003); heart failure patients use two-way video devices to participate in a congestive heart failure program from home (Chetney, 2003); and interactive devices such as "Health Buddy" allow adolescents with asthma to better manage their condition (Guendleman et al., 2002).

Future telehealth applications will build communication links between the patient, clinics, hospital, and primary care providers enhancing the continuum of care by linking the patient and family to the provider. A health "smart" home will allow the disabled and the elderly to live independently using automatic devices linked to emergency and support services (Raille et al., 2002). The Aware Home Research Initiative project (Mynatt et al., 2004) is one such example of smart systems designed to allow aging in place. Noninvasive sensors applied directly on the body or via a wearable clothing will improve the management of chronic health conditions, allowing the measurement of such things as vital signs, but also body posture, microcirculation, falls (Sixsmith and Johnson, 2004), movement, and pressure. These sensors will automatically detect serious situations and send alarms to a remote control center (Lymberis and Olsson, 2003; Rialle et al., 2002).

Healthwear, as described by Pentland (2004) are wearable systems with sensors that can continuously monitor vital signs, physical activity, social interactions, and sleep patterns. "By personalizing healthwear to the end-user, a truly personal medical record can revolutionize health care" (Pentland, 2004). Memory glasses (DeVaul, Corey, and Pentland, 2003) is another device being tested to aid the elderly. DiBetNet, a computerized game for young diabetics using a belt with motion sensors (Kumar, 2004) is another example. Both examples were generated from work at Massachusetts Institute of Technology's Media Lab. Another groundbreaking experiment at the Atlanta Veterans Affairs Rehabilitation Research and Development Center examined the use of cyber crumbs for elderly patients with vision loss. "Cyber crumbs, an electronic equivalent of a bread crumb trail, provides support for independent travel and an in situ awareness of the surroundings" (Ross, 2004, p. 30).

As Global Positioning Services (GPS) become more accurate they could assist the visually impaired with sounds or remind the Alzheimer patient about what to do in a certain location (Rodriquez and Cabrera, 2004). Wireless patient tracking will utilize satellite-based systems enhancing the safety of patients with such things as dementia. Satellite links and real-time video are being developed to deliver trauma services to rural patients (Gillespie, 2004). Wireless health outcome monitoring using cell phone technology is one such example that healthcare management group uses to assess cancer patients (Bielli et al., 2004).

Developments in microsystems and nanotechnologies will allow miniaturization and noninvasive monitoring of physiologic data (Lymberis and Olsson, 2003). Today, small capsules taken by mouth transmit video images that are stored on a recorder belt worn by the patient. The physician views saved images in an imaging station. Wireless embedded systems using mote technology that involves miniature sensors with two-way radios, microprocessors, and software that find each other and form a wireless network are currently being researched. Such networks could monitor glucose levels, pulse or oxygen saturation sending data to a remote location. The goal is for these sensors to be the size of a dust particle (Bloch, 2004).

Robotics and three-dimensional imaging will increasingly be used in surgical settings. Robots are being studied as a potential solution to such things as the nursing shortage (Bloch, 2004; Jossi, 2004).

Applications for Advanced Practice: Transforming the Way We Learn

Web-based educational programs are changing the way consumers and healthcare providers learn. These programs continue to proliferate providing the opportunity for interactive learning and simulations with the ability to have multiuser discussions and presentations in a learning collaboratory environment. Faced with limited funds nursing schools now have the ability to form partnerships and share their resources via the virtual classroom. The Internet allows nurses and students alike access to the most up-to-date research and knowledge facilitating evidence-based practice. Technological innovations such as video streaming, and virtual reality three-dimensional displays are providing more sophisticated formats in which to deliver educational materials. Web-based educational programs can reach remote students who otherwise would be unable to attend class (Sakraida and Draus, 2003; Smith-Stoner, 2003, Simpson, 2003; Brantley, Laney-Cummings, and Spivack, 2004).

The role of the nurse as a patient/consumer educator in the digital age is evolving as well. Computer-based education programs are becoming an effective method to present information and improve outcomes. Online educational materials can be tailored to an individual's literacy level and presented in a bilingual format (Lewis, 2003). Remote interactive telehealth networks have been shown to be effective in providing preoperative patient education to rural locations and are increasingly being used for disease management (Thomas et al., 2004; Roupe, 2004).

Applications for Advanced Practice: Transforming How We Conduct Research

The decoding of the human genome in February 2001 showcased the central role IT play in advanced research. A collaborative international decoding effort involving over 1,000 researchers saw chemical sequences sent over high-speed networks into data repositories for other scientists to examine and use. This work culminated in a raw sequence of calculations numbering over 22 billion (Interagency, 2003).

In 2001, the federal government combined the 21st Century Initiative (IT2) and the Next Generation Internet Initiative (NGI) into The Networking and Information Technology Research and Development (NITRD) program. The NITRD has set its focus on foundations for national security, scientific leadership, research, and learning. Investigation of complex phenomena requires many people, skills, and state-of-the-art tools. The NITRD enables major research agencies to coordinate plans and activities and to leverage strengths and avoid duplication maximizing investments. NITRD funds support research efforts in federal laboratories, universities, and in partnerships with private industry. The cost-effectiveness of such collaboration and resource sharing is key to exploring and prototyping complex technologies (Interagency, 2003).

These collaborative efforts have resulted in digital libraries that are today invaluable tools in research, and vital components for medical practice, healthcare, education, and training. Allow a distant user to manipulate a high-voltage transmission electron microscope, with real-time streaming video to the desktop, and help medical students experience surgical techniques via a "heptic" instrument connected to a computer that simulates the sense of touch (Interagency, 2003).

The process of conducting research is also enhanced by technologies, and telehealth applications with a research focus are flourishing in this virtual research environment. Lederberg and Uncapher (1989) first mentioned the use of these virtual research environments when they introduced the concept of a research collaboratory. The National Council of Research (1993) defined a collaboratory as a "center without walls in which the nation's researchers can perform research without regard to geographic location— interacting with colleagues, accessing instrumentation, sharing data and computational resources, and accessing information from digital libraries." There are numerous collaboratories already established, and

growth of these will continue as data mining, visualization techniques, and knowledge repositories become more prevalent. A recent review by Skiba (2004) highlighted the growing number of research collaboratories in the healthcare arena.

Challenges and Issues

If this transformation is to occur, the healthcare profession must tackle some key challenges and issues. These issues center on legal, ethical, and public policy arenas.

Legal Issues

The predominant legal issues concerning telehealth are licensure and liability and malpractice. The National Conference of State Legislatures (2004) identified legislation concerning telehealth in 37 of 50 states, with most of the activity occurring in the year 2000 and beyond. The following paragraphs explore the practice implications of each of these issues.

Licensure

The lack of infrastructure for interstate licensure has been a key impediment to the growth of telehealth. Currently, each state has established practice acts for medical, nursing, and allied health professionals that dictate the procedures for obtaining and renewing a license to practice within that state. In April 1996, the Federation of State Medical Boards proposed creation of a limited interstate license for teleconsulting physicians, which was rejected by the American Medical Association in June 1996. The issues contributing to the defeat of the measure included a concern that rural patients would leave their rural primary care provider for a specialist, the cost of telehealth equipment, and payment for provision of telehealth services (*Medical Economics*, 1997).

The U.S. Congress contracted with the Center for Telemedicine Law for a background paper concerning telehealth licensure issues in early 1997 (*http://www. ntia. doc.gov/reports/telemed/legal.htm*). Alternative approaches to licensure outlined in that report include consulting exceptions, endorsement, mutual recognition, reciprocity, registration, limited licensure, national licensure, and federal licensure. In the following paragraph, each approach is briefly defined, and implications for the current practice environment are identified.

Consulting exceptions are common to most states. They allow an out-of-state physician to provide services at the request of and in consultation with a referring physician. However, these exceptions were developed for rare occurrences and not expected to be used on a full-time basis, as they would be for telehealth. **Licensure by endorsement** is currently used to permit providers licensed in one state to apply for licensure in another state in which they would like to practice. Unfortunately, in operationalizing telehealth, this could require providers to apply for licensure in all 50 states. **Mutual recognition** is a licensure system used in Europe and Australia in which licensing bodies agree to accept the policies of the licensee's home state. This method would require agreement by the states on standardized rules and regulations governing healthcare across the states. **Reciprocity** is an approach that would allow states to grant practice privileges to a provider of another state without further credential review. This would require states to develop agreements with several other states. In a **registration** system, a provider is required to notify another state of intent to practice. The provider would be required to follow the rules of the state but not to meet the state's entrance requirements. **Limited licensure** is an option in which providers are required to obtain a license in every state in which they practice. The provider would have the option of applying for a limited license in subsequent states that would specify a limited scope of practice. An assumption of this approach is that application requirements would be less burdensome for a limited scope of practice. **National licensure** involves standardized requirements for licensure throughout the United States. This option would create a centralized administration for licensure resulting in lost revenue for states, questions regarding legal authority of the states, logistical challenges, and funding concerns. A final approach is **federal licensure** in which providers are issued one license by the federal government that would be valid throughout the United States. The system would be administered through federal agencies at the national, state, or local level.

The National Council of State Boards of Nursing has developed a mutual recognition model of licensure (Simpson, 1998). This would allow nurses licensed in their home state to practice in other states under their respective state's Nurse Practice Act, when that state is part of the interstate compact (Hardin and Langford, 2001). Nurses would remain accountable to their home state board of nursing. As of March 2004, 17 states have enacted the nurse licensure compact, with three additional states having legislation signed by their governor and pending implementation (National Council of State Boards of Nursing, 2004).

The State Licensure Committee of the American Telemedicine Association (ATA, 1998) issued recommendations for a policy statement (*http://atmeda.org/news/policy.html*) that:

- Preserves the right of each state to regulate medicine in traditional face-to-face physical setting
- Preserves licensure authority at the state level
- Avoids unnecessary restraints on interstate commerce
- Ensures that all patients have access to the healthcare expertise necessary to protect and promote their health, regardless of the location of the provider
- Advances telemedicine as a valuable service delivery strategy that can play a critical role in overcoming time and distance barriers that often limit access to quality healthcare.

The ATA report continues with proposed "rules of engagement" for telemedicine

- A telemedicine request originates from a physician who is fully licensed in the patient's state.
- The patient and requesting physician must have a real physician-patient relationship.
- The patient and requesting physician must have a real face-to-face encounter.
- The out-of-state physician using telemedicine must be fully licensed in the state in which the physician is located.
- The responsibility of medical care for the patient must remain with the requesting physician.

Liability and Malpractice

The second major legal issue that must be addressed with telehealth is liability and malpractice. "Currently, malpractice cases hinge on two legal questions: (1) whether a physician-patient relationship existed and (2) whether the physician breaches his or her duty of care" (Saltzman and Lammers, 1997, p. 24). Part of the challenge concerning telehealth and liability is that there is a lack of statutory and case law (Saltzman and

Lammers, 1997; Physician's Insurers Association of America, 1998). In addition, since medical liability originates when there is injury due to a breach in the standard of care, the fact that the standard of care in telehealth has not been defined is another area of concern (Physician's Insurers Association of America, 1998). The ANA does not believe that telehealth will impact the scope of practice, however. "Scopes of practice should be driven by decisions about allowable services based on the profession's or legislature's obligation to ensure ethical and high quality service" (American Nurses Association, 1999).

"During the discussion at the PIAA Telemedicine Colloquium, consensus emerged that the liability resulting from a telemedicine encounter between a physician and patient would likely be direct liability as opposed to vicarious (liability imposed upon a person even though he is not a party to the specific occurrence)" (Physician's Insurers Association of America, 1998, p. 13). Two liability issues that may require consideration for telehealth encounters include equipment malfunction and failure to use the technology. With regard to the former, clinicians may be at increased risk if equipment malfunction leads to an adverse event. In addition, if telehealth permits high-quality care, it is possible that clinicians may be held liable for failure to deliver it.

One advantage of telehealth applications from a liability perspective is that use of the technology generates an electronic medical record. "The existence of a recorded copy of the actual consultation, rather than (or in addition to) a summary note in the patient record should have major implications" (Ostbye and Hurlen, 1997, p. 270). Not only will the provider have a complete record, but the interaction may be used for educational sessions as well.

The PIAA (1998, p. 19) developed risk management recommendations for providers engaged in telehealth applications. A summary of the recommendations is provided below.

- Become proficient with the technology.
- Ensure that the use of telemedicine is appropriate for the situation.
- Educate the patient regarding options and limitations in the use of telemedicine.
- Become familiar with referring physicians and their credentials.
- Inform your insurance carrier of the nature and scope of your telemedicine practice.

- If technology does not provide a clear assessment or if results are equivocal, see the patient in person or refer him/her for face-to-face or follow-up consultation.
- Make sure there are realistic expectations of all parties. This technology is not perfect or appropriate for all types of interactions.
- Clarify roles and responsibilities of all practitioners. Make sure the division of responsibilities is clear and complete.
- Make sure contractual issues are reviewed and clarified.
- Maintain an archive of each system in use.
- Make every attempt to personalize the telemedicine encounter.
- Document, document, document.

Ethical Issues

The predominant ethical issues concerning telehealth are privacy, confidentiality, and security. The following definitions have been set forth by the American Society for Testing and Materials Committee E31 on Healthcare Informatics, Subcommittee E31.17 on Privacy, Confidentiality, and Access (1997):

Privacy   "The right of individuals to be left alone and to be protected against physical or psychological invasion or the misuse of their property. It includes freedom from intrusion or observation into one's private affairs, the right to maintain control over certain personal information, and the freedom to act without outside interference."

Confidentiality   The "status accorded to data or information indicating that it is sensitive for some reason, and therefore it needs to be protected against theft, disclosure, or improper use, or both, and must be disseminated only to authorized individuals or organizations with a need to know."

Data security   "The result of effective data protection measures; the sum of measures that safeguard data and computer programs from undesired occurrences and exposure to accidental or intentional access or disclosure to unauthorized persons, or a combination thereof; accidental or malicious alteration; unauthorized copying; or loss by theft or destruction by hardware failures, software deficiencies; operating mistakes; physical damage by fire, water, smoke, excessive temperature, electrical failure or sabotage; or a combination thereof. Data security exists when data are protected from accidental or intentional disclosure to unauthorized persons and from unauthorized or accidental alteration."

System security "The totality of safeguards including hardware, software, personnel policies, information practice policies, disaster preparedness; and oversight of these components. Security protects both the system and the information contained within from unauthorized access from without and from misuse from within. Security enables the entity or system to protect the confidential information it stores from unauthorized access, disclosure, or misuse, thereby protecting the privacy of the individuals who are the subjects of the stored information."

Buckovich et al. (1999) conducted a comparative review and analysis of 28 independent draft principles on privacy, confidentiality, and security. Eleven consistent principles were identified.

1. Individuals have a right to the privacy and confidentiality of their health information.

2. Outside the doctor-patient relationship, health information that makes a person identifiable shall not be disclosed without prior patient informed consent and/or authorization.

3. All entities with exposure or access to individual health information shall have security/privacy/confidentiality policies, procedures, and regulations (including sanctions) in place that support adherence to these principles.

4. Individuals have a right to access in a timely manner their health information.

5. Individuals have a right to control the access and disclosure of their health information and to specify limitations on period of time and purpose of use.

6. Employers have a right to collect and maintain health information about employees allowable or otherwise deemed necessary to comply with state and federal statutes (e.g., ERISA, drug testing, and workers' compensation). However, employers shall not use this information for job or other employee benefit discrimination.

7. All entities involved with healthcare information have a responsibility to educate themselves, their staff, and consumers on issues related to these principles.

8. Individuals have a right to amend and/or correct their health information.

9. Health information and/or medical records that make a person identifiable shall be maintained and transmitted in a secure environment.

10. An audit trail shall exist for medical records and be available to patients on request.

11. Support for these principles needs to be at the federal level.

The Health Insurance Portability and Accountability Act of 1996 (HIPAA) is designed to protect the privacy of all individually identifiable health information obtained by providers and other covered entities, regardless of whether the information is or has been in electronic form. "The requirements for the use and disclosure of personally identifiable health information are applicable regardless of how the information is recorded or stored, how the information is transmitted, the time sequence of its creation and use, or the way it is communicated" (Denton, 2003, pp. 320–321). A major challenge for clinicians involved in telehealth is having working knowledge of the state privacy laws in every state in which they practice. Protections afforded by HIPAA preempt state law only when state law is less restrictive. Therefore, clinicians using the general provisions outlined by the federal law may not be meeting the requirements in the states in which they practice (Denton, 2003).

Public Policy

The Western Governors Association (WGA, 1998) identified three key policy barriers to the growth of telehealth initiatives. Those three issues include infrastructure planning and development, telecommunications regulation, and lack of reimbursement for telehealth services. In addition, the recent National Telecommunications and Information Administration (2000) report highlights a persistent problem called the digital divide . . . Internet "have-nots."

The WGA discovered that state policy makers failed to consider telecommunication needs across various state activities, resulting in missed opportunities for cost-sharing and reducing redundancy in states' networks. They proposed "tighter integration of strategic planning efforts for telemedicine and telecommunications" (Western Governors Association, 1998, p. 2). In addition, they proposed inviting private sector telecommunications companies, equipment manufacturers, and medical service providers to discussions.

One of the greatest issues in the regulation of telecommunications concerns the ability of communities to obtain the types of services necessary at affordable rates. The Telecommunications Act of 1996 leveled the playing field by requiring discounted services for rural health providers. Unfortunately, this program has been off to a slow start, but individual states are beginning to dedicate support for state-operated networks to support telehealth (Western Governors Association, 1998).

The historical funding sources for development of telehealth applications rested largely with the National Aeronautics and Space Administration and the Department of Defense (Grigsby and Sanders, 1998). Initially, Medicare reimbursement was generally not available (with the exception of certain Health Professional Shortage Areas (HPSAs)) since telehealth applications do not meet the Healthcare Financing Administration requirement for in-person, face-to-face contact. The Medicare, Medicaid, and SCHIPS Balanced Benefits Improvement and Protection Act of 2000 provided for new regulatory rules by the Center for Medicare and Medicaid Services (CMS) that expanded the list of Current Procedural Terminology CPT codes, the geographic areas, and the eligible originating sites (Antoniotti and Armstrong, 2003).

The digital divide is still a persistent public policy issue. For the last 5 years, data were collected to address the penetration of telephone and computers in consumer homes. These analyses were directed to examine the haves and the have-nots in the information age. Here are some of the highlights of the most recent report (National Telecommunications and Information Administration, 2000). The penetration rates have increased nationwide in terms of people entering into the information age. Computer penetration has grown substantially with the following changes in penetration: more than half of households (51%) have computers; households with Internet access increased by 58–41.5%; and the proportion of individuals using the internet increased by one-third to 44.4% (National Telecommunications and Information Administration, 2000).

Despite these increases, there has been a widening in the gap between lower and higher income families. The "digital divide" between certain groups of Americans has increased between 1994 and 2000. According to the NTIA (2000) report, large gaps remain for Internet access among Black (23.5% penetration) and Hispanic (23.6% penetration) households when compared to the national average of 41.5% penetration. Single female heads of households and rural poor, the disabled, and rural and central city minorities constitute the profile of the least connected group of Americans. Significant populations still remain unconnected and will be unable to take advantage of the numerous telehealth applications highlighted in this chapter. Telehealth applications, particularly interactive health communications, may help to reduce health disparities through their potential for promoting health, preventing disease, and supporting clinical care for all; however, those with health problems are least likely to have access (Eng et al., 1998). Thus, this is another public policy issue that needs to be tackled if telehealth applications are to provide the maximum benefits to all.

Conclusion

Without a doubt, telehealth applications will proliferate in the future. Healthcare professionals need to seize the opportunities made possible by advanced technologies and create powerful and human-centered telehealth applications. To start this process, healthcare professionals need to become actively involved in resolving challenges and shaping public policy.

References

2001 Report to Congress on Telemedicine. (2002). *Office for the Advancement of Telehealth.* Available at *http://telehealth.hrsa.gov/pubs/report2001/intro. htm#overview*

Antoniotti, N. M., Armstrong, T. M., and the ATA Policy Committee. (2003). *American Telemedicine Association: Report on Reimbursement.* Available at *http://www.americantelemed.org/news/newres.htm*

American Nurses Association. (1999). *Core Principles of Telehealth.* Washington, DC: American Nurses Publishing.

American Nurses Association. (1997). Telehealth, a tool for nursing practice. *Nursing Trends & Issues* 2(4):1–7.

American Society for Testing and Materials Committee E-31 on Healthcare Informatics, Subcommittee E-31.17 on Privacy, Confidentiality, and Access. (1997). *Standard Guide for Confidentiality, Privacy, Access, and Data Security Principles for Health Information Including Computer-based Patient Records.* Philadelphia, PA: ASTM (Designation E-1869-97).

American Telemedicine Association. (1998). *ATA State Medical Licensure Committee Draft Report to ATA Board of Directors.* Available at *http://atmeda. org/news/policy.html*

Bielli, E., Carminati, F., La Capra, S., Lina, M., Brunelli, C., and Tamburini, M. (2004). A wireless health outcomes monitoring system (WHOMS): Development and testing with cancer patients using mobile phones. *Medical Informatics and Decision Making* [electronic version] 4:7.

Bloch, C. (2004). *University and State Activities: Telemedicine, Telehealth, Informatics, and Research*. Kalamazoo, MI: Bloch Consulting Group.

Bloch, C. (1999). *Federal Telemedicine Activities and Internet Sites*. Potomac, MD: Bloch Consulting Group.

Borowitz, S. M. and Wyatt, J. C. (1998). The origin, content, and workload of e-mail consultations. *The Journal of the American Medical Association* 280(15):1321–1324.

Brantley, D., Laney-Cummings, K., and Spivack, R. (2004). *Innovation, Demand and Investment in Telehealth*. U.S. Dept. of Commerce: Office of Technology Policy. Retrieved April 25, 2004, from *http://www.technology.gov/reports/TechPolicy/Telehealth/2004Report.pdf*

Brennan, P., Moore, S., Bjornsdottir, G., Jones, J., Visovsky, C., and Rogers, M. (2001). HeartCare: An Internet-based information and support system for patient home recovery after coronary artery bypass graft (CABG) surgery. *Journal of Advanced Nursing* 35(5):699–708.

Brennan, P., Moore, S., and Smyth, K. (1995). The effects of a special computer network on caregivers of persons with Alzheimer's disease. *Nursing Research* 44:166–172.

Brennan, P. and Ripich, S. (1994). Use of home-care computer network by persons with AIDS. *International Journal of Technology Assessment in Health Care* 10:258–272.

Brennan, P., Ripich, S., and Moore, S. (1991a). The use of home-based computers to support persons living with AIDS/ARC. *Journal of Community Health Nursing* 8(1):3–14.

Brennan, P., Moore, S., and Smyth, K. (1991b). ComputerLink: Electronic support for the home caregiver. *Advances in Nursing Science* 13(4):14–27.

Buckovich, S. A., Rippen, H. E., and Rozen, M. J. (1999). Driving toward guiding principles: A goal for privacy, confidentiality, and security of health information. *Journal of the American Medical Informatics Association* 6:122–133.

Cherry, J. C., Moffat, T. P., Rodriguez, C., and Dryden, K. (2002). Diabetes disease management program for an indigent population empowered by telemedicine technology. *Diabetes Technology & Therapeutics*. 4(6):783–791.

Chetney, R. and Sauls, E. (2003). A picture speaks louder than words . . . but a digital camcorder tells the whole story. *Home Healthcare Nurse* 21(10):694–695.

Chetney, R. (2003). The cardiac connection program: Home care that doesn't miss a beat. *Home Healthcare Nurse* 21(10):680–686.

Constantelou, A. and Karounou, V. (2004). Skills and competencies for the future of eHealth. *The IPTS Report, European Commission Joint Research Center* 81. Retrieved March 3, 2004, from *http://www.jrc.es/home/report/english/articles/vol81/welcome.htm*

Demarest, L. and Acoraci, L. (2004). Choosing and using a digital camera in home care. *Home Healthcare Nurse* 22(1):61–63.

Denton, D. R. (2003). Ethical and legal issues related to telepractice. *Seminars in Speech and Language* 24(4):313–322.

DeVaul, R., Corey, V., and Pentland, A. (2003). The memory glasses: Subliminal vs overt memory support with imperfect information. In *Proceedings of the 7th International Symposium on Wearable Computers* (pp. 146–153). Piscataway, NJ: IEEE Press.

Diepgen, G. and Eysenbach, T. (1998). Responses to unsolicited patient e-mail request for medical advise on the World Wide Web. *The Journal of the American Medical Association* 280(15):1333–1335.

Eng, T., Maxfield, A., Patrick, K., et al. (1998). Access to health information and support (policy perspectives). *The Journal of the American Medical Association* 280(15):1371–137.

Ferguson, T. and Frydman, G. (2004). The first generation of e-patients (editorial). *British Medical Journal* [electronic version] 328:1148–1149.

Fox, S. and Fallows, D. (2003). *Internet Health Resources*. Pew Internet & American Life project. Available at *http://www.pewinternet.org*

Fridsma, D., Ford, P., and Altman, R. (1994). A survey of patient access to electronic mail, attitudes, barriers, and opportunities. In J. Ozbolt (Ed.), *Proceeding of the Annual Symposium on Computer Applications in Medical Care* (pp. 15–19). Philadelphia, PA: Henly & Belfus.

Forkner-Dunn, J. (2003). Internet-based patient self-care: The next generation of health care delivery. *Journal of Medical Internet Research* 5(2):e8. Available at *http://www.jmir.org/2003/2/e8*

Gillespie, G. (2004). The I.T. of tomorrow: Is it here today? *Health Data Management* [electronic version].

Gray, J., Pompilio-Weitzner, G., Jones, P. C., Wang, Q., Coriat, M., Safran, C. (1998). Baby CareLink: Development and implementation of a WWW-based system for neonatal home telemedicine. In *Proceedings of the American Medical Informatics Symposium* (pp. 351–355).

Gray, J., Safran, C., Davis, R. B., et al. (2000). Baby CareLink: Using the Internet and telemedicine to improve care for high-risk infants. *Pediatrics* 106:1318–1324.

Grisby, J. and Sanders, J. (1998). Telemedicine: Where it is and where it's going. *Annals of Internal Medicine* 129(2):123–127.

Guendelman, S., Meade, K., Benson, M., Chen, Y. Q., and Samuels, S. (2002). Improving asthma outcomes and self-management behaviors of inner-city children: A randomized trial of the Health Buddy interactive device and an asthma diary. *Archives of Pediatric and Adolescent Medicine* 156(2):114–120.

Hardin, S. and Langford, D. (2001). Telehealth's impact on nursing and the development of the interstate compact. *Journal of Professional Nursing* 17(5): 243–247.

Hersh, W., Helfand, M., Wallace, J., Kraemer, D., Patterson, P., Shapiro, S., and Greenlick, M. (2001). Clinical outcomes resulting from telemedicine interventions: A systematic review. *Medical Informatics and Decision Making* [electronic version] 1:5.

Interagency Working Group on Information Technology Research and Development. (2003). *Advanced Foundations for American Innovation: Supplement to the President's FY 2004 Budget*. Arlington, VA: National Coordination Office for Information Technology Research and Development. Retrieved April 28, 2004, from *http://www.nitrd.gov/pubs/blue04/04BB-final.pdf*

Institute of Medicine, Committee on Quality Health Care in America. (2001). *Crossing the Quality Chasm: A New Health System for the 21st Century*. Washington, DC: National Academy Press.

Institute of Medicine. (1996). *Telemedicine: A Guide to Assessing Telecommunications in Health Care*. Washington, DC: National Academy Press.

Johnson, B., Wheeler, L., and Deuser, J. (1997). Kaiser Permanente medical center's pilot telehome health project. *Telemedicine Today* 8:16–19.

Jossi, F. (2004). *Robostaff. Healthcare Informatics—On-Line*. Retrieved April 27, 2004, from *http://www.healthcare-informatics.com/issues/2004/04_04/jossi.htm*

Kane, B. and Sands, D. Z. (1998). AMIA Internet Working Group, Task Force on Guidelines for the Use of Clinic-Patient Electronic Mail: Guidelines for the clinical use of electronic mail with patients. *Journal of the American Medical Informatics Association* 5(1):104–111.

Kassirer, J. P. (1995). The next transformation in the delivery of health care. *The New England Journal of Medicine* 332(1):52–54.

Kerkenbush, M., and Lasome, C. (2003). The emerging role of electronic diaries in the management of diabetes mellitus. *AACN Clinical Issues* 14(3):371–378.

Kinsella, A. (1998). *Home Healthcare, Wired & Ready for Telemedicine . . . The second generation*. Sunriver, OR: Information for Tomorrow.

Kumar, V. (2004). The design and testing of a personal health system to monitor adherences to intensive diabetes management. Master's Thesis. Harvard-MIT Health Sciences and Technology Program, 2004 cited in A. Pentland. Healthwear: Medical technology becomes wearable. *Computer* 37(5):42–49.

LaFramboise, L. M., Todero, C. M., Zimmerman, L., and Agrawat, S. (2003). Comparison of Health Buddy with traditional approached to heart failure management. *Family and Community* 26(4):275–288.

Lederberg, J. and Uncapher, K. (1989). *Towards a National Collaboratory*. New York: The Rockefeller University.

Lewis, D. (2003). Computers in patient education. *Computers, Informatics, Nursing* 21(2):88–96.

Loane, M. and Wootton, R. (2002). A review of guidelines and standards for telemedicine. *Journal of Telemedicine and Telecare* 8(2):63–71.

Lymberis, A. and Olsson, S. (2003). Intelligent biomedical clothing for personal health and disease management: State of the art and future vision. *Telemedicine Journal and e-Health* 9:379–386.

Mosby. (1998). *Medical & Nursing Dictionary* (5th ed., p. 895E). St. Louis, MO: Author.

Mynatt, E., Melanhorst, A.S., Fisk, A., and Rogers, W. (2004). Aware technologies for Aging in Place: Understanding users needs and attitudes. *Pervasive Computing* 3(2):36–41.

National Conference of State Legislatures. (2004). *Telemedicine Legislation*. Available at *http://www.ncsl.org/programs/health/teleleg.htm*

National Council of Research. (1993). *National Collaboratories: Applying Information Technology for Scientific Research*. Washington, DC: National Academy Press.

National Council of State Boards of Nursing. (2004). *Nurse Licensure Compact Implementation*. Available at *www.ncsbn.org/nlc/rnlpvncompact_mutual_recognition_state.asp*

National Telecommunications and Information Administration. (2000). *Falling Through the Net: Toward Digital Inclusion. Falling Through the Net Series on the Telecommunications and Information Technology Gap in America* (4th report). *http://www.ntia.doc.gov/pdf/fttn00.pdf*

Ostbye, T. and Hurlen, P. (1997). The electronic house call: Consequences of telemedicine consultations for physicians, patients, and society. *Archives of Family Medicine* 6(3):266–271.

Pentland, A. (2004). Healthwear: Medical technology becomes wearable. *Computer* 37(5) 42–49.

Peterson, J. (2004). Breakthrough Technology Conference Welcome. Retrieved on July 16, 2004, at *http://www.arlingtoninstitute.org/springseminar2004/2aprilCon_home.asp*

Physicians Insurers Association of America (1998). *Telemedicine: A Medical Liability White Paper*. Rockville, MD: Physicians Insurers Association of America.

Phipps, R. and Merisotis, J. (1999). *What's the Difference? A Review of Contemporary Research on the Effectiveness of Distance Learning in Higher Education*. Washington, DC: The Institute for Higher Education Policy.

President's Information Technology Advisory Committee. (1999). *Information Technology Research: Investing in our Future*. Arlington, VA: National Coordination Office for Computing, Information and Communications.

Raille, V., Duchene, F., Noury, N., Bajolle, L., and Demongeot, J. (2002). Health "smart" home: Information technology for patients at home. *Telemedicine Journal and e-Health* 84:395–409.

Rempher, K., Lasome, C., and Lasome, T. (2003). Leveraging Palm technology in the advanced practice-nursing environment. *AACN Clinical Issues* 14(3):363–370

Rodriquez, C. and Cabrera, M. (2004). Location-based healthcare services. *The IPTS Report, European Commission Joint Research Center 81.* Retrieved March 3, 2004, from *http://www.jrc.es/home/report/english/articles/vol81/welcome.htm*

Ross, D. (2004). Cyber crumbs for successful aging with vision loss. *Pervasive Computing* 3(2):30–35.

Roupe, M. (2004). Interactive home telehealth: A vital component of disease management programs. *Case Management* 9(1):47–49.

Sakraida, T. and Draus, P. (2003). Transition to a Web-supported curriculum. *Computers, Informatics, Nursing* 21(6):309–315.

Saltzman, K. and Lammars, K. (1997). Telemedicine: Where health care services meet technology. *Infusion* 4(2):23–26.

Schlachta, L. M. and Pursley-Crotteau, S. (1997). Leveraging technology, telemedicine in disease management and implications for infusion services. *Infusion* 4(2):36–40.

Simpson, R. (2003). Welcome to the virtual classroom: How technology is transforming nursing education in the 21st century. *Nursing Administration Quarterly* 27(1):83–86.

Simpson, R. (1998). Long-distance nursing kindles multistate licensure debate. *Nursing Management* 29(12):8–9.

Sixsmith, A and Johnson, N. (2004). A smart sensor to detect the falls of the elderly. *Pervasive Computing* 3(2):42–47.

Skiba, D. (2004). Research collaboratories: Using technologies to advance science. In J. Fitzpatrick and K. Montgomery (Eds.), *Internet and Nursing Research: A Guide to Strategies, Skills, and Resources.* New York: Springer.

Skiba, D. and Mirque, D. (1994). The electronic community: An alternative health care approach. In S. Grobe and E.S.P. Plutyer-Wenting (Eds.), *Nursing Informatics, An International Overview for Nursing in a Technological Era* (pp. 388–392). Amsterdam, The Netherlands: Elsevier.

Smith-Stoner, M. and Willer, A. (2003). Video streaming in nursing education: Bringing life to online education. *Nurse Educator* 28(2):66–70.

Sparks, S. (1992). Exploring electronic support groups. *American Journal of Nursing* 92(12):62–65.

Spielberg, A. R. (1998). On call and online, sociohistorical, legal, and ethical implications of e-mail for the patient-physician relationship. *Journal of the American Medical Association* 280(15):1353–1359.

Telemedicine Editorial. (1997). Obstacles to telecomedicine's growth. *Medical Economics* 74(23):69.

Telemedicine Report to Congress. (1997). *Legal Issues—Licensure and Telemedicine. http://www.ntia.doc.gov/reports/telemed/legal.htm*

Thomas, K., Burton, D., Withrow, L., and Adkisson, B. (2004). Impact of a preoperative education program via interactive telehealth network for rural patients having total joint replacement. *Orthopaedic Nursing* 23(1):39–44.

Western Governors Association. (1998). *Telemedicine Action Update.* Denver, CO: Western Governors Association.

Widman, L. E. and Tong, D. A. (1997). Requests for medical advise from patients and families to health care providers who publish on the World Wide Web. *Archives of Internal Medicine* 157(2):209–212.

Witherspoon, J., Johnston, S., and Wasem, C. (1994). *Rural TeleHealth, Telemedicine, Distance Education and Informatics for Rural Health Care.* Boulder, CO: Western Interstate Commission of Higher Education Publications.

Zimmerman, L., Barason, S. Nieveen, J., and Schmaderer, M. (2004). Symptom management intervention in elderly coronary artery bypass graft patients. *Outcomes Management* 8(1):5–12.

PART **9**

Research
Application

35

Computer Use in Nursing Research

Veronica D. Feeg

Sarah E. Sheehan

Asher E. Beckwitt

Betty L. Chang

OBJECTIVES

1. Describe general data and computer applications related to proposal development and project implementation in both quantitative and qualitative research.

2. Discuss an overview of computer-based applications that facilitate or support the steps of the research process, including data collection, data management and coding, data analysis, and results reporting.

3. Compare and contrast select computer software applications that can be used in quantitative and qualitative research data analysis related to the steps of the research process.

4. Discuss examples of specific computer applications that have been used in quantitative and qualitative research studies.

KEY WORDS

research process
research methodology
quantitative
qualitative
data collection
data management
data analysis
research applications
computer applications

The uses of computers and software applications are ubiquitous throughout the research process, from the inception of ideas through the selection of approaches, refinement of each of the stages, capturing the data, synthesizing the results, and presenting it to the world through dissemination. This chapter will provide an overview of the research process for two separate and dissimilar research approaches—quantitative and qualitative—and discuss select computer applications and uses relative to these approaches and specific to the universally understood research steps that are unique to each approach.

The computer has been a tool for researchers in various aspects of the research process and has gone beyond its historic application once limited to number crunching. Personal computers, laptops, tablets, and even handheld PDAs (personal digital assistants) have become part of the researcher's necessary resources in mounting a research project or study. From word-processing proposals and manuscripts to database management of subjects, contacts, or logistics, nurses have used a range of hardware and software applications that are generic to operations in addition to the tools and devices that are specific to research data collection, analysis, results reporting, and dissemination.

In today's electronic healthcare environments, numerous advances have been made with the sources of data collection relative to general clinical applications in nursing, health, and health services. System implementations for large clinical enterprises have also provided opportunity for nurses and health service researchers to identify and extract information from existing computer-based resources, although the ethical ramifications of using patient data must be always considered. In addition, the era of Web-based applications has produced a plethora of innovative means of entering data and, subsequently, collecting data in ways that were not possible before. With the advancements in the implementation of clinical systems, acceptable terminology and vocabularies to support nursing assessment, interventions, and evaluation, computers are increasingly being used for clinical and patient care research. Although research is a complex cognitive process, certain aspects of carrying out research can be aided by software applications. For example, examination of patient outcomes of nursing care and the effect of interventions would have been prohibitive in the past, but with the aid of computers and access to large data sets, many health outcomes can be analyzed quantitatively and qualitatively.

The objective of this chapter is twofold: (1) to provide an overview of general computer and software applications related to the stages of the research process and (2) to describe how computers facilitate the work of the researcher or serve in some capacity as the foundation of the research itself. To begin, the chapter will focus on some of the considerations related to the logistics and preparation of the research proposal, project planning, and budgeting, followed by the implementation of the proposal with data capture, data management, data analysis, and information presentation. The use of literature search systems and online bibliographic retrieval and management applications are discussed in detail in the Chapter 36. The general steps of proposal development, preparation, and implementation are applicable to both quantitative and qualitative approaches.

Proposal Development, Preparation, and Implementation

All research begins with a good idea. The idea is typically based on the nurse researcher's identification of a problem that is amenable to study using a philosophical and theoretical orientation. The philosophical aspect sets the stage for selecting one's approach to investigating the problem or developing the idea. Good clinical ideas often come from

personal experiences, based on the researcher's foundation of knowledge that aids in drawing inferences from real clinical situations. These unfold by way of iterative consideration of problem and process—leading the investigator to evolve an approach to the problem, and subsequently a theoretical paradigm to address the problem. Because the theoretical paradigm emerges from these iterative considerations, and because the theoretical perspective will subsequently drive the organization of the research study, it is important to distinguish between these two distinct approaches separately. Each theoretical paradigm directs how the problem for study will unfold. The researcher uses a selected theoretical approach and operationalizes each step of the research process that will become the research design and methodology, either qualitative, quantitative, or some combination of both. Each approach can be facilitated at different points along the proposal development process with select computer applications. These will be described as they relate to the theoretical approach.

Quantitative and Qualitative Approaches

The important distinction to be made between the quantitative and qualitative approaches is that for a quantitative study to be successful, the researcher is obliged to develop fully each aspect of the research proposal *before* collecting any data, whereas, for a qualitative study to be successful, the researcher is obliged to allow the data collected to determine the subsequent steps as it unfolds in the process and/or the analysis. Quantitative research is derived from empiricism and logical positivism philosophical orientations (Weiss, 1995), with multiple steps bound together by precision in quantification. The requirements of a hypothesis-driven or numerically descriptive approach are logical consequences of, or correspond to, a specific theory and its related tenets. The hypothesis can be tested statistically to support or refute the prediction selected a priori or in advance.

The qualitative approaches are a collection of different research traditions (e.g., phenomenology, hermeneutics, and grounded theory) that share a common view of reality, which consists of the meanings ascribed to the data such as a person's lived experiences (Creswell, 2003). With this view, theory is not tested, but rather, perspectives and meaning from the subject's point of view are described and analyzed. For nursing studies, knowledge development is generated from the patient's experiences and responses to health, illness, and treatments. The requirements of the qualitative approach are a function of the philosophical frames through which the data unfold and evolve into meaningful interpretations by the researcher.

General Considerations in Proposal Preparation

Several computer applications have become indispensable in the development of the research proposal and generally in planning for the activities that will take place when implementing the study. The word-processor applications for microcomputers have become the necessary clerical tool to manage the text from numerous sources and assemble them in a cogent and organized package. Microsoft Word (Microsoft Corporation, 2000) and WordPerfect (Corel Corporation, 2000) provide capabilities and a platform into which other off-the-shelf applications can be integrated. Tables, charts, and figures can be inserted, edited, and moved as the proposal takes shape. Personal computer applications that allow inserting simple graphic designs give the researcher a powerful means of expressing concepts through art. Line art and scanned images with programs such as Illustrator or Photoshop 7 can be integrated into the document for clear visual effects. References and call outs can be managed with additional software add-ons, including bibliographic managers such as Reference Manager (Institute Information Systems, 1997), Procite (Niles Software, 2003), and Endnote (Niles Software, 2004). Searching online is one function of these applications, and then working between the reference database and the text of the proposal document is efficient and easy, calling out citations when needed with "cite as you write" capability.

Research applications and "call for proposals" are often downloadable from the Internet into a fillable Adobe Acrobat form where individual fields are editable and the documents can be saved, printed, or submitted from the Web. The Web also allows the researcher to explore numerous opportunities for designing a proposal tailored to potential foundations for consideration of funding. Call for proposals, contests, and competitive grants plays a role in developing the idea in one direction or another, and the links from Web sites give the researcher a depth of understanding of what is expected in the proposal.

Research Study Implementation

A funded research study becomes a logistical challenge for most researchers in managing the steps of the process, maintaining the integrity of the procedures, managing the information and paper flow, and keeping confidential and secure the data collection and storage, which culminates in analyzing and reporting the results. Several software applications exist and have evolved to assist the researcher in the overall process of study implementation. These applications are operations oriented, used in nonresearch programs and projects as well, but can assist the researcher in management of time, personnel, money, products, and ultimately dissemination.

General database applications including Microsoft Access, FileMaker Pro 7 (FileMaker, Inc., 2004), and more sophisticated, integrated, and proprietary database management applications such as Oracle and Lotus provide the researcher with mechanisms to operationalize the personnel, subjects, forms, interviews, dates, times, and/or tracking systems over the course of the project. Most of these applications require specially designed screens that are unique to the project if the research warrants complicated connections such as reminders, but simple mailing lists and zip codes of subjects' addresses and contact information in a generic form can also be extremely useful for the researcher.

Several other generic computer programs can aid the researcher in daily operations and project management. Spreadsheet applications are invaluable for budgeting and budget planning, from proposal development through project completion. One multipurpose off-the-shelf application from Microsoft is Excel (2004a). Universally understood and easy to use, Excel allows the researcher to manage costs and calculate expenses over the course of the project period, producing a self-documenting plan by categories to track actual spending and money left. Templates can be developed for repetitive tasks. Scheduling and project planning software is also available from Microsoft (Project Manager) that allows the project director to organize the work efficiently and track schedules and deadlines over the lifetime of the project.

In summary, the general considerations of developing and conducting a research study are based on philosophical approaches and will dictate which methodology the researcher will use to develop the study. Although this will subsequently influence the research and computer applications to be used in carrying out the project, the steps of proposal preparation are less specific, and the computer applications are useful in both quantitative and qualitative studies. After identifying the research problem, however, the researcher must proceed through the steps of the research, where computers play an important role that is unique to each of the methodologies.

◼ The Quantitative Approach

Data Capture and Data Collection

Data capture and data collection are processes that are viewed differently from the quantitative and qualitative perspectives. Nurses may already be familiar with data collection that is focused on the management of patient care.

Patient monitoring, patient care documentation, and interview data are collected by nurses, although not always for research purposes. Data collection can take a number of forms depending on the type of research and variables of interest. Computers are used in data collection for paper-and-pencil surveys and questionnaires as well as to capture physiologic and clinical nursing information in quantitative or descriptive patient care research. There are also unique automated data capturing applications that have been developed recently that facilitate large group data capture in single contacts or allow paper versions of questionnaires to be scanned directly into a database ready for analysis.

Questionnaires/Paper and Pencil   Surveys and questionnaires, traditionally administered in paper-and-pencil forms, can be programmed into a computer application either in a microcomputer or on a Web site accessed through the Internet. Computers are being used for direct data entry in studies where subjects enter their own responses via a computer and simultaneous coding of response to questions and time "on-line" can be captured (Brennan and Ripich, 1994). The use of notebook microcomputers has gained popularity in recent years for allowing the user to enter the data directly into the computer program at the time of the interview with a subject, with innovations emerging in touch screens, light pens, and even wireless data entry with PDAs (Bakken et al., 2003). Responses to questions can be entered by the respondent or a surrogate directly into the computer or Web site through Internet access. General Web-design software such as Microsoft Frontpage and customized Java script programming allows using a database interface for the extraction of Web-based data to transform the multiple steps that would otherwise be part of data capture, data extraction, and data cleaning into an automated and accurate single-step process. The data from the Internet can then be downloaded for analysis.

Several special applications have been used in nursing research that can facilitate large group data capture. Group use applications in specially designed facilities have been developed to engage an audience in simultaneous activity, recording their impressions through electronic keypads located proximal to the users, and capturing that information for display or later analysis. One type of application, Team Expert Choice (Expert Choice, 2004) uses the analytic hierarchy process, a mathematical technique, with handheld keypad technology to elicit group responses and automatically score, analyze, prioritize, and present information back to the group graphically. This kind of groupware can supplement data collection from a focus group to add a quantitative component to the subjective question as it elicits and captures opinion via pairwise comparisons (Feeg, 1999).

Software packages also exist that can be integrated with the researcher's scanner to optically scan a specially designed questionnaire and produce the subjects' responses in a database ready for analysis. OmniPage (OmniPage, 2004) is a top rated OCR (optical character recognition) program that converts a scanned page into plain text. Programs such as Remark Office or Remark Classic (Principia, 2004) can facilitate scanning large numbers of questionnaires speed and accuracy. These products, enhanced even more with the Web-based products such as Remark Web Survey (Principia, 2004), increase the accuracy of data entry with very low risk of errors, thereby improving the efficiency of the data capture, collection, and entry processes.

Physiologic Data   The collection of patient physiologic parameters has long been used in physiologic research. Some of these parameters can be measured directly from patient devices such as cardiac monitoring of heart rhythm, rate, and fluid or electrolytes. Now that many measurements taken from various types of imaging (e.g., neurologic, cardiovascular, and cellular) have become digitized, they can also be entered directly from the patient into a computer program for analysis. Each of these applications is unique to the measures, such as systems to capture cardiac functioning and/or pulmonary capacity, devices that relay contractions, or monitors that pick up electronic signals. Numerous measurements of intensity, amplitude, patterns, and shapes can be characterized by computer programs and used in research. Each of these measurement systems have evolved with the unfolding of research specific to their questions, and within each community of scholars, issues about the functionality, accuracy, and reliability of electronic data extracted from these physiologic devices are debated.

Along with the proliferation of clinical diagnostic measurement systems, there has been a rapid expansion of unique computer applications that have emerged for the data analysis aspects of these clinical systems, physiologic and record sources. Millions of gigabytes of data are stored in machines that can be tapped for multiple studies on the existing data. Data mining is a powerful tool in the knowledge discovery process that can now be done with a number of commercial and open-source software packages (Berger and Berger, 2004). Data mining is a mechanism of exploration and analysis of large quantities of data in order to discover meaningful patterns and rules, applied to large physiologic data sets as well as clinical sources of data. The nature of the data and the research question determine the tool selection, i.e., data-mining algorithm or technique. Tools and consultants exist to help researchers unfamiliar with data-mining algorithms to use data mining for analysis, prediction, and reporting purposes (see MSDN Library, 2000). Many of the first commercial applications of data mining were in customer profiling and marketing analyses. Today, many special technologies can be applied, for example, to predict physiologic phenomena such as genetic patterns in tumors that might respond to therapy based on classification of primary tumor gene expression or tissue rejection post-heart transplantation from blood samples and biopsies (Berger and Berger, 2004).

Unique Nursing Care Data in Research   Scientists and technologists from a variety of disciplines are working hard to identify the domain of data and information that is transferable across situations, sites, or circumstances that can be captured electronically for a wide array of analyses to learn how the health system impacts the patients it serves. The American Nurses Association (ANA) has supported the need to standardize nursing care terms for computer-based patient care systems. The clinical and economic importance of structured recording to represent nursing care was recognized by the acceptance of the nursing minimum data set (Werley, Lang, and Westlake, 1986). The ANA has accepted seven systems of terminology for the description of nursing practice: the North American Nursing Diagnosis Association (NANDA) taxonomy of nursing diagnosis, Georgetown Home Health Care Classification (McCormick et al., 1994; Saba, 1997; Zielstorff et al., 1995), Nursing Interventions Classification (Bulechek and McCloskey, 1997), Nursing Outcomes Classification (Daly et al., 1997), patient care data set (Ozbolt, 1999), Omaha Home Health Care (Martin and Norris, 1996), and the International Classification of Nursing Practice (Saba, 1997; Zielstorff et al., 1995). Other terminology that may encompass issues of major interest to nursing is the minimum data set (MDS and MDS+) which is part of the residence assessment inventory (RAI) used for the documentation of resident problems in nursing homes (Hansebo et al., 1999a, Zulkowski, 1999).

Although none of the above has emerged as a standard, a structured coding system is needed for recording patient care problems that are amenable to nursing actions, the actual nursing actions implemented in the care of patients, and the evaluation of the effectiveness of these actions. Outcomes research and quality indicators have become the data end-points that justify healthcare

services. The use of structured terms across healthcare settings would provide for comparability of patient care using patient records. There is new emphasis in the federal government to produce electronic health records (EHRs) and cross-platform compatibility through the development of collaborative efforts across organizations in the government and the information technology industry (Thompson and Brailer, 2004).

Data Coding

In quantitative studies, the data for the variables of interest are collected in a numerical form. These numerical values are entered into designated fields in the process of coding. Coding may be inherent in software programs for the physiologic data and many of the electronic surveys. The coding may be generated (by a computer program) from measurements directly obtained through imaging or physiologic monitoring or entered into a computer by a patient or researcher from a printout or a questionnaire/survey into a database program. Most statistical programs contain data editors that permit the entry of data by a researcher as part of the statistical application. In such a situation, fields are designated and numerical values can also be entered into the appropriate fields without the use of an extra program. For mechanisms that translate and transfer source data to prepare it for analysis, generic programs such as Excel (Microsoft, 2004a) again serves multiple needs. In addition to allowing simple transfers of data from source to a statistical analysis package, Excel has its own powerful, but simple, analysis capabilities and exceptionally easy to use graphic translators that can turn statistics into visual graphs and charts.

Coding data is a precise operation that needs careful consideration and presents the researcher with challenges that warrant technical or cognitive applications. Coding data is a combination of cognitive decisions and mechanical clerical recording of responses in a numerical form with numerous places for error to occur. There are several ways of reviewing and "cleaning" the data prior to analyses. Some computer programs allow for the same data to be entered twice (preferably by different people to check for errors) with the premise that if the double entry does not match, one entry is wrong. One also must check for missing data and take them into consideration in the coding and analyses. Reviewing data for values outside of those allowable is another way of examining the data for errors. It can best be done by examining the multiple printouts produced by the statistical software packages and by perusing for outliers or artifacts carefully. While coding data is a process activity in quantitative research to get results, it is a substantive activity for the qualitative researcher as it becomes the essence of the interpretation of data collected.

Data Analysis

Data analysis in a quantitative study combines a variety of techniques that apply statistical procedures with the researcher's cognitive organization of research questions, results, and visual or textual information, translated into tables, charts, and graphs to make the data meaningful. It translates the numeric and conceptual elements of the inquiry into meaningful representations of information. In general, the statistical analyses are ordered by the conceptual arrangement of hypotheses, variables, measurements, and relationships, and ultimately answers the research questions. There are myriad ways to consider data analysis. The presentation below is organized around the broad types of research of interest in nursing and general research goals or questions. The researcher may use different types of analyses depending on the goal of research. These goals may require different statistical examinations: descriptive/exploratory analyses, hypothesis testing, estimation of confidence intervals, model building through multivariate analysis, and structural equation model building. Various types of nursing research may contain a number of these goals. For example, to test an intervention using an experimental or quasi-experimental design, one may first perform descriptive/exploratory analyses followed by tests of the hypotheses. Quality improvement, patient outcome, and survival analysis studies may likewise contain a number of different types of analyses depending on the specific research questions.

In general, the statistical analysis steps of the research process rely heavily on the functions specific to a variety of statistical software applications. Two of the most popular programs in use today are the Statistical Package for Social Sciences (SPSS Version 13; SPSS Inc., 1999) and Statistical Analysis Services (SAS Version 9; SAS Institute, 1999), however a variety of other packages and programs exist such as STATA (Statistical Software for Professionals, 2004) and are often supported by libraries or unique to particular scientific disciplines. Which package one selects depends on the user's personal preference, particular strengths, and limits of the applications including number of variables, options for analyses, and ease of use. These packages have given the user the power to manipulate large data sets with relative ease and test out statistical combinations that have exponentially improved the analyses possible in a fraction of time that it once took.

The different types of analyses required by goals of the research will be addressed further. This description will be followed by examples of types of nursing research that incorporate some of these types of analyses.

Descriptive and Exploratory Analysis The researcher may first explore the data means, modes, distribution pattern, and standard deviations, and examine graphic representations such as scatter plots or bar graphs. Tests of association or significant differences may be explored through chi-squares, correlations, and various univariate, bivariate, and trivariate analyses, and an examination of quartiles. During this analysis process, the researcher may recode or transform data by mathematically multiplying or dividing scores by certain log or factor values. New variables can also be created by combining several existing variables. These transformations or "reexpressions" allow the researcher to analyze the data in appropriate and interpretable scales (Behrens and Smith, 1996). The researcher can then easily identify patterns with respect to variables as well as groups of study subjects of interest. Both commercial statistical packages provide the ability to calculate these tests and graphically display the results in a variety of ways.

SPSS 13 (SPSS Inc., 1999) provides the user with a broad range of capabilities for the entire analytical process. SPSS is a modular, tightly integrated, and full-featured software comprised of SPSS base and a range of add-on modules. With SPSS, the researcher can generate decision-making information quickly using a variety of powerful statistics, understand and effectively present the results with high-quality tabular and graphical output, and share the results with others using various reporting methods, including secure Web publishing. SAS 9 (SAS, 1999) provides the researcher with tools that can help code data in a reliable framework, extract data for quality assurance, exploration or analysis, perform descriptive and inferential data analyses, maintain databases to track, and report on administrative activities like data collection, subject enrollment or grant payments, and deliver content for reports in the appropriate format. SAS allows for creating unique programming within the variable manipulations. Stata 8 (Statistical Software for Professionals, 2004) is also a fully integrated statistical package with full database management capabilities and a range of sophisticated statistical tests particularly useful for epidemiologists and physical scientists. All of these statistical packages have evolved to provide an integrated collection of tools that assist in aspects of the research study management—from planning to dissemination—in addition to the reputable statistical

SAS 9.1.3[a]	SPSS (version 13.0)[b]
Created for business intelligence needs	Designed for academic use
Create and design forms that can be used for data entry via the Web, the Internet, or paper	Create a variety of charts including bar graphs, three-dimensional bar graphs, pie charts, dot graphs, paneled charts, and population pyramids
Store research data	Ability to export tables and charts directly into Microsoft PowerPoint
Create analysis files in repeatable fashion	
Perform descriptive and inferential data analysis	Allows text data strings of more than 256 bytes
Maintain databases to track and report on data collection and subject enrollment	Ability to perform calculations with data and time
Manage data with predictive and descriptive modeling, forecasting, simulation, and optimization	Ability to share data between SPSS and SAS
	Provides a variety of add-on modules for customization
Software is available on Microsoft Windows. Linux and Apple MacIntosh platforms	
Comprehensive installation instructions available on the SAS Website	

[a]SAS and research. SAS Homepage. Retrieved September 30, 2004, from *http://www.sas.com/govedu/education/research.html*
[b]What's new in SPSS 13 for Windows. SPSS Homepage, Retrieved September 30, 2003, from *http://www.spss.com*

Figure 35.1
Comparison of SPSS and SAS general features and functions.

analyses and data manipulation capabilities that they have provided for many years (see Fig. 35.1).

As part of exploratory analysis, simple and multiple regression analyses can be used to examine the relationships between selected variables and a dependent measure of interest. Certain models can be developed to determine which collection of variables provides the best prediction of the dependent measure. Printouts of correlation matrices and regression analysis tables provide the researcher with condensed, readable statistical information about the relationships in question. An example of a template taken from a commonly used program can be seen in Fig. 35.2.

Hypothesis Testing or Confirmatory Analyses
Hypothesis testing or confirmatory analyses are based on an interest in relationships and describing what would occur if a hypothesis were true. The analysis of data allows us to compare the actual outcomes with the hypothesized outcomes. Inherent in hypothesis testing is the probability (*P* value) of an event occurring given a certain relationship. These are conditional relationships based on the variables selected for study, and the typical mathematical tables and software for determining *P* values are accurate only insofar as the assumptions of the test are met (Behrens and Smith, 1996). Certain statistical concepts such as statistical power, type II error, selecting alpha values to balance type II errors, and sampling distribution are decisions that the researcher must make regardless of the type of computer software. These concepts are covered in greater detail in research methodology courses and are outside the scope of the present discussion.

Model Building
An application used for confirmatory hypothesis testing approach to multivariate analysis is structural equation modeling (SEM) (Byrne, 1984). Byrne describes this procedure as consisting of two aspects: (1) the causal processes under study are represented by a series of structural (i.e., regression) equations and (2) these structural relations can be modeled pictorially to enable a clearer conceptualization of the theory under study. The model can be tested statistically in a simultaneous analysis of the entire system of variables to determine the extent to which it is consistent with the data. If goodness of fit is adequate, the model argues for the plausibility of postulated relationships among variables (Byrne, 1984). Most researchers may wish to consult a statistician to discuss the underlying assumptions of the data and plans for testing the model.

```
CONGESTIVE HEART FAILURE
MODEL  NCare = Rural, Urban, Hospsiz1, Hospsiz2, Hospsiz3, Char1, Char2, Char3, Char4
```

Model: MODEL1
Dependent Variable: NCare

Analysis of Variance

Parameter Estimates

Variable	DF	Parameter Estimate	Standard Error	T for Ho: Parameter= 0	Prob > |T|	Variable Label
INTERCEP	1	1.99	0.11	18.29	0.0001	Intercept
RURAL	1	-0.31	0.17	-1.77	0.08	RURAL
URBAN	1	-0.16	0.11	-1.50	0.14	URBAN
HOSPSIZ1	1	0.69	0.17	4.17	0.00	LESS THAN OR EQUAL TO 100 BEDS
HOSPSIZ2	1	0.25	0.13	1.89	0.06	101-200 HOSPITAL BEDS
HOSPSIZ3	1	0.22	0.11	1.92	0.06	201-400 HOSPITAL BEDS
CHAR1	1	0.21	0.13	1.60	0.11	EQUIPMENT
CHAR2	1	0.44	0.13	3.30	0.00	NURSE/PATIENT RATIO
CHAR3	1	0.52	0.13	3.84	0.00	AUTONOMY IN DECISION MAKING
CHAR4	1	0.12	0.13	0.92	0.36	LICENSED

Figure 35.2
Example of regression analysis.

Different types of modeling programs, such as LISREL (Joreskog and Sorbom, 1978) or EQS (Byrne, 1984), are commercially available. The researcher will identify latent (unobservable) variables of interest (e.g., emotions) and link them to those that are observable (direct measurement) and plan with the statistician to specify and examine the impact of one latent construct on another in the modeling of causal direction.

SPSS 13 (SPSS Inc., 1999) offers Amos, a powerful SEM and path analysis add-on to create more realistic models than if using standard multivariate methods or regression alone. Amos is a program for visual SEM and path analysis. User-friendly features such as drawing tools, configurable toolbars, and drag-and-drop capabilities, help the researcher build structural equation models. After fitting the model, the Amos path diagram shows the strength of the relationship between variables. Amos builds models that realistically reflect complex relationships because any variable, whether observed (such as survey data) or latent (such as satisfaction or loyalty) can be used to predict any other variable.

Meta-analysis   Meta-analysis is a technique that allows researchers to combine data across studies to achieve more

focused estimates of population parameters and examine effects of a phenomenon or intervention across multiple studies. It uses the effect size as a common metric of study effectiveness and deals with the statistical problems inherent in using individual significance tests in a number of different studies. It weights study outcomes in proportion to their sample size and focuses on the size of the outcomes rather than on whether or not they are significant.

Although the computations can be done with the aid of a reliable commercial statistical package such as Meta-Analysis (Comprehensive Meta-Analysis, 2004), the researcher needs to consider the following specific issues in performing the meta-analysis (Behrens and Smith, 1996): (1) justify which studies are comparable and which are not, (2) rely on knowledge of the substantive area to identify relevant study characteristics, (3) evaluate and account for differences in study quality, and (4) assess the generalizability of the results from fields with little empirical data. Each of these issues must be addressed with a critical review prior to performing the meta-analysis.

Meta-analysis offers a way to examine results of a number of quantitative research that meet meta-analysis researchers' criteria. Meta-analysis overcomes problems encountered in studies using different sample sizes and instruments. The software application Meta-Analysis (Biostat, 2000) provides the user with a variety of tools to examine these studies. It can create a database of studies, import the abstracts or the full text of the original papers, or enter the researcher's own notes (see Fig. 35.3). The meta-analysis is displayed using a schematic that may be modified extensively as the user can specify which variables to display and in what sequence. The studies can be sorted by any variable including effect size, the year of publication, the weight assigned to the study, the sample size, or any user-defined variables to facilitate the critical review done by the researcher (see Fig. 35.4).

Graphical Data Analysis There are occasions when data need to be displayed graphically as part of the analysis and interpretation of the information or for more fundamental communication of the results of computations and analyses. Most statistical packages including SPSS, SAS, and STATA, and even spreadsheets such as Excel, provide the user with tools for simple to complex graphical translations of numeric information thus allowing the researcher to display, store, and communicate aggregated data in meaningful ways. Special tools for spatial representations exist, such as mapping and geographic displays, so that the researcher can visualize and interpret

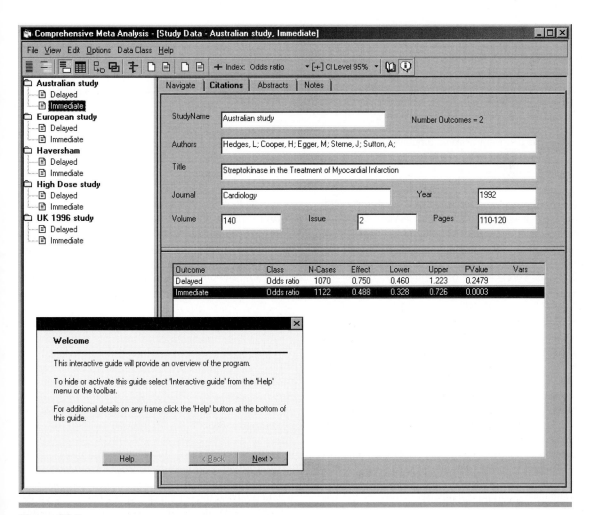

Figure 35.3
Meta-analysis study database interface.

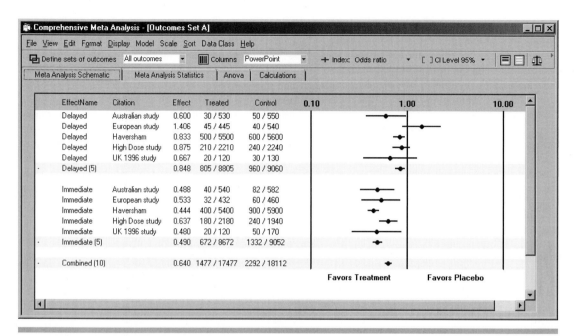

Figure 35.4
Meta-analysis program graphic display.

patterns inherent in the data. Geographic information system (GIS) technology is evolving beyond the traditional GIS community and becoming an integral part of the information infrastructure of visualization tools for researchers. For example, GIS can assist an epidemiologist map data collected on disease outbreaks or a health services researcher can communicate graphically areas of nursing shortages. GIS technology illustrates relationships, connections, and patterns that are not necessarily obvious in any one data set, enabling the researcher to see overall relevant factors. The Geographic Resources Analysis Support System (GRASS) is a popular public-domain GIS software product (see *http://www.cecer. army.mil/grass/GRASS.main.html*). ArcGIS 9 (ESRI, 2004) system is a GIS for management, analysis, and display of geographic knowledge, which is represented using a series of information sets. The information sets include maps and globes with three-dimensional capabilities to describe networks, topologies, terrains, surveys, and attributes (see Fig. 35.5).

In summary, the major emphasis of this section has provided a brief discussion about the range of traditions, statistical considerations, and computer applications that aid the researcher in quantitative data analysis. As

computers have continued to integrate data management functions with traditional statistical computational power, the researchers have been able to develop more extensive and sophisticated projects with data collected. Gone are the days of the calculator or punch cards as the computing power now sits on the researchers' desktops or laptops, and with speed and functionality at their fingertips.

The Qualitative Approach

Data Capture and Data Collection

The qualitative approach focuses on activities in the steps of the research process that differ greatly from the quantitative methods in fundamental sources of data, collection techniques, coding, analysis, and interpretation. Thus, the computer becomes a different kind of tool for the researcher in most aspects of the research beginning with the capture and recording of narrative or textual data.

In terms of qualitative research requiring narrative content analysis, the computer can be used to record the observations, narrative statements of subjects, and memos of the researcher in initial word-processing applications for future coding. Software applications that aid

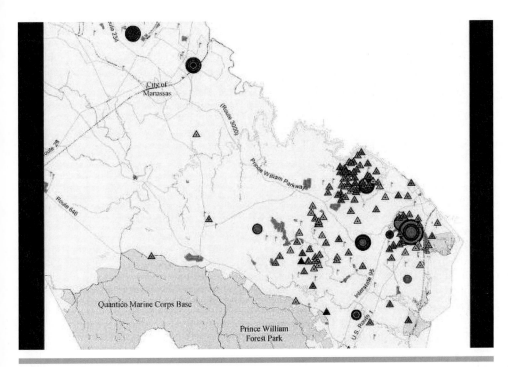

Figure 35.5
ArcGIS 9 mapping system of epidemiologic data.
(Spread of measles in Prince William County, Prince William County Fire and Rescue, Virginia. By
Dr. Jared Florence and David J. Simms. Retrieved on October 2, 2004, from
http://www.esri.com/mapmuseum/mapbook_gallery/volume16/health4.html.)

researchers in transcription tasks include text scanners, such as OmniPage (Scansoft, 2004b). Other devices include vocal recorders or speech recognition software such as Dragon Naturally Speaking 7 (Scansoft, 2004a), where the researcher can input the information into text documents by speaking into a microphone without typing. Some questions can elicit responses from subjects that can be captured directly. These narrative statements, like the quantitative surveys, can be either programmed for use in microcomputers or on the Internet's World Wide Web (WWW) so that subjects' responses can be entered directly into the computer.

Qualitative Data Collection   In most interviews, simple electronic audiotaping is often used during interviews, whereby the interviews are entered into a word-processing program by clerical assistants in preparation for analysis. The narrative statements entered into a word processor are stored for subsequent coding and sorting according to

one's theoretical framework. Through analysis, categories from the data emerge as interpreted by the researcher. It is important to point out that for both quantitative and qualitative data, the computer application program is only a mechanical, clerical tool to aid the researcher in manipulating the data. Using the Internet for indirect and direct data collection in qualitative studies can also provide a vehicle for data analysis that yields a quantitative component as well as the qualitative analysis. Computers are not only able to record the subject's responses to the questions but also routinely record the number of minutes the subject was "online" and the number of times they "logged in."

Data Coding

Historically, qualitative researchers have relied on narrative notes that may often be first audio recorded then transcribed by a typist. Coding qualitative text data was a time-consuming task, often involving thousands of pages of typewritten notes and the use of scissors and tape for the development of coding and categories. With the advent of computer packages, the mechanical aspects of the coding and sorting have been reduced. The researcher must decide on which text may be of interest and use a word-processing program to search for words, phrases, or other markers within a text file using any number of word-processing software packages.

Some specific software packages developed for qualitative research coding and analysis interface directly with the most popular word-processing software packages. The application program Ethnograph (Seidel and Clark, 1984; Seidel, Friese, and Lenard, 1994) was one of the first packages developed specifically for the purpose of managing some of the mechanical tasks of qualitative data analysis. Another qualitative package commonly used is NUD.IST (Non-numerical Unstructured Data Indexing Searching and Theorizing) (Gahan and Hannibal, 1998; Richards and Richards, 1993). This program has been described by Richards and Richards (1993) as assisting the researcher to establish an index of data codes and seek relationships among the coding categories. The ease with which researchers can code and recode large amounts of data with the aid of computerized programs encourages the researcher to experiment with different ways of thinking

about data and recategorizing them. Retrieval of categories or elements of data is facilitated by computer storage. Newer technologies have evolved from Ethnograph and NUD.IST with improved user interfaces, including NVivo and N6 (QSR, 2004).

In Ethnograph, the narrative text is first imported and each line is numbered. The text is then "coded" by indicating segments that pertain to a particular code. Once the codes are entered, the Ethnograph program can be instructed to search the text (individually or across multiple cases) for specific coded segments. These segments are then generated as output and can be incorporated into a word-processing program or printed directly from Ethnograph for review. Figure 35.6 presents the result of a search for the codes "history" (history of the injury) and "signs" (signs and symptoms associated with injury) in one individual case. The results show that the code history consists of a 15-line segment, while the code signs consists of an 8-line segment embedded within the history segment.

Qualitative Data Analysis

Qualitative research, like quantitative research, is not a single entity, but a set of related yet individual traditions,

---

```
SEARCH CODE: HISTORY, SIGNS

#-HISTORY
    :    As you reconstruct the history, when      24 -#ᵃ
    :    he fell -- this guy fell off the back      25  #
    :    of his truck.  The first thing that        26  #
$-SIGNS
    :    happened he had -- he had weakness or       27  # -$ᵇ
    :    paralysis and numbness in both his          28  # |
    :    legs.  Couldn't move for almost an          29  # |
    :    hour.  And it began to come back.  And      30  # |
    :    ever since that time he's had these --      31  # |
    :    these weird sensations and pain --          32  # |
    :    pain has gone from his legs.  Bladder       33  # |
    :    and bowel disturbance.  Had a GU work-      34  # -$
    :    up.  They can't document that he has a      35  #
    :    (------------).  I think he does.           36  #
    :    Impotence.  And I think he contused         37  #
    :    the spinal cord is what he did.             38 -#
a = # indicates the primary code in this segment "history".
b = $ indicates the secondary code in this segment "signs"; this code is also
      a sub-segment of the "history" segment.
```

Figure 35.6
Example of coding using Ethnograph.

aims, and methods. Some individual traditions within qualitative research are ethnography, grounded theory, phenomenology, and hermeneutics. The distinguishing feature of qualitative research is that the goal is to understand the qualities or essence of phenomena and/or focus on the meaning of these events to the participants or respondents in the study. The forms of data are usually the words of the respondents or informants rather than numbers. Computerization is especially helpful to the researcher in handling large amounts of data.

Computer Application Programs   A number of general-purpose or specific software packages can be used in qualitative analysis: one package can be used is a free text retrieval program such as that available in a word-processing program; another is any number of standard database management or indexing programs; third is a program specifically developed for the purpose of qualitative analysis. Four of the commonly used special-purpose programs for qualitative analysis are Ethnograph (Seidel and Clark, 1984); NUD.IST (Richards and Richards, 1993); NVivo, an evolution of NUD.IST (QSR, 2004); and Atlas.ti (Atlasti.com, 2004), a comprehensive application that supports text, graphics, video, and audio data. In addition, logic-based systems that use "if-then" rules for representation of relationships and conceptual network systems are also available (Huberman and Miles, 1999).

General-Purpose Software   Word-processing programs in current use offer a number of features useful to the qualitative researcher. The ability to search for certain key words allows the researcher to tag the categories of interest. In addition, such features as cut and paste; linking texts; insertion of pictures, tables, and charts; and the inclusion of video and audio data enhance the application. Add-on applications specific to integrating multiple elements help the researcher organize a range of data and materials for analysis. A comprehensive program is ATLAS.ti (Version 5.0; Atlasti.com, 2004), a powerful workbench for the qualitative analysis of large bodies of textual, graphical, audio, and video data. It offers a variety of tools for accomplishing the tasks associated with any systematic approach to "soft" data, such as material that cannot be analyzed by formal and statistical approaches in meaningful ways (Atlasti.com, 2004).

Data management programs (e.g., Excel) can be used to categorize data, link categories, and address a number of queries within categories, domains, or themes of interest. For example, the researcher can list all early adolescents who smoked more than one pack (of cigarettes) per day who gave birth to preterm babies. These programs

work better for discrete rather than unstructured texts (Chang, 2001).

Special-Purpose Software   Several software products have evolved and improved for the specific purpose of analyzing qualitative data. Ethnograph is one such program, which is used after the data have been entered using a word-processing program and converted to an ASCII file. Each file can be designated by its context and identifying features with markers provided by the computer program. The researcher can have the program produce a file that numbers each line of the narrative data. From this line file, the researcher can begin to assign each line or paragraph a category. The researcher keeps track of the category definitions and is alert to dimensions that emerge. Recoding can be done to provide for inductive thinking and iterative comparisons. Through the use of a "search command," the computer program can be made to search for data segments by categories throughout the typed document.

Ethnograph provides a column format, permitting numbered lines in the first column and categorical notations in the second column. Using a command entered by a researcher, it can selectively or globally delete or replace coding categories and produce an output file containing sorted, cross-referenced coded segments from the original text data sets entered via a word-processing program. The split screen allows the researcher to view more than one file at a time, so is useful in constant comparison and contrasting of data. Researcher memos and theoretical notes written by the researcher during analysis can also be stored and retrieved with Ethnograph.

Another application for qualitative analysis is NUD.IST (Richards and Richards, 1993). With this program, the researcher establishes an index of data codes and seeks relationships among the coding categories. NUD.IST uses a hierarchical tree structure to provide a graphic representation of the relationships between and among codes/categories. The ability of the NUD.IST program to search for co-occurring codes and identifying relationships among codes helps the researcher to gain new insight from the data. Computer enhancements that build connections between categories of data may suggest relationships between concepts, but it is up to the researcher to establish the meaning and significance of the suggested relationships through intensive analysis (Taft, 1993).

NVivo and N6 from QSR (QSR, 2004) provide a new generation of software tools beyond Ethnograph and NUD.IST with multiple advantages for researchers. Because qualitative research takes many forms, these two applications can be selected based on the user's specific methodological goals, the nature and scale of the study, and the computer equipment. While NVivo supports fluid, rich data, detailed text analysis, and theory building, N6 supports small or large projects with automatic merge and multisite use capabilities. NVivo can manage documents or nodes in visual displays that show structure and properties of the document (see Fig. 35.7). N6 management tools can handle shifting nodes, rearranging trees, and changing addresses and titles, with fully integrated document and node operations.

Logic-Based Systems   These applications use rules for representation of hypotheses. Although some of the retrieval patterns are boolean, such as looking for one code or another in combinations in a text, they may also search

for positive and negative cases of a code (Huberman and Miles, 1999). The program may also be used to print out matrices if the researcher determines a set of codes for columns (e.g., ages), and another set for rows (e.g., categories of statements indicating a range of depression). Each cell in the matrix then will contain the text segments indexed by both the column and row codes for the cell (Huberman and Miles, 1999).

Conceptual Network Systems   A system known as concept diagrams, semantic nets, or conceptual networks is one in which information is represented in a graphic manner. The objects in one's conceptual system (e.g., age and experiences) are coded and represented by a box diagram (node). The objects are linked (by arcs) to other objects to

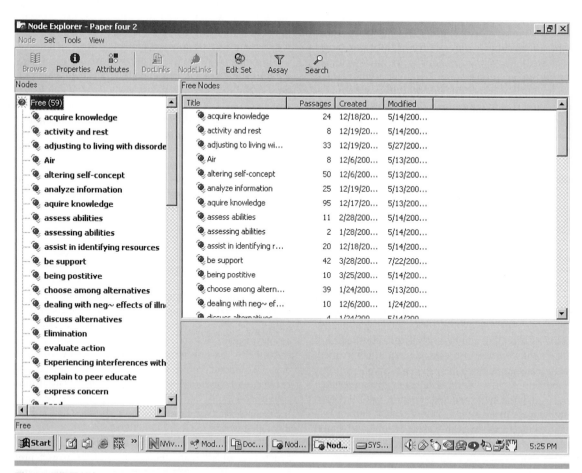

Figure 35.7
Example of NVivo display.

show relationships. Like rule-based systems, semantic nets have been widely used in artificial intelligence work. In order to view the relationships of an object in the system, the researcher examines the node in the graph and follows the arcs to and from it (Huberman and Miles, 1999). Semantic network applications may be useful in model building and providing a pictorial overview. Decision Explorer (Banxia, 2004) offers the user a powerful set of mapping tools to aid in the decision-making process. Ideas can be mapped and the resulting cognitive map can be further analyzed. The software has many practical uses, such as gathering and structuring interview data and as an aid in the strategy formulation process. The software is primarily described as being a recording and facilitation tool for the elicitation of ideas, as well as a tool to structure and communicate qualitative data. It allows the user to gather and analyze qualitative data and thus makes sense of many pieces of qualitative data in order to achieve a coherent picture of a given issue or problem (OR/MS Today, 1999, *http://www.lionhrtpub.com/orms/orms-10-99/swr.html*).

Data Analysis for Qualitative Data
Qualitative data analyses often occur on an ongoing basis with data collection in a reflexive and iterative fashion. There is no clear demarcation of when data collection should end and analysis begin. The process of obtaining observations, interviews, and other data over a period of time results in a vast body of data that may be hundreds or thousands of pages of field notes and researcher memos. Although computer applications can aid considerably in organizing and sorting this massive data, the theoretical and analytical aspects of decision-making about concepts and themes must be made by the researcher (Chang, 2001).

As an example, some of the tasks the computer can facilitate in data analysis using grounded theory (one approach to qualitative research) are as follows. Once a researcher has determined which parts of the interviews and observations can be tagged as categories, certain properties or dimensions can be determined and coded. The researcher may engage in "constant comparison" to compare every incident that has been categorized by the same code and compare its meaning with other incidents similarly categorized. This process should continue until the researcher determines that the categories are internally consistent, fit with the data, and are saturated. Saturation is achieved when the researcher can find no more properties for a category and new data are redundant with the old (Cresswell, 2003).

Strauss and Corbin (1990) suggest that, in the later stages of research, the researcher may engage in axial coding. In this stage, the research elaborates and explains key categories considering the conditions under which the event occurs, the processes that take place, and possible consequences. Glaser (1978) indicates that the researcher may engage in theoretical sampling, which is a deliberate search for episodes in incidents that enlarge the variances of properties and place boundaries around categories.

Uses and Caution   Software programs for qualitative research save time for the researcher in terms of file management, reducing the manual labor of cutting, pasting, sorting, and manual filing. They may also encourage the researcher to examine the data from different perspectives, recoding and reorganizing the data in different frameworks.

One must be mindful that qualitative analysis is a cognitive process, not a mechanical one (Chang, 2001). The essence of qualitative research is the meaning and interpretation of the data within context. Taft believes that there may be cause for concern when researchers assume the reality of the concepts identified and emphasize their frequency rather than their meaning (1993). The ability of software enhancements to generate quasi-frequency distributions and cross-tabulations may tend to further increase the investigator's confidence in believing such findings and relationships when in fact these may be an artifact of the way in which the data are manipulated. While computer programs facilitate coding, organization of data, and preparation of the data for interpretation, they cannot replace the thinking and decision-making that is at the heart of qualitative analysis. As in all research, the burden of analysis and interpretation rests on the researchers (Chang, 2001).

Dissemination of Results

While dissemination of results continues to occur by traditional means such as presentations at professional meetings and publication in journals and monographs, online reporting is becoming increasingly common. Some Web sites frequented by nurses are peer review journals such as *Online Journal of Nursing Informatics* (*http://www.cisnet.com/*) and selected nursing articles on various Web sites such as that of the ANA (*http://www.nursingworld.org*). Nursing forums sponsored by various professional nursing organizations (e.g., *American Journal of Nursing*, Sigma Theta Tau, and National League for Nursing) often allow participants to chat online with presenters or authors of certain articles on designated dates during scheduled times. Nearly all organizations have their own Web sites. Some examples are the Alzheimer's

Disease Education and Referral Center (*http://www. alzheimers.org*), American Heart Association (*http:// www. americanheart.org*), American Medical Informatics Association (*http://www.amia. org*), and RAND Corporation (*http:// www.rand.org*). The Cochran Collection has numerous centers all over the world (e.g., for San Francisco: *sfcc@sirius.com*; Canada: *http://hiru.mcmaster. ca/cochrane/centres/canadian/*; Dutch: *http:// www.amc. uval.nl*; Italian: *http://www.areas.it*; Germany: *httpi://www. cochrane.de*; Providence, RI: *http://www. cochrane.org*). As with all publications, online as well as hardcopies, the information accessed must be evaluated by the users for their appropriateness for the purpose for which it was retrieved.

Reports to some agencies may be submitted online. In fact, there is a trend for all paper submissions to be accomplished online. For many agencies within the federal government, the grant application, submission, and reporting are all performed online. Regardless of the method of submission and medium for publication, the published article may be incorporated into one or several online bibliographic retrieval systems.

This chapter has summarized the processes of quantitative and qualitative research and described select computer applications that can assist the researcher in proposal preparation, data collection, data coding, data analysis, and dissemination for both types of research. The following section presents examples of research in which the nurse researchers used a variety of software applications in several steps of the proposal development, data collection, and analysis.

Examples of Research Studies

Examples of Quantitative Research

In a study by Atherton, Feeg, and El-Adham (2003), a secondary analysis was done on a publicly available data set from the federal government. The researchers hypothesized that race, ethnicity, and insurance coverage would be determinants of pregnant women receiving epidural anesthesia during delivery. They designed the study as an exploratory examination of the Agency for Healthcare Research and Quality (AHRQ) Medical Expenditure Panel Survey (MEPS) HC-046 (1996–2000 Pregnancy Files), a nationally representative survey of the U.S. civilian noninstitutionalized population. This data set includes specific variables of interest collected by interviewers through a series of five rounds of interviews over a 2.5-year period. Using computer-assisted personal interviewing (CAPI) technology, data were collected from

each household as part of the larger project cosponsored by AHRQ and the National Center for Health Statistics. The sampling frame for the MEPS HC is drawn from respondents to the National Health Interview Survey (NHIS), which provides a nationally representative sample of the United States with over-sampling of Hispanics and Blacks (MEPS HC-046, 2003). Based on predictions formed from the literature, the researchers predicted differences in race/ethnicity, and health insurance coverage for use of epidural during normal, vaginal, uncomplicated delivery.

The data were downloaded from the Internet and imported into a spreadsheet data file using Excel. After intensive cleaning and matching of the data with the panels containing full sets of demographic information available from the NHIS data on the subjects, the usable set of MEPS data was coded to control for extraneous variables that might have confounded the findings, including complications associated with childbirth. The clean data set was submitted to a logistic regression analysis to identify determinants of epidural use. With some patch coding between the files and logistic regression within the SAS options on the final data set, the researchers were able to determine that ethnicity and insurance coverage significantly influenced whether or not a woman received an epidural during childbirth.

In another study using several quantitative techniques and software applications, Kodadek and Feeg (2002) presented subjects with two rounds of questions eliciting their values and preferences for treatment of a loved one at end of life. Using vignettes, the researchers randomly assigned subjects to one of three identical situations where they were asked to assume the role of a caregiver of a dying loved one. The scenarios were exact in the severity of the loved one's illness, likelihood of dying, and respiratory-related clinical conditions with the exception of age, relationship, and type of disease. The subjects first recorded their responses to open-ended questions, which were collated and recorded on index cards. The index cards were sorted by three research assistants, identifying groups or categories, and achieving adequate interrater reliability of the categories for the card sort.

The situations were re-presented to the subjects with a quantitative questionnaire that elicited numeric comparisons for each of the categories on "relative importance" and to the final question of "preference of options." These data were entered into the Expert Choice software (Expert Choice, 2004) for each subject by the researcher, and the profile output yielded a score that was used to compare the three groups. Each subject's score was entered into SPSS and analyzed using correlation, ANOVA, and posthoc comparisons to determine if age and relationship made a difference for the subjects' values and preferences related to end-of-life decisions.

Examples of Qualitative Research

A phenomenological approach was used to examine parents' experiences of conflict with healthcare providers (Moore and Beckwitt, 2003). Researchers interviewed 18 parents of children with cancer, audiotaped, and transcribed the interviews verbatim, and obtained participants' verification of the transcripts. Using NVivo, a qualitative analysis software program, the researchers separately coded the transcripts. In NVivo this process involves establishing "nodes" that are similar to categories or codes. The researchers in the study used NVivo to deductively code the conflict experiences of participants according to Rubin, Pruitt, and Kim's (1994) five strategies for dealing with conflict. These strategies included problem solving, yielding, withdrawing, inaction, and contending. After coding the data separately, the researchers compared coding to verify consensus. A new NVivo project was created to represent the researchers' consensus coding. Using this new project, the researchers were able to abstract themes and identify passages associated with each conflict strategy to use in their final report.

A second approach to data analysis in this study was narrative analysis or examination of participants' stories. The researchers employed Ginsburg's (1998) approach to narrative analysis to identify turning points or transformations in parents' narratives of their approaches to conflict, in which they became advocates for their children. For this narrative analysis, the researchers used NVivo to organize the transcripts and search for the occurrences of turning points. The researchers found that NVivo was a valuable tool for the deductive coding (selection of nodes) section of the study. It was not as useful for conducting the narrative analysis portion of the analysis.

In another qualitative study, Moore and Beckwitt (2004) examined the self-care practices of children with cancer and the dependent-care practices of their parents. One researcher interviewed 9 children and 18 parents in this purposive sample. The interviews were audiotaped, transcribed, and confirmed by participants. Using NVivo, one researcher and one graduate student individually reviewed the data using a deductive approach to code practices by self-care requisites or needs, according to Orem's (2001) theory of self-care. These requisites included universal, developmental, and health deviation self-care requisites. After individual reviews, the researchers evaluated the coding until they reached agreement.

NVivo was used in this study to (a) deductively assign nodes to practices and (b) inductively create nodes to identify nursing interventions related to the practices. They determined that both children and parents performed self-care or dependent-care practices, respectively. Findings were that participants performed a smaller number of activities related to the requisites interferences with development and health deviation than with other self-care practices. The researchers concluded that there is a need for more supportive-educative nursing interventions to assist families with these activities. NVivo was found to be an effective tool in organizing codes and identifying the areas where nursing interventions were needed.

■ Summary

This chapter has reviewed two research paradigms and philosophical orientations that specify different underlying approaches to research and the use of computers in various stages of the research process. Examples of some quantitative and qualitative studies that have utilized computers and various commercial application packages have also been provided. Hopefully, the plurality of approaches derived from different philosophical orientations and the computer applications briefly described will be a beginning for further exploration for the reader. With the facilitation of the mechanical and clerical aspects of research by computers, the researcher will be freed to interpret new relationships and gain added insight never before available.

■ References

Atherton, M., Feeg, V., and El-Adham, A. (2003). Racial, ethnic and insurance determinants of epidural use in childbirth: Analysis of a National Sample Survey. *Nursing Economic$* 22(1):6–13.

Bakken, S., Cook, S., Curtis, L., Soupios, M., and Curran, C. (2003). Informatics competencies pre- and post-implementation of a Palm-based student clinical log and informatics for evidence-based practice curriculum. In *Proceedings of the American Medical Informatics Association Symposium* (pp. 42–46).

Behrens, J. T. and Smith, M. L. (1996). Data and data analysis. In D. Berliner and R. Calsee (Eds.), *Handbook of Educational Psychology* (pp. 945–989). New York: MacMillan Library Reference.

Berger, A. M. and Berger, C. R. (2004). Data mining as a tool for research and knowledge development in nursing. *Computers, Informatics, Nursing* 22(3):123–131.

Biostat. (2000). *Comprehensive MetaAnalysis* (*www.meta-analysis.com/html/biostat.html*).

Brennan, P. F. and Ripich, S. (1994). Use of a home-care computer network by persons with AIDS. *International Journal of Technology Assessment in Health Care* 10:258–272.

Bulechek, G. M. and McCloskey, J. (1997). All users of NIC encouraged to submit new interventions, suggest revisions. Iowa Intervention Project Research Team. *Image: The Journal of Nursing Scholarship* 1:10–20.

Byrne, B. M. (1984). *Structural Equation Modeling with EQS and EQS/Windows: Basic Concepts, Applications, and Programming*. Thousand Oaks, CA: Sage.

Chang, B. L. (2001). Computer use in nursing research. In V. Saba and K. McCormick (Eds.), *Essentials of Computers for Nurses: Informatics for the New Millennium*. New York: McGraw-Hill.

Corel Corporation. (2000). *Wordperfect 9 (2000)*. Ottawa, ON.

Cresswell, J. W. (2003). *Research Design: Qualitative, Quantitative, and Mixed Methods Approaches* (2nd ed.). Thousand Oaks, CA: Sage.

Daly, J. M., Maas, M. L., and Johnson, M. (1997). Nursing outcomes classification: An essential element in data sets for nursing and health care effectiveness. *Computers in Nursing* 15:S82–S86.

ESRI. (2004). *ArcGIS® 9*. Redlands, CA (*www.esri.com*).

Expert Choice, Inc. (2004). *Team Expert Choice®*. Arlington, VA (*www.expertchoice.com*).

Feeg, V. D. (1999). Using the analytic hierarchy process as an alternative weighting technique to magnitude estimation scaling. *Nursing Research* 48(6):207–214.

FileMaker, Inc. (2004). *FileMaker Pro® 7*. Santa Clara, CA (*www.filemaker.com*).

Gahan, C. and Hannibal, M. (1998). *Doing qualitative Research using QSR NUD.IST*. Thousand Oaks, CA: SCOLARI Sage Publications Software.

Ginsburg, F. D. (1998). *Contested lives: The abortion debate in an American community* (2nd ed.). Berkeley, CA: University of California Press.

Glaser, B. G. (1978). *Theoretical Sensitivity*. Mill Valley, CA: Sociological Press.

Hansebo, G., Kihlgren, M., Ljunggren, G., and Winbald, B. (1999a). Staff views on the Resident Assessment Instrument, RAI/MDS, in nursing homes, and the use of the Cognitive Performance Scale, CPS, in different levels of care in Stockholm, Sweden. *Journal of Advanced Nursing* 3:642–653.

Huberman, A. M. and Miles, M. B. (1999). Data management and analysis methods. In N. K. Denzin and YSL (Ed.), *Handbook of Qualitative Research* (pp. 428–440). Thousand Oaks, CA: Sage.

Institute Information Systems. (1997). *Reference Manager* (Version 8). Carlsbad, CA: Thomson ISI ResearchSoft. Available at *http://www.refman.com/pr-rm11.asp* (accessed: May, 2005).

Joreskog, K. G. and Sorbom, D. (1978). *LISREL IV's User's Guide*. Chicago, IL: National Educational Resources.

Kodadek, M. and Feeg, V. D. (2002). Using vignettes to explore how parents approach end-of-life decision making for terminally ill infants. *Pediatric Nursing* 28(4):333–343.

Martin, K. S. and Norris, J. (1996). The Omaha system: A model for describing practice. *Holistic Nursing Practice* 11:75–83.

McCormick, K. A., Lang, N., Zielstorff, R., et al. (1994). Toward standard classification schemes for nursing language: Recommendations of the American Nurses Association Steering Committee on databases to support clinical nursing practice. *Journal of the American Medical Informatics Association* 1:421–427.

Microsoft Corporation. (2004a). *Excel®*. Redmond, WA.

Microsoft Corporation. (2004b). *Microsoft Word®*. Redmond, WA.

Microsoft Corporation. (2004c). *Microsoft Frontpage®*. Redmond, WA.

Moore, J. B. and Beckwitt, A. (2003). Parents' reactions to conflict with healthcare providers. *Western Journal of Nursing Research* 25:30–44.

Moore, J. B. and Beckwitt, A. (2004). Children with cancer and their parents: Self-care and dependent-care practices. *Issues in Comprehensive Pediatric Nursing* 27:1–17.

MSDN Library. (2000). *Building and Using Data Mining Models*. Microsoft Corporation. [online]. Available at *http://msdn.microsoft.com/library/default.asp?url=/libr ary/en-us/olapdmad/agdatamining_686r.asp* (accessed May, 2005).

Niles Software Inc. (2003). *ProCite®* (Version 5.0).Berkeley, CA: ISI ResearchSoft.

Niles Software Inc. (2004). *Endnote®* (Version 8.0). Berkeley, CA: ISI ResearchSoft.

Orem, D. E. (2001). *Nursing: Concepts of Practice* (6th ed.). St. Louis, MO: C. V. Mosby.

OR/MS Today. (1999). *Decision Explorer®* Banxia Software Ltd., Kendal, Cumbria, U. K. (*http://www.lionhrtpub.com/orms/orms-10-99/swr.html*).

Ozbolt, J. G. (1999). *Testimony to the NCVHS Hearings on Medical Terminology and Code Development*. School of Nursing and Division of Biomedical Informatics, School of Medicine, Vanderbilt University.

Principia. (2004). *Remark Office®, Remark Classic®, Remark Web Survey®* (*www.principia.com*).

Qualitative Solutions and Research Pty. Ltd. (1999). *NVivo, NUD*IST, NUD*IST Vivo, NUDIST, NUDIST VIVO* software products. Retrieved October 2, 2004, from *http://www.qsrinternational.com*

Richards, L. and Richards, T.J. (1993). *QSR NUD.IST*. Victoria, Australia: Qualitative Solutions and Research Pty. Ltd.

Rubin, J. Z., Pruitt, D. G., and Kim, S. H. (1994). *Social Conflict: Escalation, Stalemate, and Settlement* (2nd Ed.). New York: McGraw-Hill.

Saba, V. K. (1997). Why the home health care classification is a recognized nursing nomenclature. *Computers in Nursing* 15:S69–S76

SAS Institute. (1999). *Statistical Analysis System*. Cary, NC: Scansoft, Inc.

Scansoft, Inc. (2004a). *Dragon Naturally Speaking® 7* (*www. scansoft.com/naturallyspeaking*).

ScanSoft, Inc. (2004b). *OmniPage Pro® 14* (*www.scansoft.com/omnipage*).

Seidel, J. and Clark, J. (1984). The Ethnograph: A computer program for the analysis of qualitative data. *Qualitative Sociology* 7(12):110–125.

Seidel, J., Friese, S., and Lenard, C. (1994). *Ethnograph* (Version 4.0). Amherst, MA: Qualis Research Associates.

SPSS Inc. (1999). *Statistical Package for Social Sciences (SPSS)*. Chicago, IL.

Strauss, A and Corbin, J.M. (1990). *Basics of Qualitative Research: Grounded Theory Procedures and Techniques*. Newbury Park, CA: Sage.

Taft, L. B. (1993). Computer-assisted qualitative research. *Research in Nursing and Health* 16:379–383.

Thompson, T. and Brailer, D. (2004). *The Decade of Health Information Technology: Delivering Consumer-centric and Information Rich Health Care*. Washington DC: Department of Health and Human Services (DHHS).

Weiss, S. J. (1995). Contemporary empiricism. In A. Omery, C. E. Kasper, and G. G. Page (Eds.), *In Search of Nursing Science* (pp. 13–17). Thousand Oaks, CA: Sage.

Werley, H. H., Lang, N. M., and Westlake, S. K. (1986). The nursing minimum data set conference: Executive summary. *Journal of Professional Nursing* 2:217–224.

Zielstorff, R. D., Lang, N. M., Saba, V. K., et al. (1995). Toward a uniform language for nursing in the US: Work of the American Nurses Association Steering Committee on databases to support clinical practice. *Medinfo* 8(pt. 2):1362–1366.

Zulkowski, K. (1999). MDS + Items not contained in the pressure ulcer RAP associated with pressure ulcer, prevalence in newly institutionalized elderly. *Ostomy/Wound Management* 1:24–33.

36

Computerized Information Resources

Diane S. Pravikoff

June Levy

OBJECTIVES

1. Identify steps in choosing appropriate databases.
2. Identify steps in planning a computer search for information.
3. Identify sources of information for practicing nurses.
4. Identify the difference between essential and supportive computerized resources.

KEY WORDS

information retrieval
MEDLINE/PubMed
CINAHL
unified medical language systems
World Wide Web
information resources
health reference databases

Introduction

This chapter presents information about electronic resources that are easily available and accessible and can assist nurses in maintaining and enhancing their professional practices. These resources aid in keeping current with the published literature, in developing a list of sources for practice, research and/or education, and in collaborating with colleagues.

As is evidenced in earlier chapters, nurses use computers for many purposes. In the past, most of the focus has been on computerized patient records, acuity systems, and physician ordering systems. One of the major purposes for which computers can be used, however, is searching for information. Many resources are available by computer, and the information retrieved can be used to accomplish different ends. It is important that the nursing professional determine her or his exact requirements beginning the search. Planning the search will be stressed throughout this chapter.

To maintain professional credibility, nursing professionals must (1) keep current with the published literature,

(2) develop and maintain a list of bibliographic and other sources on specific topics of interest for practice, research, and/or education, and (3) collaborate and network with colleagues regarding specifics of professional practice. Electronic resources are available to meet each of these needs. This chapter addresses each of these requirements for professional credibility and discusses both essential and supportive computerized resources available to meet them. *Essential* computerized resources are defined as those resources that are vital and necessary to the practitioner to accomplish the specific goal. In the case of maintaining currency, for example, these resources include bibliographic retrieval systems such as MEDLINE or the CINAHL database, current awareness, or review services, and may be accessible in various formats: CD-ROM, Internet, or World Wide Web. *Supportive* computerized resources are those that are helpful and interesting and supply good information but are not necessarily essential for professional practice. In meeting the requirement of maintaining currency, supportive computerized resources include document delivery services, electronic publishers, and metasites on the

World Wide Web. There are many resources available to meet each of the above requirements for professional credibility. For the purposes of this chapter, selective resources are identified and discussed as examples of the types of information available. Web site URLs of the various resources are included as well.

Maintaining Currency with the Published Literature

It is obvious that one of the most important obligations a nurse must meet is to maintain currency in her or his field of practice. With the extreme demands in the clinical environment—both in time and amount of work—nurses need easily accessible resources to answer practice-related questions and ensure that they are practicing with the latest and most evidence-based information. Information is needed about current treatments, trends, medications, safety issues, business practices, and new health issues, among other topics.

The purpose of the information retrieved from the sources listed below is to enable nurses to keep abreast of the latest and most evidence-based information in their selected field. Both quantity *and* quality must be considered.

When using a resource, check that:

1. The resource covers the required specialty/field
2. The primary journals and peripheral material in the field are included
3. The resource is updated regularly and is current
4. The resource covers the appropriate period
5. The resource covers material published in different countries and languages
6. There is some form of peer review, reference checking, or other means of evaluation

Essential Computerized Resources

Essential computerized resources for maintaining currency include bibliographic retrieval systems for the journal literature, current awareness services, and review services of the journal literature and currently published books. All of these assist the nurse in gathering the most current and reliable information.

Bibliographic Retrieval Systems   One of the most useful resources for accessing information about current practice is the journal literature. Although there may be a delay between the writing and publishing of an article, this time period is seldom more than a few months. The best way to peruse this literature is through a bibliographic retrieval system, since there is far too much literature published to read it all. Bibliographic retrieval systems also allow filtering and sorting of this vast amount of published material.

A bibliographic retrieval system database allows the nurse to retrieve a list of citations containing bibliographic details of the material indexed, subject headings, and author abstracts. The nurse can search these systems using specific subject headings or key words. Most bibliographic retrieval systems have a controlled vocabulary, also known as a thesaurus or subject heading list, to make electronic subject searching much easier. For this reason, the vocabulary is geared toward the specific content of the database. These controlled vocabularies are made available online as part of the database. Key word searching is necessary when there are no subject headings to cover the concepts being searched. The nurse can also search by specific fields including author, author affiliation, journal title, serial number (ISSN), grant name or number, or publication type. In bibliographic retrieval systems, most fields in the records are word-indexed and can be searched individually to retrieve specific information.

Previously available as print indexes, these systems are now available electronically on CD-ROM, through online services, or via the World Wide Web. To access them, a computer with a CD-ROM drive, a modem, and/or Internet access is required.

Since each of these bibliographic retrieval systems has its own specific content, a nurse may have to search several systems to retrieve a comprehensive list of citations on a particular topic. Directories of descriptions of bibliographic retrieval systems can be found on the World Wide Web, e.g., DoCDat, directory of clinical databases in the U.K. (*http://www.lshtm.ac.uk/docdat/*), Database Descriptions by Dykes Library (*http://library.kumc.edu/*), and the National Library of Medicine (NLM) databases (*http://www.nlm.nih.gov/databases/*).

The main bibliographic retrieval systems that should first be considered are MEDLINE, the CINAHL database, ERIC, PsycINFO, and the Social SciSearch database.

MEDLINE/PubMed   The NLM provides free access to many online resources (Table 36.1). One of these, MEDLINE, covers 4,700 journals in 40 languages with over 12 million references from 1966 to the present in the fields of medicine, nursing, preclinical sciences, healthcare systems, veterinary medicine, and dentistry. The nursing subset in MEDLINE covers over 200 nursing

Table 36.1   A List of Online Databases

Database	URL	Subject	Type
		General databases	
AIDSinfo	*http://aidsinfo.nih.gov*	HIV/AIDS clinical trials	Factual and referral
ClinicalTrials.gov	*http://clinicaltrials.gov*	Patient studies for drugs and treatment	Factual and referral
DIRLINE	*http://dirline.nlm.nih.gov*	Directory of organizations providing information services	Referral
HSRProj (health services research projects in progress)	*http://gateway.nlm.nih.gov*	Ongoing grants and contracts in health services research	Research project descriptions
HSRR Health Services and Sciences Research Resources	*http://wwwcf.nlm.nih.gov/ hsrr_search/ home_search.cfm*	Research datasets and instruments used in health services research	Factual
HSTAT Health Services Technology Assessment Tests	*http://hstat.nlm.nih.gov*	Clinical practice guidelines, technology assessments, and health information	Full text
Locator Plus	*http://locatorplus.gov*	Catalogs of books, audiovisuals, and journal articles held at National Library of Medicine	Bibliographic citations
MEDLINE/PubMed	*http://www.ncbi.nlm.nih.gov/* or *http://gateway.nlm.nih.gov*	Biomedicine. Includes the following databases/ subsets now: AIDS, BIOETHICSLINE, NURSING, HealthSTAR, HISTLINE, POPLINE, SPACELINE, CANCERLIT, and so forth	Bibliographic citations
MedlinePlus	*http://medlineplus.gov/* Spanish: *http://medlineplus.gov/esp/*	Consumer health information	Factual, bibliographic citations
MeSH Vocabulary File	*http://www.nlm.nih.gov/mesh*	Thesaurus of biomedicine-related terms	Factual
OLDMEDLINE	*http://gateway.nlm.nih.gov/* or *http://www.ncbi.nlm.nih.gov*	Biomedicine	Bibliographic citations

(Continued)

Table 36.1   A List of Online Databases (*Continued*)

Database	URL	Subject	Type
TOXNET databases (NLM database and electronic resources): toxicology data network			
CCRIS (Chemical Carcinogenesis Research Information Systems)	*http://toxnet/nlm.nih.gov*	Chemical carcinogens, mutagens, tumor promoters, and tumor inhibitors	Factual
ChemIDplus	*http://sis.nlm.nih.gov/ chemidplus*	Identification of chemical substances	Factual
DART/ETIC (Developmental and Reproductive Toxicology/ Environmental Teratology Information Center	*http://toxnet/nlm.nih.gov*	Test results Developmental and reproductive toxicology	Bibliographic citations
GENE-TOX (genetic toxicology)	*http://toxnet/nlm.nih.gov*	Genetic toxicology test results on chemicals	Factual
Haz-Map	*http://hazmap.nlm.nih.gov*	Effects of exposure to chemicals. Links jobs and hazardous tasks with occupational diseases	Factual
HSDB (hazardous substances data bank)	*http://toxnet/nlm.nih.gov*	Hazardous chemical toxic effects, environmental fate, safety, and handling	Factual
IRIS (Integrated Risk Information Systems)	*http://toxnet/nlm.nih.gov*	Potentially toxic chemicals	Factual
ITER (international toxicity estimates for risk)	*http://toxnet/nlm.nih.gov*	Data of human health risk assessment	Factual
NCI-3D	*http://chem.sis.nlm.nih.gov/nci3d/*	Two- and three-dimensional information about substances	Factual
Tox Town	*http://toxtown.nlm.nih.gov*	Toxic chemicals and environmental health risks	Interactive guide
TOXLINE (toxicology information online)	*http://toxnet/nlm.nih.gov*	Toxicologic, pharmacologic, biochemical, and physiologic effects of drugs and other chemicals	Bibliographic citations
TRI (toxic release inventory)	*http://toxnet/nlm.nih.gov*	Annual estimated releases of toxic chemical to the environment, amounts transferred to waste sites, and source reduction and recycling data	Numeric

Source: National Library of Medicine. (2004). *NLM Databases and Electronic Resources*. Retrieved June 8, 2004, from *http://www.nlm.nih.gov/ databases/*.

journals. The database is updated weekly on the World Wide Web and monthly on CD-ROM (National Library of Medicine, 2004).

The NLM's databases use a controlled vocabulary (thesaurus), called MeSH (Medical Subject Headings) (MeSH: *http://www.nlm.nih.gov/mesh/introduction2004. html*). These index terms facilitate subject searching within the databases.

MEDLINE and the nursing subset are available free over the World Wide Web through the NLM's home page at *http://www.nlm.nih.gov*. There are two ways to search this database: PubMed and the NLM Gateway. The NLM Gateway is a Web-based system that allows users to search multiple NLM retrieval systems simultaneously. The database is also available through the commercial vendors mentioned below. All of these options allow the nurse to search by subject, key word, author,

title, or a combination of these. An example of different searches with a display using the Cinahl Information Systems interface is shown in Figs. 36.1 and 36.2.

Loansome Doc allows the nurse to place an order for a copy of an article from a medical library through PubMed or the NLM Gateway. The full text of articles for some journals is available via a link to the publisher's Web site from the PubMed abstract or record display. Some of the full text is available free of charge. The links indicating free full text display on the Loansome Doc order page prior to order placement and on the Loansome Doc Order Sent page immediately after the order is finalized. As of May 12, 2004, a total of 117 providers supplied free full text for 455 journals. A list of these titles is available on the NLM Web site *(http://www.nlm.nih.gov/loansomedoc/loansome_home. html)*.

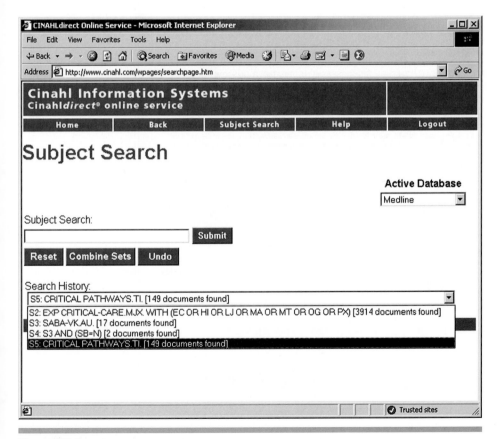

Figure 36.1
MEDLINE search.
(Courtesy of Cinahl Information Systems.)

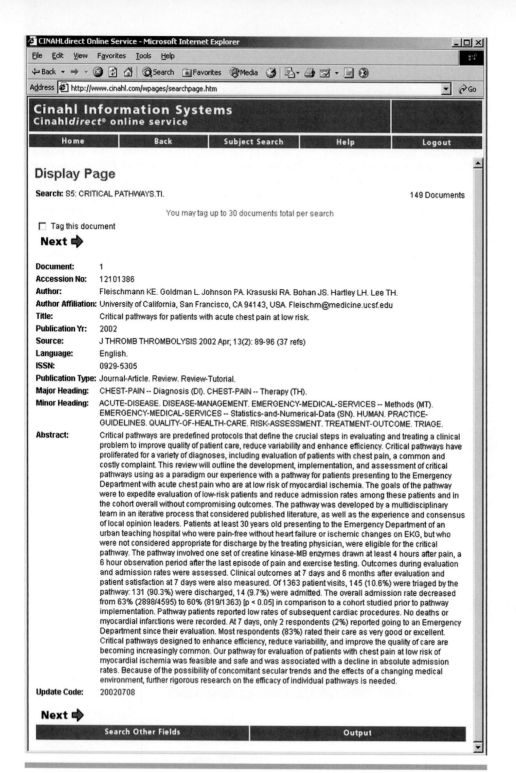

Figure 36.2
MEDLINE search result.
(Courtesy of Cinahl Information Systems.)

CINAHL   The CINAHL database, produced by Cinahl Information Systems, a division of EBSCO Publishing, Inc., provides comprehensive coverage of the literature in nursing and allied health from 1982 to the present. It also covers chiropractic, podiatry, health promotion and education, health services administration, biomedicine, optometry, women's health, consumer health, and alternative therapy (Cinahl Information Systems, 2004b). Over 1,700 journals and books, pamphlets, dissertations, audiovisuals, software, and proceedings are indexed. Some journals covered are published in other countries. Full text is available for some critical paths, research instruments, practice acts and standards of practice, drugs, legal cases, patient education handouts, accreditation and clinical innovation documents, and Web site descriptions. It is updated weekly.

The CINAHL database also uses a controlled vocabulary for effective subject searching. The CINAHL *Subject Heading List* uses the NLM's MeSH terms as the standard vocabulary for disease, drug, anatomic, and physiologic concepts (Cinahl Information Systems, 2004a). There are approximately 4,686 (40%) unique CINAHL terms for nursing and the allied health disciplines. Specific field searching and quality filters are available in the CINAHL database and are similar to those found in MEDLINE. An essential part of research papers is the list of references pointing to prior publications. Cited references from selected nursing and allied health journals are searchable in the CINAHL database.

This bibliographic retrieval system and the others mentioned below are available through commercial vendors on CD-ROM, through online services, or via the World Wide Web. Some of the main commercial vendors are Dialog Corporation, Ovid Technologies, EBSCO Publishing, and Proquest Information and Learning. It is possible to check on the Web sites of these commercial vendors to find which databases are available and if there are any new ones.

ERIC   The ERIC (Educational Resources Information Center) database is published by the United States Department of Education and contains more than 1,200,000 citations covering education-related literature (Educational Resources Information Center, 2003). It covers virtually all types of print materials, published and unpublished, from 1966 to the present day. It is updated monthly. This database gives the nurse a more comprehensive coverage of education than any other bibliographic retrieval system. The database underwent reengineering in 2004 but during the transition period it could be searched at *http://www.eric.ed.gov* or at

http://eduref.org. A controlled vocabulary of more than 10,000 terms, *Thesaurus of Eric Descriptors*, assists with computer searches of this database on the Internet through the World Wide Web (see the URLs mentioned previously) (United States Department of Education, n.d.). As with the other two bibliographic databases mentioned, nurses are able to access all of the data in each record on ERIC by searching, using subject headings or key words or by searching for a word(s) in a specific field (Barrett and Colby, 1995).

PsycINFO   The PsycINFO database, produced by the American Psychological Association, provides access to psychologically relevant literature from journals, dissertations, reports, scholarly documents, books, and book chapters with more than 1.9 million references from the 1880s to the present. Updated weekly, most of the records have abstracts or content summaries from material published in over 50 countries (American Psychological Association, 2004b). Using the *Thesaurus of Psychological Index Terms* of more than 7,000 controlled terms and cross references, the nurse can search for specific concepts effectively. Key word and specific field searching are also available (American Psychological Association, 2004a).

Social SciSearch   Produced by the Institute for Scientific Information (ISI), the Social SciSearch database is an international multidisciplinary bibliographic retrieval system that covers 1,500 journals in the social, behavioral, and related sciences. Since the database contains all of the records published in the Social Sciences Citation Index, the nurse can search the cited references as in the citation index in the CINAHL database. The database covers from 1972 to the present and is updated weekly (Thomson ISI, 2004c).

A few other bibliographic retrieval systems to keep in mind are databases such as CHID online (Combined Health Information Database), produced by the federal government, the American Association of Retired Persons (AARP) database AgeLine, the Excerpta Medica database EMBASE, the National Technical Information Service NTIS database, and the UMI Proquest Digital Dissertations.

Current Awareness Services   Most bibliographic retrieval systems are updated monthly or quarterly. Some are even updated weekly. In addition to the delay between the writing and publishing of the material that is indexed in the database, there is also a delay between the receipt of material, the indexing, and finally the inclusion of the citations for the indexed material in the database. To obtain access to more current material than that available in a bibliographic database, the nurse should use a current awareness service.

Current awareness services are helpful when used in addition to bibliographic retrieval systems. These services provide access to tables of contents of journals and allow individuals to request articles of interest. They may include not only journal articles but also proceedings from conferences, workshops, symposia, and other meetings. Often, hospital or university librarians may provide these services as well.

Unlike the bibliographic databases, where subject searching using controlled vocabulary is available, only key word searching for the subject, author, title, or journal is available in current awareness services or databases.

Some current awareness services or databases are Current Contents Connect, Reference Update, UnCover, the in-process database for MEDLINE (formerly PRE-MEDLINE), the CINAHL*direct* current awareness database, and PreCINAHL on EBSCOHost.

Current Contents Connect from ISI provides a current awareness service to over 8,000 journals and 2,000 recently published books and conference proceedings in the fields of science, social science, technology, and arts and humanities. Complete bibliographic information together with English language author abstracts and publisher names and addresses are provided (Thomson ISI, 2004a).

Weekly issues covering 1,100 publications of Reference Update, also compiled by ISI, can be received via diskette or the Internet. Reference Update uses the references provided in the ISI subscription service covering more than 60 disciplines, including pharmacology, clinical medicine, cardiovascular systems, physiology, psychiatry, behavioral sciences, and public health (Thomson ISI, 2004b.).

UnCover, from the UnCover Company, is an online current awareness alerting service covering nearly 25,000 English language periodicals. Searching this database is free at Ingenta's Web site *http://www.ingenta.com/*.

PubMed's in-process records (formerly PREMED-LINE) provide basic information and abstracts before the citations are indexed. These records are added daily (National Library of Medicine, 2004).

The current awareness service offered by Cinahl Information Systems, a division of EBSCO Publishing, Inc., publishers of the CINAHL database, is available on the CINAHL*direct* online service and EBSCOHost (PreCINAHL). This service is similar to that described

above which contains citations of those articles received but not yet indexed with CINAHL subject headings from the CINAHL thesaurus. The fields that are key word searchable include the article title, author, and journal title. There is no additional charge to subscribers to use this database. Once indexed, the records are included in the CINAHL database and deleted from the current awareness database. An example from this database is shown in Figs. 36.3 and 36.4.

The second type of current awareness provided by Cinahl Information Systems is within the bibliographic database itself, where the searcher is able to choose from a group of over 30 specific or special interest categories, which actually function as "virtual" databases. Possibilities include such areas as advanced nursing practice, case management, home healthcare, or military/uniformed services. By selecting one of these categories, documents are retrieved that are either in specific journals in the field or have been selected by indexers as being of interest to those in that field. The results can be limited by any of the available limits on the database, e.g., publication type such as research, journal subset such as blind peer-reviewed, and presence of full text. A nurse with limited time can peruse the latest literature in one of these fields in this way (Figs. 36.5 and 36.6).

Review Services   Although the bibliographic retrieval systems and the current awareness services and databases act as filters to the ever-exploding volume of literature, sometimes the information retrieved needs to be evaluated to determine whether or not it is appropriate. For example, a monthly literature search might be done on a bibliographic and current awareness database and then a review service checked for commentaries on the sources retrieved. Supportive computerized resources that synthesize the literature include the *Online Journal of Clinical Innovations* (*http://www.cinahl.com*), *the Joanna Briggs Institute for Best Practice* (*http://joannabriggs.edu.au/*), *Clinical Evidence* (*BMJ Publishing at http://www.clinicalevidence.com*) or the *Cochrane Library Database of Systematic Reviews* (*http://www.cochrane.org/reviews*). Review services such as Doody's Review Service or reviews noted in bibliographic databases or review journals, such as *Bandolier, Evidence-Based Nursing, Evidence-Based Practice, Best Practice*, and *ACP Journal Club*, can also be used to evaluate sources. Review services provide information to searchers about recently published books, journal articles, audiovisuals, and software. These reviews may also include ratings, opinions, or commentaries about the material.

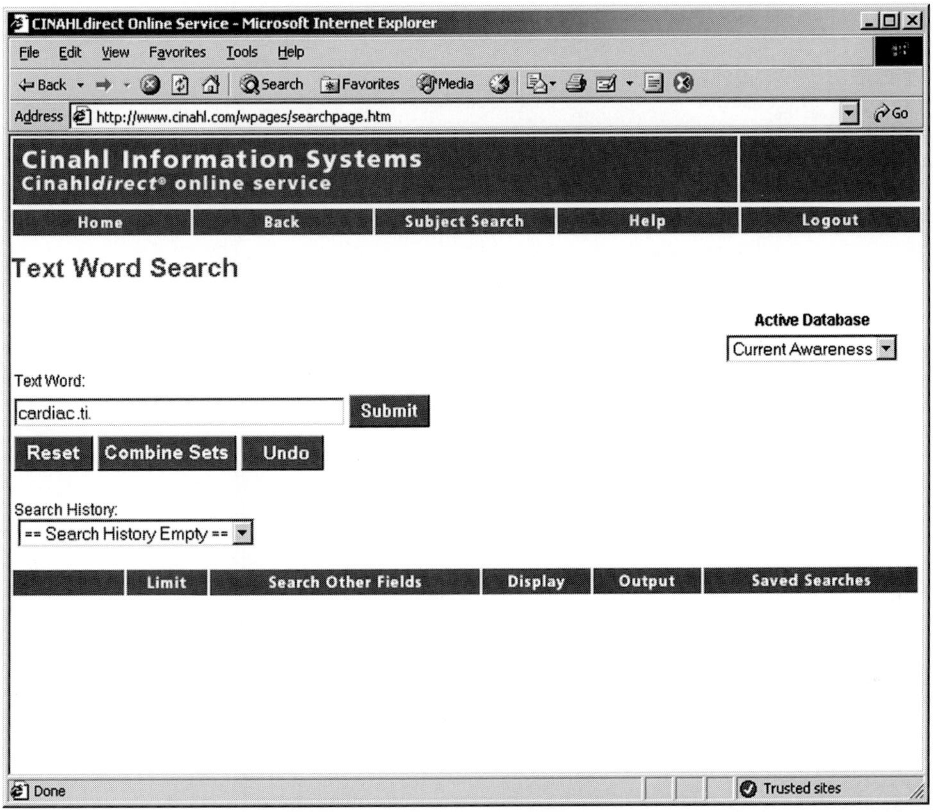

Figure 36.3
Current awareness search.
(Courtesy of Cinahl Information Systems.)

Doody's Review Service *(http://www.doodyenterprises.com/)* is a service offered as a membership benefit to those belonging to Sigma Theta Tau and other nursing professional groups. Doody's Book Review Service develops a profile on its members and sends a weekly electronic mail (e-mail) bulletin describing books and software that meet the parameters of the profile. The service currently contains over 70,000 print and electronic titles. The searcher can use author names, title, specialty, publisher, and key words to find books of interest. The results show price, ISBN, and publisher as well as a rating, when available. Materials are rated using a star system and a questionnaire that assesses the extent to which objectives are met and the appropriateness of the work's readability, among other criteria. (Approximately half of the titles are rated.) The information presented allows serious consideration of the book along with information to assist in making choices. Another Web site, *http://www.nursingbooks.com*, described as designed for nurses by nurses, allows for searching by key word, author, and title. Tied to the Barnes & Noble Web site and search engine, the site categorizes books into various areas, including those intended to help clients, increase knowledge, or shape one's career. Although reviews are not always present, the tables of contents for individual books, along with synopses, are included.

It is well known that books are generally long in the development stage and are not as current as journal articles or documents on the World Wide Web; however, the *depth* of material presented in books must be considered. An in-depth discussion of *all* aspects of cardiac rehabilitation, for example, may be valuable in planning

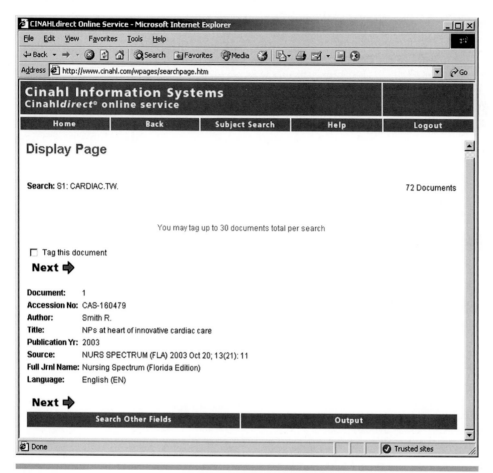

Figure 36.4
Current awareness search result.
(Courtesy of Cinahl Information Systems.)

care and would probably not be examined in a journal article where space is a consideration. Yet it would still be necessary for maintaining currency in the field.

Supportive Computerized Resources

Supportive computerized resources that assist the nurse in maintaining currency provide additional information and enhance the value of the essential computerized resources described previously.

Document Delivery Services   Obtaining a bibliographic list of citations is only the first step in obtaining

information on a particular topic. After carefully evaluating the citations, either from the title and/or the abstracts, or after using one of the review processes described previously, the nurse will need to get the full text of the sources retrieved. A local library would be the first place to go to locate the items retrieved in a search. Publishers of journals or books, database vendors and providers (NLM, American Psychological Association, Ovid Technologies, EBSCO Publishing, Proquest Information and Learning), and document delivery services (UnCover, ISI, Cinahl Information Systems) are secondary sources through which full text of items can be obtained for a fee. Fees differ depending

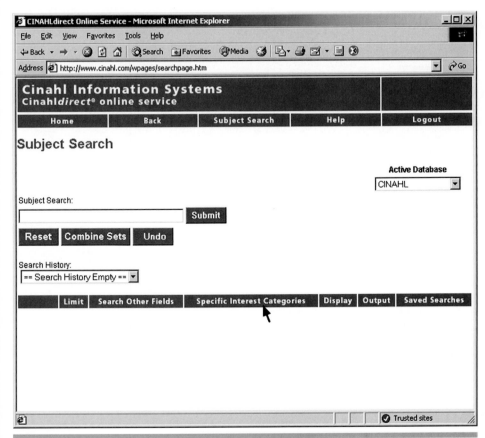

Figure 36.5
Specific interest category initial screen on the CINAHL database.
(Courtesy of Cinahl Information Systems.)

on the service, the urgency of the request, and the publisher's charges. Hard copy is usually sent via fax, mail, or electronic delivery (Stricker, 1998).

Electronic Publishers   Another resource option is publications, such as electronic journals and Morbidity and Mortality Weekly Report (MMWR), that are available on the World Wide Web. Sparks (1999) presents an excellent case for the importance of including electronically published information in a search for information. It offers several advantages over print material, including the speed of publishing, the comparatively small amount of space required for publishing, and the ease of availability of the documents. These advantages are important; however, because a document is published quickly it does not necessarily mean it is accurate. The credibility and accuracy of the source of electronically published material must always be considered. The criteria mentioned along with additional criteria discussed later can be useful in evaluating this material. Some of the main electronic-only nursing journals are *the Online Journal of Issues in Nursing*, published by Kent University School of Nursing in partnership with the American Nurses Association; *Online Journal of Clinical Innovations*, published by Cinahl Information Systems; *On-Line Journal of Nursing Informatics*, published in Pennsylvania; and *Australian Electronic Journal of Nursing Education*, published at Southern Cross University in Australia. Other journals such as *Nursing Standard Online* have print counterparts but may have portions that are only electronic.

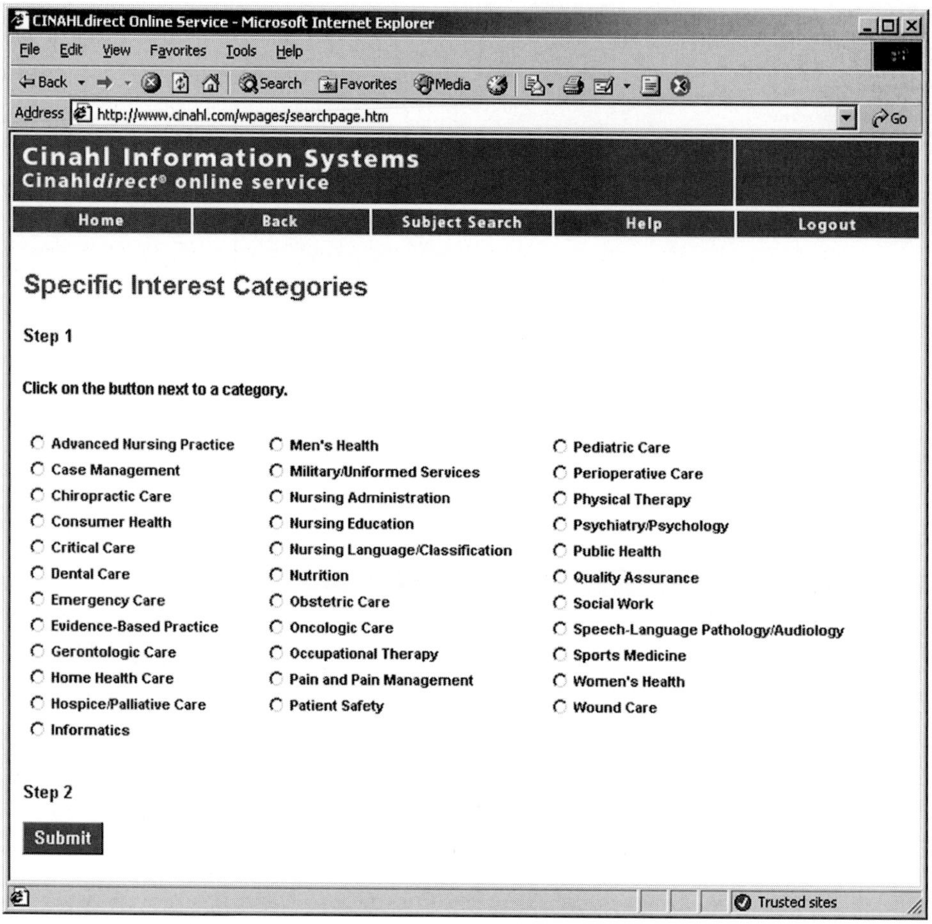

Figure 36.6
Available 2004 specific interest categories.
(Courtesy of Cinahl Information Systems.)

Nursing publishers and organizations have their own Web sites, which have details about new publications, sometimes full text of some of the latest journal articles, official position statements of organizations, and/or practice guidelines. To identify the Web sites of nursing publishers and organizations, search Web site indexes such as Yahoo (*http://www.yahoo.com*) or Google (*http://www.google.com*), or browse Web site lists on Web sites such as that of the University of Buffalo Library (*http://ublib.buffalo.edu*) or the Allnurses.com site (*http://allnurses.com*) have been provided. On a Web site index such as Yahoo, do a general search for "nursing and publishers," "nursing and organizations," or "nursing and associations" or under the specific names

of the publishers and organizations (e.g., Delmar). Advanced searches are also available.

Lippincott Williams & Wilkins (*http://www.nursing-center.com*) has placed over 30 journals including the *American Journal of Nursing, Nursing Research, CIN: Computers, Informatics, Nursing,* and *JONA: Journal of Nursing Administration,* among others, on their journals page with issues from January 1996 to the present. The site has search capability that allows key word searching of the contents of the journals on the site. Articles are available for a fee.

Many nursing organizations provide a significant amount of support to practicing nurses. Many publish journals and provide these as a member benefit. They also provide access to the full text of their position statements and/or practicing guidelines. Some of these publications are the American Nurses Association's Web site NursingWorld (*http://www.nursingworld.org/*) and the Web sites of the American Academy of Nurse Practitioners (*http://www.aanp.org/*), American College of Nurse Practitioners (*http://www.nurse.org/acnp/*), the Association of Pediatric Oncology Nursing (*http://www.apon.org/*), and many others. Details regarding new publications and ordering items can be found on the Web sites of most publishers.

Metasites on the World Wide Web   Since there is so much information on the World Wide Web, identification and evaluation of Web sites is very important to determine which provide valid information. One of the ways to identify Web sites is to consult a metasite. There are several Web sites that can be classified as metasites concerning the same specific topic. The Hardin Meta Directory of Internet Health Sources, sponsored by the Hardin Library for the Health Sciences at the University of Iowa (*http://www.lib.uiowa.edu/hardin/md/*) is one of these as is the National Information Center on Health Services Research & Health Care Technology (NICHSR) (*http://www.nlm.nih.gov/nichsr/hsrsites.html*), a government site. These sites basically function as lists of lists that provide links to other subject-specific Web sites.

Other sites function as metasites within their own Web site. CINAHL*Sources* on the Cinahl Web site (*http://www.cinahl.com*) contains an indexed selection of Web sites that are described both in terms of the organization and the contents of the Web site itself. These Web sites can also be reached directly from the table of contents page if the nurse has no need for the additional information presented in the description.

Once the Web sites have been identified, it is very important to evaluate them. At minimum, the nurse should ask the following questions: (1) Who created the site? (2) Is the purpose and intention of the site clear? (3) Is the information accurate and current? (4) Is the site well-designed and stable? (Schloman, 1999).

There are also Web sites that can be used to evaluate other Web sites. OMNI (Organising Medical Networked Information) (*http://omni.ac.uk/*) is a collaborative British effort to identify, select, evaluate, describe, and provide access to biomedical network resources. HON (Health on the Net Foundation) (*http://www.hon.ch/*) is an international initiative to promote effective Internet development and use in the areas of medicine and health. HealthWeb (*http://www.healthweb.org*) is a collaborative project of several health sciences libraries including the National Network of Libraries of Medicine. Other Web sites that

critically evaluate are National Council Against Health Fraud (*http://www.ncahf.org*), a voluntary health agency that focuses on health fraud; and Quack Watch (*http://www.quackwatch.com*), a member of the Consumer Federation of America (Schloman, 1999; Durkin, 1997). Additionally, Web sites providing information or discussions concerning specific diseases should be evaluated in this way (e.g., the Web sites of the American Diabetes Association [*http://www.diabetes.org/*], American Heart Association [*http://www.amhrt.org/*], and the Multiple Sclerosis Foundation [*http://www.msfacts.org/*]).

 Developing and Maintaining a List of Sources for Research/ Practice/Education

Essential Computerized Resources

The purpose of the information retrieved from these information resources is to enable nurses to answer specific questions that relate to research, practice, and/or education. For example:

- A staff nurse needs to find information to share with her or his colleagues on oral care and the prevention of pneumonia.
- A nursing student has to finish a term paper and needs to find five nursing research studies on caring for a Hispanic patient with a myocardial infarction.
- A nurse manager needs to find research studies and anecdotal material showing the best way to prevent patient falls in her or his health facility.

Bibliographic Retrieval Systems   Resources essential in answering this type of question again include bibliographic databases as well as various Web sites. Once again, the resources need to be carefully evaluated for coverage and currency. Once a resource has been selected, the nurse breaks down her or his needs into a search statement such as, "I need information on oral care and prevention of pneumonia." The information on this topic would best be found in a bibliographic database. On such a database, the best method of searching is to do a subject search using a controlled vocabulary (MeSH headings in MEDLINE, CINAHL subject headings in the CINAHL database, and so forth).

Search Strategies   One of the most important aspects of searching the literature is formulating the exact strategy to obtain the information from a resource, whether from a bibliographic retrieval system or a Web site. There are six steps in planning the search strategy.

1. Plan the search strategy ahead of time.

2. Break down the search topic into components. To find information on oral care and the prevention of pneumonia, remember to include synonyms or related terms. The components of the above search would be oral hygiene or mouth care and prevention of pneumonia. Sometimes the terms for the search will be subject headings in the database's subject heading list (often called a thesaurus); in other cases, they will not be (Fig. 36.7).

3. Check for terms in a subject heading list, if available. If the concept is new and there are no subject headings, a text word or key word search is necessary. For example, before the term "critical paths" or "critical pathways" was added to MeSH or the CINAHL *Subject Heading List*, it was necessary to do a text word search for this concept. A search using the broad term "case management" would have retrieved many articles that would not necessarily discuss or include critical paths.

4. Select "operators," which are words used to connect different or synonymous components of the search. The "and" operator, for example, makes the search narrower or more specific as the results of the search for two different terms will only result in records that include *both* terms as subject headings (Fig. 36.8) (Verhey, Levy, and Schmidt, 1998).

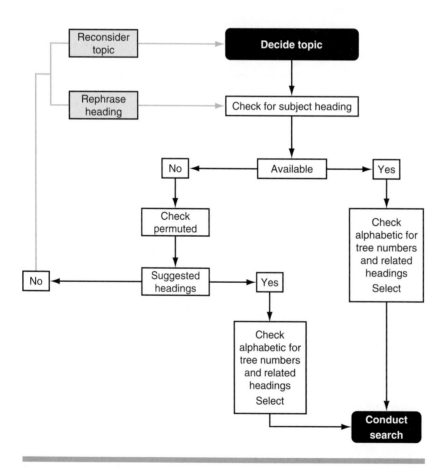

Figure 36.7
Strategy for a successful literature search.
(Courtesy of Cinahl Information Systems.)

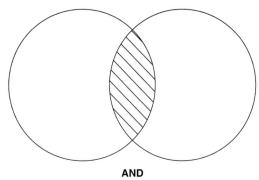

AND

Concept 1 "AND" Concept 2 = This means that only articles with both concept 1 and concept 2 are searched for.

Figure 36.8
Venn diagram **AND**.

The "or" operator can be used to connect synonymous or related terms, which broadens the search (Fig. 36.9). An example combining subject headings using "or" and "and" operators is shown in Fig. 36.10.

The "not" operator can be used to exclude terms (Fig. 36.11).

5. Run the search. For the search on oral care and pneumonia, select the option "explode" for the subject headings oral hygiene and mouth care. This would ensure the retrieval of articles on the broad heading and the more specific headings. For example, the specific headings under oral hygiene are "dental devices, home care" and "toothbrushing."

6. View the results.

Practice Guidelines and Position Statements
Organization-specific practice guidelines, position statements, and standards of practice can often be accessed and obtained from the Web site of an individual's professional organization. These are extremely useful documents that present information on the scope of practice, qualifications, and education among other important details. Additionally, Cinahl Information Systems currently includes nurse practice acts as one of its publication types in the CINAHL database. These appear in full text and can be read online or printed.

Continuing Education and Computer-Assisted Learning   Many nurses do not have the time or money to attend conferences and workshops to keep abreast of the latest information in their specialties or to complete the necessary units or credits for continuing education (CE) for relicensure or recertification. The World Wide Web is a wonderful source for nurses that can be used to satisfy their requirements for CE. The sites are easy to access, and there is no travel time or great expense involved (Plank, 1998). To identify CE Web sites visit Nursing Network (*http://www.nursingnetwork.com/webconted.htm*) or the Nurse Friendly Nationwide Directory (*http://www.nursefriendly.com/ceu/*), or use one of several search engines (Alta Vista at *http://www.altavista.com*, Google at *http://www.google.com*, or Ask Jeeves at *http://www.askjeeves.com*) to obtain CE nursing sites. There are many nursing sites that offer online CE and CEU certificates, such as RnCeus.com at *http://www.rnceus.com* and the CE Connection at Lippincott Williams & Wilkins site at *http://www.nursingcenter.com/prodev/ce_online.asp/*.

As mentioned at the beginning of this chapter, nurses use computers for many purposes. Computer-assisted instruction (CAI), computer-assisted learning (CAL), and interactive videodisc (IVD) provide easy learning experiences using a computer.

Supportive Computerized Resources

Supportive computerized resources that assist in practice, research, and education contain all types of health information including drug and treatment information, anatomy, and physiology. Specific products such as the

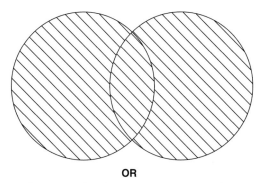

OR

Concept 1 "OR" Concept 2 = This means that articles with either concept 1 or concept 2 are searched for.

Figure 36.9
Venn diagram **OR**.
(Courtesy of Cinahl Information Systems.)

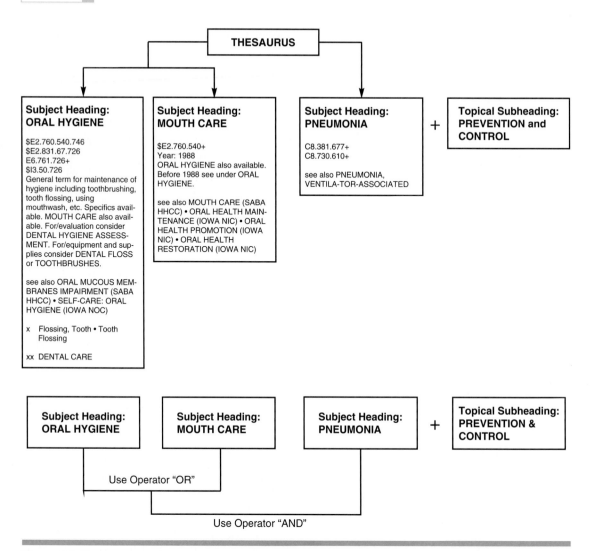

Figure 36.10
Subject headings using **OR** and **AND** operator.

Merck Manual of Diagnosis and Therapy (*http://www. merck.com*) or the *Physician's Desk Reference* available as *PDRhealth* (*http://www.pdrhealth.com/ drug_info/*) are also available on the World Wide Web. The Visible Human Project includes complete, anatomically detailed, three-dimensional representations of the male and female human bodies. The National Library of Medicine itself claims the "largest collection of medical knowledge in the world." The Cochrane Library's *Database of*

Systematic Reviews, available online and on CD-ROM, is another excellent source.

Web sites of particular interest in this category include the Nursing Theories Page (*http://www.sandiego.edu/nursing/theory*) and the Virginia Henderson International Library and Research Registry (*http://www.stti.iupui.edu/ library/*) as well as the Interagency Council on Information Resources for Nursing (ICIRN) *(http://icirn.org)*. ICIRN prepares "Essential Nursing References" published

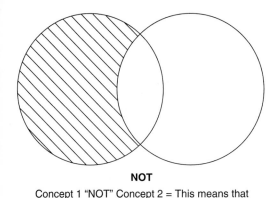

NOT

Concept 1 "NOT" Concept 2 = This means that
articles with concept 1 that do not include
concept 2 are searched for.

Figure 36.11
Venn diagram **NOT**.

biannually by the National League for Nursing in *Nursing Education Perspectives*.

Collaboration and Networking Regarding Issues of Professional Practice

Nurses frequently gather information from their personal networks—either at the worksite or at professional meetings. The increased availability of computers makes contact with other professionals much easier, resulting in networking and collaboration possibilities heretofore impossible. Information retrieved by this method enables nurses to learn from their colleagues' experiences. When considering with whom to network, the specialty of the person should be evaluated along with experience, the material they have published in their field, and the research undertaken by the institution with which they are affiliated. Most of this information is not published and would be unavailable through traditional information resources.

Computerized resources for collaboration and networking vary in several technical details (e.g., their focus, the presence or absence of a moderator to monitor messages, the number of participants, and their level of interactivity).

Essential Computerized Resources

Electronic Mail and Listservs An important fundamental computerized resource for collaboration and networking is e-mail, which is at the core of almost any electronic communication. Necessary components for e-mail are an Internet service provider (ISP) such as America OnLine or Earthlink and an e-mail software such as Eudora or those provided by Web browsers (NetScape or Internet Explorer). E-mail allows one-to-one communication between individuals and can provide immediate response to practice-related questions.

A second essential computerized resource for collaboration is an electronic discussion group or "listserv." Listservs allow individuals to subscribe free of charge and to read and respond to messages via e-mail. Since the messages are posted to all of the members, the listserv allows sharing and dissemination of information with colleagues. Some listservs have a closed membership for a specific group (e.g., librarians or specific nursing groups), and some are moderated. In a moderated group, an individual or group of individuals reads the messages prior to distribution to the group (Hayden, 1997). Subject-specific listservs include NURSENET (general nursing), Nrsing-L (nursing informatics), NRSINGED (education issues/faculty), and NurseRes (research). Specialty listservs are very helpful in increasing dialogue between individuals within the same specialty.

Supportive Computerized Resources

Electronic Bulletin Boards, Forums, Newsgroups, and Chat Rooms Bulletin boards, forums, newsgroups, and chat rooms are examples of supportive computerized resources. Similar to a traditional bulletin board, the electronic version has an administrator who sends the discussion to various Web sites, where nurses visit to read and participate in the discussion (Hayden, 1997). This format for electronic networking has almost entirely been replaced by forums and newsgroups, which have become more and more sophisticated in their interactivity and design. The premise behind each of them is similar. An individual posts a message concerning a topic (known as a "thread") for others to read and respond to. Lippincott's Nursing Center (*http://www.nursingcenter.com*), for example, has many different forums under broad nursing categories such as roles, care settings, and areas of practice. Participants can respond to a previously posted thread or begin a new one in any of these broad areas or the subtopics within them. Newsgroups operate in much the same way but have a tendency to be less focused. All of these resources are interactive but on a delayed basis. An individual may respond to a message immediately or wait several days. Chat rooms, on the other hand, are interactive in "real time." Conversations in chat rooms can be compared to telephone conversations—without the benefit of sound. Examples of chat rooms can be found at *http://virtualnurse.com* or *http://www.nursechat.com/.*

Each of these methods of collaboration and networking provides an option for nurses to contact and build relationships with other professionals concerning issues important to them.

Summary

While these three categories of information needs have been discussed as if they were independent of one another, a nurse might often find that she or he has needs that transcend all three categories or that fall under a different category each time, depending on the task. For example, a staff nurse may need to investigate the best methods to assess and manage pain. The process of retrieving appropriate information would be to first search for research studies and anecdotal material on the topic of pain management and pain measurement. This would involve a search for pain measurement or pain with therapy, drug therapy, and diagnosis using essential computerized resources such as bibliographic retrieval systems like MEDLINE or the CINAHL database.

Networking with other professionals facing the same task would be an additional step in this process. The nursing listservs mentioned under the "Collaboration and Networking Regarding Issues of Professional Practice" section would be an important and essential resource, while e-mailing colleagues who are specialists in the field of pain would be a supportive resource. To locate specialists, a bibliographic retrieval system could be searched for research studies on pain measurement or management. The author affiliation field in the records retrieved would help track the institution with which the author is affiliated.

Making sure to keep current on any new material published on pain measurement and pain management, by using current awareness services or Web sites, would also be vital in locating information on this topic. Bibliographic retrieval systems, already used as an essential resource, could be searched each month to assess what new material had been published on the topic. Supportive computerized resources might include a similar search for papers on the Cochrane Library's *Database of Systematic Reviews*, or consulting electronic publications such as *Worldviews on Evidence-Based Nursing* or the *Online Journal of Clinical*
Innovations. The articles in the latter journal have corresponding summaries that are indexed and appear in full text on the CINAHL database, making them easily accessible in a traditional literature search to answer practice questions.

An important part of identifying and using these essential and supportive computerized resources is the evaluation of each of them to assess whether or not they contain the information needed. Therefore, the nurse must determine what she or he is looking for, identify the most appropriate resources to locate the information needed, and, using the criteria discussed throughout this chapter, evaluate the resources to assess if they are valid, current, and accurate.

Finally, it is important to realize that computerized information resources are like a "moving target," in that technology is changing so quickly that resources used today may be gone, unavailable, or outdated tomorrow. The use of bibliographic retrieval systems, search engines, and metasites encourages searching by *subject* or *concept*, which is the most reliable way to cope with the ever-changing nature of technology. This is vital to maintaining currency with the published literature, developing and maintaining a list of sources of topics of interest for practice, research, and/or education, and collaboration and networking with colleagues regarding issues of professional practice.

References

American Psychological Association. (2004a). *Guide to the Fields in Our Database Records.* Retrieved June 8, 2004, from *http://www.apa.org/Psycinfo/about/fieldguide.html*

American Psychological Association. (2004b). *PsycINFO Database Information.* Available at *http://www.apa.org/psycinfo/products/psycinfo.html*

Barrett, L. and Colby, A. (1995). Eric's indexing and retrieval: 1995 update. In J. E. Houston (Ed.), *Thesaurus of ERIC descriptors* (13th ed., pp. xiii–xvii). Phoenix, AZ: Oryx Press.

Cinahl Information Systems. (2004a). *CINAHL 2004 Subject Heading List.* Glendale, CA: Cinahl Information Systems.

Cinahl Information Systems. (2004b). *Cumulative Index to Nursing & Allied Health Literature 49(part B).* Glendale, CA: Cinahl Information Systems.

Durkin, C. (1997). Tracking and evaluating Web sites. *National Network* 21(2):8, 11.

Educational Resources Information Center. (2003). *A Little about ERIC.* Retrieved June 8, 2004, from *http://searchERIC.org/abit.htm*

Hayden, K. A. (1997). Internet tools and resources in continuing health education. *Journal of Continuing Education in the Health Professions* 17:121–127.

National Library of Medicine. (2004). *NLM Databases and Electronic Resources*. Retrieved June 8, 2004, from *http://www.nlm.nih.gov/databases/*

Plank, R. K. (1998). Nursing on-line for continuing education credit. *The Journal of Continuing Education in Nursing* 29:165–172.

Schloman, B. F. (1999). Whom do you trust? Evaluating Internet health resources. *Online Journal of Issues in Nursing*. Retrieved June 8, 2004, from *http://www.nursingworld.org/ojin/infocol/info_1.htm*

Sparks, S. M. (1999). Electronic publishing and nursing research. *Nursing Research* 48:50–54.

Stricker, U. D. (1998). Deliver me: When subscribing is not an option. *Information Highways* 5(4):20–25.

Thomson ISI. (2004a). *Current Contents Connect®*. Retrieved June 8, 2004, from *http://www.isinet.com/products/cap/ccc*.

Thomson ISI. (2004b). *Reference Update*. Retrieved June 8, 2004, from *http://www.isinet.com/products/cap/ru*.

Thomson ISI. (2004c). *Social SciSearch® ONTAP® Social SciSearch® (File 207)*. Retrieved June 8, 2004, from *http://library.dialog.com/bluesheets/html/ bl0007.html*

United States Department of Education. (n.d.). 2004. *Thesaurus of ERIC Descriptors*. Retrieved June 8, 2004, from *http://www.ericfacility.org/resources.html*

Verhey, M. P., Levy, J. R., and Schmidt, R. (1998). *Information RN*. Glendale, CA: Cinahl Information Systems.

Recommended Readings

Allen, M. and Levy, J. R. (2002). Evidence-based searching for nursing and allied health. *Biblioteca Medica Canadiana* 23(3):90–95.

Bird, D. (2003). Discovering the literature of nursing: A guide for beginners. *Nurse Researcher* 11(1):56–70.

Bowen, D. M. and Forrest, J. L. (2003). Solving puzzling clinical questions. *RDH* 23(5):34, 36, 38, passim.

Conn, V. S., Isaramalai, S., Rath, S., Jantarakupt, P., Wadhawan, R., and Dash, Y. (2003). Beyond MEDLINE for literature searches. *Journal of Nursing Scholarship* 35(2):177–182.

Ebbert, J. O., Dupras, D. M., and Erwin, P. J. (2003). Concise review for clinicians. Searching the medical literature using PubMed: A tutorial. *Mayo Clinic Proceedings* 78(1):87–91.

Garg, A. and Turtle, K. M. (2003). Effectiveness of training health professionals in literature search skills using electronic health databases—a critical appraisal. *Health Information and Libraries Journal* 20:33–41.

Gillespie, L. D. and Gillespie, W. J. (2003). Finding current evidence: Search strategies and common databases. *Clinical Orthopaedics and Related Research* 413:133–145.

Harris, G. (2003). Web search alert. Search query saving tips. *Information Highways* 10(5):21.

Jacso, P. (2003). Savvy searching. Using controlled vocabulary (content part). *Online Information Review* 27(4):284–286.

Levy, J. R. (2002). Effective literature searching. *Online Journal of Clinical Innovations* 5(4):1–2.

Levy, J. R. (2002). Searching the CINAHL Database part 1: Evidence-based practice. *CINAHL News* 21(1):10, 12, 15.

Lindell, C. and Chew, K. (2003). Internet research for the health care professional: Wading through the Web. *Nursingmatters* 14(3):7.

Parker, M. D. (2003). The Internet . . . as a research tool: Finding the balance. *RDH* 23(9):78–81.

Poynton, M. R. (2003). Information technology and the clinical nurse specialist. Recall to precision: Retrieving clinical information with MEDLINE. *Clinical Nurse Specialist* 17(4):182–184.

Pravikoff, D. (2000). On the information highway, or sitting on the curb. *Journal of Nursing Education* 39(3):99–100.

Pravikoff, D. S. and Donaldson, N. E. (2001). Online journals: Access and support for evidence-based practice. *AACN Clinical Issues: Advanced Practice in Acute and Critical Care* 12(4):588–596.

Rogers, B. (2004). Research & ethics corner. Research utilization—putting the research evidence into practice. *AAOHN Journal* 52(1):14–15.

Shelling, J. (2003). CPD: Searching the literature: Advanced techniques for exhaustive searching. *Collegian* 10(3):36–38.

White, B. (2004). Making evidence-based medicine doable in everyday practice. *Family Practice Management* 11(2):51–58, 72–73.

Witchell, L. (2003). Seven steps to online literature searching. *Ophthalmic Nursing* 6(4):24–26.

PART 10

International
Perspectives

37

Nursing Informatics in Canada

Kathryn J. Hannah

Nora Hammell

Lynn M. Nagle

OBJECTIVES

1. Describe nursing's role in information systems in Canada.
2. Identify major organizational structures that have led to standards in Canada.
3. Understand the organizational factors influencing information system development in Canada.
4. Describe the Canadian Nursing Components for Health Information Systems.

KEY WORDS

information systems
standards
hospital information systems
nursing minimum data set (NMDS)
public policy

Introduction

Nursing's role in managing information in health service organizations and care facilities in Canada is similar to that of other developed countries. The Canadian Nurses Association (CNA) has taken the position that "registered nurses and other stakeholders in healthcare delivery require information on nursing practice and its relationship to client outcomes. A coordinated system to collect, store and retrieve nursing data in Canada is essential for health human resource planning, and to expand knowledge and research on determinants of quality nursing care. . . . CNA believes that registered nurses should advocate and lead in implementing the collection, storage and retrieval of nursing data at the national level" (Canadian Nurses Association, 2001). CNA, the provincial and territorial nurses associations and nursing informatics interest groups across Canada have been instrumental in supporting nurses' involvement with innovations in health informatics by disseminating information and promoting standards and ethics in the development of nursing informatics. Current

applications of nursing informatics cover many kinds of clinical, education, administrative, research, and health-care systems initiatives (e.g., telehealth, electronic health records [EHRs], decision support systems, workload measurement, and virtual education).

Nevertheless, the focus of nursing informatics in Canada is on the role of nursing within healthcare organizations. In most healthcare organizations, nurses manage both patient care and patient care units within the organization. Usually nurse clinicians manage patient care and nurse managers administer the patient care units within the organization. Therefore, for some time, nursing's role in the management of information has been considered to include both the information necessary to manage patient care using the nursing process and the information necessary for managing patient care units within the organization.

With regard to the nursing management of patient care, nursing practice is information intensive. Nurses constantly handle enormous volumes of patient care information. In fact, nurses constantly process information mentally, manually, and electronically. Nurses have long been recognized as the interface between the patient and the healthcare organization. Like nurses in other countries, Canadian nurses integrate information from many diverse sources throughout the organization to provide patient care and to coordinate the patient's contact with healthcare services and facilities. In addition, they manage patient care information for purposes of providing nursing care to patients.

There is also a long-standing tradition that nurses have the role of custodians of information on behalf of other caregivers and users of patient information. For almost 40 years it has been widely recognized that nurses spend enormous amounts of time engaged in information handling; the seminal study, in three New York hospitals, found that registered nurses spend from 36 to 64% of their time on information handling, with those in administrative positions spending the most time (Jydstrup and Gross, 1966). Nurses must be able to manage and process nursing data, information, and knowledge to support patient care delivery in diverse care delivery settings (Graves and Corcoran, 1989). There is an essential linkage among access to information, client outcomes, and patient safety. "As Lang has succinctly and aptly described the present situation: If we cannot name it, we cannot control it, finance it, teach it, research it or put it into public policy" (Clark and Lang, 1992). Access to information about their practice arms nurses with evidence to support the contribution of nursing to patient outcomes. Outcomes research is an essential foundation for evidence-based nursing practice. Evidence-based practice is a means of promoting and enhancing patient safety.

Among the factors that influence nursing's role in managing patient care environments is the patient assignment methodology in use in the hospital or on individual patient care units (see Hannah and Shamian, 1992). Each of these patient assignment methodologies requires a different nursing role in managing patient care information and consequently different information management skills for the nurses involved. Similarly, nursing's role in managing information for purposes of administering patient care units is influenced by the role of the nurse managers within the organization. Variations in decision-making, patient assignment, documentation protocols, and institutional governance style all affect nursing's role in information management for administrative purposes. However, the single most important element that determines nursing's role in information management for administrative purposes is the governance model in use in the hospital (Hannah and Shamian, 1992).

Contextual Factors Influencing the Development of Health Information in Canada

Canadians have a unique healthcare system, one that is the envy of many countries. One of the things that makes the Canadian healthcare system unique is the belief in health as a right not as a privilege, or an economic commodity, but rather as a right for Canadians. This philosophy is reflected in the principles on which the provincial health systems in Canada are based and it is legislated through the Canada Health Act by which all Canadian provinces abide. These principles include universality, portability, accessibility, comprehensiveness, and public administration. In addition, health is a provincial responsibility in Canada, not a federal one. Conformity on health matters between provinces is by mutual consent and agreement not legislation.

Unfortunately, like other healthcare systems, in Canada the provincial health systems are presently in a box analogous to the room in which Alice in Wonderland found herself when she began to grow. The system is under enormous pressures as depicted in Fig. 37.1. These factors are well described and documented elsewhere (Hannah, Ball, and Edwards, 2005; Hannah and Anderson, 1994).

The overall picture is one in which the expenses and costs associated with healthcare are rising and the resources available to pay for healthcare in Canada have been reduced. Canadian nurses need to find ways to be more efficient and more effective and can maximize the quality of care that is available to Canadians with the available resources. We must identify strategies to provide enhanced information management to facilitate the management of our ever-diminishing health resources.

These, then, are some of the factors that are influencing the drive toward the identification of essential data needs of nurses. In Canada, the information revolution has prompted initiatives by healthcare organizations to develop or acquire automated information systems focused on the utilization of data for the purposes of resource allocation, patient specific costing, and outcomes of services. The information revolution has also been a driving force in the evolution of national health information through the formation of the Canadian Institute for Health Information (CIHI).

During the 1990s, Canadian healthcare systems underwent profound reform initiated by action at the federal and provincial level in response to numerous reports and commissions (Epp, 1986; Angus, 1989; Wilk, 1991; Information Highway Advisory Council, 1995; CANARIE, 1996; Health Canada, 1997; National Forum on Health, 1997). Roles of healthcare

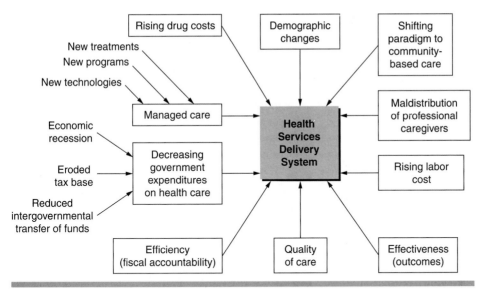

Figure 37.1
Pressures on health services delivery systems.

providers and organizations were examined with a view to eliminating duplication of services and functions as well as providing efficient delivery of quality healthcare. New models of care delivery are emerging, such as "patient-focused care" and "hospitals without walls," directed at elimination of inefficiency in the structure and approach to healthcare. De-institutionalization of care and changes in the scope of medical practice are occurring. In addition, there is an increasing trend toward consumerism in which self-help groups, disease-specific groups, and other special interest groups expect to be involved in their own care. Another common outcome of the reviews most provinces conducted of their healthcare systems was recognition of information systems as a key enabler (and lack of quality information as a key barrier) to health sector reform.

Literally, every study of healthcare services in Canada, including such seminal Canadian works as the Hall Commission (Royal Commission on Health Services [Hall Commission, 1964] and the Lalonde Report (Lalonde, 1974), has pointed out the importance of good information to manage healthcare systems. Overarching concern about the effectiveness and efficiency of the Canadian healthcare systems, beginning in the mid-1980s, led to a growing recognition that health information in Canada was in a sorry state. As shown in Table 37.1, over the past 5 years, the need for better information with which to

manage the healthcare systems in Canada and the health of Canadians has become an increasing national priority and a consistent theme of the various federal and provincial studies of the Canadian health systems (National Forum on Health, 1997; Clair, 2000; Advisory Committee on Health Human Resources, 2000; Fyke, 2001; Mazankowski, 2002; Romanow, 2002; Standing Senate Committee on Social Affairs Science and Technology, 2002).

The inevitable conclusion is that information and information management will become increasingly important in the future. Canadian nursing must ensure that information related to the nursing contribution to patient care is available in local and national data sets. Thus, the data elements from which this information is derived must be collected and stored in a retrievable format.

 National Health Information Organizations

Canadian Institute for Health Information

The establishment of the National Health Information Council in the late 1980s lead to the National Task Force on Health Information, also known as the Wilk Task Force, which presented comprehensive goals and a

Table 37.1   Canadian Institute for Health Information (CIHI) Health Information Data Elements and Proposed Nursing Components

Care items

Medical diagnosis
   (Most responsible, primary, secondary)
Procedure and dates
Client status*
Nursing interventions*
Nursing intensity*
Client outcomes*

Patient demographics

Health care number
Date of birth and age
Sex
Weight
   (Newborns and infants 28 days or less)
Postal code
Race/ethnicity*
Unique geographical location*
Unique lifetime identifier*

Service items

Province/institution number/chart number
Most responsible consultant
Admission date and hour
Institution from
Admission category
Admit by ambulance
Discharge date and hour
Length of stay
Institution to alive/death code
Responsibility for payment
Main patient service
Unique nurse identifier*
Principal nurse provider*

*Proposed Nursing Components of Health Information (HI:NC) elements.

strong vision for a nationwide health information system (National Task Force on Health Information, 1990). Subsequently, the recommendations of the Wilk Task Force (National Task Force on Health Information,

1991) resulted in the merger of four existing entities to create the CIHI in 1992 (Project Team for the Planning of the Canadian Institute for Health Information, 1991; Canadian Institute for Health Information, 2002). CIHI is an independent, pan-Canadian, not for profit organization, established jointly by federal and provincial/territorial ministers of health, with a mandate (Canadian Institute for Health Information, 2002) to:

■ Coordinate the development and maintenance of a comprehensive and integrated approach to health information for Canada

■ Provide and coordinate the provision of accurate and timely data and information required for:
   ▪ Establishing sound health policy.
   ▪ Effectively managing the Canadian health system.
   ▪ Generating public awareness about factors affecting good health.

The core functions of CIHI (Canadian Institute for Health Information, 2002) are to:

■ Identify and promote national health indicators

■ Coordinate and promote the development and maintenance of national health information standards

■ Develop and manage health databases and registries

■ Conduct analysis and special studies and participate in research

■ Publish reports and disseminate health information

■ Coordinate and conduct education sessions and conferences

During the decade of its existence, CIHI has become an acknowledged and trusted source of quality, reliable and timely aggregated health information for use in understanding and improving the management of the Canadian health systems and the health of the population of Canada.

Canada Health Infoway Inc.

As CIHI, and its various aggregated databases, evolved and matured, their focus was on health indicators and population health as well as information to manage the healthcare system. The healthcare community came to realize that there was still limited information available to support decision-making related to clinical care of individuals and groups of patient/clients of the health systems. The need for a pan-Canadian EHR gradually emerged during the later half of the 1990s beginning with the report of the National Forum on Health (National Forum on Health, 1997). The recommendations in this report (National Forum on Health, 1997) resulted in commitment in October 2000 by the federal government of $500 million to support the development and coordination of pan-Canadian health information systems necessary to achieve an EHR. This funding was recognition, by federal, provincial, and territorial governments, of the potential of information and communications technologies to improve the efficiency, cost-effectiveness, access, quality, and safety of health services in Canada. The Federal/Provincial/Territorial Advisory Committee on Health Infostructure (Advisory Committee on Health Infostructure, 2001) set its top priority on the development of EHR and telehealth. It identified the need to begin working immediately on the building blocks for the next stages in development of EHRs.

Canada Health Infoway Inc. (Infoway) was incorporated in January 2001 and began its first year of operation in April 2001. The Infoway Mission (Canada Health Infoway Inc., 2002) is "To foster and accelerate the development and adoption of electronic health information systems with compatible standards and communication technologies on a pan-Canadian basis with tangible benefits to Canadians. The Corporation will build on existing initiatives and pursue collaborative relationships in pursuit of its mission." Specific objectives of Infoway (Canada Health Infoway Inc., 2002) are to:

- Accelerate the development and adoption of modern systems of health information and communication technologies (ICTs)

- Define and promote standards governing shared data to ensure the compatibility of health information networks

- Support the adoption of such standards for health information and compatible communications technologies for the health sector in Canada

- Enter into collaborative arrangements as required with the governments of Canada, the provinces and territories, corporations, not-for-profit organizations [sic], and other public and private partners for the development and adoption of standards and technologies

- Incorporate standards that protect personal privacy, confidentiality of individual records, and the security of health information

- Carry out the work of *Infoway* in both official languages

The emerging EHR will ultimately incorporate data related to patient assessment and interventions contributing to patient outcomes and providers' patterns of practice. It is imperative that nursing assessments, interventions, and practice patterns are included in the EHR because nursing is the single largest group of healthcare providers.

Standards Council of Canada

The Canadian Advisory Council (CAC) on Health Informatics (Z295) advises the Canadian Stands Association arm of Standards Council of Canada (SCC) on matters related to Health Informatics Standards. SCC is the official Canadian member of International Standards Organization (ISO). The CAC provides representation on behalf of Canada at the ISO's Technical Committee 215 (ISO/TC 215) on Health Informatics Standards where CAC representatives speak on behalf of Canada. The CAC has a dual role: first, to provide technical input to SCC on Health Informatics standards development in Canada and second, to provide feedback about the utility in Canada of ISO health informatics standards. The goal of the CAC is to harmonize national with international health information standards, specifically those addressed by the ISO/TC 215 on Health Informatics. The CAC chair is determined by CIHI. The Canadian Standards Association (CSA) provides secretariat support. Members of CAC represent key stakeholder groups in the area of health information and health informatics in Canada, and reflect a balance of interest from industry, governments, users, and general interest groups.

 ## Obstacles to Effective Nursing Management of Information in Canada

In Canadian hospitals, like most U.S. or European hospitals, the major obstacles to more effective nursing management of information are the sheer volume of information, the lack of access to modern information handling techniques and equipment, and the inadequate information management infrastructure. The volume of information that nurses manage on a daily basis, either for patient care purposes or organizational management purposes, is enormous and continuing to grow. Nurses continue to respond to this growth with incredible mental agility. However, human beings do have limits and a major source of job dissatisfaction among Canadian nurses is information overload resulting in information induced job stress.

Antiquated manual information systems and outdated information transfer facilities are information redundant and labor-intensive processes, to say nothing of an inappropriate use of an expensive human resource. Modern information transfer and electronic communication systems allow rapid and accurate transfer of information along electronic communication networks.

Software and hardware for modern electronic communication networks are only two aspects of an information infrastructure. The other major aspect is lacking in most hospitals and health services organizations, that is, the absence of appropriate infrastructure to facilitate information management. Infrastructure includes but is not limited to data management policies and procedures, methods for data stewardship and custodianship, user training, and information management support staff. Support staff are necessary to support nurses in analyzing and interpreting information appropriately.

 ## Issues Related to Effective Nursing Management of Information

Primary among the nursing issues related to information management in Canada is the lack of adequate educational programs in information management techniques and strategies for nurse clinicians and nursing managers. At the time of writing, there are only a few preservice nursing education programs in Canada offering a course in modern information management techniques and strategies related to nursing. At a minimum, such a program must include advanced study of information management techniques and strategies such as information flow analysis, the use of spreadsheets, databases, and word processing packages. Ideally such courses would also introduce concepts and provide hands-on experience related to the use of patient care information systems.

Another major issue is that nursing is frequently underrepresented in the selection and installation of patient care information systems and financial management systems in Canada. Regrettably, many senior nurse managers fail to recognize the importance of this activity and opt out of the process. They then complain when the systems do not meet the needs of nursing. Canadian senior nursing executives must recognize the importance of allocating staff and money to participate in the strategic planning process for information systems in their organizations. Other senior management personnel must also recognize the importance of nursing

input into the strategic planning process for information systems. In any hospital, nurses are the single largest group of professionals using a patient care system and nursing represents the largest part of the budget requiring financial management. Nursing, therefore, represents the single largest stakeholder group in Canada related to either a patient care information system or a financial information system.

Nurses have been involved in the management of nursing information since the initial systems for gathering minimum uniform health data which can be traced back to systems devised by Florence Nightingale over a century ago (Verley, 1970). This early role in the management of nursing information began to change dramatically with the introduction of computers into healthcare and nursing environments. The role evolved as nurses became more involved in the selection and utilization of information systems. These developments have been well documented elsewhere (Hannah, Ball, and Edwards, 2005) along with detailed information on the nursing responsibilities, roles, and contributions to the selection and implementation of information systems in healthcare organizations. The issues for nurses no longer relate to computers or management information systems but rather information and information management. The computer and its associated software are merely tools to support nurses as they practice their profession. Far too much attention has been directed to the technology rather than its content. Current hospital information systems do little to assist nurses in their real role, which is providing nursing care. Canadian nurses must be able to manage and process nursing data, information, and knowledge to support patient care delivery in diverse care delivery settings. To accomplish this goal, Canadian nurses are increasingly focusing on the contents (the data) contained in information systems instead of being distracted by the glamour and romance of the technology.

Unfortunately, despite Nightingale's early attempts to develop a nursing database, nurses in Canada have yet to reach consensus on the minimum set of data elements essential to the practice of nursing and the coding of those elements. In fact, at present in Canada, there are absolutely no nursing data elements that are collected and stored provincially or nationally for use in decision-making related to health policy or resource allocation. Nurses in Canada who have developed a heightened awareness of the importance of collection, storage, and retrieval of nursing data have recognized these data gaps. In 1990, attention began to be directed at initiating the process by which the nursing profession in Canada will begin to address the essential data needs of nurses in all practice settings in Canada (Canadian Nurses Association, 1990).

The patient discharge abstracts prepared by medical records departments across Canada and the United States currently contain no patient care delivery information. The abstracts therefore fail to acknowledge the contribution of nursing during the patient's stay in the hospital. This is important because the abstracts are used by many agencies for a variety of purposes including funding allocation and policy making. Presently, much valuable information is being lost. This information is important in determining the actual costs of hospitalization and the effectiveness of nursing care in achieving appropriate patient outcomes.

At a time when considerable emphasis is being placed on the development of a national health database in Canada, it is important that a minimum number of essential nursing elements be included in that database. In Canada these nursing data elements are beginning to be referred to as the Nursing Components of Health Information (HI:NC). Such a set of data elements would be similar to the uniquely nursing elements included in the Nursing Minimum Data Set (NMDS) currently being tested in the United States. The nursing profession in Canada must provide the leadership in defining appropriate nursing data elements to be included in the national health database, specifically through the patient discharge abstract. In Canada, there is a need to extend the use of the concept of the HI:NC.

Thus the salient issue in information management for nurses in Canada is that of identification of nursing data elements that are essential for collection and storage in a national health database. These data elements must reflect the data that nurses use to build information that is the foundation for clinical judgement and management decision-making in any setting where nursing is practiced. The remainder of this chapter will focus on the issue of defining those data elements that are essential to the practice of nursing.

Initiatives Directed at the Development of Nursing Components of Health Information for Use in Canada

In Canada, nurses are in the fortunate position of recognizing the need for nursing data elements at the time when the status of national health information is under review. The challenge for nurses is to capitalize on this timing and define those data elements required by nurses in Canada. To prevent losing control of nursing data, Canadian nurses must take a proactive stance and mobilize resources to ensure the development and implementation of a national health data base that is congruent with the needs of nurses in all practice settings in Canada. Some initiatives intended to promote the vision of a national health data base becoming a reality in Canada are in progress.

Prompted by the work of our U.S. colleagues on the NMDS, and in response to contextual factors influencing nursing in Canada, nurses in Canada have recognized the importance of the collection and storage of essential data elements (CNA, 1990). Initiatives are currently underway directed at building awareness and consensus regarding the definition and coding of these essential data elements. Amongst these initiatives are strategic plans for the development of HI:NC for use in Canada.

CNA responded to a resolution calling for a national consensus conference "to develop in Canada a standardized format (NMDS) for purposes of ensuring entry, accessibility, and retrievability of nursing data" (Canadian Nurses Association, 1990). The Nursing Minimum Data Set Conference was held in Edmonton, Canada, October 27–29, 1992. The overall objective of this working conference was to develop a NMDS in Canada to ensure both the availability and accessibility of standardized nursing data. Due to recognition of the paucity of dialogue that had taken place on the topic among Canadian nurses and the inappropriateness of attempting to achieve consensus on the topic at such an early stage, the invitational conference brought together those individuals best able to formulate a plan for initiating the development of a NMDS in Canada. The Canadian NMDS conference culminated in the identification of five elements:

- Client status is broadly defined as a label for the set of indicators that reflect the phenomena for which nurses provide care, relative to the health status of clients (McGee, 1993). Although client status is similar to nursing diagnosis, the term client status was preferred because it represents a broader spectrum of health and illness. The common label "client status" is inclusive of input from all disciplines. The summative statements referring to the phenomena for which nurses provide care (i.e., nursing diagnosis) are merely one aspect of client status at a point in time, in the same way as medical diagnosis.

- Nursing interventions refer to purposeful and deliberate health affecting interventions (direct and indirect), based on assessment of client status, which are designed to bring about results which benefit clients (Alberta Association of Registered Nurses [AARN], 1994).

- Client outcome is defined as a "clients' status at a defined point(s) following health care [affecting] intervention" (Marek and Lang, 1993). It is influenced to varying degrees by the interventions of all care providers.

- Nursing intensity "refers to the amount and type of nursing resource used to [provide] care" (O'Brien-Pallas and Giovannetti, 1993).

- Primary nurse identifier is a single unique lifetime identification number for each individual nurse. This identifier is independent of geographic location (province or territory), practice sector (e.g., acute care, community care, and public health), or employer.

Group deliberations on each of the data elements are summarized elsewhere (Canadian Nurses Association, 1993). These nursing data elements were proposed for addition to existing national data sets as a next step toward a cross-sectoral, multidisciplinary, longitudinal national health database in Canada (Canadian Nurses Association, 1993). However, some individuals and national organizations in Canada perceived the Canadian use of the term "NMDS" to portray a stand-alone nursing data set such as that in the United States. In Canada, this was not the intent. It is essential in Canada that the nursing data elements constitute one component of fully integrated health information data, e.g., the CIHI Discharge Abstract Data Set (Canadian Institute for Health Information, 2002) or an EHR such as that being developed under the leadership of Infoway. Therefore, the five nursing data elements were identified collectively as the Nursing Components of Health Information (Health Information: Nursing Components, HI:NC) (Canadian Nurses Association, 1993).

Following the conference in 1992, CNA's Working Group on the Nursing Components of Health Information (HI:NC Working Group) continued to build on the work that had been started, and in 1997 a national consensus was reached on three clinical nursing care data elements: *client status, nursing intervention,* and *client outcome* as well as *nursing resource intensity* and *nurse identifier* (Canadian Nurses Association, 2001).

Identifying those data elements that represent the most important aspects of nursing care is only the first step. In Canada, nurses face an immediate challenge to determine the most effective and efficient means to collect and code data elements that reflect nursing practice. To collect the data reflecting nursing contributions

within the larger health information system, *there is a need for consistent data collection using standardized languages to aggregate and compare data* (Canadian Nurses Association, 1998).

In October 1999, a meeting was held at CIHI in Toronto. Representatives of CIHI and CNA, as well as nurse researchers and nursing informatics specialists, from across the country, discussed the gaps and opportunities for nursing data in the national health databases held by CIHI. A number of nursing informatics leaders representing CNA supported ICNP® in principle as the most universal, generic, and comprehensive foundational classification system for nursing at the time. CIHI representatives committed to exploring the inclusion of the five data elements comprising the HI:NC in their national data bases. Regrettably, CIHI's investigation of the version of ICNP® available at the time (the early Beta Version) revealed that the lack of a coding structure was a significant barrier to implementation at that time. This barrier has now been eliminated in the Beta 2 Version. Another barrier was the apparent lack of awareness and consensus among nurses about the need for and importance of capturing nursing data nationally. As discussed in the following paragraph, the second barrier has been substantially reduced in the intervening 4 years since the CIHI analysis of ICNP®.

In March 2000, CNA completed a discussion paper (Canadian Nurses Association, 2000), which proposed that registered nurses in Canada support ICNP®, in principle, as the foundational classification system for nursing practice in Canada. Responses and feedback received from the consultation related to this discussion paper indicated strong support from CNA's member jurisdictions for investigating how ICNP® might be adapted for use in Canada (Canadian Nurses Association, 2001). The result was the CNA Position Statement: Collecting Data to Reflect the Impact of Nursing Practice (Canadian Nurses Association, 2001).

In Canada, nurses have come to recognize the need to incorporate the HI:NC into the national health information infostructure (national data bases and EHR) as federal and provincial health information systems are being re-structured. To ensure that nursing data are incorporated into the national health infostructure, nurses must participate in the design, standards development, and pilot studies to ensure the capture of data that are essential to reflect the contribution of nursing to healthcare in Canada.

As nurses in Canada pursue the development of the HI:NC, several issues germane to the development of minimum data sets emerge. The first need is to ensure that data are available, reliable, valid, and comparable, i.e., data standards are established. To this end the CNA has endorsed the ICNP® for use in Canada. It is also important to define the scope of the compiled data set to ensure that only those essential data elements are collected and to avoid proliferation of data. In addition, it is essential to promote the concept to ensure widespread use and educate the nurses to ensure the quality of the data that are collected.

Implications of the Nursing Components of Health Information

In the absence of a national system for the collection, storage, and retrieval of nursing data elements, it is evident that much valuable information is being lost. In Canada, as in other countries, this information is important to demonstrate the contribution nursing makes to the care of the patient and to demonstrate the cost effectiveness of nursing care (Werley et al., 1988, 1991). As we move away from nursing specific models of patient care delivery to models that focus on the patient emphasizing collaboration of disciplines, multi-skilling of healthcare providers, standardization of care, and streamlining of documentation through charting by exception, it is imperative that nurses be able to articulate what is and is not nursing's role. Further nurses will be asked to demonstrate nursing's contribution to patient care in terms of outcome measures that are objective and measurable. Nurses require nursing data to identify outcomes of nursing care, defend resource allocation to nursing, and justify new roles for nursing in the healthcare delivery system (Gallant, 1988; McPhillips, 1988; Werley et al., 1991). Similarly, nurses need to understand and value nursing data so that in the selection and implementation of information systems for their organizations, nurse administrators insist that they or their designate play a major role and that nursing data needs are incorporated into the selection and implementation criteria. For greater detail on selection and implementation, the reader is referred to Hannah, Ball, and Edwards (2005).

While on the one hand we must preserve our professional nursing identity, Canadian nurses must balance this against professional ghettoization. The collection and storage of essential nursing data elements that are not integrated as components of a national EHR and national patient care data sets will serve to ghettoize nursing especially in a socialized health case system such as Canada's. This is dangerous at a time when significant emphasis is being placed on multidisciplinary collaboration, patient-focused care, and patient outcomes. In Canada, contributions to the only national health database are voluntary rather than legislated and the elements are established by consensus rather than by legislation. In view of priorities in Canadian healthcare as well as the culture of negotiation and consensus, the nursing participation in the determination of the integrated data elements could not be clearer.

Nurse clinicians need to know what nursing elements are essential for archival purposes so that nursing documentation is inclusive of these elements. With the move toward standardization of care through the use of care maps it is essential that outcomes of nursing care are determined and included in the care maps. As healthcare organizations embrace the concept of charting by exception in an effort to decrease the valuable hours spent by healthcare workers in documentation, nurses must be sure that those tools that outline the inherent patient care delivered are not devoid of nursing in contribution to patient care. For in the absence of data that reflect nursing activities there is no archival record of what nurses do, what difference nursing care makes, or why nurses are required. At times of fiscal restraint, objective nursing data is required to substantiate the role of nurses and the nurse:patient ratios required in the clinical setting.

Nurse researchers need a data base of essential data elements to facilitate the identification of trends related to the data elements for specific patient groups, institutions, or regions and to assess variables on multiple levels including institutional, local, regional, and national (Werley et al., 1988). The collection and storage of essential nursing data elements will facilitate the advancement of nursing as a research-based discipline (Werley and Zorn, 1988). Nurse educators need these essential nursing data elements to develop nursing knowledge for use in educating nurses and to facilitate the definition of the scope of nursing practice (McCloskey, 1988).

Finally, the definition of HI:NC is essential to influence health policy decision-making. Historically health policy has been created in the absence of nursing data. At a time when we are in the midst of profound healthcare reform it is essential that nurses demonstrate the central role of nursing services in the restructuring of the healthcare delivery system.

Meeting the Challenge: Canadian Nursing Informatics Association (CNIA)

Although the cadre of Canadian nurses working in informatics roles has increased over the past decade, it is clear that efforts are needed to increase awareness of all nurses of the relevance of informatics to the profession. In particular, our nurse leaders in practice and education need to embrace and assist in advancing the health informatics agenda and assure that nurses are engaged. Throughout the 1990s, a few nursing informatics interest groups emerged in various parts of the country; some have endured while others have not. Specifically, in 1999, a Board decision was made to disband the COACH (Canada's Health Informatics Organization) Nursing Informatics Special Interest Group (NI-SIG). Despite the numerous accomplishments and leadership within this group, the nurse membership was low and few nurses perceived the benefits of joining the group. Suffice it to say that a minority of nurses perceived any relevance of informatics to the scope of their daily work. Moreover, the multiplicity of forces compelling governments and healthcare leaders to adopt technology solutions today, were less evident even then.

Today health informatics in Canada has been propelled to the forefront of healthcare management strategies with substantial, focused investments in ICTs by the federal and provincial governments (Irving, 2003). In general, healthcare provider organizations are beginning to appreciate the strategic and clinical value of care transformation through the use of ICTs. Providers are also being challenged by the need for cost-containment and a clear demonstration of the effective inputs and outputs of clinical care delivery. In this regard, the importance of capturing, interpreting, and profiling the significant contribution of nurses to the health outcomes of Canadians has never been more profound.

With the dissolution of the COACH NI-SIG, a group of nurses committed to the importance of informatics for all nurses began to formalize a new national nursing informatics organization. In 2002, the CNIA was established under the leadership of Dr. Lynn Nagle. The CNIA represents a national nursing perspective on issues of health informatics and provides opportunities for nurses to network and lead on issues of nursing informatics. The mandate of the CNIA is to engage nurses in all sectors and is inclusive of nurses in practice, administrative, educational, or research roles. In a very short time, the CNIA has been deemed an essential structure to assure the positioning of Canadian nurses to influence national and provincial ICT strategies.

CNIA Objectives

The need to harness the existing nursing informatics expertise, address the required informatics competencies of all nurses, and extend the profession's understanding of the significance of health informatics are key priorities for the CNIA. The overall objectives include the following:

- To provide nursing leadership for the development of nursing/health informatics in Canada.
- To establish national networking opportunities for nurse informaticians.
- To facilitate informatics educational opportunities for all nurses in Canada.
- To engage in international nursing informatics initiatives.
- To act as a nursing advisory group in matters of nursing and health informatics.
- To expand awareness of nursing informatics to all nurses and the healthcare community.

The achievement of these objectives is being operationalized through a number of initiatives; some of which will be subsequently described.

CNIA Membership and Affiliations

The CNIA membership is constituted primarily by registered nurses, but is also open to vendor and non-nurse participation. The Board of Directors is comprised of nursing informatics leaders representative of each provincial and territorial region. The CNIA has leveraged its position and formalized linkages with regional nursing informatics interest groups previously in existence and is working to support the emergence of new regional groups.

In establishing the CNIA, the interim board of directors sought the support of CNA. A clear alignment with the national professional organization was viewed as a strength for the future sustainability of the group. At its inception, the CNIA was supported by the CNA as an "Emerging Group." In 2004, the scope and growth of CNIA's national membership and compliance with the CNA criteria, afforded CNIA "Associate Group" status. This status brings further credence to the CNIA and opportunities to review and influence relevant national nursing policy and strategic directions.

The emergence of the CNIA was also strongly supported by COACH and a formal strategic alliance was established at the outset. In recent years, COACH has provided the association with instrumental support at the annual eHealth conferences; affording the CNIA publicity and recognition as a supporting organization of the conferences. In addition, the CNIA has the option to submit content and updates to the COACH e-Newsletter on a regular basis.

CNIA's formal alliance with COACH has also facilitated the appointment of the Canadian nurse nominee to the International Medical Informatics Association—Nursing Informatics Working Group (IMIA-NI WG). The IMIA-NI WG provides an opportunity to engage with international nursing informatics colleagues and extend our learnings beyond our national borders. Opportunities to further leverage respective expertise and experiences are already under discussion with colleagues in the United States, Europe, South America, and Australia.

CNIA is also participating in a collaborative forum designed to engage key Canadian health informatics and health professional organizations in discussions regarding the national ICT strategies being supported by Canada's Health Infoway Inc. Members of this collaborative include Infoway, COACH, CNA, Canadian Medical Association (CMA), Canadian Health Information Management Association (CHIMA), and the Canadian Telehealth Society.

CNIA Initiatives

In May 2002, the CNIA secured funding from the federal agency, Office of Health Information Highway (OHIH) to undertake a national study of Canadian Schools of Nursing. This study was directed to deriving a better understanding of the informatics education being provided to nurses in basic education programs across the country. In particular, the study focused on the availability of informatics expertise among nursing faculty, informatics content within core curricula, and the state of technology infrastructure to support informatics in schools of nursing. Completed in 2003, the study findings highlighted the significant gaps in the informatics knowledge of nursing faculty, the lack of informatics integration into core curricula, and the need for investment in ICT infrastructure in Canadian Schools of Nursing. Recommendations have been directed to a number of professional nursing organizations, but particularly the Canadian Association of Schools of Nursing (CASN), the Association of Canadian Executive Nurses (ACEN), the Office of Nursing Policy (ONP), CNIA, and CNA. A copy of the final report is posted on the CNIA Web site (*www.cnia.ca*) (Clarke, 2003). Several presentations have been made to a number of nursing groups and the study findings have been published (Nagle and Clarke, 2004).

CNIA's is currently focused on addressing the need for education and communication on issues of nursing informatics. In June 2004, with the support of the CNA, the CNIA held a full day preconference workshop for nurse leaders attending the CNA Biennium in St. John's, Newfoundland. The workshop introduced basic informatics concepts and provided the participants with demonstrations of informatics in practice and education. The content of this workshop has been captured for the purpose of future replication in a variety of forums.

In the fall of 2004, CNIA launched "Nursing Informatics Rounds" online. Supported by Longwoods Publishing and a gift-in-kind from Bell Canada, these rounds are being Webcast to nurse participants across the country. The topics are varied but focus primarily on case illustrations of interest to administrators, educators, and practitioners. These sessions are designed to demonstrate the impact and relevance of informatics for Canadian nurses. This educational initiative is concurrently under evaluation and its success yet to be determined. Members of the CNIA will be provided with a certificate of completion for their attendance in these rounds.

At the time of this writing, members of the CNIA also receive regular updates through the Web site and a quarterly newsletter. Members also have the opportunity to dialogue with other nurse colleagues online with regard to any topics of interest. Plans are currently in progress to hold the first Canadian Nursing Informatics Conference in the fall of 2005.

 ## Conclusion

It is clear that a priority for nursing in Canada is the identification of the HI:NC, those essential nursing data elements that must be collected, stored, and retrieved from a national health information database. Nursing leaders must respond to the challenge to identify those data essential for the management of patient care and patient care units. The HI:NC have the potential to provide nurses with the data required to build information for use in reshaping nursing, as a profession prepared to respond to the health needs of Canadians in the twenty-first century; however, the window of opportunity to have nursing data elements included in a national data set is narrowing. We must ensure that the vision of nursing components in our national health information system becomes a reality for nursing in Canada.

 ## References

Advisory Committee on Health Human Resources. (2000). *The Nursing Strategy for Canada*. Conference of Deputy Ministers, Ottawa.

Advisory Committee on Health Infostructure. (2001). *Tactical Plan for a Pan-Canadian Health Infostructure: 2001 Update*. Office of Health and the Information Highway, Health Canada, Ottawa.

Alberta Association of Registered Nurses (AARN). (1994). *Client Status, Nursing Intervention and Client Outcome Taxonomies: A Background Paper*. Edmonton: Author.

Angus, D. E. (1989). *Review of Significant Health Care Commissions and Task Forces*. Ottawa: CNA.

Canada Health Infoway Inc. (2002). *Annual Report: Accelerating the Development of Electronic Health Information Systems for Canadians*. Montreal, Author.

Canadian Institute for Health Information. (2002). *http://www.cihi.ca/*. Accessed September 20, 2004.

Canadian Network for the Advancement of Research, Industry, and Education (CANARIE). (1996). *Towards a Canadian Health Iway: Vision, Opportunities, and Future Steps*. Ottawa: Author.

Canadian Nurses Association. (1990). Report of the Resolutions Committee. Unpublished.

Canadian Nurses Association. (1993). *Papers from the Nursing Minimum Data Set Conference*. Ottawa: Author.

Canadian Nurses Association. (1998). *Policy Statement: Evidence-Based Decision-Making and Nursing Practice*. Ottawa: Author.

Canadian Nurses Association (CNA). (1999). *http://www.cna-nurses.ca*.

Canadian Nurses Association. (2000). *Collecting Data to Reflect Nursing Impact: A Discussion Paper*. Ottawa: Author.

Canadian Nurses Association. (2001). *Making Nursing Evident: Nursing Informatics Strategy Session*. Ottawa. Unpublished.

Canadian Nurses Association. (2001). *Position Statement: Collecting Data to Reflect the Impact of Nursing Practice*. Ottawa: Author.

Clair, M. (2000). *Emerging Solutions Report of Commission d'étude sur les services de santé et les services sociaux*. Government of Quebec, Quebec.

Clark, J. and Lang N. (1992). Nursing's next advance: An international classification for nursing practice. *International Journal of Nursing* 39(4):102–112, 128.

Clarke, H. (2003). *Assessing the Informatics Education Needs of Canadian Nurses—Educational Institution Component*. Report Submitted to Health Canada, Office of Health Information Highway. Project G3-6B-DP1-0054.

Epp, J. (1986). *Achieving Health for All: A Framework for Health Promotion*. Ottawa: Health and Welfare Canada.

Fyke, K. J. (2001). *Caring for Medicare Sustaining a Quality System*. Government of Saskatchewan, Regina.

Gallant, B. J. (1988). Data requirements for the nursing minimum data set as seen by nurse administrators. In H. H. Werley and N. M. Lang (Eds.), *Identification of the Nursing Minimum Data Set* (pp. 165–176). New York: Springer.

Graves, J. R. and S. Corcoran (1989). The study of nursing informatics. *Image: Journal of Nursing Scholarship* 21(4):227–231.

Hannah, K. J. and Anderson, B. (1994). Management of nursing information. In J. Hibbert and M. Kyle (Eds.), *Canadian Nursing Management*. Toronto: W.B. Saunders.

Hannah, K. J. and Shamian, J. (1992). Integrating a nursing professional practice model and nursing informatics in a collective bargaining environment. In *Nursing Clinics of North America*. Philadelphia, PA: W. B. Saunders.

Hannah, K. J., Ball, M., and Edwards, M. J. A. (2005). *Introduction to Nursing Informatics* (3rd ed.). New York: Springer-Verlag.

Health Canada. (1997). *Health and the Information Highway (News Release)*. Ottawa: Health Canada.

Information Highway Advisory Council. (1995). *Final Report of the Information Highway Advisory Council*. Ottawa: Industry Canada.

Irving, R. (2003). *2003 Report on I.T. in Canadian Hospitals: Top Issues, Applications and Vendors*.

Jydstrup, R. A. and Gross, M. J. (1966). Cost of information handling in hospitals: Rochester region. *Health Services Research* 1:235–271.

Lalonde, M. (1974). *A New Perspective on the Health of Canadians*. Ottawa: Queen's Printer.

Marek, K. and N. Lang (1993). Nursing sensitive outcomes. *Papers from the Nursing Minimum Data Set Conference* (100–120). Canadian Nurses Association. Ottawa: Canadian Nurses Association.

Mazankowski, D. (2002). *Framework for Reform Report of the Premier's Advisory Council on Health*. Edmonton: Alberta Queen's Printer.

McCloskey, J. C. (1988). The nursing minimum data set: Benefits and implications for nurse educators. In *National League for Nursing, Perspectives in Nursing 1987–1989* (pp. 119–126). New York: National League for Nursing.

McGee, M. (1993). Response to V. Saba's paper on Nursing Diagnostic Schemes. *Papers from the Nursing Minimum Data Set Conference* (pp. 64–67). Canadian Nurses Association. Ottawa: Canadian Nurses Association.

McPhillips, R. (1988). Essential elements for the nursing minimum data set as seen by federal officials. In H. H. Werley and N. M. Lang (Eds.), *Identification of the Nursing Minimum Data Set* (pp. 233–238). New York: Springer.

Nagle, L. M. and Clarke, H. (2004). Assessing the informatics education needs of Canadian nurses. In M. Fieschi, E. Coiera, and Y. J. Li (Eds.), *Proceedings of the 11th World Congress on Medical Informatics*. Bethesda, MA: AMIA.

National Forum on Health. (1997). *Canada Health Action: Building on the Legacy. The Final Report of the National Forum on Health* (Vol. I). Ottawa: Prime Minister's Office.

National Task Force on Health Information. (1990). An opportunity to renew Canada's health information systems. M. Wilk. Ottawa, National Health Information Council, Health Canada. Unpublished Manuscript.

O'Brien-Pallas, L. and Giovannetti, P. (1993). Nursing intensity. *Papers from the Nursing Minimum Data Set Conference* (pp. 68–76). C. N. Association. Ottawa: Canadian Nurses Association.

Project Team for the Planning of the Canadian Institute for Health Information. (1991). Canadian Institute for Health Information Planning Report to the Conference of Deputy Ministers of Health (Hannah Report). K. J. Hannah. Ottawa, National Health Information Council, Health Canada. Unpublished.

Romanow, R. J. (2002). *Building on Values: The Future of Health Care in Canada*. Ottawa: Queen's Printer.

Royal Commission on Health Services (Hall Commission). (1964). *Royal Commission on Health Services*. Ottawa: Queen's Printer.

Standing Senate Committee on Social Affairs Science and Technology (Chair: The Honourable Michael J. L. Kirby). (2002). *Final Report: The Health of Canadians—The Federal Role*. Ottawa: Queen's Printer.

Verley, H. (1970). *Florence Nightingale at Harley Street*. London: Dent & Sons.

Werley, H. H., Devine, E. C., Zorn, C. R., Ryan, P, and Westra, B. L. (1991). The nursing minimum data set: Abstraction tool for standardized, comparable, essential data. *American Journal of Public Health* 81:421–426.

Werley, H. H., and Zorn, C. R. (1988). The nursing minimum data set: Benefits and implications. In *National League for Nursing, Perspectives in Nursing—1987–1989* (pp. 105–114). New York: National League for Nursing.

Wilk, M. B. (1991). Health Information for Canada 1991: Report of the National Task Force on Health Information. Ottawa: National Health Information Council.

38

Nursing Informatics in Europe

Margareta Ehnfors

Anna Ehrenberg

Rolf Nikula

OBJECTIVES

1. Describe elements of the European Union (EU) e-Health action plan.
2. Reflect on electronic patient records (EPRs).
3. Describe nursing terminology work in Europe.
4. Give examples of initiatives to develop nursing minimum data sets in Europe.
5. Give examples of European models of terminology/information.
6. Explain the difference between technical installation, functional implementation, and organizational implementation.
7. Give examples of future developments.

KEY WORDS

overview on Europe, IT, and nursing informatics
electronic patient records (EPR)
terminologies
implementation of health information systems

In Europe, as in many countries worldwide, the main rational for implementing a greater use of information technology (IT) in the healthcare sector is to improve safety and quality, improve patient outcomes, and at the same time try to reduce costs of healthcare. Europe is a continent with over 750 million inhabitants in about 50 countries with many different languages, cultures, social systems, and other living conditions. This makes it obvious that it is not possible to provide the entire picture of nursing informatics in the area. Instead, this presentation will give a couple of examples from Europe with emphasis on the situation in Scandinavia; however, many of the issues that will be mentioned are common for many countries both within and outside Europe.

Widespread use of IT in the healthcare services is very limited in comparison to other areas of society. Informatics or computerized solutions were accepted and fully integrated first by manufacturers and production of services in the 1980s, next in business services such as banking, and only in the 1990s was it introduced in the healthcare sector. It will probably not be developed to its optimum in supporting core processes in patient care for another 10 years. Part of the reason is the fact that managing peoples' illness and health is very complex. In many areas we have found that the use of knowledge and applications in nursing, quality assurance, and nursing informatics in Europe mostly starts 5–10 years after the same development in the United States, although the gap is slowly decreasing partly due to the development of IT.

The main mission, in Europe, is to establish a stable infrastructure that improves healthcare quality, facilitates the reduction of errors, and the delivery of evidence-based and cost-effective care. Some core building blocks of this are electronic health records (EHRs), nursing informatics education at all levels, communication and terminologies, and standards for technology, communication, and patient care.

IT in the European Union (EU)

Within the growing EU the informatics issues have a central position. The European Commission (EC) is a driving force of healthcare informatics development by funding projects that are all cross-cultural involving healthcare professional users, educators, and administrators, always with three or more countries participating. In May 2004, the EC adopted an action plan, the "e-Health Action Plan" aiming at delivering better quality healthcare throughout Europe. The plan covers many aspects of informatics such as electronic prescriptions, computerized patient records, and information systems to cut waiting time and reduce errors. The plan sets out the objective of a "European e-Health Area" and many practical steps to reach this are identified; among other things a high-speed Internet access for health systems is needed. One goal is that by 2005 member states (in EU) should develop their own roadmaps for e-Health, and an EU public health portal should be up and running to provide a one-stop shop to access health information. They also agreed that work needs to progress to allow measurement of the impact of e-Health technologies on the quality and efficiency of services as well as productivity. Europe is strong on healthcare and electronic business and this will be used for the benefit of patients. The goal is that four out of five European physicians have access to Internet and one out of four European citizens use the Internet to get information on health and illness. More information on e-Health can be found at *http://europa.eu.int/information_society/qualif/health/index_en.htm.*

National IT Strategy

There are many European countries that have developed national IT policies and strategies. The government's IT policy in Sweden has three objectives: confidence in IT, competence to use IT, and information about society services available to all citizens. One goal is that all households and companies in all parts of Sweden within a few years should have access to an IT infrastructure with high-speed connections. The government supports the private enterprises to reach this and other IT-related goals. Confidence in IT also implies that citizens must trust that information retrieved is secure and invisible to others when needed. The use of electronic signatures will facilitate this. Another goal is the ability to communicate between systems. The directors of all the regional healthcare services in Sweden have agreed to develop their hospital systems so that they can communicate with each

other nationwide and still keeping confidentiality rules. This is different from the fragmented information management currently in place in many instances. The first phase of the project is focused on the admitting data that should be possible to share among different healthcare professionals and geographical areas to enhance the security and also adhere to the idea of data once entered are used many times. Most of the staff in hospitals or other healthcare agencies is not (due to security reasons) connected to the Internet where a lot of knowledge is found. Another problem is that the information and knowledge available on the Internet most frequently is presented in English, which is not the first language in most European countries.

There are not enough data standards agreed on or implemented to allow comparison of information based on aggregation of data from different sites. This deficiency hampers the current ability to build knowledge from patient care data.

Patient Participation

One of the grounds for the e-Health Action Plan in the EU is that the ministers have identified the potential for citizen empowerment through widespread availability of high quality appropriate health information on the Internet. This is in line with the focus of Nordic nursing research on patient participation. Studies have found that improved patient participation and the consideration of patient preferences have improved outcomes and treatment adherence, as well as increased patient satisfaction with their care.

Continuity of Care and Availability of Information

Key concepts in Europe are continuity of care and care providers, and to meet the healthcare needs of a more mobile population. This is supported by many projects aiming at making data available in different settings including the patient's home and also by practicing telemedicine. Telemedicine or telehealth, which is the practice of medicine and nursing over a distance where data and documents are transmitted through telecommunication systems, is widely disseminated in parts over Europe. There are some established systems, and a number of developments under way. According to their own reporting, many countries, such as Austria, Germany, Greece, Slovenia, France, United Kingdom, Ireland, Belgium, Denmark, Norway, Finland, Sweden, Iceland, Portugal, Spain, and Italy are practicing telemedicine, but the practice by other allied health professions is rare. Some countries have a special legislation regulating telemedicine (Äärimaa, 2003).

Electronic Patient Records

Although most nurses by their professional behavior make notes on patient care, such as their assessments, decisions, and evaluations, only a few European countries have a law forcing nurses to record nursing. All registered nurses (RNs) in Sweden are by law, since 1986, obliged to document nursing care (SFS, 1985). Regulations emphasize that RNs have an autonomous responsibility for planning, implementing, and evaluating nursing care and that nursing diagnoses in the patient record is a part of that responsibility (SOSFS, 1990). Nurses gradually have accepted the idea of nursing diagnoses, but there are no agreed standardized expressions or routinely implemented nursing diagnoses in practice. Swedish nurses prefer the use of problem statements.

A Swedish study by the National Board of Health and Welfare (2000) can be used to illustrate the increasing amount of information in healthcare: In 1971 a 4-week hospital stay generated three sheets of paper, in 1984 it generated 18 sheets, and in 1999 a shorter stay of 10 days generated 34 sheets of record information. The solution is not to write more and more, but instead to focus on the relevant information. The nursing diagnosis is the weakest link in the nursing process, and thus it is promising that some projects have shown that educational efforts have positive effects on both quantity and quality of nursing diagnoses. Common flaws found in studies in nursing recording are unspecific notes, systematic assessment and nursing diagnoses are rare, and a lack of planned and prioritized interventions.

Dissemination of Electronic Patient Records

In Norway and Sweden EPRs are quite common both in primary healthcare and in hospitals. In Sweden the estimated occurrence of EPR in primary healthcare is 85–90% while the percentage for hospitals is about 40%. In Norway there are EPRs for 81% of the hospital beds (Laerum, 2004).

Development of Common Terminology for Nursing Practice in Europe

Because of the heterogeneity of European countries and their healthcare systems, it is not easy or straightforward to present an overview of the development of common terminologies for nursing practice. Our attempt is to give a few examples from the European arena, without laying claims to give a comprehensive survey of this field so full of nuances.

There is probably a great variety in reasons for the development of uniform terminologies for nursing in different European countries. Some of the common factors that may have contributed are the increasing cost constraints in the mostly publicly financed healthcare systems, which have raised demands for cost-effective care and quality improvement. The professionalization of nursing, the effort to make nursing visible and aspirations for greater accountability have been additional influencing factors. One of the early initiatives that laid a foundation for terminology work in nursing was the concerted action on "People's needs for nursing care" by the World Health Organization that was accomplished in many European countries in the 1980s (WHO, 1987). This was an important milestone in European nursing, which raised the awareness about the need to make nursing care more visible. The nursing process was used as a framework for the project, a framework which has continuously provided a foundation for many terminology initiatives within nursing in Europe. During the 1990s, the activities in many European countries on quality assurance/improvement and the introduction of the electronic health record, pushed for standardization and accessibility of nursing information.

Belgium, undoubtedly, is the European country that has made nursing care most visible and where early on the contribution of nursing in healthcare has been acknowledged by national level policy makers. Since 1988, it is mandatory for all hospitals in the country to collect data four times per year, using the Belgian nursing minimum data set (B-NMDS). The NMDS consists of 23 nursing interventions, medical diagnoses, patient demographics, nurse variables, and institutional characteristics (Sermeus et al., 1994; Sermeus and Deleis, 1997). The 23 nursing interventions have been derived from extensive testing, and cover areas such as hygiene, mobility, elimination and feeding assistance, and wound care. There have only been a few additional initiatives on NMDS in Europe, as for example, the Swiss CH-NMDS (Berthou and Junger, 2000).

In the Netherlands, a nursing information reference model (NIRM) has been developed to accommodate both the information needs of nurses at the clinical level and for aggregating data at higher levels (Goossen, Epping, and Dassen, 1997a,b). The model identifies a base level of patient data; a second level of interpretations and decisions by the nurse, including nursing diagnoses, interventions, and outcomes; a third level of aggregated data on nursing diagnoses, interventions, and outcomes for institutional purposes; and a fourth level of information aggregated for international sharing.

The development of terminology work in the Nordic countries holds some common features. The national nursing associations worked jointly on quality assurance during the late 1980s, which was one of the foundations for the awareness of the need for common terminology in nursing. The level of computerization is generally high in society, which also may have been a contributing incentive for development. Nurses in Denmark were early pioneers in the development of common terminology and informatics in Europe. In the early 1990s, Danish nurses initiated the joint project, "Telenurse," within the EU to promote standardization of nursing data in electronic health records (Mortensen, 1999). This project was later linked to the International Council of Nurses' (ICN) project for development of an International Classification for Nursing Practice (ICNP) (Clark and Lang, 1992; ICN, 2001), which has had an impact on the interest for the ICNP in Europe.

In Sweden it became mandatory for nurses to keep patient records in 1986, which sparked local efforts to apply the nursing process for recording. The VIPS model (acronym for the Swedish spelling of Well-being, Integrity, Prevention, and Safety) was developed with the purpose of conceptualizing the essential elements of nursing care, clarifying and facilitating systematic thinking and nursing recording (Ehnfors, Thorell-Ekstrand, and Ehrenberg, 1991; Ehrenberg, Ehnfors, and Thorell-Ekstrand, 1996). The nursing documentation model is based on the structure of the nursing process, and in addition includes other areas for which the nurse has responsibility and is accountable for recording. The focus of the model is on patients' functioning in daily life activities rather than on pathophysiologic problems. Experience has shown that the model has good content validity in different areas of nursing care (Ehrenberg, Ehnfors, and Thorell-Ekstrand, 1996). The VIPS model is used throughout Sweden as well as in Finland, Norway, Denmark, Estonia, and Latvia. The model has proven to be useful in nursing practice of different specialties. It has been fully computerized and is used in all higher level nursing education programs in Sweden.

The diversity of initiatives depicted can be seen as a mirror of the multiplicity of European cultures and healthcare. There is probably no single terminology that can serve all the different purposes and needs in health-care. How then, can all these terminology efforts in different countries be linked and what are the possible next steps to enhance the development of nursing for the benefit of better patient care in Europe? As the links between the European countries are being tied more closely, the need for collaboration within the nursing community is evident. One such effort is the work of the Association for Common European Nursing Diagnoses, Interventions and Outcomes (ACENDIO), which was established in 1995 (*www.acendio.net*). The aim of the association is to support the development of standardized classifications, terminologies, and data sets for sharing and comparing nursing data. ACENDIO (1) supports the development of nursing informatics by biannual conferences, publications, and presentations to advance understanding and work in this area; (2) serves as a network for nurses in different European countries so that they can share knowledge about developments; and (3) provides resources such as reference lists and sample methodologies for developing and evaluating nursing vocabularies and by providing interpretation of international standards for terminologies and classifications.

In addition, the European standardization organization (CEN) initiated a project to develop a common system of concepts and semantic categories for nursing. The European standardization organization is called CEN from the French name "Comite'Europeén de Normalisation" and is the European body similar to the International Standardization Committee (ISO). The CEN in turn meets with national healthcare standardization bodies in the different European countries. Some of the work in CEN lays the foundation for further work in ISO. Recently, the CEN initiated work on common concepts and semantic categories to build a nursing reference terminology. This work was transferred to ISO and was later developed internationally, based on the work in CEN. The final draft of International Reference Terminology was submitted to ISO by the International Medical Informatics Association—Nursing Special Interest Groups (IMIA-NI) and the ICN (ISO bulletin, 2003). All of these collaborative endeavors have formed a foundation for a reference terminology, which will enable nurses all over Europe to translate and communicate their national terminologies and nursing data on the European and international level.

International Council of Nurses (ICN)

Professional organizations are also working in some areas of nursing informatics. One example is the ICN that is built up by national nursing organizations. ICN has initiated the development of the ICNP, which has been translated into at least 12 European languages and tested in several countries. Many European nursing associations have also been active participants in the development of the ICNP. At the Web site of ICNP, *www.icn.ch/icnp*, updated information on the classification itself and of ongoing projects in different countries can be found.

Concept and Process Modeling

The method of concept and information modeling has been carried out in many countries during the last decennium. Today, there are many models of different parts of the healthcare system as a result of these activities. In Sweden, one model on care processes is called the SAMBA model (Structured Architecture for Medical Business Activities). The mission of SAMBA was to develop a process model for the workflow of Swedish healthcare when dealing with one individual subject of care. The work aimed at including all health professionals and it comprised analysis of process models previously developed by several counties. At an early stage it was evident that it is difficult to create a uniform model corresponding to the variations which the former models present. The differences between the former models proved to be due to the fact that they had been created from different perspectives. It was therefore of the utmost importance to identify a common perspective and purpose of the process model. The model was divided into three parts. One is a core process, which is the *clinical process* in healthcare. The model also consists of a *management process*, which monitors and evaluates the clinical process based on the mandate to provide healthcare, and a *communication process* dealing with information and interaction with the surrounding world as documents or messages. The model seems useful in most situations in healthcare and can be used to describe the enterprise on different levels of detail. A short version is available in English at *http://www.sfmi. se/samba/dokument/samba_en_1_8.ppt*.

Implementation of IT in Healthcare

In Europe, and specifically in the Nordic countries, the tradition of participatory design, when developing applications, has created a tradition for user involvement and participation that has impact not only on design, but also on project management (PM) and implementation. In this part, the issue of implementation and aspects regarding this will shortly be presented and discussed.

Through the text, EPRs will be used as an example. The reason for using EPR is that with this, or similar applications, healthcare attempts for the first time to implement a major application into its core processes.

Implementation—A Tricky Term

First of all it is important to settle on the meaning of the concept of implementation. It is also necessary to differentiate between often-used (misused) terms as implementation and installation. In a technical context, implementation most often stands for the process of installation of a computer code/program into a hardware environment. When the term implementation is used in an organizational context this will indicate a different understanding of the concept. When, after a long period, the decision to invest in an IT solution has been taken and the actual application has been purchased or developed, the process of introducing the IT application into healthcare begins, a process including many steps and phases. The first step, most often being the *technical installation* of hardware (e.g., local net, servers, PCs, and printers) and the chosen software, is the actual application (e.g., EPR/EHCR, PAS, and HIS). Following the technical installation, after a period of tests, comes the *functional implementation*. This phase includes activities to introduce the users to the application and its functionality. Typically, this includes basic computer skills (if necessary) and application training, i.e. how to use the functionality within the application (e.g., to order an x-ray and register nursing notes). In many cases this would be seen as the completion of the implementation, as the application is up and running and all users know how to use it. But in recent years, there has been a growing awareness of what has been named *organizational implementation*, a process where the change of workflow and organizational structure are important factors (Walsham, 1993; Nikula, Svedberg, and Elberg, 1999; Atkinson and Peel, 1998; McDonald and Barett, 1990).

Organizational Implementation

Healthcare managers on all levels now focus on effects, not merely due to the shift of medium for the patient record, i.e., primary effects, but effects *made possible* by the implementation of the EPR, i.e., indirect effects (Tang, 2003). This means that the actual use of the application and its functionality is not enough to accomplish the objectives. In many instances the objectives of implementing EPR is not merely to alter the routines of documentation of patient care. The objectives are often described as seamless care, supporting clinical and nursing protocols, better service to patients, and increased medical safety (van Bemmel and Musen, 1997). To be able to realize the possibilities embedded in the EPR as a technology, the implementation has to induce organizational changes. These changes most often comprise changes in the workflow, how the actual daily tasks are performed, and changes in the way clinical work and cooperation are organized. The organizational implementation is more about how the application supports planned and wanted changes in workflow and organizational structure.

Project Management

The Scandinavian model for participatory design has had the biggest impact on PM. Project teams are mostly selected to be representatives of different categories of clinicians and organizational parts of the healthcare enterprise. This is to ensure that as many perspectives as possible will be considered during the process of, for example, stating required functionality. In many countries this is also a way to deal with the demands for participation and influence raised by unions. This participatory and representative policy is not completely without problems. The belief that the representative selection of project teams will ensure "user involvement" is to a degree a deception. Selecting a group of clinicians from a total workforce of perhaps several thousand in a complex organization will most certainly involve some sort of compromise. Another problem is that this group will not be genuine users, but will be spokespersons for the "users," for a very long time. During the project the team will develop a culture of its own with specific skills and knowledge. When the application will eventually be implemented within the whole enterprise (hospital, HMO, and so forth), very few (real) users will be really involved. The alternative option is to select members for project teams from a knowledge perspective, focusing on those who can contribute the most.

Clinical and Nursing Implementation

When implementing IT applications concerning medical and/or nursing processes there is a growing attention on the issues of development and maintenance of the databases. To realize the advantages of EPR when the application is used in the everyday clinical setting there is a "price to pay," i.e., actions have to be taken, by clinicians, before and during the implementation, and later

on. Textbooks on medical informatics present lists of potential advantages of EPR and describe prerequisites for obtaining all these advantages in general terms (Shortliffe, 1990; van Bemmel and Musen, 1997). Not all the advantages have a "price tag" fixed to them, but in most cases there is a certain amount of effort, inconvenience, or compromise "to pay" before each of the advantages can be realized (Nikula, Svedberg, and Elberg, 1999; Nikula, Elberg, and Svedberg, 2000).

The price to pay concept illustrates that it takes human effort to create better healthcare and that clinicians therefore play a very important role when implementing EPR systems. To exemplify this it is necessary to focus on some of the essential advantages of the EPR opposed to paper-based patient record (PPR), namely the possibility to present data in various views, decision support, and sharing data between different parties.

Variety of views on data appears to be a very attractive advantage. The clinician may decide to read the record the same way as reading the PPR or to adjust the presentation to the clinical situation, but this feature requires structured data entry, common terminology, and that the clinician learns how to retrieve the needed information. *The structure of data* is important if data are to be reused and presented in several different ways. All data (tests, notes, nursing diagnoses, physical findings, and so forth) entered into the system has to be clearly "marked," the terminology has to be agreed on, and the clinicians' discipline when entering data has to be rigid. An EPR application may be designed to support this behaviour, e.g., by providing online guidelines.

Decision support is advantageous if the clinician enters the data. There would be limited use of a sophisticated alert system proposing, e.g., nursing protocols or pointing out a potential risk for medication interaction, if a medical record clerk enters the record. Decision support facilities also demand structured data entry, if the data should be automatically recognized and responded to by the EPR system.

Support of other data analysis may prove an important feature for quality control, quality improvement, and resource management. This feature may enable rapid information retrieval; however, without restrictions on data entry structure and terminology, a data analysis would be difficult or even impossible to perform or interpret.

Electronic data exchange and sharing care support assumes reuse of data, i.e., data are entered only once. When this feature is applied to the already structured data, such as name, date of birth, or addresses, it is simple. Though it would be more interesting to share clinical information between professions, e.g., when nurses have entered information about patients' social situation (family, type of housing, profession: job, and so forth), physicians could view this as part of their notes. This form of cross-clinician sharing of patient information demands an agreement between clinicians on rules, standards, and most of all, on common terminology.

Future Development

The future development needed for nursing informatics in Europe is implementation of decision support systems, integration of research-based knowledge in patient records, and feedback of clinical experience by aggregated data from patient records, as well as emphasis on educating practicing nurses, students, and educators (Ehnfors and Grobe, 2004). Most of all we need nurses educated in NI that can take a lead in the development of NI in different countries in Europe.

Conclusion

One of the main challenges for Europe and the rest of the world is the process of getting standards for EPR. The possibility of aggregating data on groups of patients requires standardized information in the individual patient record. This is the same idea as atomic-level patient data collected once, used many times (Zielstorff et al., 1993).

Generally speaking, there is a beginning of development of NI in Europe. Signs of this are doctoral work in NI, scientific papers, research funding available (some very large from the EU), research groups in many countries, support from professional organizations in nursing in many countries, European and international networks are at hand, and there are possibilities to study NI both in graduate and undergraduate schools.

References

Äärimaa, M. (2003). ICT, eHealth Telemedicine. Policy perspectives of European doctors. Presentation at the Ministerial Conference and Exhibition: The contribution of ICT to Health, Brussels.

Atkinson, C. J. and Peel, V. (1998). Transforming a hospital through growing, not building, an electronic patient record system. *Methods of Information in Medicine* 37(3):285–293.

Berthou, A. and Junger, A. (2000). *NURSING Data: Final Report (Short Version) 1998–2000 Period.* Lausanne: ISE.

Clark, J. and Lang, N. (1992). Nursing's next advance: An International Classification for Nursing Practice. *International Nursing Review* 39(4):109–112, 128.

Ehnfors, M. and Grobe, S. J. (2004). Nursing curriculum and continuing education: Future directions. *International Journal of Medical Informatics.* 73:591–598.

Ehnfors, M., Thorell-Ekstrand, I., and Ehrenberg, A. (1991). Towards basic nursing information in patient records (Vard i Norden). *Nursing Science and Research in the Nordic Countries* 21(3/4):12–31.

Ehrenberg, A., Ehnfors, M., and Thorell-Ekstrand, I. (1996). Nursing documentation in patient records: Experience of the use of the VIPS-model. *Journal of Advanced Nursing* 24:853–867.

Goossen, W. T. F., Epping, P. J. M. M., and Dassen, T. W. N. (1997a). Criteria for nursing information systems as a component of the electronic patient record: An international Delphi study. *Computers in Nursing* 15(6):307–315.

Goossen, W. T. F., Epping, P. J. M. M., and Dassen, T. W. N. (1997b). Nursing information in electronic patient records: Criteria established in a Delphi study. In U. Gerdin, M. Tallberg, and P. Wainwright (Eds.), *Nursing Informatics: The Impact of Nursing Knowledge on Health Care Informatics* (pp. 161–166). Amsterdam, The Netherlands: IOS Press.

International Council of Nurses. (2001). *International Classification for Nursing Practice: Beta 2 Version.* Geneva, Switzerland: International Council of Nurses.

ISO Bulletin. (September, 2003). Nursing language. *Terminology Models for Nurses* (pp. 16–18). Available at *http://www.iso.ch/iso/en/commcentre/isobulletin/articles/2003/pdf/terminology03-09.pdf.*

Laerum, H. (2004). *Evaluation of Electronic Medical Records* [doctoral thesis]. Trondheim, Norway: Faculty of Medicine, Norwegian University of Science and Technology.

McDonald, C. J. and Barnett, O. (1990). Medical-record systems. In E. H. Shortliffe and L. E. Perreault (Eds.), *Medical Informatics, Computer Applications in Health Care* (pp. 181–218). New York: Addison-Wesley.

Mortensen, R. (1999). *ICNP and Telematic Applications for Nurses in Europe: The Telenurse Experience.* Amsterdam, The Netherlands: IOS Press.

Nikula, R. E. (1999). Organizational and technological insight as important factors for successful implementation of IT. In N. M. Lorenzi (Ed.), *JAMIA Symposium Proceedings* (pp. 585–588). Philadelphia, PA: Hanley & Belfus.

Nikula, R. E., Elberg, P., and Svedberg, H. (2000). Informed decisions by clinicians are fundamental for EPR implementation. *International Journal of Medical Informatics* 58–59:141–146.

Nikula, R., Svedberg, H., and Elberg, P. (1999). Clinicians must invest resources when implementing electronic patient records. In P. Kokol, B. Zupan, J. Stare, M. Premik, and R. Engelbrecht (Eds.), *Medical Informatics Europe '99; 1999* (pp. 824–827). Ljubljana, Slovenia: IOS Press.

Sermeus, W. and Deleise, L. (1997). Development of a presentation tool for nursing data. In R. A. Mortensen (Ed.), *ICNP in Europe: Telenurse*. Amsterdam, The Netherlands: IOS Press.

Sermeus, W., Delesie, L., Van Landuyt, J., Wuyts, Y., Vandenboer, G., and Manna, M. (1994). *The Nursing Minimum Data Set in Belgium: A Basic Tool for Tomorrow's Health Care Management*. Leuven: Katholieke Universiteit Leuven.

Shortliffe, E. H. and Perreault, L. E. (1990). *Medical Informatics, Computer Applications in Health Care*. New York: Addison-Wesley.

Tang, P. H. (2003). Key capabilities of an electronic health care record system. In *Committee on Data Standards for Patient Safety*. Washington, DC: National Academies Press.

van Bemmel, J. H. and Musen, M. A. (1997). *Handbook of Medical Informatics*. Heidelberg: Springer Verlag.

Walsham, G. (1993). Implementation. In *Interpreting Information Systems in Organizations* (pp. 210–231). Cichester: John Wiley & Sons.

WHO. (1987). *Peoples Need for Nursing Care: A European Study*. Copenhagen: World Health Organization Regional Office for Europe.

Yura, H. and Walsh, M. B. (1988). *The Nursing Process. Assessing, Planning, Implementing, Evaluation* (5th ed.). Norwalk: Appleton & Lang.

▮ Recommended Readings

Berg, M. (2001). Implementing information systems in health care organizations: Myths and challenges. *International Journal of Medical Informatics* 64(2–3):143–156.

Berg, M. (ed). (2004). *Health Information Management—Integrating Information Technology in Health Care Work*. London: Routledge.

Clark, J. (Ed.) (2003). Naming nursing. In *Proceedings of the First ACENDIO Ireland/UK Conference, Swansea, Wales, U.K.* Bern: Verlag Hans Huber.

Kaplan, B., Brennan, P. F., Dowling, A. F., Friedman, C. P., and Peel, V. (2001). Toward an informatics research agenda: Key people and organizational issues. *Journal of the American Medical Informatics Association* 8(3):235–241.

Lorenzi, N. M. and Riley, R. T. (1994). *Organizational Aspects of Health Informatics—Managing Technological Change*. New York: Springer-Verlag.

Scholes, M., Tallberg, M., and Pluyter-Wenting, E. (2000). *International Nursing Informatics: A History of the First Forty Years 1960–*. Swindon: British Computer Society.

39

Pacific Rim

Evelyn J.S. Hovenga
Robyn Carr
Michelle Honey
Lucy Westbrooke

OBJECTIVES

1. Describe the development of nursing informatics (NI) in some Pacific Rim countries.
2. Identify historical milestones, changes, and trends influencing nurses to embrace informatics.
3. Discuss NI leadership, international links, education, research, and their impact on the development of NI as a nursing discipline or specialty.

KEY WORDS

information systems
standards
hospital information systems
public policy

The evolution of NI has varied in each of the Pacific Rim countries. The adoption of informatics usually began as a vision by one or more individuals. Such people used any number of opportunities plus their leadership skills to promote and disseminate the use of information technologies (ITs) to support nurses in all areas of nursing practice. This occurred in healthcare, educational, and government organizations, as well as within the IT industry and via any number of new and existing professional organizations. Events external to the nursing profession frequently became the catalyst stimulating some type of activity by nurses toward the adoption of informatics. International and multidisciplinary links have assisted these beginnings and its progression. Australia, New Zealand, and Hong Kong have made considerable progress since the early 1980s, South Korea since the 1990s in this regard, although much remains to be done. Nurses in a number of other countries in this region have only just begun or have yet to learn about NI although the introduction and use of these technologies in the health industry is progressing rapidly especially in Malaysia and Japan.

The Asia Pacific Medical Informatics Association (APAMI) was formed in 1993 as a regional group of the International Medical Informatics Association (IMIA). APAMI has helped launch national healthcare informatics associations in Malaysia, Indonesia, and the Philippines and has generated awareness about the field in India, Pakistan, Sri Lanka, and Fiji. Other member nations are Australia, Hong Kong, Japan, Korea, New Zealand, the People's Republic of China, Singapore, Taiwan, and Thailand. Nurses in these countries who are interested in promoting informatics to their profession need to link up with this network.

Evidence suggests that many nurses continue to have some difficulty in embracing these technologies to support their practice (Ho and Hovenga, 1999, 2003). Furthermore, it continues to be a challenge for many nurses to obtain appropriate education in informatics both during their initial nurse education and as a component of post-nurse registration specialist courses. Notwithstanding these conditions, an increase in computer use by practicing nurses in Australia, New Zealand, and other Asia Pacific countries is creating an awareness of the opportunities and gains to healthcare resulting from an increase in the use of computers, information, and telecommunication technologies. Thus, nurses in all health environments are becoming more dependent on electronic information.

This chapter aims to provide an overview of these historical events, primarily from Australia and New Zealand, and to highlight critical success factors for the benefit of those who have yet to embark on such a journey. The chapter concludes by summarizing significant events and examining their impact on the evolution of NI in this region.

Health and Nursing Informatics in New Zealand

New Zealand's total population is just over 4 million. These people are predominantly found in the urban areas, with the greater Auckland area having over a third of the total population. In 2003, there were 32,687 active registered nurses and midwives working in nursing and midwifery in New Zealand. With most of the nurses and midwives practicing in Auckland, this city by default becomes the focus of the drive for greater health informatics awareness. Notable changes have occurred within New Zealand nursing legislation that impact on the roles and future of nurses. Firstly, in line with international trends in nursing workforce development, the Nursing Council of New Zealand established the new role of nurse practitioner. Then in 2003, legislation was passed permitting nurse prescribing. At this early stage there are only a few Nurse Practitioners and fewer nurses prescribing, but there is clearly a move toward further postgraduate education to attain these new nursing roles. The impact of globalization has seen an increase in the movement of nurses in and out of New Zealand, which increases the challenges for the Nursing Council in terms of ensuring safety to practice at the level expected in New Zealand while not providing unnecessary barriers for overseas nurses.

As part of ensuring standards of practice the government passed the Health Practitioners Competence Assurance (HPCA) Act (2003). This Act came into force in 2004 and replaced the Nurses Act of 1977. The HPCA Act 2003 requires each health practitioner group to describe its profession in terms of scopes of practice. The purpose of scopes of practice is to ensure the safety of the public by defining the health services that health practitioners can perform.

Changes are continuous in the informatics arena and there are many sources and pressures for these. The overview diagram describes the major influences in

informatics in New Zealand (Fig. 39.1). Each item shown is summarized in more detail further.

The hub labeled "Informatics Influences" represents information collection, since this is seen as central to nursing, informatics, and healthcare. The other entities identified are significant players in New Zealand's healthcare system, which influences NI and its development.

Health and Nursing Informatics in Australia

Australia is a federation of eight states and territories. It has a population of just fewer than 20 million. Approximately 71% of all its households are located in inner and outer urban and provincial areas, mostly near cities on the coast. In 2001, the national census indicated that there were 1,259 nursing workers per 100,000 population where 51% worked less than 35 hours per week (AIH&W, 2004a, p. 229).

Around 225,000 registered (80%) and enrolled (20%) nurses are employed in acute care hospitals (65%), aged and community care (35%) in Australia. Of these 89% are employed as clinical nurses, mostly within the following specialties: medical/surgical (30%), geriatrics and gerontology (17%), operating theatre and related nursing (7%), midwifery, obstetrics and gynecology (7%), and mental health (7%) (Karmel and Li, 2002). The trend suggests we increasingly need a greater proportion of nurses in the aged and community care sectors as a result of projected population demographic changes.

As a consequence of the globalization of the profession, Australia's contribution to international education, the resultant workforce mobility, economic growth, and changes in the healthcare industry resulting from technology and informatics advances, changes are being witnessed in the nursing workforce. Credentialing and accreditation of nursing specialties is now being promoted. Nursing specialty and other organizations have developed and adopted practice standards, competencies, guidelines for curricula development, and various professional development programs. Australia has more than 50 such specialty national nursing organizations (NNOs), where the Health Informatics Society Australia's nursing informatics special interest group (HISA NI Sig) is one of these. We meet twice each year to discuss current issues impacting on the nursing profession. Most have developed a set of specialty competencies and they provide credentialing services.

Following the November 2003 Australian Health Ministers' Conference it was announced that a national nursing taskforce would be established to drive major

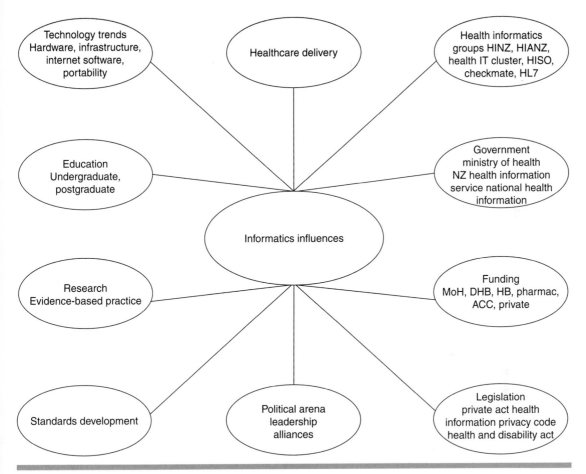

Figure 39.1
Overview diagram—major influences in informatics in New Zealand.

nursing education and workforce reforms as recommended by a previously undertaken national review of nursing education. Consequently the HISA NI Sig has been funded to develop a strategic plan for NI capacity building, and a plan for the nursing profession's engagement with the Australian government and its informatics agenda.

Healthcare Funding Framework

The government, through the Ministry of Health chiefly funds healthcare in New Zealand. Overall, the funding of healthcare in New Zealand is driven by business requirements, where information is used as the basis for cost-effective quality care, given limited resources.

Healthcare is available for all resident New Zealanders via a national system. The cost of every consultation with the general practitioner is subsidized by the government. Tertiary care is almost totally publicly funded. There remains in New Zealand an impression that if you have an accident or are acutely sick, then good quality public hospital care will be available. There is, however, competition between private and public healthcare in the primary and secondary arena. Elective surgery is more often provided in the private sector, although it may be funded by the public sector, as the public hospitals struggle to cope with long waiting lists and beds full of acutely ill and injured people. The role of the private sector has increased significantly. In 1999, private insurance funded about 6% of healthcare compared with just 2% 10 years ago, and given the ageing population, improved options of health treatments, and increasing demands yet limited public budgets, this trend is likely to continue. The cost of private health insurance is rising with premiums predicted to increase faster than the general cost of living. This means health insurance costs the individual more and there is a widening gap between those who need and those who can afford private healthcare.

The government also controls healthcare provision and funding through agencies such as the Accident Compensation Corporation (ACC). The ACC provides a range of health benefits and subsidies to assist individuals in the event of an accident. The establishment of the ACC has virtually eliminated suing for compensation in the event of an accident covered by the ACC. Information is collated about the nature and costs associated with accidents. ACC funding is provided through a levy on employers and employees. More recently ACC has targeted accident prevention and as an incentive has weighted levies, charging more to those companies and organizations that have employee/member accidents.

All prescription-related medicines are regulated by the government though Pharmac. Subsidies are available on a range of medicines, although only a few options within each drug classification may be subsidized by Pharmac. The public can purchase an increasing number of over-the-counter remedies, and there is an increasing need for drug information for medical practitioners, nurses, and the public.

In Australia work began in collaboration with Professor Fetter from Yale University during the 1980s to develop patient classification systems to describe the case-mix serviced by healthcare organizations. Since 1992, the Australian Refined Diagnosis Related Group (AR-DRG) standard has been in use first for the purpose of monitoring and comparison of hospital activity and later for costing and funding purposes. This Australian Hospital Information, Performance Information Program relies on data obtained from individual patient records, including the ICD-10-AM codes. A number of case-mix systems are in use to suit a variety of patient populations. Service weights to reflect the cost of providing various hospital-based services including nursing were developed and are currently in the process of being updated. These are included in various funding formulas adopted. This case-mix system has been adopted by Germany and is being considered for adoption by other countries.

Health spending continues to increase. By 2001–2002 this amounted to 9.3% of the gross domestic product (GDP) compared with 8.9% in 1999–2000. In 2001–2002, the Australian government spent 46.3% primarily on health research, aged care, and medical services. All taxpayers contribute a 1.5% Medicare levy and high-income earners who do not have private health insurance, pay an additional 1%. State, territory and local governments spent 22.3% mainly on community and public health services. The cost of public hospitals is shared by all governments in accordance with specifically negotiated healthcare agreements. Nongovernmental sources such as third party payers and individual contributions amount to 31.4%. This funds all private hospital care. The Australian government manages a Pharmaceutical Benefits Scheme (PBS) which is jointly funded by them and non-government sources (AIH&W, 2004a, pp. 242–247).

Information Governance

The NZ Ministry of Health is interested in information collection, and much of this occurs through the auspices of the New Zealand Health Information Service (NZHIS). This body controls the national database, which holds registration for 95% of New Zealanders. The NZHIS database uses a unique identifier, which is assigned at birth, and is designed to follow the individual through each healthcare event in his or her life. The unique identifier is called the national health index number or the NHI. The NHI allows easier tracking of information through healthcare episodes.

The national minimum dataset (NMDS) is a single integrated collection of health data, developed in consultation with health sector representatives and required at the national level for policy formulation, performance monitoring, evaluation, and research. This data is to be reported by all hospitals, including private hospitals. Statutory requirements govern the reporting of certain diseases such as cancer and tuberculosis and other communicable diseases.

All information collection, storage, access, and retrieval in New Zealand is governed by the Privacy Act (1993) and the Health Information Code (1994) and subsequent amendments. This act is one of the most comprehensive pieces of privacy legislation anywhere in the world.

The Australian Institute for Health and Welfare (AIH&W) provides research and statistical support to the Australian state and territory governments. In 1993, all public health authorities, the Australian Bureau of Statistics, and the AIH&W signed an agreement to improve the quality of and cooperation in the development of national health information. This now provides the national infrastructure needed to provide high quality health data. It includes the National Health Data Dictionary of established data definitions and data standards to support electronic health records (EHRs) development in Australia, as well as the National Health Data Collection and Reporting Guidelines, national minimum data standard edits, and data policy guidelines. The Health Data Standards Committee has the responsibility for data standards and it oversees the work of the Classifications and Terminology Working Group through the AIHW.

Australia's health sector governance is fragmented as decision-making occurs across 21 different jurisdictions (Boston Consulting Group Report, 2004, p. 26). A recent review undertaken on behalf of the newly established National Health Information Group (NHIG) and the Australian Health Information Council (AHIC) identified this as a significant impediment to the provision of better healthcare outcomes, safety, quality, and cost efficiencies. The adoption of health informatics principles is seen as an enabler of coordination between the stakeholders. The review undertaken in early 2004 was a first step in the development of a revised national health information management and communications technology strategy. The trend is toward greater coordination between providers with a strong emphasis on improving health outcomes. The current structure is shown in Fig. 39.2. This structure optimizes cross-jurisdictional effort, and provides a clearer distinction between accountabilities and it facilitates appropriate resourcing. It was noted that there was a strong case for decisive national action following years of underinvestment.

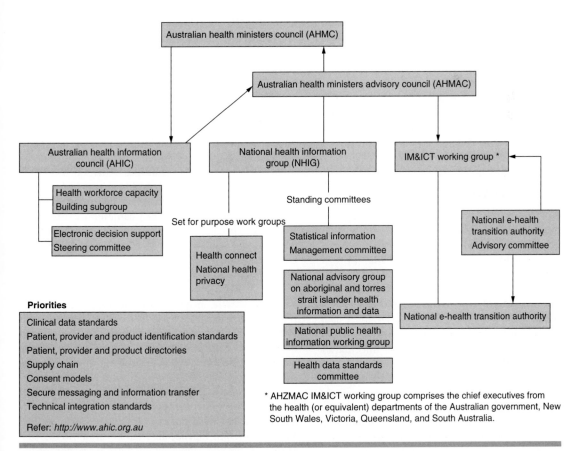

Figure 39.2
Current Australian AHMAC IM & ICT governance structure, May 2005.

The Boston Consulting Group (2004, p. 13) recommendations include the establishment of a new entity with full-time staff to provide the necessary leadership and drive the IM & ICT agenda forward as well as promote the adoption of common standards to provide a national interoperability platform to maximize system connectivity, integrated decision support functionality, clinical information transfer, secure messaging, and broadband rollout. These recommendations are now being implemented.

The AIH&W has developed the National Health Information Knowledgebase, an Internet- based interactive electronic storage site for national health metadata. It includes a powerful query tool and is regarded as a world benchmark in data/_metadata registries (NHWI, 1998). The existing metadata items are now being reengineered to align them with the new international metadata standards (METeOR project) (AIH&W, 2004b).

Professional Organizations and Government Advisory Groups

Both New Zealand and Australia have many health informatics and related professional organizations and groups advising various government departments and specific projects. There tends to be a considerable overlap of members between these.

 ## New Zealand Health Informatics Groups

There are a number of informatics interest groups in New Zealand, each with a slightly different focus. Table 39.1 identifies and gives a high-level definition of these groups. Health Informatics New Zealand (HINZ) is a national, not-for-profit organization whose focus is to facilitate improvements in business processes and patient care in the health sector through the application of appropriate information technologies. HINZ, a new organization, emerged in September 2000 from two health informatics organizations: Nursing Informatics New Zealand (NINZ) and New Zealand Health Informatics Foundation (NZHiF). NI was originally formed in 1990 and NZHiF was originally formed in 1994. The executive committee works to maintain our purpose and service for the members, through dynamic goals. HINZ does not compete with existing organizations or activities, but assists network key and influential partners to improve the effectiveness of health informatics business in New Zealand.

HINZ acts as a single portal for the collection and dissemination of information about the New Zealand Health Informatics Industry. Membership is for anyone who has an interest in health and informatics and wants to be part of an organization that can provide relevant up-to-date information about health informatics. HINZ holds an annual conference in collaboration with other main health IT organizations.

HINZ, in conjunction with other professional health-related groups such as New Zealand Health Information Technology Cluster, New Zealand Institute of Health Management, and New Zealand Health Level 7 (NZHL7) Users Group (NZHUG), jointly organizes an annual national conference as well as seminars throughout the year.

 ## Health Informatics Groups in Australia

The history of the formation of medical, health, and NI groups reflects the difficulties experienced as a consequence of a federal system of government and vast distances between population centers.

Australia has had a representative to IMIA's Working Group 8 (WG8) (now NI Sig) since 1984. Nurses were the second group of health professionals to organize themselves to promote health informatics in Australia. The general practitioners were first, beginning in the late 1970s although the Health Information Managers Association (HIMAA) has been in existence since 1949 but the integration of informatics is more recent. NI is now a Sig of the HISA, which came into existence in 1993. It has been a long and torturous path to reach this position.

Historical Developments

NI in Australia began with the Royal Australian Nursing Federation (now ANF) in 1984. A year later a small group of midwives in Victoria, including Joan Edgecumbe, who is now the executive officer of the HISA decided to call a general meeting of nurses interested in computer use. About 70 nurses agreed to establish the Nursing Computer Group Victoria (NCGV). This group continued to flourish and hosted the Fourth International Symposium on Nursing Use of Computers and Information Science in Melbourne in 1991. The profits of this conference enabled the formation of the HISA. These and other associated events are summarized in Table 39.2.

Table 39.1   New Zealand Health Informatics Groups

Group	Description
HINZ	Health Informatics New Zealand (HINZ) is a national, not-for-profit organization whose focus is to facilitate improvements in business processes and patient care in the health sector through the application of appropriate information technologies. HINZ has established working groups to mirror those within the International Medical Informatics Association Special Interest Group in Nursing Informatics (IMIA-NI). The HINZ Nursing Informatics Working Group is most active of HINZ groups.
NZHUG	New Zealand Health Level 7 User Group (NZHUG) is the New Zealand arm of the international Health Level 7 (HL7) organization, which has a proven and widely used methodology for standards development. The organization is comprised of technical committees and Sigs. The technical committees are directly responsible for the content of the standards. Sigs serve as a test bed for exploring new areas that may need coverage in HL7's published standards.
NZHITC	The NZ Health IT Cluster Inc. (NZHITC) is a consortium of 37 organizations with a common interest in improving healthcare delivery. The cluster was formed as part of Industry New Zealand's cluster development program and has been formally working together to provide mutual support for local and international business development.
MoH	The Ministry of Health plays an important role for the formal intra- and intergovernment liaison work it undertakes, its influence on sector policy and strategy, and its funding capability.
DHB's	District Health Boards New Zealand (DHBNZ) is a national organization that has been set up by the 21 DHBs to assist with representation, help coordinate joint DHB processes and activities, and undertake work that can be done more effectively and efficiently on a national basis.
DHB forums	The NZ CIO/CEO/CFO forums comprise members who are chief information officers (CIOs), chief executive officers (CEOs), and chief financial officers (CFOs) from DHBs. Through sharing information, the forum members aim to advance respective strategies (business and technical).
HIGB	The Health Intranet Governance Board (HIGB) is responsible for the governance of the Health Intranet, the New Zealand national health information network, and has been responsible for the development of the Health Network Code of Practice.
IPAC	Independent Practitioners Association Council (IPAC) has a group of key technical people "GEEK" who work within the IPAC structure and who have established a regular forum to discuss issues and share information. This group includes some vendor representatives.
HISO	A proactive ministerial committee with responsibility for direction setting together with the overall governance of the New Zealand health and disability sector standards agenda.
Standards NZ	Standards NZ are heavily involved in the development and application of national, regional, and international standards, many of which are developed in partnership with Australia. Standards NZ is the New Zealand's representative in the International Organization for Standardization (ISO) and its sister organization, the International Electrotechnical Commission (IEC).
NZCA	The New Zealand Coding Authority (NZCA) exists to promote excellence and coding consistency in clinical coding through advice and support for the New Zealand clinical coder workforce and related organizations.
Statistics New Zealand	Statistics New Zealand (Stats NZ) administers the Statistics Act (1975) producing the official statistics for the nation.
ACC	The Accident Compensation Corporation (ACC) administers New Zealand's accident compensation scheme, which provides accident insurance for all New Zealand citizens, preventing injury, buying health and disability support services to treat, care for, and rehabilitate injured people.

(Continued)

Table 39.1 New Zealand Health Informatics Groups (*Continued*)

Group	Description
NDPG	The National Data Policy Group (NDPG), originally the Data Definitions Working Group, was formed to ensure consultation with the health sector on the data elements that are collected in the national minimum dataset (NMDS) and their definitions. The NDPG in its present form has been in existence since 1997 and has been chaired by NZHIS staff during that period.
ILG	Information Liaison Group (ILG) provides input to the Ministry's current short-term information projects that are designed to provide DHBs with access to information from the systems managed by the business units. The ILG has an impact on the decision-making processes of all DHBs and the MoH, in that it is a forum where these parties can be represented when changes to business rules and reporting requirements from the business units can be discussed and prioritized.
CLANZ	Clinical Leaders Association of New Zealand (CLANZ) manages issues critical to health such as clinical safety, quality of care, and resource management demands also embracing competent and effective clinical leadership. CLANZ seeks to grasp opportunities evident within the New Zealand health system for clinicians willing to take responsibility and to show leadership, by building strategic partnerships and alliances with other health organizations and agencies.
CHECKMATE	Collaboration for Health and Clinical Knowledge Management and Technology (CHECKMATE) is somewhat unique in being academically led but having a multisectoral membership including academics, software developers, and end users. This group is primarily focused on knowledge systems rather than technology and the main objective is to bring together people from throughout the health IT sector who have interests in research and training.
HIANZ	Health Information Association of New Zealand (HIANZ) is involved with medical records and medical libraries.

It has been a tortuous path toward the recognition and professionalization of health (and nursing) informatics as a discipline. We have not managed to achieve a unity or consensus regarding how best to operate as one national professional organization to date although increasingly joint activities are being organized.

Nursing Informatics in Hong Kong

Hong Kong nurses established NURSINFO (HK) Ltd. in 1991, and this organization has enjoyed a consistent increase in membership. They have as their motto "Nursing Informatics for Excellence in Patient Care." They organize regular educational activities, use a communication network, produce a regular newsletter, and are actively involved with the Hong Kong Society of Medical Informatics and the Hong Kong Computer Society. Together they participate in the organization of trade exhibits and regular conferences. The Hong Kong Hospital Authority is responsible for over 40 hospitals and over 50 specialist clinics that are part of a large multisite, multiprotocol intelligent data network to provide seamless data communications throughout. Implementation began in 1993. It includes a clinical management system focusing on patient-oriented data sharing. This provides longitudinal medical profile for patients and can be accessed by healthcare professional on a need to know basis. Telemedicine and videoconferencing are in use and multimedia enhancement in the clinical setting with voice recording and imaging now helps to speed up the work process and strengthens services in the clinical areas.

Nursing Informatics in South Korea

A Sig of the Korean Society of Medical Informatics, the premier organization in Korea dedicated to the development and application of medical and health informatics in the support of patient care, education, research, and administration of healthcare arena in general. The Society was established in October 1989. KOSMI is hosting the next International Nursing Informatics Symposium to be held in Seoul, August 2006, under the auspices of IMIA NI (*http://www.ni2006.org/*).

Table 39.2 History of Australian Health Informatics Professional Groups and the Promotion of this Discipline

Year	By Whom	Purpose
1949	Health Information Managers Association (HIMAA)	Established: refer *http://www.himaa.org.au*
1984	Royal Australian Nurses Federation (RANF)	Adoption of position statement on "Computerization in Health Services—Implications for Nursing" (RANF, 1984)
1985	Royal College of Nursing Australia (RCNA)	Seventh National Conference theme, "Information Processing—Challenges and Choices for Nurses," Melbourne. This inspired a small group of midwives.
1985	Midwives Association	General meeting of nurses interested in computer use—70 nurses attended. The Nursing Computer Group Victoria (NCGV) was established.
1986	Royal Adelaide Hospital Nurses Education Fund	Sponsored a National Nursing Conference with the theme: "From Lamp to Light Pen—Computers in Nursing" to celebrate their 150th Jubilee. Nurses from Queensland and Western Australia computer groups established the previous year, networked.
1986	Health Commission of Victoria	Government funded the then senior nursing advisor to undertake a world tour to investigate the likely impact on nurses of computer use in the health industry.
1986	Royal Australian College of General Practitioners (RACGP)	National computer committee established following the formation of several state-based medical computing interest groups.
1986	Australian participants at Medinfo '86	Around 20 Australians met in Washington DC and decided to form a network with the aim of promoting health informatics among health professionals. This resulted in the formation of a number of computer groups in several states over the years that followed. Meanwhile the Australian Computer Society (ACS) Inc. was the organization that represented Australia at IMIA.
1987	RACGP	Computer Fellow position established in conjunction with Monash University's Department of Community Medicine.
1988	RACGP	Standards for computerized medical records systems released.
1989	Australian Medical Informatics Association (AMIA)	A Western Australia initiative to form AMIA with state-based branches. The inaugural meeting of AMIA (Victorian Branch) was held in Melbourne in 1991. AMIA secured an affiliation with the ACS and became the ACS medical informatics Sig.
1990	Australian Health Informatics Association SA	Sixteen health informatics enthusiasts met in South Australia and established AHIA SA. They published six issues of the Health Informatics News and Technology (HINT) annually.
1991	ACS medical informatics Sig	The ACS MI SIG organized a 1-day health track at the ACS annual conference held in Adelaide that year. This was seen as an opportunity for members of the many disparate groups to meet and discuss the possibility of forming one national organization. Disagreement regarding the name (medical vs. health) and the entry requirements remained unresolved.
1991	Australian Health Informatics Association Qld	A group of health professionals organized regular educational meetings in Brisbane and formed AHIA Qld.
1991	Health Informatics Association New South Wales (HIANSW)	HIANSW was established by 36 people representing a wide range of health and IT professionals, including nurses. They produce a regular newsletter, Computers in Health Information Processing (CHIP)

(Continued)

Table 39.2   History of Australian Health Informatics Professional Groups and the Promotion of this Discipline (*Continued*)

Year	By Whom	Purpose
1991	NCGV	International Nursing Informatics Symposium held in Melbourne hosted by the NCGV under the auspices of the IMIA NI working group.
1991	NI '91 postconference meeting	Nurses from all states and territories discussed the formation of a National Nursing Informatics group. Everyone agreed to work together, but the formalization of a new national organization was problematic due to differences between the state-based groups regarding affiliations with other professional nursing organizations. Subsequently, the NCGV changed its name to Nursing Informatics Australia (NIA).
1992	NIA	Postconference profits were used to establish a secretariat and launch a new look magazine.
1992	Australian Nursing Informatics Council (ANIC)	One representative from each state-based nursing informatics group was appointed to form ANIC
1992	Standards Australia (SA)	Health Informatics Standards Committee—IT-14 established
1992	HIANSW conference	Another attempt at uniting the 23 distinct groups was made at the first HIANSW conference held in Laura, New South Wales, to discuss how to best work together and how health (medical) informatics should be represented at IMIA. This resulted in a resolution to: 1. Form a National Council of Health Informatics Groups. 2. Combine three newsletters/journals, CHIP, HINT, and Nursing Informatics Australia, into one national and multidisciplinary magazine with a national editorial board. The first issue of Informatics in Healthcare Australia came out in May 1992, funded by NIA.
1992	AMIA meeting, Melbourne	Discussion paper summarizing deliberations and a scenario for the development of one new national organization to represent the field of health informatics in Australia was circulated widely.
1992	ANIC	Initiated the idea to organize a national conference in 1993. Several groups supported this idea, and since NIA was the only organization with the necessary funds, this group managed this inaugural conference. This became an annual event known as HIC—Health Informatics Conference.
1993	Health Informatics Society of Australia (HISA)	A special meeting of representatives from interested groups, facilitated by Dr. Ian Graham, who was the Director, Centre for Health Informatics at the Austin Hospital, was held in Sydney. This meeting produced a draft Constitution for HISA, reflecting an agreed set of principles. (refer *www.hisa.org.au*)
1993	HISA Victoria	NIA was reconstituted as the HISA Victoria branch
1993	HISA Inaugural general meeting	The draft constitution was presented to potential HISA members at its inaugural general meeting held in conjunction with the inaugural Health Informatics Conference (HIC '93), and they voted for its adoption. Conference profits were then used to fund the further development of the constitution and incorporation.
1994	HISA constituted	The NIA (now HISA Vic) secretariat became HISA's secretariat.
1994	HISA standards SIG	HISA's representative to IT-14 informed the committee of the recommendation for the adoption of HL7 messaging standards, this was accepted.
1995	HISA	HISA became the official group to represent Australia at IMIA

(*Continued*)

Table 39.2 History of Australian Health Informatics Professional Groups and the Promotion of this Discipline (*Continued*)

Year	By Whom	Purpose
1996	HISA NI Sig	HISA nursing informatics Sig established.
1997	General Practice Computing Group (GPCG)	Established by GPs, funded by the Australian Government Department of Health and Ageing to provide a strategic and cooperative approach to Australian GP informatics (refer *www.gpcg.org/*)
2000	HISA	A new constitution was adopted making HISA a company limited by guarantee of its members
2001	Australian College of Health Informatics (ACHI)	Meeting of seven health informaticians funded by the Australian Department of Health and Aged Care resulted in the formation of ACHI in 2002 with 18 invited Fellows selected via a peer review and consensus regarding the country's 20 top health informaticians to act as the peak reference body for health informatics in Australia. By 2004 there were 30 Fellows and Members (refer *www.achi.org.au*)
2002	HL7 Australia	A Health Level Seven (HL7) user group established.
		An HL7 International Affiliates meeting held in Melbourne (refer *www.hl7.org.au*)
2002	HISA	Hosted an international ISO TC215 meeting in Melbourne
2003	HISA	A pathology SIG established
2004	HISA	An aged care SIG established

Trends in Healthcare

The changes in responsibility for healthcare provision in New Zealand have seen a more collaborative approach resulting in integrated care being seen as a priority. Integrated care is being supported by technology, enabling information to flow. Electronic health event summaries, laboratory and radiology data are now being transmitted between providers across primary and secondary sectors (Chu et al., 2002). The Internet and Intranet are providing a wealth of information to health providers as well as consumers.

The Web environment and the use of powerful integration engines, is now providing contextual views of data that is browser-based and single logon. Placed over multiple hospital information systems this connection provides a "single patient view" of data across all medical applications. At last we are seeing applications that can be used by the clinicians. We have tools that allow ease of messaging and mapping and products to support the clinical workflow process. Online technologies provide products and services that enhance patient care and improve clinical outcomes through evidence-based health information and decision support systems.

Although New Zealand is a small country it has a surprising number of health IT companies who are pro-ducing software that is not only being used locally but also internationally (i-Health).

Technology Trends

The healthcare environment is changing at an ever-increasing pace due to the proliferation of new and emerging technologies. Embracing the advances in technology enables us to deliver healthcare in new and innovative ways. Basic hardware has advanced into multiple components of input and output devices. Development of infrastructures has enabled this technology to be networked and the Internet to provide a medium to transmit information nationally and internationally. The physical constraints and boundaries are now so blurred that healthcare delivery can occur at any time or place.

New Zealand has been embracing these changes in technology and has particularly benefited from the development of infrastructure. No longer is information restricted to individuals and organizations. Higher speed networks including wireless and broadband are enabling information in a variety of formats to be shared. Digital images are becoming the norm and picture archiving and communication systems (PACS) abound. Exploration into telehealth has occurred in a number of fields including teledermatology, teleradiology, telepsychiatry, and telepediatrics (Oakley, 2001). This has been made possible by the infrastructure that improves transmission in both speed and quality.

Improvements in portability are now allowing the use of technology in a greater range of settings. Both personal digital assistants (PDAs) and tablets are being used or trialed in the clinical setting by students and healthcare professionals. One of the nursing schools has issued PDAs to its students and the success of this has been evidenced by the reluctance of the students to relinquish them. Some Australian nurses are using PDAs for point-of-care information and clinical documentation for community and acute hospital nursing, hospital-based infection control and wound management.

Funding for the use of the technologies is probably one of the biggest limitations imposed in embracing new technologies to enhance care delivery. Unfortunately for New Zealand, its size does not allow economies of scale but this does not prevent efficient use of the available resources. Although the cost for individual items of technology decreases, our demands for this technology, and therefore our overall spending, increases. Nurses need to be prepared to work alongside and use technology to best care for clients. Healthcare organizations are now looking to implement clinical information systems and electronic patient records.

Current National Initiatives

The New Zealand Ministry of Health, in 2001, prepared a 5-year broad strategic directive for information and technology developments, referred to as "The WAVE Report" that was largely driven and developed by the key stakeholders. The report was produced by means of collaboration among industry, clinicians, government, and healthcare managers. It identified New Zealand's most pressing health IT needs and significant issues that will continue to form barriers to improved health outcomes and reducing delivery costs over the next 5 years. The report has been the cornerstone of activity for getting things working better and has also formed the foundations for long-term issues such as EHRs. While it is not necessarily unique in its content or conclusions, the collaborative approach to developing the report heralded a new way of getting whole of sector buy in for a range of national initiatives, changing the focus from debating direction to unifying action.

Following the WAVE report, the drive for collaboration from the bottom-up has consolidated as the district health boards (DHBs) replace their isolated departmental

systems with more integrated and dynamic Web-based technologies that support a more connected delivery network. Already, over half of the 21 DHBs have entered into some form of shared service arrangements for information systems. Such arrangements have reduced duplication and contributed to more effective and efficient management of infrastructure with greater interoperability. It has also made the development of a national EHR based on key components more of a reality.

The development of national technology infrastructure has proved useful; however, securing appropriate access to relevant clinical and administrative information throughout the health sector remains the greatest challenge. Early progress has been made in the areas of claims systems and laboratory results. For example, approximately 70% of laboratory results are sent from community laboratories to general practitioners by electronic messaging. Practice management software for patient administration is currently estimated to be in use by 80% of general practices. Approximately 50% of general practitioners are using software for clinical purposes such as electronically generating prescriptions and electronically recording details of patient health encounters. Electronic claims from primary care providers number approximately 66 million per year.

New Zealand government's health policies have been driving toward a population health management approach. Accordingly, the sector has been slowly moving away from a "bricks and mortar" hospital-centric approach to an integrated healthcare. Although significant gaps remain, the move has proved heavily reliant on collaboration between government, contracting agencies, and delivery units.

The national health information agreements and the establishment of the National Health Data Dictionary in 1993 laid the foundation for consistent health data sets in Australia. In 1999, the first national strategic information action plan, Health Online was initiated. This was followed by a number of projects initiated by the Australian government: Health*Connect*, Medi*Connect*, the provision of quality health information for consumers known as Health*Insite*, and the national supply chain initiative along with more than 360 projects such as the integration of primary health and hospital care, several shared and coordinated care projects, and the establishment of health call centers.

In 2005 it is expected that a strengthened governance model with greater central leadership will be implemented to enable better use of information technologies through a better-connected health system. The overall aim is to improve health outcomes whilst containing cost increases driven by advances in medical technologies and an ageing population.

Standards Development and Adoption

Following the 2001 WAVE Report, the minister of health directed that a WAVE working group, the Ministerial Committee on a Health Information Standards Organization (HISO), be established to investigate the implications of establishing a nonstatutory organization to manage health information standards (NZ Ministerial Committee on Health Information Standards Organisations, 2002). HISO drew together hitherto disparate health-related groups with specific interest in producing IT standards for New Zealand. HISO's role includes identifying, developing, publishing, and monitoring New Zealand's health information standards (Cressey, 2003). The scope of development activities that HISO will be involved with includes standards associated within the following categorization scheme:

- Records structure and content—data formats.
- Vocabulary—codes for medical and other healthcare terms.
- Messaging—standards used for the interchange of data.
- Security and privacy—how access to information is managed.

HISO (governed by the Health Information Standards Committee—HISC), and supported by the Ministry of Health produced the New Zealand Draft National Health Standards Information Plan (NZHSP) to assist in its role of developing health information standards for the health and disability sector. HISO enhances the New Zealand e-Government Interoperability Framework (e-GIF) direction.

The NZHSP recognizes there is an urgent need to progress work on national standards. It analyses the key sector drivers, requirements, and issues and sets a foundation to rapidly advance the sector information standards agenda. It proposes a framework for describing the sector priorities, standards development processes, governance and leadership, and presents a clear statement of the proposed plan for the development and adoption of national health information standards. NZHSP anticipates HISO undertaking the constituent parts of that framework.

A key driver for HISO's role—consistent use of standards—is aimed at the acceptance throughout the health and health-related industries of such standards.

This requires enabling real-time access to information about the standards (i.e., what standards are agreed, what are being developed or proposed, what initiatives are taking place, and what are the downstream implications) including where the information may be freely accessed. The availability of detailed and clinically relevant data is essential for clinical care decisions and for oversight groups making decisions related to the quality of that care. Today health information systems are expected to meet a variety of changing demands for data and information to support many purposes (e.g., automated alerts, decision support, quality monitoring, payment policy, and outcomes research).

Standardized terminology systems are essential to permit the use and exchange of clinical data across applications and IT systems. Given point-of-care documentation, technology is now available to build electronic health information systems that will efficiently meet a variety of needs. This includes providing immediate feedback to care providers by, for example, issuing alerts related to relevant best practice guidelines, generating data needed for internal and external quality monitoring, exchanging critical patient information in a timely manner across the healthcare continuum, and reducing provider burden associated with current documentation requirements.

Currently one of the most significant challenges to implementing electronic health information systems is the current lack of standards for electronic patient medical record information, especially standards around the terminology that expresses clinical documentation.

Standards New Zealand and HISO, working partnership with Standards Australia (SA), were persuaded to establish a health informatics committee in 1992. The SA IT-14 committee now has several active technical subcommittees and works closely with other similar groups such as HL7 Australia, the ISO Technical Committee 215 (TC215) and the Comite Europeen de Normalisation (CEN) TC251. Nurses are represented via the Royal College of Nursing and Central Queensland University. The focus in Australia has been in the area of standards development to facilitate data interchange to first of all support all types of e-commerce and now to support the interchange of clinical data. This is putting a greater emphasis on the need for a standard architectural structure for patient records and terminologies.

A number of Australian IT-14 committee and subcommittee as well as Health Level Seven (HL7) Australian members have been instrumental in influencing many international standards to ensure that they meet Australian and New Zealand needs. Particularly the development of new ISO standards for requirements for an EHR architecture (ISO/TS 18308) and the EHR definition, scope, and context (ISO/DTR 20514), plus the HL7 EHR System Functional Model (EHR-S) and the revision of the four-part CEN/TC 251 EHRcom standard (ENV 13606). The latter will now include an additional part detailing the archetype interchange format. Archetypes are constraint-based models of domain entities and were first defined by the Australian-based OpenEHR group, an international not-for-profit foundation working toward interoperable lifelong EHRs. We are working toward the harmonization of all related HL7 version 3, CEN and ISO standards so that we will be able to have fully interoperable clinical records.

Two IT-14 members represent that committee at the national ICT Standards Committee and the Health Data Standards Committee who report to the NHIG and the AHIC who currently make up the Australian government governance model. In July 2004, NHIG endorsed HL7 as the standard for healthcare messaging in Australia. This represents a small step toward the implementation and an increase in the adoption of available standards.

Research

Australia and New Zealand now have a number of Masters and PhD students who are conducting research in areas of health informatics. Health-related information has a number of uses. Apart from the direct use of information in the care of clients, there is a growing awareness of the need for timely and accurate data for research. Two specific areas that are currently gaining more attention within NI are clinical pathways and evidence-based practice. In New Zealand, this is demonstrated by The Centre for Evidence Based Nursing—Aotearoa (CEBNA) and the New Zealand Guidelines Group (NZGG). CEBNA is a partnership between the Auckland District Health Board and the University of Auckland, School of Nursing. CEBNA collaborates with the Joanna Briggs Institute for Evidence Based Nursing and Midwifery, the lead centre, in an Australasian-wide collaboration, that includes centers throughout Australia, Hong Kong, and Singapore. These centers are committed to an evidence-based approach to healthcare and to promoting an evidence-based culture in nursing.

The New Zealand Guidelines Group (NZGG) was set up in 1996 by the National Health Committee (NHC) as an informal network of expertise and information on guidelines development and implementation.

NZGG is funded by the Ministry of Health and through contracts with other health agencies such as ACC.

Numerous clinical pathway projects have been established and their findings disseminated. Of particular note in New Zealand is the main national children's hospital (Starship Hospital, which provides a wide range of complex medical, surgical, and mental health services for children throughout New Zealand and the South Pacific.) "Clinical Guidelines for Common Pediatric Conditions." Such projects are strongly supported by the New Zealand Ministry of Health (2002) as part of a policy level strategy signaled through The New Zealand Health Strategy, the Health and Disability Sector (Safety) Act 2001 and health professionals' competency assurance legislation, which provide clear direction toward quality improvement in healthcare.

HISA organizes an annual conference where between 40 and 60 papers are presented each year. These are indexed in CINAHL and provide a good overview of progress in health informatics in Australia. Health informatics does not exist as a research category for the major government research funding organizations such as the Australian Research Council or the National Health & Medical Research Council, which makes it difficult to obtain research funds from these organizations. It is anticipated that this will change in the near future as part of the Australian government's health workforce capacity building initiative.

Education

In New Zealand, NI has been recognized as significant by the Ministries of Health and Education since the early 1990s. A national "Guidelines for Teaching Nursing Informatics" curriculum was introduced into the undergraduate preparation of nurses programs in 1991. Nursing Council of New Zealand does not identify any specific computer skills within the competencies that registered nurses are required to attain; yet the competencies involve information management and communication that may be achieved using computer technology. Much of NI is integrated into the undergraduate curriculum under the guise of other subjects. For example, law and ethics covers the Privacy Act (1993), which emphasizes the importance of the collection, storage, and use of client information, whether stored on paper or computer; evidence-based practice which includes the discernment of evidence to ascertain its worthiness to base nursing practice on; and research which includes literature searches, and therefore the use of the Internet and access to international nursing literature databases. Undergraduate nurse education therefore reflects the need for computer literacy. The new nursing student, most commonly from secondary school, enters with increased computer skills than ever before. Rather than compulsory computer skills training, optional classes are available for those students that require additional assistance in this area.

Changes have taken place in undergraduate nursing education, including the computer literacy of entering students and the credentials with which new nurses qualify. Since the mid-1990s nurses registering for practice in New Zealand also complete an undergraduate degree. The impact of these changes on undergraduate nursing education has a flow-on effect within postgraduate education. Furthermore, the changes in health service delivery in New Zealand and the establishment of new roles and career opportunities for nurses are drivers for an increased demand for postgraduate nursing education. These new advanced nursing roles require postgraduate qualifications. Yet there have been barriers to nurses accessing postgraduate education, which is generally based in urban areas. Nurses are found throughout the country and the nature of nursing necessitates shift work. Nurses in New Zealand are predominantly women and there are gender issues that make access to postgraduate education problematic. Learning that uses the benefits of technology is becoming increasingly common with flexible learning, e-learning, and online courses available for postgraduate nursing education.

Whilst NI as a postgraduate specialist subject has not been recognized in New Zealand, nurses are favoring the health informatics options. In 1998, the University of Otago, in conjunction with Wellington Medical School, offered for the first time a diploma in health informatics. The University of Auckland commenced offering postgraduate programs that include courses in health informatics in 2001. Both tertiary education providers have given nurses the opportunity to study informatics in a broad context alongside other health professionals.

The first Australian experiences of nurses using computers were compiled into an edited text by Graham MacKay and Anita Griffin in 1989. The first Australian textbook on health informatics was published in 1996 (Hovenga, Kidd, and Cesnik, 1996). Much of NI education continues to be provided by nursing computer/informatics groups via study days, seminars, and conferences. The Lincoln Institute of Health Sciences (now Latrobe University) provided registered nurses undertaking postregistration degrees with opportunities to include computer studies in their course as early as 1979. Central Queensland University introduced nurses to computers in 1989 with a strong commitment to a computer-assisted-managed learning project (Zelmer et al., 1991). A 1990 survey of all tertiary nursing programs in Australia found that 27% (10 out of 37 respondents) had more than 5 years' experience of teaching computing to nurses, and 73 % (27) included computing within their nursing programs most frequently as a core unit (Hancock and Henderson, 1991). There has been little progress since then. Informatics education for nurses in Australia varies considerably from one university to another (Hovenga et al., 1999; Soar et al., 2003). Most have one person attempting the impossible, often in environments where fellow nurse academics have little or no knowledge of informatics. In some instances, there is active resistance to its introduction.

Some schools of nursing integrate informatics into their undergraduate nursing program to some extent. Most universities offer one unit of study within their undergraduate nursing pre- and postregistration programs as an elective. Central Queensland University offers an undergraduate degree program in NI as a post registration program. This enables all registered nurses either to obtain a double degree or to convert their hospital-based certificate or University-based diploma into a Bachelor's degree. CQU also offers a certificate, postgraduate diploma, and Master's degree in health informatics. Some of these graduates are now pursuing PhD studies, others are actively engaged in promoting the use of IT in the workplace, and many work in hospital-based NI positions.

◼ Summary

It is clearly evident that the professional health, medical, and nursing organizations play a major role in the awareness raising, education, and dissemination of knowledge about the field of health informatics. This is becoming increasingly complex with the proliferation of government initiatives spanning multiple government departments. This is a reflection of the multidisciplinary nature of health informatics. Nurses, as the largest group of health professionals, have a major role to play. This requires a sound knowledge about the many stakeholders so that nurses can play a role in coordinating their efforts to ultimately benefit the healthcare consumer, patients, communities, and society as a whole.

References

Asia Pacific Medical Informatics Association (APAMI), an IMIA Regional Group, *http://www.apami.net/index. php*, accessed August 6, 2004.

Australian Government Department of Health and Ageing eHealth initiatives, *http://www.health.gov.au/ ehealth.htm*, accessed August 6, 2004.

Australian Government: National Supply Chain initiative, *http://www.healthsupplychain.gov.au/events.htm*, accessed August 6, 2004.

Australian Government: GP (Primary Health Care) and Hospital Care Integration, *http://www.health.gov.au/ pcd/programs/gphi/index.htm*, accessed August 6, 2004.

Australian Government: Aboriginal and Torris Strait Islander coordinated care trials, *http://www.health. gov.au/oatsih/pubs/coord.htm*, accessed August 6, 2004.

Australian Government: Health Call Centres Program, *http://www.health.gov.au/pcd/programs/hcc/index.htm*, accessed August 6, 2004.

Australian Health Care Agreements, *http://www.health. gov.au/ahca/agreements.htm*, accessed August 6, 2004.

Australian Hospital Information, Performance Information Program (formerly the Casemix Development Program), *http://www.health.gov.au/ casemix/*, accessed August 7, 2004.

Australian Institute of Health and Welfare (AIHW). (2004a). *Australia's Health 2004*, *http://www.aihw. gov.au/publications/index.cfm/title/10014*, accessed August 6, 2004.

Australian Institute of Health and Welfare (AIHW). (2004b). AIHW Access No. 16, May 20, 2004, Project Report—METeOR is coming *http://www.aihw.gov.au/ publications/hwi/access16/access16-c01.pdf*, accessed August 6, 2004.

Australian Institute of Health and Welfare (AIHW), *Knowledgebase*, *http://www.aihw.gov.au/ knowledgebase/index.html* accessed August 6, 2004.

Boston Consulting Group Report. (2004). *National Health Information Management and Information & Communications Technology Strategy*. NHIG & AHIC Australian Department of Health and Ageing. *http://www.health.gov.au/healthonline/docs/bcg.pdf*, accessed August 6, 2004.

Chu, S., Mair, M., and Hobson, C. (2002). Developing the health event summary system. In *Proceedings of Health Informatics New Zealand Congress 2002*. Auckland.

Cressey, P. (2003). Building the Health System of the Future: IT and IM as Building Blocks, Health Care and Informatics Review Online December 1, 2003. Enigma Publishing, *http://www.enigma.co.nz/hcro/website/ index.cfmhttp://enigma.co.nz/*, accessed August 6, 2004.

Health Level Seven (HL7). *Electronic Health Record Functional Model and Standard*, *http://www.hl7.org/ ehr/*, accessed August 6 2004.

Ho, M. Y. and Hovenga, E. J. S. (1999). What do nurses have to say about information technology in their workplace? In J. Walker, S. Wheaton, M. Wise, and K. Stark (Eds.), *HIC 99 Handbook of Abstracts*. Full Paper on CD-ROM of Proceedings, HISA, Melbourne, Australia.

Ho, M. Y. and Hovenga, E. J. S. (2003). The study of Queensland nurses' attitude and behaviour towards computerisation at the workplace In H. de Fatima Marin, E. P. Marques, E. Hovenga, and W. Goossen (Eds.), *Proceedings of Nursing Informatics, Rio de Janeiro*.

Hovenga, E. J. S., Kidd, M., and Cesnik, B. (1996). *Health Informatics, An overview*. South Melbourne: Churchill Livingstone.

Hovenga, E. J. S., Luck, J., Plummer, A., and Ho, M. (1999). *An Australian Survey of Informatics Education in Health, Medical and Nursing Programs*. Unpublished Working Paper.

ICT Standards Committee. (2004). Foundations for the Future: Priorities for health information standardisation in Australia, 2004–2008. Unpublished Working Paper.

i-Health Ltd, *http://www.i-healthviews.com/overview_ profile.aspx*

Karmel, T. and Li, J. (2002). The Nursing Workforce 2010 —National Review of Nursing Education, *http://www. dest.gov.au/archive/highered/nursing/pubs/nursing_ worfforce_2010/nursing_workforce_default.htm*, accessed August 7, 2004.

MacKay, G. and Griffin, A. (1989). *Nurses Using Computers: Australian Experiences*. Armidale, New South Wales: A.C.A.E Publications.

National Nursing Organisations, *http://www.anf.org.au/ nno/*, accessed August 6, 2004.

New Zealand Ministerial Committee on Health Information Standards Organisations. (2002). *Setting up a New Zealand Health Standards Organisation*. Wellington: Ministry of Health.

New Zealand Ministry of Health. (2001). *From Strategy to Reality: The WAVE Report*. Wellington: Ministry of Health.

New Zealand Ministry of Health. (2003). *From Present to Future: A Draft National Health Information Standards Plan for New Zealand*. Wellington: Ministry of Health.

NHWI News International Recognition for the Knowledgebase. (1998). *AIH&W Newsletter*, No.14, p. 3.

Oakley, A. (2001). Teledermatology in New Zealand. *Journal of Cutaneous Medicine and Surgery* 5(2):111–116.

OpenEHR Community, *http://www.openehr.org/*, accessed August 6, 2004.

Orion Systems International *http://www.orion.co.nz/*

Royal Australian Nurses Federation. (1984). *Computerised Patient Data and Nursing Information Systems: Some Considerations*. Melbourne, Australia.

Soar, J., Marsault, A., Sara, T., Mount, C., Hardy, J., Swinkels, W., and Yearwoord, J. (2003). *Health Informatics Education, HISA & Australian Department of Health and Ageing, http://www.health.gov.au/healthonline/docs/hiefrept.pdf*, accessed August 6, 2004.

Wilson, S. (2002). Development of a personal digital assistant (PDA) as point-of-care technology in nursing education. In *Proceedings of Health Informatics New Zealand Congress 2002*. Auckland.

Wilson, S. K. and Roy, D. (2003). KIWI Nurs: An automated documentation solution for nursing education. In *Proceedings of 8th International Congress in Nursing Informatics, Rio de Janeiro*.

Zelmer, A. C., Lynn, B., McLees, M. A., and Zelmer, A. E. (1991). A Progress Report on the Use of CAL/CML in a Three Year Pre-Registration Diploma Program. In E. Hovenga, K. Hannah, K. McCormick, and J. Ronald. (Eds.), *Nursing Informatics '91; Proceedings of the Fourth International Conference on Nursing Use of Computers and Information Science*. Melbourne: Springer-Verlag.

40

Nursing Informatics in Asia

Hyeoun-Ae Park

OBJECTIVES

1. To describe the development of nursing informatics (NI) in selected Asian countries.
2. To identify historical milestones, changes, and trends influencing how nurses embrace informatics, such as government initiatives and international collaborations.
3. To discuss NI practice, education, and research.

KEY WORDS

information systems
standards
health informatics
government initiatives

Since computers were first introduced into the healthcare sectors of Asian countries in the 1970s, there have been exciting developments in healthcare informatics associated with the rapid growth in information and communication technology. The first applications of information technology in healthcare in Asian countries were in administration, billing, and insurance. Now these countries are moving toward implementing paperless electronic health records. This chapter provides an overview of the current status of the field of NI in South Korea, Japan, China, Taiwan, and Thailand. It describes the history of NI, the use of informatics in clinical practice, informatics education, informatics research, and government initiatives and professional outreaches.

The short histories of NI have varied between Asian countries, but all governments have played a very important role in introducing information technology into the healthcare sector by providing funds, developing infrastructure, and introducing policies to promote its use. Professional organizations have also played an important role. In most of these countries computers were first used in nursing during the early 1970s, although the terms health informatics and NI were not introduced until the 1980s or early 1990s following the establishment of professional organizations for health informatics.

The adoption of informatics in Asian countries usually began as a vision by a group of individuals in the government or a professional organization, who promoted the use of information technologies to support nurses in all areas of nursing practice. This occurred in nursing care practice, education, and research organizations, as well as within the information technology industry and via related government departments and existing professional organizations.

As information technology has become indispensable to the daily activities of healthcare professionals, more and more nursing schools are beginning to realize the importance of providing informatics courses to nurses. Basic computer literacy education is now a part of nursing education in most Asian countries, and graduate programs majoring in NI are also available now in some countries, such as South Korea and Taiwan.

Reports of research into NI began to appear in the domestic Asian nursing journals in 1990s, but such research is still in its infancy. In most countries, information technology first appeared as an educational tool, following by its use in clinical practice in applications such as expert systems and electronic nursing records. This use in clinical practice lead to the development of standards becoming a favorite research topic.

Events external to the nursing profession frequently catalyzed the adoption of informatics by nurses. International multidisciplinary informatics links have assisted these beginnings and their progression. The progress in Japan, China, and South Korea has been expedited by the hosting of the International Medical Informatics Association (IMIA) triannual conferences in 1980, 1989, and 1997, respectively. Moreover, the formation of the Asia Pacific Medical Informatics Association in 1993 helped launch national healthcare informatics associations in China, Japan, South Korea, Taiwan, and Thailand due to the hosting of triannual conferences in the Pacific Rim. The China, Japan, and Korea Medical Informatics Association (formed in 1999) organizes conferences, seminars, and workshops once a year and creates forums for the sharing of experience and knowledge among both experts and users in these three countries. Asian Nurses who are interested in promoting informatics to their profession need to link up with this network.

This chapter provides an overview of the historical events in South Korea, Japan, Taiwan, China, and Thailand, and highlights factors that are critical to success for the benefit of those who have yet to embark on such a journey. The chapter concludes by summarizing significant events and examining their impact on the evolution of NI in this region.

Korea

South Korea comprises eight provinces with seven metropolitan cities, and the total population was about 47 million in 2002. The population is predominantly in urban areas, with 21% living within the Seoul metropolitan area. There are currently 190,720 licensed midwives and nurses, of whom 81,478 are practicing and 23,331 of these are situated in the Seoul metropolitan area.

Health informatics in South Korea has grown considerably in recent years with the professional outreach activities of the Korean Society of Medical Informatics (KOSMI) as well as with the help of government, private businesses, academic institutions, and medical and nursing organizations.

History of Nursing Informatics in Korea

The use of computers in South Korean healthcare began in the late 1970s in hospital finance and administration systems to expedite insurance reimbursements. Soon thereafter, the national health insurance system expanded to cover the whole population, and computers became necessary equipment in healthcare organizations. The terms *health informatics* and *NI* were first introduced in Korea when the KOSMI was founded in 1987.

In contrast, computers were not used in nursing education and research until 1993, and NI was not taught in universities until 1994. In 1993, the Nursing Informatics Special Interest Group was organized as one of the five special interest groups in the KOSMI, since the Nursing Informatics Group has held its own session at the biannual conferences of the KOSMI. Nursing has been highly visible in the KOSMI by the presentation and publishing of papers on the use of computers in nursing at these conferences and in the Journal of the KOSMI. The IMIA conference MEDINFO98, held in Seoul, provided an excellent opportunity for Korean nurses to become acquainted with NI. Currently, there are more than 200 active nurse members in the KOSMI out of 1,000 active members.

Further momentum for NI has been coming from funding for a NI study group provided by the Korean Science and Engineering Foundation since 1998. Activities of the study group include journal reviews and research activities such as survey studies of NI education and computer applications in nursing practice in Korean hospitals.

Korean nurses have attended and participated in many international conferences promoted or supported by IMIA or IMIA-NI since 1989. Korean nurses represented the country at the IMIA-NI Group in 1995, since then Korea has sent a representative to the group and participated actively in developing and furthering NI.

Use of Information Technology in Clinical Practice

According to a report published by the Korea Health Industry Development Institute in 2000, 100% of teaching hospitals, 96% of general hospitals, and 75% of private clinics now have hospital information systems (Korea Health Industry Development Institute, 2000). Such a high implementation rate is believed to have been initially driven by financial factors associated with medical insurance claims, with the focus subsequently shifting to all areas of patient care when clinicians began to use computers in their practices. A recent study shows that all of the teaching hospitals and about 40% of general hospitals in Korea are using order communication systems (Kwak, 2000), which enable physicians to communicate with other departments for practice-related requisitions and the retrieval of data. In addition, about 95% of teaching hospitals and 20% of general hospitals are equipped with picture archiving and communication systems (PACSs). There has been a great deal of interest among healthcare organizations in acquiring these systems since the government announced high reimbursement rates for diagnostic radiology examinations using PACSs in 2000, and PACSs are now one of the most common information technology systems in South Korean hospitals. Hospitals in South Korea are now beginning to implement paperless electronic medical record systems.

The use of computers in clinical nursing practice in Korea began first in medium-sized hospitals. These hospitals initially used computers mainly for administration and billing, as did most hospitals in other countries, but later a patient-care component was added. These systems allowed physicians to enter medical orders directly into the computer, and major ancillary departments could receive requisitions and enter test results. The nurses' work lists could be viewed on screens or printed so that nurses did not need to copy medication schedules or care activities onto the Kardex, or write paper messages. Other Korean hospitals were also pursuing this level of automation. Nursing information systems proliferated when large hospitals (with more than 1,000 beds) began opening in the mid-1990s. These new hospitals were equipped with nursing information systems when they first opened. They included unique nursing activities such as nursing assessments, nursing care plans, and patient classifications, in addition to nursing activities related to billing, managerial and coordinating activities, and physician-delegated tasks.

A home healthcare system for community-based clinical practice was developed by the Home Healthcare Team at the College of Nursing, Seoul National University (Park et al., 2000). Home healthcare nurses use laptop computers to note and check medication and progress in electronic patient records, and to communicate electronically with other home healthcare team members.

Health Informatics Education

As information technology has become indispensable in healthcare and its impact on the daily activities of healthcare professionals has become significant, schools are beginning to realize the importance of health informatics education for clinicians. According to a recent survey on health informatics and computer education programs in South Korean medical and nursing schools, about 25% of medical schools and 21% of nursing schools offer health informatics courses, while the remainder offer introductory computer courses (Park, 2002). The course contents vary a great deal from school to school, and the instructors are mostly self-taught in these subjects. This indicates that there is a need for standardization of health informatics courses for baccalaureate programs based on the tasks

of healthcare professionals, together with graduate programs to produce qualified health informatics educators.

Most nursing schools in Korea are adding informatics to graduate curricula so that graduate students can take informatics courses as an elective. The graduate specialization program in NI in Korea was first introduced at Seoul National University in 2001. This program is the only one in Korea that awards a master's degree in NI.

Research

Most papers presented at KOSMI conferences and published in the Journal of the KOSMI since 1991 have addressed the application of commercially available programs, with more recent papers discussing the use of computers as a tool for nursing education. Distance education using the Internet has also been described (Park, Cho, and Kim, 1998; Cho and Park, 1998; Kim et al., 2000; Choi et al., 1999). The trend toward system integration in the health industry in the late 1990s lead to more articles and presentations on standardization. Papers on the standardization of nursing vocabulary and nursing documentation forms have also appeared (Park et al., 1999; Park and Cho, 2000; Coenen et al., 2001).

Another popular research area is the use of artificial intelligence in nursing diagnosis (Park, Lee, and Song, 1995; Kim, 1998; Yoo et al., 1998). The use of personalized digital assistants (PDAs) in hospital and home healthcare settings along with the standardization and the use of Web-based electronic patient records are current areas of interest (Hyun et al., 1999, Cho and Park, 2003).

Standardization Activities

There are current efforts to implement a single, integrated healthcare and nursing terminology in South Korea, the primary motivation for which is compatibility of data, clinical documentation, and research outcomes across the country. There are Korean representatives actively involved in several international initiatives toward this end, such as International Organization for Standardization/Technical Committee 215 (ISO/TC215) and Health Level Seven (HL7).

Administrative information systems in the healthcare sector essentially use the Korean Standard Classification of Diseases (the Korean version of the International Classification for Disease [ICD] 10), while clinician information systems are beginning to use more concept-oriented terminology such as the SNOMED (Systematized Nomenclature of Medicine). The majority of existing nursing terminologies, such as the North American

Nursing Diagnosis Association (NANDA) Taxonomy I and II, Nursing Interventions Classification (NIC), Home Healthcare Classification (HHCC), the Omaha system, Nursing Outcomes Classification (NOC), and International Classification for Nursing Practice (ICNP), have been translated into Korean and standardized. Among these terminologies, the NANDA is the most frequently used in nursing education, and the 3N (NANDA-NIC-NOC) and ICNP are most frequently used in clinical practice for electronic nursing record systems in Korea.

Government Initiatives

The Korean government has contributed to the development of health informatics by providing funding or other incentives and guidelines in telemedicine, emergency medical systems, infectious diseases reporting systems, and standardization. The Korean government has contributed to the implementation of a nationwide information highway, with the Ministry of Information and Communication having funded information highway projects since the early 1990s. There are two information highways available: (1) the South Korea Advanced Research Network, which is mainly used for research activities; and (2) a nationwide commercialized network built by telecommunication companies (Korea Ministry of Information and Communication, 2002). These networks interconnect 12 metropolitan areas in South Korea at 622 Mbps, and smaller surrounding cities are connected at 155 Mbps. Individual users at their homes can use ADSL (asynchronous digital subscriber line) to connect to the Internet at a speed of 1–8 Mbps, and currently more than 50% of South Korean homes have ADSL connections. This is the highest percentage among all countries of the world.

The Korean Ministry of Health and Welfare established a long-term plan for a national health and welfare network (NHWN) in 1993. The NHWN covers six areas: public health, hospitals and clinics, health insurance, food and drugs, national pension, and health and welfare administration. Public health was selected as the top-priority project in 1994, to be carried out in three phases. The first phase (from 1994 to 1997) computerized the administrative and patient-care activities of health centers. The second phase (from 1998 to 2001) developed infrastructure for the public health network, integrating network systems among health centers, health subcenters, and primary healthcare posts. An electronic data interchange system between the public healthcare facilities and the health insurers was developed for health insurance claims. Possible ways of linking the NHWN to the city, county,

and district networks of the Ministry of Governmental Affairs and Home Affairs were studied. The current third phase, which started in 2001, involves the development of data warehousing at the level of major cities and provinces. Once this system is implemented successfully, it will be expanded to the whole of South Korea.

Professional Outreach

Since its foundation in 1987, the KOSMI has played a very important role in promoting and developing health informatics by holding biannual academic conferences, various seminars, workshops, and open forums, and by publishing journals. KOSMI has also offered educational programs for beginners in health informatics.

Organizations such as the Korean Medical Association and the Korean Nurses Association have also played significant roles by including health informatics in their continuing education programs. Another healthcare informatics expert group, the Health Informatics Standardization Committee, serving as the South Korean technical advisory group of the ISO/TC215, has held open forums and published health information standards.

The IMIA has contributed significantly to furthering the knowledge of South Korean healthcare professionals about worldwide trends in health informatics. These individuals have attended and participated in many international conferences promoted or supported by the IMIA since 1989.

Technology Trends

The rapid growth in the number of mobile telephone users (currently estimated to be around 65% of the total population) and the advances in wireless local area network (LAN) technology have lead to mobile computing in healthcare becoming a popular issue in South Korea, with many healthcare organizations testing its feasibility in special wards. The main users of the systems currently are nurses attending patients at bedsides, but this will soon be extended to other healthcare professionals. Although PDAs, Web pads, and notebook and tablet computers are all suitable mobile computing platforms, users favor notebook computers with wireless LAN connections because of their larger screen size and easier-to-use interface.

The need for telemedicine continues to grow in Korea with the increasing numbers of elderly, patients with chronic diseases, and patients who are discharged early. Many telemedicine systems have been tested over the past 10 years, one of which is a teleconsultation system initiated by the government. Such systems allow, for example, a generalist doctor at a health center in a remote area to have a telepathology or a teleradiology consultation with the specialists of a tertiary hospital. Another example of telemedicine is telecare at home, with the telecare center of Seoul National University Hospital and the telemedicine center of Gil Hospital being among the most active telecare-at-home clinics (Yoo, 2002). Telepractitioners at these centers maintain special schedules for their remote clients. They set aside 1–2 days per week to take care of their clients using virtual reality technology via the Internet. Currently, the teleconsultation fee is reimbursed by health insurance, whereas the use of telecare-at-home clinics is not yet covered.

Summary

The Korean healthcare environment is becoming inhospitable due to high healthcare costs, increasing competitions among healthcare organizations, decreased funding from the government, and customers with more sophisticated demands. The introduction of information systems and information technology can help healthcare organizations to survive under these difficult conditions.

Health informatics and the usage of information technology have seen rapid progress in South Korea. Most of the Korean healthcare organizations were computerized following the introduction of the national health insurance system. Over the past few years there have been exciting developments in the areas of PACS, electronic medical records, information highways, mobile computing, telemedicine, and health informatics education. All of these developments have improved, either directly or indirectly, the productivity of healthcare professionals, the efficiency and effectiveness of the healthcare industry, and also the education of healthcare professionals.

Japan

The population of Japan is about 127 million, which is about twice that of the United Kingdom and half that of the United States. There are about 10,000 hospitals in Japan, of which about 430 have more than 400 beds. About 750,000 nurses work at these hospitals, including about 220,000 nurse aides, and there are about 260,000 medical doctors, 90,000 dentists, and 230,000 pharmacists (Ministry of Health, Labour and Welfare, 2004).

The healthcare delivery system in Japan provides easy access to healthcare. All citizens can choose healthcare institutions and doctors freely, and their financial contribution to health insurance is proportional to their income. The insurance fee is deducted from the monthly salary, and pooled by each insurance union. Insured individuals and families pay 20 and 30%, respectively, of all health expenditure, and the publicly funded health insurance pays the rest when a patient receives medical treatment in a hospital. The hospital receives reimbursement for the balance from the national health insurance. The Japanese government will contribute a maximum of 70,000 yen to the medical treatment of a person over 1 month. Both the easy access to healthcare and low out-of-pocket cost in Japan help to provide the populace with a sense of security.

The total health expenditure of Japan remains lower than that in some other advanced nations, which is partially attributable to healthier dietary habits. The relatively small number of healthcare professionals working in Japan also helps to contain healthcare expenditure. The average length of hospital stays has recently been shortened, and thus many newly hospitalized patients are in the acute phase. This increases the probability of medical accidents, which can be offset by utilizing health informatics to improve medical safety.

Health Informatics in Japan

Japan began to pay attention to the use of computers in healthcare during the late 1970s following the increased use of computers in other industries. Japan hosted the IMIA conference MEDINFO80 in 1980. The Japanese Association of Medical Informatics (JAMI) was founded at that time with the aim of supporting health informatics in Japan. Since then JAMI has held 24 annual and biannual academic conferences, and these conferences have contributed considerably to the progress of health informatics in Japan (JAMI, 1996; Kamiizumi and Ota, 2004). Initially research was focused on computerized billing systems for medical fees, and the development of the use of personal computers at an individual level (JAMI, 2004). The focus then shifted to research and development of systems at the organizational level, such as hospital and regional information systems, and research into basic information technology for healthcare such as database design, network security, and data-switching technology. The current focuses are ethical issues in health informatics, medical finances, and quality assurance. This illustrates that the scope of health informatics has gradually expanded since it was first introduced into Japan during the 1980s.

Medical information departments in about 50 national university hospitals have made the largest contribution to the development of health informatics in Japan. Each organization has been developing its own hospital information systems for its own applications to clinical practice, education, and research (Supplement of national university medical information processing department liaison conference, 1995–2003). This work helped Japan to determine the information, information technology, and mechanisms that were needed for healthcare applications, but their independence has hindered standardization in many healthcare fields. Standardization is one of the many problems in the use of healthcare information technology that needs to be resolved.

History of Nursing Informatics in Japan

The Third International Congress on Medical Informatics, MEDINFO80, organized by the IMIA, was held in Tokyo in 1980. This congress included a special interest group on NI, which represented the beginning of NI in Japan (JAMI, 1996; Kamiizumi and Ota, 2004). This did not result in immediate progress in Japanese NI education, due to schools being vocationally oriented. However, in the late 1990s nursing education in Japan rapidly shifted to a more academic orientation, and there are now more than 100 universities offering baccalaureate programs and 40 universities offering graduate programs. Some baccalaureate programs and graduate schools include NI courses in their curricula. NI was applied more in clinical practice than in academic fields during the 1990s, with more nurses learning about utilizing computers in nursing practice through the activities of medical information department settings in the national university hospitals. It was also evident that clinical nurses presented more papers than academic researchers at the annual meetings of the JAMI. The Annual Meeting for Nursing Information Systems that was established as a task force of the JAMI also supports clinical practice, and most of its members are clinical nurses. The Nursing Division of the JAMI was established in 2000 and is managed by a team of clinical nurses and academic researchers. Several textbooks on NI have been published, but systematized NI education has not yet been implemented. The Japanese Nurses Association prepared a course on nursing information management as a first step of a continuing education curriculum for ward managers. The standard textbook was published on March 2004 (Kamiizumi and Ota, 2004), and the lecturers are researchers of health informatics and NI, and clinical nurses working at the hospitals where hospital information systems were introduced.

Nursing Informatics Education

As on April 2004, there were 486 professional schools, 31 junior colleges, 120 universities, and 45 graduate schools in Japan (Tokyo Academy, 2004), compared to 461 professional schools, 74 junior colleges, and 30 universities in 1994 (Japanese Nursing Association, 2002). This comparison illustrates that nursing education in Japan has shifted from professional schools to universities and postgraduate education during the last 10 years. However, there are still very few universities with separate NI programs. The increasing development of hospital information systems in Japan has lead to discussions on the utilization of information technology in clinical nursing practice. Continuous education of NI is being emphasized, along with the promotion of electronic health records. However, it is difficult to conclude that the curricula of nursing schools have reflected the changes in society and clinical fields. Rather, it appears that clinical practice is now more advanced than nursing education.

Universities provided elementary computer literacy education during the first half of the 1990s, but this became unnecessary thereafter due to the introduction of computer education into elementary and junior high schools. Overall, the teaching of computer literacy on document retrieval, utilization of statistical processing, and Web utilization has increased, but barriers to the development of the NI remain in Japan: (1) there are few researchers and educators in NI, (2) there is little development of educational tools, and (3) the cost of improving the network and computer environments is high. However, the importance of universities providing a satisfactory curriculum is being recognized due to the increasing importance of NI, with this being more so in graduate schools than in baccalaureate education.

Nursing Informatics Research

The amount of NI research is increasing in Japan, the two main purposes of which are improving the quality and standardization of nursing practice. NI was one of the main subject areas of paper presentations at a recent annual meeting of the Japanese Academy of Nursing (Japan Academy for Nursing Science, 2003), indicating that it is becoming one of the major areas in nursing. There were many reports on research into the use of information technology as an education tool during the 1990s (Ochiai, Sota, and Ezumi 1997; Kanai-Pak et al., 1997; Muranaka et al., 1997; Yamanouchi, Nakano, and Nojiri, 1997; Majima, 1997; Ezumi, Sota, and Ochiai, 1997), and on the use of information technology in clinical practice, especially on decision support systems for nursing in hospital information systems and electronic health records (JAMI, 2003). There has also been research into the use of information to prevent nursing-related accidents (Tsuru et al., 2004) and into telenursing (Kawaguchi, Azuma, and Ohta, 2004). Research into nursing-practice algorithms using thinking-aloud methods have begun in Japan.

Nursing Informatics Practice

Becoming a specialist in NI is useful when hospital information systems and electronic health records are introduced. However, the accreditation program of the Japan Nursing Association does not recognize the training for such specialists. Instead, the training of informatics nurses mainly occurs in hospital settings. In each hospital, nurses working on medical information are active in committees and working groups. Most of them involve not only nursing-related work but also medical-information-related work. Their lack of formal technical education often causes difficulties, and hence it is predicted that the importance of nurses with NI education will increase. The JAMI began an accreditation program for "healthcare information technologists" in 2003. Hospitals are looking for new healthcare staff with knowledge of both healthcare and information technology who can control information flow. Although a healthcare information technologist is a healthcare professional with such training, it is necessary to distinguish between the roles of the NI clinical nursing specialist and a healthcare information technologist. Informatics nurses will be expected to expand their activities in healthcare when both professions are introduced to hospitals.

Japanese Government Initiatives and Standards Development in Japan

An "e-Japan" strategy encompassing all Japanese ministries and related agencies is progressing now in Japan. The standardization of medical information is one of the main themes in the healthcare sector. The Ministry of Health, Labor, and Welfare announced a grand design for healthcare, and set the following achievement goals for 2006 (Panel on Healthcare and Medical Information Systems, 2002): (1) electronic health records will be introduced into 60% of hospitals with more than 400 beds and into 60% of clinics and (2) the electronic health expenditure payment system will be introduced into 70% of all hospitals. Standardization of the terminology used in electronic health records is a requirement for achieving this goal, and the Ministry of Health, Labor, and Welfare has begun a project for developing a national standard, which is publicly available on the Internet (The Medical Information Systems Development Center, 2004). This is especially useful for hospitals introducing hospital information systems for the first time. The following five standards have already been

completed: (1) 581 facilities now perform medical diagnoses using the ICD 10, (2) 330 facilities have surgical and medical treatment standards, (3) 5,700 clinical tests have been registered in the clinical laboratory test standard, (4) about 38,000 drug names have been registered by 203 enterprises, and (5) about 210,000 medical supplies have been registered by 336 enterprises. Standardized symptoms, physiologic function examinations, imaging tests, dental terminology, and nursing terminology are currently under development, and nursing actions and observation items in nursing terminology are available to the public since the middle of 2004. The terminology used in nursing practice has been collected, analyzed, and redesigned. About 260 fundamental nursing practices have been identified and named in Japan. They have been categorized into daily-life care, family support, guidance and education, adjustment during organization, care in the usage of equipment, care for the terminally ill and the bereaved family, and others. The two hospitals where electronic health records using this nursing terminology were developed have utilized the terminology describing nursing care plan and nursing order, and in the implementation of care; and differences in the nursing care offered to patients became clear. Continuous 24-hour observation of nursing care can be shared, indicating that the use of such a system is very useful for the medical profession.

 ## China

According to the Fifth National Census reported by the National Bureau of Statistics, the population of China was almost 1.3 billion in 2000. The population is aging fast, with those 65 years old and older representing 6.96% of the population in 2000, compared to 5.57% in the 1990 census. Comparison of the two censuses also reveals that the population is now more educated, with college, high school, middle school, and elementary school education increasing between 1990 and 2000 by 154, 39, 45, and 4%, from 1,422 to 3,611, 8,039 to 11,146, 23,344 to 33,961, and 37,057 to 35,701 per 100,000, respectively (National Population and Family Planning Commission of China, 2001). There were 17,764 hospitals, 5,275,000 healthcare professionals, and 1,266,000 registered nurses in China in 2003. This translates into approximately 1 nurse per 1,000 people (Ministry of Health, China, 2003). Only 5 and 20% of registered nurses in China have baccalaureates and 3-year diplomas, respectively (Nursing School of Weizhou Medical College, 2004).

In China, the majority of the population is found in rural areas, and thus the overall healthcare level, stability of society, and economic development of the whole of China is influenced by healthcare services in rural areas (Hao et al., 2000). The primary healthcare systems in rural China typically involve cooperation at county, town, and village levels. These systems include providing medical services, the training of healthcare staff, hygiene education, and the development of a patriotic health campaign (Ma, 2000).

The SARS epidemic in China lead to reconsiderations of the current healthcare systems in rural areas. Some Chinese consider that the system is not moving forward and that more effort should be devoted to epidemic prevention, and that a new system of cooperative medical care and new salvation system of the poor should be set up to ensure health in rural areas and enhance the stability of society and economic development of country (Zong, 2004). The SARS epidemic also led to suggestions of an integrated system for responding to public health emergencies and for disease control and prevention (Luo, Feng, and Zhang, 2004).

The health information infrastructure has improved dramatically in China since the initiation of the National 95 Plan. This plan includes implementation of a National Medical Information Network, advances in constructing hospital information systems as well as advances in community healthcare, health supervision, disease control, maternal and child healthcare, telemedicine, and distance medical education (Ministry of Health, China, 2003).

The China Medical Informatics Association (CMIA) was founded in 1981. This is an academic group and is a member of the IMIA. The CMIA hosted the sixth international MEDINFO89 meeting in Beijing (CMIA, 2004). There are two other professional societies related to medical informatics in China: the Chinese Society of Medical Information (under the China Medical Association) and the Chinese Hospital Information Management Association (under the Chinese Hospital Association). The Chinese Society of Medical Information was founded in 1993, and its activities include holding academic conferences and seminars, continuing education, and training. There have been nine academic conferences since 1993 (Liu, Wang, and Du, 2003). The Chinese Hospital Information Management Association was founded in 1996, and its activities include holding national and international academic collaborations and exchanges, establishing rules and standards of national hospital management, and training hospital information management staff. In 2004, the Chinese Society of Medical Information hosted a conference on hospital information systems in collaboration with the American Healthcare Information and Management Systems Society (CHIMA, 2004).

Nursing Information Systems in China

The development of nursing information management systems began in China in late 1970s (Li et al., 2001), and they were first used in 1987 (Nursing Center, Ministry of Health, China, 1995; Li et al., 1999; Fu, 2000). The first software implementation was a computer-assisted primary nursing care system (Nursing Center, Ministry of Health, China, 1995). The development of information management systems for nursing in Chinese traditional medicine began in 1994 (Li et al., 2001). Many hospitals in China now use nursing information systems, although there are no official statistics available. Some examples include a nursing information system for the management of nursing staff, nursing operation work, continuing education, scientific research, and finance and economics (Zhang, Fu, and Fan, 1999); nursing information systems for nursing records and nursing management based on an army satellite project called the No. 1 Project of PLA (Qi et al., 2000; Zhang, Cheng, and Qi, 2003; Wang, Wu, and Xu, 2003; Fang, Wang, and Han, 2004; Liu et al., 2004); and an Internet-based nursing information management system (Wang et al., 2001; Zhang et al., 2004).

History of Nursing Informatics in China

The Nursing Informatics Special Interest Group with 20 hospital nurses was founded as a branch of the CMIA in 1991. A year later an expert group for nursing information technology was founded by the Nursing Department of the Chinese Ministry of Health, its mission being to establish criteria for nursing management and the training of nurse administrators for nursing information management (Nursing Center, Ministry of Health, China, 1995).

The first article referring to the term "nursing information science" appeared in China in 1999, and this led to the application of information technology in the field of nursing science for education and research (Fan and Fu, 2000; Fan and Li, 2000). The term NI was first used in the Chinese literature in 2002 (Jiang, 2002).

Nursing Informatics Education

Higher nursing education was introduced in 1983, and by 2001 there were 120 schools with 3-year diploma programs, 62 schools offering a baccalaureate, and 11 schools with master's programs (Nursing School of Weizhou Medical College, 2004). At least one computer course is required at the baccalaureate level, and nursing students can select other computer courses as elective courses.

According to a literature review, computer-assisted instruction began at nursing institutes in China during the mid-1990s, since then it has been used in baccalaureate and continuing education courses in the clinical nursing field (Zhu, Lu, and Yin, 1995; Jiang et al., 1998; Li et al., 2002). Distance learning is also being used for nursing continuing education in China. The first distance learning program in China is a collaboration between China and Canada run by the School of Nursing, Tianjin Medical University in 1999 (Zhou and Song, 2001).

Nursing Informatics Research

NI research is at its infancy in China, with only 30 research articles published in domestic nursing journals from 1994 to 2004 (with key words related to the use of computers in nursing and nursing information with the research areas of nursing practice, nursing management, and nursing education).

Nursing Informatics Practice

The use of NI in clinical practice in China includes nursing quality management, staff management, nursing information management, and training clinical skills for staff nurses (Zhang, Cheng, and Qi, 2003). Several expert systems for nursing diagnoses, nursing care plan, and nursing assessment have been reported (Ji et al., 1994; Wang, 1995; Zhang, Fu, and Fan, 1999).

The major weakness of nursing information management systems in China is the lack of national standards and the low level of computer literacy and informatics skill exhibited by nurses (Nursing Center, Ministry of Health, China, 1995).

■ Thailand

Thailand is located in Southeast Asia with Burma, Cambodia, Laos, and Malaysia as neighboring countries. The country has a population of about 65 million living in 76 provinces. The life expectancy of males and females is 71.6 and 74.7 years, respectively. Ninety-five percent of the population is Buddhist and 3.8% is Muslim (CIA, 2004). Even though most people work in agriculture, major revenue of the country comes from service and industry (Economy, 2004). There were 92 regional/general hospitals, 707 community hospitals, and 9,559 health centers across Thailand in 2004 (Country Health Profile, 2004). The government is currently launching a Universal Healthcare Coverage policy in order to improve the access to and quality of healthcare, as well as to contain health-

care expenditure. The Thai government is restructuring its healthcare system by placing more emphasis on primary care and health promotion. Recently the government has also attempted to develop a healthcare hub for international clients. These policies require changes in human resources including nurses, since the demand for nurses in primary care settings across the country is increasing to serve the population at large, as is that for nurses competent at working in hospitals serving international clients.

NI was first introduced as small special interest groups and later expanded to the national level through the support of the Nurses' Association of Thailand, the World Health Organization, and the Ministry of Public Health (MOPH). This section describes the development of NI in Thailand between 1997 and 2004.

The Development of a Health Information System

In 1997, the Thai MOPH began to implement a national health information system, which included the development of a nursing component. The former director of the MOPH Nursing Division, Mrs. Areeya Suppalak, considered it important to provide nurses with the means of using information technology. Funding was received from the World Health Organization in 1999 as a result of a collaborative effort between the Center for Nursing Research at the Department of Nursing, The Faculty of Medicine, Ramathibodi Hospital, Mahidol University, and the MOPH Nursing Division to develop the ideal nursing minimum data set (NMDS) and a preliminary nursing classification system (Phuphaibul et al., 1999). The NMDS was identified as essential for developing an efficient nursing database. The project was expanded and the development of the nursing classification system was later merged with the project of the Nurses' Association of Thailand for validating the alpha version of the ICNP developed by the International Council of Nurses (ICN) (International Council of Nurses, 1999).

Development of an NMDS

The first step in developing a nursing information system is to identify an essential NMDS, and here the process of developing an NMDS specific to Thailand is discussed. In the survey study of Phuphaibul et al. (1999), questionnaires were sent to nurses from 500 randomly selected hospitals, 378 of which were returned and analyzed. That survey study identified 23 items of nursing data, including patient name, hospital number, ID number, admission number, patient's address and phone number, address and phone number of significant person, gender, birth date, religion, education, health insurance, patient and family medical history/allergy, admission date, medical diagnosis, laboratory test, nursing problem, nursing intervention, nursing outcome, discharge/expired date, discharge plan, condition before discharge, referral, and home visit.

ICNP Translation and Validation

A resolution on developing an international nursing language was adopted during the 1989 ICN meeting in Seoul, Korea. The ICN therefore committed itself to the development of an international nursing taxonomy (i.e., the ICNP). The Nurses' Association of Thailand, under the former president Dr. Tassana Boontong, endorsed the development of the ICNP and agreed to translate it into Thai and validate an alpha version thereof. A steering committee of 24 experts from various nursing institutes was appointed, and the Thai translation of the ICNP was supervised by Dr. Siriporn Khampalikit and Ms. Angkana Siriyaporn with financial support from the MOPH Nursing Division in 1998.

The first NI conference was held in Bangkok in 1999, supported by the World Health Organization with additional support for a guest speaker, Dr. Amy Coenen from the ICN. More than 200 nurses across the country were invited to validate and comment on the alpha version of the translated ICNP. After the meeting, the Nursing Informatics Society of Thailand (TNI) was established with an initial membership of 114. The information gathered from the meeting was analyzed and reported to the World Health Organization and the Nurses' Association of Thailand. Later, in October 1999, the translation of the beta version of the ICNP was completed, validated, and disseminated (Phuphaibul et al., 2000). The content was further revised for improvement as the Nurses' Association of Thailand continued to further develop the nursing classification. The ICNP is currently used as a basis for the data set describing the nursing care of patients and their families. However, many issues, such as the need for concept-based translation and increasing nursing involvement in the process, still need to be addressed in order to implement the data set successfully (Volrathongchai, Delaney, and Phuphaibul, 2003).

Nursing Information System

A further attempt to implement the ICNP in the Thai nursing environment was the developed, a collaborative software program called "Healthware 2000" by the MOPH Nursing Division for the collection and retrieval of nursing care data. Several hospitals served as pilot hospitals. However, the usefulness of the program was limited by it not being sufficiently user friendly and many nurses having limited knowledge of the ICNP. The unsuccessful implementation of Healthware 2000 lead to the MOPH Division of Nursing further developing standard care plans using the ICNP, which were later adapted to computer implementation. This project is still in progress.

Recently the Nurses' Association of Thailand under the leadership of Dr. Jintana Unipan provided seed money for the development of a database including nursing diagnoses, nursing interventions, and nursing outcomes in 10 leading diagnostic-related groups using the beta version of the ICNP. The steering committee for this project comprised nurses from seven specialty areas: medical nursing, surgical nursing, pediatric nursing, maternal and child nursing, mental health and psychiatric nursing, community nursing and home healthcare, and cancer nursing.

Although a preliminary Thai NMDS has been identified, challenges associated with its development and implementation within the Thai national health information system remain. The evident continuity of the development of NI in Thailand demonstrates the commitment of the national nursing organizations. However, stronger collaborations between all concerned parties and a strategic plan are necessary for further achievement.

Professional Outreach

The first Medical Consortium meeting in 1991 lead to the establishment of the Thai Medical Informatics Society (TMI), who introduced the concept of medical informatics into Thailand. The founders were a group of medical professors whose original idea was to apply computer technology to medical care, and currently the TMI has 300 active members (Thai Medical Informatics Society, 2003).

The main objectives of the TMI are as follows:

1. To be the center for coordinating and distributing medical information.

2. To develop means for the management of medical information in administration and academic areas.

3. To exchange information and experience in medical informatics.

4. To support those who practice medical informatics.

5. To provide suggestions and recommendations for medical information sectors both within and outside the MOPH.

6. To not be involved in any commercial or political activities.

The main activities of TMI are as follows:

1. Holding an annual conference.

2. Supporting the meeting, training, and information sharing for the development of medical informatics in Thailand.

3. Publishing and distributing four issues of documents per year as approved by the board.

4. Being the center for the coordination of the medical information exchanges.

5. Being the center for information and ideas focused on the development of medical informatics.

The TMI includes a clinical informatics special interest group, a NI special interest group, and the HIS/LIS Club. The clinical informatics group aims to motivate those who are interested in health information systems, such as system managers, medical administrators, and clinical practitioners, to collaboratively build a national plan for a better health information system. Examples of a clinical information system are a population health risk appraisal system, a clinical management supporting system, a clinical management system, a medical management system, and clinical telemedicine. The NI interest group focuses on the classification of nursing data and the development in nursing databases. Several hospitals have been working on the development of nursing databases. The HIS/LIS Club is the forum for those interested in software development for specific clinical applications (HIS/LIS Club Thailand, 2004).

The TNI supports the development of NI, especially nursing databases using the ICNP. The society has collaborated with the Nurses' Association of Thailand and the MOPD Nursing Division in validating and developing the ICNP. The Nurses' Association of Thailand currently aims to develop a standard nursing care plan for clinical applications using the ICNP (Volrathongchai, Abbott, and Phuphaibul, 1999).

The activities of TNI are as follows:

1. Holding a joint annual meeting with the Nurses' Association of Thailand and the Medical Informatics Society.

2. Publishing and distributing its newsletter every 4 months.

3. Supporting other academic and research activities in NI.

4. Responding to the NI training needs of Thai nurses.

Standards Development

The development of Thai nursing standards is related to the development of the ICNP, although for medicine the ICD 10 has been used in all health service facilities. The use of a diagnostic-related group classification system is required for reimbursements from the National Health Care Fund, since the Thai healthcare system is moving toward a national health insurance policy. Additionally, the HL7 has been employed in many hospitals as the standard interface for the Web-based hospital information systems (Narawong, 2004).

Taiwan

There were 610 hospitals and 175,000 healthcare professionals in Taiwan in 2002, serving a population of 22.5 million (Health and National Health Insurance Annual Statistics Information Service in Taiwan, 2004). The healthcare professionals included 34.3% registered nurses and 17.7% licensed practicing nurses.

History of Nursing Informatics in Taiwan

The term NI was first used in Taiwan in 1990. At that time the focus was on hospital information systems providing nursing data such as nursing personnel information, care planning, and scheduling. However, computers had been used in nursing education since the 1980s, and the related nursing research into patient classification supported by the National Science Council began in the 1990s (Hsu et al., 1996). Although a formal master's program focusing on NI was not available until 2001, the elective courses in baccalaureate and master's programs had started in the late 1990s. All baccalaureate programs included at least one or two computer courses. Currently, some nursing students act as assistants for faculty in designing distance-learning classes.

Nursing Information Systems in Taiwan

Based on the unpublished results of a 2002 national survey, only 27% of hospitals had implemented nursing information systems, 9% were developing them, and 24% were making plans to develop them, whereas 40% were not planning to make any investment in nursing information systems in the near future. The pattern for long-term-care information systems was similar, in that almost 50% of long-term-care institutes were not planning any investment in information systems and only 19% had installed information systems.

Nursing Informatics Education

Computer-assisted instruction programs have been developed by the Ministry of Education for nursing vocational education programs since 1986. The content includes diet education for diabetic patients, biostatistics, maternal child health, stress management, and patient nutrition (Chen, 1992). The growth of the Internet has lead to the integration of distance education into nursing curricula. Online courses are available for baccalaureate programs in counseling, teaching principles and strategies, and long-term care. In addition, some schools provide multimedia self-testing systems. Students are videotaped when tested for nursing skills such as injections or enemas, and then the content is sent online to the instructor for grading. Schools provide an environment with simulated patients for students to practice before taking the test (Chang, Shu, and Chang, 2002).

At least six graduate programs in health or medical informatics provide informatics trainings at master's level for students with nursing backgrounds: the National Yang-Ming University, the National Taipei College of Nursing, the National Chung-Cheng University, Taipei Medical University, Chang-Gung University, and Tzu-Chi University. A total of around 10 master's students with nursing backgrounds will graduate from these informatics programs every year. Among these six universities, the National Yang-Ming University, the National Chung-Cheng University, Taipei Medical University, and Tzu-Chi University have PhD programs with a current total of around 10 students with nursing backgrounds, but no PhDs have been awarded yet.

Nursing Informatics Research

NI research is still at its infancy in Taiwan, with only around 40 papers published in domestic nursing journals in the period 1994–2003. The first formal academic association on NI was set up in 2004, when a NI working group was organized within the Taiwan Association of Medical Informatics, which had been established in 1991. Hopefully, the Taiwan Nursing Informatics Association will be set up by early 2005 with a strong consensus, given that a series of seminars and training courses in NI have been successfully run nationwide since the mid-2003 by the National Yang-Ming University, the Taipei College of Nursing, the National Union of Nurses' Associations, and the Chang-Gung Institute of Technology.

Standardized terminology such as existing nursing diagnosis classification systems and the ICNP have been

translated for clinical use, and tests of their reliability and validity have been proposed in Taiwan (Lu, 1998; Chiang, 1998). Users' perceptions and satisfaction toward computer use in daily practice have been analyzed. Qualitative approaches such as interviews have been used to explore how well nurses will accept the change from manual charting to computerized documentation (Lee, Yeh, and Ho, 2002). Quantitative approaches such as surveys have been applied to investigate the attitude and satisfaction toward the use of personal digital assistants (PDAs) for charting and the storage of nursing records (Lai and Chen, 2003).

Nursing Informatics Practice

Computerized care plans are now common in clinical use. Moreover, decision support systems to test the integration of medical diagnoses and nursing diagnoses, and expert systems implemented on PDAs for the emergency triage system have been reported (Chang, Tzeng, and Sang, 2003; Lai et al., 2001). Patient classification systems have also been applied for patient assessment, nursing interventions, and staff workload assignments (Hsu et al., 1996). These systems are designed to be integrated with costings so as to accurately define nursing fees. In addition, PDAs have been used recently by nurses in their daily practice. Nurses can chart vital signs and input and output other data at the point of care, and also access patient laboratory data, medication, or medical history without having to go back to nursing stations (Li et al., 1998; Lin and Laio, 2003).

Standardization and the National Health Information Infrastructure

The ROC Biological and Medical Engineering Association and the Taiwan Association of Medical Informatics successfully obtained approvals from the international DICOM and HL7 organizations to become the members in 2000. The HL7 and DICOM have been widely adopted as the national standards by governmental, academic, and industrial institutes, notably by the Ministry of Health in Taiwan.

A national "e-Taiwan" program has been promoted by the Ministry of Health to promote the development of health informatics in Taiwan since 2002. Another, larger program (the National Health Information Infrastructure Program) is expected to start in early 2005. Both programs will enhance the development of NI in Taiwan.

Summary

The Healthcare environment in Asian countries is becoming inhospital due to high healthcare costs, increasing competition amongst healthcare organizations, decreased funding from governments, and customers with more sophisticated demands. The introduction of information systems and information technology can help healthcare organizations to survive under these difficult conditions.

Healthcare informatics and the use of information technology has proceeded rapidly in Asian countries, with exciting developments in the areas of clinical practice, informatics research, and informatics education over the past decade. All of these developments have improved—either directly or indirectly—the productivity of healthcare professionals, the efficiency of the healthcare industry, and also the education of healthcare professionals.

It is clear that professional organizations play a major role in raising awareness, education, and dissemination of knowledge in health informatics. This is becoming increasingly complex with the proliferation of government initiatives spanning multiple government departments, which is a reflection of the multidisciplinary nature of health informatics. Nurses, as the largest group of health professionals, have a major role to play. A sound knowledge of the many stakeholders will ensure that nurses can coordinate their efforts to ultimately benefit the healthcare consumer (our patients), communities, and society as a whole.

Acknowledgments

I would like to thank Satoko Tsuru for contributing NI in Japan, Ting-Ting Lee and Polun Chang for contributing NI in Taiwan, Luo Zhimin for contributing NI in China, and Rutja Phuphaibul and Siriporn Khampalikit for contributing NI in Thailand.

References

References for Nursing Informatics in Korea

Cho, I. S. and Park, H. A. (1998). Development of a web-based CAI program for maternity nursing practice. In Cesnik, B., McCray, A. T., and Scherrer, J. R. (Eds.), *Proceedings of MEDINFO 98* Vol. 9, pt. 2, pp. 736–739).

Cho, I. S. and Park, H. A. (2003). Development and evaluation of a terminology-based electronic nursing record system. *Journal of Biomedical Informatics* 36(4/5):304–312.

Choi, W. J., Park, H. A., Cho, I. S., Park, I. S., and Cho, M. S. (1999). Development of a web-based educational program for clinical medication errors. *The Seoul Journal of Nursing* 13(2):164–173.

Coenen, A., Marin, H. F., Park, H. A., and Bakken, S. (2001). Collaborative efforts for representing nursing concepts in computer-based systems: International perspectives. *Journal of the American Medical Informatics Association* 8(3):202–211.

Hyun, S. K., Lee, S. G., Chun, J. H., Choi, J. W., Lee, I. H., Kim, K. U., Lee, S. J., and Park, J. Y. (1999). Development of nursing information system using personal digital assistance. In C. K. Hong (Ed.), *Proceedings of the Fifteenth Biannual Academic Conference of Korean Society of Medical Informatics* (p. 85). Taegu, Korea: KOSMI.

Kim, J. A. (1998). A comparative study on the effects of the nursing diagnosis systems using neural network and expert system. *Journal of Korean Society of Medical Informatics* 1:75–81.

Kim, H. S., Kim, I. S., Cho, W. J., and Kim, M. I. (2000). The effects of internet-based distance learning in nursing. *Computers in Nursing* 18:19–25.

Korea Health Industry Development Institute. (2000). *ISP Report for Medical Information Sharing*. Korea Health Industry Development Institute.

Korea Ministry of Information and Communication. (2002). *IT Korea Guide*.

Kwak, Y. S. (2000). Impact of medical informatics on healthcare in Korea. In T. Longzheng, M. Kimura, and H. Cho (Eds.), *Conference Proceedings: The Second China-Japan-Korea Joint Symposium on Medical Informatics* (pp. 7–9). Seoul, Korea: KOSMI.

Park, H. A. (2002). Nursing informatics in Korea. *Computers Informatics Nursing* 20(3):101–107.

Park, H. A. and Cho, I. S. (2000). Standardization of nursing classification systems in Korea. In V. Saba, R. Carr, W. Sermeus, and P. Rocha, (Eds.), *One Step Beyond: The Evolution of Technology and Nursing* (pp. 277–282). Auckland, New Zealand: Adis International.

Park, H. A., Cho, I. S., and Kim, J. E. (1998). Development of the in-service education program for nurses on the internet using multimedia teaching materials. *Journal of Korean Society of Medical Informatics* 2:59–68.

Park, H. A., Cho, I. S., Yoon, S. J., Han, J. R., Choi, W. J., Chun, Y. I., Yoo, K. S., Lee, Y. S., Park, J. S., Kim, S. H., Kim, K. D., and Kuen, H. K. (1999). Development of standardized nursing documentation forms for nursing information standard. *The Korean Nurse* 2:75–90.

Park, H. A., Lee, E. O., and Song, M. S. (1995). Development of nursing diagnosis system using back-propagation neural network model: An application to stomach cancer patients. In R. A. Greenes, H. E. Peterson, and D. J. Protti (Eds.), *Proceedings of the MEDINFO 95* (Vol. 8, pt. 2, pp. 1399–1403).

Park, J. H., Kim, M. J., Hong, K. J., Han, K. J., Park, S. A., Yoon, S. Y., Park, H. T., and Kang, Y. K. (2000). Implementation of homecare nursing network system. In T. Longzheng, M. Kimura, and H. Cho (Eds.), *Proceedings of the Second China-Japan-Korea Joint Symposium on Medical Informatics* (pp. 129–130). Cheju, Korea: KOSMI.

Yoo, T. W. (2002). Introducing home tele-care in Korea. In KMA (Ed.), *Conference Proceedings: The 30th General Congress of Korean Medical Association* (pp. 46–52). Seoul, Korea: KMA.

Yoo, J. S., Ryou, H. B., Park, J. W., and Ko, I. S. (1998). Development of the information system for nursing process: An implementation of nursing diagnosis system using neural network. *Journal of Korean Society of Medical Informatics* 2:49–58.

References for Nursing Informatics in Japan

Ezumi, H., Sota, Y., and Ochiai, H. (1997). Teaching method and evaluation of information education in Shimane Nursing College. In U. Gerdin, et al. (Eds.), *Nursing Informatics* (p. 601). Amsterdam, The Netherlands: IOS Press.

Japan Academy of Nursing Science. (2003). *The 23rd Annual Meeting of Japan Academy of Nursing Science Supplement* [in Japanese].

Japan Association of Medical Informatics. (1996). *Nursing Information System Workshop. Information System for Nursing* [in Japanese]. Tokyo: Japanese Nursing Association Publishing Company.

Japan Association of Medical Informatics. (2003). *Japan Journal of Medical Informatics Supplement* [in Japanese] 23.

Japan Association of Medical Informatics. (1980–2003). *Japan Journal of Medical Informatics Supplement* [in Japanese] 1–23.

Kamiizumi, K. and Ota, K. (2004). *Nursing Information Management* [in Japanese]. Tokyo: Japanese Nursing Association Publishing Company.

Kanai-Pak, M., Hosoi, R., Arai, C., Ishii, Y., Seki, M., Kikuchi, Y., Kabasawa, K., and Sato, K. (1997). Innovation in nursing education: Development of computer—assisted thinking. In U. Gerdin, et al. (Eds.), *Nursing Informatics* (pp. 371–375). Amsterdam, The Netherlands: IOS Press.

Kawaguchi, T., Azuma, M., and Ohta, K. (2004). Development of a telenursing system for patients with chronic disease. *Journal of Telemedicine and Telecare* 10(4):239–44.

Majima, Y. (1997). Application of the Internet for Nursing Education, in Nursing Informatics. In U. Gerdin, et al. (Eds.), *Nursing Informatics* (pp. 587). Amsterdam, The Netherlands: IOS Press.

Ministry of Health, Labour and Welfare. (2004). *http://www.mhlw.go.jp/english/index.html* (Welcome to Ministry of Health, Labour and Welfare).

Muranaka, Y., Fujimura, R., Yamashita, K., Furuhashi, Y., Yamamoto, S., and Arita, K. (1997). Development of a CAI program entitled "Introduction to Nursing Process." Requirement for nursing education in Japan. In U. Gerdin, et al. (Eds.), *Nursing Informatics* (pp. 487–491). Amsterdam, The Netherlands: IOS Press.

Ochiai, N., Sota, Y., and Ezumi, H. (1997). Self-study program on HTML browser—application to clinical nursing general remarks course. In U. Gerdin, et al. (Eds.), *Nursing Informatics* (pp. 360–363). Amsterdam, The Netherlands: IOS Press.

Panel on Healthcare and Medical Information System. (2002). *Final Report of Grand Design for Informatization in Healthcare and Medical Field* [in Japanese].

Supplement of National University Medical Information Processing Department Liaison Conference. (1995–2003) [in Japanese].

The Medical Information System Development Center. (2004). *http://www.medis.or.jp/* [in Japanese]. (MEDIS-DC.)

Tokyo Academy. (2004). *http://www.tokyo-ac.co.jp/med/index.html* [in Japanese]. ((Data of Nursing Educational Facility.)

Tsuru, S., Aida, H., Takahashi, H., and Iizuka, Y. (2004). Design of assessment sheet to estimate risk of accidents depending on patient, in supplement of 74th meeting for reading research papers of the Japanese Society for Quality Control [in Japanese].

Working Group for Nursing Issue. (2002). In Japanese Nursing Association Publishing Company (Eds.), *Statistical Data on Nursing Service in Japan* [in Japanese] The author is the Working Group for Nursing Issue.

Yamanouchi, K., Nakano, M., and Nojiri, M. (1997). A Small Intranet for Teaching How to Use Internet. In U. Gerdin, et al. (Eds.), *Nursing Informatics* (pp. 585). Amsterdam, The Netherlands: IOS Press.

References for Nursing Informatics in China

Chinese Hospital Information Management Association. (2004). *News on CHIMA 2004 and CHITA 2004.* http://www.chima.org.cn/

China Medical Informatics Association. (2004). *The Introduction of CMIA.* http://www.cmia.info/AboutUs.asp.

Fan, D. L. and Fu, Y. X. (2000). Talking about necessity of study "Nursing Information Science". *Shanxi Nursing Journal* 14(2):47–48.

Fan, D. L. and Li, Z. Z. (2000). Attempting to develop "nursing information science" continuing education. *Journal of Nursing Science* 15(11):684.

Fang, J. H., Wang, F., and Han, Y. H. (2004). Development and application of "The data base of information archives of nursing staff". *Modern Hospital* 4(4):98–99.

Fu, G. F. (2000). Application and development of nursing information system. *Anthology of Medicine* 19(5):798–799.

Hao, M., et al. (2000). An introduction of project policy analysis on issues, mechanism and development strategies of three-tier health care network in rural China. *Chinese Health Resources* 3(6):253–255.

Ji, H., Qu, W. X., He, Y. S., and Liu, J. E. (1994). Study on computer assisted nursing diagnosis system. *Chinese Hospital Management* 10(9):568–570.

Jiang, A. L. (2002). Meeting the challenges of information age: The rise and development of nursing informatics. *Nanfang Journal of Nursing* 10(5):1–2.

Jiang, A. L., et al. (1998). Application study on computer assisted instruction courseware of nursing process. *Chinese Journal of Nursing* 33(2):97–98.

Li, F. F., Jiang, A. L., and Shi, Q. (2002). Development of multimedia courseware "Care of oral cavity". *Chinese Journal of Nursing* 35(5):295–296.

Li, Z. Z., Zhang, L. L., and Wang, Z. C. (2001). Development and application of "Chinese Traditional Medicine Nursing" information management system. *Today nurse*, August 2001 23–24.

Li, Y .J., Zhang, L. L., Wen, M. G., and Zhao, Z. R. (1999). Development and application of nurse information management system. *The First Military Medical University* 19(1):10–12.

Liu, W. J., Wang, T. C., and Du, Y. X. (2003). Historical review of 10 anniversaries of the Chinese Society of Medical Information of China Medical Association. *Chinese Journal of Medical Library Information Sciences* 12(6):1–4.

Liu, Y. L., et al. (2004). A study on the development and application of nursing information in military hospital. *Chinese Hospital Management* 24(1):44–46.

Luo, L. X., Feng, Z. C., and Zhang, J. (2004). Research on the hospital function of response to public health emergency. *Chinese Hospital Management* 24(3):3–5.

Ma, Z. J. (2000). Primary health cares system with Chinese characteristics of the rural areas. *Chinese Health Economics* 19(50):51–52.

Ministry of Health, P. R. China. (2003). *National Health Information Developmental Essential (2003–2010)*. http://www.moh.gov.cn/tjxxzx/gjwsxxhjs/1200304140011.htm.

Ministry of Health, P. R. China. (2003). *Statistics of Chinese Health Care Enterprise in 2003*. http://www.moh.gov.cn/tjxxzx/tjsj/tjgb/1200404270011.htm

National Population and Family Planning Commission of China. (2001). *The Changes of the Population of China in the Fifth National Census*. http://www.chinapop.gov.cn/rkzh/zgrk/tjgb/t20040326_2819.htm

Nursing Center, Ministry of Health, P. R. China. (1995). Status and development of nursing information management system in China. *Chinese Journal of Nursing* 30(6):381–383.

Nursing School of Weizhou Medical College. (2004). *How to Connect with the World: Interviewing with Secretary of Chinese Nursing Association*. http://www.wzmc.net/hlxy/duijiedian.htm

Qi, L. Y, Zeng, F., Tang, X. D., F, L. L., Bai, F., and Liu, C. X. (2000). Application of nursing record information management based on "No. 1 Project of PLA". *Medical Information* 13(9):499–500.

Wang, P. H. (1995). Computer expert system for nursing specialty level assessment. *Journal of Nursing Science* 10(2):96–97.

Wang, D. Z., Wu, Y., and Xu, A. H. (2003). The whole nursing management based on nursing information system of "No.1 Project of PLA". *ACTA Academiae Medicinae Militaris Tertiae* 25(9):835–836.

Wang, S. Y., Zhang, G. P., Hao, B. L, and Jiang, H. (2001). Design and performance of net-base nursing information management system. *Journal of the Fourth Military Medical University* 22(Suppl.): 136–137.

Zhang, Q. (2003). Application of computer in Chinese hospital nursing management. *Journal of Nursing Science* 18(2):156–157.

Zhang, P., Cheng, W., and Qi, W. D. (2003). Application of nursing management information system. *Medical Information* 16(6):317–319.

Zhang, L. L, Fu, Y. X., and Fan, D. L. (1999). Applying of nursing department information managing system in nursing management. *Shanxi Nursing Journal* 13(5):204–205.

Zhang, L. L., Li, Y. J., Chen, L., and Wen, M. G. (2004). Design and application of net-based nurses information management system. *Nanfang Journal of Nursing* 11(1):54–55.

Zhang, X. H., Liang, J. L., and Zhang, Q. (1999). Computerized nursing diagnostic intelligence system. *Shanxi Nursing Journal* 13(2):49–50.

Zhou, D. H. and Song, L. X. (2001). Developing distant nursing education in China. *Chinese Journal of Nursing* 36(5):369–371.

Zhu, D., Lu, Y. J., and Yin, L. (1995). Computer assisted instructor for fundamental nursing teaching. *Chinese Journal of Nursing* 30(8):480–481.

Zong, X. S. (2004). SARS call out a new system of country medicare in China. *Medicine and Society* 17(2):51–52, 55.

References for Nursing Informatics in Thailand

CIA-The World Factbook, Thailand. (2004). http//www.cia.gov/cia/publications/factbook/geos/th.htm

Country health profile: Thailand. (2003). *http://w3.whosea.org/cntryhealth/Thailand/thaistatus.htm*

Economy. (2004). *http://www.amazing-thailand.com/economy.html*

HIS/LIS Club Thailand. (2004). *http://www.his-lis.worlsmedic.com/*

International Council of Nurses. (1999). *The International Classification for Nursing Practice: The Beta Version. http:www.icn.ch*

Narawong T. (2004). A review from SNM meeting. *http://www.thaisnm.org/*

Phuphaibul, R., Kumpaliki, S., Sriyaporn, A., Suppalek, A., Sawaengdee, K., and Vatjanavisit, T. (1991). *The Royal Thai Government/The World Health Organization: Nursing Minimum Data Set and Preliminary Nursing Classification Development.* Bangkok: Mahidol University, Department of Nursing, Center of Nursing Research.

Phuphaibul, R. and Sumranvejaporn, K. (1999). *Nursing Informatics.* Bangkok: Nitibunnakarn.

Phuphaibul, R., Suppalek, A., Sawangdee, K., and Vadjanavisit T. (2000). Nursing minimum data set survey. *Thai Journal of Nursing* 49(3):180–185.

The Nurses' Association of Thailand. (1999). *International Classification for Nursing Practice: Beta version* [Thai translation]. Bangkok: Samcharearnpanich Press.

The Thai Medical Informatics Society. (2004). *http://www.tmi.or.th/*

Volrathongchai, K., Abbott, P., and Phuphaibul, R. (1999). Nursing Informatics: Improving nursing in Thailand. *Ramathibodi Nursing Journal* 5(3):263–272.

Volrathongchai, K., Delaney, C. W., and Phuphaibul, R. (2003). Nursing minimum data set development and implementation in Thailand. *Journal of Advance Nursing* 43(6):588–594.

References for Nursing Informatics in Taiwan

Chang, P. J, Shu, T. H., and Chang, C. B. (2002). Current status and future development of multimedia web-based learning in the nursing department of the National Taipei College of Nursing. *Journal of Health Science* 4(3):265–272.

Chang, P., Tzeng, Y. M., and Sang, Y. Y. (2003). The development of wireless PDA support systems for comprehensive and intelligent triage in emergency nursing. *Journal of Nursing* 50(4):29–40.

Chen, W. L. (1992). Application of computer assisted instruction in nursing education. *Journal of Nursing* 39(4):118–123.

Chiang, L. C. (1998). Nursing diagnosis development in Taiwan: Now and future. *Journal of Nursing* 45(2):28–39.

Health and National health Insurance Annual Statistics Information Service in Taiwan. (2004). *Number of Medical Care Institutions and Registered Medical Personnel by Locality, Taiwan Area, 1988–2002. http://www.doh.gov.tw/statistic/index.htm*

Hsu, N. L., Feng, R. C., Lo, H. Y., and Wang, P. W. (1996). The establishment of factor type patient classification systems. *Journal of Nursing* 43(3):23–35.

Lai, H. and Chen, L. (2003). Nurse satisfaction with the clinical use of personal digital assistant. *Tzu Chi Medical Journal* 15(2):97–103.

Lai, Y. H., Liu, L., Hsu, C. Y., and Chen, J. S. (2001). Medical diagnosis assisted nursing process support system. *New Taipei Nursing Journal* 3(1):67–78.

Lee, T. T., Yeh, C. H., and Ho, L. H. (2002). Application of a computerized nursing care plan system in one hospital: Experiences of ICU nurses in Taiwan. *Journal of Advanced Nursing* 39(1):61–67.

Li, T. Z., Wang, R. H., Hsu, S. S., Chen, L. F. and Chang, H. Y. (1998). Information technology and nursing: Using PDAs in clinical nursing care. *Journal of Nursing* 45(1):69–76.

Lin, J. S. and Liao, Y. C. (2003). A study of nurses' attitude and satisfaction toward using personal digital assistant in nursing practice. *New Taipei Journal of Nursing* 5(2):3–12.

Lu, Z. Y. (1998). Current status and future development of ICNP. *Journal of Nursing* 45(2):35–39.

CHAPTER

41

Nursing Informatics in South America

Heimar F. Marin

OBJECTIVES

1. Describe nursing informatics development in the region.
2. Identify the use of information technology in clinical practice.
3. Describe educational and distance learning efforts.

KEY WORDS

nursing informatics
clinical informatics
training and education
NIEn/UNIFESP
terminology
ICNP-Brazilian version

Nursing informatics in 13 South American countries has been based more on activities of individuals than on a policy established by governments or national efforts. Each country has varied levels of development and deployment of technological resources; however, the use of technology has been a visible tendency in health and nursing education, practice, research, and administration. The growth of information technology in Latin America and the Caribbean has been consistently the world's highest for 20 years; however, significant differences exist among countries and regions in each country.

The use of technology by nurses follows the evolution of technology use in the region. Most developed parts of the country have better access and ability to implement services and applications in nursing.

Computers are considered an important tool to help nurses take care of patients and to organize nursing service and nursing education. In addition, the Internet and wireless comunication are also a trend in this field. Consequently, health institutes and universities are exploring ways to introduce news resources in order to facilitate the process of patient care and promote quality and safety.

The objective of this chapter is to present an overview of the development of nursing informatics in South America, identifying some initiatives in the field,

including discussion on the current use of terminologies, and initiatives to dissiminate nursing informatics resources in the region.

 Background

Nursing has been identified around the world as an emerging profession for over a 100 years. The professional evolution has been a continuous process influenced by science and technology, which has been the driving force to further nursing development. Several examples of use and development of computer applications in healthcare impact nursing profession. For many years, nurses were considered as the primary users of technology in healthcare (Safran, Slack, and Bleich, 1989).

Historically, nurses are used to facing challenges, adapting new tools into the practice to improve their performance, and creating new models to enhance patient care. Technology can represent a unique instrument to help nurses face further challenges and discover how to use its resources to innovate and maybe to redesign their way of taking care of people (Marin, 1996).

Today's technology causes significant modification of human activities and, consequently, of the way we learn and work. Traditional methods of teaching, managing, and practicing a profession do not support the requirements of modern life anymore.

Furthermore, information is the key element for decision-making process in the healthcare area. The more specific information in place to support clinical decisions, the better care can be delivered to the patient. The quality of care is related to the scope of knowledge and information that health providers can access on which to base their clinical decisions. Thus, technology plays an important role in facilitating access to the information because for the information to be useful and meaningful, it has to be timely.

Recognizing computers and all information technology resources available as powerful instruments, gradually, each country became more aware of the possibilities to apply information technology to enhance activities in taking care of clients/patients.

There is a clear trend in the direction of the computerization of health records. In addition, more people are able to connect to the Internet that is a telecommunication resource with no parallel to fast exchange data and information. As a result we can expect to see better-informed healthcare providers and consumers (Pan America Health Association/World Health Organization, 2001).

Considering trends and tendency in healthcare informatics, and to facilitate the process in South American countries, the Pan American Health Organization (PAHO) has published guidelines and protocols to orient the development and deployment of information and communication technology in Latin America and the Caribbean (Pan America Health Association/World Health Organization, 1998, 2001, 2003).

It is also important to emphasize that Latin America and the Caribbean region rank third in information technology expenditure. A study performed by the Pan America Health Organization/World Health Organization (1998) showed that the Information Society Index, based on the use of information, computer, and social infrastructure, is evolving rapidly.

■ Nursing Informatics Initiatives

In South American countries, as in any other country in the world, the initial motivation to develop computer systems in the healthcare area was driven by financial and administrative concerns. The hospital sector can be considered the area better served by information systems. Countries like Brazil, Mexico, Argentina, Colombia, Chile, and Paraguay have clinical information systems in hospitals or health institutes.

Although clinical information systems are being used in some ways to support clinical care and management, a few hospitals or healthcare institutes developed applications for nursing documentation where nursing data

can be processed. In general, patient data that are also used for nursing administration are integrated in the system or nurses have to collect and analyse nursing data separately.

Hospitals have been working to design their own systems in order to attend to specific needs and policies. More recently, national and international software industry became more represented in the South America healthcare market. Consequently, they provide a broader range of solutions with systems that address patient care documentation.

Many additional initiatives are spread throughout the Latin American countries. It can be observed that the use of computers as an instrument to support nurses' activities in taking care of patients still needs a lot of investment of human and material resources. Clinical systems based on the nursing process are not common in these countries. Most of the computer systems implemented are intended to control administrative data. The most frequently implemented and used applications still are the nursing orders.

In spite of this, nurses are becoming even more involved with the design, implementation, and evaluation of clinical information systems. Vendors and developers recognize that the success of a computer system requires nursing input and collaboration.

In addition, as an open and evolving market, international developers are making investments to sell and implement computer systems in South America, because South America represents one of the most promising market in the world of technology.

Even so, it is necessary to emphasize that the inclusion of nursing elements of practice in the patient record is under the responsibility of nurses. They need to be involved with the programmers, vendors, and developers to drive the professional requirements. Taking care of patients is what nurses know how to do. Therefore, it is essential to assure that all information required to perform nursing care is present in the health information systems.

Congresses, conferences, workshops, education, and training programs are being organized in the countries to share experiences and information in nursing informatics searching for solutions that could enhance the delivery of patient care.

Distance Learning and the Educational Perspectives in Nursing Informatics

Technology is transforming not only nursing practice but also nursing training and education models. With the introduction of computers in the healthcare area, nurses became primary users, responsible for data input. Consequently, they had to become computer-literate in order to use computer technology in an efficient manner. To meet educational and training needs, nursing schools and hospitals initiated programs to prepare nurses to use computers. In addition to teaching how to use computer applications, course instructors also considered the use of computers to teach nursing content.

Computer applications in nursing education are also changing nursing education from a passive teaching to an active learning process. Computers allow students to work at the time that best meets their specific needs. Usually, the programs are very interactive and easy to use and offer immediate feedback about students' performance.

Formal education programs in nursing informatics, such as a specific nursing informatics specialization and master or doctoral course is also being provided. The Núcleo de Informática em Enfermagem at the Universidade Federal de São Paulo (NIEn/ UNIFESP) was the first center to offer the specialization degree (certificate) in South America. NIEn/UNIFESP also provides, since 1989, the nursing informatics discipline in its graduate and undergraduate nursing programs. The research "line" in nursing informatics is attended by professionals from different regions of the country and has been responsible for the preparation of several masters and doctoral students in nursing informatics. The students after graduation return to their own institutes to implement education and research programs and to participate in the development of patient care systems.

Latin American countries are investing a significant effort to prepare professionals in health informatics. An example of this was recently implemented in Brazil. A 4-year grant from the Fogarty International Center of the National Institutes of Health (U.S.), promoted the establishment of a bilateral consortium of health informatics faculty. A program was designed to enhance training in Brazil by augmenting the teaching resources of local faculty. This training program was based on the experience of the Brazilian faculty and some lessons learned from an existing training program in Boston (U.S.), which involved faculty from Harvard University and its affiliated hospitals: Massachusetts Institute of Technology (MIT), Boston University, and Tufts University (Marin et al., 2004).

The program started in October 1999. Since then, it has sponsored 10 onsite courses in Brazil, which were subsequently made available on the Internet and CD-ROM, together with regular medical informatics courses taught yearly at Harvard and MIT. The program started, in years 1 and 2, with activities targeted at

faculty from leading universities in southern Brazil, which are better equipped with staff and material resources than universities in other parts of the country. There were short courses in Brazil, which were taught by a mix of Brazilian and U.S. faculty, as well as support for faculty enrichment via participation in international scientific events. In years 3 and 4, the training program was responsible for the organization of several scientific meetings in Brazil and continued to promote student and faculty participation in national and international conferences, short-term courses, and workshops.

During the development and implementation of this training program, different regions of Brazil were reached, delivering courses that were previously given in São Paulo or Rio de Janeiro. By the end of 2003, it was found that around 1,724 professionals were involved as either a faculty member or a student in the program.

There has been a trend toward distance learning program development in South America. Computer technology is providing students living in distant regions and having difficulties in accessing the main educational centers the opportunity to improve their personal knowledge base. A contributing factor to the development and success of these programs is the distance between countries and cities due to the geographic characteristics of South America.

In Brazil, the Brazilian Council of Telemedicine was established in 2002. It is developing several educational programs. The council includes the telenursing group. Presently, this group organized two teleconferences in the country with more than 400 participants, each from different regions that discussed nursing topics such as pressure ulcers, catheters, and home care.

Nursing Terminology and Documentation

Sharing and communicating information is essential to make decisions and deliver care. Exchange of information requires the communicating parties to agree on a communicating channel, an exchange protocol, and a common language. The language includes an alphabet, words, phrases, and symbols that express and assign meaning, understood by all users (Pan America Health Association/World Health Organization, 1997).

Clark (1995) pointed out that "communicating among ourselves has always been important but communicating with other people about nursing has acquired a new urgency since we are forced to recognize that the value of nursing is no longer apparent to those who have the power to influence our practice" (p. 25).

Other issues to be considered are reimbursement policies, cost containment, and technological development in recent years.

However, it is the nurses' responsibility to decide not only what kind of data are important to describe the contribution of nurses in the healthcare process and to assure continuous care, but also to decide how these data could be described. What kind of language will be useful to support the several different activities performed by nurses? In fact, the use of a vocabulary in nursing must assure both communication among the nurses and communication between nurses and the other providers responsible for patient care.

Efforts have been made in this area, and now different clinical vocabularies are available; however, building a vocabulary that standardizes the clinical nomenclature for use in clinical practice and that fulfills all requirements is a challenge.

In 1990, the International Council of Nurses (ICN) initiated a long-term project to develop an International Classification for Nursing Practice (ICNP) with the objective to establish a common language about nursing practice to be used for describing nursing care for people in a variety of settings (Mortensen, 1996). The development of this classification is being improved through analysis and several field tests performed by different countries.

In Brazil, the dissemination of the ICNP started around 1996, when NIEn/UNIFESP became a sponsoring partner in the Telenurse Consortium, a project led by Randi Mortensen, director of the Danish Institute for Health and Nursing Research. The paper and electronic forms of the ICNP-Brazilian version (*http://www.epm.br/enf/nien/cipe*) have been available since September 1997. The ICNP Beta 2 is also available in Brazilian Portuguese version (Conselho Internacional de Enfermagem, 2003).

Other terminologies are also being used in the country, including Home Health Care Classification (HHCC) system developed by Saba (1992), which is also available on the Internet (*http://www.sabacare.com*) in Brazilian Portuguese version.

The most frequently used vocabularies may not necessarily be the best ones, but they may reflect the demands of insurance companies and other payers. Although there are quantitative differences in terms of breadth of coverage and internal representational structure, no clinical vocabulary has been elected so far as the ultimate solution for clinical documentation automated retrieval and rapid communication. Several obstacles have yet to be passed before nursing communities embrace a standardized vocabulary that proves useful in

a variety of tasks and settings: regional, national, and international (Marin and Machado, 1996).

The task is a challenge, and continuous studies must be done to reach the balance that will facilitate nursing practice documentation around the world.

Historically, nurses have several problems in obtaining nursing documentation. Currently, with the expansion of health knowledge and information, the quantity of nursing documentation has certainly increased; however, the same cannot necessarily be said about the quality of the information documented. Health data rarely become health information.

Considering these statements, the Pan American Health Organization/World Health Organization decided to sponsor an expert meeting to produce a guidebook that could provide information about how nursing informatics and standards can improve practice and management. The main goal was to characterize how nursing informatics and the use of standards can improve nursing practice and management, taking advantage of resources.

The recommendations from the experts were merged into a textbook edited by the Division of Systems at the Pan America Health Association/World Health Organization. The book (Building Standards-based Nursing Information System) (PAHO, 2001) was published in English and Spanish and distributed to universities, professional organization, and technical cooperation agencies.

Summary

Nursing informatics as an integrated part of healthcare follows the progress that has been made in the whole sector of health informatics. Because of the wide variety among countries and even inside larger countries, the development of nursing informatics is conducted on a case-by-case basis, taking into consideration the specific requirements of each region. Furthermore, the development and deployment of nursing informatics is dependent on national priorities and human capabilities.

This situation represents a great opportunity for nursing. The future is exciting, because with technological advances nurses have the chance to drive their own professional destinies. Adapting technological resources to their practice help nurses to see emerging trends in the healthcare field as challenges and unique opportunities for career growth. There are new roles, new areas, and new jobs demanding experts. Opportunities are wide open for those who have decided to incorporate information technology into their daily practice in the process of taking care of patients.

References

Clark, J. (1995). An International Classification for Nursing Practice (ICNP). In S. B. Henry, W. L. Holzemer, M. Tallberg, and S. J. Grobe (Eds.), *Informatics: The Infrastructure for Quality Assessment and Improvement in Nursing* (pp. 25–31). San Francisco, CA: University of California Nursing Press.

Conselho Internacional de Enfermagem. (2003). *Classificação Internacional para a Prática de Enfermagem Beta 2*. traduação: Heimar de F. marin, São paulo, SP.

Marin, H. F. (1996). Nursing informatics applications. In N. Oliveri, M. Sosa-Iudicissa, and C. Gamboa (Eds.), *Internet, Telematics and Health* (p. 265). Amsterdam, The Netherlands: IOS Press.

Marin, H. F. and Machado, L. O. (1996). Introduction to clinical vocabularies: What does the clinician need to know? In *Proceedings of the Eight National Conference on Clinical Computing in Patient Care: Capturing the Clinical Encounter*, Boston.

Marin, H. F., Massad, E., Marques, E. P., and Machado, L. O. (2004). International training in health informatics: A Brazilian experience. In *MEDINFO 2004*. San Francisco, USA (accepted for oral presentation, September).

Mortensen, R. (1996). *The International Classification for Nursing Practice ICNP with TELENURSE Introduction*. Copenhagen: Danish Institute for Health and Nursing Research.

Pan America Health Association/World Health Organization. (1997). *Health Technology Linking the Americas. Moving Towards a Vision: Implementing and Using Information Systems and Technology to Improve Health and Healthcare in Latin America and the Caribbean*. Washington, DC: Series Health Services Information Systems.

Pan America Health Association/World Health Organization. (1998). *Information Systems and Information Technology in Health: Challenges and Solutions for Latin America and the Caribbean*. Health Services Information Systems Program. Washington, DC: Division of Health Systems and Services Development.

Pan America Health Association/World Health Organization. (2001). *Building Standard-Based Nursing Information Systems*. Washington, DC: Division of Health Systems and Services Development.

Pan America Health Association/World Health Organization. (2003). *O Prontuário eletrônico do paciente na assistência, informação e conhecimento médico*. Washington, DC: Division of Health Systems and Services Development.

Saba, V. K. (1992). The Classification of Home Health Care Classification of nursing diagnoses and interventions. *Caring Magazine* 11:50–56.

Safran, C., Slack, W. V, and Bleich, H. (1989). Role of computing in patient care in two hospitals. *M.D. Computing* 6:141–148.

PART 11

The Future of Informatics

42 Future Directions

Kathleen A. McCormick

OBJECTIVES

1. Describe the future vision of nursing informatics in the first decade of the twenty-first century.
2. Identify some of the key components of information technology (IT).
3. Describe some of the key scientific influences on the informatics future.
4. Define the potential of genetics, genomics, and proteomics in healthcare and the need for bioinformatics.
5. Understand some of the core competencies nurses in informatics will need in the future.

KEY WORDS

future hardware and software applications
demographic shifts
infection and chronic diseases
genetics/genomics/proteomics/bioinformatics

This fourth edition contains much that points the reader to the foundations of the future. The excitement of the electronic health record (EHR), open source, international standards, biodefense, Internet, handheld, and PDAs are a few of the peeks into the future. The authors are experts in these areas and have dedicated an entire chapter to describe their application to the nursing profession. This chapter aims to synthesize a vision of what healthcare might have for information system needs in the future years.

■ The New Twenty-First Century Scenario

The nurse of this decade has much more evidence to point to in the patient's genes, genomes, and proteomes. The new science is revolutionizing the way we conduct science and the way we will prevent disease and diagnose and treat patients. The new science will also allow the nurse to point to the particular patient's reason for

This chapter is based on a keynote presented at HIMSS to the First Nursing Informatics Task Force, February 22, 2004. Orlando, Florida.

myocardial infarction, whether the person can regulate calcium, sodium, and potassium compared to normal persons, or whether the ultimate of their food digestion leads to more cholesterol production or more glycogen storage. They will have the mechanism identified on the way that enzymes such as lipase either work correctly or incorrectly in the metabolic processes. Metabolic maps will link the biochemistry of the cell, with the genes and proteins regulating them, with the clinical conditions manifested.

The nurse needs new resources to monitor evidence for conducting genetic screening on children born with autism. Nurses may need environmental, agricultural, and health data combined. Are the genetic biomarkers appropriate for the region that the nurse is working in? For example, is there evidence that water, chemicals in the environment or in medications, or lead in the environment are causing more or less of a particular condition in their geographic catchment? Will the data support genetic counseling, genetic profiling, or microarray studies of the person's genes and tissues, compared to animals with the same condition produced by genetically engineered models of disease?

The scenario begins and ends with the genetic information. Whether the concerns of the nurse are prevention, diagnosis, cure, or rehabilitation, the evidence will come from the genetic profiles. Once a condition is diagnosed, the patient's blood or tissue will be subjected to candidate drugs that might suppress or enhance the genes regulating their disease. Before the medication is even administered to the patient, the possible impact of the drug on the condition and adverse reactions will be known. What is not known is the patients' responses. What host defenses will they bring to bear on the drug or the altered genes? Will they have the genes that make them fast healers or slow healers from surgical procedures? Will they have the racial and genetic profiles that bestow on them certain genetic traits that protect them from developing certain diseases or toxic effects of noxious chemotherapies? Will they be able to accept medication that suppresses their immune response to allergens? What proteins are showing in their blood, urine, plasma, and tissues that indicate that they are susceptible to certain environmental exposures or mutations in their genes? The types of IT needed to support these new approaches to healthcare are grid technologies, high performance computers, and robust integrated information systems based on standards.

Population data will be supported by genetic profiles in groups of patients who do or do not have a population condition. When identical twin children are exposed to a virus, pathogen, or pesticide, why does one develop a neurologic or immunologic condition? Why does the other one who was similarly exposed to environmental stressors never develop the condition?

Obviously, those of you who read the scenario in the third edition (McCormick, 2001) want to know how close we are to achieving the vision that was described almost 5 years ago. The vision is close to reality if you visit the exhibits of the voice recognition companies, hold a handheld, or talk and e-mail people day in and day out from almost any point on the globe.

The vision is close to reality if you have global satellite in your automobile and can report an urgent health condition to someone who is sending an ambulance to your site based on geographic locators and telephone rapid response. The scenario is almost real to those who have decision support capabilities. The scenario is nowhere near real to those who are continuing to practice in an environment devoid of information systems.

For those of you who are disappointed, do not be. In the 30 years of a simple nursing career several incredible technological advances have occurred. In a book entitled *King of Hearts*, the author G. Wayne Miller (2000)

reminds us that 25 years ago a child died of surgery from congenital defects and adults died needing a heart valve. What often appears to be the lack of progress is happening in front of us in IT technology. When we step back to look, much of what we take for granted in IT today was not present 10 years ago.

 ## A President and a Secretary of Health Decree Acceleration

There is reason for optimism for a shortened future toward achieving the informatics goals described in this book. The primary reason is a President who in his State of the Union Address said:

"By computerizing health records, we can avoid dangerous medical mistakes, reduce costs, and improve care." (George W. Bush—State of the Union Address—January 20, 2004.) On April 27, 2004, the announcement of President Bush's groundbreaking Health Information Technology (HIT) Plan was made during his speech at the American Association of Community Colleges Annual Convention in Minneapolis, MN. Saying modern technology has not caught up with a major aspect of healthcare and we have got to change that, the President set a **10-year goal for a majority of Americans to have** EHRs when and where they are needed; EHRs that are designed to share information privately and securely among and between healthcare providers when authorized by the patient. To accomplish this goal and to coordinate federal HIT efforts, the creation of a new, sub-Cabinet level post at the Department of Health and Human Services (HHS) is another major tenet of the President's HIT Plan. An announcement was made of a National Health Information Technology Coordinator who would guide ongoing work on health information standards and work to identify and implement the various steps needed to support and encourage HIT in the public and private sector healthcare delivery systems. President Bush appointed David J. Brailer, MD, PhD to be the nation's first National Health Information Technology Coordinator, a sub-Cabinet level post at the Department of Health and Human Services (HHS) on May 6, 2004. Bipartisan support seems to be present for such advancements in the EHR. In May 2005, the Secretary of DHHS, Michael Leavitt indicated he will unveil a plan to lead collaborative state efforts to create a digital health care environment.

We have entered the new decade of the EHR. But to achieve that goal, Dr. Charles Safran, the former President of the American Medical Informatics Association (AMIA), has said that we will need 6,000 more physicians and 6,000 more nurses prepared in information sciences to move in this direction.

A Nation's Health Information Technology Plan

President Bush's HIT Plan also called for:

- The federal government to accelerate the identification and adoption of voluntary standards necessary for the safe and secure sharing of health information among health providers

- Increased money for demonstration projects involving modern electronic records systems that test IT and establish best practices for wider adoption, including a doubling of demonstration project funding to $100 million in the President Bush's budgets.

- Creating federal incentives and opportunities that encourage healthcare providers to use electronic medical records.

Under the HIT Plan, federal agencies must review their policies and programs and propose modifications and new actions to the President.

National Standards Endorsement on July 1, 2003

Prior to these announcements, on July 1, 2003, former secretary of HHS, the Honorable Tommy Thompson, announced two new steps in building a national electronic healthcare system that allowed patients and their doctors to access complete medical records anytime and anywhere they are needed, leading to reduced medical errors, improved patient care, and reduced healthcare costs. First, the former Secretary announced that the Department had signed an agreement with the College of American Pathologists (CAP) to license the College's standardized medical vocabulary system (SNOMED) and make it available without charge throughout the United States. This action opens the door to establishing a common medical language as a key element in building a unified electronic medical records system in the United States. Secondly, the former Secretary announced that HHS had commissioned the Institute of Medicine (IOM) to design a standardized model of an EHR. The healthcare standards development organization known

as HL7 had also been asked to evaluate the model once it had been designed. HHS will share the standardized model record at no cost with all components of the U.S. healthcare system. The HL7 standards group released a model for balloting in 2004, and it was approved.

 ## IT in Relationship to People, Organization, and Policies

In April 2004, a conference convened by the AMIA brought together experts in the design, implementation, and evaluation of EHRs. During this conference there was a general consensus among the presenters and participants, that in the past 25 years of implementing systems, people, organizations, and policies are dominant forces 90% of the time and the IT is only 10% of the implementation. They recommended attention be paid to business process reengineering, organizational dynamics, and changing strategy when planning and implementing systems. Training was oftentimes more important than the IT in several real scenarios of hospital information system implementation.

Several Drivers of More Information Technology Today

There are several drivers creating more IT in healthcare today. A recent American Hospital Association and Cap Gemini study forecasts top issues. Healthcare and hospitals are increasingly investing in IT to deal with several issues. Among their issues are rising costs and limited access to capital. The scarce labor pool of nurses (and in the future doctors) is driving changes in the way that healthcare is delivered. The consumer and patient have shifted focus away from the hospital toward a focus on the consumer and patient themselves. Patient safety is a national issue in the United States and abroad. The complexities of the healthcare conditions and the complexities of medical reporting are also driving more utilization of IT.

Still another focus is a result of September 11, 2001, which pointed to deficiencies in public health reporting, the lack of a public health information infrastructure, and a critical need for integrated systems (Snee and McCormick, 2004). Competition is also eroding profits, which is driving more competitive healthcare environments, while the consumer is becoming more knowledgeable and demanding.

HIMSS Leadership Healthcare CIO Surveys

Another way to monitor the trends in U.S. healthcare IT is from the Healthcare Information Management Systems Society (HIMSS) annual survey of healthcare Chief Information Officers (CIOs). In the most recent survey released in February 2004, the CIOs said that the main IT issue facing them was patient safety and medical errors and developing IT systems to support measuring and monitoring safety and errors (HIMSS, 2004). Upgrading security on IT systems to meet Health Insurance Portability and Accountability Act (HIPAA) requirements followed that issue. The top technologies that the CIOs predict for the future were:

- High speed networks
- The Internet
- Client server systems
- Wireless information systems

Over half of the respondents mentioned the use of personal digital assistants (PDAs), bar coding, and speech recognition as technologies that their facilities plan to implement in the near future. Sixty percent of the respondents in 2004 said they had planned to implement an EHR or they had already begun installing one. Additional needs included patient scheduling, additions to their Web sites, and IT outsourcing of functions.

Table 42.1 lists some of the technologies that may be important drivers in the future.

Trends Toward 2030

Major trends in healthcare that will influence the IT developments are those listed in Table 42.2. Each of these will be described briefly in the remainder of this chapter.

Demographic Trends

The U.S. population will shift toward an aged population in the next decade, thus shifting the focus from a youth-centric to an aged-centric culture (Dychwald, 2003). Aged persons have more health conditions, take more medications, and require more procedures and devices than younger persons.

Thus, there will be an increased focus on preventing, diagnosing, and delivering care to this population. More programs that monitor information flow in the home, in rehabilitation facilities, and in extended care or nursing home environments will be necessary. But new predictions

Table 42.1   Future Trends in IT

Bar coding

Bioinformatics/Biomedical Informatics/Computational Biology

Claims Processing

Client server systems

Data Warehousing

Decision Support

Disease Management/Outcomes

Electronic Health Record—Clinical Information Systems—Computer-Based Patient Records-Hospital/Healthcare Information Systems

High speed networks

HIPAA compliance

Identify management—Smart Cards

Laboratory Information Management Systems

Medication error prevention/Patient Safety

Mobile computing/technology/wireless

Outsourcing services

Personal Digital Assistants (PDAs)

Point-of-Care Computing

Practice management

Prescription management

Scheduling

Security upgrades

Speech recognition

Standards

Supply ordering/management

Telecommunications/Telehealth/Telemedicine

Vocabulary integration/interface

Web portals/Internet access to/from staff/professionals/consumers

Table 42.2   Trends in Health affecting IT in the Future

Demographics—the graying of America

Growth in chronic disease

Emerging infectious disease threats

Changes in health-seeking behavior toward the Internet

Focus on quality = focus on IT

Security and biodefense

Genetic revolution

by Olschansky (2004) warn us that this influx of aged persons might cease and the mortality rate might actually decline in the new century because of infectious diseases and obesity that claim lives at any age.

Growth in Chronic Diseases

With an aging population comes the more frequent occurrence of chronic diseases. Among the chronic diseases expected in the future are Ischemic Heart Disease, Unipolar Major Depression, Road Traffic Accidents, Cerebrovascular Disease, Chronic Obstructive Pulmonary Disease, Chronic Obstructive Pulmonary Disease, Lower Respiratory Infections, Tuberculosis, War, Diarrheal diseases, and HIV. Newly added to this list is Obesity that has the same devastating effect as other chronic diseases on mortality and morbidity predictions for the new century.

However, the volume of children will also increase because of population growth. As we look at the aging population, the data on children balances the additional need for IT resources to monitor and prevent causes of their deaths. The following are reasons children will continue to die in the next decade (When Children Die, 2003, p. 4):

- Mixed causes: 33%
- Unintentional injuries: 22%
- Congenital anomalies: 12%
- Homicide and suicide: 8%
- Short gestation: 8%
- SIDS: 5%
- Cancer: 4%
- Respiratory Distress: 2%
- Heart Disease: 2%
- Placental cord membranes: 2%
- Complications of pregnancy: 2%

Emerging Infectious Disease Threats

Threats from emerging infectious diseases are given in Table 42.3. These are naturally occurring threats from infectious diseases without a bioterrorism event (described by Weiner and Phillips in their chapter). These infectious diseases and new strains of the flu can cause worldwide devastation due to our global lives and our mobile society. New IT resources will be required to alert health professionals, to operationalize resources, and to provide timely reporting of findings between

Table 42.3   Emerging Infectious Diseases

The flu
Respiratory infections
HIV/AIDS
Diarrheal diseases
Tuberculosis
Malaria
Measles
Pertusis
Tetanus
Meningitis
Syphilis
Antibiotic resistant diseases

government agencies and within public health personnel. Smart technologies of many kinds will be called on to keep vaccination records and to document exposures in various parts of the globe (Simpson, 2004). Information systems such as PathPort and MIDAS will be ready for deployment. These technologies, now being developed and used in research environments, will be ready for national use. Nurses with IT backgrounds are currently being enlisted to work on teams for surveillance in large cities, states, and regions of the civilian and military components of the country. The use of geographic information system (GIS) technology will be required by nurses in practice and in public health areas (Riner, Cunningham, and Johnson, 2004).

Changes in Health-Seeking Behavior on the Internet

Three chapters in this book have focused on consumers. Consumers are moving to the Internet to obtain information. They are also obtaining information from TV ads, health magazines, and pharmacy sites (IOM, 2003a).

Focus on Quality = Focus on Informatics

There have been almost a dozen reports from the IOM that have stressed the importance and need for IT in improving the quality of healthcare, demonstrating that outcomes can be achieved, efficiencies delivered, and costs decreased (IOM, 1997, 2000, 2001a,b, 2003 b,c,d, 2004 a,b). These landmark reports all recommend: (1) employing evidence-based practice and clinical practice guidelines, (2) applying quality improvement methods, and (3) utilizing informatics. In her report resulting from her Scholar-in Residence program at the IOM, Angela McBride summarizes the effects of these recommendations on reshaping the practice of nursing, but warns that barriers to achieving them include our academic institutions. Nursing academics still do not have faculty knowledgeable about IT, and the competencies needed in nursing are not systematically incorporated by educational levels into accreditation standards and performance appraisals (McBride, in press).

Security and Biodefense

To protect, mitigate, respond, and recover from acts of bioterrorism, there are several IT technologies that nurses in public health and practice will become more familiar with in the future. Securing the homeland will continue to be one of the highest priorities of the nation in the decade ahead. Technologies will be required to prevent, detect, treat, remediate, and attribute acts to terrorism. Inherently secure infrastructures will be important technological capacities. They are:

- Surveillance systems
- Preparedness planning and readiness management programs
- Control and disease prevention guidance embedded in decision supports
- Vaccine and drug delivery registries, adverse drug reporting systems, and stockpile warehouses
- National education and health alert networks
- Emergency response operational plans and systems
- Quarantine databases and logistics planning
- Mobilization and workforce systems
- Field reporting via wireless and PDAs
- Remote education and training Web-based and distance education facilities
- Real-time decision support systems
- Database integration and interoperability
- Assurance of services
- Sustainment and improvement in delivery systems
- Adverse drug reporting and hazard monitoring
- User registration and workforce deployment registration systems
- Data standards with specific terminology for biosafety and security

- Information security assurance
- Automatic access to policies, reporting requirements, and practices of multiple government agencies

Whether threats are biologic (particularly genetically modified), chemical, radiologic, and nuclear or high explosive resulting in trauma, all threats result in morbidity, mortality and diseases better supported by a robust information infrastructure. Similar to the integrative needs in hospital information systems, the public health and security of the country depend on a critical infrastructure that links our food, water, agricultural resources (plant and animal), public health, government, defense, information and communication networks, border control energy, transportation, finance and banking, chemical and hazardous materials, postal and shipping, and national monuments. Laboratory networks across federal, state, and local systems will be required. Nurses could also become involved in pursuing social and behavioral consequences to bioterrorism incidents to anticipate, counter, and diffuse psychosocial consequences from events. These psychosocial consequences occur in natural events such as hurricanes, tornadoes, and earthquakes, as well as bioterrorism-induced events.

Genetic Revolution

Advances in today's science have resulted in growth in the computer systems that analyze and link data from the testing of genes, genomes, and proteomes to different parts of the EHR. The advances in genomics and proteomics have emerged as a result of the Human Genome Project at the National Institutes of Health. New ways of collecting and analyzing data will continue to be a priority for at least 10 more years. These new IT tools will help to elucidate treatments to prevent and treat infectious diseases in plants, animals, and humans and to address complex areas of health such as obesity, environmental influences on health, and the neuronal/biochemical/behavioral/environmental basis of many behaviors such as depression, addiction, and schizophrenia.

- Genes are the segment of the chromosome that regulate the fundamental physical and functional units of heredity. Genes regulate the synthesis of proteins.
- Genomics is the identification and functional characterization of multiple genes. Microarray technologies help to decipher the functional

implications of gene expression and unravel some of the information related to the gene function.

■ Proteomics is the analysis of a set of proteins in a cell that in turn is determined by gene expression at the protein level.

These advances have taken place, not only in research and healthcare, but also in industrial manufacturing and agriculture. For years, our food sources have been modified and protected from environmental contaminants through genetics. Animal strains have been developed to improve industrial production of animals free of genetic diseases, thus lowering the production costs of our agricultural production processes. In the United States, biotechnology is a $34 billion industry with 16% compounded annual growth in revenue (Ernst and Young, 2003a).

By studying the genetics of diseases, viruses, fungi or bacteria, the United States is discovering ways to develop new drugs, antibiotics, vaccines, and therapeutics to target specific diseases. Genetic advances have allowed breakthroughs in producing 150 new medications in less than three decades (Ernst and Young, 2003b). The robust bioinformatics computers support developed to keep pace with these discoveries helped focus attention on the proteins, antibodies, and enzymes regulating treatments; on genes and protein biomarkers in identifying medical diagnostics; and on new vaccines and other treatments through recombinant DNA methods in preventing disease.

Combining the information known in biology about genetics with digital technology, future electronics will try to replicate and heal themselves in a way similar to what the human body does with genetics. These new advanced electronic engineering systems will seek to be more like human biology in their functions. Future developments need to give healthcare the potential of monitoring an individual molecular level analysis to achieve instantaneous drug design resulting from the malformations in protein folding resulting in individualized diagnosis and treatments.

Nanotechnology

Nanotechnology refers to the interaction of cellular and molecular components of engineered materials—typically clusters of atoms, molecules, and molecular fragments—at the most elemental level of biology. Typically, the dimensions of molecules are 100 nm or smaller.

Nanotechnology involves shrinking to the atomic scale, the diagnostics and treatments of our future, and studying the simplest parts of biology like the flow of water, calcium, sodium, and potassium into and out of cells. Nanoscience allows the opportunity to gain access to the living cell for diagnostic and treatment purposes. This in turn allows opportunities for both clinical and basic research in prevention, diagnosis, and treatment.

The opportunity to go inside the cell allows the simultaneous interaction of multiple proteins and nucleic acids at the molecular level and should provide a better understanding of the regulatory and signaling networks that govern the behavior of the normal cell as they undergo transformations in disease. It is the most promising science to allow:

1. Scientific investigation into the molecular nature of disease

2. Simultaneous measurement of gene and protein expression

3. Recognition of specific protein structures and structural domains

4. The following of protein transport among different cellular compartments (NCI, 2004)

Nanotechnology is said to be the biggest natural bridge between life sciences and physical sciences and requires interdisciplinary research and applications. It is the hope of government agencies that the new nanodevices, now in research and development, will help detect diseases such as cancer at its earliest stages and hopefully devise treatments that prevent it. If one can pinpoint the disease before it manifests itself or becomes malignant, then new treatments can be developed. The goals of early detection nanotechnologies are to develop molecular sensors that can detect disease-associated biomarkers and transmit the information via wireless technology to clinicians. Smart platforms for collecting input from multiple mass spectrometry machines will help in faster disease recognition. Cell imaging tools also will be considered in nanotechnology. Individual cells will be labeled with fluorescent material during surgery and the escape of cells will be monitored. Subsequent metastasis into regional areas will be predicted and risks identified. Some of the treatments will involve nanotechnology devices that control the spatial and temporal release of therapeutic agents (such as chemotherapies), while monitoring the effectiveness in vivo of the diseased cells. Nanoscale devices might help nurses manage the consequences of diagnosis and treatment of many diseases such as pain, nausea, loss of appetite, depression, and difficulty breathing. A knowledge of the societal implications of these technologies will also be required and nursing is a healthcare professional partner to facilitate those studies.

Table 42.4   Genetic Academic Programs and Other Resources

University of Iowa College of Nursing MSN Genetics Nursing Programs

Cincinnati Children's Hospital Medical Center Genetics Program for Nursing

Genetic Health Nursing, College of Nursing, Rush University, Chicago

University of Washington/Seattle Advanced Practice Genetics Nurse Program

University of California/San Francisco, Genomics Specialty Options, Department of Physiological Nursing

The National Coalition of Health Professional Education in Genetics

The International Society of Nurses in Genetics

Nursing and the Core Competencies for the Future

Nurses have been involved as genetic counselors and have defined the core curriculum for this specific domain. The entry in genetic nursing in the future will require nurses to complete graduate degree programs and clinical practice requirements in genetic medicine, human genetics, and/or genetic counseling according to the International Society of Nurses in Genetics (ISONG) (Silbertein, 2003). Genetic academic programs and other resources can be found in Table 42.4.

Ethical, Social, and Legal Issues

Nurses will be involved in the ethical, social, and legal issues resulting from these new genetic discoveries. They will have to use information systems to (Silberstein, 2003):

- Assure patient informed consent
- Assure confidentiality and security of information
- Assure that patients are not discriminated against
- Assure access to genetic technologies from vulnerable and minority populations
- Assure culturally sensitive genetic counseling

Decision support tools are needed in the future for nurses in general practice. They will have to be as knowledgeable as genetic counselors in making decisions in prevention, diagnosis, and treatment of diseases.

Summary

The next decade offers the nurse involved in informatics many exciting challenges. Graduate nurses in informatics may assist in developing several of these new systems. Others may be involved in implementing and evaluating them (McCormick et al., in press). The faculty might have to educate the students about the challenges and ethical, legal, and social issues arising out of the discoveries. If we succeed in preparing more nurses in informatics, we will also have contributed to this future. Several of the authors of this book have become experts in developing and implementing the future. The next decade provides many challenging issues to hold in balance while delivering healthcare based on advanced IT systems. The advanced IT systems offer the most promise in delivering quality care, assuring patient safety, preventing errors, measuring outcomes, and controlling costs in healthcare.

References

Dychwald, M. (2003). *Cycles: How we will Live, Work and Buy*. New York: Simon & Shuster.

Ernst and Young. (2003a). *Resilience: Americas Biotechnology Report*.

Ernst and Young. (2003b). *Beyond Borders: The Global Biotechnology Report*.

HIMSS. Leadership Survey. (2004). *Healthcare CIO Results*. Final Report.

IOM. (1997). In R. S. Dick, E. B. Steen, and D. E. Detmer (Eds.), *The Computer-Based Patient Record. An Essential Technology for Health Care*. Washington, DC: National Academy Press.

IOM. (2000). In L. T. Kohn, J. M. Corrigan, and M. S. Donaldson (Eds.), *To Err is Human: Building a Safer Health System*. Washington, DC: National Academy Press.

IOM. (2001a). *Crossing the Quality Chasm: A New Health System for the 21st Century*. Washington, DC: National Academy Press.

IOM. (2001b). In GS Wunderlich and PO Kohler (Eds.), *Improving the Quality of Long-Term Care*. Washington, DC: National Academy Press.

IOM. (2003a). In J. Aungst, A. Haas, A. Ommaya, L. W. Green (Eds.), *Exploring Challenges, Progress and New Models for Engaging the Public in the Clinical Research Enterprise: Clinical Research Roundtable Workshop Summary*. IOM. Washington, DC: The National Academies Press.

IOM. (2003b). In J. M. Corrigan, A. Greiner, and S. M. Erickson (Eds.), *Fostering Rapid Advances in Health Care: Learning from System Demonstrations*. Washington, DC: National Academies Press.

IOM. (2003c). In K. Gebbie, L. Rosenstock, and L. M. Hernandez (Eds.), *Who Will Keep the Public Healthy? Educating Public Health Professionals for the 21st Century*. Washington, DC: National Academies Press.

IOM. (2003d). In A. C. Griner and E. Knebel (Eds.), *Health Professions Education: A Bridge to Quality*. Washington, DC: National Academies Press.

IOM. (2004a). In A. Page (Ed.), *Keeping Patients Safe. Transforming the Work Environment of Nurses*. Washington, DC: National Academies Press.

IOM. (2004b). In K. Adams, A. C. Greiner (Eds.), *The 1st Annual Crossing the Quality Chasm Summit: A Focus on Communities*. Washington, DC: National Academies Press.

McBride, A. (2004). A year as an Institute of Medicine scholar-in-residence. *Nursing Outlook* 52(4):219–220.

McCormick, K. A. (2001). Future directions. In V. K. Saba and K. A. McCormick (Eds.), *Essentials of Computers for Nurses: Informatics for the New Millennium*. New York: McGraw-Hill.

McCormick, K. A., Sensemier, J., Delaney, C., and Bickford, C. (in press). Introduction to informatics and nursing. In L. Kun (Ed.), *Biomedical Engineering Handbook*, 3d ed. Boca Raton, FL: CRC press.

Miller, G. W. (2000). *King of Hearts*. New York: Crown Publishers.

(2003). *When Children Die*. Washington, DC: National Academy Press.

NCI. (2004). *Cancer Nanotechnology: Going Small for Big Advances*. NIH Publication No. 04-5489.

Olschansky, S. J. (2004). Institute of Medicine Lecture, Annual Meeting Lecture.

Riner, M. E., Cunningham, C. J., and Johnson, A. (2004). Public health education and practice using geographic information system technology. *Public Health Nursing* 21(1):57–65.

Silberstein, N. (2003). Genetic Technology Training. In *www.advanceweb.com* (Vol. 5, No. 23).

Simpson, R. L. (2004). No-borders nursing: How technology helps global ills. *Nursing Administration Quarterly* 28(1):55–59.

Snee, N. and McCormick, K. A. (2004). The case for integrating Public Health informatics Networks. *IEEE Engineering in Medicine and Biology* 23(1):81–88.

Clinical Care Classification (CCC) System Version 2.0*

Two Terminologies: CCC of Nursing Diagnoses and CCC of Nursing Interventions Classified by 21 Care Components

Virginia K. Saba

A complete description of the CCC of Nursing Diagnoses and CCC of Nursing Interventions classified by the 21 Care Components including their definitions, indexing, and coding. Internet address: http://wwwsabacare

Table A.1 Clinical Care Classification (CCC) (Version 2.0)—21 Care Components: Alphabetic Index with Codes

A	ACTIVITY COMPONENT	L	RESPIRATORY COMPONENT
B	BOWEL/GASTRIC COMPONENT	M	ROLE RELATIONSHIP COMPONENT
C	CARDIAC COMPONENT	N	SAFETY COMPONENT
D	COGNITIVE COMPONENT	O	SELF-CARE COMPONENT
E	COPING COMPONENT	P	SELF-CONCEPT COMPONENT
F	FLUID VOLUME COMPONENT	Q	SENSORY COMPONENT
G	HEALTH BEHAVIOR COMPONENT	R	SKIN INTEGRITY COMPONENT
H	MEDICATION COMPONENT	S	TISSUE PERFUSION COMPONENT
I	METABOLIC COMPONENT	T	URINARY ELIMINATION COMPONENT
J	NUTRITIONAL COMPONENT	U	LIFE CYCLE COMPONENT
K	PHYSICAL REGULATION COMPONENT		

 Clinical Care Classification (CCC) of Nursing Diagnoses with Expected and/or Actual Outcomes and Coding Structure

The coding structure for the CCC of Nursing Diagnoses with Expected and/or Actual Outcomes are described.

The coding structure consists of five alphanumeric characters.

Coding Structure

- ■ Care component—1st Alpha Code A–U
- ■ Nursing diagnosis major category—2nd/3rd digit: 01–61
- ■ Nursing diagnosis subcategory—4th decimal digit: 1–9
- ■ Expected/actual outcome—5th digit: 1–3 (use only one)

Note: 1 = improved, 2 = stabilized, and 3 = deteriorated

Table A.2 Clinical Care Classification of Nursing Diagnoses (Version 2.0) and Coding Scheme for 59 Major Categories and 123 Subcategories[1]

CCC of Nursing Diagnoses (Version 2.0) includes the following changes: new terms with new codes, revised terms with old codes, and revised/new codes with old terms. Changed and/or missing code/terms represent a revised/new and/or deleted code/terms. See Appendix A2 for a detailed list of changes on Web site www.sabacare.com

A Activity Component
- 01 Activity Alteration
  - 01.1 Activity Intolerance
  - 01.2 Activity Intolerance Risk
  - 01.3 Diversional Activity Deficit
  - 01.4 Fatigue
  - 01.5 Physical Mobility Impairment
  - 01.6 Sleep Pattern Disturbance
  - 01.7 Sleep Deprivation
- 02 Musculoskeletal Alteration

B Bowel/Gastric Component
- 03 Bowel Elimination Alteration
  - 03.1 Bowel Incontinence
  - 03.2 Colonic Constipation
  - 03.3 Diarrhea
  - 03.4 Fecal Impaction
  - 03.5 Perceived Constipation
  - 03.6 Unspecified Constipation
- 04 Gastrointestinal Alteration
- 51 Nausea

C Cardiac Component
- 05 Cardiac Output Alteration
- 06 Cardiovascular Alteration
  - 06.1 Blood Pressure Alteration

D Cognitive Component
- 07 Cerebral Alteration
  - 07.1 Confusion
- 08 Knowledge Deficit
  - 08.1 Knowledge Deficit of Diagnostic Test
  - 08.2 Knowledge Deficit of Dietary Regimen
  - 08.3 Knowledge Deficit of Disease Process
  - 08.4 Knowledge Deficit of Fluid Volume
  - 08.5 Knowledge Deficit of Medication Regimen
  - 08.6 Knowledge Deficit of Safety Precautions
  - 08.7 Knowledge Deficit of Therapeutic Regimen
- 09 Thought Processes Alteration
  - 09.1 Memory Impairment

E Coping Component
- 10 Dying Process
- 52 Community Coping Impairment
- 11 Family Coping Impairment
  - 11.1 Compromised Family Coping
  - 11.2 Disabled Family Coping
- 12 Individual Coping Impairment
  - 12.1 Adjustment Impairment
  - 12.2 Decisional Conflict
  - 12.3 Defensive Coping
  - 12.4 Denial
- 13 Posttrauma Response
  - 13.1 Rape Trauma Syndrome
- 14 Spiritual State Alteration
  - 14.1 Spiritual Distress

- 53 Grieving
  - 53.1 Anticipatory Grieving
  - 53.2 Dysfunctional Grieving

F Fluid Volume Component
- 15 Fluid Volume Alteration
  - 15.1 Fluid Volume Deficit
  - 15.2 Fluid Volume Deficit Risk
  - 15.3 Fluid Volume Excess
  - 15.4 Fluid Volume Excess Risk

G Health Behavior Component
- 17 Health Maintenance Alteration
  - 17.1 Failure to Thrive
- 18 Health Seeking Behavior Alteration
- 19 Home Maintenance Alteration
- 20 Noncompliance
  - 20.1 Noncompliance of Diagnostic Test
  - 20.2 Noncompliance of Dietary Regimen
  - 20.3 Noncompliance of Fluid Volume
  - 20.4 Noncompliance of Medication Regimen
  - 20.5 Noncompliance of Safety Precautions
  - 20.6 Noncompliance of Therapeutic Regimen

H Medication Component
- 21 Medication Risk
  - 21.1 Polypharmacy

I Metabolic Component
- 22 Endocrine Alteration
- 23 Immunologic Alteration
  - 23.1 Protection Alteration

J Nutritional Component
- 24 Nutrition Alteration
  - 24.1 Body Nutrition Deficit
  - 24.2 Body Nutrition Deficit Risk
  - 24.3 Body Nutrition Excess
  - 24.4 Body Nutrition Excess Risk
  - 24.5 Swallowing Impairment
- 54 Infant Feeding Pattern Impairment
- 55 Breastfeeding Impairment

K Physical Regulation Component
- 25 Physical Regulation Alteration
  - 25.1 Autonomic Dysreflexia
  - 25.2 Hyperthermia
  - 25.3 Hypothermia
  - 25.4 Thermoregulation Impairment
  - 25.5 Infection Risk
  - 25.6 Infection Unspecified
  - 25.7 Intracranial Adaptive Capacity Impairment

L Respiratory Component
- 26 Respiration Alteration
  - 26.1 Airway Clearance Impairment
  - 26.2 Breathing Pattern Impairment
  - 26.3 Gas Exchange Impairment
- 56 Ventilatory Weaning Impairment

(Continued)

M Role Relationship Component
27 Role Performance Alteration
  27.1 Parental Role Conflict
  27.2 Parenting Alteration
  27.3 Sexual Dysfunction
  27.4 Caregiver Role Strain
28 Communication Impairment
  28.1 Verbal Impairment
29 Family Processes Alteration
31 Sexuality Patterns Alteration
32 Socialization Alteration
  32.1 Social Interaction Alteration
  32.2 Social Isolation
  32.3 Relocation Stress Syndrome

N Safety Component
33 Injury Risk
  33.1 Aspiration Risk
  33.2 Disuse Syndrome
  33.3 Poisoning Risk
  33.4 Suffocation Risk
  33.5 Trauma Risk
34 Violence Risk
  34.1 Suicide Risk
  34.2 Self-Mutilation
57 Perioperative Injury Risk
  57.1. Perioperative Positioning Injury
  57.2 Surgical Recovery Delay
58 Substance Abuse
  58.1 Tobacco Abuse
  58.2 Alcohol Abuse
  58.3 Drug Abuse

O Self-Care Component
35 Bathing/Hygiene Deficit
36 Dressing/Grooming Deficit
37 Feeding Deficit
38 Self-Care Deficit
  38.1 Activities of Daily Living (ADLs) Alteration
  38.2 Instrumental Activities of Daily Living (IADLs) Alteration
39 Toileting Deficit

P Self-Concept Component
40 Anxiety
41 Fear
42 Meaningfulness Alteration
  42.1 Hopelessness
  42.2 Powerlessness
43 Self-Concept Alteration
  43.1 Body Image Disturbance
  43.2 Personal Identity Disturbance
  43.3 Chronic Low Self-Esteem Disturbance
  43.4 Situational Self-Esteem Disturbance

Q Sensory Component
44 Sensory Perceptual Alteration
  44.1 Auditory Alteration

  44.2 Gustatory Alteration
  44.3 Kinesthetic Alteration
  44.4 Olfactory Alteration
  44.5 Tactile Alteration
  44.6 Unilateral Neglect
  44.7 Visual Alteration
45 Comfort Alteration
  45.1 Acute Pain
  45.2 Chronic Pain
  45.3 Unspecified Pain

R Skin Integrity Component
46 Skin Integrity Alteration
  46.1 Oral Mucous Membranes Impairment
  46.2 Skin Integrity Impairment
  46.3 Skin Integrity Impairment Risk
  46.4 Skin Incision
  46.5 Latex Allergy Response
47 Peripheral Alteration

S Tissue Perfusion Component
48 Tissue Perfusion Alteration

T Urinary Elimination Component
49 Urinary Elimination Alteration
  49.1 Functional Urinary Incontinence
  49.2 Reflex Urinary Incontinence
  49.3 Stress Urinary Incontinence
  49.4 Total Urinary Incontinence
  49.5 Urge Urinary Incontinence
  49.6 Urinary Retention
50 Renal Alteration

U Life Cycle Component
59 Reproductive Risk
  59.1 Fertility Risk
  59.2 Infertility Risk
  59.3 Contraception Risk
60 Perinatal Risk
  60.1 Pregnancy Risk
  60.2 Labor Risk
  60.3 Delivery Risk
  60.4 Postpartum Risk
61 Growth and Development Alteration
  61.1 Newborn Behavior Alteration (first 30 days)
  61.2 Infant Behavior Alteration (31 days through 11 months)
  61.3 Child Behavior Alteration (1 year through 11 years)
  61.4 Adolescent Behavior Alteration (12 years through 20 years)
  61.5 Adult Behavior Alteration (21 years through 64 years)
  61.6 Older Adult Behavior Alteration (65 years and older)

---

1. Adapted from NANDA: Taxonomy I: Revised 1990.
2. Adapted with Permission from NANDA Nursing Diagnoses & Classification 2003–2004.

Clinical Care Classification (CCC) of Nursing Interventions with Type Intervention Actions and Coding Structure

The coding structure for the CCC of Nursing Interventions with Type Intervention Actions are described.

The coding structure consists of five alphanumeric characters.

Coding Structure

- Care component—1st Alpha Code A–U
- Nursing diagnosis major category—2nd/3rd digit: 01–72
- Nursing diagnosis subcategory—4th decimal digit: 1–9
- Type intervention action—5th digit: 1–4 (use major one or more)

Note: 1 = assess, 2 = care, 3 = teach, 4 = manage

Table A.3   Clinical Care Classification of Nursing Interventions and Coding Scheme: 72 Major Categories and 126 Subcategories

CCC of Nursing Diagnoses (Version 2.0) includes the following changes: new terms with new codes, revised terms with old codes, and revised/new codes with old terms. Changed and/or missing code/terms represent a revised/new and/or deleted code/terms. See Appendix A2 for a detailed list of changes on Web site *www.sabacare.com*

A   Activity Component
- 01   Activity Care
  - 01.2   Energy Conservation
- 02   Fracture Care
  - 02.1   Cast Care
  - 02.2   Immobilizer Care
- 03   Mobility Therapy
  - 03.1   Ambulation Therapy
  - 03.2   Assistive Device Therapy
  - 03.3   Transfer Care
- 04   Sleep Pattern Control
- 05   Musculoskeletal Care
  - 05.1   Range of Motion
  - 05.2   Rehabilitation Exercise
- 61   Bedbound Care
  - 61.1   Positioning Therapy

B   Bowel/Gastric Component
- 06   Bowel Care
  - 06.1   Bowel Training
  - 06.2   Disimpaction
  - 06.3   Enema
  - 06.4   Diarrhea Care
- 07   Ostomy Care
  - 07.1   Ostomy Irrigation
- 62   Gastric Care
  - 62.1   Nausea Care

C   Cardiac Component
- 08   Cardiac Care
  - 08.1   Cardiac Rehabilitation
- 09   Pacemaker Care

D   Cognitive Component
- 10   Behavior Care
- 11   Reality Orientation
- 63   Wandering Control
- 64   Memory Loss Care

E   Coping Component
- 12   Counseling Service
  - 12.1   Coping Support
  - 12.2   Stress Control
  - 12.3   Crisis Therapy
- 13   Emotional Support
  - 13.1   Spiritual Comfort
- 14   Terminal Care
  - 14.1   Bereavement Support
  - 14.2   Dying/Death Measures
  - 14.3   Funeral Arrangements

F   Fluid Volume Component
- 15   Fluid Therapy
  - 15.1   Hydration Status
  - 15.2   Intake/Output
- 16   Infusion Care
  - 16.1   Intravenous Care
  - 16.2   Venous Catheter Care

G   Health Behavior Component
- 17   Community Special Services
  - 17.1   Adult Day Center
  - 17.2   Hospice
  - 17.3   Meals-on-Wheels
- 18   Compliance Care
  - 18.1   Compliance with Diet
  - 18.2   Compliance with Fluid Volume
  - 18.3   Compliance with Medical Regimen
  - 18.4   Compliance with Medication Regimen
  - 18.5   Compliance with Safety Precautions
  - 18.6   Compliance with Therapeutic Regimen
- 19   Nursing Contact
  - 19.1   Bill of Rights
  - 19.2   Nursing Care Coordination
  - 19.3   Nursing Status Report

(Continued)

Table A.3   Clinical Care Classification of Nursing Interventions and Coding Scheme: 72 Major Categories and 126 Subcategories (*Continued*)

20 Physician Contact	33.3 Pulse
20.1 Medical Regimen Orders	33.4 Respiration
20.2 Physician Status Report	**L Respiratory Component**
21 Professional/Ancillary Services	35 Oxygen Therapy Care
21.1 Home Health Aide Service	36 Pulmonary Care
21.2 Medical Social Worker Service	36.1 Breathing Exercises
21.3 Nurse Specialist Service	36.2 Chest Physiotherapy
21.4 Occupational Therapist Service	36.3 Inhalation Therapy
21.5 Physical Therapist Service	36.4 Ventilator Care
21.6 Speech Therapist Service	37 Tracheostomy Care
H Medication Component	**M Role Relationship Component**
22 Chemotherapy Care	38 Communication Care
23 Injection Administration	39 Psychosocial Care
23.1 Insulin Injection	39.1 Home Situation Analysis
23.2 Vitamin B_{12} Injection	39.2 Interpersonal Dynamics Analysis
24 Medication Care	39.3 Family Process Analysis
24.1 Medication Actions	39.4 Sexual Behavior Analysis
24.2 Medication Prefill Preparation	39.5 Social Network Analysis
24.3 Medication Side Effects	**N Safety Component**
24.4 Medication Treatment	40 Substance Abuse Control
25 Radiation Therapy Care	40.1 Tobacco Abuse Control
I Metabolic Component	40.2 Alcohol Abuse Control
26 Allergic Reaction Care	40.3 Drug Abuse Control
27 Diabetic Care	41 Emergency Care
65 Immunologic Care	42 Safety Precautions
J Nutritional Component	42.1 Environmental Safety
28 Enteral Tube Care	42.2 Equipment Safety
28.1 Enteral Tube Insertion	42.3 Individual Safety
28.2 Enteral Tube Irrigation	68 Violence Control
29 Nutrition Care	**O Self-Care Component**
29.2 Feeding Technique	43 Personal Care
29.3 Regular Diet	43.1 Activities of Daily Living (ADLs)
29.4 Special Diet	43.2 Instrumental Activities of Daily
29.5 Enteral Feeding	Living (IADLs)
29.6 Parental Feeding	**P Self-Concept Component**
66 Breastfeeding Support	45 Mental Health Care
67 Weight Control	45.1 Mental Health History
K Physical Regulation Component	45.2 Mental Health Promotion
30 Infection Control	45.3 Mental Health Screening
30.1 Universal Precautions	45.4 Mental Health Treatment
31 Physical Health Care	**Q Sensory Component**
31.1 Health History	47 Pain Control
31.2 Health Promotion	47.1 Acute Pain Control
31.3 Physical Examination	47.2 Chronic Pain Control
31.4 Clinical Measurements	48 Comfort Care
32 Specimen Care	49 Ear Care
32.1 Blood Specimen Care	49.1 Hearing Aid Care
32.2 Stool Specimen Care	49.2 Wax Removal
32.3 Urine Specimen Care	50 Eye Care
32.5 Sputum Specimen Care	50.1 Cataract Care
33 Vital Signs	50.2 Vision Care
33.1 Blood Pressure	
33.2 Temperature	

(Continued)

Table A.3   Clinical Care Classification of Nursing Interventions and Coding Scheme: 72 Major Categories and 126 Subcategories (*Continued*)

R **Skin Integrity Component**	59 Dialysis Care
51 Pressure Ulcer Care	60 Urinary Catheter Care
51.1 Pressure Ulcer Stage 1 Care	60.1 Urinary Catheter Insertion
51.2 Pressure Ulcer Stage 2 Care	60.2 Urinary Catheter Irrigation
51.3 Pressure Ulcer Stage 3 Care	72 Urinary Incontinence Care
51.4 Pressure Ulcer Stage 4 Care	73 Renal Care
53 Mouth Care	**U** **Life Cycle Component**
53.1 Denture Care	74 Reproductive Care
54 Skin Care	74.1 Fertility Care
54.1 Skin Breakdown Control	74.2 Infertility Care
55 Wound Care	74.3 Contraception Care
55.1 Drainage Tube Care	75 Perinatal Care
55.2 Dressing Change	75.1 Pregnancy Care
55.3 Incision Care	75.2 Labor Care
S **Tissue Perfusion Component**	75.3 Delivery Care
56 Foot Care	75.4 Postpartum Care
57 Perineal Care	76 Growth and Development Care
69 Edema Control	76.1 Newborn Behavior Care (first 30 days)
70 Circulatory Care	76.2 Infant Behavior Care (31 days through 11 months)
71 Neurovascular Care	76.3 Child Behavior Care (1 year through 11 years)
T **Urinary Elimination Component**	76.4 Adolescent Behavior Care (12 years through 20 years)
58 Bladder Care	76.5 Adult Behavior Care (21 years through 64 years)
58.1 Bladder Instillation	76.6 Older Adult Behavior Care (65 years and older)
58.2 Bladder Training	

INDEX

Page numbers followed by italic *f* or *t* denote figures or tables, respectively.